ELSEVIER'S COMPREHENSIVE REVIEW

for the Canadian PN Examination

Second Edition

ELSEVIER'S COMPREHENSIVE REVIEW

for the **Canadian**

PN Examination

Karen Katsademas, RN, BScN, MN
Fanshawe College, London, ON

Marianne Langille, RN, BScN, MEd
Fanshawe College, London, ON

ELSEVIER

Notice

Senior Editor (Acquisitions, Canada): Roberta A. Spinosa-Millman
Content Development Manager: Lenore Spence
Content Development Specialist: Theresa Fitzgerald
Publishing Services Manager: Deepthi Unni
Senior Project Manager: Manchu Mohan
Senior Book Designer: Margaret M.Reid

Last digit is the print number: 9 8 7 6 5 4 3 2 1

 Working together to grow libraries in developing countries

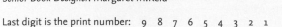 www.elsevier.com • www.bookaid.org

To my parents Fred and Cathy Smith, who would be so very proud of this book

Karen Katsademas

To my family for their enormous support and encouragement

Marianne Langille

CONTRIBUTOR

Janice Henty, RN, BScN, MEd
Toronto, ON
(REx-PN Question Item Writer)

Joscelyne Bergen, RN, BScN
Instructor, Practical Nurse Program
School of Health, Education and Human Services
Yukon University
Whitehorse, YT

Natasha Fontaine, RN, BN, PID
Faculty of Health Programs/Program Coordinator
Practical Nursing
College of the Rockies
Cranbrook, BC

Sandy Madorin, RN, MSCN
Program Coordinator, Practical Nursing
School of Health, Wellness and Sciences
Georgian College
Barrie, ON

Lorraine G. McInnis, RN, BN CPN(C)
Professor/Instructor Nursing and Health Studies
Algonquin College of Applied Arts and Technology
Ottawa, ON

Cindy Pallister, RN, BScN, MScN, Simulationist
Nursing Professor
St. Clair College
Chatham, ON

Lisa Jo Russell, RN, BScN, BEd, MEd(c)
Sessional Instructor, Nursing
Thompson Rivers University
Kamloops, BC

Valerie Sokolowski, RN, MN
Faculty, Practical Nursing
College of New Caledonia
Prince George, BC

Kari Dawn Ubels, CD, HBScN, RN
Associate Chair of Practical Nurse Curriculum
Faculty of Health and Community Studies
NorQuest College
Edmonton, AB

Lana Wadman, RN, BScN
Faculty, Practical Nursing
Health and Human Services
Nova Scotia Community College
Sydney, NS

Jess White, RN, BN, ENC(C), CAE
Faculty, School of Nursing
Assiniboine College
Winnipeg, MB

Elsevier's Comprehensive Review for the Canadian PN Examination, Second Edition has been designed to provide a rapid reference with easily obtainable information for the student who is preparing for either the Regulatory Exam-Practical Nurse (REx-PN®) or the Canadian Practical Nurse Registration Examination (CPNRE®). It is uniquely Canadian, with content created specifically for the Canadian market. Expert contributors from across Canada have joined with editors to ensure that the text reflects current Canadian nursing practice and trends. The content, based on the test plan of the REx-PN and the blueprint for the CPNRE, is a refresher of learned knowledge, with a focus on the role of the practical nurse, health promotion, professional practice, preventive and primary health care, teaching–learning, nursing judgement, and critical thinking. Gerontological considerations, evidence-informed practice, community focus, and nontraditional settings are included, as appropriate. Appendices include the Entry-Level Competencies for Licensed (or Registered) Practical Nurses in Canada, Medical Terminology, Abbreviations, Common Laboratory and Diagnostic Tests, and Mathematical Formulae.

Beyond requiring a broad knowledge of nursing theory, students also need to feel confident tackling the particular types of questions found in the REx-PN or CPNRE. For many, it is not a lack of nursing knowledge that affects their performance on the examination but difficulties in applying their knowledge in the exam situation. Chapters that introduce and describe the examinations and that offer tips for mastering the types of questions found on the examinations provide valuable guidelines. Each chapter in this comprehensive review includes practice questions representative of those found on either the CPNRE or the REx-PN and are authored within the framework of practical nursing practice in Canada. The case-based questions are representative of the CPNRE questions, and the independent questions have been revised to include alternate format question types that are found in the REx-PN. All questions provide the student with an opportunity to apply learned knowledge to the test situation, particularly at the critical thinking and application cognitive levels.

In addition to the practice questions that appear in the chapters, two CPNRE practice exams and two REx-PN practice exams are included at the end of the book. Questions have been authored by nursing experts in the field of exam preparation and referenced to established resources. Answers and rationales, as well as the Client Needs which correspond to the REx-PN format, alongside the competency and taxonomy tag which correspond to the CPNRE format for the practice exams, are also provided.

We have included a NEW specialized chapter on end-of-life care, with topics including caring for the dying client, palliative care, hospice care, medical assistance in dying (MAiD), grief and bereavement management, and organ donation.

In some provinces, the term *RPN* refers to "registered psychiatric nurse"; however, for the purposes of this textbook, the term *RPN* refers to "registered practical nurse."

The authors and contributors of the text recognize and acknowledge the diverse histories of the first peoples of the lands now referred to as Canada. It is recognized that individual communities identify themselves in various ways; within this text, the term *Indigenous* will be used to refer to all First Nations, Inuit, and Métis people within Canada.

Knowledge and language concerning sex, gender, and identity are fluid and continually evolving. The language and terminology presented in this text endeavour to be inclusive of all people and reflect what is, to the best of our knowledge, current at the time of publication.

ACKNOWLEDGEMENTS

We would like to acknowledge and thank the following individuals for their time, support, and expertise in the preparation of this text: Roberta Spinosa-Millman and Theresa Fitzgerald, of Elsevier, and Janice Henty, for her nursing expertise in contributing to the REx-PN examination question item writing and as a consultant. We would like to acknowledge and thank Karen Lowry for expertise and guidance with the copy editing of the text.

We would also like to recognize the contribution of Janice Marshall-Henty, Cheryl Sams, and Jonathon Bradshaw, authors of *Mosby's Comprehensive Review for the Canadian RN Exam*, along with its numerous contributors. Their original work served as a foundation for our writing and set a standard of excellence we conscientiously followed.

CONTENTS

DETAILED CONTENTS

Introduction

To practise as a practical nurse in Canada, you must be registered or licensed. A component of the registration is successful completion of a registration exam. To write the exam, you must have completed an approved practical nursing program or have foreign qualifications that have been assessed as being equivalent to a Canadian nursing education. Until 2022, all practical nursing applicants across Canada except Quebec completed the Canadian Practical Nurse Registration Examination (CPNRE®). Beginning in January 2022, eligible candidates in British Columbia (BC) and Ontario complete the Regulatory Exam–Practical Nurse (REx-PN®). If you pass the exam in your home province or territory and meet all other requirements for registration, you qualify to apply for registration in all jurisdictions (with the exception of Quebec). Questions on the exam are designed to evaluate the knowledge of an entry-level practical nurse who has just finished their education. Nursing specialties are not tested. Testable material is applicable to all Canadian settings: large cities, small towns, the East Coast or West Coast, community clinics, acute care hospitals, and nontraditional settings. When writing the examination, you need to be able to answer based on the knowledge, skills, and behaviours of a model nurse, not just based on what you or your colleagues might have experienced in a particular setting.

BACKGROUND TO THE CANADIAN PRACTICAL NURSE REGISTRATION EXAMINATION

The CPNRE is a multiple-choice, computer-based examination. The exam, offered in English and French, is the same for all practical nursing applicants across Canada with the exception of Ontario, BC, and Quebec. The CPNRE is developed by practical nurse educators, clinicians, and administrators from across Canada with the assistance of Meazure Learning-Yardstick. There are several exam windows per year. Applicants may choose from a number of secure test centres in more than 100 cities and towns in Canada. The examination is delivered in Pearson VUE's network of proctored test centres across Canada. To search for Pearson VUE test centres, visit http://www.pearsonvue.com/cpnre/.

The examination is based on a specific blueprint, or framework. Individual questions were authored by a team of nursing experts from across Canada, and all are referenced to at least two published or reliable on-line resources. All questions were tested experimentally and analyzed statistically to determine their suitability for inclusion in the examination.

A complex scoring system is used to mark the exam, but essentially you receive a mark for all correct responses. Marks are not deducted for incorrect answers. The results of the examination are reported as "Pass" or "Fail." Students who are about to write the examination often worry, "What happens if I fail?" With proper preparation, including management of "test stress," this should not happen. If you do not pass the first time you write the CPNRE, you may rewrite the exam. All provinces and territories that administer the CPNRE allow a candidate to write the exam a total of three times.

BACKGROUND TO THE REGULATORY EXAM – PRACTICAL NURSE (REx-PN)

The REx-PN is a new computer adaptive test (CAT) that candidates in Ontario and BC complete. The examination is offered in English (Ontario and BC) and in French (Ontario only). The REx-PN was developed by nurse educators, clinicians, and administrators from Ontario and BC with the assistance of National Council of State Boards of Nursing (NCSBN). NCSBN issues a *REx-PN Examination Candidate Bulletin* that provides information on registering to take the REx-PN. It is important for all candidates to read this bulletin, found at www.rexpn.com.

The examination is based on a specific test plan, or framework. Individual questions were authored by Canadian nurse educators in Ontario and BC. All questions were tested experimentally and analyzed statistically to determine their suitability for inclusion in the examination.

A complex scoring system is used to mark the exam. You receive a mark for all correct responses and no partial marks are given. Marks are not deducted for incorrect answers. The results of the examination are reported as "Pass or "Fail." You will be administered a minimum of 90 questions, and in order to pass you must be above the passing standard. The passing standard is met when you have answered enough questions that the computer is able to determine that you can provide safe nursing care. The *REx-PN Examination Candidate Bulletin* provides additional information on passing and failing the REx-PN. The bulletin can be found at www.rexpn.com. Students who are about to write the examination often worry, "What happens if I fail?" With proper preparation, including management of "test stress," this should not happen. If you do not pass the first time you write the REx-PN, you may rewrite the exam. The NCSBN allows a candidate to write the exam an unlimited number of times after a 60-day waiting period between each examination.

ELSEVIER'S COMPREHENSIVE REVIEW

Elsevier's Comprehensive Review for the Canadian PN Examination is designed to provide a rapid reference with easily obtainable information for the student who is preparing for the CPNRE or the REx-PN. It is the only comprehensive review text that contains content specific to these Canadian examinations. Each chapter is a refresher of previously learned knowledge that provides need-to-know information focused on nursing judgement, actions, critical thinking, and the role of the practical nurse. Necessary medical terminology, relevant math formulae, and common laboratory and diagnostic tests are included as appendices at the end of the text.

Chapter 2 presents a description of the CPNRE so that you may become familiar with the format of the test and the types of questions it includes. Tips for studying and taking the multiple-choice examination are provided. Chapter 3 presents a description of the REx-PN so that you may become familiar with the format of the CAT and the types of questions it includes. Tips for studying and taking the CAT are provided. Each subsequent chapter contains a review of a major clinical area, followed by multiple choice and alternate format questions that test the practical nurse's knowledge of principles and theories underlying nursing care in a range of different situations and settings. Rationales for correct answers for these practice questions are provided, as are the competencies (CPNRE), client needs (REx-PN), and identification of question taxonomies.

In addition, this text includes two practice examinations that are similar in format and content to the CPNRE and two practice examinations that provide students with content and question types similar to the REx-PN. These practice exams give you the opportunity to apply your knowledge to the particular types of questions you will experience in the CPNRE or the REx-PN. You can choose to write an entire exam to mimic true test conditions or to answer particular sections or questions.

After you have answered the questions, review the correct answers and rationales for each item. Analyze your mistakes. Were there knowledge gaps? Did you misread the question? Did you assume information that wasn't given in the question? Did you misunderstand what the question meant? Identify the frequency with which you made particular errors and use this information as a reference database for further study. Perhaps you need to review certain topics, practise your math skills, or increase your reading comprehension.

Do not attempt to memorize any of the information from the practice questions or to use any of the questions to study content. All test items on the CPNRE and REx-PN are secure and have never been published; questions in this text will *not* be on the CPNRE or REx-PN.

Remember, you are not expected to get a perfect score. If you correctly answer about 65% of the practice questions in this text, you are likely to succeed on the actual registration examination.

BIBLIOGRAPHY

Meazure Learning - Yardstick. (2021). *The Canadian Practical Nurse Registration Examination prep guide* (6th ed.).

Yardstick Assessment Strategies. (2019). *Examination blueprint (2022–2026) Canadian Practical Nurse Registration Examination (CPNRE)*.

WEBSITES

- Canadian Practical Nurse Registration Examination (CPNRE) (http://cpnre.ca): This site includes information about the CPNRE.
- National Council of State Boards of Nursing (www.ncsbn.org): This site includes information about the REx-PN and other exams.
- RExPN (www.rexpn.com): This site includes information specific to the REx-PN.

Tips for Writing the CPNRE®

DESCRIPTION OF THE EXAMINATION AND TEST-TAKING TIPS

The Canadian Practical Nurse Registration Examination (CPNRE) consists of 160 to 170 questions, including experimental questions that are not counted toward your examination score. Some of the experimental questions may be in a format other than multiple choice. An experimental question is one that has not been statistically validated and is undergoing trial evaluation with exam candidates. You will not know which questions are the experimental questions, so answer all questions as though they count toward your grade. The writing time for the exam is 4 hours.

Multiple-Choice Questions

The multiple-choice test items are written as either case-based or independent questions. Case-based questions present a health care scenario along with approximately three to five questions related to the scenario. Independent, or stand-alone, questions contain all the information necessary to answer the question. In the CPNRE, 40 to 60% of the questions are case based.

Each multiple-choice question is made up of two components. The part that asks the question or poses a problem is called the *stem*. The alternatives from which you are asked to select the best answer are called the *options*. There are four options, and *only one* of the options is the correct answer. The other three options are called *distractors*. Distractors may seem to be reasonable answers but are, in fact, incorrect or incomplete. All questions are worth one mark. Marks are not deducted for wrong answers.

2.1 Sample Question

While receiving a blood transfusion, Mr. Ryan develops chills and a headache. What would be the nurse's initial action?

1. Notify the physician stat.
2. Stop the transfusion immediately.
3. Cover Mr. Ryan with a blanket and administer ordered acetaminophen (Tylenol).
4. Slow the blood flow to keep the vein open.

The correct answer is 2. Mr. Ryan is experiencing a transfusion reaction. Thus, the blood infusion must be stopped immediately.

Examination Blueprint

The CPNRE is written according to a blueprint that includes competencies; levels of cognitive ability called *taxonomies*;

and the variables of client type, client age, client culture, client diversity, and work environment. It is not organized into sections on maternal–newborn nursing, medical–surgical nursing, pediatric nursing, mental health nursing, and so on.

Competencies

Competencies include knowledge, skills, behaviours, and clinical judgements that a practical nurse is expected to demonstrate in order to provide safe, professional care. In the exam, competencies are applied to various health situations and clients. For example, what are the safety hazards for the mental health client, the infant, or the older person? How do you prevent the spread of infection in a hospital, in a day care centre, or to an immunocompromised client? Practical nurses learn these competencies in their education programs. There are 76 competencies in five categories. See Appendix A for a complete list of the CPNRE competencies.

Competency categories

Professional, ethical, and legal practice

Licenced practical nurses (LPNs) adhere to practice standards and an ethical framework. They are responsible and accountable for safe, competent and ethical nursing practice. They are expected to demonstrate professional conduct as reflected through personal attitudes, beliefs, opinions and actions. Licensed practical nurses focus on personal and professional growth. Licensed practical nurses are expected to utilize knowledge, critical thinking, critical inquiry and research to build an evidence-informed practice.

They are guided by a Code of Ethics when making professional judgments and practice decisions. They engage in critical thinking and critical inquiry to inform decision-making. They use self-reflection to understand the impact of personal values, beliefs and assumptions in the provision of care.

They adhere to applicable provincial/territorial and federal legislation and regulations, professional standards and employer policies that direct practice. They engage in professional regulation by enhancing their competence, promoting safe practice and maintain their fitness to practice. Licenced practical nurses recognize that safe nursing practice includes knowledge of relevant laws and legal boundaries within which the licensed practical nurse must practice.

(Yardstick Assessment Strategies, 2019, p. 6)

Approximately one quarter of the questions on the exam (15–25%) concern professional, ethical, and legal practice.

Sample Competency and Related Sample Question:
PR-34—Documents according to established legislation, practice standards, ethics, and organizational policies.

2.2 Sample Question
Mrs. Leung was found by the nurse at 0100 hours lying on the floor beside her bed. What should the nurse document in the health record?
1. Mrs. Leung fell out of bed at 0100.
2. At 0100 hours, Mrs. Leung was found by the nurse on the floor beside her bed.
3. Mrs. Leung got out of bed at 0100 hours, slipped, and fell on the floor.
4. Mrs. Leung apparently fell out of bed at approximately 0100 hours.

    The correct answer is 2. This notation provides factual and objective documentation about the nurse's observation.

Foundations of practice
Licensed practical nurses use critical thinking, reflection, and evidence integration to assess clients, plan care, implement interventions and evaluate outcomes and processes. Foundational knowledge includes nursing theory, health sciences, humanities, pharmacology and ethics.

    (Yardstick Assessment Strategies, 2019, p. 6)

Over half of the questions (60–70%) relate to this competency.

Sample Competency and Related Sample Question:
- FP-60.2—Engage in safe infusion therapy practices.

2.3 Sample Question
The physician order reads, "IV TKVO." What does this mean?
1. Intravenous infusion rate of 10 mL per hour
2. Intravenous infusion rate of 15 mL per hour
3. Intravenous to be locked with saline
4. Intravenous rate that will maintain the patency of the infusion

    The correct answer is 4. *TKVO* means "to keep vein open."

Collaborative practice
Licensed practical nurses work collaboratively with clients and other members of the health care team. They recognize that collaborative practice is guided by shared values and accountability, a common purpose or care outcome, mutual respect and effective communication.

    (Yardstick Assessment Strategies, 2019, p. 6)

Nearly one quarter of the questions on the exam (10–20%) relate to collaborative practice.

Sample Competency and Related Sample Question:
- CP-67—Determines own professional and interprofessional role within the team by considering the roles, responsibilities and scope of practice of others.

2.4 Sample Question
The nurse checks on a client who was admitted to the hospital with pneumonia. They have been coughing profusely and has required nasotracheal suctioning. They have an intravenous infusion of antibiotics. The client is febrile. Which of the following tasks may the nurse delegate to the support worker assigned to the client today?
1. Assessing vital signs
2. Changing intravenous dressing
3. Nasotracheal suctioning
4. Administering a bed bath

    The correct answer is 4. The nurse may delegate this task to the support worker.

Taxonomies of Questions
To test your thinking abilities, questions are written at different cognitive levels: knowledge and comprehension, application, and critical thinking. Knowing the percentage of questions on the exam pertaining to each cognitive level will help guide your studying.

Knowledge and Comprehension
The knowledge and comprehension level requires recollection of facts. For these types of questions, you are required to define, identify, or select remembered information. Knowledge questions require basic memorization. A maximum of 5% of the questions on the CPNRE are of the knowledge and comprehension type.

2.5 Sample Question
Which of the following is an adverse effect of digoxin?
1. Tachycardia
2. Bradycardia
3. Diarrhea
4. Urticaria

    The answer is 2, bradycardia. To answer this question correctly, you need to have memorized the adverse effects of digoxin and the terms *tachycardia* and *bradycardia*.

Application
The application level of the intellectual process requires not only knowing and understanding information but also being able to apply it to a new situation. This level includes modifying, manipulating, or adapting information when providing client care. A minimum of 50% of the questions on the CPNRE are application based.

2.6 Sample Question
Before taking Mr. Singh's vital signs, the nurse asks him if he is taking any medications. He answers, "Digoxin every morning and Tylenol in the evening." Which of the following vital sign changes might the nurse anticipate?
1. Increased blood pressure to 140/85 mm Hg
2. Decreased pulse to 53 beats per minute
3. Decreased respiratory rate to 10 breaths per minute
4. Increased temperature to 38.5°C

The answer is 2, decreased pulse. This question requires knowledge about several drugs, interpretation of vital signs, and application of this information to a particular client.

Critical Thinking

Critical-thinking questions require the most complex level of cognitive function. They ask you to analyze, evaluate, problem-solve, or interpret data from a variety of sources before you respond to them. This often involves prioritizing nursing actions. Many refer to critical-thinking questions as "tricky" or "unfair" because the options may all be correct, but only one option is considered the most important or comprehensive response. A minimum of 45% of the questions on the CPNRE are critical-thinking questions.

2.7 Sample Question

Mr. Singh has asthma and is experiencing acute shortness of breath and wheezing. What should the nurse do first?
1. Administer his ordered "rescue inhaler"
2. Administer his ordered combination inhaled drugs
3. Notify the physician
4. Encourage increased fluid intake

The answer is 1, administer his rescue inhaler. All the options could be correct, but administering the rescue inhaler is the first thing the nurse should do. Consider the nursing process: validate your data.

Other Blueprint Variables

Client Type

In the CPNRE, a *client* is defined as "an individual (or their designated representative), family, and group" (Yardstick Assessment Strategies, 2019, p. 10).

Client Age

Questions reflect the statistical representation of Canadians in relation to age, from birth to older person.

Client Diversity

"Items will be included that measure awareness, sensitivity and respect for diversity, without introducing stereotypes" (Yardstick Assessment Strategies, 2019, p. 11). Because Canada comprises a variety of cultural backgrounds, the CPNRE integrates sensitivity and respect for diverse beliefs and values. It does not specifically test knowledge of individual cultures, other than that of Indigenous peoples in Canada.

Work Environment

"Practical nurses work in a variety of practice settings and contexts where health care is delivered. As a result, the work environment is *only* specified where necessary" (Yardstick Assessment Strategies, 2019, p. 11).

STUDY AND EXAMINATION TIPS

Although you may be academically well prepared to write the CPNRE, strategies for studying, stress management, and test-taking will increase your chances of success and help alleviate test anxiety.

Study Tips

It is easy to become overwhelmed as you prepare to study for the CPNRE. Remember, though, that you know a lot more than you think you do. While studying is crucial, much learning is not a conscious activity. The first key to developing successful study strategies is to be realistic. Identify where you have incomplete knowledge or the need to refresh your learning.

Keep in mind that most of the questions on the exam do not merely test recalled facts, so you should try to understand the material that you read rather than memorize it. The focus of your studies should be on principles of care and nursing interventions within a particular health situation; that is, what should the nurse do or say?

Because the exam will likely include approximately one or two questions per competency, make sure you do not get bogged down in one particular content area. For example, there may be only one competency related to assessment and monitoring of central venous catheters (CVCs), so you should not spend too much time studying CVCs.

One of the best strategies for learning is to form a study group. Self-testing and peer testing have proven to be the most effective methods for consolidating material. Have each member of the group choose a topic to teach the other members. This way, you stimulate discussion and get different perspectives on the subjects, which will help you in understanding and remembering them. If you are unable to participate in a study group, try teaching yourself the information. Rephrase or reword the written information to aid in understanding rather than memorizing.

Repetition works well for many people. If you are having trouble remembering some knowledge material, it may help to record it so that you can play it aloud while performing other activities.

Schedule your studying. Start reviewing content several months prior to the exam so that you do not feel rushed or panicked at the volume of material you need to learn. Cramming or "all-nighters" may be useful for memorizing facts, but the CPNRE is an exam that requires problem-solving based on a comprehensive knowledge base. It is better to think through and analyze the material, make judgements, and determine how the subject relates to nursing. By performing these analytical and reflective processes, you are more likely to commit the information to long-term memory, which is much more reliable than your short-term memory.

To remember the strategies for studying, you can use the initialism PQRS, which stands for *p*lanning, *q*uestions practice, *r*epetition, and *s*elf- and peer testing.

While you study, remember to stay hydrated, eat sensibly, build in exercise breaks, and get plenty of sleep. It is also important to pursue other activities and not be involved solely in study. Research has shown that both sleep and "time out," in the form of exercise, social activities, or nutrition breaks, help consolidate learned information.

Managing Test Stress

If I take one more multiple-choice test, I think I may become physically ill. I won't be able to help myself. Can't they think of any other way of assessing how much we know?

The student quoted above is setting themselves up for failure because of their negativity toward the format of the test.

It is perfectly normal to feel nervous and anxious about the CPNRE. You have worked hard to be successful in your nursing program, and now all that effort comes down to passing a 4-hour exam. As you prepare for the CPNRE, empower yourself by developing a positive mental attitude. Henry Ford said, "Whether you think you can or think you can't … you're right." Challenge your negative thoughts! Do not let them guide you.

Stress Management Tips

Become active and positive about your learning and your preparation. The more actively you plan and prepare, the more likely you will be successful. The following tips will help you manage stress:

- Try to avoid fellow students who feel overly anxious about the exam. Anxiety is like a communicable disease. You can catch it.
- Use the power of positive thinking. Build up your self-confidence by repeating to yourself, "I am well prepared. I will pass this exam."
- Practise yoga or other forms of exercise; they are great stress relievers.
- Try aromatherapy—lavender works well to promote relaxation. Sometimes just the smell will help you remember to relax and breathe.
- Eat a well-balanced diet and get plenty of rest.

The evening before the examination
The night before a test, I can't sleep. Then I worry because I can't sleep. Then I can't sleep because I'm worrying that I'm worried that I can't sleep. By morning, I'm glad to get out of bed just to stop the terrible racket in my head.

The evening before the exam, organize your clothes and exam supplies. Make sure you know the location of the exam and have arranged your transportation to the exam.

Then, be nice to yourself. Do something you enjoy and get a good night's sleep. Information is processed during sleep, so sleep will help you retain what you have studied. Last-minute cramming may have aided you in past test situations, but it is helpful only for memorizing facts. It actually decreases your ability to problem-solve the application and critical-thinking types of questions that are on the CPNRE.

The day of the examination. Eat a healthy breakfast of protein and complex carbohydrates. If you absolutely cannot eat, try drinking a sports electrolyte solution. Although you need to be adequately hydrated, do not drink too many fluids or cups of coffee. Dress in comfortable clothes, preferably in layers, so that you can add or take off articles depending on the temperature of the exam room. If possible, try to make time for light exercise, even if it is walking the last few blocks to the exam centre.

Plan to arrive at the test location at least 30 minutes ahead of the exam start time. This cushion will allow you time to relax, visit with friends, and prepare yourself mentally. However, avoid talking about the exam with your friends, as conversations about it will only make you more anxious. Arriving early also gives you time for that last-minute washroom trip—stress is a potent diuretic. When you sit down in the exam room, make a conscious effort to relax and continue your positive thinking.

During the examination. Remember to keep that positive focus during the exam. Repeat to yourself: "I know this information, and I can answer these questions. I will pass the exam." Reading and keeping focused is essential. Take mini "brain breaks" by performing relaxation exercises in your seat, such as slow deep breaths, shoulder shrugs, neck rolls, and arm and leg rotations.

After the examination. After the exam, you will likely feel a sense of relief that it is over, but you may also feel the need to review questions in your head and discuss answers with your peers. Try not to dwell on this activity for too long. These postmortems can bring you down. Remember, you have probably done better than you think!

Tips for Writing Multiple-Choice Exams

Listed below are some tips for completing the multiple-choice questions particular to the CPNRE:

A. Read and listen to the exam instructions carefully.
B. Plan your time and pace yourself. Although it is important not to speed through questions, do not spend more than 1 to 1.5 minutes on any question. Keep track of time. You should answer approximately 25 to 30 questions in each half hour.
C. Do not spend a lot of time on one question if you do not know the answer. If you are stuck on a question, leave it and return to it later. Go on to a question that you find easy. The feeling of success will give you confidence.
D. Reading comprehension is crucial to success. Read the stem of each question carefully and make sure that you understand exactly what it asks. One of the most common test-taking errors is misreading the question. In the CPNRE, important words are not highlighted, so you should identify words such as *initial*, *most important*, or *priority*. Take special note of any negatives such as *never* or *except*.

2.8 Sample Question
The nurse discovers that Ms. Chang has received twice the dose of an ordered medication. What is the most important initial action for the nurse to perform?
1. Complete an incident report.
2. Notify the ordering health care provider.
3. Assess Ms. Chang for adverse effects of the overdose.
4. Report the error to the nurse administrator.
    The key word is *initial*; thus, the correct answer is 3.

E. Because the majority of the questions are either at the application or critical-thinking cognitive levels, you must be prepared to problem-solve *every* question. There are no rules for answering questions. Each question must be approached with a view to solving the problem based on your nursing judgement in this particular situation.

F. Try to answer the question before looking at the multiple-choice options.

G. Read all the options before choosing one. Do not immediately assume that a response is correct without looking at all the other options; another answer may be *more correct* than the one you choose first.

H. Read each option carefully, mentally crossing out the options you know are incorrect. Choose the best option out of the ones remaining.

I. Some questions that appear to be trick questions may, in reality, measure your ability to think critically. If you believe all the options are correct, choose the one that is most comprehensive, makes the most common sense, or is the most professional answer.

2.9 Sample Question

Which of the following is most important when performing a preoperative assessment?
1. Physical assessment
2. Cardiac assessment
3. Assessment of vital signs
4. Auscultation of breath sounds
   All options are valid, but answer 1 is the most inclusive.

J. To choose the most important nursing action when all of the answers appear to be correct, use the following guidelines:
   - Read the situation and question very carefully.
   - In many cases, consider the mnemonic *ABC* (*a*irway, *b*reathing, *c*irculation).
   - Remember the nursing process: collect and validate information before acting.
   - Consider safety—for the client and for yourself.
   - Choose an action that can be completed quickly and safely, almost at the same time as other actions.
   - Do not necessarily look for fancy answers.
   - Choose simple, common-sense, safe actions.
   - Choose the sickest, most unstable client as the priority.

K. A common error students make is choosing a response that might have been applicable in a specific client situation that they have experienced. Always answer according to "textbook," or standard, nursing principles.

L. Answer as you believe the perfect "textbook nurse" would answer.

M. Do not assume any information that is not given. Choose your answer based only on information in the question asked.

N. Do not panic if you have never heard of a particular disease or client situation. Apply general nursing principles to each question—you may be able to answer the question by doing so. Candidates for the exam come from various academic backgrounds, and curricula are not identical in all programs. You are not expected to know all the answers, nor are you expected to write a perfect exam!

2.10 Sample Question

Ms. Townsend is suffering from Hick's asymmetrical dementia. Which of the following activities would be appropriate for her condition?
1. Vigorous exercise
2. Competitive games
3. Social stimulation in group activities
4. Solitary reading
   Hick's asymmetrical dementia is a fictitious disorder. The care needs for a client with dementia are fundamental, so the correct response is answer 3. This is a "trick question" for the purpose of illustration. The CPNRE, however, contains no trick questions.

O. Your first answer choice is usually correct. You may have learned some information subconsciously, and your first impression is often an automatic response to what you have learned. Do not second-guess yourself unless you are absolutely sure that you have misunderstood the question or provided a wrong answer.

P. Select answers that are therapeutic, show respect, involve the client in care, and focus on nursing judgement rather than hospital rules or orders from other health team members.

2.11 Sample Question

Jessica tells the nurse, "I am tired of waiting for you to comb my hair. You're never here when I want you." Which of the following responses is the most appropriate for the nurse to give?
1. "I'm sorry you've had to wait. I'll get your comb out for you and be back in 15 minutes to do your hair."
2. "That's not fair. I spent my lunch break with you yesterday."
3. "Jeremy down the hall is really sick, and he needs me more than you do right now."
4. "I'm doing my best, but I have a really busy assignment today."
   Option 1 acknowledges the client's feelings, shows respect, and provides a clear, factual response.

2.12 Sample Question

Ms. Steele asks the nurse when she can start eating after bowel surgery. What is the most appropriate response for the nurse to give?
1. "You'll have to ask the doctor."
2. "Tell me about your appetite."
3. "You'll likely start on clear fluids once bowel sounds can be heard."
4. "I'll have the dietitian consult with you about the most nutritious postsurgery menus."
   Option 3 involves nursing judgement and directly answers the client's question.

Q. Most questions will ask about actions that are based on nursing judgement rather than physicians' orders. However, some questions may test your knowledge of the scope of nursing practice and have as a correct response "contact the health care provider." Examples of such situations include unclear or illegible orders, a specific request from a client, deteriorating client condition, or a client emergency.

R. In the case of communication questions, answers that demonstrate the nurse asking the client open-ended questions are most often correct.

2.13 Sample Question

Which of the following would elicit the best information from Mr. Loates about his pain?
1. "Do you have severe pain?"
2. "Do you have any pain?"
3. "Is your pain throbbing or stabbing?"
4. "Describe your pain to me."

Option 4 is open-ended—that is, it requires the client to give more than a one- or two-word answer. Phrasing questions in an open-ended fashion is a key component of therapeutic nursing communication.

S. Do not choose an answer because you have seen that question before and think you recall the answer. Questions on the exam may look similar to ones you have encountered during practice but will not be exactly the same. Therefore, the answer may also not be the same.

T. If all else fails, guess. Never leave a question unanswered. You have at least a 25% chance of getting it correct.

Tips for Guessing

1. If two of the options are similar except for one or two words, choose one of those.
   Example:
   Take the apical pulse
   Take the radial pulse
2. If two options have opposite meanings, choose one of those.
   Example:
   Vasodilation
   Vasoconstriction
3. If two quantities or mathematical calculations are similar, choose one of those.
   Example:
   0.14 mL
   0.014 mL

U. Answering 160 to 170 questions can be boring, stressful, and tiring. You may find yourself becoming confused about what information relates to the question. Throughout the exam, take a mini-exercise break every 20 minutes; sip water, do neck rolls, and flex your arms and legs.

V. Do not panic if someone leaves when you have completed only 20 questions. Most "early leavers" do not do better than exam writers who use the entire allotted time.

SUMMARY

Preparing for the examination well in advance, ensuring comprehensive content review, following the test-taking tips, developing your reading comprehension, and maintaining a positive outlook will equip you with the necessary abilities to be successful in the CPNRE.

REFERENCES

Yardstick Assessment Strategies. (2019). *Examination blueprint (2022–2026) Canadian Practical Nurse Registration Examination (CPNRE)*. Author.

BIBLIOGRAPHY

Bradley, P., & Page-Cutrara, K. (2024). *Elsevier's Canadian comprehensive review for the NCLEX-RN examination*. (3rd ed.) Elsevier.

Dickson, K. (2021). *Overcoming exam anxiety*. Athabasca University. https://www.athabascau.ca/support-services/tutoring-learning-support/learning-tools/overcoming-exam-anxiety.html

Hanoski, T. (2002). *Exam anxiety*. https://drthanoski.com/exam-anxiety

Learning Development and Success. (n.d.). *Managing test anxiety*. Western University. https://studentexperience.uwo.ca/remote/docs/LDS-Tip-Sheet--Test-Anxiety.pdf

Learning Development and Success. (n.d.). *Writing multiple choice tests*. Western University. https://learning.uwo.ca/selfhelp/skill_building_handouts/pdfs/Exams%20-%20Preparing,%20Writing,%20and%20Beyond/Writing%20Multiple.pdf

Yardstick Assessment Strategies. (2021). *The Canadian Practical Nurse Registration Examination (CPNRE) prep guide* (6th ed.). Author.

WEBSITES

- Association for Applied Psychophysiology and Biofeedback (http://www.aapb.org): This site contains information and resources concerning biofeedback and its benefits.
- Test Anxiety (https://www.heretohelp.bc.ca/workbook/test-anxiety): This site was developed by HeretoHelp in BC to help with test anxiety.

Tips for Writing the REx-PN®

DESCRIPTION OF THE EXAMINATION AND TEST-TAKING TIPS

The REx-PN exam is a computer adaptive test (CAT), which means that the test is built as the candidate answers questions. The computer determines the next question to administer based on the candidate's answer. If a candidate answers a question correctly, the computer will select a somewhat more challenging question. If a candidate answers a question incorrectly, the computer will select a somewhat less challenging question. Each question requires the candidate to submit an answer before the next question is given and the candidate will not be able to go back to review a question or change an answer. You will answer from 90 to 150 questions, including 30 pretest items that are not counted toward the examination score. A pretest item is a question that has not been statistically validated and is undergoing trial evaluation with exam candidates. You will not know which questions are the pretest items, so answer all questions as though they count toward your grade. The writing time for the exam is 4 hours. The National Council of State Boards of Nursing (NCSBN) has created the website https://www.rexpn.com/ where candidates can obtain detailed information about the REx-PN and the registration process. The regulatory body for the province you intend to obtain licensure in (e.g., British Columbia [BC] or Ontario) will determine your eligibility, and if you meet the exam eligibility requirements, it will allow you to complete the registration process. The College of Nurses of Ontario website https://www.cno.org/ provides information on the exam and the registration process for candidates intending to obtain licensure in Ontario. The BC College of Nurses & Midwives website https://www.bccnm.ca provides information on the exam and the registration process for candidates intending to obtain licensure in BC. The regulatory body will release the exam results to the candidate.

Types of Questions

Candidates completing the REx-PN will receive several question types. Many of the questions will be multiple choice. Other question types include multiple-response, fill-in-the-blank calculation, exhibit, and graphics.

Multiple-Choice Questions

Most of the questions that you will receive on the REx-PN will be in multiple-choice format. Each multiple-choice question is made up of two components. The part that asks the question or poses a problem is called the *stem*. The alternatives from which you are asked to select the best answer are called the *options*. There are four options, and *only one* of the options is the correct answer. The other three options are called *distractors*. Distractors may seem to be reasonable answers but are, in fact, incorrect or incomplete. All questions are worth one mark. Marks are not deducted for wrong answers.

3.1 Sample Question

A client develops chills and a headache while receiving a blood transfusion. What would be the nurse's initial action?
1. Notify the health care provider stat.
2. Stop the transfusion immediately.
3. Cover the client with a blanket and administer ordered acetaminophen.
4. Slow the blood flow to keep the vein open.
   The correct answer is two. The client is experiencing a transfusion reaction. Thus, the blood infusion must be stopped immediately.

Multiple-Response Questions

Some questions on the exam will be multiple response. When answering a multiple-response question, you will need to select more than one option. There may be two or more options that are correct. You will not be given credit for a correct answer unless all of the correct options are selected.

3.2 Sample Question

The nurse is teaching a client with gastroesophageal reflux disease (GERD) about foods that can worsen acid reflux. What foods should be included in the teaching session? **Select all that apply.**
1. Chocolate
2. Carrots
3. Spicy foods
4. Peppermint
5. Whole wheat bread
   The correct answers are 1, 3, and 4. Avoidance of certain foods that exacerbate acid reflux (e.g., chocolate, caffeine, citrus, tomatoes, alcohol, peppermint, spicy, or fried foods) can improve mild gastroesophageal reflux symptoms. Carrots and whole wheat bread will not exacerbate acid reflux.

Fill-in-the-Blank Calculation

Some items on the exam will require you to calculate an answer using numbers. The answer may need to be submitted as either a whole number or using decimal places. These instructions will be provided in the item. You will have access to a calculator on the computer screen. Rounding, if required, should be completed at the end of the calculation.

3.3 Sample Question

A health care provider prescribes ibuprofen liquid 250 mg PO every 8 hours prn for a client with pain. The medication label states: Ibuprofen 100 mg/5 mL. The nurse prepares to administer one dose. How many millilitres should the nurse prepare to administer one dose? **Fill in the blank. Record your answer using one decimal place.**

Answer: 12.5 mL

Formula:

$$\frac{\text{Dosage ordered}}{\text{Dosage available}} \times \text{Drug form} = \text{Amount of drug to administer}$$

$$\frac{250\text{ mg}}{100\text{ mg}} \times 5\text{ mL} = 12.5\text{ mL}$$

The formula for calculating a medication dose is used to complete this question. Your answer will need to be typed into the answer box to one decimal place as directed in the instructions.

Exhibit Questions

Some items on the REx-PN are exhibit questions. In exhibit questions, you will be presented with a problem and an exhibit with additional client information.

3.4 Sample Question

The nurse reviews the health record of a client requesting pain medication for premenstrual syndrome. The nurse determines that nonsteroidal anti-inflammatory drugs (NSAIDs) are contraindicated based on which of the following information?

History and physical	Allergy: Aspirin Hyperthyroidism
Medications:	Vitamin B6 50 mg daily
Laboratory results:	Hemoglobin 150 g/L

1. Allergy to Aspirin
2. Hyperthyroidism
3. Vitamin B6 50 mg daily
4. Hemoglobin 150 g/L

Answer: 1. This exhibit question provides you with data from the client's health record and asks you to identify the contraindication to the use of NSAIDs. NSAIDs are contraindicated in clients with a history of any of the following: allergy to Aspirin, allergy to NSAIDs, conditions that place the client at risk for bleeding, current hemorrhagic stroke, or severe kidney or liver disease.

Graphic Questions

In a graphic question, an image will be used as either part of the stem or as options.

3.5 Sample Question

At what age would the nurse expect a child to be able to perform the fine motor behaviour depicted in the following image?

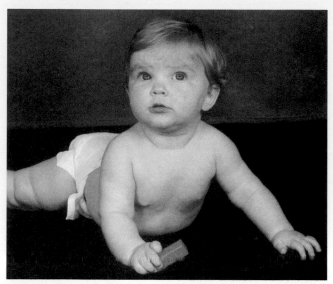

Photo by Paul Vincent Kuntz, Texas Children's Hospital, Houston, TX.

1. 6 months
2. 10 months
3. 18 months
4. 24 months

Answer: 2. The image shows the pincer grasp (using the thumb and index finger). Infants use a crude pincer grasp by 8 to 9 months and by 10 months of age, the pincer grasp is sufficiently established to enable infants to pick up finger foods.

Examination Test Plan

The REx-PN is written according to a test plan that includes client needs and integrated processes. It is not organized into sections on maternal–newborn nursing, medical–surgical nursing, pediatric nursing, mental health nursing, and so on.

Client Needs

There are four major client needs categories that the NCSBN (2020) has identified as the base of the test plan structure. These client care needs provide the framework for the nursing actions and competencies that a practical nurse is expected to demonstrate in order to provide safe, professional care. The client needs categories include safe and effective care environment, health promotion and maintenance, psychosocial integrity, and physiological integrity. The safe and effective care environment category has two subcategories including management of care, and safety and infection control. The physiological integrity category has four subcategories including basic care and comfort, pharmacological and parenteral therapies, reduction of risk potential, and physiological adaptation.

Safe and effective care environment. The safe and effective care environment category includes the two subcategories of management of care and safety and infection control. According to NCSBN, management of care means that *"the nurse provides and directs nursing care that enhances the care delivery setting to protect the client and health care personnel"*

(NCSBN, 2020, p. 7). Approximately 18 to 24% of the questions concern management of care. The NCSBN indicates that safety and infection control means that *"the nurse protects clients and health care personnel from health and environmental hazards"* (NCSBN, 2020, p. 12). Approximately 10 to 16% of the questions relate to safety and infection control.

3.6 Sample Question: Management of Care

The nurse assesses a client who was admitted to the hospital with pneumonia. The client has been coughing profusely and has required nasopharyngeal suctioning. They have an intravenous infusion of antibiotics. The client is febrile. Which of the following tasks may the nurse delegate to the unregulated care provider assigned to the client today?
1. Assessing vital signs
2. Changing intravenous dressing
3. Nasopharyngeal suctioning
4. Administering a bed bath

The correct answer is 4. The nurse may delegate administering a bed bath to the unregulated care provider (UCP). Changing the intravenous dressing is not a skill that can be delegated to a UCP. Assessing vital signs and performing nasopharyngeal suctioning of an unstable client cannot be delegated to a UCP.

3.7 Sample Question: Safety and Infection Control

A toddler with varicella is hospitalized for cardiac investigations. What type of isolation precautions should the client be placed on?
1. Contact
2. Protective
3. Airborne
4. Droplet

The correct answer is 3. Airborne-infection precautions are used for clients with varicella. Small airborne particles caught on floating dust in the room can be inhaled from anywhere in the room.

Health promotion and maintenance. According to NCSBN, health promotion and maintenance means "the nurse provides and directs nursing care of the client that incorporates knowledge of expected growth and development, prevention and early detection of health problems, and strategies to achieve optimal health" (NCSBN, 2020, p. 16). Approximately 6 to 12% of the questions relate to health promotion and maintenance.

3.8 Sample Question

The nurse is developing an exercise program for a client with moderate osteoarthritis of the knees. Which of the following forms of exercise would the nurse include in this program?
1. Step aerobics
2. Running
3. Water aerobics
4. Bike riding

The correct answer is 3. Water activities are good exercise alternatives for people with musculo-skeletal limitations.

Psychosocial integrity. According to NCSBN, psychosocial integrity means that "the nurse provides and directs nursing care that promotes and supports the emotional, mental and social well-being of the client experiencing stressful events, as well as clients with acute or chronic mental illness" (NCSBN, 2020, p. 21). Approximately 8 to 14% of the questions relate to psychosocial integrity.

3.9 Sample Question: Psychosocial Integrity

A nurse is teaching guided imagery to a group of clients with coronary artery disease. Which of the following is an example of guided imagery?
1. Singing
2. Back massage
3. Sensory peaceful words
4. Listening to music

The correct answer is 3. Guided imagery is used as a means to create a relaxed state through the person's imagination, often with the use of sensory words. Imagination allows the person to create a soothing and peaceful environment. Singing, back massage, and listening to music are other types of stress management techniques.

Physiological integrity. The physiological integrity category includes the four subcategories of basic care and comfort, pharmacological and parenteral therapies, reduction of risk potential, and physiological adaptation. According to NCSBN, basic care and comfort means "the nurse provides comfort and assistance in the performance of activities of daily living" (NCSBN, 2020, p. 27). Approximately 6 to 12% of questions concern basic care and comfort.

3.10 Sample Question: Basic Care and Comfort

The nurse is caring for a client on the medical–surgical unit with a wound that has a drain and a dressing that needs changing. Which of these actions should the nurse take first?
1. Put on sterile gloves.
2. Provide analgesic medications as ordered.
3. Avoid accidentally removing the drain.
4. Gather supplies.

The correct answer is 2. Because removal of dressing is painful, it often helps to give the client an analgesic at least 30 minutes before the wound is exposed and the dressing is changed.

According to NCSBN, pharmacological and parenteral therapies means "the nurse provides care related to the administration of medications and parenteral therapies" (NCSBN, 2020, p. 31). Approximately 14 to 20% of the questions concern pharmacological and parenteral therapies.

3.11 Sample Question: Pharmacological and Parenteral Therapies

Which type of drugs can have an adverse interaction with corticosteroids?
1. Nonsteroidal anti-inflammatory drugs (NSAIDs)
2. Antibiotics

3. Narcotic analgesics
4. Oral anticoagulants
   The answer is 1. The use of corticosteroids with NSAIDs produces adverse gastro-intestinal effects.

According to NCSBN, reduction of risk potential means that "the nurse reduces the likelihood that clients will develop complications or health problems related to existing conditions, treatments or procedures" (NCSBN, 2020, p. 35). Approximately 8 to 14% of the questions concern reduction of risk potential.

3.12 Sample Question: Reduction of Risk Potential

Which of the following topics is most important for the nurse to discuss preoperatively with a client who is scheduled for a colon resection?
1. Care for the surgical incision
2. Medications used during surgery
3. Deep-breathing and coughing techniques
4. Oral antibiotic therapy after discharge home
   The answer is 3. Preoperative teaching, demonstration, and redemonstration of deep breathing and coughing are needed for clients having abdominal surgery to prevent postoperative atelectasis.

According to NCSBN, physiological adaptation means that "the nurse manages and provides care for clients with acute, chronic or life-threatening physical health conditions" (NCSBN, 2020, p. 39). Approximately 6 to 12% of the questions concern physiological adaptation.

3.13 Sample Question: Physiological Adaptation

Which is a symptom of early hypokalemia?
1. Seizures
2. Paralytic ileus
3. Stomach cramps
4. Muscle weakness
   The correct answer is 4. Muscle weakness is an early symptom of hypokalemia. Paralytic ileus is a late symptom of hypokalemia. Seizures and stomach cramps are not symptoms of hypokalemia.

Integrated Processes

There are six processes that are fundamental to the practice of nursing that the (NCSBN, 2020) has identified and included throughout the client needs categories. The integrated processes are nursing process (assessment, analysis, planning, implementation, and evaluation), caring, communication and documentation, teaching and learning, culture and spirituality, and client safety.

3.14 Sample Question: Integrated Process of Caring

An 85-year-old has difficulty walking after a knee replacement. The client tells the nurse, "It's awful to be old. Every day is a struggle. No one cares about old people." Select the nurse's best response.

1. "Everyone here cares about old people. That's why we work here."
2. "It sounds like you're having a difficult time. Tell me about it."
3. "Let's not focus on the negative. Tell me something good."
4. "You are still able to get around, and your mind is alert."
   The answer is 2. The nurse uses empathic understanding to permit the client to express frustration and clarify their 'struggle' for the nurse.

Level of Cognitive Ability

To test your thinking abilities, questions are written at different cognitive levels: knowledge and comprehension, application, and critical thinking. Many questions on the REx-PN are at the application level

__Knowledge and comprehension.__ The knowledge and comprehension level requires recollection of facts. For these types of questions, you are required to define, identify, or select remembered information. Knowledge questions require basic memorization.

3.15 Sample Question

Which of the following is a possible therapeutic effect of nonsteroidal anti-inflammatory drugs (NSAIDS)?
1. Anxiolytic effects
2. Diuretic effects
3. Antipyretic effects
4. Antimicrobial effects
   The answer is 3, antipyretic. To answer this question correctly you need to have memorized the therapeutic effects of NSAIDs and the terms *anxiolytic*, *diuretic*, *antipyretic*, and *antimicrobial*.

__Application.__ The application level of the intellectual process requires not only knowing and understanding information but also being able to apply it to a new situation. This level includes modifying, manipulating, or adapting information when providing client care.

3.16 Sample Question

Before taking a client's vital signs, the nurse asks the client if they are taking any medications. The client answers, "Digoxin every morning and Tylenol in the evening." Which of the following vital sign changes might the nurse anticipate?
1. Increased blood pressure to 140/85 mm Hg
2. Decreased pulse to 53 beats per minute
3. Decreased respiratory rate to 10 breaths per minute
4. Increased temperature to 38.5°C
   The answer is 2, decreased pulse. This question requires knowledge about several drugs, interpretation of vital signs, and application of this information to a particular client.

__Critical thinking.__ Critical-thinking questions require the most complex level of cognitive function, asking the candidate to analyze, evaluate, problem-solve, or interpret data from various sources. This often involves prioritizing nursing actions. Often all of the options may be correct, but one action will be the most correct in a particular situation.

3.17 Sample Question

A client has asthma and is experiencing acute shortness of breath and wheezing. What should the nurse do first?
1. Administer the ordered "rescue inhaler."
2. Administer the ordered corticosteroid inhaled drugs.
3. Notify the health care provider.
4. Encourage increased fluid intake.

The answer is 1, administer the rescue inhaler. All the options could be correct, but administering the rescue inhaler is the first thing the nurse should do.

STUDY AND EXAMINATION TIPS

Although you may be academically well prepared to write the REx-PN, strategies for studying, stress management, and test-taking will increase your chances of success and help alleviate test anxiety.

Study Tips

It is easy to become overwhelmed as you prepare to study for the REx-PN. Remember, though, that you know a lot more than you think you do. While studying is crucial, much learning is not a conscious activity. The first key to developing successful study strategies is to be realistic. Identify where you have incomplete knowledge or the need to refresh your learning.

Keep in mind that most of the questions on the exam do not merely test recalled facts, so you should try to understand the material that you read rather than memorize it. The focus of your studies should be on principles of care and nursing interventions within a particular health situation; that is, what should the nurse do or say?

One of the best strategies for learning is to form a study group. Self-testing and peer testing have proven to be the most effective methods for consolidating material. Have each member of the group choose a topic to teach the other members. This way, you stimulate discussion and get different perspectives on the subjects, which will help you in understanding and remembering them. If you are unable to participate in a study group, try teaching yourself the information. Rephrase or reword the written information to aid in understanding rather than memorizing.

Repetition works well for many people. If you are having trouble remembering some knowledge material, it may help to record it so that you can play it aloud while performing other activities.

Schedule your studying. Start reviewing content several months prior to the exam so that you do not feel rushed or panicked at the volume of material you need to learn. Cramming or "all-nighters" may be useful for memorizing facts, but the REx-PN is an exam that requires problem-solving based on a comprehensive knowledge base. It is better to think through and analyze the material, make judgements, and determine how the subject relates to nursing. By performing these analytical and reflective processes, you are more likely to commit the information to long-term memory, which is much more reliable than your short-term memory.

To remember the strategies for studying, you can use the initialism PQRS, which stands for *p*lanning, *q*uestions practice, *r*epetition, and *s*elf- and peer testing.

While you study, remember to stay hydrated, eat sensibly, build in exercise breaks, and get plenty of sleep. It is also important to pursue other activities and not be involved solely in study. Research has shown that both sleep and "time out," in the form of exercise, social activities, or nutrition breaks, help consolidate learned information.

Managing Test Stress

If I take one more multiple-choice test, I think I may become physically ill. I won't be able to help myself. Can't they think of any other way of assessing how much we know?

The student quoted above is setting themselves up for failure because of their negativity toward the format of the test.

It is perfectly normal to feel nervous and anxious about the REx-PN. You have worked hard to be successful in your nursing program, and now all that effort comes down to passing one exam in a format that may be different from the types of exam you are most familiar with. As you prepare for the REx-PN, empower yourself by developing a positive mental attitude. Henry Ford said, "Whether you think you can or think you can't … you're right." Challenge your negative thoughts! Do not let them guide you.

Stress Management Tips

Become active and positive about your learning and your preparation. The more actively you plan and prepare, the more likely you will be successful. The following tips will help you manage stress:

- Try to avoid fellow students who feel overly anxious about the exam. Anxiety is like a communicable disease. You can catch it.
- Use the power of positive thinking. Build up your self-confidence by repeating to yourself, "I am well prepared. I will pass this exam."
- Practise yoga or other forms of exercise; they are great stress relievers.
- Try aromatherapy—lavender works well to promote relaxation. Sometimes just the smell will help you remember to relax and breathe.
- Eat a well-balanced diet and get plenty of rest.

The evening before the examination

The night before a test, I can't sleep. Then I worry because I can't sleep. Then I can't sleep because I'm worrying that I'm worried that I can't sleep. By morning, I'm glad to get out of bed just to stop the terrible racket in my head.

The evening before the exam, organize your clothes and exam supplies. Make sure you know the location of the exam and have arranged your transportation to the exam.

Then, be nice to yourself. Do something you enjoy and get a good night's sleep. Information is processed during sleep, so sleep will help you retain what you have studied. Last-minute cramming may have aided you in past test situations, but it is helpful only for memorizing facts. It actually decreases your ability to problem-solve the application and critical-thinking types of questions that are on the REx-PN.

The day of the examination. Eat a healthy breakfast of protein and complex carbohydrates. If you absolutely cannot eat, try drinking a sports electrolyte solution. Although you need to be adequately hydrated, do not drink too many fluids or cups of coffee. Dress in comfortable clothes, preferably in layers, so that you can add or take off articles depending on the temperature of the exam room. If possible, try to make time for light exercise, even if it is walking the last few blocks to the exam centre.

Plan to arrive at the test location at least 30 minutes ahead of the exam start time. This cushion will allow you time to relax, visit with friends, and prepare yourself mentally. However, avoid talking about the exam with your friends, as conversations about it will only make you more anxious. Arriving early also gives you time for that last-minute washroom trip—stress is a potent diuretic. When you sit down in the exam room, make a conscious effort to relax and continue your positive thinking.

During the examination. Remember to keep that positive focus during the exam. Repeat to yourself: "I know this information, and I can answer these questions. I will pass the exam." Reading and keeping focused is essential. Take mini "brain breaks" by performing relaxation exercises in your seat, such as slow deep breaths, shoulder shrugs, neck rolls, and arm and leg rotations.

After the examination. After the exam, you will likely feel a sense of relief that it is over, but you may also feel the need to review questions in your head and discuss answers with your peers. Try not to dwell on this activity for too long. These postmortems can bring you down. Remember, you have probably done better than you think!

Tips for Writing the REx-PN Exam

Listed below are some tips for completing the questions particular to the REx-PN:

A. Read the exam instructions carefully.
B. Read and focus on each question before moving on to the next. Remember, you will not be able to go back and change an answer once it has been submitted.
C. Plan your time and pace yourself. Although it is important not to speed through questions, do not spend more than 1 to 1.5 minutes on any question. Keep track of time. You should answer approximately 25 to 30 questions in each half hour.
D. Do not spend a lot of time on one question if you do not know the answer.

E. Reading comprehension is crucial to success. Read the stem of each question carefully and make sure that you understand exactly what it asks. One of the most common test-taking errors is misreading the question. In the REx-PN, important words are not highlighted, so you should identify words such as *initial*, *most important*, or *priority*. You will be given a whiteboard that can be used to jot down these important words.

3.18 Sample Question

The nurse discovers that the client has received twice the dose of an ordered medication. What is the most important initial action for the nurse to perform?
1. Complete an incident report.
2. Notify the ordering health care provider.
3. Assess the client for adverse effects of the overdose.
4. Report the error to the nurse administrator.
   The key word is *initial*; thus, the correct answer is 3.

F. Be prepared to problem-solve *every* question. There are no rules for answering questions. Each question must be approached with a view to solving the problem based on your nursing judgement in this particular situation.
G. Try to answer the question before looking at the options.
H. In multiple-choice questions or multiple-response questions, read all the options before choosing.
I. Read each option carefully, mentally crossing out the options you know are incorrect. Choose the best option or options out of the ones remaining.
J. Some questions that appear to be trick questions may, in reality, measure your ability to think critically. If you believe all the options are correct, choose the option or options that are most comprehensive, make the most common sense, or are the most professional response or responses.

3.19 Sample Question

Which of the following is most important when performing a preoperative assessment?
1. Physical assessment
2. Cardiac assessment
3. Assessment of vital signs
4. Auscultation of breath sounds
   All options are valid, but answer 1 is the most inclusive.

K. To choose the most important nursing action when all of the answers appear to be correct, use the following guidelines:
   • Read the situation and question very carefully.
   • In many cases, consider the mnemonic *ABC* (*a*irway, *b*reathing, *c*irculation).
   • Remember the nursing process: collect and validate information before acting.
   • Consider safety—for the client and for yourself.
   • Choose an action that can be completed quickly and safely, almost at the same time as other actions.
   • Do not necessarily look for elaborate answers.
   • Choose simple, common-sense, safe actions.
   • Choose the sickest, most unstable client as the priority.

L. A common error students make is choosing a response or responses that might have been applicable in a specific client situation that they have experienced. Always answer according to "textbook," or standard, nursing principles.

M. Answer as you believe the perfect "textbook nurse" would answer.

N. Do not assume any information that is not given. Choose your answer based only on information in the question asked.

O. Do not panic if you have never heard of a particular disease or client situation. Apply general nursing principles to each question—you may be able to answer the question by doing so. Candidates for the exam come from various academic backgrounds, and curricula are not identical in all programs. You are not expected to know all the answers, nor are you expected to write a perfect exam!

3.20 Sample Question

A client is suffering from Hick's asymmetrical dementia. Which of the following activities would be appropriate for her condition?

1. Vigorous exercise
2. Competitive games
3. Social stimulation in group activities
4. Solitary reading

Hick's asymmetrical dementia is a fictitious disorder. The care needs for a client with dementia are fundamental, so the correct response is answer 3. This is a "trick question" for the purpose of illustration. The REx-PN, however, contains no trick questions.

P. Your first answer choice is usually correct. You may have learned some information subconsciously, and your first impression is often an automatic response to what you have learned. Do not second-guess yourself unless you are absolutely sure that you have misunderstood the question or provided a wrong answer.

Q. Select answers that are therapeutic, show respect, involve the client in care, and focus on nursing judgement rather than hospital rules or orders from other health team members.

3.21 Sample Question

The client Jessica tells the nurse, "I am tired of waiting for you to comb my hair. You're never here when I want you." Which of the following responses is the most appropriate for the nurse to give?

1. "I'm sorry you've had to wait. I'll get your comb out for you and be back in 15 minutes to do your hair."
2. "That's not fair. I spent my lunch break with you yesterday."
3. "Jeremy down the hall is really sick, and he needs me more than you do right now."
4. "I'm doing my best, but I have a really busy assignment today."

Option 1 acknowledges the client's feelings, shows respect, and provides a clear, factual response.

3.22 Sample Question

A client asks the nurse when they can start eating after bowel surgery. What is the most appropriate response for the nurse to give?

1. "You'll have to ask the health care provider."
2. "Tell me about your appetite."
3. "You'll likely start on clear fluids once bowel sounds can be heard."
4. "I'll have the dietitian consult with you about the most nutritious postsurgery menus."

Option 3 involves nursing judgement and directly answers the client's question.

R. Most questions will ask about actions that are based on nursing judgement rather than health care providers' orders. However, some questions may test your knowledge of the scope of nursing practice and have as a correct response "contact the health care provider." Examples of such situations include unclear or illegible orders, a specific request from a client, deteriorating client condition, or a client emergency.

S. In the case of communication questions, answers that demonstrate the nurse asking the client open-ended questions are most often correct.

3.23 Sample Question

Which of the following would elicit the best information from a client about their pain?

1. "Do you have severe pain?"
2. "Do you have any pain?"
3. "Is your pain throbbing or stabbing?"
4. "Describe your pain to me."

Option 4 is open-ended—that is, it requires the client to give more than a one- or two-word answer. Phrasing questions in an open-ended fashion is a key component of therapeutic nursing communication.

T. Do not choose an answer because you have seen that question before and think you recall the answer. Questions on the exam may look similar to ones you have encountered during practice but will not be exactly the same. Therefore, the answer may also not be the same.

U. In multiple-response questions, each response is a true or false statement; select all the choices that are true.

V. In fill-in-the-blank calculation questions, read the question carefully and complete the required calculation to the decimal place instructed; ensure you confirm your answer with the on-screen calculator.

W. An exhibit question will contain relevant information required to answer the question. It may also contain information that is not relevant. Use your knowledge and judgement to choose the correct response.

X. If all else fails, guess. Consider all the choices and select your best answer to allow you to proceed to the next question.

Tips for Guessing

1. If two of the options are similar except for one or two words, choose one of those.

   Example:

   Take the apical pulse

   Take the radial pulse

2. If two options have opposite meanings, choose one of those.

   Example:

   Vasodilation

   Vasoconstriction

3. If two quantities or mathematical calculations are similar, choose one of those.

Example:

0.14 mL

0.014 mL

Y. Answering up to 150 questions can be boring, stressful, and tiring. You may find yourself becoming confused about what information relates to the question. Throughout the exam, take a short break every 20 minutes; sip water, do neck rolls, and flex your arms and legs.

Z. Do not panic if someone leaves when you have completed only 20 questions. Most "early leavers" do not do better than exam writers who require a longer period of time.

SUMMARY

Preparing for the examination well in advance, ensuring comprehensive content review, following the test-taking tips, developing your reading comprehension, and maintaining a positive outlook will equip you with the necessary abilities to be successful in the REx-PN.

REFERENCES

National Council of State Boards of Nursing (NCSBN). (2020). *2022 REx-PN® test plan.* Author.

BIBLIOGRAPHY

Bradley, P., & Page-Cutrara, K., (2024). *Elsevier's Canadian comprehensive review for the NCLEX-RN examination* (3rd ed.). Elsevier.

Dickson, K. (2021). *Overcoming exam anxiety.* Athabasca University. https://www.athabascau.ca/support-services/tutoring-learning-support/learning-tools/overcoming-exam-anxiety.html

Hanoski, T. (2018). *Exam anxiety.* https://drthanoski.com/exam-anxiety

Keenan-Lindsay, L., Sam, C. A., & O'Connor, C. (2022). *Perry's maternal child nursing care in Canada* (3rd ed.). Elsevier.

Learning Development and Success. (n.d.). *Managing test anxiety.* Western University. https://studentexperience.uwo.ca/remote/docs/LDS-Tip-Sheet--Test-Anxiety.pdf

Learning Development and Success. (n.d.). *Writing multiple choice tests.* Western University. https://learning.uwo.ca/selfhelp/skill_building_handouts/pdfs/Exams%20-%20Preparing,%20Writing,%20and%20Beyond/Writing%20Multiple.pdf

WEBSITES

- Association for Applied Psychophysiology and Biofeedback (http://www.aapb.org): This site contains information and resources concerning biofeedback and its benefits.
- British Columbia College of Nurses & Midwives (https://www.bccnm.ca): This site contains links to information on all aspects of being a licensed practical nurse in BC.
- College of Nurses of Ontario (https://www.cno.org/): This site contains links to information related to all aspects of being a registered practical nurse in Ontario.
- Test Anxiety (https://www.heretohelp.bc.ca/workbook/test-anxiety): This site was developed by HeretoHelp in BC to help with test anxiety.

Professional Practice and the Nurse–Client Relationship

Practical nurses in Canada are major contributors to and an essential part of the health care system. Changes in health care delivery have occurred in health care organizations over the past years to meet the changing needs of client populations and the health care system. Practical nurses are adapting to these changes to provide a highly competent workforce. Practical nurses work either independently or collaboratively with registered nurses (RNs) to provide care to clients of varying complexity in acute and long-term care, as well as in community and mental health care settings. Practical nurses are valuable members of the health care team in providing quality client care.

An understanding of the unique and overlapping scopes of practice within nursing and how nursing teams function effectively contributes to safe, competent care and quality outcomes for clients. Nursing care delivery models are based on principles of collaboration and partnership, allowing for optimal teamwork, respect, and knowledge sharing.

The Canadian Council for Practical Nurse Regulators (CCPNR, 2020) outlines the practice expectations of licensed practical nurses and registered practical nurses (LPNs and RPNs). Practical nurses are expected to uphold ethical standards, meet standards of practice, and have the required skills, abilities, and entry-to-practice competencies that ensure consistently safe and competent care. The practical nurse provides care to the individual, family, group, community, and larger populations. The scope of practice of a practical nurse depends on the complexity of knowledge, critical thinking, and judgement required in the practice environment.

REGULATION AND LICENSING OF NURSING IN CANADA

In Canada, nursing is a profession that is self-regulated and consists of different groups of nurses. These groups are as follows:

- Registered practical nurses (RPNs) in Ontario or licensed practical nurses (LPNs) in the rest of Canada
- Registered nurses (RNs)
- Registered psychiatric nurses who practise only in British Columbia, Alberta, Saskatchewan, Manitoba, and Yukon
- Nurse practitioners (NPs)

Provincial and territorial regulatory bodies are responsible for the licensing and registration of all nurses in Canada. These regulatory bodies are responsible for defining the scope of practice, standards of practice, and ethical standards that nurses must meet in their particular jurisdiction. Self-regulation also means that the regulator or licensing organization is responsible for disciplining nurses who do not meet the established standards of practice (Astle & Duggleby, 2024).

NURSING LEGISLATION

Nursing practice acts and health professions acts regulate the registration and licensing of nurses, describe continuing competency requirements and any restricted or controlled acts, and explain discipline procedures for the profession. Nursing practice acts have been revised across the country to reflect the growing autonomy and expanding roles of the nurse. The legislative acts exist primarily to protect the public in terms of health, safety, and welfare. Most provinces and territories provide a registration certificate, while others provide a licence. Legislation also provides title protection for nurses. Using the titles RN, LPN, RPN, and, in some provinces and territories, NP, is limited to only those nurses who are authorized to do so by their legislative and regulatory bodies.

Practical Nursing Scope of Practice

In Canada, the practical nurse's scope of practice is determined by legislation and regulatory and licensure requirements. Standards of nursing practice define the expectation for practical nurses in various practice settings and situations, and generally guide nursing practice.

Practical nurses must be able to practise entry-level competencies using knowledge, skill, and judgement. The practical nurse is determined to be competent if they successfully complete an approved Canadian practical nursing educational program (or an equivalent non-Canadian nursing program) and pass either the Regulatory Exam-Practical Nurse (REx-PN) in British Columbia and Ontario or the Canadian Practical Nurse Registration Examination (CPNRE) in all other provinces and territories except Quebec. Internationally prepared nurses must meet specific regulatory requirements, including passing a registration examination and meeting academic standards, to be eligible to become a practical nurse (Astle & Duggleby, 2024).

Reciprocity between provinces and territories may allow qualifying practical nurses to practise in different provinces and territories. This reciprocity becomes available once the practical nurse has completed the registration process. Practical nurses in most provinces are required to write a jurisprudence examination before becoming registered. The jurisprudence examination assesses an applicant's knowledge and understanding of the laws, regulations, bylaws, practice standards, and guidelines that govern the practice of nursing (visit the website of your jurisdiction's regulatory body for more information on the jurisprudence examination).

A regulatory body is mandated by the province or territory to set minimum entry-to-practice requirements to promote public safety and professional accountability. Jurisdictions typically include the following entry-to-practice requirements for practical nursing:

- Graduation from an approved postsecondary program for practical nursing
- A clear criminal record check
- Knowledge of the nursing process (assessment, planning, implementing, and evaluating nursing care) for clients of differing ages
- Ability to work independently as well as collaboratively with other health care providers in acute, unpredictable situations
- Ability to work with a range of clients: individuals, families, groups, and (if need be) communities
- Understanding of and ability to apply ethical practice standards
- Ability to collaborate and communicate with others, including the client and other health care providers
- Ability to be accountable and responsible for one's own actions
- Ability to work within the scope of practice
- Willingness to learn on an ongoing basis
- Ability to cope with change (Astle & Duggleby, 2024)

EDUCATION

For the practical nurse, the entry-level educational requirement in Canadian jurisdictions is a 2-year diploma program (Astle & Duggleby, 2024). Many academic institutions in Canada are beginning to offer pathways that bridge practical nursing and registered nursing programs. Practical nurses have many opportunities to further their education through certification in specialty areas such as operating room technique and management, geriatric nursing, dialysis, women's health, and mental health (Astle & Duggleby, 2024). It is important that practical nurses continually update their knowledge and skills. In today's rapidly changing health care workplace, there are frequent advances in research, technology, and practice. It is essential for practical nurses to be lifelong learners and to expand their knowledge base as well as keep current with practice standards.

PRACTICE ENVIRONMENTS

Practical nurses work in a multitude of practice environments across Canada. Practice environments range from chronic care to acute care, and they include nontraditional settings such as businesses and governmental organizations. Most practical nurses work in long-term/geriatric care, rehabilitation, acute care, and community health. Practical nurses may also be employed as administrators, educators, and researchers.

Long-Term Care Facilities and Rehabilitation Centres

Long-term care facilities are mostly residential. They provide nursing care for individuals with chronic illnesses who require 24-hour nursing care and support services for individuals who cannot care for themselves at home but do not require hospital care. The facilities also provide respite care. Geriatric care will depend on the individual's health status and care requirements.

Rehabilitation centres focus on helping clients become as independent as possible so that they can take care of their own needs. Practical nurses work as part of an extensive health care team that plans clients' rehabilitation and their return to the community. These clients may have a chronic illness or may have experienced an acute illness.

Acute Care Facilities

Acute care settings provide health care for a short time in which an immediate health concern is assessed, treated or both. Clients in acute care settings may have complex, multisystem conditions with many health care needs. Practical nurses in these settings must possess a wide variety of technical skills and must meet the physical and psychological needs of these acutely ill clients and their families.

Community and Other Settings

Many community practical nurses are involved in important roles such as performing health assessments and direct care to clients or groups (e.g., families that need parenting skills) within a community setting. The scope of community nursing practice includes population-focused health promotion, protection, maintenance, and restoration. The term *community nursing* is broad and encompasses public health nursing, community health nursing, and community-based nursing.

In recent years, clients are being sent home earlier from acute care facilities. This trend has increased the need for community-based nurses. The required nursing services are more complex because the level of care needed in these community populations is increasingly acute. This acuity is in part due to the earlier discharges from hospitals. However, in addition, more clients are being cared for at home rather than being admitted to long-term care facilities. For example, practical nurses now require the skills to provide home care for clients with tracheostomies, central venous lines, and home dialysis.

NURSING ROLES

The Role of the Practical Nurse

Most provinces now have two categories of nurses: (a) registered nurses (including nurse practitioners) and (b) practical nurses. The title of a practical nurse is "registered practical nurse" (RPN) in Ontario and "licensed practical nurse" (LPN) in the rest of the provinces and territories. Most jurisdictions recognize that practical nursing is a separate category within the wider field of professional nursing. Most jurisdictions also recognize that practical nurses and RNs learn approximately the same body of nursing knowledge. RNs study this content in more detail and over a longer period of time, while practical nurses study for a shorter period, resulting in more focused knowledge (Astle & Duggleby, 2024).

Practical nurses may work independently or they may work collaboratively with RNs. "While specific scopes of practice may differ among jurisdictions, it is common to find that as the complexity and unpredictability of the patient's condition and risk of negative outcomes increase, practical nurses will need more collaboration and support from RNs" (Astle & Duggleby, 2024, p. 67).

The Role of the Registered Nurse

For the RN, the entry-level educational requirement is a 4-year baccalaureate degree in nursing, with the exception of Quebec, which accepts a 3-year college diploma. Many nurses go on to further their education and study for a master's or doctoral degree in nursing or other disciplines. A master's degree in nursing is necessary for nurses seeking positions as clinical nurse specialists, nurse practitioners, nurse administrators, or nurse educators. RNs are caregivers, client and family advocates, clinical educators, administrators, professors, and researchers, and fulfill many other roles.

The Role of the Unregulated Care Provider

"Unregulated care providers (UCPs) are not regulated through legislation and are not members of an organization or professional college that governs their role" (Wilk et al., 2022). There are many other titles for this role, such as *health care aide*, *personal support worker*, or *nursing attendant*. These support workers are usually employees of a facility or an agency and are bound to perform in their role as per the terms of their employment agreement. Registered or licensed staff working with these individuals must be aware of the role expectations set by the employer for this category of worker and of the level of competence of the individual worker. Registered or licensed staff are not accountable for the care provided by the support worker (Astle & Duggleby, 2024).

NURSING PRACTICE AND THE LAW

It is important for nurses to know the legal parameters they work within to protect their clients' rights as well as their own. They need to know the specific nursing laws of the jurisdiction in which they practise and be familiar with the federal *Canada Health Act* (1985), which applies to health care across Canada. Provincial and territorial legislatures create laws that apply to only their jurisdictions. For example, *The Nursing Act* in Ontario describes the boundaries of nursing practice within that province only. Provincial and territorial laws also give authority to their nursing regulatory bodies (Astle & Duggleby, 2024).

Nursing regulatory bodies are responsible to the public. Their mandate is to ensure that the nursing care delivered to the public is safe and competent and meets standards of care and a code of ethics. In addition, regulatory bodies set nursing examinations and grant registration or licensure.

These regulatory bodies also can revoke or suspend a nurse's licence if a nurse violates the parameters of the registration statute. An investigation of public complaints or misconduct is carried out by the regulatory body, and a hearing may be held. The nurse must be informed of the charges. Further legal action may occur if the nurse's registration is revoked or removed from the jurisdiction's register and there are criminal or civil wrongs (Astle & Duggleby, 2024).

Most health care organizations are accredited by Accreditation Canada. The accreditation requires that these organizations have clear, written nursing policies and procedures that meet the standards of care and guide a nurse's practice. If a charge of negligence is brought against an individual nurse that results in a lawsuit, the nurse's actions and practice are compared with the organization's standards of care and the provincial or territorial nursing standards of practice. If an organizational policy violates the jurisdictional standards of practice, then the organizational policy is overridden by law. It is the nurse's responsibility to know the jurisdictional law and standards of practice (Astle & Duggleby, 2024).

Legal Liability

A tort is "a civil wrong committed against a person or property" (Astle & Duggleby, 2024, p. 123). A tort is not a criminal act, but if it is serious enough, a nurse may be charged with a criminal offence. Most lawsuits involving nurses are for negligence or malpractice, which comes under the "unintentional" classification. The terms *negligence* and *malpractice* are sometimes used interchangeably (Irvine et al., 2013).

Intentional Torts

Intentional torts are deliberate actions that violate another's rights and include assault, battery, invasion of privacy, and false imprisonment (Astle & Duggleby, 2024):

- Assault is a physical or verbal threat that creates apprehension or a fear of being harmed. No contact is necessary. For example, if a nurse threatens to start an intravenous (IV) line without a client's consent, then the nurse could be sued for assault. Consent would negate the possibility of a lawsuit (Fridman, 2012; Irvine et al., 2013).
- Battery is intentional physical contact with an individual without that person's consent. The contact may not necessarily be harmful but may be offensive (Astle & Duggleby, 2024; Fridman, 2012; Osborne, 2015). If the nurse started the IV line without consent, the nurse could be sued for battery.
- Invasion of privacy protects the client's rights to be free from intrusion into their private affairs. For example, a nurse would be liable if the nurse released confidential information about a client to an unauthorized individual without the client's consent.
- False imprisonment is intended to protect an individual's freedom and basic rights. For example, a nurse may be liable if the nurse prevents a client from leaving a health care agency voluntarily. Also, a nurse who uses restraints (chemical or physical) inappropriately may be considered liable (Astle & Duggleby, 2024).

Unintentional Torts

Negligence is a failure to take the care that a reasonable nurse in similar circumstances would have taken (Canadian Nurses

Protective Society [CNPS], 2022). Negligence can be considered a liable act if it causes injury, even if there was no intent. Nurses are negligent if they do not meet the standards of practice that are set by their regulatory body and cause injury to the client because of a lack of nursing care or prevention of injury (Astle & Duggleby, 2024). Usually, the courts consider negligence to be the failure to use that degree of skill or learning ordinarily used under the same or similar circumstances by other nursing professionals (Astle & Duggleby, 2024). In order for a nurse to be found negligent, the court must have evidence that the nurse:

- *Did not meet the duty of care*, a term meaning that the client relies on the nurse's professional skills and knowledge and the nurse has a legal duty to take reasonable care.
- *Breached the standard of care*, meaning that the court will determine what constituted reasonable nursing care in the circumstances.
- *Caused foreseeable harm through a breach in the standard of care*, meaning that the client was actually harmed. It must be proven that the nurse's negligent act caused the harm (Osborne, 2015).

Nurses are accountable for their own actions. An agency may also be found jointly liable with the nurse if the agency does not ensure that standards of nursing practice are being met in its facility. Common negligent acts are listed in Box 4.1.

Criminal Prosecution

Nurses may be reported to the police if involvement in criminal activity is suspected. The police may investigate, and charges will be laid under the *Criminal Code of Canada* if there is sufficient evidence. Nurses are interviewed by the investigators, and a formal statement will be requested. Any information given by the nurse can be used as evidence in the trial proceedings. Therefore, it is important for a nurse to consult with a criminal lawyer before giving any statement or answering questions (CNPS, 1999).

BOX 4.1   Common Negligent Acts

- Medication errors that result in injury to patients
- Intravenous therapy errors that result in infiltrations or phlebitis
- Burns caused by equipment, bathing, or spills of hot liquids and foods
- Falls resulting in injury
- Failure to use aseptic technique as required
- Errors in sponge, instrument, or needle counts in surgical cases
- Failure to give a report, or giving an incomplete report, to an incoming shift
- Failure to monitor a patient's condition adequately
- Failure to communicate a significant change in a patient's status
- Failure to properly delegate or supervise

From Astle, B., & Duggleby, W. (2024). *Potter and Perry's Canadian fundamentals of nursing* (7th ed.). Elsevier.

Some examples of criminal activities that nurses could be charged with include the following:

- Theft of narcotics
- Theft of client or agency property
- Assisted suicide
- Criminal negligence
- Battery by threatening or inflicting bodily harm
- Sexual assault

NURSING PROFESSIONAL PRACTICE

Nursing Accountability

Practical nurses are responsible and accountable for their decisions and actions. The CCPNR includes Professional Accountability and Responsibility in the standards of practice for practical nurses (CCPNR, 2020). This standard includes the following indicators for LPNs:

- Practice within applicable legislation, regulations, bylaws, and employer policies.
- Self-assess their professional practice and competence and participate in continuous learning.
- Share knowledge and expertise to meet client needs.
- Practice within LPN scope of practice and individual level of competence and consult and collaborate when necessary.
- Have a duty to report any circumstances that potentially or actually impede professional, ethical, or legal practice.
- Adhere to established client safety principles and quality assurance measures to anticipate, identify, evaluate, and promote continuous improvement of safety culture.
- Advocate for continuous improvements in health care through policies and procedures that support evidence-informed practice.
- Are accountable and responsible for their own practice, conduct, and ethical decision making.
- Document and report according to established legislation, regulations, laws, and employer policies.
- Provide leadership to support and participate in mentoring and preceptorship. (CCPNR, 2020, p. 5)

Ethical Nursing Practice

Ethics is "concerned with determining what is good or valuable for all people" (Astle & Duggleby, 2024, p. 109). Nursing regulatory bodies are tasked with establishing and upholding ethical standards. Ethical standards provide practical nurses with guidance on ethical practice, decision making, behaviour, and relationships. Most ethical standards for practical nurses promote the following values:

- Being accountable for one's actions
- Upholding the patient's rights to privacy and confidentiality
- Providing care that maintains the patient's dignity
- Demonstrating respect for the client at all times
- Promoting integrity by providing safe, competent, and ethical nursing care
- Evaluating one's work and maintaining competency (Astle & Duggleby, 2024)

NURSING PROFESSIONAL RELATIONSHIPS AND COMMUNICATION

The Therapeutic Nurse–Client Relationship

The nurse–client relationship is central to nursing. A professional relationship is created through the nurse's application of knowledge, communication theory, understanding of human behaviour, and commitment to ethical behaviour. Helping relationships are at the foundation of clinical nursing practice. The nurse is considered the helper and interacts with the client in consideration of the client's unique health needs, human responses, and patterns of living (Astle & Duggleby, 2024). The key points in this relationship are as follows:

- The relationship is based on trust, respect, empathy, and professional intimacy and requires the appropriate use of power.
- The purpose of the relationship is to meet the needs of the client.
- Nurses establish, maintain, re-establish, and terminate relationships with clients.
- Nurses use a client-centred care approach to ensure that all professional behaviours and actions meet the therapeutic needs of the client.
- Nurses are responsible for effectively establishing and maintaining the boundaries in the relationship.
- Nurses protect the client from harm by ensuring that abuse is prevented or stopped and reported (Astle & Duggleby, 2024).

The nurse–client relationship goes through a series of developmental phases. The four phases are pre-interaction, orientation, working, and termination:

1. The *pre-interaction phase* begins before the nurse meets the client and may involve accessing information about the client, a diagnosis, or a procedure. It includes identifying a suitable setting and anticipation of the client's needs, issues, or concerns.
2. The *orientation phase* involves the meeting of the nurse and the client. This stage begins with a social exchange and expands to include decision making regarding the client's goals, the role of both the client and the nurse in facilitating fulfillment of the goals, and the expected length of the relationship.
3. The *working phase* consists of the nurse and the client working together to facilitate the accomplishment of the client's goals. It is important for the nurse to use therapeutic communication skills to encourage the client to self-explore and take action to meet their goals.
4. The *termination phase* is a time to evaluate the achievement of goals and for the nurse and the client to separate and make the transition whereby the client or another caregiver assumes responsibility for the care (Astle & Duggleby, 2024).

Communication

It is critical that nurses develop and use effective communication skills to facilitate optimum relationship building. Communication is an ongoing, dynamic, and multidimensional process that consists of a variety of interactions between a sender and a receiver. The referent (e.g., a message, perception, or sound) motivates a person to share information with another person. The sender encodes a message, the content of the communication, and sends it to a receiver (through a particular channel), who decodes the message. The message may be influenced by many factors, including the environment in which the communication occurs and interpersonal variables, such as the educational, developmental, or cultural background that each individual brings to the communication. Feedback is the message returned by the receiver. For effective communication, both the sender and the receiver need to be sensitive and open to each other's message. In the nurse–client relationship, the nurse needs to take primary responsibility for ensuring that communication is open, purposeful, and therapeutic. Fig. 4.1 illustrates the concepts in active communication.

Nurses use a wide range of effective communication strategies and interpersonal skills to guide their interactions with clients and with all members of the interprofessional team. They must have an awareness of cultural factors that influence communication. Nurses plan and provide care by recognizing and respecting the diversity of different cultures. Positive interpersonal communication is vital for creating a positive therapeutic environment and includes the following:

- The use of warmth and genuineness as the nurse ensures confidentiality, connects with clients, and demonstrates respect for spiritual, psychological, and physical aspects of care
- Being respectful of clients and other members of the interprofessional team
- Being empathetic to the client experience
- Using self-disclosure appropriately

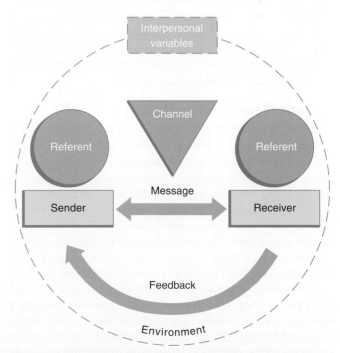

Fig. 4.1 Communication is an active process between a sender and a receiver. (From Astle, B., & Duggleby, W. (2024). *Potter and Perry's Canadian fundamentals of nursing* (7th ed.). Elsevier.)

Communication involves the use of verbal and nonverbal means. Verbal communication includes the spoken word, and nonverbal communication includes factors such as tone, rate, and volume of the voice, as well as facial expression, mannerisms, and appearance. When delivering or receiving communication, it is important to consider both the verbal and nonverbal aspects of the message.

A key factor associated with communication is the use of effective listening skills. Listening is an active process that involves paying attention to both verbal and nonverbal cues and is required by the nurse when interacting with clients, other nurses, and members of the interprofessional team.

Conflict Resolution

The health care team is composed of many different people. Each team member has a different background and brings his or her own professional knowledge, expertise, values, beliefs, and goals into the workplace. Sometimes, differences between people can lead to conflict and disagreements.

Conflict occurs at four levels:
- Intrapersonal conflict that occurs within the individual
- Interpersonal conflict that occurs between two or more individuals
- Intragroup conflict that occurs within a group
- Intergroup conflict that occurs between two or more groups, departments, or organizations

Many factors contribute to conflict, such as unclear roles and responsibilities, limited resources, unresolved prior conflicts, and ineffective communication. It is important to resolve conflicts when they occur.

Effective conflict resolution begins with an acknowledgement that there is a conflict and that it needs to be positively addressed. Collaboration is the best approach to conflict resolution. It satisfies the interests of most parties because it requires that they work together to find a common solution. Collaboration involves the use of active listening and defining a clear agreement to resolve the conflict.

Practice Standard Documentation

Accurate documentation by nurses is an important standard of care from a legal as well as an ethical perspective. Nurses document important details of client care on the client health record. Accurate and detailed documentation improves client outcomes because the health care team can better plan care, improve assessment, and evaluate the effectiveness of care interventions. Verbal documentation such as verbal physician's orders should be avoided except in specific—usually emergency—situations because of the increased risk of error or misinterpretation. People who have the authority to write orders, including physicians and NPs, need to sign any verbal order they made as soon as possible after the event. Individual health care facilities have telephone communication policies in place to facilitate this process. Nurses should refer to agency policy for issues relating to late entries, correcting errors, or completing an omission. Late entries are often documented by writing the current date and time in the next available space and writing "late entry for [date and shift]" (Astle & Duggleby, 2024).

Documentation is important in all other aspects of nursing practice as well. Documentation formats have changed; electronic records and fax transmissions are replacing paper records. Electronic and fax records must also be kept confidential. Confidentiality of health records is integral to documentation, accountability, and nurses' ethical standards.

From a legal and ethical perspective, nurses must keep all client information confidential and can only release the information with the written consent of the client or authorized designate, such as a guardian or someone who has power of attorney or power of care. Clients or other authorized designates and other members of the specific client's health care team can access and read the client health record. Individual health care facilities all have systems in place and specific policies to ensure that client confidentiality is maintained. The College of Nurses of Ontario (CNO) practice standards regarding documentation stress the importance of maintaining confidentiality of client health information, including passwords or information required to access the client health record. Nurses are not allowed to share their password to access the electronic health record (EHR) with anyone else and must log off the EHR when not using it.

Nurses must understand and adhere to policies, standards, and legislation related to confidentiality when using the EHR. Access only information for which you have a professional need to provide care (CNO, 2019). "Maintaining the confidentiality of medical records is an essential responsibility of all members of the healthcare team" (Astle & Duggleby, 2024, p. 237). It is important to safeguard any information regarding personal health information as well. Do not leave such information around for unauthorized people to view. You must destroy anything that is printed when the print information is no longer required. Most agencies have shredders or locked receptacles for shredding or later incineration (Astle & Duggleby, 2024).

Some institutions have a prescribed order entry. The prescriber enters an order directly into the computer, which avoids need for the transcription of orders. Computer interfaces transfer the order to the medication administration record (MAR), the pharmacy record, and the automated dispensing system (Astle & Duggleby, 2024). Nurses are accountable to determine whether the medication ordered is the correct medication. Administering medications requires knowledge and skill to prevent medication errors.

Accreditation Canada has developed key criteria for providing good documentation. Documentation should include information that is factual, accurate, complete, and current and complies with the standards of Accreditation Canada (Astle & Duggleby, 2024), as outlined below:
- Documentation should include factual records that contain descriptive and objective information.
- It should be accurate, with exact measurements, the agency's approved abbreviations, correct spelling, date and

time, and the recorder's name and role, such as "Cheryl Sams, LPN [or RPN]," which confirms that the nursing care has been delivered.

- Current records need to be recorded with timed entries on a regular basis and always as soon as possible in the following instances:
  - When vital signs are monitored
  - Preparation for tests or surgeries
  - Change in client status and who was notified of the change
  - Admission, transfer, discharge, or death of a client
  - Treatment for a sudden change in status.
- It should be organized, with the information presented in a logical order.
- It must comply with standards set by the Accreditation Canada as well as jurisdictional legislation and regulatory bodies.

Each health care facility also has its own policies that need to be followed to ensure consistency and complete information recording. Some examples include the following:

- Subjective-objective-assessment-plan (SOAP)
- Problem-intervention-evaluation (PIE), which can be added to the SOAP format
- Narrative notes that describe the nursing care delivered and the client's response
- Focus charting, which includes *data* (subjective and objective), *action* or nursing interventions, and *response* from the client (DAR)
- Charting by exception (CBE) systems, in which the practical nurse only records abnormal findings and trends in clinical care (Astle & Duggleby, 2024)

Table 4.1 describes the legal guidelines for information recording.

TABLE 4.1   Legal Guidelines for Documentation

Guidelines for Electronic and Written Documentation	Rationale	Correct Action
Do not document retaliatory or critical comments about a client or care provided by another health care provider. Do not enter personal opinions.	Statements can be used as evidence of nonprofessional behaviour or poor quality of care.	Enter only objective and factual descriptions of a patient's behaviour or the actions of another health care provider. Quote all client statements.
Correct all errors promptly.	Errors in recording can lead to errors in treatment or may imply an attempt to mislead or hide evidence.	Avoid rushing to complete documentation; be sure that information is accurate and complete.
Record all facts.	Record must be accurate, factual, and objective.	Be certain entry is factual and thorough. A person reading your documentation needs to be able to determine that a client received adequate care.
Document as close as prudently possible to the time of the event.	Most accurate method of recalling details. Details can be lost and discrepancies can arise the longer the wait to the documentation of the event.	Document as soon after the event as possible to ensure accuracy.
If an order is questioned, record that clarification was sought.	If you perform an order known to be incorrect, you are just as liable for prosecution as the prescriber is.	Do not record "physician made error"; instead, chart that "Dr. Wong was called to clarify order for analgesic." Include the date and time of phone call, whom you spoke with, and the outcome.
Document only for yourself.	You are accountable for information you enter into a patient's record.	Never enter documentation for someone else. Check agency policy for circumstances when a third party may document for another nurse (e.g., designated recorder for emergency situations).
Avoid using generalized, empty phrases such as "status unchanged" or "had good day."	This type of documentation is subjective and does not reflect client assessment.	Use complete, concise descriptions of assessments and care so that documentation is objective and factual.
Begin each entry with the date and time and end with your signature and credentials.	Ensures that the correct sequence of events is recorded; signature documents who is accountable for care delivered.	Do not wait until end of shift to record important changes that occurred several hours earlier; sign each entry according to agency policy (e.g., Mei Lin, LPN).
Avoid "precharting" (documenting an entry before performing a treatment or an assessment or before giving a medication).	Invites error and thus endangers the health and safety of the client; it is also illegal and can constitute falsification of health care records.	Document during or immediately after giving care or after administering a medication.
Protect the security of your password for computer documentation.	Maintains security and confidentiality.	Once logged in to a computer, do not leave computer screen unattended. Log out when you leave the computer. Make sure the computer screen is not accessible for public viewing.

Continued

TABLE 4.1 Legal Guidelines for Documentation—cont'd

Guidelines Specific to Written Documentation	Rationale	Correct Action
Do not erase, apply correction fluid to, or scratch out errors made while recording.	Charting becomes illegible: It may appear as if you were attempting to hide information or deface record.	Draw a single line through error; write "error" above it, sign your name or initials, and date it. Then record note correctly.
Do not leave blank spaces or lines in written progress notes.	Allows another person to add incorrect information in open space.	Chart consecutively, line by line; if space is left, draw a line horizontally through it and place your signature and credentials at the end.
Record all entries legibly and in black ink. Do not use felt-tip pens or erasable ink.	Illegible entries can be misinterpreted, thereby causing errors and lawsuits; ink from felt-tip pens can smudge or run when wet and may destroy documentation; erasures are not permitted in clinical documentation; black ink is more legible when records are photocopied or scanned.	Never use pencil to document in a written clinical record. Never erase entries or use correction fluid. To indicate an error in written documentation, place a single line through the inaccurate information and write your signature with credentials at the end of the text that has been crossed out.

From Astle, B., & Duggleby, W. (2024). *Potter and Perry's Canadian fundamentals of nursing*, (7th ed.). Elsevier.

TABLE 4.2 Dos and Don'ts for Change-of-Shift Reports

Dos	Don'ts
Do provide only essential background information about client (i.e., name, sex, age, physician's diagnosis, and medical history).	Don't review all routine care procedures or tasks (e.g., bathing, scheduled changes).
Do identify patient's nursing diagnoses or health care problems and their related causes.	Don't review all biographical information already available in written form.
Do describe objective measurements or observations about patient's condition and response to health problem, and do emphasize recent changes.	Don't use critical comments about patient's behaviour, such as "Mrs. Wills is so demanding."
Do share significant information about family members as it relates to patient's problems.	Don't make assumptions about relationships between family members.
Do continuously review ongoing discharge plan (e.g., need for resources, patient's level of preparation to go home).	Don't wait until near discharge to discuss the plan.
Do relay to staff significant changes in the way therapies are given (e.g., different position for pain relief, new medication).	Don't describe basic steps of a procedure.
Do describe instructions given in teaching plan and patient's response.	Don't explain detailed content unless staff members ask for clarification.
Do evaluate results of nursing or medical care measures (e.g., effect of back rub or analgesic administration), and describe results specifically.	Don't simply describe results as "good" or "poor."
Do be clear about priorities to which incoming staff must attend.	Don't force incoming staff to guess what to do first.

From Astle, B., & Duggleby, W. (2024). *Potter and Perry's Canadian fundamentals of nursing* (7th ed.). Elsevier.

The change-of-shift report is very important in settings where one nurse takes over care responsibilities from another nurse. The communication about the client's condition is only a small part of the report. The change-of-shift report needs to be concise but comprehensive so that the nurse starting the new shift will be able to provide a level of continuity of care. However, the change-of-shift report is not a part of the legal permanent client health record. Table 4.2 provides a comparison of dos and don'ts of the change-of-shift report. SBAR (*sit*uation, *b*ackground, *a*ssessment, and *r*ecommendation) is one example of a communication tool that enables information to be transferred accurately between nurses. It uses a simple, structured framework that allows nurses to produce hand-off reports that are standardized and clear. Effective communication is a vital factor in the delivery of safe, quality client care. It also helps provide continuity of care among nurses (Astle & Duggleby, 2024). Box. 4.2 describes the Identification, Situation, Background, Assessment, Recommendation, Repeat back (I-SBAR-R) technique, a reformulation of SBAR, that is used in many different reporting situations.

BOX 4.2   The Identification, Situation, Background, Assessment, Recommendation, Repeat Back (I-SBAR-R) Technique

When calling the physician, follow the I-SBAR-R process as follows:

Identification: Who is calling and who are you calling about?
- Identify yourself and your role
- Identify the unit, the client, and the room number

Situation: What is the situation you are calling about?
- Briefly state the problem: What it is, when it started, and the severity

Background: Provide background information as necessary related to the situation, including the following:
- The admitting diagnosis, date of admission, and pertinent medical history
- List of current medications, allergies, intravenous fluids, and laboratory tests
- Laboratory results (date and time each test was performed and results of previous tests for comparison)
- Other clinical information
- Code status

Assessment: What is your assessment of the situation? Examples include the following:
- Most recent vital signs
- Changes in vital signs or assessment from previous assessments

Recommendation: What is your recommendation, or what do you think needs to be done? Examples include the following:
- Client to be admitted or transferred
- New medication or further tests
- Client to be seen now
- Orders to be changed

Repeat back:
- Repeat back orders that have been given
- Clarify any questions

From Astle, B., & Duggleby, W. (2024). *Potter and Perry's Canadian fundamentals of nursing* (7th ed., p. 247, Box 16.10). Elsevier. Adapted from Joint Commission on Accreditation of Healthcare Organizations. (2005, February). The SBAR technique: Improves communication, enhances patient safety. *Joint Commission Perspectives on Patient Safety, 5*(2), 2; Enlow, M., Shanks, L., Guhde, J., & Perkins, M. (2010). Incorporating interprofessional communication skills (ISBARR) into an undergraduate nursing curriculum. *Nurse Educator, 35*(4), 176–180; and Grbach, W., Struth, D., & Vincent, I. (2008). *Reformulating SBAR to "I-SBAR-R."* Quality and Safety Education for Nurses. http://qsen.org/reformulating-sbar-to-i-sbar-r/

CONSENT

Ethical Implications

Consent to treatment is a very important aspect of ethical care. It is critical that clients are fully informed and fully understand the implications of the treatment before authorizing the care, whether via signed consent or verbal consent. Practical nurses assist and support client participation in making decisions about their health and well-being when factors reduce their capacity for making decisions, in accordance with applicable legislation and regulation (CCPNR, 2013).

CCPNR provides guidance to practical nurses on the ethical responsibilities affecting informed consent. According to the CCPNR code of ethics, LPNs:

2.1 Respect the right and responsibility of clients to be informed and make decisions about their health care.

2.1.1 Respect and support client choices.

2.1.2 Assist and support client participation in making decisions about their health and well-being when factors reduce their capacity for making decisions, in accordance with applicable legislation and regulation.

2.1.3 Respect and adhere to the jurisdictional legislation on capacity assessment and substitute decision-making when the client is incapable of consent.

2.1.4 Consider with other healthcare professionals and substitute decision-makers the best interests of the client and any previously known wishes or advanced directives that apply in situations where the client is incapable of consent.

2.6 Provide care to each client recognizing their individuality and their right to choice. (CCPNR, 2013, p. 5)

Legal Implications

There are also legal implications in relation to informed consent. Clients must fully understand the implications of the consent and receive full disclosure on all the risks, benefits, alternatives, and consequences of refusal of treatment or care (Tyerman & Cobbett, 2023). The legal obligation falls to the physician or health care provider to disclose the information in such a way that the client can understand all the information that is being delivered. The consent form must specify the details of the procedure, including the name of the person who is performing the procedure. The person who will perform the procedure should obtain consent from the client. It is essential to remember that except in emergency situations, failure to obtain consent for treatment (whether written or verbal) could result in a lawsuit with charges of battery.

Nurses cannot obtain informed consent for surgery because they do not perform surgery. The same is true for other procedures that require consent that will not be performed by the practical nurse. It is the physician's responsibility to obtain consent for the procedure they will be performing. Nurses may sign as witnesses to the client's written consent, proving that the client appears to be mentally competent and confirming the identity of the signature and that the client signed voluntarily, although some agency policies may not support this practice. The nurse should ask the client if they understand the procedure before the consent is witnessed. If there is a suspicion that the client does not understand, the physician needs to inform the client further. If a client refuses to provide consent, the nurse needs to explore and determine the reason for refusal and discuss it with the health care team.

Currently, nurses rarely require written consent from a client to perform a particular procedure. However, they must obtain verbal consent before starting the procedure. Doing so ensures that the client understands the care goals and reduces the risk that a battery lawsuit could occur against the nurse (Keatings & Adams, 2024). Consent can be verbal, written, or implicit. For example, if a client lifts up a leg for the nurse to provide wound care, then it is implicit that the client is giving consent.

If the client is unable to understand the nature of the consent, then a substitute decision maker with the appropriate authority will need to provide consent for care, which may involve signing a consent form. The substitute decision maker may receive the authority by proxy or power of attorney or power of care or may be appointed through court guardianship. Clients with mental illness or cognitive impairment may still have the ability to provide informed consent and to refuse treatment unless the court has ruled that they are legally incompetent to make personal health care decisions (Keatings & Adams, 2024).

RESTRAINTS

Restraints are physical, chemical, or a restricted environment. There has been much controversy over the past few years concerning the risks and benefits of restraints. The ethical question of consent for restraints has also arisen, as well as the possible liability issues of lack of consent. The ideal situation is not to use restraints, but it may be necessary for clients, particularly those with mental illness, who are at risk of harming themselves or others. Statistics clearly indicate that personal injuries are higher when a client is restrained (Astle & Duggleby, 2024).

Clients have been asphyxiated by physical restraints. Other complications from the use of restraints include pressure injuries, constipation, pneumonia, urinary and fecal incontinence, and urinary retention. There is also the issue of the anxiety and fear experienced by clients under restraint, as well as the impact on the client's self-esteem (Astle & Duggleby, 2024). A policy of least restraint is the usual agency approach, which ensures that all care alternatives have been attempted prior to restraint. It is important for nurses to know the restraint policies of their agencies and the legal implications of these.

If restraints are used, nurses need to check the restraints and the client's condition frequently to make sure that the client's circulation is not impaired and that no other injuries or potential risks are present. It is always recommended that nurses try alternative methods of intervention to address difficult behaviour, such as frequent toileting to reduce agitation or utilizing a "sitter."

RESUSCITATION GUIDELINES

Cardiopulmonary Resuscitation

CPR is the standard treatment for respiratory or cardiac arrest in many health care facilities. CPR is commonly performed as it has the potential to revive clients. Because CPR is considered a treatment, client consent may be required before initiating the resuscitation, although emergency situations are unique (CNPS, 2006).

When a capable client does not want to have CPR performed, the refusal must be documented in the client health record. This refusal is often documented by the physician. Some provincial or territorial legislation allows nurses to accept the refusal for CPR and document the refusal in the client's health record as do not resuscitate (DNR). If the client is legally capable of making decisions, then the family cannot overrule the client's treatment or care wishes.

Health care facilities should have DNR policies in place that guide the health care team in the decision-making process surrounding the DNR issue.

Jurisdictions and agencies have different sets of resuscitation protocols from legal and regulatory bodies. DNR orders are necessary in some jurisdictions, and in others, CPR requires consent. It is essential that nurses know the protocols in their jurisdictions.

It is the responsibility of the health care team to discuss the potential care requirements with the client and his or her family, including providing CPR, and together to devise a comprehensive plan of treatment. This plan needs to be documented in the client health record. Health care providers do not have to provide CPR if it will not benefit the client. CPR may, in fact, be harmful in some situations by increasing pain and suffering and prolonging the dying process. The plan of care must include the client's current condition and the expectation for the future condition. The plan must be based on current best practices and treatment goals. The client must consent to the treatment plan. If the client requests CPR and the health care team does not think that CPR will benefit the client, then the health care team must discuss this decision with the client and his or her family. Variations of the DNR order can allow for partial resuscitation in accordance with the client's request. The DNR order can be suspended at any time and then reinstated when the client would like it reordered (CNPS, 2006).

Nurses play an important role in making certain that the client's wishes are identified and communicated clearly to the health care team. In addition, nurses must encourage the client to be the decision maker in the treatment plan, document communication about end-of-life and resuscitation concerns in the health record, review the resuscitation wishes, advocate on behalf of the client, and implement the client's wishes (Tyerman & Cobbett, 2023). It is critical that nurses discuss the presence of advance directives and meet the legislation requirements of their jurisdiction. It is important that nurses follow the capable client's wishes whether or not there is a written order on the client's health record.

Nurses are expected to be competent in providing CPR if required for their role. Some health care facilities require a formal credential such as health care provider and automated external defibrillator (AED) certification.

MEDICATION ADMINISTRATION

Medication administration is an important role for nurses. Medication is used for a variety of purposes, including diagnosis, treatment, cure, relief, or prevention of health conditions. Nurses give medications in many practice settings with many nursing responsibilities. Nurses are responsible for delivering medication accurately and safely to the client, teaching the client about the medication, and evaluating the effect of the medication on the client (Astle & Duggleby, 2024).

Implications for Administering Medications

The scope of practice of practical nurses is determined by legislative acts at the federal and provincial/territorial levels. Practical nurses must know their own jurisdictional laws that affect medication administration. In addition, practical nurses must be aware of their own practice agencies' medication policies before they administer medications. They must have the knowledge, skill, and judgement before they give medications. This knowledge is particularly necessary in the case of controlled substances that are regulated by law. Violations of the *Controlled Drugs and Substances Act* may lead to a loss of nursing licence or registration, fines, or imprisonment (Astle & Duggleby, 2024).

Medication Actions

There are many variables in how medications act and their types of actions. There are factors other than the characteristics of the medication that affect its actions. For example, individuals react very differently to medications and may not react the same way to successive doses. It is very important for nurses to understand all the effects of the medications on individuals so that impact can be evaluated. Types of medication effects are listed below:

- Therapeutic effect is the expected or predicted physiological response from the medication and is the desired outcome.
- Side effects are unintended, secondary effects that a medication predictably will cause. The side effects can be harmless or can harm the individual.
- Toxic effects can develop after taking a medication for a long time or when the level of a medication increases in the blood because of impaired metabolism and medication clearance. Toxic effects can be lethal depending on the medication action.
- Adverse effects are generally severe, negative responses to medication that were unexpected and not seen during medication testing. These effects should be reported to the Health Products and Food Branch of the federal government. Reporting is voluntary.
- Idiosyncratic reactions are unpredictable and occur when an individual overreacts to a medication or has a different reaction from the norm.
- Allergic reactions are unpredictable responses to a medication after repeated doses. The medication is perceived by the body as an allergen, causing a release of antibodies. The reaction can be mild or severe and cause an anaphylactic reaction leading to airway obstruction from swelling of the larynx and pharynx, severe wheezing, and shortness of breath. Urticaria, angioedema, and the delayed action of a rash and fever are other possible symptoms. Allergic reactions can be life-threatening, particularly when the individual becomes hypotensive from vasodilation.
- Medication interactions can occur when one medication potentiates (increases) or decreases the action of another. This commonly occurs when several medications are

taken. Two medications can have a synergistic effect, and the medications together cause more of a effect than if they had been given separately (Astle & Duggleby, 2024).

Medication Dose Responses

After a medication is taken, it breaks down in the body and is absorbed, distributed, metabolized, and excreted. The individual's metabolism, weight, gender, and body size affect the medication response. Many medications take some time to be absorbed, with the exception of IV medications, which are absorbed directly into the bloodstream. It is important that the medication is kept at a constant level in the blood—one within the therapeutic range between the peak high (the highest serum concentration) and a trough low. The therapeutic level prevents toxicity and resultant damage to the body. In order to keep the medication at a therapeutic level, the nurse needs to administer the medication at regular times throughout the day. With IV infusions, the peak concentration occurs quickly, but the serum level also begins to fall immediately. It is important for the nurse to teach the client to take the medications on the prescribed schedule to maximize their effect. Refer to Fig. 4.2 to see a picture of the different forms of oral medication.

Nursing Roles in Medication Administration

Nurses must have the knowledge necessary to administer and evaluate medications effectively. This knowledge comes from the life sciences and includes an understanding of pharmacokinetics (the study of drug concentrations), human growth and development, human anatomy, nutrition, and mathematics. In addition to knowledge, nurses and employers need to assess nurses' ability to carry out their roles relating to medications competently and safely in each situation. Nurses need the knowledge, skill, and judgement to independently meet the medication standard of practice. Nurses must also hold the competencies and resources to provide interventions during

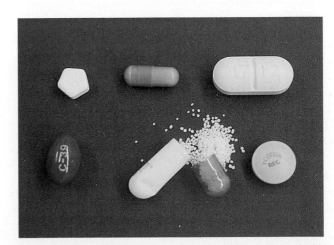

Fig. 4.2 Forms of oral medications. *Top row:* Uniquely shaped tablet, capsule, scored tablet. *Bottom row:* Gelatin-coated liquid, extended-release capsule, enteric-coated tablet. (From Astle, B., & Duggleby, W. [2024]. *Potter and Perry's Canadian fundamentals of nursing,* [7th ed., Fig. 35.1, p.726]. Elsevier.)

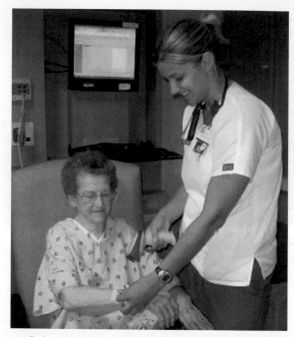

Fig. 4.3 Before administering any medication, the nurse checks the bar code on the client's bracelet and on the medication packet. (From Astle, B., & Duggleby, W. [2024]. *Potter and Perry's Canadian fundamentals of nursing* [7th ed., Fig. 35.12, p. 741]. Elsevier.)

an adverse drug event. The nurse needs a working knowledge of the medication action.

A critical role for nursing in medication administration is client teaching. The nurse needs to assess the client's ability to safely administer his or her own medication. The situations can be complex, and the nurse needs to be able to assess for client attitude, knowledge, physical and mental status, and responses.

In order to accurately and safely administer medications, nurses must learn to use the "10 rights" to ensure accuracy. These rights are as follows:
- Right medication
- Right dose
- Right client (see Fig. 4.3)
- Right route
- Right time and frequency
- Right documentation
- Right reason
- Right to refuse
- Right client education
- Right evaluation

A nurse meets the medication standard of practice by doing the following:
- Verifying that the prescription is complete and accurate or following up with the prescriber to get a complete prescription
- Assessing the appropriateness of the medication as prescribed for the client in the particular situation
- Not implementing or giving a medication order that is incomplete, illegible, or misinterpreted, and following up with the prescriber

- Considering the medication when scheduling dosing times, if not specified
- Knowing the trade and generic medication names
- Knowing the accepted abbreviations for their agency
- Processing the prescription as written or computerized physician order entry and not substituting generic or therapeutic interchanges
- Making any necessary changes to the MAR or electronic medication administration record (eMAR) to record the medication name
- Requesting written orders or computerized physician order entries when the prescriber is present and avoiding the use of verbal orders except in emergencies
- Repeating verbal or telephone orders in their entirety for accuracy and documenting them in the health record
- Assessing if the medication is ordered appropriately for that particular situation
- Retaining faxed and printed email orders and refusing unsecured email orders
- Consulting with colleagues and presenting a clear, evidence-informed rationale explaining their concerns is a must if nurses disagree with a medication order. The nurses then present their concerns to the prescriber, discuss the situation with their immediate nursing authority if the concern is unresolved, and contact the prescriber for more discussion. If the concern is still unresolved, then they must contact a higher nursing authority and inform the prescriber. Next, nurses document their concerns in the health record and fill out an unusual occurrence form or incident report.

Routes of Medication Administration

The route of the medication is prescribed according to the medication properties and desired effect on the client's condition. The nurse collaborates with the prescriber to decide on the best route. The medication administration routes are as follows:
- Oral medications are given by mouth. This is the most common and easiest route and has the slowest and most prolonged effect.
- Sublingual medications are placed under the tongue and absorbed. This medication should not be swallowed.
- Buccal route medications are placed against the mucous membrane of the cheek until the solid medication dissolves. They should not be swallowed or chewed.
- Parenteral medications are injected into body tissues. The four main sites are intradermal, subcutaneous (only for volumes of 0.5–1 mL), intramuscular (for volumes of up to 3 mL), and IV. Other sites for injections into body cavities include epidural, intrathecal, intraosseous, intraperitoneal, intrapleural, and intra-arterial. Additional education would be needed to administer medications at these extra sites and may be beyond the scope of practice of the practical nurse.
- Topical medications are applied by spreading them on the skin, applying moist dressings, soaking body parts in a solution, flushing the affected part, or giving medicated baths. The effects can be systemic if the client's skin is thin or broken down, if the concentration is too high, or if contact with the skin is prolonged. Transdermal discs or

patches can also be used. Instilling drops or ointment to the mucous membranes can also be done.

- The inhalation route can be used to administer medications through nasal passages, orally, by endotracheal tube, or via a tracheostomy.
- Using the eye route involves inserting a medication directly into the client's eye.
- Nasal sprays and drops are common forms of medications administered in the nostrils.
- Ear installation involves placing a solution into the ear canal for product dissolving and absorption.
- Intravaginal or intra-anal medications (suppositories) are inserted into the anal or vaginal cavities and melt when they reach body temperature, releasing the medication for absorption (Astle & Duggleby, 2024).

NURSING ISSUES AND TRENDS

The Nursing Process

A nurse uses the nursing process to guide, plan, organize, provide, and evaluate nursing care. A practical nurse must use the nursing process in combination with an ability to think critically and the ability to synthesize relevant knowledge, clinical experiences, and standards of practice. Fig. 4.4 outlines critical thinking and the nursing assessment process.

Assessment

Assessment is a collection of personal, sociocultural, physiological, and psychological health status data, as well as general information. It is a determination of current health status from the physical assessment.

Analysis

Analysis is a classification of data: screening, organizing, and grouping significant, related information. It is also a definition of a client's problem: determining an appropriate nursing diagnosis that is a definitive statement of the client's actual or potential difficulties, concerns, or deficits that can be altered through nursing interventions.

Planning

Planning involves the client, family or significant others, and practical nurse, who collaborates with the appropriate health team members to formulate the plan. Planning also establishes client outcomes. Outcomes are expected changes in the client's behaviour, activity, or physical state. Outcomes must be objective, realistic, and measurable and include a realistic period for accomplishment.

Implementation

Implementation is the actual administration of the planned care.

Evaluation, Outcome, and Revision of Care

If an outcome is not reached in the specified time, the client is reassessed. Reordering of priorities may be necessary because the process of evaluation is ongoing.

Evidence-Informed Practice and Best Practice Guidelines

Evidence-informed practice is the systematic application of the best available evidence to decision making in relation to clinical management and policy setting. Nurses are using evidence-informed practice as they manage the need for

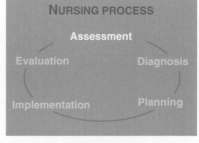

Fig. 4.4 Critical thinking and the assessment process. *CNA*, Canadian Nurses Association. (From Astle, B., & Duggleby, W. [2024]. *Potter and Perry's Canadian fundamentals of nursing* [7th ed., Fig. 14.2, p. 189]. Elsevier.)

efficiency and improved client outcomes along with increasing demands for accountability.

Best Practice Guidelines (BPGs) are evidence-informed tools that when implemented improve client, nurse, and organizational outcomes. These guidelines are systematically developed statements, based on the best available evidence, that assist nurses to make decisions about appropriate care. Goals for using BPGs include the following:

- Improved client care
- Reduction in the variation in care
- Transfer of research evidence into practice
- Assistance with clinical decision making
- Reduction of cost

Advocacy

All nurses are expected to take on advocacy roles within the Canadian health care system. They are expected to advocate for the best health interest for their clients and families and to advocate for the client's wishes and expectations, especially when clients are unable to express their needs clearly.

Nurses advocate for organizational or system changes that will improve quality care for clients. When nurses advocate, they give their clients a voice. When done correctly, advocacy leads to empowered clients. Empowered clients ask questions to gain a better understanding of all the options available within their plan of care. Nurses are expected to be client advocates within all practice areas and within the health care team.

Political Activism

Nurses may become politically active within their profession and communities. Political activism is usually seen as nurses advocating for the Canadian public in general or involving themselves in current health care issues that clients are experiencing (e.g., access to services).

Political activities can include lobbying all levels of government to introduce policies, laws, and regulations that benefit the health of Canadians, such as increased funding for community care or cancer treatment centres.

A nurse's involvement in nursing organizations is based on the province or territory in which the nurse is employed as well as individual choice. In all cases, if the individual is employed as a practical nurse, they must be a member of the appropriate nursing regulatory body (e.g., CNO). In addition, in most provinces or territories, the practical nurse must also join the professional nursing association. In those situations, the regulatory body and professional association are one entity (such as the College of Licensed Practical Nurses of Manitoba). The regulatory function, whether part of the professional association or not, involves registering or licensing individuals to the profession, setting standards of practice, and disciplining nurses who do not meet the standards (Astle & Duggleby, 2024). When the regulatory body is separate from the nursing professional association, the individual practical nurse has the choice to join or not join the professional nursing association (such as Registered Practical Nurses Association of Ontario, [WeRPN]). The regulatory body registers the nurse and has a mandate of public protection. The professional association represents the nursing profession and promotes the role and use of nurses in the health care system.

Labour organizations (often termed *unions*) are separate from both the professional association and the regulatory organization. Unions assist nurses with workplace issues, including the application and interpretation of labour laws and health and safety issues. When a nurse is employed by an organization that has an established union contract, the nurse must then pay associated fees to the union. Membership in the union is voluntary, but payment of union fees becomes mandatory.

PRACTICE QUESTIONS

Case 1

A nurse educator has revised the hospital's orientation program in anticipation of the hospital orientating many new graduate nurses within the next 3 months. The nurse educator decides to use sample client health records to highlight areas of professional practice. The educator conducts their first education session with the new graduates.

Questions 1 to 5 refer to this case.

1. During the documentation session, one of the new nurses asks what abbreviations can be used within the client's health record. What abbreviations should the nurse use?
   1. Abbreviations learned in nursing school
   2. Abbreviations that have been approved by the Canadian Nurses Association
   3. Abbreviations that have been approved by the hospital
   4. Abbreviations that are in common use on specific units within the hospital

2. Which of the following statements is the most accurate information with regard to client consent?
   1. Nurses are responsible for ensuring that clients sign all consent forms on the health record.
   2. The health care provider proposing the procedure requiring written consent is the person who must ensure that written client consent is obtained.
   3. Verbal consent for an operative procedure is acceptable, and signed consents are not always necessary.
   4. When a client is admitted to the hospital, the client signs a written consent that covers all treatments.

3. In the sample client's health record, the new graduate nurses discover that a nurse has written "Verbal Order, acetaminophen (Tylenol), 325 mg, PO, prn, for pain." There is no evidence that this was an emergency situation. Which of the following describes best practice in relation to verbal medication orders?

1. Verbal orders are to be avoided, except in an emergency situation.
2. Nurses should follow the same practice for verbal orders as for telephone orders.
3. Verbal orders should never be accepted, including in emergency situations.
4. Only registered nurses may receive verbal orders for medications from a physician.

4. The new graduate nurses review a variety of orders on the sample health records. Which of the following is a correct medication order?
   1. Acetaminophen 325 mg PO for pain
   2. Acetaminophen 325–650 mg PO for pain q4–6h prn
   3. Acetaminophen 325–650 mg PO for pain as needed
   4. Acetaminophen 325 or 650 mg q4–6h prn

5. During the orientation, the nurse educator explains that the hospital uses evidence-informed practice to guide clinical decision making. Which of the following statements best describes evidence-informed practice?
   1. An opportunity to obtain funding from the government
   2. An opportunity to transfer research findings into practice
   3. A chance for professionals to trial untested research findings
   4. A way to promote enhanced assessment skills

Case 2

A manager of home care nurses has noticed over the past 3 months a lack of clarity about the roles of the team members, poor team morale, increasing negative communication, and team conflict. The manager decides to support the staff by providing an education session.

Questions 6 to 9 refer to this case.

6. One of the new team members is a nurse practitioner (NP). How should the manager describe the level of education for the NP?
   1. A nurse who has specialty certification from the Canadian Nurses Association
   2. A nurse who has taken a special interest course in a unique field
   3. A nurse who has an undergraduate degree in a discipline other than nursing
   4. A nurse educated at the master's level with a specialization in a particular practice area

7. The manager is preparing the education session for the staff group. Which of the following is true in relation to the teaching and learning process?
   1. It is important to use the same approach with all types of learners.
   2. It is better to introduce all new knowledge instead of connecting it to previously learned knowledge.
   3. Learning occurs best when the individual has an identified need to learn.
   4. It is always best to deliver education quickly and at the same time of day.

8. The manager explains that effective interpersonal communication with clients and team members includes which of the following?
   1. The use of "you" statements when interacting with clients and colleagues
   2. The use of warmth and genuineness in interactions
   3. The use of questions that elicit single-word responses in order to promote efficient communication
   4. The use of frequent self-disclosure to ensure that others will share your point of view

9. In situations in which a team conflict has arisen, what would be the best statement by the manager to the staff?
   1. "We should put aside our differences and work together as a team."
   2. "I think we should employ a conflict-resolution specialist to help us."
   3. "Let's have a discussion about what we can agree is expected team behaviour."
   4. "These are the guidelines for team behaviour in this agency."

Case 3

A nurse works in a long-term care facility where many of the residents experience acute agitation.

Questions 10 to 12 refer to this case.

10. The facility follows a "least-restraint policy." What is the most important consideration with a "least-restraint policy"?
    1. That a family conference is organized prior to the implementation of a restraint
    2. That all possible alternative interventions have been exhausted before a restraint is implemented
    3. That the client has no manifestations of delirium or dementia
    4. That the client has signed consent for the application of restraints

11. The nurse charts the behaviour of a client. Which of the following statements would be the most appropriate documentation?
    1. "The client was agitated today."
    2. "The client was confused this morning."
    3. "The client was shaking his fist at the practical nurse at 1100 hours."
    4. "The client was behaving inappropriately during the evening shift."

12. The nurse consults the provincial or territorial standards of nursing practice when contemplating the use of restraints. What is the most important purpose for using standards of nursing practice?
    1. Standards will help the nurse make decisions about ongoing learning needs.
    2. Standards will act as a guide to the nurse's clinical decision making.
    3. Standards will help the nurse in malpractice situations.
    4. Standards will guide the nurse to be aware of protection of personal health, safety, and welfare.

Case 4

Anna, a nurse from Poland, has immigrated to Canada. She received her nursing education in Poland and is now studying for the Canadian Practical Nurse Registration Examination (CPNRE). She has discovered many differences in terms and meaning between nursing practice in Canada and nursing practice in Poland.

Questions 13 to 15 refer to this case.

13. Anna knows she must be able to articulate the differences and similarities between various nursing organizations. The mandate of nursing regulatory organizations is which of the following?
    1. Protection of the public
    2. Protection of nurses
    3. Protection of nursing employers
    4. Protection of all regulated health care providers

14. Anna is trying to distinguish the difference between standards of nursing practice and the nursing Best Practice Guidelines. What are the Best Practice Guidelines?
    1. Classifications that assist in the analysis and grouping of data
    2. Advance directives that clearly indicate the client's wishes and needs
    3. Tools based on proven criteria that improve client, nurse, and organizational outcomes
    4. Policies that guide compassionate care and ethical nursing decisions

15. Anna has noticed the term *DNR* in one of the sample questions in the exam preparatory book. What does DNR mean?
    1. Do not perform cardiopulmonary resuscitation.
    2. Do not administer cardiac compressions.
    3. Do not perform any life-saving actions.
    4. Do not perform any form of resuscitation that has not been agreed upon by the client or substitute decision maker.

Independent Questions

Questions 16 to 29 do not refer to a particular case.

16. When communicating with a client's physician, the nurse states that the client is experiencing dyspnea and suggests ordering a STAT chest X-ray. This is an example of which components of the I-SBAR-R technique for communicating with the client's physician? **Select all that apply.**
    1. Situation
    2. Assessment
    3. Recommendation
    4. Identification
    5. Background

17. Which of the following is the nurse responsible for knowing when administering medications? **Select all that apply.**
    1. Purpose of the medication
    2. Effect of the medication
    3. Cost of the medication
    4. Potential adverse effects of the medication
    5. Contraindications of the medication

18. A nurse is temporarily employed in a family physician's office while the regular nurse is on vacation. The physician has left a note for the temporary nurse to complete a referral to a gynecologist for a client requesting a therapeutic abortion. The temporary nurse has strong religious values against abortion, and was unaware that working with clients requesting abortions would be part of the role in the office. What is the best action for the temporary nurse?
    1. Leave a note for the physician indicating refusal to make the referral for an abortion.
    2. Complete the referral to the gynecologist as part of the obligation to provide care for the client in the absence of the regular office nurse.
    3. Notify the physician that they will not be working in the office after today's shift.
    4. Tell the client that the usual nurse will make the referral when they return from vacation next week.

19. A nurse hears an unregulated care provider (UCP) tell a client: "If you don't stay quiet in your bed while I help this other client, I won't feed you your supper." What would be the priority action for the nurse?
    1. Ask the client to repeat what the UCP stated.
    2. Make sure that the UCP is not assigned to that client when future assignments are developed.
    3. Remove the UCP from the client situation and report the incident to the nurse manager the next morning.
    4. Determine whether the UCP needs help with the clients.

20. A resident in a long-term care facility tells the nurse that their leg hurts from the fall they had an hour ago. The nurse was unaware of the fall and obtains details about the fall from the unregulated care provider (UCP) who cared for the resident at the time of the fall. Which statement related to accountability is correct?
    1. The nurse is accountable in all situations for the actions of the UCP.
    2. The nurse is not accountable for the actions of the UCP because they nurse was on lunch break at the time of the fall.
    3. The nurse is accountable for the resident's fall because the nurse was the only registered/licensed staff on duty at the time of the fall.
    4. The nurse is not accountable for the care or actions of the UCP.

21. A nurse has been asked by their manager to work an extra 4 hours after their 12-hour shift because three nurses have called in sick. The nurse has worked four 12-hour shifts consecutively. The nurse admits to being tired and not sure whether they are too fatigued to work the extra 4 hours. Which of the following is the most appropriate?
    1. The nurse cannot refuse to work the additional 4 hours as their manager has made the request and there are no other replacements.
    2. The nurse has no obligation to work the additional 4 hours, and he should report their decision to the union representative.

3. The nurse must be offered time and a half for the extra 4 hours.
4. The nurse's first priority in deciding to work the extra 4 hours is whether they are competent to provide safe care.

22. Which of the following are components of informed consent? **Select all that apply.**
    1. The consent must be voluntary.
    2. The consent must be given in writing.
    3. The client must be legally capable.
    4. The consent must be specific to the proposed treatment or procedure.
    5. The client must be told of the risks and benefits of the proposed procedure.

23. A client is ordered 325 mg of acetylsalicylic acid (ASA) prn for headache. The nurse is aware that this client is also receiving warfarin (Coumadin). Which of the following actions is the most appropriate for the nurse to take?
    1. Contact the doctor for clarification of the orders.
    2. Ask the client if he has taken ASA before while also taking Coumadin.
    3. Contact the pharmacist about the potential medication interaction.
    4. Consult with nursing colleagues about whether to give the ASA to the client.

24. A second-year nursing student has asked the nurse about the use of restraints. Which of the following are considered a restraint category? **Select all that apply.**
    1. Chemical
    2. Physical
    3. Hazardous
    4. Environmental
    5. Natural

25. A student nurse has forgotten their computer password. The student asks a nurse to share their password in order to access a client's chart. What should the staff nurse do?
    1. Share the password since the student nurse provided direct client care.
    2. Ask the student nurse to write the care on a piece of paper, and the staff nurse will enter it later.
    3. Do not share the password and direct the student nurse to the policy on retrieving forgotten passwords.
    4. Explain the situation to the charge nurse, who will locate a password.

26. A client is ordered venlafaxine (Effexor) for depression. The client refuses to take the medication, stating that it causes headaches. What should the nurse do?
    1. Do not give the medication because the client has withdrawn consent.
    2. Tell the charge nurse the situation to see if they can convince the client to take the medication.
    3. Administer the medication because the client has been diagnosed with depression.
    4. Insist that the client take the medication but offer acetaminophen for the headache.

27. Which of the following are examples of a tort? **Select all that apply.**
    1. A nurse threatens to insert a urinary catheter without client consent.
    2. A nurse gives a prn dose of an antipsychotic drug to an agitated client because the unit is short-staffed.
    3. The plan of care for a client is not completed within 24 hours of the client's admission.
    4. A nurse starts an IV line without client consent.
    5. An advanced-practice nurse recommends hospitalization for a client who is dangerous to self and others.

28. The nurse is not able to read the obstetrician's handwriting for postpartum orders for a client. What should the nurse do?
    1. Ask the client what the obstetrician ordered for postpartum pain relief.
    2. Contact the obstetrician for clarification of the orders.
    3. Ask the unit clerk for clarification of the obstetrician's handwriting.
    4. Consult other postpartum charts for this obstetrician to compare similar orders.

29. Which of the following actions by a nurse constitutes a breach of a client's right to privacy? **Select all that apply.**
    1. Documenting the client's daily behaviour during hospitalization
    2. Releasing information to the client's employer without consent
    3. Discussing the client's history with other staff during care planning
    4. Asking family to share information about a client's prehospitalization behaviour
    5. Placing papers with client information in a standard trash can after ripping into small pieces

REFERENCES

Astle, B., & Duggleby, W. (2024). *Potter and Perry's Canadian fundamentals of nursing* (7th ed.). Elsevier.

Canadian Council for Practical Nurse Regulators (CCPNR). (2013). *Code of ethics for licensed practical nurses in Canada*. https://ccpnr.ca/wp-content/uploads/2021/03/IJLPN-CE-Final.pdf

Canadian Council for Practical Nurse Regulators (CCPNR). (2020). *Standards of practice for licensed practical nurses in Canada*. https://ccpnr.ca/wp-content/uploads/2021/03/StandardsofPracticeEnglishFinal-1-1.pdf

Canadian Nurses Association (CNA). (2017). *Code of ethics for registered nurses*. https://cna-aiic.ca/en/nursing-practice/nursing-ethics

Canadian Nurses Protective Society (CNPS). (1999). Legal risks in nursing. *InfoLAW*, 8(1).

Canadian Nurses Protective Society (CNPS). (2006). Consent for CPR. *InfoLAW*, 15(2). https://cnps.ca/article/consent-for-cpr/

Canadian Nurses Protective Society (CNPS). (2022). Negligence: When would a nurse face an allegation of negligence? *InfoLAW*, 3(1). https://cnps.ca/article/negligence/

College of Nurses of Ontario (CNO). (2022). *Practice standard: Medication.* http://www.cno.org/globalassets/docs/prac/41007_medication.pdf

Fridman, G. (2012). *Introduction to the Canadian law of torts* (3rd ed.). LexisNexis Canada.

Irvine, J., Osborne, P., & Shariff, M. (2013). *Canadian medical law* (4th ed.). Carswell.

Keatings, M., & Adams, P. (2024). *Ethical and legal issues in Canadian nursing* (5th ed.). Elsevier Canada.

Osborne, P. H. (2015). *Essentials of Canadian law: The law of torts* (5th ed.). Irwin Law.

Tyerman, J., & Cobbett, W. (2023). *Lewis's medical-surgical nursing in Canada: Assessment and management of clinical problems* (5th ed.). Elsevier, Inc.

Wilk, M. (2022). *Sorrentino's Canadian textbook for the support worker* (5th ed.). Elsevier.

BIBLIOGRAPHY

College of Nurses of Ontario (CNO). (2006). *Practice standard: Therapeutic nurse–client relationship.* http://www.cno.org/globalassets/docs/prac/41033_therapeutic.pdf

College of Nurses of Ontario (CNO). (2018). *Practice guideline: RN and RPN practice: The client, the nurse and the environment.* http://www.cno.org/globalassets/docs/prac/41062.pdf

College of Nurses of Ontario (CNO). (2019). *Practice standard: Documentation.* http://www.cno.org/globalassets/docs/prac/41001_documentation.pdf

WEBSITES

- **Association of New Brunswick Licensed Practical Nurses** (http://www.anblpn.ca): This site contains links to information on all aspects of being an LPN professional in New Brunswick.
- **British Columbia College of Nurses & Midwives** (https://www.bccnm.ca): This site contains links to information on all aspects of being an LPN professional in British Columbia.
- **Canadian Council for Practical Nurse Regulators** (http://ccpnr.ca): This site contains information on the four standards of practice that govern the ethical principles of LPNs and RPNs as well as the legal and professional expectations of LPNs and RPNs.
- **College of Licensed Practical Nurses of Alberta** (http://www.clpna.com): This site contains links to information on all aspects of being an LPN professional in Alberta.
- **College of Licensed Practical Nurses of Manitoba** (http://www.clpnm.ca): This site contains links to information on all aspects of being an LPN professional in Manitoba.
- **College of Licensed Practical Nurses of Newfoundland and Labrador** (http://www.clpnnl.ca): This site contains links to information on all aspects of being an LPN professional in Newfoundland and Labrador.
- **College of Licensed Practical Nurses of Prince Edward Island** (https://clpnpei.ca): This site contains links to information on all aspects of being an LPN professional in Prince Edward Island.
- **College of Nurses of Ontario** (http://www.cno.org): This site contains links to information related to all aspects of being a RPN professional in Ontario.
- **Nova Scotia College of Nursing** (http://www.clpnns.ca): This site contains links to information on all aspects of being an LPN professional in Nova Scotia.
- **Ordre des infirmières et infirmiers auxiliaires du Québec** (http://www.oiiaq.org): This site contains links to information on all aspects of being an LPN professional in Quebec.
- **Registered Practical Nurses Association of Ontario** (https://www.werpn.com): This site contains information on the professional association representing the voice of practical nurses in Ontario.
- **Saskatchewan Association of Licensed Practical Nurses** (http://www.salpn.com): This site contains links to information on all aspects of being an LPN professional in Saskatchewan.

Health Assessment Across the Lifespan

Health assessment is the collection of information about an individual's well-being. The information can come from a variety of sources: verbal information from the person or the person's family; physical information that the practical nurse obtains through inspection, palpation, and auscultation; and laboratory testing. All of these and any other sources of information are gathered to assist the practitioner to obtain a complete picture of the individual's well-being.

For the purpose of easy access, this chapter is divided into site-specific sections. Normally, the nurse must consider the person as a whole rather than as the sum of many individual parts. However, this chapter focuses on one system or area at a time. One of the arts of nursing is to paint the whole picture once all the parts are known. Imagine an artist's palette; the areas of information are the colours on the palette, and the care for the client will be determined once the picture has been painted.

As a member of the health care team, it is imperative that the nurse assess the client and that the assessment be recorded. The nurse must believe what they hear and report it, especially if it is abnormal. The nurse, especially the novice nurse, must not second-guess and ignore the findings due to feelings of doubt. If you are in doubt, report the findings and ask a more experienced member of the team to verify them.

The most important aspect of health assessment is the history. Not only is what is said important, but how it is said is also key. The role of the nurse is to get the whole story by asking pertinent questions and steering the conversation in a way that is productive and time-efficient. The physical examination will confirm or refute the story and assist the nurse in obtaining the information needed to help make the diagnosis. Whether the result is a nursing diagnosis or a medical diagnosis, the story is a vital component.

INTERVIEWING SKILLS AND HISTORY-TAKING

Communication Techniques

To take a history, or to listen to a history, the nurse must use a variety of question types, as summarized in Table 5.1.

How the nurse responds to the answers can be as important as the questions themselves. Table 5.2 provides a number of responses, descriptors, and examples.

It is not just the spoken word of an interview that can give you the complete story. It is important to observe the client's posture, eye contact, facial expressions, voice, language, the use of touch, and any gestures. All of these factors enhance the depth and meaning of the spoken word.

A complete history can take up to an hour or even longer to obtain, which is not always practical even at the best of times. The nurse must therefore decide what information is a priority in a shortened amount of time. Over the course of caring for the client, the nurse can continue to ask questions and listen to the whole story. Another reason to do a complete history is to find out any areas of concern in which health teaching and health promotion would be beneficial.

It is not always possible for the history to come from the client. For an infant or young child, the history will come from the child's caregiver (parent, grandparent, or guardian). In the case of an adult who is comatose or too ill to engage in conversation, the information may come from a spouse, a child, or a friend. Understand that information gathered in these circumstances is modified by the person relaying it. Watch the child closely for nonverbal communication. Be inclusive and call the person by name. You must build up a therapeutic relationship not just with the client but also with the provider of information.

Interviewing adolescents can present its challenges. Teens want to be considered as adults but can revert to wanting a parent close by, especially when they are in a stressful situation. Certain information will not be shared unless a good trusting relationship has been built, which may happen only if the parent is not present. Not all adolescents are the same. Levels of maturity, understanding, and the ability to express oneself can range widely. Starting with the easiest questions can be helpful, and when there is a greater sense of trust, the more sensitive questions can be broached.

Interviewing the older person can be a much slower process. Giving the client more time to answer will decrease the potential for frustration and stress. Open-ended questions might take longer to answer because they may cover a lengthy life history. If the client has a deficit in short-term memory, the nurse will need to rely on the family members to fill in the gaps.

If a client has a hearing impairment, sit directly in front of the client. Speak clearly and loudly enough for the client to hear and understand what you are saying.

If the impairment is significant, make sure that the person is wearing hearing aids if appropriate or that a sign-language interpreter is available.

If there is a language barrier, if possible, use an interpreter who is not a family member. The family member might not translate all the information, thinking that they are protecting the client from difficult information.

TABLE 5.1   Communication Techniques

Type of Question	Description of Question	Examples
Open-ended questions	• They are good at the beginning of the interview. • They can lead to a lot of information. • Questions are unbiased. • The practical nurse to be an active and interested listener and encourage the story; for example, using "Tell me more" promotes more information. • They can lead clients to go off on many tangents.	"How are you feeling today?" "Tell me about your health concerns." "Why have you come to the clinic today?"
Closed or direct questions	• They are good for specific details. • They are useful to fill in the gaps from the open-ended response. • They can be used to expedite the interview. • Nurses should ask one question at a time only. • Nurses should use culturally appropriate language. • Client answers are quite often "yes" or "no."	"Do you have any medication allergies?" "Do you get short of breath climbing a flight of stairs?" "When was the last time you ate anything?"

TABLE 5.2   Examples of Responses and Descriptors

Response	Description of Response	Examples
Facilitation	• It encourages further information. • It shows an interest in the information being shared, which will promote storytelling.	Nurse: "Yes" Nodding your head Good eye contact "Mm-hmm" or "Uh-huh" "Go on, I'm listening."
Silence	• It is useful after open-ended questions. • Maintain good eye contact. • Try not to interrupt. • Watch the client for nonverbal clues.	
Reflection	• Repeat part of what the client said to allow them to expand on it. • Expand on an important concept. • Specifically focus on an emotional aspect of what the client has said.	Client: "I don't understand how to do it. I feel so scared." Nurse: "You feel scared?" Client: "I suffered from this last year and now it's back." Nurse: "You had this last year?"
Empathy	• It gives the client a sense of feeling understood. • It can promote the therapeutic relationship. • It gives the green light to the client to talk about their thoughts and feelings.	Nurse: "This is probably very scary for you to go through." "I can imagine that if that happened to me I would also be scared, frightened, upset ..." etc. "I can understand how frustrating this must be for you."
Clarification	• Seek clarification when you do not understand what the client is saying or when you think that what they are saying can be interpreted in more than one way. • Use information the client has shared as a point of clarification. Are you on the right track?	Client: "My job is very heavy." Nurse: "You do a lot of heavy lifting in your job?" Nurse: "Let me get this straight: the pain occurs only in the morning, you get relief when you drink three cups of coffee, and the pain does not return until the following morning. Is that correct?" Client: "Yes, that's right."
Confrontation Interpretation Explanation Summary	• Leave these responses to the end and use as a wrap-up of the interview. • If you do not agree with something that the client has said, question them on it. • Using interpretation helps the client identify with an emotion or explanation as to why something has happened. • Using explanation literally explains the why and what of some notion. • Using summarizing can clarify the issues, put them into sequence, restate your client's perceptions and your own, and validate the information with the client.	Nurse: "You say that you are okay with being in the hospital, but you seem to be so sad and worried." "Do you realize that every time you come to the emergency department with abdominal pain, your mother-in-law is visiting from out of town?" "You must drink the CT dye so that the X-ray will be clear for the physician to interpret."

If the client starts to cry during the interview process, let the person cry. Crying is an important expression of grief and release. Do not move on to another topic to avoid the painful issue. Offer a tissue and perhaps a hand on the shoulder, if this is culturally acceptable.

Be careful if you sense a threat of violence. Nurses can be very vulnerable in the workplace to clients who are under the influence of drugs and alcohol or who are very angry. Recognizing these factors and positioning yourself accordingly can prevent possible physical abuse that might be directed at you. Do not stay in a closed room alone with such a client. Always make sure that other members of the health care team can see you. If you suspect there is a potential for violence, protect yourself, do not take any risks, and think of safety first. Talk calmly and quietly; do not raise your voice and argue with the client. Verbal abuse from clients or toward clients is also not acceptable. Nurses must make it known that they are health professionals and must be treated accordingly.

Ethnocultural and sociohistorical differences in client care can be a learning experience for both parties but can also be a deterrent to complete care. Be careful to try to understand cultural differences. What are the codes of behaviour? Who can be touched or not, and who can be in a room without a chaperone? If there is a language barrier, such differences might be more difficult to interpret. What are the client's perceptions of health care workers, the system, and the treatments? In order to build a trusting therapeutic relationship with clients from some cultures, you may have to divulge some information about yourself, too. It is best to start the interview process formally. Stand to greet the client, let them know how you would like to be referred to, and elicit the same from them. Keep a good distance apart; 1.5 to 3 metres is acceptable. Be tolerant of different cultural beliefs and adjust your questions and responses accordingly.

Consider the client's gender and sexual identify and expression when communicating. During the interview process, allow the client to self-identify their own sex and gender identity.

The Complete Health History

A complete history includes many aspects. Keep in mind who is providing the information, which may be the client, a parent, the spouse, a friend, or someone else. If the client is very ill or if it is an emergency situation, stress will be an added factor in the presentation of the story. The following is a list of the different areas of information to be collected:

- Biographical data
- Reason for seeking care
- Present health or history of the present illness
- Past history
- Family history
- Review of all systems
- Functional assessment or activities of daily living

If there is pain, further information is needed. Use the mnemonic "OPQRSTUV" (Jarvis et al., 2024) to explore all areas:

O: Onset: When did the pain begin?

P: Provocative or Palliative: What makes the pain worse? What makes it better?

Q: Quality or Quantity: How does it feel? How severe is it?

R: Region or Radiation: Where is the pain? Does it spread?

S: Severity scale: On a scale of 0 to 10, where 0 is no pain and 10 is the most severe pain that you can imagine, where is your pain?

T: Timing: When did the pain start? How often does the pain occur, and how long does it last?

U: Understanding client's perception of the problem. What do you think that it means?

V: Values: What is your acceptable pain level?

Keep in mind social or cultural differences. Consider how the social determinants of health may impact the client. For example, consider the fact that people's dietary intake may be impacted by their income or access to food resources. Some clients will be survivors of trauma such as Indigenous clients who are residential school survivors or are family members of people who attended residential schools. If the client is not native to Canada, determine when they arrived, the country or region of origin, and the conditions in that location. Are there any religious considerations that would affect blood-product transfusions, dietary options, the need for clergy, or perhaps the necessity of a chaperone during an examination?

If the client is an infant, include details of pre- and postnatal health and labour and delivery. Also ask about the developmental history. It is challenging at times to get a complete history from adolescents. Keep in mind that it is important to include a psychological assessment as adolescents can be very vulnerable to depression and suicide.

The Mental Status Examination

A person's mental status is defined as their emotional and cognitive function assessed through behaviour. By assessing mental status first, the nurse can establish a baseline, and reassessment can monitor any changes, especially in response to the stress of illness and feeling of being unwell. Serious health conditions such as alcoholism, renal failure, diabetes, liver disease, or brain disease might alter the mental assessment. Various medications can also alter the assessment, as will low educational levels.

It is difficult to assess mental status in a child, but the older the child, the easier it is as the cerebral cortex matures and the attention span increases with age. Assessing the older person client often takes longer because the client may need more time to answer the questions, and there may also be recent memory loss. As well as memory loss, sensory losses of sight and hearing can cause frustration, social isolation, and apathy. The older client might also have experienced a number of losses, such as loved ones, friends, job, income, or health, giving rise to an added risk of depression and despair.

The behaviour assessment should include the following factors:

- Consciousness
- Facial expression
- Speech

- Mood and affect
- Orientation to time, place, person, and self
- Attention
- Memory
- Higher intellectual function
- Insight and judgement
- Thought process
- Thought content
- Perceptions

For the average client, the mental assessment can be incorporated into the rest of the health history. The four main headings are *appearance*, *behaviour*, *cognition*, and *thought process* (ABCT) (Jarvis et al., 2024). The Mini-Mental State Examination (MMSE) can be performed if a more thorough assessment is needed (Folstein et al., 1975).

ASSESSMENT TECHNIQUES

The practical nurse uses the following techniques when objectively assessing the client:
- Inspection
- Palpation
- Auscultation

The techniques are performed in order with the exception of the examination of the abdomen, when auscultation is done immediately after inspection. Note that percussion is part of the assessment technique but is not a required competency of the entry-level practical nurse.

The Technique of Inspection

Inspection is the most powerful of all the technical skills. It yields the most data because the nurse's physical examination is guided by the observation of any abnormalities. The inspection starts as soon as the practitioner sees the person and continues throughout the whole encounter. Nurses must learn to be astute in the art of looking. It is very difficult at first not to touch the client. So just stand back and observe. Perform a general body scan. Watch for behaviour, as well as generalized symmetry. Then move on to more specific observations.

The Technique of Palpation

Palpation is the art of touching the body to assess the skin and the underlying organs, as well as any abnormalities. The sense of touch can be used to feel texture; temperature; moisture; vibration; pulsation; swelling; rigidity; spasticity; organ location; crepitations; the presence of any lumps, bumps, or lesions; and the presence of any pain or tenderness.

Generally, the pads of the fingertips are used. Make sure that your hands are warm. Be careful not to poke the skin but to gently rub the fingertips in a circular motion.

The dorsa of the hands are used for assessing temperature and moisture. The skin on the back of the hand is thinner and more sensitive. The base of the fingers or the ulnar edge of the hand is used to detect vibrations. Bimanual palpation is the use of both hands at the same time.

The Technique of Auscultation

Auscultation is listening to body sounds through a stethoscope. The earpieces should be comfortable and directed toward the nose. As you bend your head to listen, the earpieces should make a perfect seal with the natural curvature of the ear canal. There are two parts to the stethoscope: the diaphragm and the bell. The diaphragm is used to listen to high-pitched sounds, such as bowel, respiratory, or heart sounds, whereas the bell is useful for hearing low-pitched sounds, such as heart murmurs or bruits. The bell must be placed on the skin very lightly, and the diaphragm should be pressed firmly down on the skin. Clean the stethoscope with an alcohol wipe between uses as it can become a vector for cross-contamination. The neck of the stethoscope should be 30 to 35 cm in length. The noise in the surrounding areas should be minimal. If the client's chest is particularly hairy, wet the hair to avoid mistaking it for "crackles" in the lungs. The sounds are more accurate if listened to over bare skin and not over clothes.

The General Survey

At your first encounter with the client, start your general survey. Establish that the airway is clear, that the client is breathing, and that there is circulation. Throughout the general survey, establish that appearance, behaviour, cognition, and thought processes are all intact.

Physical appearance: Does the client look their stated age? Is the client oriented to time, place, and person? Is the sexual development appropriate for the client's age and gender? Do a general scan of the colour and condition of the skin. Are there any signs of acute distress?

Body structure: Check height and weight. Are these the expected values? Look at body symmetry and posture. How comfortable is the client sitting or lying down? Is the body proportionate?

Mobility: Assess gait if possible. Note the range of motion of the limbs and joints.

Vital signs: Take the pulse, respiratory rate, blood pressure, temperature, and oxygen saturation.

For infants, measure the circumference of the head and the length of the body.

HEAD AND NECK WITH REGIONAL LYMPHATICS ASSESSMENT

The Anatomy and Landmarks of the Head and Neck

Keep in mind that there are two halves to the body: the left and the right. Remember to examine both sides of the body and always assess for symmetry. The symmetry is not perfect, but, for the most part, it is very close.

The skull is composed of cranial bones; sutures separate the frontal, temporal, parietal, and occipital bones. At birth, the sutures have not approximated completely to allow room for the brain to grow. The areas where they have not joined together are called *fontanelles*. The posterior fontanelle closes within the first 2 months of birth, and the frontal fontanelle closes sometime between 9 months and 2 years of age.

There are 14 facial bones, and the head sits upon the vertebrae of the cervical spine. The first vertebra, C1, is located at the base of the spine and is called the *atlas*; the second, C2, is called the *axis*. The cervical vertebrae continue down to C7, which is called the *vertebra prominens*. The prominens is highly palpable when the neck is flexed forward as it has a long spinous process.

Many muscles control the face and facial expressions. The motor component to cranial nerve VII, or the facial nerve, innervates most of the muscles. Cranial nerve V, the trigeminal nerve, controls the movement of the masseter muscles—which assist in talking and chewing—from the mandible and the temporomandibular joint. The sensory component of the trigeminal nerve is responsible for feeling light touch along the areas controlled by the three sections of the nerve: the forehead, the cheek, and the chin. The sensory component of the facial nerve is taste on the anterior two thirds of the tongue.

The pulsation of the temporal artery can be felt anterior to the ear. This artery supplies blood and nutrients to the face and head.

Salivary glands protect the teeth and mucosa by rinsing them and aid digestion by containing enzymes to start the digestive process and providing lubrication for the food bolus. The parotid gland is located anterior to and slightly below the tragus of the ear on either side of the face. The submandibular gland is located at the angle of the jaw and below the mandible. The sublingual glands are under the tongue at the front of the mouth. None of the glands are normally palpable.

The muscles of the neck are the sternomastoid, the trapezius, and the omohyoid. They are innervated by cranial nerve XI, the spinal accessory nerve. These muscles are responsible for holding the head up and providing the range of motion of the head. At the base of the neck is the clavicle. Down along the neck there are a variety of structures: the hyoid bone, the thyroid cartilage, the cricoid cartilage, the trachea, and the manubrium at the bottom.

The thyroid gland is an endocrine gland that synthesizes and secretes thyroxine (T_4) and triiodothyronine (T_3), hormones that regulate cellular metabolism and growth. The thyroid gland is also responsible for calcitonin, which regulates the amount of calcium in the bloodstream and stimulates growth. The gland has two lobes and should be smooth, without lumps or bumps. The cricoid cartilage is just above the thyroid.

The Anatomy and Landmarks of the Regional Lymphatic System

The lymphatic system plays a vital role in the body. It is responsible for cleaning the blood, returning fluid to the blood from the tissues, and fighting infection. The lymph nodes that are situated along the pathways of the lymphatic system filter bacteria and foreign particles from the lymph fluid. If there is an infection, the lymph nodes become swollen and sore. If they become cancerous, they are fixed, nontender, and firm.

Subjective Data Specific to the Head and Neck
*Questions specific to the older person
- Are you experiencing any headaches? If yes, describe the headache.
- What types of stress do you have in your life?
- What coping strategies have you been using?
- Are you taking any medications?
- Do you have any allergies?
- Have you had a recent head injury?
- Did you lose consciousness?
* **Do you have any illnesses now, such as diabetes or lung or heart disease?**
* **Are you experiencing vertigo or dizziness? If yes, does it interfere with your daily routine?**
- Do you have any neck pain?
* **Have you noticed any decrease in the range of motion of your neck? If yes, does it restrict your ability to do your daily activities or work?**
- Have you had any trouble breathing?
- Have you had any trouble swallowing?
- Do you smoke? If so, how many cigarettes per day and for how many years?
- How often do you drink alcohol?
- Have you noticed any lumps or bumps in your neck?
- Have you had a cold recently?
- Have you ever had surgery to the head or neck region?
- If the client is an infant, ask the adult: Were there any difficulties with the pregnancy, labour, or delivery? Has your baby been following a normal growth pattern?

Objective Data Specific to the Head and Neck
- Inspect and palpate the head and hair. Look at and feel the head for redness, swelling, lumps, bumps, and lesions. Check the hair for texture and the presence of lice. The eggs are white ovals that stick to the hair strands and will not brush off easily. They come off individually when they are pulled off with fingernails, as opposed to dandruff, which will flake off or blow off the hair quite easily. The nits are black and can jump around the head. They tend to migrate to the base of the hair at the back of the neck and around the posterior of the ears. They can be very irritating to the skin.
- Palpating the head should be relaxing to the client. At every opportunity, make the examination process a relaxing and calm one for the client and for you.
- For an infant, measure the circumference of the head. Assess for any tenderness over any of the cranial bones.
- Palpate the temporal artery pulse.
- Palpate the temporomandibular joint, assessing for tenderness, cracking, or crepitus. Test for range of movement, as well as smooth movement when the mouth is opened.
- Test the movement of the mandible against resistance for strength.
- Inspect the face, looking at the skin condition, facial expressions, and symmetry. Note any tics or fasciculation.
- Inspect and palpate the neck. Assess for symmetry and that the trachea is midline.

- Look for the client's ability to perform voluntary head movements. Perform a series of range-of-motion exercises with the neck and assess for strength using movement against resistance. With an infant, assess the head posture and control. By 4 months, an infant should have head control.
- Using the fingertips and creeping down the skin, not poking it, feel for all the lymph nodes in the neck. If there is a palpable node, note its size and consistency and feel for tenderness. Check both sides simultaneously for symmetry.

EYE ASSESSMENT

Landmarks of the Eye

- Palpebral fissures are the space between the upper and lower eyelids. When the eye is closed, the eyelids approximate with no distance between them. When open, the eye is partially covered to the upper part of the iris by the upper eyelid.
- The limbus is where the sclera and cornea come together.
- The canthus can be found where the eyelids meet in the corners of the eye. The lateral (outer) canthus is toward the ear, and the medial (inner) canthus is toward the nose. At the inner canthus is the caruncle, a fleshy area that contains sebaceous glands.
- The upper lids contain Meibomian glands within the tarsal plate. The tarsal plates contain connective tissue that gives the eyelid its shape. In the older person, the connective tissue loses elasticity, thus not maintaining the eyelid's shape. The Meibomian glands secrete an oily substance that lubricates the eye, prevents the tears from overflowing, and maintains a good seal when the eyes are closed.
- The palpebral conjunctiva is a thin mucous membrane. It lines the inside of the eyelids and is clear with many blood vessels. The bulbar conjunctiva covers the eyeball, overlying the sclera. The bulbar conjunctiva merges with the cornea at the limbus, where the cornea covers and protects the iris and pupil.
- The lacrimal apparatus provides protection to the eye by providing an irrigation system to keep the cornea and the conjunctiva moist and lubricated. Tears form in the lacrimal gland and wash over the eyes. The tears drain out of the eye through the puncta at the inner canthus into the lacrimal sac and down the lacrimal duct into the inferior meatus and turbinates of the nose.
- Eye movement is controlled by six extraocular muscles attached to the eye and the orbit. The muscles provide straight and rotary movement. The muscles of the eyes are coordinated so that the eyes move in a parallel fashion (called *conjugate movement*). This movement is important as the brain can only perceive one image at a time. Cranial nerves III, IV, and VI (oculomotor, trochlear, and abducens) innervate the muscles of the eye to produce various movements.

The Internal Anatomy of the Eye

The outer layer of the eye is called the *sclera*. It is made up of a white fibrous tissue and should have a smooth consistency. It serves as a protective shield and is continuous with the transparent cornea that protects the iris and pupil.

The cornea bends (refracts) the incoming light rays, which are then directed back to the retina. The cornea is very sensitive to touch. The corneal reflex is tested by touching the cornea with a wisp of cotton. If the reflex is normal, the fifth cranial nerve (the trigeminal nerve) sends a message to the brain and cranial nerve VII sends a message to the eye to blink.

The eye's middle layer consists of the choroid, iris, pupil, lens, and anterior and posterior chambers. The choroid protects the retina by supplying blood to it and by decreasing the amount of light that reflects internally. Anteriorly, it is continuous with the muscle of the ciliary body, which controls the thickness of the lens. The muscle fibres in the iris contract, or dilate, the pupil to vary the amount of light admitted into the eye. This is called the *papillary reflex*. A direct reflex occurs when the light is shone into the eye; a consensual light reflex is the constriction of the contralateral pupil—in other words, when the light is shone into one eye, the pupil of the other eye also constricts. Accommodation occurs when the pupils constrict to help the eye to focus on close objects. The lens lies posterior to the pupil. It flattens to see distant objects and bulges to see close objects. After the age of 40 years, a person's lens starts to lose elasticity and the ability to see close objects diminishes; this is called *presbyopia*. By 70 years of age, the lens begins to thicken due to a clumping of proteins and yellow deposits called *nuclear stenosis* or *senile cataract*.

The posterior chamber contains the aqueous humour. It provides nutrients and removes waste products to the surrounding tissues. The anterior chamber, which sits between the cornea and the lens and iris, allows the outflow of the aqueous humour. Intraocular pressure measures the balance between the amount of aqueous humour produced and the resistance to its outflow. Increased intraocular pressure, or glaucoma, increases with age and is three to six times more likely to occur in people of African descent.

The inner retinal layer is responsible for changing the waves of light into nerve impulses. When you are looking through an ophthalmoscope, the optic disc, where the optic nerve lies, is located toward the nose. The disc is yellow-orange to pink, is oval to round in shape, and is where fibres from the retina converge to form the optic nerve. The physiological cup inside the optic disc is a brighter yellow than the disc and is the location of the entrance and exit of the retinal blood vessels. The blood vessels drain through the cup. The macula is grey in colour and is responsible for central vision. Through an ophthalmoscope, it can be located by looking toward the ear. It is at the macula that the sharpest vision can be seen. Age can decrease the effectiveness of the macula, decreasing central vision. The retinal vessels converge into the optic disc. The arteries are redder and smaller than the veins. The background of the fundus depends on the person's skin colour. Generally, it has a reddish-orange hue.

Subjective Data Specific to the Eye

- Do you have any difficulty with your vision?
- Have you noticed any difficulty reading or seeing close objects?
- Do you have any difficulty with night vision?
- Do you have any pain in your eyes?

- Do you see double?
- Have you ever had "crossed eyes"?
- Do you have any redness or swelling in your eyes?
- Do you have any discharge or watering in your eyes?
- Do your eyes feel dry or burning?
- Do you have any past history of eye problems?
- Do you have any past history of glaucoma?
- When was the last time you were checked for glaucoma?
- Do you have any family history of glaucoma?
- Do you use glasses or contacts? If yes, do they work well for you?
- When was your last eye examination?
- Were you given a prescription for glasses?
- Have you ever had any surgery on your eyes?
- Do you take any medications or drops for your eyes?

Objective Data Specific to the Eye

- Test for vision. Test the function of cranial nerve II, the optic nerve.
- Use a Snellen eye chart. The person should stand 6 metres (20 ft) away from a 6-metre chart or 3 metres (10 ft) from a 3-metre chart, cover one eye with a shield, and read the letters aloud, starting from left to right, top to bottom. Ask the person not to use a hand to cover the eye as this can compress the eyeball and distort its vision. The client should read the lowest line that they can without making more than two mistakes. Switch to the other eye, this time asking the person to read from right to left. Reading glasses must be removed, but glasses with corrective lenses for distance should stay on. Normal vision is 6/6 in metric (20/20 in the United States); in other words, the person can read at 6 metres what a person with normal vision can read at 6 metres. The numerator is the distance from the client to the chart, and the denominator is the distance from which a person with normal vision can read the same line.
- For children who do not know the alphabet or for those who cannot read English letters, use a picture chart or an E chart.
- Newborn infants can be tested for visual acuity using light perception. The infant should blink when you shine a light into the eyes.
- To test for presbyopia, use the Jaegar chart. The person should hold the card 35 cm away from the eye and be able to read it. Test each eye separately.
- Test visual fields for peripheral vision loss. The confrontation test is a broad or gross examination of peripheral vision. Stand 60 cm (2 ft) from the client and at their level. Cover your right eye and the client's left eye with opaque cards. Tell the client to look straight at your uncovered eye. Wiggle your finger and move it slowly from the periphery into the centre between you and the client. Assuming that your own peripheral vision is good, the client should see the finger at the same time you do. Then switch to the other eye.
- Test cranial nerves III, IV, and VI (oculomotor, trochlear, and abducens).

- Test the corneal light reflex (Hirschberg test). Shine a light from a distance of 30 cm (12 in) into the client's eyes and ask them to look straight ahead. There should be a symmetrical reflection of the light in both eyes. If not, then perform the cover test.
- The cover test: Ask the person to look forward and stare at your nose. Cover one eye while the person is staring; the other eye should maintain the stare and not jump around to fixate again. Repeat the test with the other eye.
- Diagnostic position test (the six fields of gaze): Direct the client to follow the movement of your outstretched finger with their eyes and without moving the head. Move your finger to the left superior oblique, left lateral, left inferior oblique, right superior oblique, right lateral, and right inferior oblique, returning to the centre each time. The eyes should move in a parallel fashion. Watch for any shaking of the eyeball (nystagmus). It is not abnormal to see it at the far lateral point.

Inspect the External Eye

- Eyebrows, eyelashes: Observe for hair distribution and the presence of scaling or lice.
- Eyelids: Observe for lid lag. The upper eyelid should cover the upper area of the iris. The lashes should approximate when closed. The skin should be without lumps, bumps, redness, or lesions.
- Eyeballs: The eyeballs should not be sunken in or protruding.
- Conjunctiva and sclera: Ask the client to look up; pull the lower lids down and inspect the conjunctiva for colour (very red may be infection, pallor may be anemia), lumps, bumps, or lesions. The sclera should be china white without lesions. In people of African descent, you may find brown macules and yellow fat deposits.
- Lacrimal apparatus: Note that the eyes are glossy and well lubricated without excess tearing. Press with your thumbs on the lacrimal gland and sac and assess for tenderness, redness, blocked ducts, and swelling.
- Cornea and lens: Shine a light on the cornea from the side and assess for any scratches or opacities.
- Iris and pupil: Note the size, shape, and equality of the pupils. Anisocoria (two different pupil sizes) occurs in 5% of the population. Test for direct and consensual pupillary light reflex. In a darkened area, shine a light into one eye and note the constriction of the pupil of that eye and the consensual constriction of that of the other eye. Repeat the test with the other eye.
- Accommodation: Ask the client to look at a distant object. The pupils will dilate. Then quickly get the client to focus on a close object. The pupils will constrict, and the eyeballs will converge. Record the findings as PERRLA: *p*upils *e*qual, *r*ound, *r*eact to *l*ight, and *a*ccommodation.

EAR ASSESSMENT

The ear is a sensory organ responsible for hearing and equilibrium. Cranial nerve VIII, the acoustic nerve, is responsible for the sense of hearing. There are three parts to the ear: the outer or external, middle, and inner ear. Behind the ear is a bony prominence called the *mastoid process*. In Fig. 5.1, the three parts of the ear are illustrated.

The Anatomy and Landmarks of the Ear
The External or Outer Ear

The outer ear consists of the auricle, the external auditory canal, and the tympanic membrane. The auricle, or pinna, consists of cartilage and skin. The tragus is the projection of skin-covered cartilage that is proximal to the opening (meatus) to the external canal. Sound waves enter the ear through the meatus and travel through the external canal. In the adult ear, the canal has a slight S-shape.

Cerumen (wax) is produced by small glands that line the canal. The cerumen is necessary to lubricate the canal and to protect it from foreign material. It is yellow and sticky. The wax is naturally excreted from the ear through the mechanisms of chewing and talking. Some people make more cerumen than the average person. The use of cotton swabs to clean out the cerumen is poor practice as the swab can impact, or compress, the cerumen, causing a buildup and blockage in the canal. It is better to dissolve excessive cerumen with a few drops of olive oil in the ear at night, sealed with a small cotton ball at the meatus.

At the end of the external canal is the tympanic membrane. Commonly known as the *eardrum*, the tympanic membrane is the dividing line between the external and middle ear. It is translucent and pearly grey in colour. It is possible to see parts of the malleus bone (umbo, manubrium, and short process) through the membrane of the middle ear. The tympanic membrane will bulge out into the external canal if there is an excess of fluid or exudate in the middle ear. If there is an infection in the middle ear, the membrane will be a red colour. A blockage of the tympanic membrane with either fluid or exudate will impair hearing. For the young child, when language development is so important, a decrease in hearing can be very detrimental.

The Middle Ear

The middle ear consists of the small ear bones and is a small cavity filled with air. The middle ear has three functions: protection of the inner ear from loud sound by reducing the amplitude; conducting sound waves through the vibration of

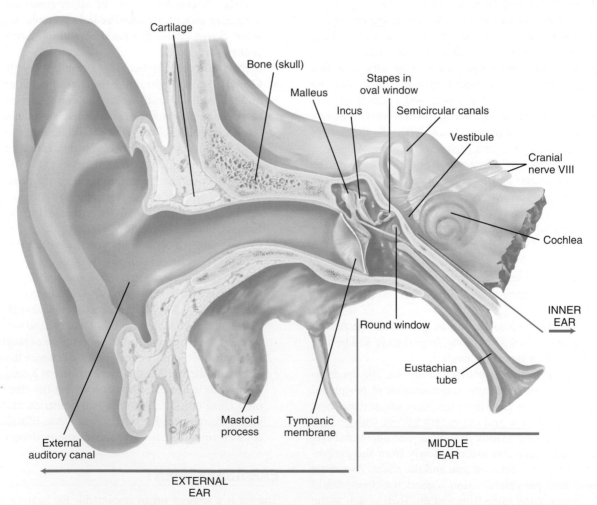

Fig. 5.1 Anatomy of the ear. (From Jarvis, C., Eckhardt, A., Browne, A. J., et al. [2024]. *Physical examination & health assessment* [4th Canadian ed., p. 360, Figure 16-1]. Elsevier.) © Pat Thomas, CMI.

the three little bones (malleus, incus, and stapes) to the inner ear through the oval window; and maintaining equalization of pressure on either side of the membrane using the eustachian tube. The eustachian tube connects the middle ear to the nasopharynx. The eustachian tube is shorter and straighter in infants and small children, giving rise to an increased risk of middle-ear infections in that population.

The Inner Ear

The inner ear consists of the bony labyrinth that contains the vestibule and the semicircular canals. The cochlea, which is the central hearing apparatus, is also present in the inner ear. The sensory organs for hearing and equilibrium are within the inner ear.

Sound vibrations continue from the middle ear into the inner ear and into the cochlea. Basilar membranes vibrate depending on the frequency of the sound. Along the basilar membrane are receptor hair cells of the organ of Corti. As the hairs bend, the vibration is transformed into electrical impulses that cranial nerve VIII (the acoustic nerve) can transmit to the brainstem. In the cortex, the sound is interpreted.

Hearing can be divided into two types: conductive hearing, through both air and bone, and sensorineural hearing. Conductive hearing loss is a mechanical dysfunction in the outer or middle ear. It might be a blockage in the canal or, in the adult, a hardening of the footplate of the stapes so that it becomes fixed and cannot vibrate. In the older person, the cilia lining the ear canal can become coarse and stiff, decreasing the conduction of sound waves through the canal.

Sensorineural hearing loss occurs when there is gradual nerve degeneration of the acoustic nerve. This starts at approximately 50 years of age and gets progressively worse. At 70 years of age, the transmission time for the sound to travel to the brain slows, which decreases the reaction time for older persons.

There can also be a mixed hearing loss. This loss is a combination of conductive and sensorineural hearing loss.

Subjective Data Specific to the Ear

- Do you have any pain in your ear?
- Do you have a history of ear infections, recent or as a child?
- Have you noticed that your child is having any difficulty hearing or is talking unusually loudly?
- Have you ever had surgery on your ear?
- Do you have any discharge coming out of your ear? If so, what colour is it? Does it have an odour?
- Do you have any trouble hearing? If so, is this new for you?
- Do you experience any excess noise at home, at work, or during leisure activities?
- Do you notice any ringing in your ear?
- Have you ever taken a medication called CISplatin (Platinol AQ)?
- Are you taking any medications?
- Do you have any allergies?
- Are you experiencing any vertigo or dizziness?
- Do you feel as if the room is spinning around or that you are spinning around?

- When was your last hearing test?
- Do you wear any hearing aids?

Objective Data Specific to the Ear
Inspect and Palpate the Outer Ear

- Assess the size, shape, and position of the ears. They should be symmetrical and positioned in line with the eye from the top of the ear. Inspect and palpate the skin for colour, lumps, bumps, or lesions. Note the edge of the helix for basal cell carcinoma.
- Assess the ear for tenderness: Press on the tragus to test for possible otitis media and wiggle the auricle for possible otitis externa. Palpate the mastoid process for any tenderness.

Tests for Hearing Acuity

There are three tests for hearing acuity: the whispered voice test, Weber test, and Rinne test. These are all crude tests, and, if positive, the client will have to be seen for more thorough tests.

- The whispered voice test: Ask the client to repeat after you two-syllable words that you whisper 30 to 60 cm from one ear while the other ear is occluded. Repeat with the other ear. A whisper is a high-pitched sound. The inability to hear it shows some high-tone loss.
- Weber test: Hit the tuning fork, taking care to hold it at the base of the handle, and place it in the middle of the head. If that is not possible, place it anywhere down the midline on a bone, such as on the forehead or chin. The sound should be heard by the client equilaterally in both ears. If there is lateralization of the sound, then the ear that hears the sound more loudly may have conductive or sensorineural loss.
- Rinne test: This test compares bone conduction with air conduction. Air conduction should take twice as long as bone conduction. To test bone conduction, hit the tuning fork, place the base onto the client's mastoid process, and say, "Can you hear this? (Yes!) Tell me when you cannot hear it anymore," and then start counting. When the client cannot hear it, place the tip of the tuning fork to the opening of the ear canal to test air conduction. Do this quickly and avoid touching the hair or skin of the client. Repeat the same question and count again. The air conduction count should be twice as long as the bone conduction count.

Testing for Balance

The Romberg test is used to assess for altered equilibrium.

- Ask the client to stand with arms at their sides and close their eyes for 20 seconds. Stand close to the client in case they lose balance (positive Romberg sign). The Romberg test also assesses the function of the cerebellum.

NOSE, MOUTH, AND THROAT ASSESSMENT
Anatomy and Landmarks of the Nose

The nose is the beginning of the airway. It has several functions apart from being a distinguishing feature on a person's face. The nose is rich in blood supply so that it can warm up the outside air before the air travels into the lungs. The hairs in the nose trap and filter large airborne particles, and the mucosal lining traps fine airborne particles before they travel into the lungs. With age, the nasal hairs can become coarse and stiff and not filter as well.

The nasal cavity is split down the centre by the nasal septum. Kiesselbach's plexus is in the anterior of the septum. It is very rich in blood supply and is the most common area for nosebleeds. The septum can be misaligned in some people, making it difficult to breathe from one nare or the other. Along the walls of each nasal cavity lie the turbinates. The sinuses and nasolacrimal duct drain into the turbinates.

The olfactory receptors are spread across the upper area of the cavity and along the upper third of the septum. The receptors merge into cranial nerve I, the olfactory nerve, which is responsible for smell. Without the sense of smell, it is difficult to taste. Over time, the number of receptors can decrease, reducing the sense of smell.

Paranasal sinuses are located in the cranium. They are air-filled spaces that aerate the head, keeping it light. When they get filled with mucus, the head feels heavy. The sinus ducts are in the nose and can get blocked, increasing the chance of sinusitis.

There are four sets of sinuses. The ethmoid sinuses are behind the orbits, and the sphenoid sinuses are deep within the sphenoid bone. These are not possible to examine without medical imaging. The maxillary sinuses, which are behind the upper cheeks under the orbits, and the frontal sinuses, which are above the medial aspect of the eyebrow, are easier to access. The frontal and maxillary sinuses are not present at birth but grow from the age of 6 to 8 years. The sphenoid sinus, although present at birth, does not grow until after puberty.

Anatomy and Landmarks of the Mouth

The mouth is also an opening for the respiratory system, but more importantly, it is the opening to and the beginning of the digestive system. Within the mouth are the tongue, gums (gingiva), buccal and lingual mucosa, teeth, and salivary glands. The lips frame the opening of the mouth.

The roof of the mouth is divided into the hard palate (anterior) and the soft palate. The uvula hangs from the soft palate at the back of the mouth. In the infant, the lip or palate might not have approximated, leaving a cleft, a condition more common in people of Asian and Indigenous descent, up to 50% of whom have a bony ridge, called the *torsus palatinus*, that runs along the hard palate.

The tongue is a mass of muscle tissue that has the ability to move and change shape. It helps in speech, chewing, swallowing, and cleaning the teeth. The taste buds are embedded into the tongue. The frenulum is a midline fold of tissue that joins the bottom of the tongue to the floor of the mouth. When children start to talk, it is noticeable if the frenulum is too short. This tongue-tied situation usually corrects itself, or the frenulum may need to be clipped to loosen it.

Over a lifetime, humans develop two sets of teeth. The first set contains 20 teeth that start to erupt between 6 months and 2.5 years and fall out between 6 and 12 years. They are replaced by 32 permanent teeth. With age, teeth or gums that are not well cared for may develop tooth decay or gingivitis, which can lead to tooth loss. Bone resorption may also occur. Without teeth, the older person may experience changes in nutrition because of an inability to chew properly.

The salivary glands provide lubrication to the mouth, which is very important in speech, cleaning the teeth, and digestion. There are three sets of salivary glands. The largest are the parotid glands. The parotid glands can be found in the cheeks, anterior to and slightly below the tragus of the ears. The duct of this gland, Stensen's duct, can be found on the upper outer area of the buccal mucosa. The submandibular gland can be found where the mandible and upper jaw meet. The opening, Wharton's duct, is on either side of the frenulum. The sublingual gland is on the anterior floor of the mouth and has many openings beside it

Anatomy and Landmarks of the Throat

Behind the mouth and the nose is the pharynx, or the throat. It is divided into the nasopharynx behind the nose, where the eustachian tubes drain and the adenoids are located, and the oropharynx, which is continuous with the mouth and contains the tonsils.

Subjective Data Specific to the Nose, Mouth, and Throat

- Are you experiencing any discharge from the nose?
- Do you get colds often? Are you experiencing any pain in the sinus area?
- Do you get nosebleeds often?
- Do you have any allergies?
- Are you taking any medications?
- Have you ever had any trauma to the nose, mouth, or throat?
- Have you ever had any surgery to the nose, mouth, or throat?
- Have you had any change in smell or taste?
- Do you have any sores in your mouth?
- Do you have a sore throat? If yes, do you have any cold symptoms?
- Do your gums bleed?
- Has there been any change to your voice?
- Do you have any difficulty swallowing?
- Is your mouth unusually dry? Do you smoke or drink alcohol? When was your last visit to the dentist?
- How often do you brush your teeth?
- Do you have any dentures or removable teeth?
- Do you grind your teeth?

Objective Data Specific to the Nose, Mouth, and Throat

Inspect and Palpate the Nose

- Inspect the nose for symmetry and to see if it is without deviation. Inspect the skin for any lumps, bumps, or lesions. Check patency by getting the client to close one nostril and breathe through the other. Repeat with the other nostril.
- Test cranial nerve I: Ask the client to close one nostril again and to close their eyes while you introduce something for

the client to smell. Ask the client to identify the scent. Repeat with the other nostril and another scent.

- Inspect the nasal cavity with a speculum and a light source. Look at the turbinates. If the client has a cold, the turbinates will be reddened, and if the client has allergies, the turbinates will have a grey-lavender hue. In some clients, the turbinates will look corroded, particularly if the client has been using cocaine. Other causes of corrosion include the overuse of decongestants, foreign objects in the nose, or nasal trauma. Note any deviation or holes in the septum, foreign bodies, polyps, swelling, or discharge.

Inspect and Palpate the Sinuses, Mouth, and Throat

- Palpate or gently tap over the sinus areas and assess for pain.
- Inspect the lips inside and out. Note any cracking, swelling, or lesions. In infants, it is normal to see a sucking tubercle caused by the friction of sucking on the breast or bottle.
- Inspect the teeth for any large caries; check for signs of bone resorption, gingivitis, or missing teeth and observe the gum line and buccal and lingual mucosa. In small children, assess for "baby bottle syndrome," in which the front teeth have been destroyed by the baby sucking on sugary fluid such as juice or sugar water. With a glove on, palpate the mucosa for lumps, bumps, and lesions. Assess the salivary ducts.
- Check cranial nerves IX and X, the glossopharyngeal and vagus nerves. Using a tongue depressor and light source, ask the client to say "Ahhh" and watch for the soft palate and the uvula to move up and back in the mouth. Then move the tongue depressor back quickly to elicit a gag response.
- Inspect the tonsils for closeness to each other and for exudate. Rate the tonsils 1+ = visible, 2+ = halfway between the tonsillar pillars and the uvula, 3+ = touching the uvula, or 4+ = touching each other.
- Test cranial nerve XII, the hypoglossal nerve. Ask the client to say "light," "tight," and "dynamite" to assess for the client's lingual speech. Instruct the client to push the tongue into the cheek against the resistance of your hand outside on the face to check tongue strength. Repeat on the other side. Ask the client to stick out their tongue and inspect it for fissures, colour, and symmetry.

RESPIRATORY ASSESSMENT

Anatomy and Landmarks of the Thorax and Lungs

The function of the respiratory system is to provide a gas exchange that supplies oxygen to the body for energy production and that removes carbon dioxide. It also maintains an acid–base equilibrium of the arterial blood. In addition, respiration helps to regulate the heat of the body, although less so in humans than in animals.

The thoracic cage is composed of the clavicle, sternum, ribs, scapulae, and vertebrae. The floor of the thoracic cage is the diaphragm. The function of the thoracic cage is to give shape to the body and to protect the organs found within, such as the lungs, heart, and liver. The chest is larger in people of European and African descent than in people of Asian and Indigenous descent.

The anterior landmarks include the clavicle on either side at the top. Between the clavicles is the top of the sternum, the manubrium. Just below the manubrium, where the sternum joins, is the manubriosternal notch, or angle of Louis. The notch protrudes slightly and is the landmark for the second rib and where the trachea bifurcates. The sternum, or breast bone, is connected to the first seven of the 12 pairs of ribs. The costal angle should be 90°. This is the angle between the costal margins; the xiphoid process is in the middle.

The posterior landmarks include the seven cervical vertebrae, the vertebra prominens, the scapulae—where the inferior border is at the level of the eighth rib—and the thoracic vertebrae. The spinous processes stick out, making it easier to count them. The twelfth, or floating, rib is not present on the anterior side. See Fig. 5.2 for illustrations of the anterior cage and the posterior thoracic cage.

It is important to imagine and understand the landmark lines on the thoracic cage. They are as follows:

- Midsternal line: the line along the sternum
- Midclavicular line: a vertical line down from the middle of the clavicle
- Anterior axillary line: a vertical line down from the anterior axillary fold
- Posterior axillary line: a vertical line down from the posterior axillary fold
- Midaxillary line: a vertical line from the apex of the axilla

The Lung Borders

Looking from the anterior, the apex of each lung is 3 cm above the clavicle. From an anterior perspective, the upper right lobe extends down to the fourth rib at the sternum and the fifth rib at the anterior axillary line. The right middle lobe extends from the fourth rib at the sternum and the fifth rib at the anterior axillary line down to the sixth rib at the midclavicular line. The right lower lobe extends from the fifth rib at the anterior axillary line down to the sixth rib at the midclavicular line and to the seventh rib at the anterior axillary line.

From a posterior perspective, the right and left upper lobes start at the level of cervical vertebra C7 and down to thoracic vertebra 10 (T10) on inspiration and T12 on expiration.

The Pleurae

There is a thin, slippery layer lining the chest wall and diaphragm called the *parietal pleura* and one lining the outside of the lungs called the *visceral pleura*. Between these linings is a very small amount of lubricating fluid to help the lungs move smoothly and noiselessly with the movement of respiration. There is normally vacuum pressure between these two layers. Any additional fluid or air between these pleural layers will compromise the expansion of the lungs and hence air exchange.

Air enters the mouth or nose and travels down the trachea, which bifurcates just below the sternal angle, and into the bronchioles, the alveolar ducts and sacs, and, finally, the alveoli. Gas exchange occurs in the alveoli. These are protected from debris by the bronchi, which have goblet cells that secrete mucus to trap debris and cilia that move the debris

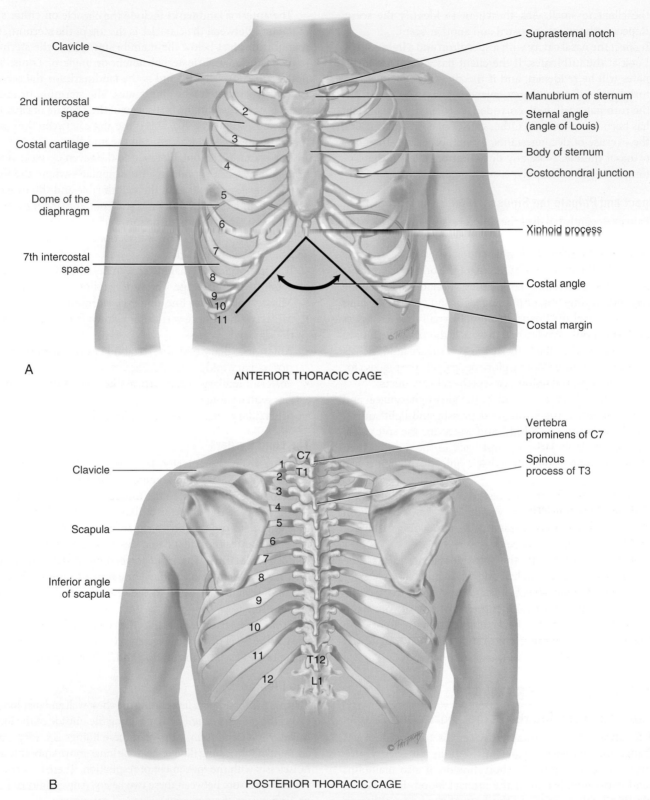

Fig. 5.2 Anatomy of the thoracic cage. **A,** Anterior view; **B,** Posterior view. (From Jarvis, C., Eckhardt, A., Browne, A., et al. [2024]. *Physical examination and health assessment* [4th Canadian ed., pp. 457–458, Fig. 19.1, 19.2]. Elsevier.) © Pat Thomas, CMI.

upward, where it can then be swallowed or coughed out of the mouth.

The control of respiration occurs in the respiratory centre in the brainstem, specifically in the pons and medulla. The need for respirations is guided by an increase in carbon dioxide in the blood and less so by a decrease in oxygen.

With each inspiration, the diaphragm moves down, causing a slight negative pressure relative to the atmosphere outside the body, which results in air rushing in to fill the vacuum. Expiration is more passive.

In infants, the rib cage is more elastic; this increases the work of breathing when the chest is recoiling and re-expanding during episodes of respiratory distress.

In the older person, there can be calcification of the costal cartilage and a loss of elasticity of the lung tissue, decreasing its ability to recoil. There is also a decrease in the number of alveoli, causing an equivalent decrease in gas exchange. This leaves the older person at a higher risk for infection, a weakened cough reflex, increased secretions, and dyspnea on exertion.

Subjective Data Specific to the Thorax and Lungs

- Do you have a cough? If so, does a change in position change the cough? If you have a cough, is the cough productive? If so, what colour is the sputum?
- Are you experiencing any shortness of breath? Can you walk up a flight of stairs without having to stop in the middle? Do you have any chest wall pain?
- Do you have any pain on breathing?
- Have you had problems with your respiratory system in the past? Was it chronic or acute?
- Do you smoke? What do you smoke? How many per day and for how many years?
- Are there any environmental irritants at work or home that can affect your breathing?
- When was your last chest X-ray, tuberculosis test, and influenza or pneumonia vaccine?

Objective Data Specific to the Thorax and Lungs
Inspection of the Anterior Chest
- Assess the level of consciousness.
- Note the size and configuration of the chest. The anterior–posterior measurement should be half the length of the transverse.
- Note the musculature of the neck and chest. Is the client using the accessory muscles or the muscles of the intercostal spaces to assist in breathing? Examine the skin for colour, texture, temperature, moisture, lumps, bumps, or lesions; observe the facial expression and the use of pursed lips to breathe. Inspect the downward slope of the ribs and the presence of a 45° costal margin angle from the ribs to the xiphoid process. Check the respiratory rate, depth, and ease.

Palpation of the Anterior Chest
- Palpate the anterior chest wall for skin temperature, moisture, texture, turgor, lumps, bumps, tenderness, or pain.
- Symmetrical chest expansion: With your hands shaped like a butterfly, rest them on the chest along the costal margins, capture a bit of skin and fat in the middle of the chest at the xiphoid process with your thumbs, and ask the client to breathe. The chest wall should move symmetrically, your thumbs should move an equal distance apart, and the fold of fat and skin should flatten.

- Assess for tactile fremitus, which is a palpable vibration, by asking the client to say "99" every time you move your hand. You can use either the ulnar edge of the hand or the bottom of the fingers on the palm to assess for vibration. Place your hands symmetrically at the area just above the clavicle and move down the chest at 5-cm intervals. You should feel vibration at the top, and it should diminish quickly as you test further down the chest wall.

Auscultation of the Anterior Chest
- Auscultate the lungs. Say to the client, "Every time that I move my stethoscope, I would like you to take a breath." This will give you control over the examination, and you will be able to hear the complete breath sound. Start at the apex of the lung about 3 cm above the clavicles. Move across and then down and repeat in 5-cm intervals down along the chest wall. In females, avoid the breast tissue.
- Listen to the complete breath sound—a complete inspiration and expiration—as a wheeze might only be audible at the end of the expiration. There should be tracheal breath sounds over the trachea, bronchovesicular sounds over the bronchi, and vesicular sounds over the rest of the chest.
- Listen for abnormal or adventitious sounds, including wheezing, stridor, crackles, and pleural friction.
- If the breath sounds are abnormal, then assess voice sounds. Bronchophony, egophony, and whispered pectoriloquy are examples of voice sounds.

Inspection of the Posterior Chest
- Inspect the posterior chest.
- Assess the curvature of the spine. Ask the client to bend over at the waist and look at the scapulae. Are the scapulae symmetrical?
- Is the client using the accessory muscles or the muscles of the intercostal spaces to assist in breathing?
- Examine the skin for colour, texture, temperature, moisture, lumps, bumps, or lesions. Carefully inspect the skin for the presence of moles. The client might not be aware of these, and they should be monitored for any change in size, shape, and appearance.

Palpation of the Posterior Chest
- Palpate the posterior chest wall for skin temperature, moisture, texture, turgor, lumps, bumps, tenderness, or pain.
- Palpate for symmetrical chest expansion: With your hands shaped like a butterfly, rest your hands on the chest along the costal margins at the level of T10, capture a bit of skin and fat in the middle of the back with your thumbs, and ask the client to breathe. The chest wall should move symmetrically, your thumbs should move apart an equal distance, and the fold of fat and skin should flatten.
- Assess for tactile fremitus by asking the client to say "99" every time you move your hand. You can use either the ulnar edge of the hand or the bottom of the fingers on the palm to assess for vibration. Place your hands symmetrically at the area of the vertebral prominens, C7, and move

down the chest in 5-cm intervals. You should feel vibration at the top, and it should diminish quickly as you test further down the back. Increased vibration can mean a density of some kind, such as a tumour.

Auscultation of the Posterior Chest

- Auscultate the lung tissue on the back. Listen from the apices at C7 to the bases at T10 and laterally from the axilla to the eighth rib. There should be bronchovesicular sounds from C7 to T5 in the centre of the back. The sounds over the rest of the lungs should be vesicular sounds. Listen for any abnormal or adventitious sounds.

ANATOMY AND LANDMARKS OF THE BREASTS AND REGIONAL LYMPHATICS

The breasts, or mammary glands, can be found anterior to the pectoralis major muscles and the serratus muscles in both males and females. They lie between the second and the sixth ribs, the sternum medially, and the tail of Spence and midaxillary line laterally.

For females, the breasts serve as part of the reproductive system. Their function is to produce milk for the newborn. The nipple is just below the centre of the breast, and around it is the areola, a darker pigmented area. Within the areola are Montgomery's glands, which lubricate the areola during lactation. An illustration of the anatomy of the breast is shown in Fig. 5.3.

Internally, the breasts are composed of glandular tissue, fibrous tissue, and adipose tissue. The glandular tissue produces the milk in lobules, and it is excreted through a series of ducts. The fibrous tissue, including Cooper's ligaments, supports the breast tissue and attaches it to the chest wall. Cooper's ligaments contract with the presence of cancer, causing a dimpling effect on the skin. With age, the elasticity of these ligaments decreases and with it the support of the breast.

There is an extensive network of lymph nodes and vessels around the breast area. There are four groups of nodes: the central axillary nodes, the pectoral nodes, the subscapular nodes, and the lateral nodes.

Breast cancer is the second cause of cancer death in females. Early detection and treatment can decrease the mortality rate. There are many risk factors for breast cancer, some of which include having dense breasts, increase in age, nulliparous, obesity, postmenopausal hormone therapy, personal or family history of breast cancer, a positive *BRCA1* or *BRCA2* blood test, and a first child born after age 30.

Subjective Data Specific to the Breasts and Regional Lymphatics
* **Specific questions for the older person**
^ **Specific questions for the adolescent**
- Do you have any pain in the breast area?
- Have you noticed any discharge from your nipple?
- Have you noticed any lumps in your breast or under your arm?
- Have you noticed any swelling in one or both of your breasts?

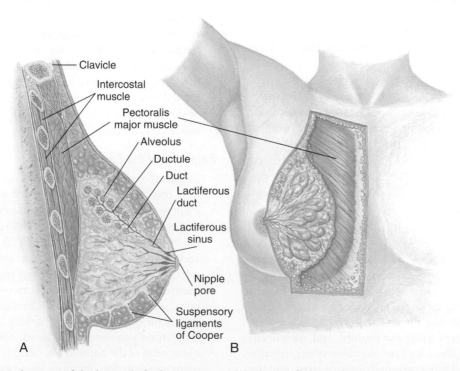

Fig. 5.3 Anatomy of the breast **A,** Surface anatomy of the breast; **B,** Internal anatomy of the breast. (From Jarvis, C., Browne, A. J., MacDonald-Jenkins, J, et al. [2019]. *Physical examination and health assessment* [3rd Canadian ed., p. 419, Figure 18-1, 18-2]. Elsevier.) © Pat Thomas, CMI.

- Have you noticed any skin changes to your breast, such as a rash or an "orange-skin" appearance?
- Has there been any recent trauma to either of your breasts?
- Do you have any history of breast disease?
- When did you experience menarche?
* **When did you start menopause?**
* **Have you taken hormone replacement therapy?**
- How many pregnancies or live births have you had?
- Did you breastfeed your children? If yes, for how long?
- Do you have any family history of breast disease?
- Did you ever have surgery to your breast or underarm?
- Do you perform breast self-examination? If yes, how often?
* **When was your last mammogram?**
^ **Have you noticed any change in your breasts?**
^ **Is there anyone you can talk to about the changes in your body?**

Objective Data Specific to the Breasts and Regional Lymphatics

Inspection of the Breast and Lymphatics

- Note the general appearance of the breasts.
- Inspect for symmetry and symmetrical movement. Ask the client to raise their arms sideways, in front, and above their head. Ask the client to place their hands together and squeeze the chest muscles. Assess for any pulling or dimpling of the skin. Inspect the skin for the look of peau d'orange ("orange-peel" skin).
- Inspect the skin for areas of redness, lumps, bumps, or lesions.
- Inspect the nipple for colour, discharge, and the presence of a supernumerary nipple (extra nipple).

Palpation of the Breast and Lymphatics

- Palpate the axilla for lymph nodes. Rest the client's right forearm on your right forearm and hold the elbow with your right hand. You now have full manoeuvrability of the right arm. Move it up, down, and side to side while palpating the right axilla with your left hand. Repeat the examination on the other side. You do not want the muscles to be taut, as a tight muscle will prevent the subtle palpation of the underlying lymph nodes. Imagine dividing the breast tissue into a pattern such as the spokes of a wheel. With the pads of your fingertips and in a circular motion, palpate throughout the entire breast. Do not poke at the tissue; a breast lump might be very difficult to feel, and poking it will only push it deeper.
- Repeat the palpation with the person lying down. Raise one arm over their head and assess the axilla again. If you find a lump, assess the size, texture, shape, position, and whether or not it is tender.
- Gently squeeze the nipple and look for any discharge.
- For the male client, inspect and palpate the breast and assess for signs of gynecomastia.

HEART AND NECK VESSEL ASSESSMENT

Anatomy and Landmarks of the Heart

The heart is a mechanical pump that pumps blood through two different circulations: the pulmonary circulation and the systemic circulation. The pulmonary circulation brings blood to the lungs via the pulmonary arteries. Here gas exchange occurs, oxygenating the blood and ridding the body of carbon dioxide. The pulmonary circulation then returns the oxygen-rich blood to the heart via the pulmonary veins. At this point, the systemic circulation takes the oxygen-rich blood and pumps it around the body via the systemic arteries. The blood leaves the heart via the aorta and returns to the heart via the systemic veins, entering the inferior and superior vena cava and re-entering the pulmonary circulation. The cycle is continuous.

The heart is upside down, with the apex at the bottom. It can be found at the fifth intercostal space, 7 to 9 cm from the midsternal border. The base of the heart, which is wider than the apex, can be found at the top of the heart by the second intercostal space. The heart is rotated slightly so that the right side is more anterior and the left side is more posterior. In an infant, the heart is more midline and assumes the adult position when the child is 6 years old.

The heart wall comprises three layers. The pericardium is the outermost and is divided into two layers with a small amount of pericardial fluid in between so that there is smooth movement of the heart muscle. The pericardium is a tough, fibrous, protective layer. The myocardium is the muscle of the heart. The endocardium is the inner lining of the heart chambers (ventricles and atria) and the valves. There are four chambers in the heart: two ventricles and two atria. Valves divide the chambers so that there is no backflow of the blood. The right atrioventricular (AV) valve is the tricuspid valve and the left is the mitral valve. The AV valves open during the diastole so the ventricles can fill. The systole occurs when the pulmonic and aortic valves (semilunar valves) open to allow the blood to be pumped out of the heart. An illustration of the heart anatomy is shown in Fig. 5.4.

The first heart sound, S_1, occurs with the closure of the AV valves. This sound can be heard loudest using the diaphragm of the stethoscope over the apex of the heart. The second sound, S_2, occurs at the end of systole, when the semilunar valves close, and can be heard best at the base of the heart. The S_3 sound is an abnormal sound that occurs with vibration at ventricular filling and can be heard immediately after S_2. S_4 occurs just before S_1 when there is resistance to the ventricles accepting the blood from the atrium.

A murmur is the sound of turbulent blood flow through the valves of the heart. This can happen from increased speed of the blood through the heart from, for example, exercise, a decrease in blood viscosity, structural defects in the valves, or structural defects on the wall of the chambers.

The heart has its own conduction system. The pacemaker is the sinoatrial node that is located near the superior vena cava

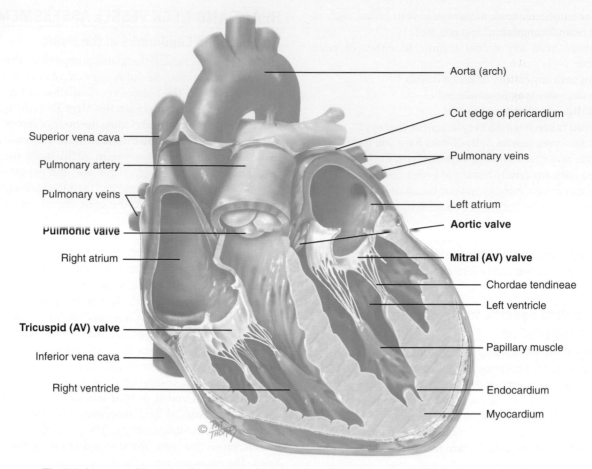

Fig. 5.4 Anatomy of the heart. (From Jarvis, C., Eckhardt, A., Browne, A., et al. [2024]. *Physical examination and health assessment* [4th Canadian ed., p. 504, Figure 20.4]. Elsevier.) © Pat Thomas, CMI.

and starts the conduction. It is then passed on over the atria to the AV node that is low in the atrial septum. After waiting for the atria to contract, the electrical current then moves on to the bundle of histidine and then over the ventricles.

Anatomy and Landmarks of the Neck Vessels

The neck vessels include the two carotid arteries that supply the brain with blood. They are considered central arteries as they are the closest to the heart. The pulsation of the carotid artery can be found at the space between the sternomastoid muscle and the trachea. Each side should be palpated separately as you do not want to cut off all blood supply to the brain.

The jugular veins bring unoxygenated blood to the heart via the superior vena cava. If they flutter or oscillate, the jugular vein pulsations may indicate a problem with the pumping efficiency of the right side of the heart. The right external jugular vein can be seen lateral to the sternomastoid muscle, just above the clavicle, and is the easiest of the jugular veins to see.

Risk factors for heart disease and stroke are smoking, high blood pressure, obesity, sedentary lifestyle, diabetes, high serum cholesterol, and stress. Indigenous people and people of African or South Asian descent have a higher risk of heart disease and stroke.

Subjective Data Specific to the Heart and Neck Vessels

* **Specific questions for the older person**
^ **Specific questions concerning the child**

- Do you experience any chest pain?
- Do you take nitroglycerin?
- Do you have any shortness of breath?
- How many pillows do you use at night to sleep?
- Do you have a cough? Is the cough worse at night?
- Do you get tired easily?
- Have you or your family noticed any change in your skin colour?
- Have you noticed any puffiness around your eyes or in your feet and ankles?
- How many times do you wake up in the middle of the night to urinate?
- Do you or any family members have a history of heart disease?

^ **Were the pregnancy, labour, and delivery normal?**
^ **Does the baby turn blue when feeding?**
^ **Have you noticed any growth or mobility problems?**
^ **Is the child able to participate in regular activities and sports at school?**

∧ Does the child have frequent nosebleeds?

∧ Has the child complained of unexplained joint or bone pain?

∧ Does the child have an increased number of colds or streptococcal infections?

* Do you have any lung disease?

* Do you have to climb stairs at home? Can you manage climbing them?

- Cardiac risk factors:
  - Please describe your normal daily diet.
  - Do you smoke? What, how many, and for how long?
  - Do you drink alcohol? How much, how often, and for how long?
  - Do you exercise? How often, what type of exercise, and for how long?
  - Do you take any cardiac medications or birth control pills? Which ones, for how long, and how much do you take?

Objective Data Specific to the Heart and Neck Vessels

Explain to the client that you are going to listen to the heart in many places and that they should not become alarmed if you are listening for a long time. Take the client's blood pressure. If you suspect orthostatic hypotension, take the blood pressure when the client is lying down and again quickly when the client sits up. Note any fall in pressure between the two positions.

Palpation of the Neck Vessels

- Palpate the carotid arteries; assess the amplitude, strength, and contour of the pulse.

Inspection of the Precordium

- Inspect the anterior chest. Look for any heaves or bulges.
- Find the apical pulse at the fifth intercostal space, midclavicular line. If you cannot see the apical pulse, palpate it. If that is difficult, ask the client to lie on their left side or to sit up and lean forward so that the heart moves closer to the chest wall and palpate again.
- Palpate the skin for lumps, bumps, lesions, and tenderness or pain.

Auscultation of the Precordium

- With the diaphragm of the stethoscope, auscultate the aortic valve at the second right intercostal space, the pulmonic valve at the second left intercostal space, the tricuspid valve at the left lower sternal border, the mitral valve at the fifth intercostal space midclavicular line, and Erb's point, located at the fourth intercostal space.
- Listen to the normal heart sounds, S_1 at the tricuspid and mitral valve region and S_2 at the aortic and pulmonic valves, and for the abnormal sounds, S_3 and S_4.
- Listen to the apical pulse for 1 minute.
- Feel the carotid pulse while listening to the S_1 sounds. They should match in rhythm and rate.

PERIPHERAL VASCULAR AND LYMPHATIC SYSTEMS ASSESSMENT

Anatomy and Landmarks of the Peripheral Vascular and Lymphatic Systems

The peripheral vascular system is made up of the blood vessels that travel away from and toward the heart. The lymphatic system runs parallel to the circulatory system. The arteries in the blood provide the tissues with oxygen and nutrients, and the veins act as a transport for the unoxygenated blood to go back to the heart and lungs to start the cycle again.

The arteries will have a pulse as the blood flows in a wavelike pattern with the recoil and expansion of the vessel. The pulse areas are brachial, ulnar, radial, femoral, popliteal, posterior tibialis, and dorsalis pedis.

Ischemia is the lack of blood flow to the tissues. It is usually caused by a blockage in the artery. When the client exercises and the tissues need a greater supply of oxygen and nutrients, more pain will occur from the ischemia. If the blockage is complete, the distal cells will die.

There are two sets of veins: the deep veins and the superficial veins. In addition, the perforators are small veins that join these two types together. As long as the deep veins are working well, the superficial, saphenous, veins can be removed safely.

The skeletal muscles assist in pushing the blood back to the heart by contracting and relaxing. There are also valves that prevent the backflow of the blood.

In the older person, the veins and arteries may occlude partially or fully due to atherosclerosis or arteriosclerosis. Prolonged bed rest, long airplane flights or sitting, cancer, and the birth control pill increase the risk of a deep vein thrombosis, which, if it breaks off, can lead to a myocardial infarction or a stroke.

The lymphatic system runs alongside the blood system. It is responsible for returning the excess fluid and proteins from the interstitial tissues to the blood. It is also responsible for collecting waste products, supporting the immune system, and collecting lipids from the intestinal tract.

The easiest lymph nodes to feel are the cervical, axillary, epitrochlear, and inguinal. The nodes should not be enlarged. If they are, assess for mobility, firmness, tenderness, and matting. Check proximally for signs of infection. Cancerous nodes are usually firm, nontender, and fixed, and if advanced, they can be matted. The spleen, tonsils, and thymus are also part of the lymphatic immune system. It is not unusual for children to have small, shoddy nodes that are not pathological.

Subjective Data Specific to the Peripheral Vascular and Lymphatic Systems

- Have you noticed any pain in your legs, especially the calves? If yes, does it become worse when you walk?
- Has there been any swelling in your legs or arms or puffiness around your eyes? If so, is the swelling worse in the evening?

- Do you have any skin sores that have not healed in a reasonable amount of time?
- Has there been any change in the temperature or hair distribution on one of your extremities?
- Have you felt any swollen glands?
- Do you have a history of cardiac disease, diabetes, high blood pressure, or pregnancy?
- Do you smoke? If so, how much and how often?
- Are you on any medication?

Objective Data Specific to the Peripheral Vascular and Lymphatic Systems

Inspection and Palpation of the Peripheral Vascular and Lymphatic Systems

- Inspect and palpate the arms for skin colour, texture, condition, temperature, and symmetry.
- Take vital signs, including brachial, radial, and ulnar pulses.
- Assess pulses for rate, symmetry, rhythm, and amplitude.
- Inspect nails for profile sign to assess for clubbing and measure the capillary refill. It should be less than 3 seconds.
- Inspect and palpate the legs for skin colour, texture, condition, and temperature, as well as for symmetry.
- Palpate the femoral, popliteal, posterior tibial, and dorsalis pedis pulses.
- Measure the calf circumference for symmetry, and if the measurement is off by more than 1 cm, refer the client for deep vein thrombosis assessment.
- Palpate the skin for edema starting from the ankle and moving your way up the leg. If edema is present, measure the distance of the edema from the knee. Inspect the backs of the legs for varicosities, especially in pregnant persons or patients who have had multiple pregnancies. Inspect the skin for hair distribution. In the older person, there may be a decrease in hair growth and peripheral pulses, and the skin can become shiny and thin. These are normal signs of aging caused by a decrease in arterial circulation.

ABDOMINAL ASSESSMENT

Anatomy and Landmarks of the Abdomen

The abdomen is a large cavity that extends from the diaphragm at the top to the pelvis at the bottom, to the vertebra and paravertebral muscles in the back, and to the lower ribs and abdominal muscles in the front.

There are four abdominal muscles, including the rectus abdominis, which is joined along the midline by the linea alba (Fig. 5.5, *A*). The umbilicus is the midpoint in the abdomen. It should be slightly inverted and uniform in colour with the rest of the skin. With abdominal bleeding, the blood can be seen around the umbilicus; it will have a blue circle around it called Cullen's sign. In the newborn, the umbilicus is very pronounced. The clamp and the extra tissue will turn black and fall off a few days after birth.

The contour of the abdomen varies. There are flat, round, protuberant, and scaphoid shapes. The first two are normal; the scaphoid shape can be a sign of malnutrition, and the protuberant shape can be a sign of obesity or ascites.

Within the abdominal cavity are many viscera. The solid viscera include the liver, which can be found in the upper right quadrant above the costal margin; the spleen, which should normally be posterior to the left midaxillary line parallel to the tenth rib; the pancreas, which is behind the stomach; the kidneys, which are retroperitoneal along the eleventh and twelfth ribs for the left one and slightly lower for the right; the adrenal glands, which are on top of the kidneys; the aorta, which is just left of the midline at the upper part of the abdomen and extends down to 2 cm above the umbilicus, where it bifurcates into the iliac arteries; and the ovaries and uterus, which are in the lower abdomen and pelvis. The liver decreases in size with age, especially after 80 years, even though the function remains normal, except for medication metabolism. In the newborn, the liver is normally felt 0.5 to 2.5 cm below the costal margin.

The hollow viscera include the stomach, which is below the diaphragm midline; the small intestine, which is in all quadrants; the large intestine (colon); the gallbladder, which is posterior to the liver at the right midclavicular line; and the bladder, which is at the top of the pelvis. In the infant, the bladder is positioned higher. The ileocecal valve, where the small intestine and the colon meet, is in the right lower quadrant.

With age, there is an increased reporting of constipation. The causes of constipation (more than three days between defecation, hard stool, straining, and the feeling of incomplete emptying) include a decrease in mobility; not enough water intake; low-residue foods; adverse effects of medication; difficulty getting to a bathroom or commode; hypothyroidism; irritable bowel syndrome; and bowel obstruction. Fig. 5.5, *B*, illustrates the abdominal organs.

Subjective Data Specific to the Abdomen

*Specific questions for the older person
^Specific questions concerning the infant

- Has there been any change to your appetite?
- What have you eaten in the last 24 hours?
- *** Who prepares your food or buys the groceries?**
- *** Do you eat alone?**
- **^ Does the child breastfeed?**
- **^ Have you introduced any new foods into the child's diet?**
- Have you gained or lost weight recently?
- Do you have any difficulty swallowing?
- Are there any foods that you cannot eat?
- Are you allergic to any foods?
- Are you experiencing any abdominal pain?
- Do you have any nausea or vomiting? What are you vomiting?
- How often do you have a bowel movement?
- Has there been a recent change to your bowel movements?
- Has there been any change to the colour or consistency of the stool?

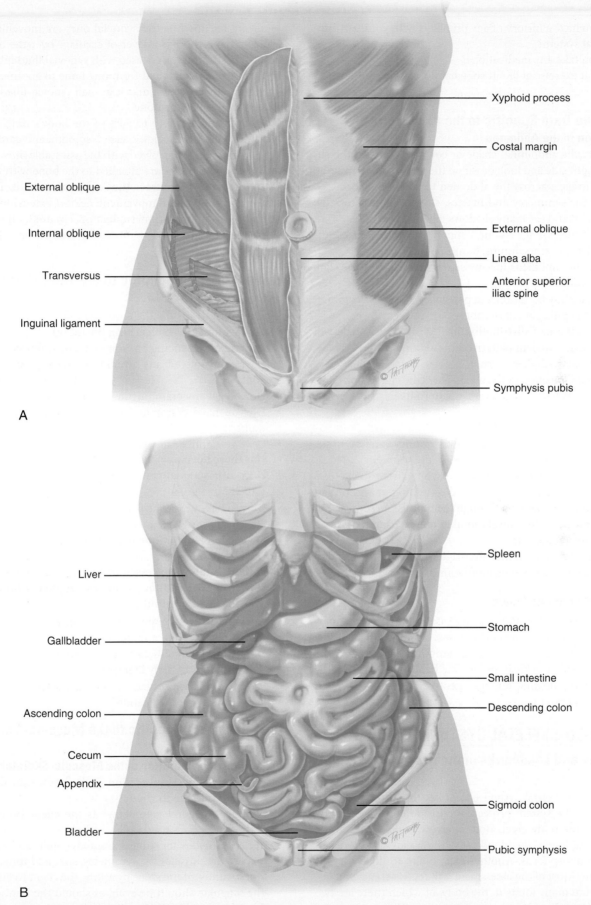

A

- External oblique
- Internal oblique
- Transversus
- Inguinal ligament
- Xyphoid process
- Costal margin
- External oblique
- Linea alba
- Anterior superior iliac spine
- Symphysis pubis

B

- Liver
- Gallbladder
- Ascending colon
- Cecum
- Appendix
- Bladder
- Spleen
- Stomach
- Small intestine
- Descending colon
- Sigmoid colon
- Pubic symphysis

Fig. 5.5 Anatomical structures of the abdominal cavity. **A,** Abdominal muscles; **B,** Abdominal organs. (From Jarvis, C., Eckhardt, A., Browne, A., et al. [2024]. *Physical examination and health assessment* [4th Canadian ed., pp. 575–576, Figs. 22.1, 22.2]. Elsevier.) © Pat Thomas, CMI.

- Do you have a history of any problems with your gastrointestinal system?
- Do you take any medications?
- Do you exercise at all? If so, what do you do and for how long?

Objective Data Specific to the Abdomen
Inspection of the Abdomen

- Inspect the abdominal shape or contour. Stand at the client's right side and look down on the abdomen, then stoop or sit to gaze across the abdomen to assess the shape. To check for symmetry and masses, shine a light across the abdomen and see if any shadows fall on the skin.
- Inspect the skin for colour, temperature, moisture, condition, texture, scars, lumps, bumps, or lesions.
- Check the umbilicus for any sign of hernia, Cullen's sign, or infection.
- Check for any pulsation and peristalsis. It is quite common to see the pulsation of the aorta.
- What is the hair distribution like? Normally, a male will have a diamond hair pattern on the abdomen, and a female will have a triangle pattern.
- Assess the position of the client. Does the client look comfortable? What is the breathing pattern like?

Auscultation of the Abdomen

Auscultate next so that the bowel sounds are accurate. Palpation and percussion will increase the sounds.

- With the diaphragm of the stethoscope, listen for up to 5 minutes in each quadrant for the tinkling sound of gas, fluid, and stool passing through the bowels. As soon as you hear and assess the bowel sound in one quadrant, move on to the next quadrant.
- Start auscultation in the lower right quadrant, the location of the ileocecal valve, as more sounds will be there.

Palpation of the Abdomen

- Lightly palpate the abdomen and assess for pain or tenderness, temperature, moisture, lumps, or bumps. Palpate any tender areas last to decrease the amount of guarding.
- If the client is ticklish, place your hand on top of the client's, start palpating, and then gently slide the client's hand out from under yours.

MUSCULO-SKELETAL SYSTEM ASSESSMENT

Anatomy and Landmarks of the Musculo-Skeletal System

The musculo-skeletal system comprises the bones, muscles, and joints. The system protects the inside core of the body and keeps the body erect. Bone marrow is produced in the bone, giving rise to the blood cells. The bones also store calcium and phosphorus. Another component to this system is movement. Most of the assessment will focus on movement.

There are many joints in the body, of which there are two types: synovial and nonsynovial joints. The nonsynovial joints are fixed, while the synovial ones are movable. In the synovial joint, there is a layer of cartilage over the opposing bones, and the joint is encased with synovial fluid lubricating it. Ligaments are attached from one bone to another, adding strength to the joint. A bursa is a small synovia-filled sac that adds protection to the bone.

Muscles make up 40 to 50% of the body's weight. There are three types of muscles: skeletal, smooth, and cardiac. The skeletal muscles are involved with the assessable movement of the body. The muscles are attached to the bone with tendons. When the muscles contract, they create movement. There are many different types of movement: flexion, extension, adduction, abduction, pronation, supination, circumduction, inversion, eversion, rotation, protraction, retraction, elevation, and depression.

Subjective Data Specific to the Musculo-Skeletal System
*Specific questions for the older person
^Specific questions concerning the infant

- Are you experiencing any joint pain or stiffness?
- Have you noticed any swelling or redness around your joints?
- Do you get any cramping in your muscles?
- Do you have cramping in your calf muscles when you walk?
- Have you noticed any weakness in your muscles?
- **Has there been any change in the weakness recently?**
- **Do you use any aids to help you walk, such as a cane or walker?**
- Do you have any bone pain?
- Have you ever broken a bone?
- Do you have any numbness or tingling sensations?
- Have you noticed any deformities in the bone?
- ^ **Has the infant progressed in a normal growth pattern?**
- * **Have you noticed that you have stumbled or fallen more over the last few months?**
- Are you involved in any exercise program?
- Are you involved in any sports?
- Do you have any difficulty getting around or maintaining your activities of daily living?
- Have you ever had surgery on your muscles, bones, or joints?
- Do you take any medication?

Objective Data Specific to the Musculo-Skeletal System
Inspection and Palpation of the Musculo-Skeletal System

- Perform a general inspection of the body. Can the client walk and support the body?
- Is there a general symmetry? Is the client protecting a limb?
- Inspect each joint for redness, size and contour, and deformity.
- Inspect the muscles for symmetry, size, and tone. Inspect for curvature of the spine by asking the client to bend over. The scapulae should be even, as should the buttocks, and the spine should follow a straight line down.

- Palpate each joint for temperature, pain or tenderness, swelling, and smoothness in movement.
- Perform a range-of-motion examination for all the muscles, both upper body and lower body. Watch closely for symmetry. Note any restrictions in the movement. Measure the flexion and extension with a goniometer if you think that there is a problem. Check the muscle strength using movement against resistance.

NEUROLOGICAL SYSTEM ASSESSMENT

Anatomy and Landmarks of the Neurological System

The Central Nervous System

The neurological system can be divided into the central system, which includes the brain and the spinal cord, and the peripheral system, which includes the 12 pairs of cranial nerves and the 31 pairs of spinal nerves.

The central nervous system is complex. The brain has two hemispheres; the right side governs the left side of the body, and the left side governs the right side of the body. It is very important to always assess both sides of the body. The four lobes that make up the brain are the frontal lobe, needed for personality, intellect, emotions, and voluntary movement; the parietal lobe, responsible for sensation; the occipital lobe, which has the visual receptors; and the temporal lobe, which is the centre for hearing. Within the temporal lobe is Wernicke's area, responsible for language comprehension. In the frontal lobe, there is Broca's area, which is responsible for motor speech.

In the aging person, there is a progressive loss of brain functioning due to a loss of neurons. Also, the speed at which information travels along the neurons decreases with age. There may also be a decrease in the amount of blood reaching the brain, as well as an increased risk of stroke, both hemorrhagic and thrombotic. The infant's nervous system is not fully developed at birth. As myelinization occurs, the nervous response increases.

The neural pathways are split between the sensory and motor pathways. The sensory ones include the spinothalamic tract, where sensations of soft touch, hot and cold, and pain are carried to the thalamus and on to the sensory cortex for interpretation. The posterior column is responsible for the sense of position, vibration, and finely localized touch.

The motor pathways are responsible for the movement and coordination of the muscles. They include the pyramidal and extrapyramidal tracts, the cerebellum, and the upper and lower motor neurons. The cerebellum is more responsible for fine motor coordination and balance.

The Peripheral Nervous System

The peripheral nervous system includes the cranial nerves, the reflexes, and the spinal nerves. There are 12 cranial nerves that enter and exit the brain. Nerves I and II extend from the cerebrum, while III to VII extend from the brainstem and diencephalons. These are both sensory and motor nerves, some of which are responsible for both.

There are 31 pairs of spinal nerves. They enter and exit from the spinal column. There are 8 cervical (arms, neck and side of the head, and top of the chest), 12 thoracic (chest and abdomen), 5 lumbar (legs), and 5 sacral (inner thigh, ankle, and groin) nerves, and 1 coccygeal nerve.

Subjective Data Specific to the Neurological System

* **Specific questions for the older person**
^ **Specific questions concerning the infant**

- Have you been experiencing frequent headaches recently?
- Did you recently have any head injury? If yes, what part of your head was hit?
- Have you been experiencing either vertigo (a spinning sensation) or dizziness (feeling faint)?
- Have you had any seizures? If so, describe them.
- Do you have any tremors? If so, are they worse with stress?
- Have you noticed any signs of tingling or numbness (pins and needles)?
- Have you noticed any weakness?
- Do you have any problems with coordination?
- Have you noticed any difficulty with speech?
- Have you noticed any difficulty with swallowing?
- Are you taking any medication?
- Do you have any allergies?
- Are there any environmental hazards at work or home?
* **Have you or your family noticed any decrease in your memory or change in your mental function?**
^ **Was the labour and delivery without difficulty?**

Objective Data Specific to the Neurological System

It is important to perform a general mental survey in the neurological examination. Include an assessment of the client's ABCT.

Cranial Nerve Testing

- Olfactory (I): Sensory nerve. Check for nasal patency and introduce a scent for each nostril while the client closes their eyes and smells.
- Optic (II): Sensory nerve. Use the Snellen chart and Jaeger test chart for eye acuity and the confrontation test for peripheral vision and examine the ocular fundus and optic disc with an ophthalmoscope.
- Oculomotor (III), trochlear (IV), and abducens (VI): Motor nerves. Perform the six fields of gaze test, watching for nystagmus (normal in the far lateral gaze), and check for PERRLA with direct and consensual light reaction.
- Trigeminal (V): Sensory and motor nerve. Assess for fine touch at the areas of the three branches of the nerve: the forehead, cheek, and chin on both sides. For the motor component, test the movement of the mandible (jaw) and also its movement against resistance.
- Facial (VII): Sensory and motor nerve. Test the anterior two thirds of the tongue for taste. For the motor component, test the movement of the face by asking the client to smile, frown, puff out their cheeks, and squeeze their eyes

shut. Watch for symmetry. The corneal reflex is used to test the sensory V and motor VII; omit doing this test unless there are abnormalities in the other tests.

- Acoustic (VIII): Sensory nerve. Assess the client's hearing using the whisper test, the Weber test, and the Rinne test.
- Glossopharyngeal (IX) and vagus (X): Both sensory and motor nerves. It is not possible to test the sensory component of the glossopharyngeal nerve as it governs taste in the posterior one third of the tongue. For the motor component, ask the client to say "Ahhh" and look in the mouth to see if the soft palate and uvula move up and back in the back of the mouth. Check the gag reflex.
- Spinal accessory (XI): Motor nerve. Check for range of motion and movement against resistance of the neck and shoulders.
- Hypoglossal (XII): Motor nerve. Check the range of motion and movement against resistance in the tongue. Ask the client to stick out their tongue and assess for any tremors and have the client repeat after you: "light," "tight," and "dynamite."

Motor, Sensory, Cerebellum, and Reflex Nerve Testing

- To test the cerebellum, ask the client to walk normally and then with a heel-to-toe tandem walk, knee bends, and Romberg test (ask the client to stand for 30 seconds with the feet together and the hands close to their sides and to close their eyes). For these tests, assess for coordination and balance. In addition, assess for fine motor coordination using rapid alternating movements. If the client cannot get out of bed, ask the client to run an ankle up and down the opposite shin.
- To assess the spinothalamic tract, use a cotton ball for soft touch and a broken tongue depressor with a sharp and dull side or, alternatively, two test tubes, one with cold water and one with hot water. For each of the tests, assess for symmetry and sensation. For soft touch, say to the client, "Every time you feel me touching you, say 'now.'" For the sensation of pain, don't follow any pattern, but apply both the sharp and dull sides of the stick and say, "Let me know if you feel sharpness or dullness when I touch you." For hot and cold, let the client feel the difference and ask the client to tell you if they feel hot or cold. Follow the dermatomes around the body, making sure to test the most distal areas.
- The posterior tract can be tested for vibration by striking a tuning fork and asking the client if they can feel the vibration as you place it on a bone of the big toes and thumbs. If not, work your way up the bony prominences until a sensation can be felt. It is normal for the older person not to feel the vibration at the outer periphery.
- For position sensation, show the client that "up" is when you lift the finger or toe upward, and "down" is when you move the finger downward. Ask the client to close their eyes and say "up" or "down" with the movement. Hold the finger or toe on the outside edges rather than on the top and bottom.

- For fine touch, use stereognosis: with the client's eyes closed, place a small object in their hand and ask the client to tell you what it is. Don't forget to repeat it with the other hand. Test for graphesthesia as well: with the client's eyes closed, draw a number or a letter on their hand and ask the client to identify it. Two-point discrimination involves using two points on the skin and asking the client to tell you if one or two points can be felt. Move the points together slowly and see at what distance the client can only feel one point.
- Check for symmetry on the other side. Extinction is the test used to assess if the client can identify whether or not they were touched with one or two points. With point location, you are testing to see if the client can point to where you just touched them. These are all testing the sensory cortex. With the older person, these sensations likely will be reduced and delayed.
- In an infant, check the rooting, grasping, Moro, sucking, stepping, and tonic neck reflexes. There should normally be a Babinski reflex up until the infant is 2 to 2.5 years of age.
- Motor nerves should be checked simultaneously whenever possible so that you can check for symmetry. Assess the muscles for tone, size, range of motion, and strength using movement against resistance. Watch for any involuntary movements.

MALE GENITOURINARY SYSTEM ASSESSMENT

Anatomy and Landmarks of the Male Genitourinary System

The male genitourinary system is composed of the bladder, penis, testicles, scrotum, prostate, and inguinal area. Fig. 5.6 illustrates these structures. The bladder is the storage area for urine. The urine leaves the bladder via the urethra, passing through the penis and out of the body.

The penis is a sexual organ as well as a functional organ. Sexually, it provides the transportation of the male sperm to the female's vaginal vault. A milky alkaline fluid that protects the sperm's viability is produced in the prostate. Prostate cancer is one of the leading cancers in males. The incidence is higher in males of African descent. Signs of benign prostatic hypertrophy (enlarged prostate) or cancer of the prostate are nocturia, frequency, decreased flow, urgency, and the feeling of not emptying the bladder.

The scrotum is a protective sac for the testicles. The testicles produce the sperm needed for reproduction. The cremaster muscle controls the elasticity of the scrotum. The muscle will permit the scrotum to shrink in cold conditions, drawing the testicles closer to the body, and to allow the testicles to descend in warm conditions to prevent them from overheating. It is important to check that the male infant's testicles are descended. Cancer of the testes is more likely to occur in males 17 to 25 years of age.

Within the inguinal area are the inguinal lymph nodes, the inguinal canal, and the femoral arteries and veins.

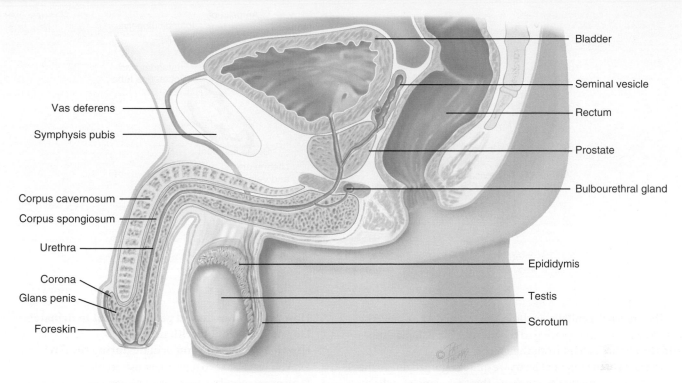

Fig. 5.6 The male pelvic organs. (From Jarvis, C., Eckhardt, A., Browne, A., et al. [2024]. *Physical examination and health assessment* [4th Canadian ed., p. 759, Fig. 26.1]. Elsevier.) © Pat Thomas, CMI.

Subjective Data Specific to the Male Genitourinary System

* **Specific questions for the older person**
^ **Specific questions concerning the infant or child**

- Do you have any burning or pain when you urinate or ejaculate?
- Do you have any trouble starting to urinate?
- What colour is your urine?
- Do you have any lumps, bumps, or lesions on your penis?
- Is there any discharge coming from your penis?
- Are there any lumps or bumps that you have noticed on your testicles?
- Are you experiencing any pain in the scrotum?
- Do you do testicular self-examination?
- Are you sexually active?
- Are you having difficulty maintaining an erection?
- Do you use condoms?
- How many sexual partners have you had in the last 6 months?
- Have you been exposed to any sexually transmitted infections?
^ **Has the child learned to use the toilet?**
^ **Is the child holding on to his genitals and crying when he urinates?**
^ **Does the child have both testicles?**
^ **Is the child urinating a lot or constantly thirsty?**
* **Do you have trouble with urine leaking?**
* **How many times do you get up at night to urinate?**
* **Do you have trouble with urgency?**
* **How many times do you urinate during the day?**

Objective Data Specific to the Male Genitourinary System

Inspection and Palpation of the Male Genitourinary System

Inspect and palpate the penis. It should be smooth and without lesions. The foreskin should retract easily. The urethral meatus should be central in the glans. The distribution, colour, and density of the pubic hair should be normal for the client's age group and should be lice-free.

Inspect and palpate the scrotum. The scrotum skin should be free of lesions. Be careful to examine the underside of the scrotum. Gently feel the testicles for any lumps. Inspect and palpate the inguinal area. Assess the femoral pulse.

FEMALE GENITOURINARY SYSTEM ASSESSMENT

Anatomy and Landmarks of the Female Genitourinary System

The female genitourinary system is made up of the external (vulva) and internal genitalia, the bladder, the urethra, and the urethral meatus. The vulva comprises the labia majora and labia minora. These are folds of skin from the mons pubis. The clitoris is at the top of the labia majora and is highly sensitive to tactile stimulation. The urethral opening is close to the vaginal opening and not far from the anus, so it is very possible for bacteria to enter this opening, giving rise to a bladder infection.

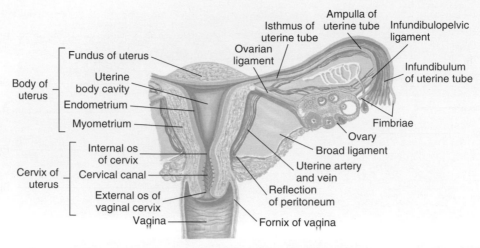

Fig. 5.7 The internal female genitalia. (From Jarvis, C., Browne, A., Mac-Donald, J., et al. [2019]. *Physical examination and health assessment* [3rd Canadian ed., p. 780, Fig. 27-2]. Elsevier.)

The internal genitalia include the vaginal vault and the cervix, which is the opening to the uterus. The fallopian tubes and the ovaries extend from the uterus.

The labia of the infant at birth are quite engorged due to the presence of the mother's estrogen. The first signs of puberty usually occur between 8.5 and 13 years of age.

In the aging person, the hormone level drops, giving rise to menopause, shrinkage and drooping of the uterus, shortening of the vagina, and decreased vaginal secretions. The internal female genitalia are illustrated in Fig. 5.7.

It is important to note that a vaccine is now available to eradicate most types of human papilloma virus (HPV), which is the major risk factor for cervical cancer.

Subjective Data Specific to the Female Genitourinary System

*Specific questions for the older person
^Specific questions concerning the infant or child

- Do you have any burning or pain when you urinate?
- Do you have any trouble starting to urinate?
- What colour is your urine?
- Are there any lumps or bumps that you have noticed on the perineum?
- ^ **Has the child learned to use the toilet?**
- ^ **Does she cry when she urinates?**
- ^ **Is the child urinating a lot or constantly thirsty?**
- * **Do you have trouble with urine leaking?**

* **How many times do you get up at night to urinate?**
* **Do you have trouble with urgency?**
* **How many times do you urinate during the day?**
- Do you or your sexual partners use condoms?
- How many sexual partners have you had in the last 6 months?
- Have you been exposed to any sexually transmitted infections?
- How old were you at menarche?
- How many times have you been pregnant?
- How old were you at the first pregnancy?
- How many live births have you had?
- How many abortions have you had?
- What was the date of your last menstrual period?
* **When did you start menopause?**
* **Do you experience any pain or bleeding during or after intercourse?**
- Do you experience any bleeding between your periods?
  * **Does sneezing or laughing cause you to urinate?**

Objective Data Specific to the Female Genitourinary System

- Place the client in the lithotomy position and examine the external genitalia.
- Inspect the pubic hair for distribution and lice; the skin for colour and the presence of any lumps, bumps, or lesions; the urethral meatus for position and condition; and the vaginal opening and the anus for discharge.

PRACTICE QUESTIONS

Case 1

A nurse is newly employed in a retirement residence. The nurse's duties include performing annual health assessments for the residents. Mrs. Clara Sloane, 86, arrives for her health assessment with the nurse.

Questions 1 to 7 refer to this case.

1. What is the most appropriate approach for the nurse to use during the interview stage of the health assessment with Mrs. Sloane?

1. Address her as Clara rather than Mrs. Sloane as older persons respond better to use of their first name.
2. Be sure to speak loudly to Mrs. Sloane if she is hard of hearing.
3. Adjust the pace of the interview to provide extra time for Mrs. Sloane to answer questions.
4. Be careful not to touch Mrs. Sloane as she may be uncomfortable with this familiarity.

2. The nurse measures Mrs. Sloane and finds her to be 110 cm. Mrs. Sloane states that she used to be 114 cm and asks why she is now shorter. What is the primary reason older persons lose height as they age?
    1. Decreased muscle mass
    2. Thinning of the vertebral discs
    3. Many older persons develop osteoporosis
    4. Most older persons have some degree of kyphosis

3. The nurse takes Mrs. Sloane's blood pressure. Which of the following is true concerning blood pressure in older persons?
    1. Both systolic and diastolic pressures are decreased.
    2. Diastolic pressure increases, while systolic pressure remains the same.
    3. Blood pressure readings become variable and unstable.
    4. There is a widening pulse pressure.

4. The nurse performs a skin survey with Mrs. Sloane. Which of the following would be a normal finding?
    1. Acrochordons (skin tags) on her eyelids and neck
    2. Edema in her lower limbs
    3. Decreased hair on her upper lip and chin
    4. Thicker skin on the dorsa of her hands and forearms

5. The nurse examines Mrs. Sloane's eyes and finds a grey-white arc around the cornea. What would the nurse say to Mrs. Sloane about this finding?
    1. "You have the beginnings of cataracts and should see an eye surgeon."
    2. "These are a normal finding in your age group and will not affect vision."
    3. "This is caused by thickening of your cornea and is probably causing some blurring of your vision."
    4. "The discoloration in your eyes is called *xanthelasma* and is caused by high levels of cholesterol."

6. Mrs. Sloane is to receive olive oil in both ears at night for cerumen impaction. What intervention should the nurse perform?
    1. Application of a small cotton ball at the meatus after instillation of the ear drops
    2. Removal of coarse ear hairs
    3. Referral to an ear, nose, and throat physician
    4. Evacuation of the cerumen using a cotton-tipped swab

7. The nurse is aware that in the older age group, neurological assessment is important. Which of the following results of Mrs. Sloane's neurological assessments would be of most concern to the nurse?
    1. Mrs. Sloane is not sure which day of the week it is today.
    2. Mrs. Sloane's Mini-Mental State Examination score has declined from 27 last year to 25 today.
    3. Mrs. Sloane states that she often misplaces her hearing aid.
    4. Mrs. Sloane believes she presently lives in her former home, which she left 2 years ago.

Case 2

Ms. Perlstein gave birth to a healthy 3 200-g boy yesterday. The nurse plans to perform a health assessment with Ms. Perlstein and the baby.

Questions 8 to 13 refer to this case.

8. When the nurse enters the room, baby Perlstein is asleep. What assessment should the nurse first perform?
    1. Respirations
    2. Apical heart rate
    3. Temperature
    4. General appearance

9. Which of the following should the nurse be aware of when examining baby Perlstein?
    1. The baby should be completely naked for the entire examination.
    2. The parents should not be present as they may be distressed by the examination.
    3. The nurse should use a soft, crooning voice.
    4. The examination is best done just before feeding.

10. Which of the following would be part of a normal respiratory assessment for neonate Perlstein?
    1. Observation of abdominal breathing
    2. Obtaining a respiratory rate of 70 breaths per minute
    3. Noting a breathing pattern that is regular, with an even rate
    4. Assessing that the baby is primarily mouth-breathing rather than nose-breathing

11. The nurse measures the head circumference of baby Perlstein. Why is this a component of a neonatal examination?
    1. The circumference indicates the degree of moulding resulting from the birth process.
    2. It is part of the Apgar score.
    3. Variations from normal may indicate a genetic abnormality or increased intracranial pressure.
    4. Abnormalities in fontanelles are more accurately assessed.

12. How would the nurse best confirm a patent rectum and anus in baby Perlstein?
    1. Confirm that the passage of meconium took place within 24 to 48 hours after birth.
    2. Stroke the anus and note a quick contraction of the sphincter.
    3. Introduce a rectal thermometer or cotton-tipped swab into the anus.
    4. Gently insert a gloved well-lubricated fifth finger into the rectum.

13. How would the nurse elicit the Moro reflex from baby Perlstein?
    1. Stroke the bottom of his feet.
    2. Hold him on his back and allow his head and trunk to drop back a short distance.
    3. Perform a sharp handclap beside his ear.
    4. Hold him vertically, allowing one foot to touch a surface.

Case 3

A nurse working in the community provides health care to students at a secondary school as part of the job.

Questions 14 to 20 refer to this case.

14. How should the nurse approach health assessments and teaching with adolescents?

1. Involve the parents, as they will be able to reinforce health teaching with their teenagers.
2. Maintain a professional and strict attitude, as adolescents will respond positively to authority.
3. Provide factual information about how students can manage specific problems they identify.
4. Provide information related to future health conditions, such as risk for heart disease and osteoporosis.

15. A thin 16-year-old female, Hilary, is worried that she has not yet begun to menstruate. What question might the nurse ask Hilary?
    1. "Tell me about your alcohol intake."
    2. "Have any women in your family had ovarian cancer?"
    3. "What kinds and amounts of food do you eat?"
    4. "How much sleep do you get each night?"

16. Bradley, age 14, states that his friends make fun of him because he is short and still looks "like a kid." Which response by the nurse is the most appropriate?
    1. "It is normal to be teased by your friends; don't let it worry you."
    2. "You are very short for your age, so perhaps the doctor should examine you."
    3. "I will show you some exercises that will help you to develop your muscles."
    4. "All boys begin puberty at different ages, so you will probably grow and become more muscular when this happens."

17. Genevieve, age 13, tells the nurse that her parents want her assessed for scoliosis. How would the nurse assess whether Genevieve has scoliosis?
    1. Have her bend at the waist to inspect for asymmetry of the scapulae.
    2. Ask her to stand sideways to them so they may measure any degree of kyphosis.
    3. Tell Genevieve to rotate sideways and observe for uneven shoulder height.
    4. Observe Genevieve from the back as she climbs a flight of stairs.

18. Sheldon, age 16, says he is very pleased that he was chosen to play for the school football team. What safety-related assessment question is important for the nurse to ask Sheldon?
    1. "Do your parents come to watch you play?"
    2. "Are you able to manage attending your games and completing your school work?"
    3. "Are you planning to play professional football one day?"
    4. "Do you use special protective equipment?"

19. Some teachers are concerned about Warren, age 18, because he has been exhibiting labile, unusual behaviours they describe as "paranoic." They wonder if he is abusing street drugs or has a mental health disorder such as schizophrenia. The nurse performs a mental health examination. What might he say to Warren to best determine his thought processes and perceptions?
    1. "What are your grades like in school?"
    2. "How do you feel today?"
    3. "I am going to ask you to remember four words, and in a few minutes, I will ask you to recall them."
    4. "Do other people talk about you?"

20. The nurse teaches a group of students about skin care. What is the most common skin condition in adolescence?
    1. Contact dermatitis
    2. Acne
    3. Eczema
    4. Rosacea

Independent Questions

Questions 21 to 30 do not refer to a particular case.

21. What of the following would indicate an abnormal finding during a health assessment?
    1. When auscultating the precordium, a third heart sound is heard.
    2. The nurse is able to palpate the apical pulse when the hand is placed over the precordium.
    3. On palpation of the nail capillary, refill is 2 seconds.
    4. The right calf measures 38 cm, while the left calf measures 38.7 cm.

22. The nurse is completing a neurological assessment on an adult client. Which of the following assessments should the nurse include when assessing the client's cerebellum? **Select all that apply.**
    1. Heel-to-toe tandem walk
    2. Gait
    3. Knee bends
    4. Romberg test
    5. Assess for PERRLA

23. Which pulse would be of most concern to the nurse?
    1. Two-month-old infant: 110 bpm at rest
    2. Ten-year-old boy: 104 bpm after exercise
    3. Seventeen-year-old athlete: 50 bpm at rest
    4. Five-day-old infant: 70 bpm after crying

24. Which of the following would be of most concern to the nurse if noted in an 8-year-old child after they fell from their bike and hit their head?
    1. Nausea
    2. Memory loss for familiar surroundings and objects
    3. Swelling and aching pain at the site of injury
    4. Blood pressure changing from 100/60 to 110/70 mm Hg

25. Which of the following changes may occur in the gastro-intestinal system of an aging person?
    1. Increased salivation
    2. Increased esophageal emptying
    3. Increased peristalsis
    4. Decreased gastric acid secretion

26. The nurse is assessing a client for possible discharge from a psychiatric facility. The nurse must assess the client's ability to make sound judgements and decisions. Which

one of the following assessment questions would best evaluate this ability?
   1. Ask the client to explain a proverb such as "a stitch in time saves nine."
   2. Ask the client to spell *moose* backwards.
   3. Ask the client what action they would take if their house caught fire.
   4. Ask the client how a train and an airplane are similar.

27. Which of the following would the nurse expect to hear when auscultating a client's breath sounds? **Select all that apply.**
   1. Wheezes
   2. Crackles
   3. Tracheal
   4. Bronchovesicular
   5. Vesicular

28. The nurse is conducting an auditory assessment with a client. Which of the following findings should the nurse document as normal? **Select all that apply.**
   1. Ability to hear low whisper at 30 cm
   2. Rinne's test results: bone conduction is better than air conduction
   3. Weber's test results: no lateralization

   4. Tympanic membrane red
   5. Symmetrical location of ears

29. The nurse is assessing a client's headache pain. Which of the following questions reflect the critical characteristics of symptoms that should be assessed? **Select all that apply.**
   1. "Where is the headache pain?"
   2. "On a scale of 0 to 10, how bad is the pain?"
   3. "How often do the headaches occur?"
   4. "What makes the headaches better?"
   5. "Do you have any family history of headaches?"
   6. "What do you think is causing these headaches?"

30. The nurse is assessing an older person and suspects elder abuse. Which of the following questions are appropriate for screening for abuse? **Select all that apply.**
   1. "Has anyone ever physically hurt you?"
   2. "Are you being abused?"
   3. "Are you alone a lot?"
   4. "Are you afraid of anybody at home or who enters your home?"
   5. "Has anyone ever failed to take care of you when you needed help?"

REFERENCES

Folstein, M. F., Folstein, S. E., & McHugh, P. R. (1975). Mini-mental state: A practical method for grading the cognitive state of clients for the clinician. *Journal of Psychiatric Research*, *12*(3), 189–198.

Jarvis, C., Browne, A. J., MacDonald-Jenkins, J., & Luctkar-Flude, M. (2019). *Physical examination & health assessment* (3rd ed). Elsevier.

Jarvis, C., Eckhardt, A., Browne, A., et al. (2024). *Physical examination & health assessment* (4th Canadian ed.). Elsevier.

BIBLIOGRAPHY

Doerflinger, D. M. (2016). *Mental status assessment of older adults: The mini-cog. Try this – general assessment series*, 3. https://hign.org/consultgeri/try-this-series/mental-status-assessment-older-adults-mini-cog

Flaherty, E. (2007). *Pain assessment for older adults. Try this – general assessment series*, 7. https://hign.org/consultgeri/try-this-series/pain-assessment-older-adults

Hartford Institute for Geriatric Nursing. (2021). *Try this: Best practices in nursing care to older adults series.* https://consultgeri.org/tools

Registered Nurses' Association of Ontario. (2013). *Nursing best practice guideline: Assessment and management of foot ulcers for people with diabetes* (2nd ed.). http://rnao.ca/bpg/guidelines/assessment-and-management-foot-ulcers-people-diabetes-second-edition

Registered Nurses' Association of Ontario. (2013). *Nursing best practice guideline: Assessment and management of pain* (3rd ed.). http://rnao.ca/bpg/guidelines/assessment-and-management-pain

Registered Nurses' Association of Ontario. (2016). *Delirium, dementia, and depression in older adults: Assessment and care* (2nd ed.). http://rnao.ca/bpg/guidelines/assessment-and-care-older-adults-delirium-dementia-and-depression

Registered Nurses' Association of Ontario. (2020). *Nursing best practice guideline: Oral health: Supporting adults who need assistance* (2nd ed.). https://rnao.ca/bpg/guidelines/oral-health-supporting-adults-who-require-assistance-second-edition

Health and Wellness

According to every theory of nursing and every nursing practice act in Canada, health promotion is considered an essential role for nurses. However, how we define health and what we consider to be priorities for health promotion have varied across time, cultures, and geography. In Canada today, there is growing recognition that health promotion involves promoting health for individuals or families (changing the person) as well as promoting changes in the community and population that result in healthier environments (changing the world). This chapter provides an overview of health, determinants of health, health promotion strategies involving individual and family action, and population health initiatives that aim to foster healthy environments in Canada.

GUIDING PHILOSOPHIES FOR HEALTH AND WELLNESS

A Definition of Health

Each individual and family has their own definition of health. The same is true for groups of people, communities, and populations. A very important goal of nursing is to help individuals and groups achieve their optimum level of health and wellness. Numerous definitions of health continue to influence how nurses attain this goal within the Canadian health care system. Some common conceptualizations of health that currently inform nursing practice are as follows:

- Health is a state of interconnected parts that include physical, mental, social, and spiritual health: "Health in part, is an individual's responsibility but also requires collective action to ensure a society and an environment in which people can act responsibily to support health. The culture and beliefs of people can influence health action" (Dames et al., 2021, p. 2).
- Health is "a state of complete physical, mental, and social well-being, not merely the absence of disease or infirmity" (World Health Organization [WHO], 1986).
- Health is a balance of biopsychological, spiritual, cultural, and environmental dimensions. In a holistic view of health, an assessment is not complete unless it is multifaceted, involving individuals, families, and communities in which individuals live and function (Clendon & Munns, 2019).
- The Ottawa Charter for Health promotion examines the concept of health as a resource or asset stating, "To reach a state of complete physical, mental, and social wellbeing, an individual or group must be able to identify and to realize aspirations, to satisfy needs, and to change or cope with the environment" (MacDonald & Jakubec, 2022, p. 85). "This distinction no longer presents health as an outcome (or state to be reached); rather health becomes

incorporated into one's activities of daily living. A patient requires health to live to their fullest potential. Canada continues to embrace the Ottawa Charter definition of health. Viewing health as a resource implies that communities and individuals can use this resource to manage and even change their surroundings" (MacDonald & Jakubec, 2022, p. 85).

Determinants of Health

Informed by studies on the factors influencing health, Health Canada has delineated 12 key determinants of health (Government of Canada, 2022a; see Table 6.1). Each determinant interacts with and has an impact on the others. Our understanding of these determinants continues to evolve, and so too does our work in addressing and influencing them (MacDonald & Jakubec, 2022).

Historical Approaches to Health

In the West during modern times, there have been three main approaches to health that influence the structure of our health care services. These approaches offer a useful framework for examining the evolution of health orientations in Canada (Astle & Duggleby, 2024; MacDonald & Jakubec, 2022)

Biomedical Approach

The biomedical approach has historically been the most prevalent in our health care system and remains the most common. In terms of health and wellness, the biomedical approach encourages health care providers to focus on disease prevention among high-risk groups. This approach is commonly considered "top down" and is directed by what some consider "expert" knowledge of the risks for disease.

The Behavioural Approach

The behavioural approach includes health teaching and awareness campaigns that help to change individual health behaviours and lifestyles. This approach became popular in the 1970s with the help of the 1974 LaLonde Report (LaLonde, 1974), a federal government report that recognized the health and economic limitations to the medical model and hospital-based care.

The Socioenvironmental Approach

The socioenvironmental approach became popular in the 1980s when a new concept of health emerged that accounted for the structural influences (poverty and appropriate housing) on health behaviours (Astle & Duggleby, 2024). It was then that we began to understand and articulate the broad determinants of health and the interrelationships among them. Health is seen as a resource and considers the

TABLE 6.1 Determinants of Health

Health Determinants	Description
Income and social status	Greatest influence on health status, behaviours, and the use of health care services. Lower-income Canadians have poorer health with more chronic illness and earlier death than higher-income Canadians, regardless of age, gender, culture, race, or residence.
Social support and coping skills	Social contacts and support networks are linked with better health by providing emotional support, caregiving, and improved management of adversity. Community, region, province, and country provide resource-sharing and social networks, which create safety nets and improve overall health for their community members.
Education and literacy	Higher education improves a person's state of health. Education increases opportunities for earning higher incomes and improves problem-solving capacity and access to health information.
Employment/working conditions	Unemployment or employment that is stressful or unsafe is linked to poorer health. Income, social contacts, and emotional health are all affected by the workplace.
Race/Racism	People exposed to racism have poorer health outcomes (particularly for mental health), as well as poor access to health care and poorer health care experiences. Indigenous people are more likely to experience health inequities due to racism and the historical and contemporary discrimination experienced as a result of colonization. The impact of these injustices has been felt for generations and continues to affect the overall health and well being of Indigenous populations in Canada.
Physical environments	Environmental contaminants in the air, soil, water, and food can cause poor health, such as respiratory conditions or other serious illnesses. Environments in the built community can impact health in many ways, such as poor air quality and unsafe building codes.
Healthy behaviours	This segment refers to those measures that individuals can do themselves to promote their own health and manage challenges. Self-sufficiency and making healthy choices will optimize their level of health.
Childhood experiences	What happens to a child during the growing years will impact the child's long-term health and the development of chronic illnesses; for example, low-birth-weight infants have almost twice the incidence of lifelong diseases.
Biology and genetic endowment	Genetics play an important role in individuals' health status. Genetic predisposition to certain conditions, as well as environmental interrelationships, puts certain individuals at risk for specific diseases.
Access to Health services	Available health services have a direct impact on individuals', families', groups', and communities' ability to prevent disease and adequately treat secondary conditions. There are still inequities in terms of accessibility to these essential services; for example, urban populations with increased access to health services have better morbidity and mortality rates than rural populations with less access.
Gender	*Gender* refers to differences in biologics, roles in society, personalities, attitudes, values, and socioeconomic position. These differences have a direct bearing on health. A gender-specific predisposition to certain disease states and treatment programs exists as well.
Culture	There are health risks related to cultural and ethnic backgrounds that affect an individual and family. Culturally specific lifestyles may influence health choices. Socioeconomic status has a major influence on health. For example, access and health care may be difficult for new immigrants who don't know the language and how to enter and manoeuvre within the health care system. It is essential that culturally appropriate care be available.

Adapted from MacDonald, S. & Jakubec, S. (2022). *Population health and the determinants of health. Stanhope and Lancaster's community health nursing in Canada* (4th ed., pp. 3–4). Elsevier Inc.

psychosocial and environmental risk factors related to the determinants of health in relation to health and health promotion (MacDonald & Jakubec, 2022).

Defining Health Promotion and Disease and Injury Prevention

Health promotion and disease and injury prevention in nursing build on our conceptualizations of and approaches to health.

Health Promotion

Health promotion is most often defined in the following ways:

- It is "the process of enabling people to increase control over, and to improve, their health" (WHO, 1986). It involves helping people optimize their sense of well-being

and health potential. It entails helping people make lifestyle changes and is considered a combination of educational and ecological supports for actions and conditions of living conducive to health (Clendon & Munns, 2019; MacDonald & Jakubec, 2022).

"Health promotion is about enabling and empowering people, communities, and societies to take charge of their own health and quality of life. It covers a wide range of social and environmental interventions that are designed to benefit and protect individual people's health and quality of life by addressing and preventing the root causes of ill health, not just focusing on treatment and cure. The three key elements of health promotion are good governance for health, health literacy, and healthy cities" (WHO, 2016).

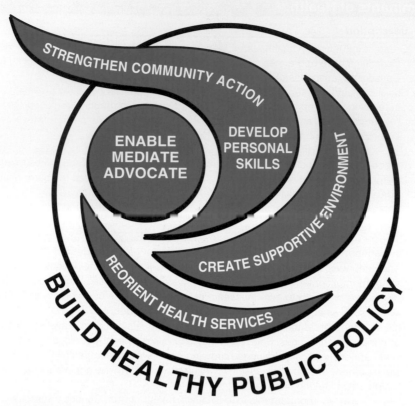

Fig. 6.1 The Ottawa Charter for Health Promotion. (From Dames, S., Luctkar-Flude, M., & Tyerman, J. [2021]. *Edelman and Kudzma's Canadian health promotion throughout the life span* [1st ed., p. 5, Fig. 1.1]. Elsevier Inc. Health Promotion Emblem, The Ottawa Charter. Source: World Health Organization [WHO]. [1986]. Ottawa Charter for Health Promotion: First international conference on health promotion, 21 November 1986. https://www.who.int/teams/health-promotion/enhanced-wellbeing/first-global-conference/emblem)

Health promotion emphasizes the importance of interventions to prevent disease and promote well-being rather than relying on remedial action to treat damaging effects. As stated in the Ottawa Charter for Health Promotion, "Health promotion is the process of enabling people to increase control over, and to improve their health. It is seen as a resource of everyday life, not just the objective of living" (MacDonald & Jakubec, 2022, p. 487).

From a socioecological perspective, health promotion is more effective if the individual as well as the organizational, community, and policy levels are targeted (Clendon & Munns, 2019).

The 1986 Ottawa Charter for Health Promotion highlights the significance of health promotion activities that extend beyond the individual level to address the context and the resources needed to promote the health of community members (Dames et al., 2021). The Ottawa Charter outlines five main strategies for health promotion (depicted in Fig. 6.1):

- Building healthy public policy through intersectoral collaborations. This strategy recognizes that collaboration among multiple sectors, such as education, industry, justice, health, and recreation, is critical to developing policies that influence health.
- Creating supportive environments through physical and social resources. This involves engaging people in creating healthy physical and social environments in their homes, organizations, and communities.

- Strengthening community action. This means that community members should be involved in sharing health-related information and capitalizing on one another's strengths and resources to foster health within their communities.
- Developing personal skills through community-based education. This involves creating opportunities for the development of the knowledge, literacy programs, and skills necessary for people to promote their own health as well as the health of their families and communities.
- Reorienting health services. This strategy means that health services should reflect the health promotion needs of the community and should be designed and operationalized with the involvement of citizens, practitioners, and decision makers from multiple sectors.

MacDonald and Jakubec (2022) provide an illustration of how the Ottawa Charter can inform interventions for the prevention of the human papilloma virus for an aggregate population of females (Fig. 6.2).

Disease and Injury Prevention

Disease prevention is also commonly referred to as *health protection*. It involves helping people reduce their risks for disease, detect disease early, or maintain optimal functioning while living with disease (Astle & Duggleby, 2024; MacDonald & Jakubec, 2022). Examples include screening for disease

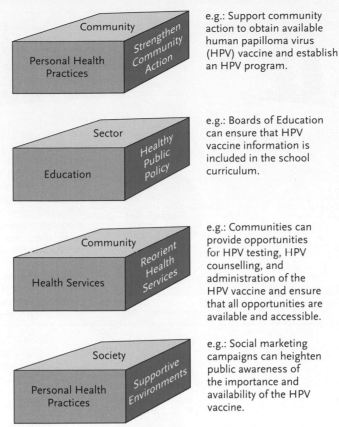

Fig. 6.2 The population health promotion model applied to a female aggregate. (From MacDonald, S., & Jakubec, S. [2022]. *Stanhope and Lancaster's Community health nursing in Canada* [4th ed., p. 95, Figure 4.3]. Elsevier Inc. Adapted and reproduced with the permission of the Minister of Health, 2016. Adapted from Public Health Agency of Canada. [2001]. *Population health promotion: An integrated model of population health and health promotion.*)

(e.g., breast self-examination and mammography), health education for behavioural change (e.g., self-care activities for clients with diabetes), and environmental intervention (e.g., ensuring that fecal occult blood tests for the early detection of colon cancer are available at local pharmacies).

According to Dames et al. (2021), to promote health, one must first assess how health is defined by the individual, family, or community and then identify realistic strategies to achieve desired health goals. Individual health cannot be separated from the health of the family, community, nation, and world. A shift to this broader perspective of health facilitates development of proactive policies to improve the health of all.

Measures of health need to encompass the complexity of health. They should characterize health by conditions that define its presence rather than its absence, identify a spectrum of health states, and reflect a lifespan developmental perspective. In addition, the social determinants of health must be taken into consideration when measuring the health of individuals and communities.

There are three main levels of prevention that distinguish nursing initiatives aimed at optimizing health and well-being, and preventing disease and injury (Clendon & Munns, 2019; MacDonald & Jakubec, 2022). These levels of prevention are as follows:

- Primary prevention: Activities that promote health and reduce risks for disease and injury. Examples include promoting healthy nutrition, rest, and physical activity by educating community members at a local health fair.
- Secondary prevention: Early detection of disease or steps taken to recover from disease and injury. An example is screening for skin cancer during regular client assessments.
- Tertiary prevention: Maintaining an optimal level of health while living with disease and injury. An example is creating exercise programs for persons with osteoarthritis.

There are five steps within the three levels of prevention: health promotion and specific protection (primary prevention); early diagnosis, prompt treatment, and disability limitation (secondary prevention); and restoration and rehabilitation (tertiary prevention).

As Dames et al. (2021) note, "the levels of prevention operate on a continuum but may overlap in practice. The nurse must clearly understand the goals of each level to intervene effectively in keeping people healthy" (p. 7).

Sometimes the terms *upstream*, *midstream*, and *downstream* are used to describe primary, secondary, and tertiary prevention interventions (Fig. 6.3). In 1979, medical sociologist Irving Zola used a river analogy, viewing the river in segments—downstream, midstream, and upstream—which

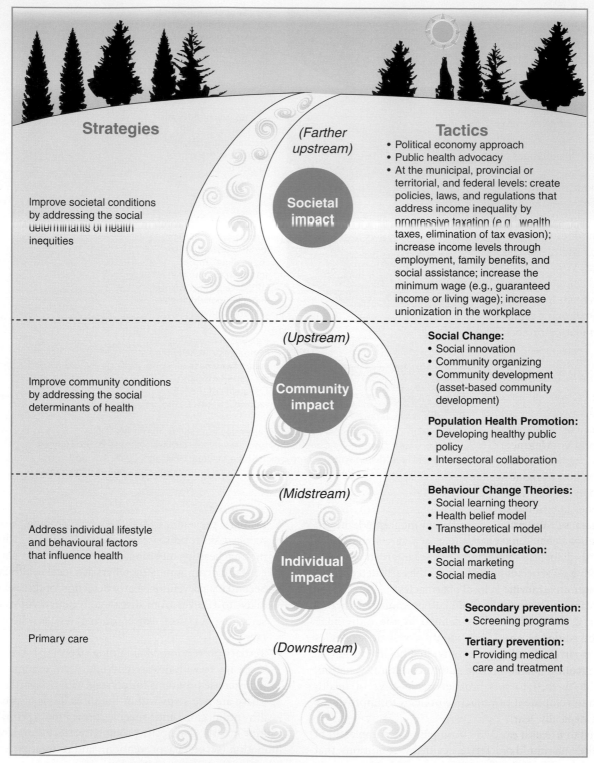

Strategies

(Farther upstream)

Improve societal conditions by addressing the social determinants of health inequities

Societal impact

Tactics
- Political economy approach
- Public health advocacy
- At the municipal, provincial or territorial, and federal levels: create policies, laws, and regulations that address income inequality by progressive taxation (e.g., wealth taxes, elimination of tax evasion); increase income levels through employment, family benefits, and social assistance; increase the minimum wage (e.g., guaranteed income or living wage); increase unionization in the workplace

(Upstream)

Improve community conditions by addressing the social determinants of health

Community impact

Social Change:
- Social innovation
- Community organizing
- Community development (asset-based community development)

Population Health Promotion:
- Developing healthy public policy
- Intersectoral collaboration

(Midstream)

Address individual lifestyle and behavioural factors that influence health

Individual impact

Behaviour Change Theories:
- Social learning theory
- Health belief model
- Transtheoretical model

Health Communication:
- Social marketing
- Social media

Secondary prevention:
- Screening programs

Primary care

(Downstream)

Tertiary prevention:
- Providing medical care and treatment

Fig. 6.3 The upstream-downstream approach to community health. (From Fournier, B., & Karachiwalla, F. [2021]. *Shah's public health and preventive health care in Canada* [6th ed., p. 62, Figure 3.1]. Elsevier Inc.).

supports a "way forward" along a flexible continuum of options. In primary prevention, upstream interventions are aimed at preventing the development of health problems before there are risks to health. In secondary prevention, midstream interventions focus on enhancing health by minimizing (low to moderate) risks to health. Tertiary prevention entails working downstream where health conditions and concerns are evident.

Socioecological System

Health promotion and disease and injury prevention occur at multiple levels within the socioecological system and require a combination of health education, advocacy, and community development, as well as political activity and policy change in the social, workplace, and community environments (Clendon & Munns, 2019).

Health education example:

- Client teaching and learning about healthy eating, healthy relationships, and physical activity (individual level)
Advocacy and community development examples:

- Collaborating with colleagues from multiple sectors to advocate for changes in hospital discharge teaching practice
- Collaborating with community health boards to advocate for the development of safe walking trails
- Enabling walk-to-school programs that encourage accessible outdoor physical activity for children (organizational and community levels)
Political activity and policy change in the social, workplace, and community environments examples:

- Involvement in hospital committees to change the organization's smoking regulations
- Reformulating protocols for preoperative teaching (policy level)

Harm-Reduction Nursing

Harm reduction is an important but controversial evidence-informed, client-centred approach to health promotion that is based on user input and demand; compassionate pragmatism; and commitment to offering alternatives to reduce the risk-behaviour consequences, to accept alternatives to abstinence, and to reduce barriers to treatment by providing user-friendly access (Astle & Duggleby, 2024). Goals are to assist clients in gaining better control over their health and enable them to take protective and proactive measures for themselves and their families (Bard et al., 2022).

Facilitating Learning Is Integral to Nursing

Health promotion inevitably involves facilitating learning. All nursing practice acts in Canada call upon nurses to be health teachers and client educators. Understanding how to teach needs to be guided by an understanding of how people learn. Teaching in professional nursing involves knowledge of content (information shared by a nurse is current, comprehensive, and evidence-informed) and process (communicating in ways that clients can understand and be enabled to learn).

Adults typically learn more successfully when they are encouraged to use past experiences to solve problems. Nurses and adult clients should collaborate on educational topics and goals. They should develop care plans that reflect what clients feel is important regarding their own health and well-being. Needs or issues that are important to the adult should be addressed early in the teaching–learning process. Ultimately, adults must accept responsibility for changing their own behaviours (Astle & Duggleby, 2024). According to the WHO (2019), "Health education is any combination of learning experiences designed to help individuals and communities improve their health, by increasing their knowledge or influencing their attitudes" (Dames et al., 2021).

According to Clendon and Munns (2019),

Heath education facilitates empowerment by showing people where to access appropriate, relevant information on health, and how to use it to build health capacity. . . . The approach of knowledge plus capacity is the contemporary approach to health education which is orientated towards improving self-efficacy and individual capacity to change. When health education is delivered in an empowering way, knowledge nurtures the self-esteem and self-confidence that is essential for developing and using health literacy. (p. 24)

Key Teaching and Learning Theories Relevant to Nursing

Paolo Freire's theory of community empowerment, 1970. Education is never neutral, and in participatory community education, community members must be involved in naming their own problems and proposing their own solutions (Freire, 1970). "Health education is an integral strategy in promoting community health. The process begins by building the knowledge base, then working with community members to identify strengths, weaknesses, assets, inequities, vulnerabilities or other aspects of community life that may impinge on health" (Clendon & Munns, 2019, p. 22).

Freire's theory of community empowerment can be applied to health education involving social action—efforts to change a whole community rather than one person at a time. A community empowerment approach also seeks to give voice to those affected by forces of oppression—including poverty, racism, and violence—which have such devastating effects on health.

Prochaska and DiClemente's model of planned behaviour change, 1998. DiClemente and Prochaska (1998) developed a transtheoretical model of behaviour change. This model describes behaviour change and involves the following stages:

- Precontemplation: There is little conscious intent to change, as well as resistance or defensiveness.
- Contemplation: The person experiences ambivalence but is more serious about changing a behaviour.
- Preparation: There are preliminary healthy behaviour attempts and conscious planning for change.
- Action: The person lives the plan.
- Maintenance: The individual employs relapse prevention strategies.

In recent years, a sixth stage entitled *relapse* has been added to describe the process of changing health-related behaviours, such as returning to an unhealthy diet or returning to substance abuse. The final stage, *termination* is not often included in the stages of change because it is difficult to achieve. It describes a period with zero temptation for relapse and the achievement of 100% self-efficacy (Raihan & Cogburn, 2022).

This model has been used to explain the process of changing behaviours that are most resistant to change, such as addictions, diet, weight control, or sexual behaviour related to HIV control (Raihan & Cogburn, 2022). In addition, nurse practitioners in the mental health setting apply this model in the management of treatment-resistant major depression (Raihan & Cogburn, 2022).

Nurses can increase an individual's motivation and capabilities to change by involving the individual in planning and goal setting, providing information that is understandable and acceptable, and assisting the person in developing new skills (Dames et al., 2021).

Alfred Bandura's social cognitive theory, 1977. Human health is a social matter, not just an individual one. This theory proposes that self-efficacy beliefs operate together with goals, outcome expectations, and perceived environmental facilitators and impediments in regulating human motivation, behaviour, and well-being (Bandura, 2004). The theory holds that people with high self-efficacy (the belief that "I can do it") can accomplish what they set out to learn or to do. Nurses can help clients to develop the following sources of self-efficacy (Bandura, 2004):

- Personal mastery: Developing awareness of past successes in similar situations
- Vicarious experiences: Observing role models, recognizing what has worked for others
- Verbal persuasion: Encouragement, receiving information, having questions answered
- Physiological feedback: Evidence of positive bodily changes
  Bandura's theory has been utilized, for example, in enhancing self-efficacy for optimized client outcomes through the theory of symptom self-management (Allegrante et al., 2019) and breastfeeding support (Razhan et al., 2021).

Ronald Rogers protection motivation theory, 1975.

- Behaviour can be influenced by intra- and interpersonal beliefs, social norms, and networks as well as policies.
- Rogers (1975) extended the health belief model, stating that the engagement in health-promoting behaviour is based on three factors: one's belief about the severity of the illness, perceived benefits of change, and barriers and confidence levels (self-efficacy) in creating change.
- Protection motivation theory also focuses on how fear influences change. One example would be stop-smoking campaigns where the threat to health is the incentive to protection motivation (Dames et al., 2021).

Nola Pender's health promotion model, 2006. Pender's health promotion model integrates knowledge from nursing with the behavioural sciences to explore motivations for health-promoting behaviours and how health care providers can promote such behaviours in the persons they serve. Her model includes the following ideas (Pender et al., 2006):

- Persons have the capacity for reflective self-awareness, including assessment of their own abilities.
- Persons commit to engaging in behaviours from which they anticipate deriving personally valued benefits.
- Perceived barriers can constrain commitment to health-promoting actions.
- Greater perceived self-efficacy results in fewer perceived barriers to a health behaviour.
- Persons can modify thoughts and emotions and their environment to create incentives for health actions.
- Families, peers, and health care providers are important sources of influence that can increase or decrease commitment to and engagement in health-promoting behaviour.

Pender's model is based on the concept of the human capacity for reflection, change, and action.

HEALTH CARE IN CANADA: POLITICAL, SOCIAL, AND ECONOMIC CONSIDERATIONS

Funding Health Care

- Publicly funded care: Universal coverage for Canadians that includes all medically necessary hospital and physician services that are funded by medicare, a national health insurance system, and governed by the *Canada Health Act*. The principles of the *Canada Health Act* are universality, accessibility, portability, comprehensiveness, and public administration (MacDonald et al., 2022).
- Privately funded care: Supplemental health services that are usually purchased from a for-profit organization as extended health coverage, either through an employer or through a policy (such as private hospital rooms, workplace medication and dental plans, and private MRI clinics).
- Voluntary services: Nonprofit organizations provide financial support and services for the prevention and detection of illness and for specific health conditions (e.g., the Heart and Stroke Foundation of Canada, Diabetes Canada, and Canadian Red Cross).

The Organization of the Health Care System

It is the responsibility of the provinces and territories to manage, organize, and deliver health care services. The federal government describes medicare as a set of 13 interlocking provincial and territorial health insurance plans, all of which have commonalities and basic standards of coverage (Astle & Duggleby, 2024). The federal government also plays a role in health care administration.

Levels of Care

There are five levels of health care: promotive, preventive, curative (diagnosis and treatment), rehabilitative, and supportive.

- Health promotion services and activities are designed to enable people to increase their control over and improve their health (e.g., the promotion of self-esteem in children and adolescents, advocacy for healthy public policy) (Astle & Duggleby, 2024).
- Disease and injury prevention services are designed to reduce risk factors for disease and injury. Prevention strategies include clinical actions (screening, immunization), environmental actions (climate control activism), and behavioural aspects (support groups).
- Diagnosis and treatment services provide diagnosis and treatment of an existing health care condition. Care provided at this level can be labelled as primary, secondary, or tertiary and is described below (Astle & Duggleby, 2024):
  - Primary care is the first contact a person makes with the health care system, which leads to diagnosis and management of the person's actual or potential health condition.

- Secondary care involves the provision of a specialized medical service by a medical specialist in their office, clinic, or hospital. The client has developed recognizable signs and symptoms that have been diagnosed or require a further diagnostic workup.
- Tertiary care is specialized consultative care, usually on referral from primary or secondary medical care providers, provided by specialists working in a setting that has personnel and facilities for diagnosing and treating complicated health conditions.
- Rehabilitation helps clients attain their optimal level of physical, mental, social, and vocational functioning. Rehabilitation generally occurs after a physical or mental illness, injury, or chemical addiction or is related to a chronic illness, disability, frailty, and aging. It focuses on improving quality of life while promoting independence and self-care (Astle & Duggleby, 2024).
- Supportive care services are provided over prolonged periods of time to clients who are disabled, who are not functioning independently, or who have a terminal illness (Astle & Duggleby, 2024). Types of supportive care include palliative and respite care.

Settings for Health Care Delivery

Institutional Sector

Institutional sector refers to hospitals, long-term care facilities, psychiatric facilities, and rehabilitation centres that provide services to inpatients and outpatients (Astle & Duggleby, 2024).

- Hospitals generally specialize in providing care over a short period of time for the purpose of diagnosis and treatment of health care problems (acute care). Examples of services within a hospital include emergency and diagnostic services, general inpatient services, critical care, outpatient services, surgical intervention, and rehabilitation facilities.
- Long-term care facilities provide accommodations for clients who require the delivery of 24-hour, on-site, supervised care, including professional health services, personal care, spiritual care, rehabilitation, and services such as meals, laundry, and housekeeping (Potter et al., 2019).
- Psychiatric facilities are located in hospitals, independent outpatient clinics, or mental health clinics and provide inpatient and outpatient care for clients with mental health disorders and or those who are experiencing emotional crisis (Astle & Duggleby, 2024; Pollard & Jacubec, 2023).
- Rehabilitation centres provide on-site therapy and restorative training to clients with the purpose of minimizing the client's dependence on care (Astle & Duggleby, 2024).

Community Sector

- There has been a shift from institution-based care to community-based care, although community-based care does not have guaranteed public funding as hospital-based care does.
- With a focus on primary and secondary care, this sector provides services for clients that are available where clients live, work, play, and learn (Astle & Duggleby, 2024).
- This sector provides surveillance and monitoring of the environment and the health of the community through the public sector.
- This sector provides specialized services that meet specific client needs (such as food banks or Meals on Wheels).
- Focus is generally on health promotion and illness prevention as well as palliative and restorative care (Astle & Duggleby, 2024).
- Common community settings include public health departments, physicians' offices, community health centres, assisted living facilities, home care, adult day care centres, community and voluntary agencies, palliative and respite care services, and parish nursing.

Challenges to the Health Care System

Two of the main challenges to the Canadian health care system are the increasing cost of care and problems with providing equal and accessible care for all Canadians (Astle & Duggleby, 2024).

Cost of Health Services

Many factors have caused an increase in health expenditures, including new and improved digital health technology (ehealth, maintenance of electronic health records, remote monitoring [robotics], nursing informatics) new pharmaceuticals, an increase in chronic and age-related diseases, an aging population, persons becoming pregnant later in life, and expectations of the health care consumer (Astle & Duggleby, 2024), as well as salary increases for health care providers and the increase in health-specific funding to deal with the COVID-19 pandemic (Canadian Institute for Health Information, 2022).

Equality and Access

There continue to be issues with accessibility to health care services, including the following (Astle & Duggleby, 2024):

- Low-income Canadians experience unequal access to those factors that determine health, such as nutritious food and safe shelter, and therefore commonly have poorer health. Also, while hospital and physician services are available to all under the terms of the *Canada Health Act*, services such as pharmacy, dental, and vision care often involve private-pay or private-insurance systems and hence are available only to those with the means to pay for them.
- Many experts believe that medicare can only be saved by privatizing certain services within the health care system.
  The federal government has a key role in the provision of health care services to Indigenous peoples. The shift in the health care structure needs to align with Indigenous peoples' beliefs.
- A shortage of nurses and physicians is compromising accessibility of health care services.
- Indigenous people are underrepresented in the health workforce. Five key strategic actions proposed for achieving a representative and culturally competent human resource cadre are integration of Indigenous ways of knowing, reduction of institutional barriers, increased

recruitment and retention for practising nurses and education, and building leadership and advocacy capacities (Astle & Duggleby, 2024).

Canada as a Diverse Society

Indigenous peoples represent an important and growing group in Canada. Indigenous peoples account for 5.0 % of the total population of Canada (Statistics Canada, 2022a). First Nations populations continue to grow both on and off reserve. In 2021, 801 045 Indigenous people were living in urban areas in Canada. This number has increased by 12.5% since 2016 (Statistics Canada, 2022b). Approximately 20% of Canada's population was born outside the country (Government of Canada, 2022b). In Toronto, Canada's largest city, this number is over 45%. Until the 1970s most immigrants came from European countries. Since then, the majority of immigrants to Canada are from Asian countries and the Middle East. Since 1999, immigration has outpaced the natural birth rate, accounting for an estimated 66% of all population growth (Astle & Duggleby, 2024; Statistics Canada, 2017).

Culture and Health

Culture has a direct impact on health and on health behaviours, including the following (Astle & Duggleby, 2024):
- Specific health problems
- Biological response to treatments
- Birth rites
- Death rites
- Dietary beliefs and practices
- Time orientation
- Attitude toward older persons
- Personal space
- Gender roles
- Social roles
- Attitude toward the health care system
- Beliefs about illness and treatments

Providing Culturally Competent Care

When working with clients who are members of groups that experience inequities, health care providers must ensure that they treat these clients in appropriate and safe ways. According to Fournier et al. (2021), a common framework that is used in many practice disciplines is the continuum of cultural awareness, sensitivity, competence, and safety.
- **Cultural awareness** means being conscious of the differences among various cultural groups.
- **Cultural sensitivity** takes cultural awareness a step further and refers to a deeper understanding of how culture shapes health and being mindful of one's own culture and cultural biases.
- **Cultural competence** refers to the skill and ability of health care providers to provide effective care to people of different cultures.
- **Cultural safety** is a step beyond cultural competence that includes self-reflection (e.g., nurses being mindful of their own cultural beliefs hend values and assessing how they may differ from the client's beliefs and how they may

influence nursing care) as well as working to reduce power imbalances through advocacy.
- **Cultural humility** is a newer concept that involves a lifelong commitment to self-evaluation and critique, to redressing the power imbalance in the health care professional–client dynamic, and to developing mutually beneficial and nonpaternalistic partnerships with communities on behalf of individuals and defined populations (Fournier et al., 2021).

The goal of culturally competent care is for nurses to provide care and services appropriate to clients' cultural characteristics. Clients include individuals, families, groups, or populations. Nurses need to value diversity, know about the cultural mores and traditions of the population they serve, and be sensitive to these when they are caring for clients. (Fournier & Karachiwalla, 2021). In order to provide culturally sensitive care, it is important for nurses to do the following:
- Bridge cultural gaps in care
- Work with cultural differences
- Enable clients and families to receive meaningful care
- Identify their own cultural beliefs and values and assess how they may differ from the client's beliefs and how they may influence nursing care
- Research information about the client's cultural background
- Assess the client's health behaviours and methods of communication
- Avoid stereotyping, generalizations, and assumptions
- Work with the individual client to develop the most culturally appropriate health interventions (Astle & Duggleby, 2024).

TRAUMA-INFORMED CARE

"Trauma-informed care refers to care focused on the client's past experience of violence and the role it currently plays in their lives. When a history of trauma is present, nurses must be aware of this and avoid situations or approaches that may retraumatize or aggravate traumatic symptoms in clients. Many clients experience a trauma related to their identity, such as marginalization based on their culture, sexual orientation, gender identity, disability, religion, and ethnicity" (Bard et al., 2022, p. 306).

Trauma-informed care is a strengths-based and person-, family-, and community-centred approach that starts with an understanding of trauma, its prevalence among service users, and its potential impacts on holistic health, behaviour, and relationships. The five main principles of trauma-informed care include awareness and validation; safety and trustworthiness; choice, control and collaboration; strengths-based and skill-building care; and cultural, historical, and identity issues (Bard et al., 2022).

Reforms in the Canadian Health Care System

Two national reports, the Kirby Report, *The Health of Canadians* (Kirby, 2002), and the Romanow Report, *The*

Future of Health Care in Canada (Romanow, 2002), have provided recommendations for reforming health care in Canada. One important recommendation includes improving and expanding primary health care (PHC).

Primary Health Care

PHC is described as the key to health care reform and sustainability. It is a philosophy and model for improving health that focuses on preventing illness and promoting health (Astle & Duggleby, 2024). PHC is based on a social justice approach (equal access for all) and addresses the factors in a person's social, economic, and physical environment that make them ill.

The five principles of PHC are accessibility, public participation, health promotion, appropriate technology, and intersectoral collaboration (MacDonald et al., 2022). The principles are interconnected.

Accessibility. As nurses, it is important to address social justice issues at all levels, from global health to individual health care needs. Inequalities in access to health care exist, and population health is strongly influenced by the social determinants of health. Nurses living and working in a community have the skills and knowledge to improve health for that community and to work with others for social justice to bring about equity. Health services are available to all Canadians, regardless of location and economic status. The WHO (2019) has reported challenges in access to health services, even in highly developed countries, between men and women, different cultures, Indigenous and non-Indigenous people, and urban and rural or remote locations. Barriers to the ability of individuals to access health care include unemployment, lack of education and health literacy, age, gender, functional capacity, and cultural or language difficulties. Barriers to community capacity include geographic features that isolate people from services or opportunities, civil conflict, and lack of structures and services (Clendon & Munns, 2019).

Public participation. Clients participate in making decisions about their own health, and they can identify health needs in the community as well as strategies to address those needs. Community partnerships are empowering: "They enhance capacity for developing social capital with mutual trust and reciprocity as well as co-operative networks for better health" (Clendon & Munns, 2019, p. 15). The focus of community partnerships is the achievement of better health, equity, justice, and good governance in health services. However, achieving these outcomes requires the political will to support good health for all community members, particularly for Indigenous-controlled community health services, which are grounded in a community participation approach (Clendon & Munns, 2019).

Health promotion. The emphasis of health promotion is on the need for health care systems to promote health and prevent disease, so their focus is on health maintenance rather than a curative approach to care (MacDonald et al., 2022). At the local level, strategies may involve instituting measures to ensure healthy lunches or access to workplace-based health services. At the global level, health promotion is being aware of problems of other countries and making sure their health issues are understood and publicized. Health promotion actions may include creating day care centres for older persons to prevent them from being socially isolated, or working with new parents to ensure they have the information and support systems they need (Clendon & Munns, 2019).

Appropriate technology. Appropriate technology includes appropriate use of health care resource methods of care, service delivery, procedures, and equipment that are socially acceptable and affordable. PHC emphasizes the right care for the right person or community at the right time to maximize efficiency and equity, rather than the most expensive technologies for all communities (Clendon & Munns, 2019; MacDonald et al., 2022).

Intersectoral cooperation. Intersectoral cooperation requires that all sectors—including government, community, and health—be committed to meeting the needs of Canadians. Ultimately, it requires that health, disability services, transportation, education, environment, and other sectors work together to respond to all the social determinants of health. Collaborative alliances encourage efficient and effective use of resources (e.g., a team of specialists from different sectors working together to ensure the long-term continuity and success of a health initiative) (Clendon & Munns, 2019; MacDonald et al., 2022).

Community Health Nursing

Changes in the health care system (including increased health spending, technology and medical advances, and client involvement in health care) have created a situation whereby clients are receiving care in their homes and communities.

- Goals for community health nursing include keeping individuals healthy, providing in-home care to those who are sick and disabled, encouraging participation in care, and cost containment. The community health nursing focus is broad, emphasizing both the community's health and direct care to subpopulations within the community (Astle & Duggleby, 2024).

- Community health nursing is a specialty nursing practice that may be carried out in a variety of settings. Examples of community health practice areas include public health nursing, home health nursing (community based), occupational health nursing, community mental health nursing, parish nursing, street or outreach nursing, and telenurse and outpost nursing. Street nurses are typically registered nurses. However, a practical nurse may work in a homeless shelter. Refer to Table 6.2.

- Community health nurses (CHNs) promote and protect the health of individuals, families, groups, and communities. Public health policy and initiative programs that coordinate care are usually managed by a registered nurse (RN). CHNs will collaborate with other health care providers on the team, such as the nurse caring for the client (Astle & Duggleby, 2024).

- CHNs must complete community assessments in order to promote client (individual, family, group, community) health and identify needs for health policy, program development, and services (Astle & Duggleby, 2024). The three

TABLE 6.2   Examples of Community Health Nursing Practice Areas

Community Health Nurses	Definition	Practice Settings	Client Group	Educational Preparation	Examples of Roles and Activities	Funding
Public health nurse (PHN)	A nurse who uses knowledge of nursing, social sciences, and public health sciences for the promotion and protection of health and for the prevention of disease among populations	• Community groups • Community health centres • Workplaces • Street clinics • Schools • Outpost settings • Homes	• Population • Aggregates and groups • Community • Families • Individuals	Baccalaureate degree in nursing or registered or licensed practical nurse (RPN or LPN)*	• Health promotion • Disease prevention • Client advocacy • Education • Direct care in clinics	Provincial and municipal governments funding
Home health nurse (HHN)	A nurse who uses knowledge and skills to provide direct care and treatment for individuals to maintain and restore health or palliation during illness	• Client's home • Schools • Clinics • Workplaces • Transition services (from hospital to home) • Older persons' housing programs • Shelter or safe house programs	• Individuals • Families • Caregivers	Registered nurse (RN) or RPN or LPN*	• Direct client care • Disease prevention • Health promotion with individual clients	Public or private funding
Occupational health nurse (OHN)	A nurse who specializes in workplace health and safety, health promotion, disease prevention, and rehabilitation for workers	• Workplaces	• Employees (individuals or groups)	RN with certificate in occupational health	• Direct care • Assessment of the workplace • Education of employees on health and safety issues	Employer
Parish nurse	A nurse who serves the health and wellness needs of faith community members	• Clients' homes • Places of worship • Hospitals	• Individuals • Families • Groups	RN	• Health promotion • Health counsellor • Liaison • Health advocate • Integrator of faith and health	Religious or faith community funding
Primary health care nurse practitioner (PHCNP)	A nurse with advanced-practice education, which allows for an expanded role, such as diagnosing episodic illnesses, prescribing medication, and ordering diagnostic tests	• Community health centres • Clinics • Physicians' offices • Emergency departments in hospitals • Nursing stations • Long-term care facilities,	• Individuals • Families • Groups • Communities	Baccalaureate degree in nursing, minimum of postbaccalaureate diploma with licensing in Extended Class (EC)	• Direct care (i.e., health assessment, diagnosis, and treatment of episodic illness) • Health promotion • Disease prevention • Community development and planning	Public or private funding
Outpost nurse	A nurse who works in an outpost or rural setting that is often geographically separated from face-to-face physician contact	• Nursing stations • Clients' homes • Community	• Individuals • Families • Groups • Rural communities	RN	• Direct care • Health promotion • Liaison with other health care providers • Referral	Provincial or federal funding

TABLE 6.2 Examples of Community Health Nursing Practice Areas—cont'd

Community Health Nurses	Definition	Practice Settings	Client Group	Educational Preparation	Examples of Roles and Activities	Funding
Military nurse	A nurse and nursing officer who is employed by the Canadian Armed Forces Health Services	• Military hospitals • Military outpatient centres • Civilian tertiary care facilities • Military operational units	• Individuals • Families	Baccalaureate degree in nursing	• Direct client care • Disease prevention • Occupational health care • Environmental health care	Federal funding
Forensic nurse	A nurse who has completed continuing education programs in the area of forensic science	• Sexual assault treatment settings, often in hospital emergency departments	• Adults and children who are victims of acute sexual assault or survivors of intimate-partner violence	RN or registered psychiatric nurse	• Direct care for collection of physical evidence • Providing crisis response, such as counselling and referral	Provincial funding
Telenurse	A nurse who provides nursing service over the telephone and computers	• Community agencies	• Individuals • Families • Caregivers	RN	• Telephone advice • Telehealth network (live video links for nurse-led telehealth clinics)	Provincial funding provided to private companies
Corrections nurse	A nurse who works in a correctional facility	• Correctional facilities,	• Inmates (individuals, groups) • Correctional facility staff	RN	• Direct care • Health promotion • Disease prevention • Inmate advocate • Crisis intervention	Provincial or federal funding
Nurse entrepreneur	A nurse who is self-employed in the provision of nursing services	• Home • Variety of workplace settings	• Individuals • Families • Groups • Communities	RN or RPN or LPN*	• Direct client care as contracted • Consultant • Advocate • Health promotion • Disease prevention	Private funding
Street or outreach nurse	A nurse who serves the health and wellness needs of marginalized populations living on the streets	• Community streets	• Individuals • Families • Communities	RN	• Direct client care (i.e., wound care; medication overdose treatment) • Disease prevention • Health promotion • Client advocate • Political activist	Provincial or municipal funding

*Some Canadian provinces and territories designate registered practical nurses (RPNs) or licenced practical nurses (LPNs) to work in some settings such as home health nursing and public health nursing. Note: In some provinces, RPN refers to registered psychiatric nurses; however, in this textbook, the abbreviation designates registered practical nurse.
From MacDonald, S. & Jakubec. S (2022). *Stanhope and Lancaster's Community health nursing in Canada* (4th ed., p. 16, Table 1.3). Elsevier Inc.

components of a community that should be assessed by the CHN include structure or locale, the people, and the social systems (Astle & Duggleby, 2024).

HEALTH PROMOTION AND DISEASE AND INJURY PREVENTION: PRACTICE FOCUS

Nutrition and Healthy Eating

Categories of Nutrients

Six nutrients are necessary for body processes and function. These nutrients are water, carbohydrates, proteins, fats, vitamins, and minerals, and they are described below (Astle & Duggleby, 2024):

Water

- Water makes up 60 to 70% of body weight.
- Water acts as a solvent for metabolic processes.
- Daily losses are through urine, feces, respiration, and perspiration; losses increase with exercise, hot weather, and fever.
- Adult intake should be approximately 1 500 mL per day to survive, including fluid and solid food sources. About 2 000 to 2 500 mL of fluid per day is needed for normal fluid balance.

Carbohydrates

- The diet should provide approximately 55% of energy in the form of carbohydrates, the major source of energy for the body.
- Sources are primarily plants and include simple forms (sugars) and complex forms (starches and glycogen).
- Complex carbohydrates are the preferred energy source.
- Fibre is an indigestible form of complex carbohydrate and is thought to be an important dietary factor in the prevention of some diseases.

Proteins

- Approximately 20% of the diet should come from proteins.
- Proteins are necessary for tissue growth, maintenance, and repair; synthesis of hormones and enzymes; composition of DNA; acid–base balance; blood clotting; and other metabolic processes.
- Complete proteins contain all the essential amino acids and come primarily from animals and seafood.
- Incomplete proteins are found in lentils, nuts, grains, soya, and peas.
- Vegetarians must ensure that they include appropriate ratios and combinations of plant proteins in order to obtain all necessary amino acids.

Fats

- The diet should include no more than 25 to 30% fat and no more than 10% as saturated fat.
- Fats or lipids are necessary as an energy source; for insulation, hormone production, vitamin absorption, nerve conduction; as a component of cell walls; and for padding and insulation of organs and the body.
- Saturated fats, found primarily in animal products, have been implicated in cardiovascular disease, cancers, and obesity.
- Unsaturated fats from plant sources (such as olive oil and flaxseed oil) are considered healthier.
- Omega-3 fatty acids from oily fish sources are believed to decrease levels of low-density lipoproteins and are recommended as part of the weekly diet.
- Plant-based unsaturated fats that have been hydrogenated to a solid form are called *trans fats*; these fats, found in solid margarines, baked goods, and table spreads, have health risks similar to those of saturated fats.

Vitamins

- Vitamins are elements obtained through dietary intake that are necessary for normal metabolism.
- Vitamins found in fresh foods are preferable to synthetic supplements.
- Vitamins are classified as water soluble (B complex and C) and fat soluble (A, D, E, K); fat-soluble vitamins can be stored by the body and are not easily destroyed in cooking or storage; water-soluble vitamins are not stored in the body and are easily lost in cooking.
- Vitamins A, C, and E and beta-carotene may act as antioxidants, neutralizing free radicals that cause oxidative damage to cells.

Minerals. Minerals are inorganic elements essential to the body as catalysts in biochemical reactions. Minerals become part of the structure of the body and enzymes (Astle & Duggleby, 2024). For example:

- Iron becomes attached to a protein globin to form hemoglobin, which enhances oxygen-carrying capacity. It plays a part in energy formation.
- Calcium is a component of bones and teeth and is needed for muscle and nerve activity and blood clotting.
- Potassium is needed to maintain fluid balance and acid–base balance in body cells. It is needed for muscle and nerve activity.
- Sodium is needed to maintain fluid balance and acid–base activity in body cells. It is critical for nerve-impulse transmission.
- Chloride aids in digestion and is needed to maintain fluid balance and acid–base balance in body cells.
- Phosphorous is a component of bone and teeth formation. It plays a part in energy formation and is needed to maintain cell membranes.
- Magnesium is a component of bones and teeth and is needed for nerve activity, energy, and protein formation. It plays a part in the immune function.
- Zinc is part of protein reproduction. It is a component of insulin and activates many enzymes. It helps transport vitamin A.
- Fluoride is a component of bones and teeth (enamel). It confers decay resistance in teeth.
- Iodine is a component of thyroid hormones that helps regulate energy production and growth (Herlihy, 2022).

Eating well helps us live and feel well. Sensible eating can provide energy for our daily tasks and protect us from many chronic illnesses, such as diabetes, obesity, and cardiovascular disease. It may even contribute to longevity (Astle & Duggleby, 2024). A number of interrelated determinants of healthy eating influence the overall well-being of individuals and the community. These determinants include physiological state; food preferences; nutritional knowledge; perceptions of healthy eating; influence of family and friends; physical, social, and economic influences; and healthy public policy (Astle & Duggleby, 2024). Promoting good nutrition is a critical concern in prevention and health promotion and an important dimension in competent self-care. Cultural and ethnic backgrounds influence eating behaviour and must be accounted for in changing eating patterns. The individual, family, and community must all be part of nutritional interventions. Research has substantiated the complexity of factors that determine eating behaviours, and all of these determinants must be part of a strategy for successful change to occur (Astle & Duggleby, 2024).

Determinants of Healthy Eating

- Physiological state: Physiological development or deterioration at both ends of the lifespan (childhood and older person) affects eating behaviour.
- Food preferences: Food preference may be individual in nature or may be affected by social and cultural norms.
- Nutritional knowledge: The amount of nutritional knowledge affects healthy eating choices in adults but has not been demonstrated to affect children and adolescents.
- Perceptions of healthy eating: Perceptions of healthy eating are influenced by current dietary guidelines and cultural influences.
- Psychological factors: Psychological factors shown to affect food choices include self-esteem, body image, chronic dieting, mood, and focus of attention.
- Interpersonal influences: Family, peers, and feelings of social isolation affect patterns of healthy eating.
- Physical environment: This determines the availability of food and access to that food, such as the proximity of supermarkets.
- Social environment: Social status and culture often influence food choice; for example, Canadian society tends to devalue preparation of food in the home and favour takeout and quick meals from the freezer.
- Economic environment: Eating behaviours are influenced by corporate-driven economic interests.
- Healthy public policy: Policies define what is considered relevant and influence our food choices, such as through the subsidization of low-energy, nutrient-dense foods.
- Household food insecurity can be defined as the inadequate or insecure access to food due to financial constraints, and is a significant social and public health issue in Canada. It has negative impacts on mental, physical, and social health and costs the Canadian health care system a considerable amount of money and resources (Dames et al., 2021).

Canada's Food Guide

The purpose of *Canada's Food Guide* (Fig. 6.4) is to assist people in making food choices that promote health and prevent nutrition-related disease through a translation of science-based nutrient into a practical pattern of food choices (Dames et al., 2021). The guide encourages the consumption of plenty of vegetables and fruits, whole-grain foods, and plant-based protein foods. Other recommendations include limiting highly processed foods, making water the drink of choice, using food labels, and being aware that food marketing can influence choices. Suggested healthy eating habits include being mindful of eating habits, cooking more often, enjoying food, and eating meals with others. The food guide provides special recommendations for children, women of child-bearing age, and adults over the age of 70 (Government of Canada, 2022c). *Canada's Food Guide* 2019 has also been translated into over 30 languages, including several Indigenous languages such as Ojibwe, Michif, and Inuinnaqtun. Health Canada and Indigenous Services Canada are committed to working with Indigenous persons in incorporating traditional food choices into their diets.

- Children: Children learn eating behaviours from adults, who serve as important role models. Children eating with their families encourages children to try new foods, develop healthier ways of eating, learn cooking skills, and explore cultural and traditional food. This practice also helps create a positive relationship with food. The food guide recommends children should be provided with small meals and snacks throughout the day.
- Child-bearing-aged clients who are planning on getting pregnant should consider taking a multivitamin with 0.4 mg of folic acid each day in addition to the amount of folate found in a healthy diet. Neural tube defects can appear within the first month of a pregnancy, so health experts recommend starting folic acid for all child-bearing persons who could become pregnant (Dames et al., 2021).
- Extra calories are required during pregnancy and lactation; an addition of an extra healthy snack each day following *Canada's Food Guide* is suggested (Government of Canada, 2022d).
- Adults over the age of 70: Vitamin D requirements increase at age 70 (to 800 IU). Vitamin D intake is associated with health benefits that include improved muscle strength, higher bone mineral density, reduced fracture rates, reduced rates of falling, and improved mobility (Dames et al., 2021).

Physical Activity

The importance of regular exercise is becoming increasingly clear as indicated by current research. The impact of physical activity on health is listed below.

- Regular physical exercise promotes health and well-being from both a physical and psychological perspective.
- Exercise increases respiratory capacity, improves digestion and fat metabolism, strengthens bones, improves joint flexibility, improves circulation, improves mood, reduces psychological symptoms, reduces the risk of heart disease, lowers body fat and reduces weight, and increases muscle strength and tone (Dames et al., 2021).
- Physical inactivity is an important public health concern for Canadians of all ages. Physical inactivity is a large

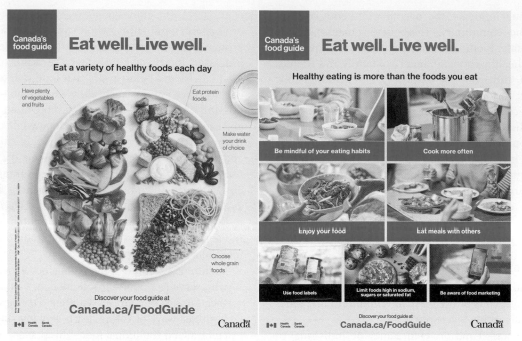

Fig. 6.4 Canada's food guide (From Canada's Dietary Guidelines: Learn about healthy eating at https://food-guide.canada.ca/en/. (All rights reserved. Canada's Food Guide: Snapshot. Health Canada, 2019. Adapted and reproduced with permission from the Minister of Health, 2020.))

influencer on mortality. Physical inactivity is linked it to a number of chronic diseases, including cardiovascular disease, cancer, and diabetes (Fournier & Karachiwalla, 2021). Other health risks of inactivity include premature death, obesity, high blood pressure, osteoporosis, stroke, depression, and colon cancer (Fournier & Karachiwalla, 2021).

- Clients should be assessed by a health care provider before starting an exercise program.
- The amount of physical activity required on a daily basis is directly correlated with the intensity of the workout (Fournier & Karachiwalla, 2021).
- A holistic approach to physical activity is required to keep the body healthy and involves exercise for cardiovascular health (endurance exercises), musculoskeletal health (flexibility activities, strength activities, bone health), and body awareness (Dames et al., 2021).
- Adults should engage in 30 minutes of moderate-intensity physical activity 5 days per week. The recommendation is for 150 minutes of moderate-to-vigorous physical activity each week, in bouts of 10 minutes or more (Fournier & Karachiwalla, 2021).
- Over half of Canadian children are not active enough for optimal growth and development. Lack of exercise among children is a major contributor to weight gain and obesity (Fournier & Karachiwalla, 2021).
- Benefits of regular physical activity for older persons include continued independent living, reduced risk of falls, improved quality of life, improved balance and posture, and prevention of bone loss (Dames et al., 2021).

Rest and Sleep

Rest and sleep are as important to health as proper nutrition and exercise (Dames et al., 2021).

- Sleep promotes tissue repair and recovery of body systems and is essential for cognitive and emotional function.
- Sleep is governed by an individual's sleep–wake cycles, or circadian rhythms; circadian rhythms are influential in controlling the pattern of major biological functions such as body temperature, heart rate, blood pressure, hormone and electrolyte secretions, and sensory acuity.
- Circadian rhythms are affected by light, temperature, and social factors (such as shift work).
- All people have individual sleep–wake cycles; hospital routines rarely take these into consideration.
- Although individual needs vary, most people require approximately 7 to 9 hours of sleep per night.
- Any disruption in the sleep–wake cycle may lead to suppressed immunity, decreased tissue repair, impaired judgement, irritability, decreased appetite, and weight loss; some accidents are believed to result from sleep deprivation, which leads to distortion of sensory perceptions. Chronic sleep deprivation may cause weight gain by altering metabolism and by stimulating excess stress hormones. It also reduces the levels of hormones that regulate appetite, which may encourage more eating (Tyerman & Cobbett, 2023).
- Sleep cycles are categorized as non–rapid eye movement (non-REM) and REM; non-REM Stage 4 is the deepest level of sleep and is believed to be important for physical restoration; heart rate and respirations are decreased in Stage 4.

- REM sleep is important for psychological restoration; dreaming occurs most often in this stage; heart rate and respirations increase in REM sleep.

Sleep Disturbances

- According to Tyerman and Cobbett (2023), "Sleep disturbances refers broadly to situations of poor-quality sleep. *Insufficient sleep* is defined as obtaining less sleep than a person requires to be fully awake or alert during the day. *Fragmented sleep* is characterized by frequent arousals or actual awakenings that interrupt sleep continuity. Sleep disturbances can be related to a variety of physical, emotional, environmental, and lifestyle factors" (p. 120).
- Changes in sleep habits and rituals may alter the ability to sleep (including shift work sleep disorder and hospital clients).
- Stress or anxiety may cause loss of sleep and less time spent in REM sleep.
- Large or spicy meals before bedtime, as well as caffeine and alcohol, may cause difficulty in sleeping.
- Excessive environmental stimulation and noise will interfere with sleep (as in critical care unit [CCU] psychosis).
- Technology devices (smartphones, computers, tablets, television) have been implicated as a potential factor in adolescent sleep deprivation. The use of technology and the number of devices used in the hour before sleep have been significantly associated with problems in daytime function, increased frequency of waking too early, waking unrefreshed, and daytime sleepiness (Tyerman & Cobbett, 2023).
- Discomfort and illness may cause difficulties in falling or staying asleep (such as pain, respiratory difficulty, restless leg syndrome).
- Enuresis (bedwetting) and nocturia (urination during the night) disrupt the sleep cycle.
- Side effects from medications, both prescription and over the counter, may lead to insomnia and disturbances in the sleep cycle; overuse of sedatives may lead to insomnia and sleep-cycle disturbances.

Sleep Abnormalities

- Insomnia is difficulty falling asleep or staying asleep; it may be temporary or chronic.
- Hypersomnia is too much sleep and may be caused by a physical illness or depression.
- Narcolepsy is excessive daytime sleepiness; the person may feel an overwhelming wave of sleepiness and fall asleep. It has an impact on REM sleep and it intensifies the emotions associated with this stage of sleep. Many individuals with narcolepsy experience hallucinations, vivid dreams, night terrors, sleepwalking, sleep paralysis and poor memory concentration, or the feeling of being unable to move or talk just before waking or falling asleep (Astle & Duggleby, 2024).

- Cataplexy is brief, uncontrollable episodes of sleep that last from a few seconds to 30 minutes. The episodes can occur any time of the day and occur occasionally to several times a day. It is a sudden bilaterally (occasionally unilateral) loss of muscle tone accompanied by an overpowering urge to sleep (Astle & Duggleby, 2024).
- Somnambulism (sleepwalking) is most common in children.
- Sleep apnea—pauses in breathing lasting over 10 seconds—is most commonly caused by upper-airway obstruction due to relaxed muscles in the oral cavity; it occurs most often in overweight, middle-aged men and postmenopausal women; loud snoring and excessive daytime sleepiness are manifestations of sleep apnea.

A Healthy Environment

The socioecological model of health described in the first section provides the theoretical basis for nurses to address individual needs as well as the social and physical environment in an effort to create conditions that support and facilitate healthy behaviours and lifestyles. More and more research is suggesting that our economic and social environment has a greater effect on our health than do advances in medicine (Fournier & Karachiwalla, 2021).

Nurses strive to promote and restore the health of individuals with an understanding that the health of individuals is inescapably tied to the health of their families, communities, and societies (Fournier & Karachiwalla, 2021). The social environment must be taken into account in health promotion and disease and injury prevention, and it must be addressed in combination with health education. "Community empowerment is a social action process by which communities, organizations and individuals gain control over their lives in the plan of changing their social and political environment to improve quality of life and equity. Participation alone is insufficient if strategies do not also build capacity of community organizations and individuals in decision making and advocacy" (Fournier & Karachiwalla, 2021, p. 77).

Social Environment

The social environment is a critical determinant of health (see Table 6.1), and researchers contend that it is as influential on health as healthy eating or physical activity (Government of Canada, 2022a). When the social environment is supportive, creating a climate of trust and mutual respect, people are more likely to be *empowered*, in control of their life, and to improve their health (Fournier & Karachiwalla, 2021). To effect changes in the social environment, nurses can do the following:

- Involve families in their own care.
- Connect clients and families to appropriate resources in the community (support groups, family resource centres, community kitchens).
- Help strengthen the social environment.

A healthy social environment is created through regulations and policies that foster cohesive, safe communities with supportive social networks and resources. To be effective and sustainable, these regulations and policies must be developed, enacted, and evaluated jointly by multiple sectors (e.g., education, housing, environment, health, justice) and community members themselves. Examples of how a healthy social environment might be created include the following:

- Example 1: In targeting smoking behaviours, nurses raise awareness of the effects of smoking and strategies for cessation, and address the social environment by advocating for no-smoking regulations in public places and for controls on media advertisements and the accessibility of tobacco.
- Example 2: In a community faced with high levels of crime, nurses educate youth and their families on minimizing risky behaviours. Nurses work with other sectors to identify high-risk areas within the community and to improve policing and supervision of those areas. Safe and accessible recreational opportunities for youth are also developed.

Physical Environment

The physical environment is an important determinant of health as well (Government of Canada, 2022a). Factors such as contaminants in the indoor and outdoor environment influence health. These contaminants, whether transmitted through air, water, food, or soil, can cause cancer, birth defects, or respiratory illness (Fournier & Karachiwalla, 2021; Government of Canada, 2022a).

Research indicates that a number of cancers are linked to environmental contaminants (Canadian Cancer Society, 2022a). Children are particularly at risk for adverse effects due to the immaturity of their metabolism and limited physiological ability to detoxify and excrete chemicals. They inhale more air in proportion to their body weight, are closer to the ground where toxins may exist, and are more apt to put things in their mouths (Dames et al., 2021). Those living in poverty are also disproportionately affected by environmental contaminants (Dames et al., 2021) because "[t]heir burden of physical, chemical and biological exposure is greater (e.g., living close to factories or expressways, and in older buildings that may have lead paint or asbestos insulation); and . . . they have less access to resources that help mitigate the negative effects of this exposure (e.g., nutritious food and high quality medical care)" (Fournier & Karachiwalla, 2021).

Nurses have a responsibility to address environmental health problems through their care for clients, families, and communities. Box 6.1 presents the CNA's recommendations on the role of nurses in environmental health.

The CNA's position statement on environmental health begins as follows: "The environment is an important determinant of health and has a profound impact on why some people are healthy and others are not. There is a role for every nurse to promote and support actions to optimize the health of the environment because of the link to human health" (Dames et al., 2021, p. 504).

BOX 6.1   Nurses and Environmental Health

The role of nurses in environmental health includes:
- Assessing and communicating risks of environmental hazards to individuals, families, and communities
- Educating patients, families, and communities about environmental health and how to address key environmental health issues
- Showing leadership in personal practices that support and reduce harm to the environment
- Collaborating with interdisciplinary colleagues to identify and mitigate environmental health risks in practice environments
- Advocating for policies that protect health by preventing exposure to those hazards and promoting sustainability
- Producing nursing science, including interdisciplinary research, related to environmental health issues
- Promoting the development of natural and built environments that support health

From Canadian Nurses Association (CNA). (2017). *Position statement. Nurses and environmental health* (pp. 1–2). https://www.cna-aiic.ca/en/policy-advocacy/policy-support-tools/position-statements.

Through a combination of health education and awareness campaigns, as well as ongoing changes to regulations and policy, nurses need to help reduce harmful exposure to environmental contaminants such as air pollutants (indoor and outdoor), pesticides, polluted water, lead, and radon. Examples of how this might be accomplished include the following:

- Example 1: Providing health education to clients, families, schools, and communities on issues such as avoiding harmful exposure to pesticides and chemicals.
- Example 2: Working with community health boards or groups to change pesticide bylaws or working with hospital-based teams to improve air quality and hospital recycling programs.

In conjunction with interventions aimed at limiting contaminant exposure, nurses need to use the ample (yet often underutilized) evidence that suggests that interacting with natural environments (in the form of gardens, plants, and animals) can have many positive spiritual, physical, and mental effects (Nisbet et al., 2020; Zhang et al., 2021) and can influence behaviours that then help to protect and sustain the health of the planet. Two examples follow; see Table 6.3 for additional examples.

- Example 1: Providing health education to clients and families about the health benefits of interacting with nature as well as ways to engage with the natural environment to promote their health, such as encouraging outdoor physical activity in green spaces.
- Example 2: Working with hospital "green teams" to redesign hospital spaces that incorporate more green plants, gardens, and window access to natural spaces. Green teams strive to create environmentally responsive health care settings and sectors (Barton et al., 2017; Rojas-Rueda et al., 2019).

TABLE 6.3	Examples of Multilevel Health Promotion and Disease Prevention Initiatives
System Level	**Intervention**
Individual level	• Health education in schools focused on healthy eating and physical activity • Health teaching with clients and families on healthy eating, physical activity, and benefits of engaging with nature • Linking clients and families to community resources and programs that support healthy living behaviours
Organizational and policy levels	• School-curriculum changes (e.g., increasing the frequency of physical education classes and banning school sales of chocolate bars and pop) • Increasing the availability of healthy foods in school and university cafeterias and vending machines • Redesigning community-based recreational areas to improve access to playgrounds and natural spaces that provide settings for physical activity • Creating community and nature-based walking trails that enable walk-to-school programs • Making changes to community environments, advocating for clean, greenspaces and climate change interventions

Promoting Client Safety

The Concept of Safety Promotion and Injury Prevention

Injuries, a leading cause of disability and death, are usually preventable. Nurses can integrate discussions of safety promotion and injury prevention into all health care encounters, particularly with more vulnerable populations, such as children, youth, and older persons. Injury prevention requires both client education and collective action to build safer environments.

Promoting Infant Safety

Most infant injuries happen in the home and are attributed to lapses in caregiver attention, the presence of household hazards, and enhanced mobility of older infants as they develop. Accidental falls are the leading cause of infant injury in Canada. Other common infant injuries include lacerations, burns, poisonings, and choking (Hockenberry et al., 2022). Approaches to reduce the risk of injury in infants include the following:

• Install smoke alarms and check them every month.
• Ensure that baby equipment, including second-hand equipment, meets Canadian safety standards, such as rear-facing infant car seats. See specific car seat safety regulations in Chapter 11.
• Keep small objects such as buttons or coins out of babies' reach. Do not feed candy, nuts, popcorn, grapes, or hot dogs to a baby, as these can cause choking.
• Avoid ribbons and ties on baby clothes and toys.
• Keep one hand on the baby at all times during care such as diaper changes. Babies can easily roll off beds and change tables.
• Do not use baby walkers with wheels.
• Know that microwaved food can be very hot on the inside while the outside is cool and can burn a baby. Stir and check the temperature before feeding.
• Always test bath water first. Hot bath water can burn a baby.
• Put the baby on their back to sleep.
  • Develop strategies to support sleep safety principles for all sleep at all times of the day and night. Provide health teaching to parents regarding sudden infant death syndrome (SIDS) and the importance of not cosleeping with the infant on noninfant surfaces such as the parents' bed, a couch, or another child's bed (Hockenberry et al., 2022).
• Keep medicines, cleaning products, alcohol, tobacco and cannabis products, and cosmetics out of reach. The most common form of poisoning involves unintentional ingestion of medicines in children (Parachute, 2022).

Safety Promotion With Children and Youth

Injuries are the leading cause of death and disability among children and adolescents (Stanwick, 2022). Leading forms of injuries include motor vehicle occupant and pedestrian accidents, drowning, falls, and residential fires (Hockenberry et al., 2022). Approaches to reduce the risk of injury in childhood and adolescence include the following:

• Teach children to swim and always maintain supervision around water.
• Teach children how to cross streets and parking lots.
• Teach children to not handle or eat items found in the street or grass.
• Teach children to not accept gifts from or go with strangers.
• Teach the safe use of equipment for play and work. Promote the use of sports helmets.
• Never allow children access to firearms.
• Encourage teens to enroll in driver education.
• Encourage teens to wear their seat belt and to avoid driving under the influence of drugs or alcohol or riding with someone who is under the influence (Hockenberry et al., 2022).
• Teach safe use of the Internet:
  • School educators can reinforce to youth the dangers of mobile technology while crossing the street, walking on the sidewalk, cycling, or driving a vehicle.
• New public safety initiatives can be created, such as phone apps to prevent texting and driving; mass media campaigns promoting the awareness of one's actions while texting, cycling, or driving; and policy and law enforcement initiatives to address dangerous texting behaviours (Stavrinos et al., 2018).

Implement traffic calming measures, such as speed bumps, to reduce speeding and aggressive driving on residential streets.
- Create more bike lanes or paths on roads.
- Change the design of products such as toys and sports equipment used by children.
- Ensure that there are padded dashboards and shatterproof windows in automobiles.
- Children should wear a seat belt or be in an age-appropriate booster seat as needed; older children should ride with a restraint system and in the back seat until age 12.
- Subsidize the costs of safety equipment such as bicycle helmets with tax credit exemptions or rebates and federal tax credits to make the purchase of bicycle helmets less expensive (Hagel & Yanchar, 2013).
- Provide health teaching and counselling on safer sex practices.
  For more information on pediatric safety, refer to Chapter 11.

Safety Promotion With Older Persons

Falls are the leading cause of injuries among older persons (Astle & Duggleby, 2024). Approaches to reduce the risk of falls include the following:
- Ensure that stairs are of uniform size, treaded, and well lit.
- Install grab rails near the toilet and tub.
- Secure all mats and carpets so they do not skid.
- Promote the wearing of skid-free footwear.
- Remove clutter.
- Provide close supervision of confused clients.
- Lock beds and wheelchairs when transferring clients.
- Use alternatives to restraints (relaxation techniques, scheduled toileting, instituting scheduled walking and ambulation routines). Restraints do not prevent falls or injury and may actually increase the severity of injury (Astle & Duggleby, 2024).

Understanding the Concept of Sexual Health

The WHO defines sexual health as "a state of physical, emotional, mental, and social well-being in relation to sexuality" (Dames et al., 2021, p. 476). Sexual health is evidenced in the free and responsible expressions of sexual capabilities that foster harmonious personal and social wellness, enriching individual and social life. It is not merely the absence of dysfunction, disease, or infirmity (WHO, 2022). Sexual health requires a positive and respectful approach to sexuality and sexual relations—one that is free of coercion, discrimination, and violence (WHO, 2022).

Components of Sexuality

Components of sexuality include the following:
- Sex: A multidimensional biological construct that encompasses anatomy, physiology, genes, and hormones, which together create a human "package" that affects how we are labelled.
- Gender: A social construct that is culturally based and historically specific and is constantly changing. *Gender* refers to the socially prescribed and experienced dimensions of "femaleness" and "maleness."

- *Gender diversity* is an umbrella term used to represent a variety of gender identities or expressions beyond masculine and feminine. They may include lesbian, gay, binary, transgender, queer, intersex, and two spirit (2SLGBTQI+). It is important to incorporate the use of gender-neutral language and the correct names and pronouns of gender-diverse people (Dames et al., 2021).
- Gender roles: The behavioural norms applied to males and females in societies, which influence individuals' everyday actions, expectations, and experiences. In some cultures, these are sharply defined; in other cultures, the lines between male and female gender roles may be more blurred.
- Gender identity: How one sees one's own gender—as male, female, or some combination, such as androgynous, intersex, or transgender (Astle & Duggleby, 2024).
- Sexual orientation: The predominant gender preference of a person's sexual attraction over time. It is independent of their sexual identity (Astle & Duggleby, 2024).
- Gender equity: refers to respecting all people without discrimination According to Dames et al. (2021), it is defined as "the fair treatment of all genders according to their respective needs and acknowledges that this treatment may be different but must be equivalent in terms of rights, benefits, obligations and opportunities" (p. 34).

Sexual Behaviours

Sexually healthy behaviours include the appreciation of one's own body; interacting with both genders in respectful ways; expressing love and intimacy in appropriate ways; avoiding exploitative or manipulative relationships; identifying and living according to one's values; effective communication with family, peers, and partners; making informed choices about family options and lifestyles; seeking prenatal and reproductive health care; avoiding contracting or transmitting a sexually transmitted infection (STI); and preventing sexual abuse (Astle & Duggleby, 2024).

The Nurse's Role in Sexual Health Promotion

- Promoting positive sexual health is essential for all health care providers, including nurses. Sexuality impacts all areas of life and human development. Growing concerns about epidemics of STIs, the impact of sexual violence on health, and sexual dysfunction also require that nurses understand the prevention of disease.
- Sensitivity is essential as nurses strive to explore and better understand clients' experiences of sexuality in health and illness. There are many different sexual cultural norms, and these norms influence attitudes toward sexual practices. The PLISSIT model may serve nurses to assess and intervene sensitively in matters related to sexual health and well-being (Astle & Duggleby, 2024):
  - *Permission*: Allowing the client to share concerns, experiences, and ask questions.
  - *Limited information*: Giving the client basic information on sexuality and sexual functioning.

- *Specific suggestions*: Making specific suggestions regarding a sexual concern or issue.
- *Intensive therapy*: Providing referral to intensive therapy; the level of intervention depends on the nurse's experience and knowledge. Examples of interventions include referral to a qualified practitioner such as a social worker or sexuality counsellor (Astle & Duggleby, 2024).

All nurses should be able to encourage clients to discuss matters related to sexual health and to give limited information and specific suggestions as entry-level competencies, depending on their own scope of knowledge. It is important for nurses to examine their own attitudes toward sexuality and be comfortable with different types of sexuality so that they can approach clients in an ethical, professional, and non-judgemental way.

Alterations in sexual health include infertility; sexual dysfunction (including dyspareunia, lack of libido, erectile dysfunction); sexually transmitted infections (STIs); lack of comfort with sexual orientation, gender identity, or gender role; body image disturbance; sexual deviation; and sexual abuse (Astle & Duggleby, 2024).

Promoting Mental Wellness and Stress Management

Emotions and Health

- Negative emotions, such as depression, anxiety, anger, or hostility, trigger neuroendocrine and immune responses, which, in turn, promote the development of a range of chronic health problems such as cardiovascular disease, certain cancers, osteoporosis, type 2 diabetes, prolonged infection, and decreased wound healing (Astle & Duggleby, 2024).
- The "fight or flight" or "stress response" to stress has been described in the literature for over 60 years. The response is a general arousal of the sympathetic nervous system, which causes increasing heart and respiratory rates, decreased intestinal perfusion and motility, increased alertness, increased blood pressure, and increased blood sugar levels.
- More recently, there was an investigation of the "tend and befriend" response, with claims that the hormone involved in the biobehaviour of nurturance and affiliation, oxytocin, causes some people experiencing stress to nurture one another rather than to run or fight and that this response is more common among women (Taylor et al., 2000).

Coping

Coping is defined as a person's effort to manage psychological stress. Coping involves some combination of problem-focused and emotion-focused strategies (Tyerman & Cobbett, 2023). For example, gathering information about a stressor focuses on the problem and what to do about it; resisting learning about a condition is a way of regulating unpleasant emotions. "The broaden and build theory of positive emotions suggest that positive emotions have the ability to fuel resilience directly, as well indirectly by promoting adaptive coping and demoting maladaptive coping strategies" (Gloria & Steinhardt, 2016). Coping approaches vary among individuals and in different situations and times. *Coping flexibility* is a common approach to successful coping. It involves the ability to assess the nature of the stressor, figure out what areas can be controlled, and change and adapt coping strategies over time and for different stressful conditions. Numerous strategies, such as regular aerobic exercise, have been shown to prevent or mitigate the effects of stress. Regular exercise results in improved circulation, increased endorphins, and an enhanced sense of well-being (Tyerman & Cobbett, 2023).

Self-Awareness Approach

Self awareness is a tool that helps people learn about interactions involving the mind, body and spirit; increases a sense of control; and counters self-defeating perceptions. Self awareness helps people recognize stress that they create through negative, unrealistic thinking and provides them an opportunity to change this negative thought pattern, which, in turn, decreases their stress and increases their control (Dames et al., 2021).

Another related concept is a nonjudgemental self-awareness called "mindfulness." It involves intentional acceptance of the unfolding experience occurring in the moment. It involves two concepts:

- The intentional self-regulation of attention: being focused on the present-moment experience, and
- Having an attitude of acceptance, openness, and curiosity toward whatever arises (Dames et al., 2021).

Approaches to Stress Management

Approaches to stress management include intrapersonal, interpersonal, and spiritual approaches, including the following (Dames et al., 2021; Tyerman & Cobbett, 2023):

- Connecting with others, developing support systems
- Regular exercise
- Getting sufficient sleep
- Learning time-management techniques
- Using guided imagery and visualization
- Practising progressive muscle relaxation
- Obtaining assertiveness training
- Journal writing
- Listening to music for relaxation
- Maintaining a clear separation between work and home life
- Maintaining humour, laughter
- Learning to accept, respect, and love oneself; letting intuition be a guide
- Stretching oneself: learning something new in order to grow
- Helping others
- Practising prayer, meditation, experiences in nature
- Seeking treatment in crisis and in mental illness

Complementary and Alternative Therapies

Canadian Context

Interest and involvement in complementary and alternative medicine (CAM) is a fast-growing trend in Canada. A nation of immigrants, we represent the world's cultures coming together, and it is estimated that more than 70% of Canadians use medicines that would be considered alternatives to conventional North American medicines (Astle & Duggleby, 2024; Dames et al., 2021). There has been a growing awareness of the limits of conventional medicine and a rise in requests for holistic care that treats the client's mind, body, and spirit. The WHO published *WHO Traditional Medicine Strategy: 2014–2023* to advance the potential use of alternative health care traditions in safe and effective ways and to help countries regulate medicines and make them safer and more accessible to their populations (Astle & Duggleby, 2024).

Key Terms Related to Complementary and Alternative Therapies

- *Complementary therapies* are those therapies used in addition to conventional (allopathic) treatment. An example would be the use of aromatherapy to lessen postsurgical anxiety.
- *Alternative therapies*, while they may include similar methods, are primarily intended to replace conventional therapies. An example would be the use of a special diet to treat cancer rather than the chemotherapy recommended by a doctor trained in conventional medicine (Bard et al., 2022).
- *Integrative therapies* involve building bridges between complementary, alternative practices, and mainstream medicine and developing clinical approaches that encourage mainstream and complementary practitioners to work together in the client's best interest. The focus is on the interrelationship among the mind, spirit, and body (Bard et al., 2022).

CAM classifications encompass diverse approaches, including alternative medical systems, such as homeopathy, naturopathy, Ayurvedic medicine from originating from India, and traditional Chinese medicine. CAM also includes manipulative and body-based therapies that focus on the body's natural abilities to heal itself such as massage, phototherapy, and chiropractic.

- **Energy-based therapies** include mind–body interventions, such as meditation, hypnotherapy, prayer and spiritual healing, or expressive therapy (art, music, or dance).
- Energy therapies include biofield therapies such as qigong, reiki, acupuncture, therapeutic touch, biofeedback, colour therapy, and bioelectromagnetic-based therapies (e.g., the use of pulsating magnetic fields) (Bard et al., 2022).
- **Biologically based therapies** include the use of herbs, foods, vitamins, and aromatherapy.
- **Indigenous healing** incorporates a holistic concept of health. The four aspects of health are spiritual, emotional, intellectual, and physical. A weakness in any of these areas causes a person to become unbalanced. Healing circles, sweat lodges, traditional medicine, and the use of medicine wheels and healing ceremonies are some of the approaches that are used to support the health and well-being of Indigenous people (Astle & Duggleby, 2024).

Technology-based practices offer a wide range of electronic communication and information using a medium that is known and comfortable to the user. With the increased use of electronic devices, mental health advice is easily accessible. It includes technology such as telemedicine, text-based counselling, and hotlines (Bard et al., 2022).

Benefits, Risks, Controversies, and Nursing Responsibilities

CAM holds much promise. Considerable research has found great efficacy in some CAM therapies, particularly in promoting relaxation and in pain relief, thereby strengthening the immune response in health and illness. More and more complementary therapies have become integrated into "traditional" approaches; for example, registered nurses certified in therapeutic touch are applying this practice with ventilated clients in CCUs. Oncology nurses practise imagery in talking children through cancer procedures. Clients are asking nurses for massage and aromatherapy and about herbal remedies not found in any Canadian textbooks. Many complementary therapies would seem to fall naturally into the practice of nursing (Bard et al., 2022), as nurses are called on to promote holistic health, prevent disease, and provide care in episodic or chronic illness.

CAM also involves controversy. Some methods are unsupported by research, and some may involve harm and risk (Bard et al., 2022). For example, herbal remedies are not standardized, and some may be toxic or interact with other medicines a person may be using. Many practitioners of CAM remain unlicensed and unregulated. Without regulation, one can call oneself a practitioner or therapist with substandard or insufficient educational preparation or supervision. Without adherence to a professional code of ethics, practitioners may exploit frightened or uninformed people for personal or financial gain. "In Canada, training standards have been set by governing organizations for specific alternative health practices. Among these licensed therapies, training standard are not necessarily 'standards.' They do vary widely from province to province/territory. There is no uniform regulation system for alternative medicine in Canada" (Hales & Lauzon, 2018, p. 365).

Professional guidelines for nurses' involvement in CAM are evolving. The 2020 Canadian Holistic Nurses Association (CHNA) has established standards of practice for CAM and integrative therapies (CHNA, 2020). The use of therapeutic touch, imagery, hypnotherapy, meditation, prayer, and art therapy by nurses can fall within conventional nursing practice if nurses are adequately prepared in their practice. With any therapy—conventional or otherwise—nurses are called on to provide ethical care, promoting genuine and voluntary consent free of duress, fraud, or misrepresentation and to ensure that sufficient information is given about the nature and expected benefits of a treatment, its side effects, consequences of refusal, and possible alternatives. It is important for nurses to be informed on Best Practice Guidelines as well as current research in the field of CAM therapies (Astle & Duggleby, 2024).

Immunization

The objectives of immunization programs are to prevent, control, eliminate, or eradicate vaccine-preventable diseases by directly protecting vaccine recipients and indirectly protecting vulnerable individuals who may not respond to vaccines or for whom vaccines may be contraindicated (Government of Canada, 2022e). Immunization enables the immune system to build up resistance to disease. Vaccines contain small amounts of viruses or bacteria that are dead (inactivated), weakened (live attenuated), or purified (subunit) components (Astle & Duggleby, 2024). Vaccines prompt the immune system to produce antibodies that will attack the virus or bacteria to prevent disease. The immune system stores the information about how to produce those antibodies and responds if there is exposure to that same virus or bacteria in the future (Herlihy, 2022). The *Canadian Immunization Guide* (Government of Canada, 2023) provides up-to-date information on the use of vaccines in Canada. It includes specific recommendations for certain population groups, including children and adults. Table 6.4 details the provincial and territorial immunization schedule for healthy adults (over 18) previously immunized. Recommended schedules for children and adolescents are provided in Chapter 11.

Vaccination and Risk Communication

Nurses must be knowledgeable not only in the principles and practices of immunization but also in risk communication as public concerns about safety continue to mount. Vaccine hesitancy is defined as a "delay in acceptance or refusal of vaccines despite availability of vaccine services" (Fournier & Karachiwalla, 2021). The WHO describes the three main factors for vaccine hesitancy as confidence, complacency, and convenience (Fournier & Karachiwalla, 2021). The Government of Canada (2021) has described four principles of effective communication that health care providers can use in their daily practice:

- Clearly communicate current knowledge using an evidence-informed approach: Have a wide variety of information formats that are tailored to different languages and levels of education. Take into account what the client knows and the information requested.
- Make the most of each opportunity to present information on vaccines and immunizations: Clarify commonly held misconceptions, encourage the client to ask questions, and provide appropriate resources based on evidence.
- Respect differences of opinion about immunization: Understand the underlying reasons for a client's refusal of a vaccine and the strength of their position.
- Represent the risks and benefits of vaccines fairly and openly: Compare the known risks associated with the vaccine with the risks associated with the vaccine-preventable infection.
- Adopt a client-centred approach: All clients have input into their decision to vaccinate and retain responsibility for their own health or the health of their children.

Workplace Safety for Nurses
Infection Control

- Nurses provide intimate bodily care to others, including those with infectious diseases.

- Hand hygiene before and after any client contact is essential to reducing transmission. Routine practices apply to blood, semen, and vaginal secretions; cerebrospinal, synovial, pleural, peritoneal, pericardial, and amniotic fluids; and any items or surfaces (such as laundry, dressings, floors, and tabletops) in contact with them. Protective barriers such as gloves, gowns, masks, and protective eyewear can reduce the risk of exposure.
- Take caution with the use and disposal of needles, scalpel blades, and other sharps. Never recap a used needle. Use special puncture-resistant containers for sharps.
- Adhere to public health recommendations for the immunization of health care workers.
- Additional isolation precautions may be necessary for airborne infections or those involving droplets, such as the use of gowns, masks, and reverse airflow engineering systems (Astle & Duggleby, 2024).

For further information about infection control related to specific diseases, refer to Chapter 7.

Safe Client Handling

Health care workers are at high risk for injury and disability from musculo-skeletal disorders. These disorders are associated with excessive back and shoulder loading due to lifting heavy loads during manual client handling or the required use of awkward postures during client care (Canadian Centre for Occupational Health and Safety [CCOHS], 2022a). Training in good body mechanics has been shown to be insufficient in reducing back injuries among nurses. Evidence supports the use of mechanical lifts and transfer devices to reduce musculo-skeletal injuries among health care workers. A reduction of injuries among nursing home staff is plausibly attributed to the introduction of a strict "no lift policy" to prevent staff from manually lifting clients. This involves having sufficient mechanical lifting equipment for all residents who need it, along with the training in its uses, and regular battery charging. In addition, most facilities have a two-person lift policy, stating that there must be two staff members present who are trained to use the mechanical lift whenever a mechanical lift is used (Wilk et al., 2022).

Preventing Workplace Violence

- The CCOHS (2022b) defines workplace violence as "any act in which a person is abused, threatened, intimidated, or assaulted, in his or her employment" (p. 1).
- Nurses work with the public, including unstable or volatile clients. Nurses have access to narcotics. Most nurses are women. Concern is growing about violent incidents in the health care workplace, including concern about the tolerance of violence as "part of the job" (International Council of Nurses [ICN], 2017).

The WHO (2019) reported health care workers, mainly nurses and those involved in direct patient care, are exposed to physical violence, mainly from clients and visitors. Many more are threatened or exposed to verbal aggression (Bard et al., 2022).

TABLE 6.4 Provincial and Territorial Routine Vaccination Schedules for Healthy, Previously Immunized Adults

Abbreviations	Description	BC	AB	SK	MB	ON	QC	NB	NS	PE (3)	NL	YT	NT	NU (4)
Tdap(1)	Tetanus, diphtheria (reduced toxoid), acellular pertussis (reduced toxoid) vaccine	With each pregnancy	Every 10 years and each pregnancy	One booster dose per adult Lifetime and each pregnancy	One booster dose per adult Lifetime and each pregnancy	One booster dose per adult Lifetime and each pregnancy	With each pregnancy	One booster dose per adult Lifetime and each pregnancy	One booster dose per adult Lifetime and each pregnancy	Every 10 years and each pregnancy	Every 10 years and each pregnancy	One booster dose per adult Lifetime and each pregnancy	Every 10 years and each pregnancy	One booster dose per adult Lifetime and each pregnancy
Td	Tetanus and diphtheria (reduced toxoid) vaccine	Every 10 years	N/A	Every 10 years	Every 10 years	Every 10 years	One dose at 50 years of age	Every 10 years	Every 10 years	N/A	N/A	Every 10 years	N/A	Every 10 years
Inf	Influenza vaccine	Annually for adults aged 65+ years	Annually for all adults	Annually for all adults	Annually for all adults	Annually for all adults	Annually for adults aged 75+ years (2)	Annually for all adults	Annually for all adults	Annually for all adults	Annually for all adults	Annually for all adults	Annually for all adults	Annually for all adults
Pneu-P-23	Pneumococcal polysaccharide (23-valent) vaccine	65+ years one dose	65+ years one dose	65+ years one dose	65+ years one dose	65+ years one dose	65+ years one dose	65+ years one dose	65+ years one dose	65+ years one dose	65+ years one dose	65+ years one dose	65+ years one dose	50+ years one dose
Zos	Herpes Zoster (Shingles) vaccine	N/A	N/A	N/A	N/A	65 to 70 years Two doses	N/A	N/A	N/A	65 years and older Two doses	N/A	N/A	N/A	N/A

(1)National Advisory Committee on Immunization (NACI) recommends that all adults should receive one dose of Tdap vaccine if they have not previously received pertussis-containing vaccines in adulthood and with every pregnancy

(2)The influenza vaccine is no longer recommended for healthy adults age 60-74. However, if you would like to get the vaccine, you can do so free of charge.

(3)The HPV vaccine is publicly funded for the adult program. The HPV is recommended for all adult males with the following risk factors: having unprotected sex with multiple partners (male and female) or with a partner who has multiple partners; history of genital warts; individuals who missed the HPV immunization in grade 6 since 2012, HPV vaccine is recommended for all men who have sex with men(MSM); and for immunocompetent males and females who have HIV regardless of age. The HPV vaccine is recommended for adult females with the following risk factors: having unprotected sex with multiple partners (male and female) or with a partner who has multiple partners; history of genital warts; an abnormal PAP test; and individuals who missed the HPV immunization in grade 6 since 2007.

(4)Anyone under the age of 27 is eligible to receive Gardasil, an HPV vaccine.

N/A -Vaccine is not publicly funded in this province/territory.

The ICN "supports the development of policies that reflect a 'zero tolerance' of violence of any form from any source, including nurses themselves, in any workplace" (ICN, 2017). Furthermore, if quality client care is to be provided, nurses must be ensured a safe work environment and respectful treatment.

Potential interventions include the following:

- Promoting comfort and reducing client frustration in health care settings. Programs like the Gentle Persuasion Approaches (GPA) train health care providers in techniques and skills to safely handle and respond respectively to clients' responsive behaviours associated with dementia. "GPA teaches workers to be self protective, respectful, and non-violent in vulnerable care situations and to prevent potential workplace injury" (Wilk et al., 2022, p. 915).
- Promotion of staff competence in dealing with violence with proper training and resources. Instituting programs such as the Nonviolent Crisis Prevention program, which is available to help nurses learn respectful, noninvasive methods for de-escalating anger and safely managing disruptive and assaultive behaviour through behaviour management while still protecting the therapeutic relationship with those in their care (Crisis Prevention Institute [CPI], 2022).
- Ensuring that staff are not alone in emergency and other high-risk settings. This includes ensuring physical security of all health care facilities (Bard et al., 2022).
- Installing and maintaining alarm systems, wearing panic alarm badges
- Liaising with local police and reporting all incidents of violence
- Incidents of workplace violence should be reported so that strategies can be developed to reduce further occurrences in the workplace (Astle & Duggleby, 2024).

Reducing the Risk of Heart Disease and Cancer
Leading Causes of Morbidity and Mortality in Canada
The leading causes of morbidity and mortality among adults in Canada are cardiovascular disease and cancer. As with other diseases, the incidence is higher among low-income Canadians (Fournier & Karachiwalla, 2021). This group is a vulnerable population that is more likely than middle-income Canadians to have poor nutrition and to experience higher levels of stress. Nurses can contribute toward building healthier communities and to educating clients about modifying controllable risk factors.

Forms of cardiovascular disease include coronary artery disease, myocardial infarction (heart attack), and cerebral vascular accidents (CVAs, or stroke). Common forms of cancer include lung and colorectal cancer in both males and females. In females, the most common cancer is breast cancer and in males the most common cancer is prostate cancer.

Risk Factors for Cardiovascular Disease
The risk factors for developing cardiovascular disease can be divided into modifiable and nonmodifiable.

Modifiable risk factors are as follows:
- A sedentary lifestyle
- High blood pressure
- Tobacco use
- Obesity
- Poor diet
- High levels of blood fats (cholesterol, low-density lipoproteins, triglycerides)
- Diabetes mellitus
- Negative emotions, such as anxiety, depression, stress and anger
- Illegal drug use (cocaine, amphetamines, hallucinogens, heroin)

Nonmodifiable risk factors include:
- Heredity: Family history of having a first-degree relative with heart disease increases the risk.
- Age: The risk factor increases with age.
- Gender: Males have a greater chance of developing heart disease and dying from it, although this gap is slowly closing. Females have an increased risk factor after menopause (Dames et al., 2021).

Prevention
- Primary prevention of cardiovascular disease involves modification of any of the above risk factors that are within one's control: eating a balanced diet, exercising more, avoiding use of illicit drugs and tobacco products, and maintaining a normal body weight.
- Secondary prevention of cardiovascular disease includes screening for hypertension, elevated blood glucose levels, and blood fat levels. With medical advice, certain medications, such as statins and Aspirin, may also limit the progression of cardiovascular disease (Fournier & Karachiwalla, 2021).

Reducing Risk Factors for Cancer
- Minimize exposure to carcinogens in the environment.
- Being more physically active
- Practising safer sex
- Cigarette smoke is a leading cause of lung cancer. Efforts to reduce or eliminate tobacco use involve smoking prevention and cessation programs.
- Promote cancer-smart nutrition: diets high in antioxidant-rich fruits and vegetables; reducing dietary fats; avoiding smoked, cured, and barbecued meats; reducing alcohol intake; and maintaining a healthy body weight (Fournier & Karachiwalla, 2021).
- Risk factors for breast cancer include female gender; advancing age; menarche prior to age 12; combined estrogen–progesterone hormone replacement therapy; and heavy use of alcohol. However, some individuals diagnosed with breast cancer have no known risks other than being female (Canadian Cancer Society, 2022a). Having a first child in one's teens or 20s (Canadian Cancer Society, 2022b) and breastfeeding at any age do provide some protection from breast cancer.
- Skin cancers are malignancies that most often develop due to chronic or sporadic but intense overexposure to both natural and artificial sources of ultraviolet (UV) light

(Canadian Cancer Society, 2022c). Fair skin colouring, freckling tendency, high nevi count, a family history of skin cancer, outdoor occupations, outdoor recreational activities, smoking, and childhood sun-exposure history influence an individual's risk for skin cancer (Tyerman & Cobbett, 2023). The most important risk factor for melanoma skin cancer is ultraviolet (UV) radiation and indoor tanning (Canadian Cancer Society, 2022c). UV radiation damages the deoxyribonucleic acid (DNA) in skin cells, causing mutations in their genetic code and altering the cells (Tyerman & Cobbett, 2023). Artificial tanning is a multi-billion-dollar industry frequented by increasing numbers of teenaged girls and young women—and contributing to rising rates of skin cancer. Sun-blocking agents reduce sunburn and other skin damage with the goal of decreasing the risk of skin cancer. The sun protection factor (SPF) index is a measure used to determine the effectiveness of various preparations and is measured by Health Canada. An SPF 30 means the sunscreen will block 97% of ultraviolet B (UVB) rays, whereas an SPF 50 blocks 98% of UVB rays. Best protection is achieved by applying a broad spectrum, water-resistant sunscreen 30 minutes before exposure to sun and reapplying every 15–30 minutes during the sun exposure. Sunscreens that block both UVA and UVB rays are more effective in preventing skin cancer then those that block only UVB rays. Applying more applications may be required for activities involving swimming, perspiration, and rubbing of the skin (Dames et al., 2021).

- Best-practice sun protection involves precautions to avoid overexposure to the sun. Individuals should not use indoor sunlamps, tanning parlours, or tanning pills. Inform clients who are on medications that make the skin more sensitive to the sun (oral contraceptives, antibiotics, antihypertensives, anti-inflammatories, immunosuppressives) to take extra precautions when spending time in the sun. Inform parents to protect their children from the sun (Astle & Duggleby, 2024). Additional important health teaching includes informing clients to wear sunglasses with both UVA and UVB protection, wear sun-protective clothing, and avoiding sun bathing between 1000 and 1400 hours since two thirds of the day's UV light comes through the Earth's atmosphere at this time (Dames et al., 2021).

In their role as health educators, nurses have a responsibility to disseminate knowledge about cancer prevention, to help enable people to choose positive health behaviours, and to contribute to reducing our "ecological footprint" in our own workplaces. Ecological changes that reduce the emission of carcinogens (such as toxic wastes and pesticides) into the air, water, and soil we share involve collective action in our communities and nations and a commitment to planetary health.

Program Evaluation

Evaluation processes are critical entry-level competencies required of licenced/registered practical nurses. In health promotion practice, evaluation is essential to assessing, improving, and sustaining effective behavioural and environmental interventions that help to promote the health of individuals, families, and communities (Pender et al., 2015). Evaluation data, such as findings from a research study, can be used to advocate for policy change and to acquire funding to support the continuation and development of health promotion initiatives.

Evaluation should be ongoing throughout the design and implementation of health promotion interventions and programs. Process and outcome evaluations are two types of evaluations aimed at understanding the effectiveness of the content, approach, and results of the health promotion interventions. Process evaluations most often target health teaching content and delivery and are therefore helpful in improving the design and implementation of the interventions. On the other hand, outcome evaluations help us to understand the effects of our interventions on health. Outcome evaluations help to pinpoint what health-related changes have occurred as a result of the health promotion intervention (Pender et al., 2015).

For example, process evaluation might entail evaluating the effectiveness of health promotion teaching interventions with a group of clients recovering from a myocardial infarction or may involve having these same people evaluate the content of what was covered, the teaching style, and the usability of the pamphlets provided. Outcome evaluations of these same interventions could be delineated by tracking the rates of readmission for cardiac-related problems.

PRACTICE QUESTIONS

Case 1

The Canadian Nurses Association has recommended that nurses be involved in efforts to promote more environmentally responsible health care. A nurse is involved in the hospital's green team. The green team's goals are to improve the hospital's recycling practices, reduce energy use, and promote more environmentally preferable health care products.

Questions 1 to 3 refer to this case.

1. The nurse understands that both the energy used and the waste produced by the health sector significantly contribute to which of the following?
   1. Global climate change and emissions of dioxins
   2. Landfill runoff
   3. Contamination of indoor air
   4. The development of wind energy alternatives
2. The green team understands that the support of all hospital staff, health care consumers, and community administrators

is critical to designing and implementing effective, sustainable disease and injury prevention initiatives. This process is best referred to as which of the following?

1. Conflict resolution
2. Advocacy and community building
3. Focus-group planning
4. Community promotion

3. How would the nurse and the green team best increase environmentally responsible behaviours within their agency?

1. Meet with administrators to outline required policy changes.
2. Assess all clients for exposure to environmental contaminants.
3. Implement educational sessions on environmentally responsible health care.
4. Promote environmentally friendly products in the hospital gift store.

Case 2

A nurse visits a homeless shelter in a large Canadian city. Many clients have substance use problems and malnutrition. All fall into the low-income bracket.

Questions 4 to 7 refer to this case.

4. The nurse approaches the local food bank to ask for donations. What types of foods would be most appropriate for clients?

1. Calorie-rich
2. Nutrient-rich
3. Inexpensive
4. Canned

5. The nurse is committed to improving the health of the clients in the shelter. What strategy has the greatest chance of sustaining improved health for the people who are homeless?

1. Treatment of addictions
2. Stable housing
3. Treatment of chronic illnesses
4. Improved nutrition

6. There is an outbreak of tuberculosis at the shelter. What is the best action by the nurse to ensure that the affected clients comply with their medication regimen?

1. Arrange for the affected individuals to be admitted to hospital.
2. Provide directly observed therapy (DOT).
3. Administer the medications in a sustained-release formula.
4. Select medications that have the lowest incidence of side effects.

7. Many of the nurse's clients have chronic open and infected wounds. What is the most likely reason for these lesions to be chronic?

1. Frequent reinjury to wounds not adequately cleaned
2. Inadequate clothes and footwear to protect the skin
3. Close association with others who have infected sores
4. Poor wound healing due to protein–calorie malnutrition

Case 3

A licenced practical nurse at City Hospital is a certified Reiki therapist. A client, Olga, has asked the nurse to practise

Reiki on her as she recovers from breast cancer. The nurse is well informed and experienced with Reiki in their native Germany. City Hospital policies support the nurse in performing complementary therapies at work.

Questions 8 and 9 refer to this case.

8. What is the nurse's responsibility in this situation?

1. Therapies such as Reiki are controversial, and the nurse must not practise Reiki in an accredited hospital.
2. The nurse may practise Reiki within their role as a certified Reiki therapist, as they are fully competent, and Olga has made an informed and legitimate request.
3. The nurse may practise Reiki at City Hospital, but only after their assigned shift and not as part of their practical nursing duties.
4. The nurse may practice Reiki, but only after Olga is discharged from hospital.

9. Reiki is considered to be a complementary therapy. What is the definition of *complementary therapy*?

1. A therapy that is used in conjunction with traditional Western medicine
2. A therapy that is used instead of traditional Western medicine
3. A therapy that is considered to be homeopathic
4. A therapy that uses only natural methods for treatment

Case 4

Mrs. Broadfoot, age 42, is admitted to a large hospital from her remote northern community. She is experiencing complications from her type 2 diabetes, including kidney failure and peripheral vascular disease. Mrs. Broadfoot is an Indigenous person.

Questions 10 to 13 refer to this case.

10. What should the nurse consider first when developing a plan of care to recognize Mrs. Broadfoot's cultural beliefs and practices?

1. Include recognized Indigenous cultural factors.
2. Value Mrs. Broadfoot's individually expressed wishes.
3. Interview Mrs. Broadfoot's family for culturally specific guidelines.
4. Refer to the unit procedure for creating care plans for Indigenous people.

11. During morning care, the nurse begins a dialogue with Mrs. Broadfoot about her illness. Mrs. Broadfoot is often silent during this interaction. What is the most likely reason for Mrs. Broadfoot's silence?

1. She does not understand English.
2. She is too tired and weak to speak.
3. She is in denial about her health and does not wish to speak about it.
4. She is using a culturally common form of communication.

12. The nurse reviews the laboratory results and discovers Mrs. Broadfoot has a low hemoglobin indicating she is anemic. Which of the following foods would be best included in Mrs. Broadfoot's diet?

1. Beef liver
2. Tofu
3. Spinach
4. Fortified cereals

13. Mrs. Broadfoot has a sudden and unexpected myocardial infarction. Her family is notified but is not able to arrive by plane before she dies. What should the nurse do prior to performing a postmortem care for Mrs. Broadfoot?
    1. Leave Mrs. Broadfoot in her bed so the family may view the body.
    2. Ensure that there is consent for autopsy.
    3. Avoid touching the body until the traditional shaman has provided permission.
    4. Identify cultural death rites that should be respected.

Independent Questions

Questions 14 to 31 do not refer to a particular case.

14. The client is ready for discharge home after giving birth to a healthy infant. Which of the following safety instructions should be given to all families with infants?
    1. Infants should be positioned on their backs to sleep.
    2. Infants should be positioned on their bellies to sleep.
    3. Infants should be prohibited from cosleeping with their mothers.
    4. Infants should be bundled up in hats and booties when they sleep.

15. Which of the following are examples of primary prevention? **Select all that apply.**
    1. Annual Papanicolaou (PAP) smears
    2. Megavitamin therapy as a complementary therapy while receiving chemotherapy
    3. Removal of an inflamed appendix before it ruptures
    4. Remaining out of direct sunlight when working outdoors in summertime
    5. Eating a variety of healthy foods each day

16. Which of the following actions demonstrates a nurse who is providing culturally competent care? **Select all that apply.**
    1. Assisting the client with discussing their health problems with their family.
    2. Asking the client to describe their traditional healing methods.
    3. Encouraging the client to take medications as prescribed.
    4. Demonstrating the proper way to administer an insulin injection
    5. Assisting the spouse of a Puerto Rican client to safely light candles.

17. The client is asking the nurse about the best way to prevent cancer. The nurse explains to the client that from a nutritional point of view, the client should do which of the following? **Select all that apply.**
    1. Increase intake of antioxidant-rich fruits and vegetables.
    2. Maintain body weight in a healthy range.
    3. Increase intake of smoked, cured and barbecued meats.
    4. Reduce alcohol intake.
    5. Keep total fat intake to 10% or less.

18. A client is admitted to the hospital following a stroke. The client weighs 132 kg and has limited mobility. What is the safest way for the nurse to move the client from the bed to sit in a wheelchair?
    1. Implement good body mechanics during the transfer from bed to wheelchair.
    2. Assign two unregulated care providers to move the client from the bed to the wheelchair.
    3. Use a mechanical lift with the assistance of another health care provider.
    4. Explain the procedure carefully to the client to ensure they stand using the support aid.

19. A client who is 9 weeks pregnant tells the nurse they have been experiencing a lot of nausea but find that chewing on crystallized ginger root alleviates the nausea. The nurse should do which of the following?
    1. Tell the client to take only medications prescribed by a medical doctor.
    2. Inform the client that there is no scientific basis for this and that they are likely experiencing a placebo effect.
    3. Review current research about ginger as an antiemetic and share this information with the client.
    4. Caution the client that no medications or home remedies are safe in the first trimester of pregnancy while the baby's organs are forming.

20. The client has had nerve-sparing surgery for prostate cancer. The nurse includes sexuality in the postoperative health teaching. Which of the following sentences would best introduce the topic?
    1. "I know that you are concerned about achieving an erection after prostate surgery."
    2. "Are you in a sexual relationship now?"
    3. "Many clients feel concerned about their sexuality after prostate surgery."
    4. "You are lucky that with nerve-sparing surgery, you will not experience sexual difficulties."

21. The nurse is developing a health teaching plan for a 60-year-old man with the following risk factors for coronary artery disease (CAD). Which of the following risks factors should the nurse focus on when teaching the client?
    1. Family history of coronary artery disease
    2. Increased risk associated with the client's gender
    3. High incidence of cardiovascular disease in older persons
    4. Elevation of the client's low-density lipoprotein (LDL) level

22. A community health nurse is preparing an educational brochure about improving the nutritional behaviours of Canadians. Which of the following topics would most likely be included in the brochure? **Select all that apply.**
    1. Explanation of the food pyramid
    2. Decreasing daily sodium intake
    3. Increasing daily intake of fruits and vegetables
    4. Decreasing daily intake of sugar-sweetened drinks
    5. Increasing daily intake of saturated fats

23. The client has been advised by a nutritionist to increase intake of vitamin D to 1 000 international units (IU). How would the client best achieve this?
    1. Increase the amount of time spent in the sunshine to at least one hour each day.
    2. Increase their intake of milk.
    3. Take a vitamin D supplement.
    4. Eat a fortified ready-to-eat cereal each morning.

24. The nurse makes a presentation about the sexual health component of the Grade 5 health curriculum at a parent–teacher meeting. The nurse explains which of the following concerning children and sexuality?
    1. All people, regardless of age, are sexual beings.
    2. It is best for children to learn the correct facts about sexuality at school rather than from family or friends.
    3. A discussion about sexuality will prepare them for sexual intercourse.
    4. In Canadian culture, society values children learning about sexuality at an early age.

25. The nurse is discussing sleep habits with a client. Which of the following activities performed before bedtime can potentially interfere with the client's sleep? **Select all that apply.**
    1. Reading novels
    2. Listening to classical music
    3. Resolving family problems
    4. Eating a large meal 1 to 2 hours before bedtime
    5. Drinking warm milk

26. Which of the following clients are participating in alternative and complementary therapies? A client who **Select all that apply.**
    1. Listens to rap music to lessen anxiety from a painful dressing change.
    2. Burns lavender-scented candles while meditating.
    3. Takes chemotherapy recommended by an oncologist.
    4. Uses prayer during a parent's hospitalization.
    5. Practises yoga to increase balance.

27. Which of the following are risk factors for the development of breast cancer? **Select all that apply.**
    1. Cigarette smoking
    2. Early menarche
    3. Fibrocystic breast changes
    4. Breast trauma
    5. Heavy alcohol use

28. Which of the following are approaches to reduce the risk of falls in the older person? **Select all that apply.**
    1. Use of restraints for confused clients.
    2. Secure all mats and carpets so they do not skid.
    3. Lock beds and wheelchairs when transferring clients.
    4. Promote the wearing of skid-free footwear.
    5. Install grab rails near the toilet and tub.

29. A child has just been prescribed three different medications by the health care provider for asthma, in addition to an over-the-counter antihistamine for allergies. Noting that the family has financial concerns, what would be important for the nurse to say to the parent related to the child's treatment?
    1. "These medications are expensive. Do you have concerns or questions for me regarding the prescribed medications?"
    2. "Your child really needs these medications. You must be sure you buy them and give them to them as directed."
    3. "If you can't afford all these medications, don't give your child the antihistamine."
    4. "There are generic forms of these medications. I will change the prescription to the less expensive forms of the medications."

30. The parent of a 5-year-old child asks the nurse how best to teach their child to cross a street safely. How would the nurse respond?
    1. Buy the child a computer game about road safety for children.
    2. Reward the child every time they cross the street in an approved manner.
    3. Talk to the child daily about the rules of crossing the road.
    4. Provide role-modelling and practise street safety.

31. Which of the following is an example of screening? **Select all that apply.**
    1. Asking if someone wears sunscreen
    2. Performing a testicular self-examination
    3. Obtaining a mammogram
    4. Undergoing a needle biopsy
    5. Checking for skin cancer during regular client assessment
    6. Creating an exercise program for women with osteoporosis

REFERENCES

Allegrante, J., Wells, M., & Peterson, J. (2019). *Annual review of public health: Interventions to support behavioural self-management of chronic diseases.* https://www.annualreviews.org/doi/pdf/10.1146/annurev-publhealth-040218-044008

Astle, B., & Duggleby, W. (2024). *Potter and Perry's Canadian fundamentals of nursing* (7th ed.). Elsevier Inc.

Bandura, A. (2004). Health promotion by social cognitive means. *Health Education & Behavior, 31*(2), 143.

Bard, B., MacMullin, E., Williamson, J., et al. (2022). *Morrison-Valfre's foundations of mental health care in Canada.* Elsevier Inc.

Barton, J., & Rogerson, M. (2017). The importance of greenspace for mental health. National Library of Medicine. *BJPsych International, 14*(4), 79–81. https://www.ncbi.nlm.nih.gov/pmc/articles/PMC5663018/

Canadian Cancer Society. (2022a). *Learn about carcinogens in your environment.* https://cancer.ca/en/cancer-information/reduce-your-risk/know-your-environment/learn-about-carcinogens-in-your-environment

Canadian Cancer Society. (2022b). *Risks for breast cancer.* https://cancer.ca/en/cancer-information/cancer-types/breast/risks

Canadian Cancer Society. (2022c). *Risk factors for melanoma skin cancer.* https://cancer.ca/en/cancer-information/cancer-types/skin-melanoma/risks#ci_ultraviolet_radiation_uvr_46_6545_02

Canadian Centre for Occupational Health and Safety (CCOHS). (2022a). *Ergonomic safe patient handing program.* https://www.ccohs.ca/oshanswers/hsprograms/patient_handling.html?=undefined&wbdisable=true

Canadian Centre for Occupational Health and Safety (CCOHS). (2022b). *Violence and harassment in the workplace.* https://www.ccohs.ca/oshanswers/psychosocial/violence.html

Canadian Council for Nurse Regulators. (2013). *Standards of practice for licensed practical nurses in Canada.* https://www.clpna.com/wp-content/uploads/2013/02/doc_CCPNR_CLPNA_Standards_of_Practice.pdf

Canadian Council for Practical Nurse Regulators (CCPNR). (2013). *Code of ethics for licensed practical nurses in Canada.* https://www.clpna.com/wp-content/uploads/2013/02/doc_CCPNR_CLPNA_Code_of_Ethics.pdf

Canadian Holistic Nurses Association (2020). *Holistic nursing standards of practice.* https://www.chna.ca/wp-content/uploads/2022/06/CHNA-HOLISTIC-NURSING-STANDARDS-OF-PRACTICE-Revised-and-approved-June-922.pdf

Canadian Institute for Health Information. (2022). *National health expenditure trends, 2021-snapshot.* https://www.cihi.ca/en/national-health-expenditure-trends-2021-snapshot

Chehreh, R., Zahrani, S. T., Karamelahi, Z., et al. (2021). Effect of peer support on breastfeeding self-efficacy in Ilamian primiparous women. *Journal of Family Medicine and Primary Care, 10*(9), 3417–3423. https://journals.lww.com/jfmpc/Fulltext/2021/10090/Effect_of_peer_support_on_breastfeeding.44.aspx

Clendon, J., & Munns, A. (2019). *Community health and wellness. Principles of primary health care* (6th ed.). Elsevier Australia.

College of Nurses of Ontario. (2019). *Practice standard: Code of conduct.* Publication No. 49040. https://www.cno.org/globalassets/docs/prac/49040_code-of-conduct.pdf

Crisis Prevention Institute. (2022). *Nonviolent crisis intervention.* https://www.crisisprevention.com/en-CA/Our-Programs/Nonviolent-Crisis-Intervention?src=homepage_programs_list

Dames, S., Luctkar-Flude, M., & Tyerman, J. (2021). *Edelman and Kudzma's Canadian health promotion throughout the life span* (1st ed.). Elsevier Inc.

DiClemente, C. C., & Prochaska, J. O. (1998). Toward a comprehensive, transtheoretical model of change: Stages of change and addictive behaviors. In W. R. Miller, & N. Heather (Eds.), *Treating addictive behaviours* (2nd ed.) (pp. 3–24). Plenum.

Fournier, B., & Karachiwalla, F. (2021). *Shah's public health and preventive health care in Canada* (6th ed.). Elsevier Inc.

Freire, P. (1970). *Pedagogy of the oppressed.* Continuum.

Gloria, C., & Steinhardt, M. (2016). Relationships among positive emotions, coping, resilience and mental health. *Stress and Health, 32*(2), 145–156. https://doi.org/10.1002/smi.2589

Government of Canada. (2021). *Communicating effectively about immunization: Canadian immunization guide. Principles of effective communication.* https://www.canada.ca/en/public-health/services/publications/healthy-living/canadian-immunization-guide-part-1-key-immunization-information/page-5-communicating-effectively-immunization.html

Government of Canada. (2022a). *Social determinants of health and health inequalities: Social and economic influences on health.* https://www.canada.ca/en/public-health/services/health-promotion/population-health/what-determines-health.html

Government of Canada. (2022b). *The Canadian people: Newcomers.* https://www.canada.ca/en/immigration-refugees-citizenship/services/new-immigrants/learn-about-canada/canadians.html

Government of Canada. (2022c). *Canada's food guide.* https://food-guide.canada.ca/en/

Government of Canada. (2022d). *Your guide to a healthy pregnancy: Prenatal nutrition.* https://www.canada.ca/en/public-health/services/health-promotion/healthy-pregnancy/healthy-pregnancy-guide.html

Government of Canada. (2022e). *Immunization in Canada: Canadian immunization guide.* https://www.canada.ca/en/public-health/services/publications/healthy-living/canadian-immunization-guide-part-1-key-immunization-information/page-2-immunization-in-canada.html

Government of Canada. (2022f). *Vaccines for COVID-19: How to get vaccinated.* https://www.canada.ca/en/public-health/services/diseases/coronavirus-disease-covid-19/vaccines/how-vaccinated.html

Government of Canada. (2023). *Provincial and territorial routine vaccination programs for healthy, previously immunized adults.* https://www.canada.ca/en/public-health/services/provincial-territorial-immunization-information/routine-vaccination-healthy-previously-immunized-adult.html

Hagel, B., & Yanchar, N. (2013). *Canadian Paediatric Society (CPS). Position statement: Bicycle helmet use in Canada: The need for legislation to reduce the risk of head injury.* Reaffirmed 2020. https://cps.ca/en/documents/position/bike-helmets-to-reduce-risk-of-head-injury

Hales, D., & Lauzon, L. (2018). *An invitation to health* (5th ed.). Nelson.

Herlihy, B. (2022). *The human body in health and illness* (7th ed.). Elsevier Inc.

Hockenberry, M., Rodgers, C., & Wilson, D. (2022). *Wong's essentials of pediatric nursing* (11th ed.). Elsevier Inc.

International Council of Nurses. (2017). *Position statement: Prevention and management of workplace violence.* Author. https://www.icn.ch/sites/default/files/inline-files/PS_C_Prevention_mgmt_workplace_violence.pdf

Kirby, M. (2002). *Vol. 6: Recommendations for reform. The health of Canadians—the federal role.* The Standing Senate Committee on Social Affairs, Science and Technology.

LaLonde, M. (1974). *A new perspective on the health of Canadians. A working document.* Government of Canada. https://www.phac-aspc.gc.ca/ph-sp/pdf/perspect-eng.pdf

MacDonald, S., & Jakubec, S. (2022). *Stanhope and Lancaster's community health nursing in Canada* (4th ed.). Elsevier Inc.

Nisbet, E., Shaw, D., & Lachance, D. (2020). Connected with nearby nature and well-being. *Frontiers in Sustainable Cities, 2*(18), 1–13. https://www.frontiersin.org/articles/10.3389/frsc.2020.00018/full

Parachute. (2022). *Poisoning: Medications.* https://www.parachutecanada.org/en/injury-topic/poisoning/

Pender, N., Murdaugh, C., & Parsons, M. (2006). *Health promotion in nursing practice* (5th ed.). Pearson Prentice Hall.

Pender, N., Murdaugh, C., & Parsons, M. (2015). *Health promotion in nursing practice* (7th ed.). Pearson Education, Inc.

Pollard, C. L., & Jakubec, S. L. (2023). *Varcarolis's Canadian psychiatric mental health nursing: A clinical approach* (3rd ed.). Elsevier Inc.

Raihan, N., & Cogburn, M. (2022). *Stages of change theory.* StatPearls Publishing LLC. https://www.ncbi.nlm.nih.gov/books/NBK556005/

Rogers, R. W. (1975). A protection motivation theory of fears and attitude change. *Journal of Psychology*, 91(1), 93–114. https://doi.org/10.1080/00223980.1975.9915803

Rojas-Rueda, D., Nieuwenhuijsen, M., Gascon, M., et al. (2019). Green spaces and mortality: A systematic review and meta-analysis of cohort studies. *The Lancet Planetary Health*, 3(11), E469–E477. https://www.thelancet.com/journals/lancplh/article/PIIS2542-5196(19)30215-3/fulltext

Romanow, R. J. (2002). *Building on values: The future of health care in Canada—final report.* Commission on the Future of Health Care in Canada. https://publications.gc.ca/site/eng/237274/publication.html

Stanwick, R. (2022). *Canadian Paediatric Society (CPS). Statements of injury: Prevention and now.* https://cps.ca/en/blog-blogue/statements-of-injury-prevention-then-and-now

Statistics Canada. (2017). *Population growth: Migration increase overtakes natural increase* (Modified 2018). http://www.statcan.gc.ca/pub/11-630-x/11-630-x2014001-eng.htm

Statistics Canada. (2022a). *Indigenous population continues to grow and is much younger than non-Indigenous population, although the pace of growth has slowed.* https://www150.statcan.gc.ca/n1/daily-quotidien/220921/dq220921a-eng.htm?indid=32990-1&indgeo=0

Statistics Canada. (2022b). *How the Census counts Indigenous people in urban areas.* https://www150.statcan.gc.ca/n1/pub/11-627-m/11-627-m2022059-eng.htm. https://www150.statcan.gc.ca/n1/daily-quotidien/171025/dq171025a-eng.htm?indid=14430-1&indgeo=0

Stavrinos, D., Pope, C., Shen, J., et al. (2018). Distracted walking, bicycling and driving; Systematic review and meta-analysis of mobile technology and youth crash risk. *Child Development*, 89(1), 118–128. http://onlinelibrary.wiley.com/doi/10.1111/cdev.12827/full

Taylor, S. E., Klein, L. C., Lewis, B. P., et al. (2000). Biobehavioral responses to stress in females: Tend-and-befriend, not fight-or-flight. *Psychological Review*, 107(3), 411–429.

Tyerman, J., & Cobbett, W. (2023). *Lewis's medical-surgical nursing in Canada: Assessment and management of clinical problems* (5th ed.). Elsevier Inc.

Wilk, M., Sorrentino, S., & Remmert, L. (2022). *Sorrentino's Canadian textbook for the support worker* (5th ed.). Elsevier Inc.

World Health Organization (WHO). (1921). *Health promotion glossary of terms 2021.* World Health Organization, 9. Licence CC. https://doi.org/BY-NC-SA3.0IGO. 9789240038349-eng.pdf

World Health Organization (WHO). (2016). *What is health promotion?* http://www.who.int/features/qa/health-promotion/en/

World Health Organization (WHO). (2019). *Review of 40 years of primary health care implementation at country level.* https://cdn.who.int/media/docs/default-source/documents/about-us/evaluation/phc-final-report.pdf?sfvrsn=109b2731_4

World Health Organization (WHO). (2022). *Overview: Sexual health.* https://www.who.int/health-topics/sexual-health#tab=tab_1

Zhang, X., Zhang, Y., & Zhai, J. (2021). Home garden with eco-healing functions benefiting mental health and biodiversity during and after the COVID-19 pandemic: A scope review. *Frontiers in Public Health*, 9(7), 1–13.

BIBLIOGRAPHY

Bandura, A. (1977). *Social learning theory.* Prentice Hall.

Canadian Cancer Society. (2022). *What is breast cancer?* http://www.cancer.ca/en/cancer-information/cancer-type/breast/breast-cancer/?region=on

DiClemente, C. C. (2007). The transtheoretical model of intentional behaviour change. *Drugs and Alcohol Today*, 7(1), 29–33.

Registered Nurses' Association of Ontario. *Environmental determinants of health.* https://rnao.ca/category/topics/environmental-determinants-health

WEB SITES

- **Canada Communicable Disease Report (CCDR)** (https://www.canada.ca/en/public-health/services/reports-publications/canada-communicable-disease-report-ccdr.html): This government journal provides information on the prevention and control of emerging and persistent infectious diseases. It publishes surveillance reports, outbreak reports, original research, rapid communications, advisory committee statements.

- **Canadian Association of Nurses for the Environment** (https://cane-aiie.ca/): The Canadian Association of Nurses for the Environment is part of the Canadian Nurses Association (CNA) Network of Nursing specialities. They represent nurses who are dedicated to the improvement of planetary health among nurses and people in Canada and globally. Contains information about research, advocacy, education, practice and policy at all levels of nursing and society regarding the links between environmental disruption and human health.

- **Dietary Reference Intakes Tables** (http://www.hc-sc.gc.ca/fn-an/nutrition/reference/table/index_e.html#rvm): This Health Canada site contains information about daily requirements for different nutrients.

- **Canada's Food Guide** (https://www.canada.ca/en/health-canada/services/canada-food-guides.html): This site includes links to the latest version of the food guide for the general population as well as the food guide for First Nations people, Inuit, and Métis; translated versions of the food guide; and a wealth of other links pertaining to nutrition in Canada.

- **Natural and Nonprescription Health Products Directorate** (https://www.canada.ca/en/health-canada/services/drugs-health-products/natural-non-prescription.html): This Health Canada site provides information on natural health products for consumers and the industry.

Nursing Fundamentals and Clinical Skills

> Nurses need a strong knowledge base that is rooted in the best evidence in order to provide high-quality and safe care to clients in the health care setting. This chapter provides a review of the fundamental knowledge that underlies all nursing care and the clinical skills that are needed to enact this care.

VITAL SIGNS

Body Temperature

Body temperature represents the balance between heat produced and heat lost by the body. Acceptable body temperatures range from 36–38°C, but there is not one temperature that is normal for all people. The average oral, temporal, or tympanic temperature is 37°C for a healthy adult and 36°C for an older person. Rectal temperatures are 0.5°C higher (37.5°C) and axillary temperatures are 0.5°C lower (36.5°C) than oral temperatures (Astle & Duggleby, 2024). See Box. 7.1 for average temperatures based on age.

Core and Surface Temperatures

- Core temperatures (temperatures of the deep tissues) are relatively constant. Examples include rectal, tympanic, esophageal, pulmonary artery, and urinary bladder temperatures.
- Surface temperatures fluctuate depending on blood flow to the skin and environmental conditions. Examples include skin, axillary, and oral temperatures.

Temperature Measurement Sites

The temperature measurement sites used routinely are the mouth, rectum, axilla, and tympanic membrane. It is the nurse's responsibility to choose the safest and most accurate site for a particular client. Listed next are advantages and disadvantages of the commonly used sites (Astle & Duggleby, 2024).

Oral temperature. Oral temperatures reflect rapid fluctuations in the core temperature. They cannot be used in infants or small children, or in confused, uncooperative, or unconscious clients. It is also necessary to wait 20 to 30 minutes before taking an oral temperature if the client has smoked or ingested hot or cold liquids or foods. Oral temperature readings can also be affected if the client is receiving oxygen therapy while taking the temperature.

Rectal temperature. Rectal temperatures are the preferred method of measurement in young children who cannot use oral thermometers, but they should not be used for newborns due to the risk of anal perforation. Some disadvantages are that rectal temperatures may lag behind a core temperature during rapid temperature changes, and they require privacy and the use of a lubricant. Other disadvantages are that obtaining a rectal temperature is an invasive procedure that may cause client discomfort, embarrassment, and anxiety.

Axillary temperature. Axillary temperature is the safest site to measure temperatures in newborns. It is an appropriate site in uncooperative or unconscious clients. Disadvantages include a longer measurement time and a lag behind core temperature during rapid temperature changes.

Tympanic membrane temperature. The tympanic membrane is an easily accessible site that provides a core temperature quickly; however, it has greater variability in results than other core temperature methods due to user variability. Inconsistencies regarding the accuracy of tympanic membrane temperature measurements in determining fever in infants and small children have been reported in the literature (Hockenberry et al., 2022).

Temporal artery temperature. The temporal artery site is easy to obtain without changing the client's position. Measurement is comfortable and eliminates the need to remove clothing. Measurement is useful in premature infants, newborns, and children. Measurement reflects rapid change in core temperature. Using this site provides a considerable reduction in required nursing time to measure, but it is inaccurate with a head covering or hair on the client's forehead, and it is affected by skin moisture such as diaphoresis or sweating (Cobbett, 2024).

Skin temperature. Skin temperature is safe and noninvasive. One example of a skin thermometer is the temperature-sensitive patch or tape applied to the forehead or abdomen. The patch changes colours at different temperatures, and if an abnormal temperature is suspected, the temperature needs to be confirmed with an electronic temperature device. Advantages are that the nurse can obtain a continuous reading on a client and the site is appropriate for newborn measurement. Disposable thermometers are not appropriate for monitoring temperature therapies (Astle & Duggleby, 2024).

Pulse

The *pulse* is the "bounding of arterial blood flow that is palpable at various points on the body" (Astle & Duggleby, 2024, p. 538). Any artery can be used for checking the pulse, but the radial and carotid arteries are most commonly used because they are easily palpable. The carotid pulse is commonly used in emergency situations.

BOX. 7.1 Average Normal Body Temperature

3–6 months: 37.5°C
1 year: 37.5°C
3 year: 37.2°C
5 year: 37°C
7 year: 36.8°C
9–11 years: 36.7°C
13 years: 36.6°C
Adults: (normal temperature ranges: 36–38°C)
  Average oral /tympanic/ temporal: 37°C
  Average rectal : 37.5°C
  Average axillary : 36.5°C

Based on Hockenberry, M., Rodgers, C., & Wilson, D. (2022). *Wong's essentials of pediatric nursing* (11th ed., p. ES2). Elsevier; Potter, P., Perry, A., Stockert, P., Hall, A., Astle, B. J., & Duggleby, W. (2019). *Canadian fundamentals of nursing.* (6th ed., p. 527, Box 30-1). Elsevier.

TABLE 7.1 Normal Resting Pulse Rates Across Age Groups

Age	Awake Rate	Sleeping Rate
Neonate (< 28 days)	100–205	90–160
Infant (1 month–1 year)	100–190	90–160
Toddler (1–2 years)	98–140	80–120
Preschool (3–5 years)	80–120	65–100
School age (6–11 years)	75–118	58–90
Adolescent (12–15 years)	60–100	50–90
Age/Condition	**Awake Rate**	**Sleeping Rate**
Well-conditioned athlete	May be 50–60	50–100
Adult	74–76	60–100
Older person	74–76	60–100

Adapted from Potter, P., Perry, A., Stockert, P., Hall, A., Astle, B. J., & Duggleby, W. (2019). *Canadian fundamentals of nursing* (6th ed., p. 546, Table 30-3). Elsevier; Hockenberry, M., Rodgers, C., & Wilson, D. (2022). *Wong's essentials of pediatric nursing* (11th ed., p. ES1). Elsevier.

Common Pulse-Rate Assessment Sites

The radial and apical locations are the most common sites for pulse-rate assessment in adults.

Radial pulse. Assessment of the radial pulse includes measurement of the rate (60–100 beats per minute in adults), rhythm (regular or irregular), strength or force (bounding, strong, weak, or thready), and equality (assessing radial pulses in both arms). If the pulse is regular, the nurse counts the pulse rate for 30 seconds and multiplies by 2. If the pulse is irregular, the nurse counts the pulse rate for 1 full minute. Refer to Table 7.1 for the normal resting pulse rates across various age groups.

Apical pulse. The apical pulse is measured with a stethoscope. It is located at the fifth intercostal space at the left midclavicular line. The apical rate is used to count the heart rate in infants and young children where the heart rates are very rapid and difficult to palpate and count accurately at a peripheral site. The apical site is also used to auscultate heart sounds when an abnormal peripheral pulse is palpated. Nurses auscultate and count the apical pulse for 1 full minute for newborns, if the heart rate is irregular, or if the client is receiving cardiac medication.

Key Terms Related to Pulse

- *Bradycardia* is a heart rate below 60 beats per minute in an adult.
- *Tachycardia* is a heart rate above 100 beats per minute in an adult.
- *Dysrhythmia* is an irregular or abnormal rhythm.
- *Sinus arrhythmia* is a normal increase in heart rate associated with inspiration. It is more common in children but often found in adults.
- *Pulse deficit* is the difference between the apical and radial pulse rates. It is frequently associated with an abnormal rhythm and is a result of ineffective heart contractions where the pulse wave is not transmitted to the periphery (Astle & Duggleby, 2024). Apical and radial rates are assessed at the same time by two nurses to determine the presence of a pulse deficit.

Respirations

Respiration is "the mechanism that the body uses to exchange gases between the atmosphere and the blood and between the blood and the cells" (Astle & Duggleby, 2024, p. 545).

Assessment of Respirations

Accurate measurement of respirations requires observation and palpation of chest wall movement. A complete assessment includes assessment of respiratory rate (10–20 breaths per minute in adults), depth (deep, normal, or shallow), and rhythm (regular or irregular). The nurse counts respirations for 30 seconds if respirations are normal and for 1 full minute if abnormalities are suspected. Refer to Table 7.2 for acceptable ranges of respirations rates by age.

Key Terms Related to Alterations in Adult Breathing Patterns

- *Bradypnea* is regular but slow breathing at a rate of less than 12 breaths per minute (Astle & Duggleby, 2024).
- *Tachypnea* is regular but rapid breathing at a rate of greater than 20 breaths per minute (Astle & Duggleby, 2024).
- *Hyperpnea* is laboured, deep respirations at a rate of greater than 20 breaths per minute. It occurs normally with exercise (Astle & Duggleby, 2024).
- *Apnea* is the temporary cessation of breathing which then resumes. Persistent cessation results in respiratory arrest (Astle & Duggleby, 2024).
- *Dyspnea* is shortness of breath resulting in laboured or difficult breathing (Astle & Duggleby, 2024).
- *Orthopnea* is an abnormal condition in which a person uses multiple pillows when lying down or must sit with their arms elevated and leaning forward to breathe deeply or comfortably. Assessment includes noting the number of pillows used by the client. Clients with orthopnea also report sleeping in recliners (Astle & Duggleby, 2024).

Pulse Oximetry

Pulse oximetry is the indirect measure of arterial oxygen saturation and pulse rate. The pulse oximeter measures pulse

TABLE 7.2 Acceptable Ranges of Respiratory Rates by Age

Age	Rate (breaths per minute)
Newborn	30–60
Infant (6 months)	30–50
Toddler (2years)	25–32
Child and preadolescent (3–12 years)	20–30
Adolescent (13–18 years)	16–19
Adult (older than 18 years)	10–20

Adapted from Astle, B., & Duggleby, W. (2024). *Potter and Perry's Canadian fundamentals of nursing* (7th ed., p. 548, Table 31.5). Elsevier Inc.

TABLE 7.3 Normal Blood Pressure Ranges By Age

Age	Blood Pressure Range (mm Hg)
Infant	Systolic 65–115
	Diastolic 42–80
7 years	Systolic 87–117
	Diastolic 48–64
14–17 years	Blood pressure will vary according to body size
Adult	Average blood pressure is 120/80
	Blood pressure over 140/90 is defined hypertension

Adapted from Wilk, M., Sorrentino, S., & Remmert, L. (2022). *Sorrentino's Canadian textbook for the support worker* (5th ed., p. 550, Table 24.4). Elsevier.

oxygen saturation (SpO₂), which is a reliable estimate of SaO₂, the percentage of hemoglobin that is bound with oxygen in the arteries or the percentage of saturation of hemoglobin (Astle & Duggleby, 2024). It is usually between 95 and 100%. Pulse oximetry below 70% is life-threatening. Some factors that affect accurate readings include peripheral vascular disease, hypothermia, hypotension, peripheral edema, jaundice, and the presence of nail polish. For clients with decreased peripheral perfusion, the nurse can apply a forehead sensor. With adults, reusable or disposable probes may be applied to the earlobe, finger, toe, bridge of nose, or forehead. In pediatric clients, pulse oximetry involves placement of a sensor and a photodetector in opposition around a foot, finger, toe, or earlobe with the sensor on top of the nail when digits are used (Astle & Duggleby, 2024; Hockenberry et al., 2022).

Blood Pressure

Blood pressure (BP) is the force of the blood under pressure pushing on the walls of an artery (Stephen & Skillen, 2021). BP depends on cardiac output and systemic vascular resistance. BP is a good indicator of cardiovascular health.

Measurement of BP

- *BP* is recorded in millimetres of mercury (mm Hg) as the systolic over the diastolic reading (e.g., 120/80 mm Hg). Optimal BP is less than 120/80 mm Hg. Refer to Table 7.3 for normal blood pressure ranges according to age.
- *Systolic BP* is the peak of maximum pressure when the left ventricle contracts and ejects blood under high pressure into the aorta.
- *Diastolic pressure* is the minimum pressure (resting pressure) exerted on the arterial walls when the ventricles relax.
- *Pulse pressure* is the difference between the systolic and diastolic pressures. For a BP of 130/90, the pulse pressure is 40 mm Hg.

Korotkoff sounds. *Korotkoff sounds* are the sounds of blood flow auscultated during BP measurement. There are five sounds; the first sound (onset of clear rhythmic tapping) and the last sound (disappearance of sound) are used for the systolic and diastolic BP readings in adolescents and adults (Jarvis et al., 2024; Stephen & Skillen, 2021).

Auscultatory gap. The *auscultatory gap* is the temporary disappearance of Korotkoff sounds during auscultation of BP. It typically occurs between the first and second Korotkoff sounds and may range from 10 to 40 mm Hg. It is more common in clients with hypertension or older person. It can cause underestimation of systolic BP or overestimation of diastolic BP (Jarvis et al., 2024; Stephen & Skillen, 2021).

Nursing considerations related to measurement of BP.
- Verify BP in both arms initially to compare and collect baseline data.
- Lower extremities (e.g., the popliteal artery behind the knee) can be used if the arms are not accessible.
- Choose a cuff with a bladder size matched to the size of the arm. For BP measurements by auscultation, the bladder width should be close to 40% of arm circumference and bladder length should cover 80 to 100% of arm circumference (Astle & Duggleby, 2024; Stephen & Skillen, 2021).
- Avoid applying the BP cuff to an arm with intravenous (IV) therapy, an arteriovenous shunt or fistula, breast or axillary surgery, a cast, or a bulky bandage.

Hypertension

Hypertension is persistently elevated BP and is often asymptomatic. It is the result of thickening and loss of elasticity of arterial walls. Hypertension is present when diastolic readings are greater than 90 mm Hg and systolic readings are greater than 140 mm Hg. The diagnosis of high normal BP is a diastolic reading between 85 and 89 mm Hg and systolic BP between 130 and 139 mm Hg. The diagnosis of high normal BP (hypertension) is made on the basis of two or more BP readings on consecutive visits (Astle & Duggleby, 2024).

Hypotension

Hypotension occurs when the systolic BP falls to 90 mm Hg or below (Astle & Duggleby, 2024). This can be a normal BP for some adults, but it is often associated with illness. Possible causes of low BP include pregnancy, medications (particularly those used to treat high BP), heart or endocrine problems, dehydration, severe blood loss, severe infection (septicemia), allergic reaction (anaphylaxis), or nutritional deficiencies.

Orthostatic Hypotension

Orthostatic hypotension, or *postural hypotension*, occurs when a person with BP within the normal range develops symptoms and low BP when moving to an upright position. Symptoms include fainting, weakness, or light-headedness, as well as a drop in BP and a rise in pulse rate. Clients at risk for orthostatic hypotension include clients with dehydration, anemia, recent blood loss, prolonged immobility, or new medications such as antihypertensives. To assess for orthostatic hypotension, the nurse records BP and pulse with the client supine, sitting, and standing (Astle & Duggleby, 2024).

INFECTION PREVENTION AND CONTROL

Infectious Process

Infection is the invasion of the body by pathogens (disease-producing organisms) and the reaction of the tissues to their presence and to the toxins generated by them. Signs and symptoms of infection may be local or systemic.

- Areas of localized infection may exhibit redness, swelling, and warmth or heat due to inflammation. Other symptoms may include discharge or exudate and pain or tenderness at the site.
- Systemic infections cause more generalized symptoms, such as fever, fatigue, and malaise. Other symptoms include enlargement of lymph nodes in the involved area, loss of appetite, nausea, or vomiting.
- Infections in older persons may not present typically as they tend to have lower body temperature, decreased pain sensation, and a reduced immune response to infection. They may have advanced infection before it is identified.

Chain of Infection

The development of an infection occurs in a cycle that depends on the presence of all of the following six elements: infectious agent, reservoir, portal of exit, mode of transmission, portal of entry, and susceptible host (Astle & Duggleby, 2024). Health care workers follow infection prevention and control practices to break the links in this chain so that infections will not develop.

1. *Infectious agent (pathogen):* an invading organism such as a bacterium, virus, fungus, or protozoan
2. *Reservoir:* an environment in which a pathogen can survive and may or may not multiply; the human body is the most common reservoir
3. *Portal of exit:* a mode of escape from the reservoir (e.g., the mouth, nose, rectum, vagina, urethra opening, or respiratory or gastro-intestinal tract)
4. *Mode of transmission:* the method by which a pathogen is transmitted to a new host (direct or indirect contact, airborne, food, and so on)
5. *Portal of entry:* the means by which the pathogen enters a new host (such as via the respiratory tract or through broken skin or mucous membranes)
6. *Susceptible host:* susceptibility depends on the individual degree of resistance to a pathogen

Health Care–Associated Infections

Health care-associated infections (HAIs) are also known as nosocomial infection or iatrogenic infection, acquired after admission to a hospital or another health care agency that were not present or incubating at the time of admission. Clients most susceptible are children and older person and individuals with severe underlying illness, a weak immune system, poor nutritional status, or loss of skin integrity. Clients in critical care settings are most susceptible because of the necessity for many invasive lines (including vascular access devices and urinary catheters) and the heavy use of antibiotics.

Medical and Surgical Asepsis
Medical Asepsis

Medical asepsis (clean technique) refers to procedures used to reduce and prevent the spread of microorganism. Common examples include hand hygiene, using clean disposable gloves to prevent direct contact with blood or body fluids, and cleaning the environment and equipment routinely (Astle & Duggleby, 2024).

Surgical Asepsis

Surgical asepsis (sterile technique) includes all procedures used to eliminate all microorganisms, including pathogens and spores, from an object or area. Examples of surgical asepsis include (a) procedures in which the client's skin is punctured (such as IV insertion or injections); (b) nonintact skin due to injury or surgery; and (c) insertion of catheters or surgical instruments into sterile body cavities (urinary catheterization, peritoneal dialysis catheters, and so on) (Astle & Duggleby, 2024).

Key principles of surgical asepsis

- A sterile object remains sterile only when touched by another sterile object.
- Only sterile objects may be placed on a sterile field. The package or container holding a sterile object must be intact and dry. A package torn, punctured, wet, or open is considered unsterile.
- A sterile object or field out of the range of vision or an object held below a person's waist is considered contaminated.
- A sterile object or field becomes contaminated by prolonged exposure to airborne microorganism.
- When a sterile surface comes in contact with a wet, contaminated surface, the sterile object or field becomes contaminated by microorganism drawn from above or below by capillary action.
- Fluid flows in the direction of gravity. A sterile object becomes contaminated if gravity causes an unsterile liquid to flow over the object's surface.
- The edges of a sterile field or container are considered to be unsterile. When the edges of a sterile drape or towel touches an unsterile surface (table, bed linen), a 2.5-cm border around the drape is considered contaminated. The edge of a sterile container becomes exposed to air after it is opened and is therefore contaminated.
- The lip of an opened bottle of solution becomes contaminated after it is exposed to air. When pouring a sterile

liquid, first pour a small amount of solution to wash away microorganism on the bottle lip. The small amount of solution is then discarded; pour a second time on the same side to fill a container with the desired amount of solution (Astle & Duggleby, 2024).

- Qualities such as conscientiousness or an "infection-control conscience," vigilance, and honesty are very important in maintaining surgical asepsis (Tyerman & Cobbett, 2023).

Infection Prevention and Control Guidelines

The risk of transmitting infection in the hospital is high, so health care workers must follow strict infection-control guidelines to prevent and control the spread of infection. Guidelines consist of two tiers: one tier of precautions to be followed for the care of all clients, called *routine practices*, and a second tier called *additional precautions* to be used to contain or isolate pathogens in one area.

Routine Practices

Routine practices (called *standard precautions* by the US Centers for Disease Control and Prevention [CDC]) are infection-control precautions designed for the care of "all clients in any setting regardless of their diagnosis or presumed infectiousness" (Astle & Duggleby, 2024, p. 698). Routine practices "apply when a health care worker is or potentially may be exposed to (a) blood; (b) all body fluids, secretions, and excretions except sweat; (c) nonintact skin; or (d) mucous membranes" (Astle & Duggleby, 2024, p. 698). Routine practices include hand hygiene; use of personal protective equipment (PPE) such as gloves, masks, eye protection, face protection, or gowns; proper disposal of sharps; routine cleaning of client equipment; waste disposal; care of laundry; and routine environmental cleaning. A key element of routine practices is to assess the risk of transmission of microorganisms before any interaction with all patients, clients, and residents, regardless of their diagnosis or infection status, and then to decide on risk-reduction strategies (Tyerman & Cobbett, 2023).

Additional Precautions

Additional precautions (called *transmission-based precautions* by the CDC) are designed to contain pathogens in one area, usually a client's room, so they are also called *isolation precautions*. These precautions are the second tier of basic infection control in addition to routine practices. There are three categories of precautions (airborne, droplet, and contact), and the category that is used depends on how a particular pathogen is spread. Some infections may require a combination of additional precautions since microorganism can be transferred by more than one route. When used either by themselves or in combination, these precautions are used in addition to routine practices (Tyerman & Cobbett, 2023).

    Airborne precautions. Airborne precautions are used for known or suspected infections caused by microbes transmitted by airborne droplets, such as measles, chicken pox (varicella), disseminated varicella zoster, and tuberculosis (TB). Barrier protection used with airborne precautions includes (a) a private negative-pressure room (door closed) and (b) a respiratory device, such as an N-95 respirator mask if the client has TB or when the client has the other conditions mentioned and the health care worker is not immune. A mask is also placed on the client if it is necessary for the client to leave the room (Astle & Duggleby, 2024).

    Droplet precautions. Droplet precautions are used for known or suspected infections caused by microbes transmitted by droplets produced by coughing, sneezing, or talking. Examples include diphtheria, rubella, influenza, pertussis, mumps, mycoplasmal or meningococcal pneumonia, scarlet fever, and sepsis. Barrier protection with droplet precautions includes (a) using a private room or cohorting clients (room door must be closed) and (b) using a mask (Astle & Duggleby, 2024; Tyerman & Cobbett, 2023).

    Contact precautions. Contact precautions are used for known or suspected infections caused by direct or indirect contact, such as colonization or infection with antibiotic-resistant organisms (AROs); major wound infections; respiratory infections such as respiratory syncytial virus; enteric infections such as *Clostridium difficile* (*C. difficile*); skin infections such as herpes simplex, impetigo, pediculosis, and scabies; and eye infections such as conjunctivitis. Barrier protection with contact precautions includes (a) using a private room or cohorting clients (the door can be open) and (b) using gloves and a mask when in contact with the client (Astle & Duggleby, 2024; Tyerman & Cobbett, 2023).

Hand Hygiene

Hand hygiene is the practice of removing or killing pathogens on the hands and maintaining good skin integrity (Astle & Duggleby, 2024). Hand hygiene consists of the use of alcohol-based hand rubs or handwashing and is the most important method of preventing HAIs.

    Alcohol-based hand rubs. Alcohol-based hand rubs or alcohol hand antiseptics are the gold standard for hand hygiene. They are quicker, easier, and more effective than handwashing if used correctly. The nurse must not use alcohol-based hand rubs of their hands are visibly soiled (e.g., with body fluids or blood).

    Handwashing. Handwashing must be performed when hands are visibly soiled. The mechanical action of washing, rinsing, and drying hands removes pathogens (Astle & Duggleby, 2024; Cobbett, 2024). Hands need to be washed with soap and water for 40 to 60 seconds with special attention to areas that are frequently missed, such as around the nails, the thumb area, and between the fingers. If the hands are visibly soiled, more time may be required to wash the hands. The decision of when and what type of hand hygiene to perform is based on the type of procedure or activity performed, the amount of time with the contaminated object or client, the degree or amount of contamination that will occur with the contact, and the susceptibility of the client or the health care worker to infection (Astle & Duggleby, 2024).

Personal Protective Equipment

PPE is clothing or equipment worn by health care providers for their protection. The use of PPE is part of routine practice when the nurse is likely to be in contact with blood, body fluids, mucous membranes, nonintact skin, body tissues, or contaminated equipment or surfaces (Astle & Duggleby, 2024). PPE includes the use of any or all of the following: masks, gloves, gowns, face protection, or eye protection. The choice of PPE is also dependent on the situation, procedure, or type of additional precautions required.

Multidrug-Resistant Organisms

Multidrug-resistant organisms (MDROs), also known as AROs or "superbugs," are "microorganisms, predominantly bacteria, that are resistant to one or more classes of antimicrobial agents" (Tyerman & Cobbett, 2023). The most common are MRSA (methicillin-resistant *Staphylococcus aureus*), CRE (carbapenem-resistant *Enterobacteriaceae*), VRE (vancomycin-resistant *Enterococci*), and *C. difficile*. During the last few decades, MDROs in hospitals have been increasing at alarming rates. Options for treating clients with these infections are extremely limited. Increased lengths of stay in hospital, costs, and mortality are associated with MDROs (Tyerman & Cobbett, 2023). There is strong evidence to suggest that MDROs are carried from client to client via the hands of health care providers (Tyerman & Cobbett, 2023).

Community-associated MRSA. MRSA infections that are acquired by persons who have not been hospitalized within the last year or undergone a medical procedure such as dialysis or surgery are known as *community-associated MRSA infections.* "Staph" or MRSA infections in the community continue to be on the rise, especially in rural, remote, and Indigenous communities in Canada. Some of the causative factors for higher risk rates include overcrowding, inadequate hygiene, poor housing conditions, pre-existing skin conditions, and high previous usage of antimicrobial medications. MRSA infection usually manifests as skin infections (pimples and boils) in otherwise healthy people (Mitevska et al., 2021).

MEDICATION ADMINISTRATION

The administration of medications is one of the primary responsibilities of nurses. It is important for nurses to have knowledge about the actions and effects of the medications that they give to clients. To safely and accurately administer medications, nurses also need knowledge about pharmacological concepts, human anatomy, growth and development, pathophysiology, psychology, nutrition, and mathematics (Astle & Duggleby, 2024).

Pharmacological Concepts
Medication Names

A medication has several different names, including a chemical, a generic, and a trade name:

1. The chemical name is a description of the medication's composition and molecular structure. This name is rarely used in clinical practice. An example of a chemical name is acetylsalicylic acid (Astle & Duggleby, 2024).
2. The generic or nonproprietary name is the first manufacturer's name for the medication, and this name is protected by law. It is the official name that is listed in the *Compendium of Pharmaceuticals and Specialties* and *Canadian Formulary.* An example of a generic name is acetaminophen (Astle & Duggleby, 2024).
3. The trade name, brand name, or proprietary name denotes the marketing name that the manufacturer uses to sell a medication. The trade name has a trademark (™) symbol beside it (as in Tempra™ or Motrin™), indicating that the name is trademarked (Astle & Duggleby, 2024).

Classification

Each medication can be categorized in one or more subcategories called *classifications.* Medications that affect the body in similar ways are in the same classification. Medication classification indicates "the effect of the medication on a body system" (Astle & Duggleby, 2024, p. 726). Medications can be in more than one classification if they have several different types of therapeutic effects, such as Aspirin, which is an analgesic, an antipyretic, and an anti-inflammatory. Other examples of medication classifications include antibiotics and antihypertensives.

Systems of Medication Administration
Metric System

The metric system involves decimals and uses divisions and multiples of 10. The basic units are metre (length), litre (volume), and gram (weight). Most countries, including Canada, use metric as their standard of measurement.

- Common metric abbreviations for volume include L (litre) and mm (millimetre).
- Common metric abbreviations for weight include kg (kilogram); g (gram); mg (milligram); and mcg (microgram).

Household Measurements

Prescriptions to be self-administered at home are often written in household measures. Examples include cups, teaspoons, or pints for volume; and ounces and pounds for weight.

Conversions and Calculations

Conversion between metric units. The metric system is a decimal system and is the most logically organized system of measurement. Metric units can be converted by simple arithmetic like multiplication and division. Each basic unit of measurement is organized into units of 10. Secondary units are formed by multiplying or dividing by 10. In multiplication the decimal point moves to the right, in division it moves to the left.

For example: 10 mg × 10 = 100 mg and 10 mg ÷ 10 = 1 mg (Astle & Duggleby, 2024).

To convert larger to smaller, multiply by 1 000 or move the decimal point three places to the right. For example, to convert 1 g to milligrams, multiply by 1 000 (1 × 1 000 = 1 000 mg). To convert smaller to larger, divide by 1 000 or move the decimal point three places to the left. For example, to convert 500 mL to litres, divide by 1 000 or move the decimal point three places to the left (500 ÷ 1 000 = 0.5 L).

Conversions between systems. The nurse may find it necessary to convert weights or volumes from one system to another. Metric units may need to be converted to household measurements for home administration. The nurse must know or refer to an equivalence table in this case. For example, if the client is to take 10 mL of brompheniramine-PPA (Dimetapp) elixir at home, the nurse must know that 1 teaspoon (tsp) equals 5 mL and that 10 mL = 2 tsp. Common conversions include the following:

$$2.2 \text{ lb.} = 1 \text{ kg}; \ 1 \text{ tbsp} = 15 \text{ mL}; \text{ and } 1 \text{ tsp} = 5 \text{ mL}$$

Dose calculations. There are several methods for calculating medication doses. The following methods are useful for either solid or liquid doses.

Example:

The health care provider has ordered 4 mg of morphine to be given subcutaneously.

The morphine is available in 10 mg/mL ampoules.

Solution using the formula method:

$$\frac{\text{Dose ordered}}{\text{Dose on hand}} \times \text{Amount on hand}$$
$$= \text{Amount to administer}$$

Using the formula, the amount to administer would be 0.4 mL (4 mg ÷ 10 mg × 1 mL = 0.4 mL)

Solution using dimensional analysis

$$x \, \text{mL} = \frac{1 \text{ mL}}{10 \ \cancel{\text{mg}}} \times \frac{4 \ \cancel{\text{mg}}}{1}$$

$$x \, \text{mL} = \frac{1 \times 4}{10} = 0.4$$

$$x = 0.4 \text{ mL}$$

Routes of Medication Administration
Oral Route

The oral route is convenient and easy, but it has a slow onset of action. This route is avoided when the client has gastro-intestinal alterations such as vomiting or reduced intestinal motility or has had gastro-intestinal surgery.

- Sublingual tablets are designed for rapid absorption when placed under the tongue.
- Buccal administration involves placing the solid medication in the mouth and against the mucous membranes of the cheek until the medication dissolves.
- Enteric-coated tablets and sustained-released capsules delay absorption until the medication reaches the small intestine, so these medications cannot be crushed.
- Liquid medications in quantities of less than 10 mL should be measured in an oral syringe for accuracy.
- If possible, tablets and capsules should be swallowed with 60–100 mL of fluid.

Parenteral Route

Parenteral administration is the injection of a medication into body tissues. There are four routes: intradermal (ID), subcutaneous, intramuscular (IM), and IV.

Intradermal route. *ID injection* refers to injection into the dermis, just under the epidermis. It is used for the tuberculin skin test or allergy testing. The most common site is the inner forearm. The bevel of the needle is pointing up during the injection so that medication is less likely to be deposited into tissues below the dermis. It is given at a 5- to 15-degree angle. A small bleb (resembling a mosquito bite) appears. The area should not be massaged.

Subcutaneous route. *Subcutaneous (subcut) injections* involve injecting medication into the loose connective tissue under the dermis at a 45- to 90-degree angle. Absorption of medication is slower via this route than via IM sites because adipose tissue is not very vascular. The most common sites are the outer posterior aspects of the upper arms, the abdomen, and the anterior aspects of the thighs. Only 0.5 to 1 mL should be given subcutaneously because subcutaneous injections can be painful. Injecting into a blood vessel during subcutaneous injections is very rare, so aspiration is not necessary. Pinch the skin before injection to elevate the skin and subcutaneous tissue above the muscle.

Typically, use a 25-gauge, 1.6-mm (5/8-inch) needle at a 45 degree angle or a 1.3-mm (1/2-inch) needle inserted at 90 degree angle to administer subcutaneous injections for normal-size adult clients. Some children may require only a 1.3-mm (1/2-inch) needle. To ensure the subcutaneous medication reaches the subcutaneous tissue, follow this rule: if you grasp 5 cm (2 inches) of tissue, insert the needle at a 90 degree angle; if you grasp only 2.5 cm (1 inch) of tissue, insert the needle at a 45 degree angle (Cobbett, 2024).

Subcutaneous medications requiring special consideration.

- Clients with diabetes who inject insulin should practise intrasite rotation (rotating injection sites within the same body part for 1 week before moving to a new location) to provide greater consistency in the absorption of insulin and prevent the development of lipodystrophy. Each injection site should be at least 1.25 to 2.5 cm away from the previous injection site (Sealock et al., 2021). Absorption rates of insulin vary based on injection site. Insulin is absorbed more quickly in the abdomen and more slowly in the thighs (Cobbett, 2024). When giving U-100 insulin, use U-insulin syringes with pre-attached 26- to 31-gauge needles.
- Injections of heparin and its derivative, low-molecular-weight heparin (LMWH), are best given in the abdomen, at least 5 cm (2 inches) from the umbilicus to prevent pain and bruising. Inject slowly to prevent bruising and pain, and do not massage these injection sites.

IM route. *IM injections* are administered directly into the muscle at a 90-degree angle. This route provides fast absorption due to the greater vascularity of muscle. The muscle can also tolerate more viscous or irritating substances. From 1 to 3 mL can be given intramuscularly, depending on the site. The Z-track method is recommended when administering IM injections because it minimizes local skin irritation by sealing the medication in the muscle tissue. IM injections are associated with more risks, and it is important that bony landmarks are used for landmarking all IM sites. The common IM injection sites are the ventrogluteal, vastus lateralis, and deltoid muscles. An IM injection usually requires an 18- to 27-gauge needle (most commonly used is 21- to 23-gauge needle), depending on the viscosity of the medication. Use longer needles (2.5 cm to 3.8 cm) for IM injections. Needle length is based on the size of the client and the location to be injected (Astle & Duggleby, 2024).

Ventrogluteal site. The ventrogluteal muscle is the safest site and the preferred site for adults and children over 7 to 12 months of age. It is free of major nerves and blood vessels and has easily palpable bony landmarks. The bony landmarks are the anterior superior iliac spine (ASIS) and the trochanter. The heel of the hand is placed over the greater trochanter with the thumb toward the groin and the fingers toward the client's head. The index finger (on the ASIS), the middle finger (on the iliac crest in the direction of the buttock), and the iliac crest form the injection site triangle (Fig. 7.1).

Dorsogluteal site. The dorsogluteal muscle was the traditional site for IM injections but is no longer recommended. There is risk of damage to the sciatic nerve as well as risk of injecting into the thicker subcutaneous tissue rather than the muscle in the area.

Vastus lateralis site. The vastus lateralis muscle is a site commonly used with infants and young children but may be used with adults as well. It is the preferred site for infants under 12 months receiving immunizations (Astle & Duggleby, 2024). The muscle is located on the anterior–lateral aspect of the thigh. Bony landmarks are the trochanter and the knee. The site for injection is the middle third of the muscle, a handbreadth below the trochanter and a handbreadth above the knee (Fig. 7.2).

Deltoid site. The deltoid muscle is an easily accessible site but is not well developed in all clients. This site should be used only for small medication volumes (less than 1 mL), when giving immunizations, or when other sites are not accessible (Astle & Duggleby, 2024). This site is not without risks as the axillary, radial, brachial, and ulnar nerves, as well as the brachial artery, lie in close proximity. The bony landmark used is the acromion process. The injection site is 3 to 5 cm below the acromion process (Fig. 7.3).

IV route. *IV injections* are administered directly into a vein. Medications are rapidly absorbed, and adverse reactions can happen immediately.

General principles for preparing parenteral injections
- When using a vial, inject air equal to the amount of medication that needs to be withdrawn into the vial to prevent negative pressure and to help with aspiration.
- When using an ampoule, tap the neck to force medication into the ampoule. Protect your fingers with an unopened alcohol wipe or a small gauze pad when snapping off the top of the ampoule.

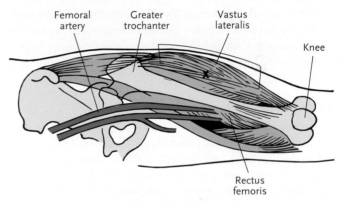

Fig. 7.2 Landmarks for the vastus lateralis site. (From Astle, B., & Duggleby, W. [2024]. *Potter and Perry's Canadian fundamentals of nursing* [7th ed., p. 794, Figure 35.31]. Elsevier Inc.)

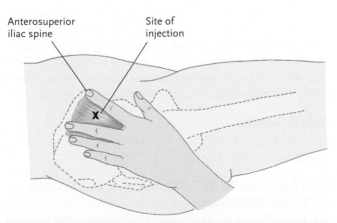

Fig. 7.1 Landmarks for the ventrogluteal site. (From Astle, B., & Duggleby, W. [2024]. *Potter and Perry's Canadian fundamentals of nursing* [7th ed., p. 793, Figure 35.30]. Elsevier Inc.)

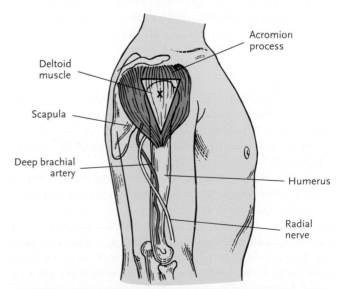

Fig. 7.3 Landmarks for the deltoid site. (From Astle, B., & Duggleby, W. [2024]. *Potter and Perry's Canadian fundamentals of nursing* [7th ed., p. 794, Figure 35.32]. Elsevier Inc.)

- Change the needle after drawing up medication from an ampoule or vial.
- Use the appropriate length needle to make sure the medication is deposited where it is intended to go.
- Inject medication slowly at a rate of 1 mL per 10 seconds to decrease pain and allow time for dispersion.
- The Z-track method is used for all substances given by IM injection. Z-track injections seal medications into muscle tissue and minimize local skin irritation. The skin and overlying subcutaneous tissues are pulled laterally prior to the injection, the needle is left in place for 10 seconds, and the skin is released after the injection. This leaves a zigzag path that seals the needle path and locks the medication in the muscle.
- Never recap needles. Use a one-handed scoop technique if it is absolutely necessary to recap.
- Use safety-engineered needles or needleless systems to eliminate the risk of needle-stick injuries. Some syringes are designed with a sheath or guard that encloses the needle after it is withdrawn from the skin to eliminate the possibility of a needle-stick injury (Astle & Duggleby, 2024). Several provinces in Canada have mandatory regulations for safety-engineered devices under their occupational health and safety acts.

Subcutaneous Butterfly Catheters

Subcutaneous butterfly catheters are used both for subcutaneous medication administration and hypodermoclysis. A subcutaneous butterfly catheter access site is used for repeated or intermittent medication doses for subcutaneous infusion of a medication. This route of administration can be used when oral routes are not possible. A fine-gauge needle (e.g., 24-gauge) is inserted into a client's subcutaneous tissue. The preferred site is the abdomen, but other sites include upper arm, upper back, anterior upper chest (avoid the breast and axilla area) and upper thigh. Only one type of medication can be injected after insertion of the catheter. The catheter must not be inserted into scar tissue, rash, a bruised area, or an area that has been recently irradiated (Astle & Duggleby, 2024).

Skin Route

Topical medications. Topical medications are applied to the skin by painting them, spreading them over an area, applying a moist dressing, soaking body parts in a solution, or giving medicated baths. These medications generally have local effects.

Transdermal medications. Transdermal medications have a systemic effect because they are applied topically via a transdermal disc or patch (such as nitroglycerine, scopolamine, or estrogen) that secures the medication to the skin and stays in place for 1 to 7 days (Astle & Duggleby, 2024). The old transdermal patch must be removed before applying the new patch, and it is important to use gloves for application of the new patch to prevent accidental absorption of the medication through the nurse's skin.

Mucous membrane medications

Eyes. Medications for eyes are available in the form of eye drops or eye ointments. Have the client look up before administering ophthalmic medications. Expose the lower conjunctiva. If using drops, place them in the lower conjunctiva near the outer canthus. If using ointment, squeeze a ribbon of ointment into the lower conjunctiva, moving from the inner to the outer canthus. Do not touch the eye with the bottle or tube. Have the client blink a few times to disperse the medication.

Ears. Otic medications are available in the form of ear drops or irrigations. If the client is supine, ask them to turn onto the unaffected side to aid gravitational flow. If they are sitting, tilt the client's head toward the unaffected side. Straighten the ear canal by pulling the pinna up and back for adults or down and back for infants and children under 3 years. Have the client remain on their side for 2 to 3 minutes to allow the medication to reach the inner ear canal. Apply gentle massage or pressure to the tragus of the ear with your finger unless contraindicated due to pain (Astle & Duggleby, 2024).

Nose. Nasal medications are available in atomizers or in drops. Clients should blow their noses first to clear any mucus. The client should be positioned with the head tilted back to aid in gravitational flow. The atomizer is squeezed quickly and firmly, or the correct number of drops is instilled in each nostril.

Vagina. Vaginal medications are available as liquid douches, creams, foam, jellies, suppositories, or tablets. The client should void prior to receiving vaginal medication. The client should be in the dorsal recumbent position with hips and knees flexed if possible. The applicator or suppository may need to be lubricated with a water-soluble lubricant. The labia are separated, and the applicator is inserted approximately 5 to 7.5 cm, angled downward and back.

Rectum. Rectal medications are available in the form of suppositories and enemas. (Refer to section on Enemas page 118 on how to administer an enema.) The client is positioned in a modified left lateral recumbent position. The suppository is lubricated with a water-soluble lubricant and inserted approximately 10 cm (past the internal anal sphincter) toward the wall of the rectum in the direction of the umbilicus. The client is encouraged to hold the suppository as long as possible for the medication to be effective.

Inhalation. Inhalants are available primarily in the form of metered-dose inhalers (MDIs) or dry powder inhalers (DPIs). They are designed to produce local effects such as bronchodilation. An MDI delivers a premeasured amount of medication with each push of the canister. A spacer may be used with an MDI for the client who is having difficulty coordinating all the steps involved in self-administration. DPIs hold dry powdered medication and create an aerosol when the client inhales.

Abbreviations

Abbreviations that are used in communicating the dosage administration schedule appear in Table 7.4.

Error-Prone and DO NOT USE Abbreviations, Symbols, and Dose Designations

The nurse should avoid unusual abbreviations and symbols and should always be familiar with the agency-approved abbreviation policy in the place of employment. Many abbreviations, symbols, and dose designations are frequently

TABLE 7.4 Common Dosage Administration Schedule Abbreviations

Abbreviation	Meaning
AC or ac	Before meals
ad lib	As desired
at bedtime	At bedtime (do not use abbreviation)
bid, BID	Twice a day
daily or every day	Daily (do not use abbreviation)
PC or pc	After meals
prn	Whenever there is a need
Qam	Every morning
qh	Every hour
q2h	Every 2 hours
qid, QID	Four times a day
STAT	Give immediately
tid, TID	Three times a day

From (Astle, B., & Duggleby, W. [2024]. *Potter and Perry's Canadian fundamentals of nursing* [7th ed., p. 732, Table 35.3]. Elsevier Inc.)

misinterpreted, have been involved in harmful medication errors (Table 7.5), and should never be used in communicating medical information.

Nursing Standards for Administration of Medication: The "10 Rights"

To administer medications safely and effectively in all practice settings, the nurse needs to be aware of provincial legislation and regulations as well as practice standards. Administering a medication requires knowledge, skill, and judgement. To ensure safe medication administration, the nurse needs to be aware of the following "10 rights" of medication administration.

Right Medication

- Administer only the medications that you prepare. Do not leave medications unattended. The nurse who administers the medication is responsible if there is an error.
- Perform three checks to compare the label on the medication package to the medication administration record (MAR). The three checks occur before removing the medication from the drawer or shelf, as the medication ordered is removed from the container or drawer, and before returning the container to the storage area (or before opening at the client's bedside for unit-dose medications).
- Compare any inconsistencies with the original health care provider's orders. Compare the MAR or computer order with the prescriber's written order.
- Listen to the client's concerns if the client states that the medication is different.
- Know both the generic and the trade name for the medication. Consult the pharmacist if you are unsure of a medication.

Right Dose

- Know the customary dose and appropriateness for different ages and sizes. Consult a reference book or pharmacist if uncertain.

- Ensure that all calculated doses or "high-alert medications" are checked by another registered nurse (RN). Make sure that double-checking is truly independent. High-alert medications are those that have a high incidence of medication errors associated with their administration. Double-checking alone will not always be the most practical strategy for error-reduction for some medication. Other special safeguards should be implemented to reduce the risk of errors. Strategies may involve standardizing orders; storage; preparation; administration of these medications; improving access to information about the medications; limiting access to special high-alert medications; and automated or independent double-checking. Some examples of high-alert medications are insulin, morphine, hydromorphone (Dilaudid), and heparin (Institute for Safe Medication Practices [ISMP], 2018a, 2021).
- Understand that pill cutters should be used to split pills and crushing devices should be used to crush pills. Enteric-coated pills or sustained-release capsules cannot be crushed or split.

Right Client

- Use two unique client identifiers to identify your client. For example, check the MAR against the client's identification bracelet and ask the client to state their full name.
- Acquire a new identification bracelet for the client if one is missing, illegible, or incorrect.
- Some facilities use a wireless bar-code scanner to help identify the right client. The bar code scans the single dose medication package and the client's armband.

Right Route

- Contact the prescriber if the route is not specified.
- Prepare injections from preparations designated "for injectable use only."
- Use special oral syringes (not compatible with IV tubing) for oral medications.

Right Time and Frequency

- Ensure that all routinely ordered medications are given within a 60-minute window around the times for which they are ordered (i.e., 30 minutes before or after the prescribed time).
- Understand why a medication is ordered for certain times of the day and whether the times can be altered. For example, a medication is ordered every 8 hours around the clock to maintain a therapeutic blood level in comparison with a medication ordered tid and meant to be given only during the hours the client is awake.
- Exercise clinical judgement in determining the proper time for administration of certain medications, such as prn medications.

Right Documentation

- Chart the time administered as well as the site for injections with your signature.

TABLE 7.5   Error-Prone and DO NOT USE Abbreviations, Symbols, and Dose Designations

Term	Intended Meaning	Misinterpretation	Correction
μg** (do not use)	microgram	Mistaken as "mg"	Use "mcg"
D/C** (do not use)	Discharge	Interpreted as "discontinue what ever medication follows" (typically discharge medications)	Use "discharge"
U or u** (do not use)	Unit(s)	Mistaken as number 0 or 4 , causing a tenfold overdose or greater (e.g., 4U seen as "40" or 4u seen as "44") Mistaken as cc. leading to administering volume instead of units. (e.g.,4u seen as 4cc)	Use "unit"
OD or od** (do not use)	Once daily	Mistaken as "right eye" (OD. oculus dexter), leading to oral liquid medications administered in the eye	Use "daily"
Q.D., ., QD, q.d., or qd** (do not use)	Every day	Mistaken as q.i.d. (four times daily), especially if the period after the q or the tail of a handwritten q is misunderstood as the letter "i"	Use "daily"
SC, sc, SQ, sub q or sq	Subcutaneous(ly)	SC and sc mistaken as SL or sl (sublingual); SQ mistaken as "5 every" The q in sub q has been mistaken as "every"	Use "SUBQ (all UPPERCASE letters, without spaces or periods between the letters or "subcutaneously"
SSRI	Sliding scale regular insulin	Mistaken as selective-serotonin reuptake inhibitor	Use sliding scale insulin
SSI	Sliding scale insulin	Mistaken as Strong Solution of Iodine (Lugol's)	
Q6PM, etc.	Every evening at 6 PM	Mistaken as every 6 hours	Use daily at 6 PM or 6 PM daily
Q1h	Daily	Mistaken as qid (four times a day)	Use daily
Qn	Nightly or at bedtime	Mistaken as qh (every hour)	Use nightly or HS for bedtime
Qhs	Nightly at bedtime	Mistaken as qhr (every hour)	Use nightly or HS for bedtime
HS	Half-strength	Mistaken as bedtime	Use half-strength
hs	At bedtime, hours of sleep	Mistaken as half-strength	Use HS (all UPPERCASE letters) for bedtime
Per os	By mouth, orally	The os was mistaken as left eye (OS, ocular sinister)	Use PO, by mouth, or orally
OD, OS, OU** (do not use)	Right eye, left eye, each eye	Mistaken as AD, AS, AU (right ear, left ear, each ear)	Use right eye, left eye, or each eye
IN	Intranasal	Mistaken as IM or IV	Use NAS (all UPPERCASE letters or intranasal
AD, AS, AU	Right ear, left ear, each ear	Mistaken as OD, OS, OU (right eye, left eye, each eye)	Use right ear, left ear, each ear
Ng or ng	Nanogram	Mistaken as mg Mistaken as nasogastric	Use nanogram or nanog
MM or M	Million	Mistaken as thousand	Use million
M or K	Thousand	Mistaken as million M has been used to abbreviate both million and thousand (Mis the Roman numeral for thousand)	Use thousand
L	Litre	Lowercase letter l mistaken as the number 1	Use L (UPPERCASE) for litre
ml	Millilitre		Use mL (lowercase m, UPPERCASE L) for millilitre
IU** (do not use)	International units	Mistaken as IV (intravenous) or the number 10	Use units(s) International units can be expressed as units alone)
Cc** (do not use)	Cubic centimetres	Mistaken as u (units)	Use mL

TABLE 7.5 Error-Prone and DO NOT USE Abbreviations, Symbols, and Dose Designations—cont'd

Term	Intended Meaning	Misinterpretation	Correction
Trailing zero after decimal point (e.g., 1.0 mg)** (do not use)	1 mg	Mistaken as 10 mg if decimal point not seen. Decimal point overlooked-resulting in 10-fold dose error.	Do not use trailing zeros
Lack of leading zero before a decimal point called a "Naked" decimal point (e.g., .5 mg)** (do not use)	0.5 mg	Mistaken as 5 mg if decimal point not seen. Decimal point is overlooked-resulting in a 10-fold dose error.	Use zero before a decimal point when the dose is less than a whole unit
Symbol @** (do not use)	at	Mistaken for "2" (two) or 5 (five)	Use "at"
Symbol >** (do not use)	Greater than	Mistaken for "7 "(seven) or the letter "L" Confused with each other	Use "greater than/ more than" "Less than/lower than"
Symbol <** (do not use)			
Abbreviations for medication names** (do not use)		Misinterpreted because similar abbreviations for multiple medications: e.g., MS, MSO4 (morphine sulphate), MgSO4 (Magnesium sulphate) may be confused for one another.	Do not abbreviate medication names.

**On the Joint Commission's "DO NOT USE" list.
Adapted from Institute for Safe Medication Practices. (2022). List of error-prone abbreviations. https://www.ismp.org/recommendations/error-prone-abbreviations-list; Institute for Safe Medication Practices Canada. (2018b). Do not use dangerous abbreviations. symbols, and dose designations. https://ismpcanada.ca/wp-content/uploads/2022/02/ISMPCanadaListOfDangerousAbbreviations.pdf

- After the client takes the medication, complete the MAR according to the agency policy to verify that the medication was administered as ordered. Chart preadministration data such as BP, pulse, or blood glucose level.
- Chart the effectiveness of certain medications, such as prn medications (such as analgesics or antiemetics).

Right Reason

- Understand why the client is getting the medication and if it makes sense.

Right to Refuse

- Be aware that in order for the client to refuse a medication, they need to be fully informed about the potential consequences of the refusal.

Right Client Education

- To ensure client safety, fully inform clients and family members about the medication and the consequences of not taking it.
- Provide information about the medication being given: the reason for taking it, its action, and possible adverse effects the client may experience while taking it.

Right Evaluation

- Before medication administration, check to make sure that the order is correct and the medication is available and accessible to the client.

- Check any special assessments required before administration of the medication.
- After the medication administration, monitor the client for medication effectiveness, adverse effects, adverse medication reactions, and medication interactions.

Medication Administration for Older Persons

- Allow extra time for administration of medications to older persons.
- Assess functional status to see whether a client will need help in taking the medications.
- Have older clients drink a little fluid before taking oral medications to ease swallowing, and encourage them to drink 150 to 180 mL after medications to prevent the medication from lodging in the esophagus.
- Have clients sit up straight in bed and tuck in their chins to decrease the risk of aspiration when taking medications.
- Request liquid medications from the prescriber if the client has trouble swallowing large pills or capsules.

Medication Errors

Medication errors are preventable events associated with the prescribing, transcribing, dispensing, or administering of medications. Many medication errors are not reported. Unreported errors mean that no one can correct their cause or reduce their incidence. Errors are rarely the fault of individual health care providers but instead stem from failures of a complicated health care system. The best approach is a

BOX 7.2 Health Care Worker Guidelines for Moving Clients Safely

- Arrange for adequate assistance when moving or transferring a client.
- Use algorithms to determine the safest equipment and client-handling technique to use for each activity or movement to be completed.
- When possible, use mechanical aids such as lifts, transfer chairs or boards, or pivot devices for lifts and transfers.
- Instruct clients about moving safely and encourage them to assist as much as possible to minimize the workload for the nurse.
- Keep the spine, neck, pelvis, and feet aligned. Avoid twisting.
- Flex the knees; keep the feet wide apart to broaden the base of support.
- Position yourself close to the client (or object being lifted) to minimize the load.
- Use the stronger, larger muscles of the arms and legs rather than those of the back.
- Slide the client toward you using a draw sheet rather than pulling or lifting.
- Tighten your abdominal and gluteal muscles in preparation for a move
- The person with the heaviest load coordinates efforts of the team involved by counting to three.

From (Astle, B., & Duggleby, W. [2024]. *Potter and Perry's Canadian fundamentals of nursing* [7th ed., p. 862, Table 37.2]. Elsevier Inc.)

nonpunitive, multidisciplinary approach in which the process is targeted rather than the practitioner. This approach focuses on why an error occurred rather than blaming the person or people involved. When an error occurs, it should be acknowledged immediately and reported to the appropriate hospital personnel. Measures to counteract the effects of the error may also be necessary. Client safety is the first concern of the nurse. It is important to first assess and monitor the client for adverse effects after a medication is administered to a client in error. The nurse is also responsible for completing an incident report for the agency about the details of the incident. The nurse follows agency policy about disclosure to the client and client's family. See Chapter 8 for a more detailed discussion of medications.

ACTIVITY AND EXERCISE

Body Mechanics

Body mechanics are "the coordinated efforts of the musculoskeletal and nervous systems to maintain balance, posture, and body alignment during lifting, bending, moving, and performing activities of daily living" (Astle & Duggleby, 2024, p. 869). Proper use of body mechanics will conserve energy, reduce stress and strain on body structures, increase safety for the caregiver and the client, and reduce the possibility of personal injury. Repeated lifting and forceful movements associated with care of clients can lead to work-related injury or illness, such as musculo-skeletal disorders. The activities of lifting, transferring, and repositioning

clients place health care workers at risk for musculo-skeletal disorders, especially back injuries. Body mechanics training has proven ineffective in preventing job-related injuries. Many facilities have found implementing "no-lift" policies and safe handling programs to be more effective.

Research has shown that sound ergonomics programs in health care facilities can lead to reductions in injuries (Astle & Duggleby, 2024). The use of technology such as lifting devices and the use of special algorithms for each client who needs help to move are crucial to the success of ergonomics programs. Box 7.2 presents guidelines for moving clients safely and avoiding back injuries.

Exercise

Exercise is physical activity for the purpose of toning the body, improving health, and maintaining fitness. It can also be used therapeutically to correct a deformity or restore the client's body to a maximal state of health. Activity tolerance (the kind and amount of exercise or activity that a client is able to perform) must be assessed prior to planning physical activity for clients with health problems. Some of the factors that influence activity tolerance include pain, lack of sleep, prior exercise pattern, anxiety, age, and muscular or skeletal impairments (Astle & Duggleby, 2024). See Chapter 6 for a more detailed discussion of physical activity.

CLIENT SAFETY

Restraints

Types of Restraints

- *Physical restraints* are any manual method or any physical or mechanical device, material, or piece of equipment that reduces the ability of the client to move freely. Examples include locked geriatric chairs, restrictive side rails, belts, hand mitts, sheet ties, and chest restraints.
- *Chemical restraints* are medications given to restrict or manage a client's behaviour or to restrict a client's movement that are not a standard therapy or dose for the client's condition.
- *Environmental restraints* control a client's mobility. Examples include a locked room, as in the case of clients placed in seclusion. A locked nursing unit is another form of environmental restraint that is designed to allow residents with dementia to wander freely and safely around the unit.

Use of Least Restraint

Least restraint means that all other possible interventions have been attempted before the decision is made to use a restraint. Restraints are a temporary or short-term intervention, and the least restrictive method for the shortest duration possible is chosen. The optimal goal is a restraint-free environment. Research indicates that restraints do not actually prevent falls and injury and may even increase the severity of injury. Restraints require a physician's order and are part of the client's individualized plan of care. Regularly reviewing the continued use of restraints is essential. It is important that the client and client's family or substitute decision maker are informed and involved in the plan of care as well.

Assessment of restraints. Routine assessment of a client in restraints is essential to prevent client injury. The restraint must be removed and the client checked and repositioned at regular intervals. Restraints should be tied with a quick-release tie rather than a knot. Proper placement of the restraint, skin integrity, pulses, and colour and sensation of the restrained part should be assessed every hour or according to agency policy. It is important to document this information.

Alternatives to restraints. Alternatives to restraints include low-height beds, bedside mats and hip guards, bed sensors or monitoring devices, and the presence of a family member or paid companion to stay with the client at risk.

Seizure Disorder Precautions

Seizures are sudden, transient alterations in brain function that result from excessive levels of electrical activity in the brain and lead to a sudden, violent, involuntary series of contractions of a group of muscles (Astle & Duggleby, 2024). Seizures can vary in severity, and the client may or may not lose consciousness.

Nursing Interventions

- Protect clients from traumatic injury: If they are standing or sitting, lay them on the floor, bed, or other flat surface. If they are in hospital, make sure the bed is in the low position, flat, and the side rails are elevated and padded. Place a pillow or folded blanket under the head. Loosen restrictive clothing. Do not attempt to restrain clients but clear the area of hazards and articles that might harm them.
- Position clients for adequate ventilation and drainage of oral secretions: Clients need to be on a flat surface. Nothing should be inserted into the mouth except in the case of status epilepticus (a medical emergency in which there are continual seizures), and then an oral airway is necessary. If possible, turn clients on their side.
- Provide privacy and support following the procedure: Stay with clients, observing and timing the seizure. Immediately following the seizure, place clients in the recovery position to prevent aspiration and remain with them until they have recovered fully. Explain what happened and answer client questions. Some clients may experience postseizure confusion and may need to have explanations repeated.

HYGIENE

Bathing

During hygienic care, the nurse incorporates other activities, such as communication, physical assessment, skin and wound care, health teaching, assessment of self-care abilities, and range-of-motion (ROM) exercises. The nurse provides hygienic care according to the client's needs and preferences, taking into consideration cultural and developmental factors.

- A complete bed bath is a bath for clients who are completely dependent and require all their care to be provided by another person.
- A partial bed bath involves bathing only certain parts of the body (such as the face, hands, underarms, and perineal area) to refresh clients and because certain areas may be more prone to skin breakdown or odour if not bathed.

Guidelines for Bathing

- Provide privacy by exposing only the areas being bathed.
- Maintain safety by keeping side rails up and providing a call bell when you are away from the bedside.
- Maintain warmth by exposing only the areas being bathed and keeping bath water warm.
- Unless contraindicated, bathe limbs from distal to proximal areas (fingers to axilla) with long, firm strokes to promote circulation and venous return.
- Promote independence by encouraging the client to participate as much as possible.
- Anticipate needs by having all your equipment at hand.

Perineal Care

Special attention to perineal care is needed for clients with in-dwelling catheters, recent rectal or gynecological surgery, recent childbirth, morbid obesity, or urinary or fecal incontinence as these clients are the most at risk for infection. In these cases, the nurse performs perineal care even if the client is able to do so, so that the nurse may assess the perineal area for skin breakdown or infection and is able to clean the area thoroughly.

Nail and Foot Care

Clients with diabetes mellitus or peripheral vascular disease require special nail and foot care as they are at risk of complications such as infection due to poor circulation, especially in their feet. Persons with diabetes also have reduced sensation to the feet. The nurse should not trim the nails of a client with impaired lower extremity circulation before checking agency policy to see if a physician's order is necessary.

Foot Care Guidelines for High-Risk Clients

- Inspect feet daily and do not allow high-risk clients to walk barefoot.
- People with diabetes should see a qualified health care provider, such as a podiatrist, for a thorough yearly foot exam.
- Wash feet daily with lukewarm water but do not soak them as that can cause maceration. Dry well and do not put cream between toes.
- Do not cut corns or calluses or use commercial removers. Consult a podiatrist.
- File the toenails straight across and square and do not use clippers or scissors. Get help to cut nails if necessary.
- Avoid crossing the legs or wearing elastic stockings and knee-high hose that can impair circulation to the lower extremities.
- Wear clean socks and stockings daily that remain dry and free of holes.
- Wear properly fitting, nonslip shoes that fully cover the feet.
- Exercise regularly to promote lower extremity circulation.

- Do not use heating pads or hot water bottles on extremities.
- Wash all cuts immediately, dry thoroughly, and treat with a mild antiseptic (Astle & Duggleby, 2024).

Oral Hygiene

Oral hygiene includes the brushing and flossing of teeth as well as care of the mouth, gums, and lips. Oral hygiene is an important practice that maintains the health of the mouth, teeth, gums, and lips; enhances comfort; and stimulates appetite.

Mouth Care for Unconscious Clients

Unconscious clients are more susceptible to drying of the mouth because they are not eating or drinking, cannot swallow oral secretions, and frequently breathe through their mouths. Oxygen therapy can also be very drying to the mouth. Proper oral hygiene reduces the incidence of pneumonia, which can be caused by Gram-negative bacteria aspirated from the mouth and into the lung (Astle & Duggleby, 2024). When giving oral hygiene, it is important to prevent the client from choking and aspiration. The client should be positioned on their side with their head turned toward the dependent side. Suction machine equipment should also be close at hand. If possible, a padded tongue blade can be used behind the back molars to separate upper and lower teeth. The mouth can be cleansed with a toothbrush or toothette moistened with water or hydrogen peroxide. A bulb syringe can be used to rinse the oral cavity; it should then be suctioned to make sure that no fluid is left in the mouth.

Stomatitis

Stomatitis is inflammation of the mouth that is caused by a variety of conditions, including viral infections, chemical irritation, radiation therapy, and chemotherapy. Gentle brushing and flossing is important. Clients with this condition should not use commercial mouthwash, drink alcohol, or smoke. Normal saline mouthwashes can be given every 2 hours if necessary, and a mild analgesic might be necessary for pain.

CARDIOPULMONARY FUNCTIONING AND OXYGENATION

Suctioning

Suctioning is the aspiration of secretions from the trachea and bronchial tree by application of negative-pressure suction. It is used to maintain a patent airway, collect sputum specimens, or stimulate a cough (Astle & Duggleby, 2024). Clients should be encouraged to cough and suctioned only when necessary, as it is uncomfortable and traumatic to the airway. Signs that the client needs to be suctioned may include one or more of the following: gurgling respirations, respiratory distress, low oxygen-saturation levels, and coarse crackles on auscultation.

Types of Suctioning

- Oropharyngeal and nasopharyngeal suctioning is used when the client is able to cough effectively but is unable to clear secretions by coughing or swallowing.
- Orotracheal or nasotracheal suctioning utilizes a catheter that is passed through the nose or mouth to the trachea. This route is used when the client is not able to cough and manage their own secretions. It is a sterile procedure.
- Tracheal suctioning is done through an artificial airway, such as an endotracheal or tracheostomy tube. Surgical asepsis is maintained for new tracheostomies and endotracheal suctioning.

Principles of Suctioning

- Suctioning should not be performed routinely but should follow a comprehensive respiratory assessment that includes chest auscultation (Astle & Duggleby, 2024).
- Lubricate the catheter with sterile normal saline, except for nasopharyngeal or nasotracheal suctioning, which requires the use of a water-soluble lubricant.
- Insert the catheter until resistance is met or the client coughs and then pull back 1 cm for tracheal suctioning Astle & Duggleby, 2024). Insert 16 cm in adults for nasopharyngeal suctioning and 16 to 20 cm in adults for nasotracheal suctioning.
- Do not apply suction while inserting the catheter.
- While removing the catheter, apply suction intermittently and rotate the catheter to prevent injury to the mucosa. Do not suction longer than 10 to 15 seconds, as this can increase the risk of mucosal damage and hypoxemia (Astle & Duggleby, 2024).
- Wait 1 to 2 minutes between passes to allow the client to rest.
- It may be necessary to hyperoxygenate the client before and after suctioning by using a manual resuscitation bag, increasing the oxygen flow rate, or having the client take deep breaths, especially if the client has had signs of cardiopulmonary compromise in the past.
- Evaluate the client's response postprocedure. Suctioning can cause hypoxemia, hypotension, arrhythmias, and possible trauma to the mucosa of the lung.

Closed (In-Line) Suctioning

Closed (in-line) suctioning is another way of suctioning an artificial airway. It requires the use of a multiuse suction catheter that is housed within a plastic sleeve and is attached to the client's artificial airway. The advantage of this method of suctioning is the association with decreased risk of hypoxia and cardiovascular complications as compared to open suctioning. It is a recommended method of suctioning clients who cannot tolerate the loss of positive-end-expiratory pressure (PEEP), such as those with severe respiratory disorders who require high amounts of PEEP or oxygen requirements (Cobbett, 2024).

Tracheostomy Care

Tracheostomy care is the removal of copious, thick, tenacious, or dried secretions from the tracheostomy tube in order to maintain a patent airway, prevent infection, and prevent irritation. Practical nurses need to check their legal scope of practice in their jurisdiction and the policies of the facility they are working in regarding whether they can perform tracheostomy care in collaboration with an RN.

Guidelines for Tracheostomy Care

- Provide tracheostomy care every 8 hours.
- Suction to remove secretions from the lumen of the tube when necessary.
- If an inner cannula is present:
  - Remove the disposable inner cannula and replace it with a new one.
  - Provide care for a nondisposable inner cannula, which involves (a) removing and placing the cannula in normal saline; (b) removing secretions from the cannula with a sterile brush; (c) rinsing the cannula with normal saline; (d) draining excess saline before inserting the cannula; and (e) locking the inner cannula in place (Astle & Duggleby, 2024; Cobbett, 2024).
- Clean around the stoma in a circular motion from the stoma site outward with saline; moving in an outward circle pulls mucus and other contaminants from the stoma periphery (Astle & Duggleby, 2024; Cobbett, 2024).
- Change the tracheostomy tape or ties if necessary, being careful not to dislodge the cannula and to secure the tracheostomy tube by holding the cannula in place by lightly pressing with one finger and using a double square knot. The knot should be located on the side rather than at the back of the neck, where it would cause pressure. Another method is the use of a tracheostomy tube holder. Leave the old tracheostomy holder in place until the new device is secure if changing it without assistance. Align the strap under the client's neck. Be sure the Velcro attachments are on either side of the tracheostomy tube. Place the narrow end of the ties under and through the faceplate eyelets. Pull ends even and secure with Velcro closures. Ensure that there is space for only one loose or two snug finger widths to be inserted under neck strap (Cobbett, 2024).
- Insert a sterile tracheostomy dressing under the ties and faceplate to absorb drainage and to prevent pressure on the clavicle (Astle & Duggleby, 2024; Cobbett, 2024).

Chest Tubes

A *chest tube* is a catheter inserted through the thorax to remove abnormal accumulations of air, fluid, or blood from the pleural space or mediastinum. The chest tube drainage system returns negative pressure to the intrapleural space. This is a skill that will require collaboration with an RN. Practical nurses need to ensure this skill is within their legal scope of practice in their jurisdiction and permitted by the policies of the facility in which they are working.

Commercial Drainage Systems

Wet suction control drainage system

- The collection chamber collects drainage from the chest tube in a series of calibrated columns.
- The water seal chamber prevents atmospheric air from entering the pleural space. The fluid level will fluctuate with respirations until the lung is fully expanded. Continuous bubbling may indicate a leak in the chest tube system.
- If gravity drainage is insufficient, the suction control chamber is used to provide suction between 10 to 20 cm of water and will drain air and fluid from the chest cavity. Gentle bubbling in this chamber indicates that there is suction.

Dry suction control drainage system

- The dry suction control chamber system contains no water. It provides higher suction pressure levels.
- It has a visual alert that indicates if the suction is not working. No bubbling is seen in the third chamber (Tyerman & Cobbett, 2023).

See Fig. 7.4 for an example of a Pleur-evac chest drainage system.

Nursing Care of the Client With a Chest Tube

- Monitor drainage; notify the physician if drainage is greater than 100 mL per hour or if drainage becomes bright red or increases suddenly.
- Mark the chest tube drainage in the collection chamber at 1- to 4-hour intervals, according to hospital policy to monitor output.
- Ensure that the tubing is not kinked, all connections are secure, and there are no dependent loops.
- Maintain the drainage system below the level of the chest to prevent reflux and decrease the risk of infection.
- Maintain a sterile occlusive dressing at the insertion site to prevent an air leak.
- Turn the client frequently to promote drainage and ventilation.
- Observe for fluctuation of fluid in the water seal chamber; the level will rise on inhalation and fall on exhalation; if there are no fluctuations, either the lung has re-expanded or the chest tube is clogged (Tyerman & Cobbett, 2023).
- Monitor the suction control chamber to make sure there is gentle bubbling in the suction control chamber. Vigorous bubbling indicates an air leak, and the physician should be notified (Tyerman & Cobbett, 2023).
- Encourage coughing and deep breathing every 2 hours with splinting of the chest area if necessary and encourage ROM exercises to the shoulder of the affected side. Encouraging incentive spirometry every hour while the client is awake may help prevent atelectasis or pneumonia (Tyerman & Cobbett, 2023).
- Determine agency policy regarding clamping of chest tubes. Chest tubes are rarely clamped, and a chest tube should never be clamped without a written order from a health care provider. Clamping can cause a tension pneumothorax where air pressure builds up in the pleural space, collapsing the lung and creating a life-threatening emergency. A health care provider may order clamping for 24 hours to evaluate for accumulation of air or fluid before discontinuing the chest tube (Astle & Duggleby, 2024, Tyerman & Cobbett, 2023).
- If the drainage system cracks or breaks, insert the chest tube temporarily into a bottle of sterile water to maintain a water seal and then replace the drainage system.

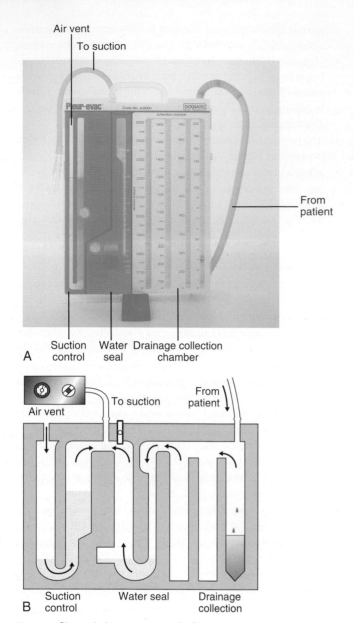

Fig. 7.4 Chest drainage system. **A,** Pleur-evac chest drainage system, a commercial three-chamber chest drainage device. **B,** Schematic of the drainage device. (From Cobbett, S. [2024]. *Canadian clinical nursing skills and techniques* [2nd ed., p. 783]. Elsevier.)

- If the chest tube is pulled out of the chest accidentally, pinch the skin together, apply an occlusive dressing, and call the physician immediately.
- Keep a clamp, a bottle of sterile water, and a sterile occlusive dressing at the bedside at all times. Clamps are kept at the bedside for special procedures, such as changing the chest drainage system.

Oxygen Therapy

Oxygen is a medication and as such can have serious adverse effects, such as absorption atelectasis or oxygen toxicity. The goal of oxygen therapy is to relieve or prevent hypoxia (reduced tissue oxygenation despite adequate perfusion). Signs of worsening hypoxia include increasing tachypnea and dyspnea, skin colour changes (pale at first, then cyanotic), increasing tachycardia, hypertension, restlessness, and disorientation (Astel & Duggleby, 2024; Tyerman & Cobbett, 2023).

Methods of Oxygen Delivery

Low-flow devices. Low-flow devices provide oxygen in concentrations that vary with the person's respiratory effort (Astel & Duggleby, 2024; Tyerman & Cobbett, 2023). When the total ventilation exceeds the capacity of the oxygen reservoir, room air is entrained. The final concentration of oxygen delivered depends on the ventilatory demands of the client, the size of the oxygen reservoir, and the rate at which the reservoir is filled. Most methods of oxygen delivery are low-flow systems. Examples of low-flow devices are low-flow nasal cannulas, oxygen -conserving nasal cannula, the simple face mask, and reservoir masks.

Nasal cannulas. The low-flow nasal cannula (nasal prongs) is a low-flow device used for a flow rate of 1 to 6 L per minute, providing oxygen concentrations of 24% (at 1 L/min) and 44% (at 6 L/min) (Astle & Duggleby, 2024; Cobbett, 2024). The oxygen-conserving cannula (Oxymizer) is a low-flow device used for a flow rate of 8 L per minute, providing oxygen concentrations of 30 to 60%. It is indicated for long-term oxygen therapy and allows for increased oxygen concentration at lower flow. This device can not be cleaned; therefore, changing the cannula weekly is recommended (Cobbett, 2024). A flow rate above 4 L per minute can be very drying for the nasal mucosa and cause irritation. The nurse also needs to be alert for skin breakdown over the ears and in the nares from nasal prongs that are too tight. The tubing can be padded to prevent necrosis over the tops of the ears.

Oxygen masks. Oxygen masks are devices used to administer oxygen, humidity, or both. Different types of face masks are as follows:

- The simple face mask delivers 40 to 60% oxygen concentrations. It is used for short-term oxygen therapy or for the delivery of oxygen in an emergency (Astle & Duggleby, 2024; Cobbett, 2024). This mask is contraindicated for clients with carbon dioxide (CO_2) retention.
- The partial rebreather mask combines a mask and a reservoir bag. It provides an oxygen concentration of 40 to 70% with a minimum flow rate of 10 L per minute (Astle & Duggleby, 2024).
- The non-rebreather mask provides the highest oxygen concentration of the low-flow systems. It has a mask and a reservoir bag and can deliver an oxygen concentration of 60 to 80%, depending on the client's ventilatory efforts. It is commonly used for the client with deteriorating respiratory status who might need to be intubated. The flow rate is 10 to 15 L/min to maintain the reservoir bag two-thirds full. The one-way valves on non-rebreather masks prevent expired air from flowing back into the bag. If it is deflated, the client may be breathing large amounts of exhaled carbon dioxide (CO_2) (Astle & Duggleby, 2024).

High-flow devices. High-flow devices deliver oxygen at rates above the normal inspiratory flow and maintain a fixed FiO_2 (fraction of inspired oxygen) independent of the client's respiratory pattern (Tyerman & Cobbett, 2023). The most common example is the Venturi mask, which entrains room air to achieve a consistent, precise oxygen concentration. Other examples include large volume nebulizer, blender masks, the high-flow nasal cannula, and aerosol devices such as the face tent and the tracheostomy collar or mask.

Venturi masks. The Venturi mask, or air-entrainment mask, delivers oxygen concentrations of 24 to 60%, with a flow rate of 2 to 12 L per minute (Astle & Duggleby, 2024). The Venturi mask is useful for delivering low, precise oxygen concentrations to clients with chronic obstructive pulmonary disease (COPD) (Astle & Duggleby, 2024; Tyerman & Cobbett, 2023).

High-flow nasal cannula

The high-flow nasal cannula is another high-flow oxygen delivery device that has an adjustable FiO_2 (2–100%) with a modifiable flow (up to 60 L/min). Having a wide range of FiO_2 and it to be used on adults, children, and infants. The FiO_2 is dependent on client respiratory pattern and input flow (Cobbett, 2024).

Oxygen Therapy for Clients With COPD

For an average adult, a high CO_2 level stimulates the brain to breathe. People with COPD and a high-CO_2 level may become less sensitive to the high-CO_2 level, reducing the drive to breathe. A client who has hypoxemia (a low oxygen level in the blood) and is a chronic CO_2 retainer may require a low level of oxygen delivery at 1 to 2 L per minute. A low arterial oxygen level will stimulate a client with COPD to breathe. Careful, ongoing assessment when administering oxygen therapy to clients with COPD is very important (Tyerman & Cobbett, 2023).

Home Oxygen Therapy

- Indications for home oxygen therapy include a partial pressure of arterial oxygen (PaO_2) of 55 mm Hg or less via arterial blood gas analysis or an SpO_2 of 88% or less via pulse oximetry on room air at rest, on exertion, or with exercise (Astle & Duggleby, 2024). This therapy improves clients' exercise tolerance and fatigue levels and may assist with the management of dyspnea.
- Home oxygen is usually delivered by nasal cannula or transtracheal oxygen (TTO); a tracheostomy collar is used in the case of the client with a permanent tracheostomy.
- Nasal cannulas, either regular or oxygen-conserving type, are usually used to deliver oxygen from a central source at home. The source may be liquid oxygen storage system, compressed oxygen in tanks, or an oxygen concentrator or extractor, depending on the home environment, insurance coverage, activity level, and proximity to an oxygen supply company (Tyerman & Cobbett, 2023).

FLUID, ELECTROLYTE, AND ACID–BASE BALANCES

Fluid and Electrolyte Balance

- Body fluids are distributed in two compartments: one containing intracellular fluid (intracerebral fluid, or all the fluid within body cells, comprising 40% of body weight) and the other extracellular fluid (ECF; extracerebral fluid, or all the fluid outside body cells, comprising 20% of body weight) (Astle & Duggleby, 2024).
- Body fluids are regulated by (a) fluid intake and the thirst mechanism; (b) hormonal controls such as antidiuretic hormone (ADH), aldosterone, and renin; and (c) fluid output through the kidneys, the skin, the lungs, and the gastro-intestinal system, with the kidneys being the most important in regulating fluid balance. This physiological balance is called *homeostasis* (Astle & Duggleby, 2024).
- Clients who are very young or very old, as well as clients with chronic or serious illnesses, are at greater risk for fluid, electrolyte, and acid–base imbalances.
- Assessment of fluid, electrolyte, and acid–base alterations includes collating data from the nursing health history and physical and behavioural assessments, as well as measuring intake and output, weighing the clients daily, and analyzing specific laboratory data, such as electrolyte results (Astle & Duggleby, 2024). See Chapter 9 for a more detailed discussion of electrolyte balance and homeostasis.

Central Venous Access Devices

Central venous access devices (CVADs) are inserted into a vein for the purpose of delivering medication or fluids directly into the bloodstream. Central venous access can be achieved by three different methods: centrally inserted catheters, peripherally inserted catheters (PICCs), or implanted ports (Tyerman & Cobbett, 2023). To determine the most appropriate type of CVAD, the nurse needs to consider the following factors: prescribed therapy, duration of therapy, physical assessment, client health history, support system and resources, device availability, and client preference (Tyerman & Cobbett, 2023). Practical nurses need to ensure this skill is within their legal scope of practice in their jurisdiction and permitted by the policies of the facility in which they are working. In some facilities, the practical nurse with the proper training may change PICC line dressing and deliver medication via PICC line and is able to remove the PICC line.

Types of CVADs

Peripherally inserted catheters. PICCs are designed for short-term use. There are two common types: short peripheral and midline. Short peripheral IVs are most commonly placed in the arm and are described in more detail under "Nursing Care of Clients with PVAD Infusion Therapy." Midline catheters range in length from 7.5 to 25 cm and lie deep in the cephalic or basilic vein with the tip not extending past the axilla. PICCs are used for clients who need vascular access for 1 week to 6 months, but they can be in place for longer periods (Tyerman & Cobbett, 2023).

Centrally inserted catheters. Centrally inserted catheters or central venous catheters (CVCs) are used to administer medications and solutions irritating to veins, deliver long-term therapy, and deliver rapid infusion of medications or large amounts of fluid. CVCs are available in single-, double-, triple-, or quadruple-lumen catheters. Multilumen catheters are useful

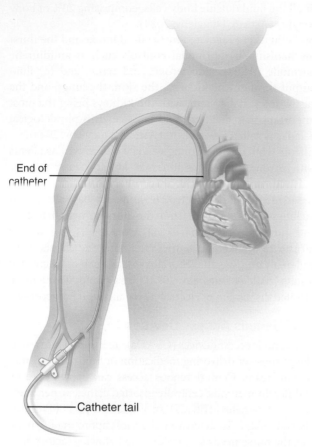

Fig.7.5 Peripherally inserted central catheter (PICC) is placed peripherally in a vein of the upper arm with the tip resting in the superior vena cava. (From Ignatavicius, D. D., Workman, M. L., & Rebar, C. [2018]. *Medical-surgical nursing: Concepts for interprofessional collaborative care* [9th ed., p. 205, Figure 13-6]. Elsevier.)

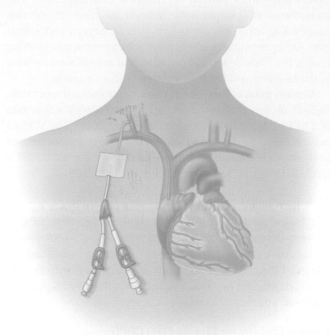

Fig.7.6 Tunnelled central venous catheter. Part of the catheter lies in a subcutaneous tunnel, separating the point where the catheter enters the vein from where it exits the skin. (From Ignatavicius, D. D., Workman, M. L., & Rebar, C. [2018]. *Medical-surgical nursing: Concepts for interprofessional collaborative care* [9th ed., p. 207, Figure 13-8]. Elsevier.)

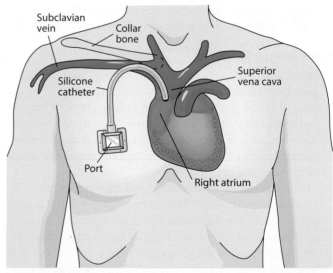

Fig. 7.7 Implanted infusion port and central venous catheter. (From Perry, A. G., Potter, P. A., & Ostendorf, W. [2018]. *Clinical nursing skills and techniques* [9th ed., p. 786, Figure 29.7]. Mosby.)

for incompatible medications that can be infused in separate lumens without mixing and a third lumen can be used for blood sampling (Tyerman & Cobbett, 2023).

Figs. 7.5 to 7.7 show examples of CVADs.

With the exception of the PICC device, CVAD catheters are inserted in the central part of the body by way of the internal jugular, subclavian, or femoral vein. All central-line devices terminate in the vena cava immediately above the right atrium, where blood flow is very rapid at 2 L per minute. There are four types of CVADs:

- Nontunnelled catheters: They are inserted by a physician, and clients with these catheters must remain in the acute care setting. There is a high rate of infection with nontunnelled catheters because they are inserted percutaneously in areas that are warm and moist, such as the neck and groin. For this reason, they are not left in place for as long as other CVADs.
- Tunnelled catheters (e.g., Hickman catheters): They are inserted in the operating room under a local anaesthetic and can be left in for years. They are hard to disguise and require daily care but can be cared for in the home setting.

- Implanted ports (e.g., Port-A-Caths): They require insertion in the operating room with local anaesthesia and also can be left in place for years. They are commonly implanted in the chest.
- PICC lines: They are placed most commonly in peripheral veins, such as the basilic or cephalic veins. They are easy to insert at the bedside either by health care providers or

specially trained nurses. They have a low infection rate because fewer bacterial colonies are present in the antecubital fossa (Tyerman & Cobbett, 2023).

Purpose of Infusion Therapy

- To correct or prevent fluid and electrolyte imbalances
- To administer medications
- To administer blood and blood products
- To provide venous access in emergency situations
- To correct or prevent nutritional imbalances

Types of Solutions

- Isotonic solutions: They have the same osmolality as body fluids. They are used most commonly for ECF replacement; for example, 0.9% saline or normal saline (NS), 5% dextrose in water (D_5W), or lactated Ringer's solution (LR) (Astle & Duggleby, 2024).
- Hypotonic solutions: They have a lower osmolality than body fluids. These solutions cause the movement of water into cells by osmosis; for example, 0.45% saline (0.5 NS) (Astle & Duggleby, 2024).
- Hypertonic solutions: They have a higher osmolality than body fluids. They concentrate ECF and cause movement of water from cells into the ECF by osmosis; for example, 10% dextrose in water ($D_{10}W$) (Astle & Duggleby, 2024).

Nursing Care of Clients With PVAD Infusion Therapy

Initiation of infusion therapy

- Common IV sites are the veins in the hand, forearm, and antecubital fossa.
- The IV infusion is started by venipuncture through the use of a butterfly an over-the-needle plastic catheter.
- The IV infusion is started distally to provide the option of proceeding up the extremity if necessary later.
- The nurse needs to check the IV solution against the prescriber's orders for the type, amount, and percentage of solution and the rate of flow.

Regulation of infusion flow rate

- The nurse must regulate the rate of infusion according to the prescriber's orders.
- The nurse calculates the infusion rate to prevent too slow or too rapid administration of IV fluids.
- Fluids that run by gravity are adjusted by means of a regulator or roller clamp. An electronic infusion pump can also regulate the rate that is preset by the nurse.
- For IV infusions running by gravity, the nurse calculates the minute-flow rate or drop rate based on the drop factor of the infusion, set using this formula:

$$\frac{\text{Amount of solution to administer}}{\text{Time for infusion in hours}} \times \frac{\text{Drip factor of tubing}}{60\,\text{min}} = \text{Drip rate (gtt/min)}$$

- For example, the minute flow rate or drop rate for an IV running at 100 mL/hr with a drop factor of 15 gtt per mL would be:

$$\frac{100\,\text{mL}}{1\,\text{hr}} \times \frac{15\,\text{gtt}}{60\,\text{min}} = 25\,\text{gtt/min}$$ Maintenance of infusion therapy

- The timing of the IV dressing change depends on the type of dressing used: Transparent semipermeable membrane (TSM) dressings must be changed every 5 to 7 days and gauze dressings are changed every 2 days. Change needle-free connectors using ANTT (aseptic non-touch technique), a minimum of every 7 days if removed for any reason, if contamination is suspected, or if it cannot be flushed clear of blood, and change the IV administration sets, including add-on devices, according to type of infusion (intermittent or continuous) and with placement of a new VAD. Always change immediately if contamination is suspected (Cobbett, 2024).
- Be aware that incompatibilities can occur between certain solutions and medications.
- Assess the "rights" for administration of medications.
- Assess the IV site and equipment regularly for complications.

Intermittent Venous Access or Saline Locks

Saline locks are used when intravascular access is desired for intermittent administration of medications by IV bolus (push) or IV piggyback (secondary administration of medications). It allows the client to be free from an IV line except when medication must be given, and it allows emergency IV access if necessary. Patency is maintained by periodic flushing with 1 to 3 mL of NS (depending on agency policy).

Complications of Infusion Therapy

Common complications of infusion therapy are infiltration, phlebitis (inflammation of the vein), infection, fluid (circulatory) overload, and bleeding or bruising at the site.

Blood Transfusions
Purpose of Blood Transfusions

- To restore blood volume after hemorrhage, surgery, or trauma
- To restore the oxygen-carrying capacity of the blood and to increase hemoglobin levels in severe anemias
- To replace specific blood components, such as clotting factors, platelets, or albumin

Nursing Care of Clients Receiving a Blood Transfusion

- Check your agency policy and your legal scope of practice with regard to blood transfusions. Some jurisdictions may prohibit the practical nurse from initiating blood products but will allow monitoring of a stable client.
- Check that the blood or blood components have been typed and cross-matched, indicating that the blood of the donor and the recipient are compatible. Check the expiration date and time on the unit of blood.
- Blood is stored in a refrigerated environment. The refrigeration unit is regulated by the blood bank. It is never

stored in refrigerators on the hospital units (Cobbett, 2024). The blood transfusion must be started within 30 minutes after receiving the blood component from the transfusion medical laboratory and it is stopped after 4 hours to minimize the risk of bacterial growth. Bags and tubing are discarded in the biohazardous waste according to agency policy (Astle & Duggleby, 2024). Take baseline vital signs (including temperature) preadministration and frequently throughout administration (check agency policy).

- Know that an IV with NS infusing through a blood administration set with a special filter is used to start the infusion.
- Maintain standard precautions/routine practices when handling blood and IV equipment.
- Know that the client needs to sign a blood administration consent form in many agencies.
- Know that before beginning the infusion, two nurses verify the blood type, Rh factor, client and blood numbers, and expiration date of the blood.
- Invert the container gently to suspend the red blood cells within the plasma.
- Stay with the client for the first 15 minutes because that is when a reaction most often occurs.
- Observe for signs of a hemolytic reaction, which generally occurs early in the transfusion (within the first 5–15 minutes). Signs include shivering, headache, lower back pain, increased pulse and respiratory rate, hemoglobinuria, oliguria, and hypotension (Tyerman & Cobbett, 2023).
- Observe for signs of a febrile reaction (usually within 30 minutes). Signs include shaking, headache, elevated temperature, back pain, confusion, and hematemesis (Tyerman & Cobbett, 2023).
- Observe for signs of an allergic reaction, such as hives, wheezing, pruritis, or joint pain (Tyerman & Cobbett, 2023).
- If any reaction occurs, stop the infusion immediately and maintain patency of the IV with NS; monitor vital signs as often as every 5 minutes; notify the physician; stay with the client; and prepare to administer emergency medications and to perform cardiopulmonary resuscitation if necessary. A urine sample may be needed to determine the presence of hemoglobin as a result of red blood cell (RBC) hemolysis. Save the blood container, tubing, attached labels, and transfusion record and return them to the laboratory.

PAIN AND COMFORT

The International Association for the Study of Pain (2021) defines *pain* as "an unpleasant sensory and emotional experience associated with, or resembling that associated with, actual or potential tissue damage" and has expanded on this with the addition of six important points:

- "Pain is always a personal experience that is influenced to varying degrees by biological, psychological and social factors.
- Although pain usually serves an adaptive role, it may have adverse effects on function and on social and psychological well-being.

- A person's report of an experience of pain should be respected.
- Through their life experiences, individuals learn the concept of pain.
- Pain and nociception are different phenomena. Pain cannot be inferred solely from activity in sensory neurons.
- Verbal description is only one of the several behaviours to express pain; inability to communicate does not negate that a human experiences pain" (International Association for the Study of Pain, 2021).

The process between an injury and perceiving pain involves four steps: transduction, transmission, modulation, and perception.

Types of Pain

Nociceptive and Neuropathic Pain

Pain is categorized as nociceptive, neuropathic, or both, according to underlying pathology. Nociceptive pain is caused by damage to somatic or visceral tissue. Examples include pain from a surgical incision, a broken leg, arthritis, or angina (Tyerman & Cobbett, 2023). Neuropathic pain is caused by damage to nerve cells or changes in spinal cord processing and is described as burning, shooting, or stabbing. This type can be difficult to treat. Examples include phantom limb pain and diabetic neuropathy (Tyerman & Cobbett, 2023).

Acute and Persistent Pain

Acute pain usually has a sudden onset and diminishes over time as healing occurs. Examples include postoperative pain, labour pain, and angina. Persistent pain persists beyond the normal time for healing. It can be disabling and is often accompanied by depression and anxiety.

Pain Scales

Descriptive scales are an objective means of measuring pain intensity. Various scales can be used for adults and children to rate pain before and after interventions. The most common one used with adults is the numeric rating scale, with which clients rate their pain on a scale of 0 to 10 (0 being no pain; 10 being the most severe pain ever experienced). Pain should be rated before and after administration of analgesics. For clients who are unable to respond to other pain intensity scales, a series of faces ranging from "smiling" to "crying" can be used. These scales can be used in a variety of client populations, including young children and older persons (Tyerman & Cobbett, 2023).

Best Practices for Pain Control

- Practice guidelines are available that recommend systematic ways of using analgesics. One example is the pain relief ladder developed by the World Health Organization (WHO) for cancer pain relief in adults. The WHO treatment plan emphasizes that different medications are administered depending on the severity of pain. The three-step ladder approach is used to determine the severity of the pain. Step 1: nonopioids are administered for mild pain; step 2: mild opioids are administered as necessary for mild to moderate pain; step 3: strong opioids are administered for moderate to severe pain. If pain persists or increases, medications from the next higher step are used to control the pain. The steps are not meant to be sequential if someone has moderate to severe pain: for this client, the analgesics given would be the stronger analgesics listed in steps 2 and 3 (Tyerman & Cobbett, 2023). The WHO has developed guidelines that focus on the physical, psychological, and pharmacological interventions for the management of primary and secondary chronic pain in children 0 to 19 years of age (WHO, 2021).

- "Current best practice guidelines suggest multimodal combination of non-opioid therapies, delivered through a multidisciplinary approach, can be often as effective as opioids in managing chronic pain while presenting far less risk of harm. People with chronic pain should have access to the appropriate individualized treatment options that are selected by the health care professional through a shared decision-making process" (Health Quality Ontario, 2018, p. 18).

- "Advocate for the most effective dosing schedule, considering the medication(s) duration of onset, effect(s) and half-life. The optimal analgesia dose is one that effectively relieves pain with minimum adverse effects" (RNAO, 2013, p. 34). "If opioids are initiated for chronic pain, start at the lowest effective dose, preferably below 50 mg morphine equivalents per day. Titrate over time to a dose of between 50 and 90 mg of morphine equivalents per day only when necessary and only after ensuring the person with chronic pain is aware of the potential harms and is willing to accept a higher risk form improved pain relief" (Health Quality Ontario, 2018, p. 25). Current best practice suggests that only one long-acting opioid is ordered at a given time for management of continuous moderate to severe pain. Examples of long-acting oral opioids are morphine sulphate controlled-release tablets (MS Contin) and morphine sulphate extended-release capsule (M-Eslon).

- It is important to give breakthrough medication doses as necessary and to consider adjuvant therapies and treatments.

- Patient-controlled analgesia (PCA) is an infusion pump that is programmed for dose and time intervals, allowing clients to control analgesic administration without overdose. The PCA pump can be IV, subcutaneous, intrathecal, transdermal, or epidural and is a good short-term option for postoperative pain. PCA offers a number of benefits. PCA empowers clients to have some control over their pain, which helps alleviate anxiety and medication use. Because clients are active participants in their care, they can medicate themselves when the pain starts. Pain relief allows clients to ambulate earlier, and, as a result, they have fewer pulmonary problems. Use of PCAs promotes healing, which leads to faster recovery and shorter hospital stays (Astle & Duggleby, 2024; Cobbett, 2024;). The RN usually has the primary responsibility for PCAs and epidural pumps. The practical nurse may be required to monitor or assist with the pump. It is important to monitor the IV site and assess for adverse effects of the medication. Many agencies require an independent double check by two nurses when initiating a PCA, changing the dose, or discontinuing the pump medications (Cobbett, 2024). The practical nurse needs to check with the agency regarding the scope of practice for PCA pumps.

Nonpharmacological Methods of Pain Relief

These methods can be used alone or in combination with pharmacological methods. Examples include progressive relaxation, guided imagery, biofeedback, transcutaneous electrical nerve stimulation (TENS), music therapy, acupressure, massage, and the application of heat or cold. Many nonpharmacological methods of pain relief in a clinical setting require a health care provider's order especially for heat and cold applications.

NUTRITION

Nutrients are the elements necessary for body processes and functions. A balanced diet with carbohydrates, fats, proteins, vitamins, and minerals provides the essential nutrients to carry out the body's normal physiological functioning.

- Carbohydrates are the main source of energy in the diet.
- Proteins are made from amino acids and are essential for the growth, maintenance, and repair of body tissue.
- Fats (lipids) are the most calorie-dense nutrient and are composed of triglycerides and fatty acids. They provide a concentrated source and stored form of energy.
- Vitamins facilitate metabolism of proteins, fats, and carbohydrates and are essential for normal metabolism. Vitamin content is usually highest in fresh foods that are used quickly and exposed minimally to cooking, storage, preparation, and processing.
- Fat-soluble vitamins A, D, E, and K can be stored in the body and are not easily destroyed by cooking or storage.
- Water-soluble vitamins (B complex and C) are not stored in the body, are easily destroyed by cooking, and can be excreted in the urine.
- Vitamin K is important in the production of prothrombin (necessary for the coagulation of blood).
- Vitamin C functions in the production of collagen, which is important in wound healing.
- Vitamin A is important in the maintenance of eyesight and epithelial linings.
- Minerals are essential to the body as catalysts in biochemical reactions. Examples include calcium, chloride, magnesium, phosphorus, potassium, sodium, iron, and zinc (Astle & Duggleby, 2024).

Canada's Food Guide

Canada's Food Guide is a tool that helps clients to make appropriate nutritional choices and healthy living decisions. The guide recommends eating plenty of fruits and vegetables, drinking water rather than sugary beverages, consuming high-protein foods, and choosing whole-grain options when available (Government of Canada, 2022). In the guide The Eat

Well Plate the proportion of each of the food groups that is recommended for healthy eating is represented. The vegetables and fruit food group fills half of the plate, emphasizing the important role these foods play. The guide also recommends switching from whole milk to skim or 1% milk and choosing a variety of protein sources such as seafood, small portions of lean meat, poultry, and beans.

"Decisions about healthy eating are influenced by many aspects of our social and physical environments, from household income and food skills to government food policies. All sectors—including agriculture, environment, education, housing, transportation, the food industry trade, child, family and social services have a role to play for Canada's Dietary Guidelines to have far reaching and longstanding effects on the nutritional health of Canadians" (Dames et al., 2021, p. 532). See Fig. 6.4 in Chapter 6 for an extract from *Canada's Food Guide*.

Therapeutic Diets

A *therapeutic diet* is a diet intended to treat disease or help to manage a medical condition. See Table 7.6 for types of therapeutic diets, indications for use of these diets, and foods permitted on the diets.

Enteral Nutrition

Enteral nutrition (EN) refers to the delivery of liquid nutrients into the gastro-intestinal tract via a tube. EN is used when the client cannot ingest food but can still digest and absorb nutrients.

Types of Feeding Tubes

- Nasogastric (NG) tubes are inserted through the nose to the stomach (see the section "Bowel Elimination" for more details).
- Nasoenteral, or small-bore, feeding tubes (such as Dobbhoff tubes) are placed through the nose into the stomach and then moved into the duodenum. Placement is checked by radiography prior to commencing tube feedings.
  Surgically placed feeding tubes.
- A gastrostomy tube (G-tube) is placed directly into the stomach through the abdominal wall and sutured in place.
- A jejunostomy tube (J-tube) is inserted directly into the jejunum for clients with pathological conditions of the upper gastro-intestinal tract.
  Feeding tubes inserted by endoscopy. In this procedure, the stomach or the jejunum is punctured during a laparotomy or an endoscopy procedure that does not require a general anaesthetic. The two types are PEG (percutaneous endoscopic gastrostomy) and PEJ (percutaneous endoscopic jejunostomy).

Nursing Care of Clients With EN

- Ensure that the head of the bed is elevated 30 to 45 degrees at all times to prevent regurgitation of feedings and aspiration into the lungs.
- Monitor the client for abdominal distension and check the residual contents of the stomach regularly to see whether the client is tolerating the feeds. Aspirate all stomach contents (residual), measure the amount, and return the contents to the stomach if the residual is less than 100 to 150 mL (depending on agency policy). If the residual volume is more than 150 mL, it indicates delayed gastric emptying, which places the client at a higher risk of aspiration, and the feeds should be withheld.
- Check placement of the tube by (a) aspirating the gastric contents and checking the pH of any gastric fluids, and (b) X-ray examination. Do not rely on the auscultation method to differentiate between gastric and respiratory placement or to differentiate between gastric and small bowel placement. To verify whether a feeding tube has sustained the proper position, mark the exit site of the feeding tube during the initial radiograph and observe for any changes in the external tube length during feedings. If a significant increase in the external length is observed, use other bedside tests to help determine whether the tube has become dislocated. When in doubt, obtain a radiograph to determine tube location (Astle & Duggleby, 2024, Tyerman & Cobbett, 2023).
- Assess bowel sounds; if absent, withhold feeds and notify the physician.
- Feeding pumps may be used for continuous feeds.
- For bolus feeds (300–400 mL of formula every 3–6 hours), leave the client in the high Fowler's position for 30 minutes after feeding.
- Change the feeding container and tubing every 24 hours to prevent bacterial growth.
- Do not hang more than 4 hours' worth of formula to prevent bacterial growth.
- Flush with 30 to 60 mL of water (according to agency policy) with an irrigation syringe after feeding.
- With feeding tubes, "monitor fingerstick blood glucose levels every 6 hours until maximum administration rate is reached and maintained for 24 hours" (Astle & Duggleby, 2024, p. 1146).

Complications of EN

Complications of EN include aspiration, diarrhea, vomiting, abdominal distension, and clogging of the feeding tube.

Parenteral Nutrition

Parenteral nutrition (PN) is a form of specialized nutrition support in which nutrients are provided intravenously to provide a positive nitrogen balance. PN can be administered in the home as well as the hospital.

Types of PN

Total PN is a nutritionally adequate hypertonic solution consisting of glucose, electrolytes, and other nutrients administered through a CVAD site.

- Peripheral parenteral nutrition (PPN) can be used for clients who are experiencing mild or moderate malnutrition for up to weeks as long as the formula has a final dextrose concentration of 5 to 10% and an amino acid content of 3%. Often PPN is administered through a

TABLE 7.6   Therapeutic Diets

Type of Diet	Uses of Diet	Foods Permitted
Clear fluids	Often a postoperative diet, also used for diarrhea or initial feeding after complete bowel rest	Broth, coffee, tea, carbonated beverages, clear fruit juices, Popsicles, Jell-O
Thickened fluids	Used for clients who have dysphagia (difficulty swallowing) and are at risk for aspiration	Any liquid can be thickened with thickening agents
Full fluids	Can be used after clear fluids following surgery. Also for clients who are unable to chew or swallow.	Clear fluids, plus smooth-textured dairy products, puddings and custards, refined cooked cereals, ice cream, and all fruit juices
Pureed	Can be used for client with dental problems or problems swallowing or chewing	All of the above, with the addition of scrambled eggs, pureed meats, vegetables, fruits, mashed potatoes, and gravy
Mechanical soft	Can be used for client with dental problems, problems swallowing or chewing, and mouth ulcerations	All of the above, with the addition of foods such as ground or finely diced meats, flaked fish, cheese, rice, potatoes, cooked vegetables, bananas, soups, etc.
Soft or Low residue	Can be used for client with inflammatory or bowel disease flares, for bowel surgery and colonoscopy prep, for clients with acute diverticultitis.	Low-fibre, easily digested foods, such as pastas, casseroles, moist tender meats, canned cooked fruits and vegetables, desserts, cakes, and cookies without nuts or coconut can be added.
High fibre	Can be used for clients with constipation or to prevent constipation	Addition of fresh uncooked fruits, steamed vegetables, bran, oatmeal, and dried fruits
Low sodium	For control of hypertension (no added salt [NAS]) and to reduce edema in clients with heart failure	Can vary from NAS to severe sodium restrictions
Low cholesterol	Used for clients with high cholesterol levels	Restrictions on foods high in cholesterol, such as eggs, regular cheese and ice cream, organ meats, fried food, and fast food
Diabetic	Used for diabetic clients	Clients with diabetes follow a healthy diet recommended for the general population as outlined in *Eating Well with Canada's Food Guide*. In hospitals, the meals are often labelled "diabetic" or "no added sugar" to indicate that the meal plan follows Diabetes Canada's current nutritional guidelines for diabetics.
Regular		No restrictions

Adapted from Astle, B., & Duggleby, W. (2024). *Potter and Perry's Canadian fundamentals of nursing* (7th ed.). Elsevier Inc.

central catheter, which may be a PICC line, implanted subcutaneous ports or a tunnelled central access device (Cobbett, 2024).

- Total parenteral nutrition or central parenteral nutrition (TPN/CPN) is administration of carbohydrates in the form of dextrose, fats in special emulsified form, proteins in the form of amino acids, vitamins, minerals, and water. High-osmolality solutions (25% dextrose) are administered in conjunction with 5–10% amino acids, electrolytes, minerals, and vitamins. TPN/CPN is administered via a central line (usually the superior vena cava) (Astle & Duggleby, 2024; Tyerman & Cobbett, 2023). CPN using concentrated dextrose solutions should not be infused into a peripheral IV or midline catheter because of the increased risk for phlebitis (Cobbett, 2024).

- Intralipid therapy is an infusion of 10 to 20% fat emulsion that provides essential fatty acids. It is usually administered at the same time as PPN or TPN. It can be administered alone through a separate peripheral catheter, through a CVAD, by Y-connector tubing, or as an admixture to TPN solution (Astle & Duggleby, 2024).

- Total nutrient admixture (TNA) is a combination of dextrose, amino acids, and lipids in one container. TNA is administered over 24 hours through a central line (Astle & Duggleby, 2024).

Indications for PN

Indications for initiation of PN include a nonfunctional gastro-intestinal tract (e.g., following bowel surgery; trauma to the head, neck, or abdomen; intestinal obstruction; chemotherapy; or radiation therapy); extended bowel rest (e.g., due to inflammatory bowel disease, severe diarrhea, or pancreatitis); or preoperative TPN (such as in the case of severe malnutrition or preoperative bowel rest).

Nursing care of clients with PN

- Infuse TPN through a large vein, such as the subclavian, due to the high osmolarity of the solution. This is done by RNs with specialized training who insert PICC lines that are started in a vein of the forearm or upper arm and threaded into the subclavian vein or superior vena cava. Physicians may insert the catheter in the superior vena cava (Astle & Duggleby, 2024).

- Ensure proper placement of the line after insertion and prior to starting TPN. Placement is confirmed by X-ray, as accidental pneumothorax can occur during insertion.
- Regulate flow carefully using an infusion pump. Rapid infusion can cause movement of fluid into the intravascular compartment, causing dehydration, circulatory overload, and hyperglycemia (Cobbett, 2024). Slow infusion can result in hypoglycemia as the body adapts to the high osmolarity by secreting more insulin; for this reason, therapy is never terminated abruptly (Cobbett, 2024).
- Use aseptic technique when handling the infusion and IV tubing or when changing dressings. Check agency policy regarding the frequency of tubing change (usually every 24 hours) and dressing change (change transparent dressings at least every 5–7 days and gauze dressings usually every 48 hours). Change dressing if damp, loosened, soiled or when inspection of site is necessary.
- Use an in-line filter to remove crystals from the TPN solution.
- Record body weights at least three times weekly and monitor blood glucose levels frequently.

Monitor fluid intake, urine, and gastro-intestinal output every 8 hours.

- Check laboratory reports daily (glucose, creatinine, blood urea nitrogen, and electrolytes); also check serum lipids and liver function if lipids are administered (Cobbett, 2024).
- Monitor temperature every 4 hours, as infection is the most common TPN complication; obtain cultures of blood, urine, and sputum (according to agency policy) to rule out other sources of infection if the client develops a fever (Cobbett, 2024).

URINARY ELIMINATION

Key Terms Related to Urinary Elimination

- *Anuria* is the absence of urine formation.
- *Diuresis* is the passage of large amounts of urine.
- *Dysuria* is painful or difficult urination.
- *Frequency* is voiding at frequent intervals (less than 2-hour intervals) or voiding more than eight times in 24 hours.
- *Hematuria* is the presence of blood in the urine.
- *Nocturia* is excessive or frequent urination after going to bed.
- *Oliguria* is urine output of less than 400 mL/day.
- *Polyuria* is voiding large amounts of urine (Astle & Duggleby, 2024).

Altered Urinary Elimination

Urinary Retention

Urinary retention is the marked accumulation of urine in the bladder as a result of the inability of the bladder to empty. Retention can occur in the postoperative period due to the effect of the anaesthetic. Prolonged retention can lead to stasis of urine in the bladder and increased risk of a urinary tract infection (UTI). Signs and symptoms of retention include any of the following: frequent voiding of small amounts, absence of urine output with palpable tender bladder, dull sound on percussion, sensation of bladder fullness, abdominal discomfort, restlessness, diaphoresis, and dribbling. A bladder scanner is a noninvasive device that creates an ultrasound image of the bladder for measuring the volume of urine in the bladder. A bladder scanner is used to assess bladder volume whenever inadequate bladder emptying is suspected (Cobbett, 2024).

Urinary Tract Infection

UTI is the most common HAI due to the frequency of urinary catheterizations. If left untreated, UTIs can spread to the kidneys, causing kidney infection and eventually kidney damage. Signs and symptoms include any of the following: dysuria, fever, chills, frequency, urgency, hematuria, and concentrated cloudy (possibly foul-smelling) urine (Astle & Duggleby, 2024).

Urinary Incontinence

Urinary incontinence (UI) is the loss of control over micturition. It may present as any of the following types (Astle & Duggleby, 2024; RNAO, 2020):

- Transient: loss of urine outside of or affecting the urinary system that resolves when the underlying cause(s), such as acute confusion or UTI, are treated
- Urge: involuntary passage of urine after a strong sense of urgency to void and the bladder contracts and empties in an involuntary fashion—for example, with alcohol or caffeine ingestion or a UTI
- Stress: leakage of small volumes of urine caused by a sudden increase in intra-abdominal pressure, such as during coughing or sneezing, laughing, rising from a chair, lifting items, or exercise
- Mixed: having features of both stress and urge incontinence
- Functional: involuntary, unpredictable passage of urine in a client with an intact urinary and nervous system, as in the case when an older person with bladder control is unable to reach the toilet. May also be referred to as disability incontinence
- UI associated with chronic retention of urine (previously overflow UI): involuntary loss of a small amount of urine (20–30 mL) when the bladder does not completely empty with a high residual urine volume or a palpable nonpainful bladder remaining after voiding
- Multifactorial UI: urine loss due to multiple interacting factors both inside and outside the urinary tract. Examples include medication, age-related changes, and environmental factors such as access to the bathroom.

Urinary Diversions

Urinary diversions divert the flow of urine from the kidneys directly to the abdominal surface via a urinary stoma. The diversion can be permanent or temporary and either continent or incontinent.

Maintaining Normal Urinary Elimination

- Promote fluid intake of 1 500 to 2 000 mL daily for the average adult and an increased intake for clients at risk of UTI and renal calculi, as well as for clients with catheters.

- Maintain normal voiding habits. Void every 3 to 4 hours to maintain a normal bladder capacity (400–500 mL) and to avoid urinary stasis.

Measuring Intake and Output

- Fluid intake should equal output. Intake is considered all dietary items that are fluid at room temperature as well as IV fluids, including blood. Output is urine, vomitus, suction drainage, bleeding, and insensible loss such as sweating.
- Normal urine output is 60 mL per hour or 1 500 mL per day. Urine outputs below 30 mL per hr (0.5 mL/kg/hr) for more than 2 hours in an adult should be reported. Also, urine outputs over 2 000 to 2 500 mL daily (polyuria) should be reported to a physician (Astle & Duggleby, 2024).
- Daily weights are the single most important indicator of fluid status. Clients should be weighed daily on the same weigh scale at the same time after voiding.

Urine Testing and Specimen Collection

Urine samples can be random (routine urinalysis), clean-catch or midstream (culture and sensitivity), or sterile (culture and sensitivity). For midstream urine specimens, the client cleans the perineum with an antiseptic solution, initiates urination to cleanse the meatus, and then urinates into a sterile specimen container. Some tests, such as the creatinine clearance test, require 24-hour collection of urine. The urine is collected in a special collection container that may have a preservative added.

Catheterization and Catheter Care

Intermittent Catheterization

A straight single-lumen catheter is introduced to empty the bladder and removed after the bladder is drained. Indications for use include relief of bladder distension and obtaining a sterile urine specimen.

In-Dwelling Catheterization (Retention or Foley Catheterization)

A catheter with an inflatable balloon is inserted into the bladder on a short- or long-term basis. Indications for use include prostate enlargement, measuring urine output in critically ill clients, or ulcers or wounds irritated by contact with urine.

Catheterization for Residual Urine

Catheterization for residual urine involves inserting a catheter after a client voids to check for the amount of urine remaining in the bladder. The bladder normally holds less than 50 mL after voiding. If the volume of urine (residual volume) is greater than 100 mL, the catheter may be left in situ. Portable bladder scanners offer a noninvasive means of assessing post-void residual volumes (Astle & Duggleby, 2024).

Catheter Care

- Keep the urinary drainage bag below the level of the bladder to prevent reflux, which can lead to UTIs.
- Secure the catheter to the client's inner thigh or abdomen with a strip of non-allergenic tape or (or multipurpose tube holders with a Velcro strap) to reduce the pressure on the urethra and the possibility of tissue injury.
- Keep the drainage tubing coiled on the bed to aid gravity drainage.
- Do not open a closed system unless absolutely necessary, to lessen the chance of UTIs.
- Perform catheter care twice daily with soap and water to cleanse the urinary meatus and encrustations on the catheter and after a bowel movement in order to reduce infections.
- Empty the drainage bag every 8 hours and record the amount, colour, odour, and consistency of urinary drainage.
- Change the urinary catheter bag and catheter regularly according to agency policy.
- Remove the catheter as soon as clinically possible to prevent UTIs.

Bladder Irrigation

Closed and open catheter or bladder irrigations are irrigations or flushes used to maintain the patency of in-dwelling catheters or to wash out the bladder and treat local infections.

BOWEL ELIMINATION

Common Bowel Elimination Challenges

- Constipation usually involves infrequent bowel movements, difficult defecation, inability to defecate at will, and hard feces (Astle & Duggleby, 2024). It can also involve abdominal distension and pain and pressure in the rectum.
- Fecal impaction is a condition in which a collection of hardened feces cannot be expelled from the rectum. The common sign is inability to pass stool for several days. Impaction should be suspected if there is a continuous oozing of diarrhea (liquid feces from higher in the bowel is seeping around the impaction).
- Diarrhea is the passage of liquid feces and an increase in the number of stools. The greatest danger from diarrhea is fluid and electrolyte imbalance.
- Fecal incontinence is the inability to control the passage of feces and gas. Skin breakdown can occur after repeated contact with liquid stool.
- Flatulence is excessive gas in the stomach and intestine. Reduction in gastro-intestinal motility, resulting from opiates, general anaesthetics, abdominal surgery, or immobilization, can cause abdominal distension due to flatulence.
- Hemorrhoids (internal and external) are dilated, engorged veins in the rectal area. They can make defecation painful.

Bowel Diversions

Bowel diversions divert the feces from the bowel directly to the abdominal surface. Surgical openings can be created in the ileum (ileostomy) or colon (colostomy) to create an artificial opening called a *stoma*. The location of the ostomy determines the consistency of the stool, with the ileostomy having more frequent liquid stools and the colostomy resulting in more solid formed stool. Proper selection and maintenance of an ostomy pouching system is important to prevent damage to the skin around the stoma.

Promoting Regular or Normal Defecation

- Understand that foods high in fibre and an increased fluid intake keep feces soft.
- Provide clients with as much privacy as possible. Lack of privacy may cause the client to ignore the urge to defecate.
- Provide clients with a position as close to normal as possible for defecation (such as on a commode chair) and give them enough time.
- Be aware of the client's normal routine and when defecation is most likely to occur, for example, 1 hour after a meal. Establishing a specific time for defecation may help to prevent constipation.
- Regular exercise within the client's physical ability is important in stimulating peristalsis and a regular bowel routine.
- Know that warm fluids and certain juices (prune) can stimulate bowel motility.

Enemas

Enemas are an instillation of a solution into the rectum and sigmoid colon. They stimulate peristalsis and initiate defecation. They are commonly used for relief of constipation but can also deliver medications that have a local effect on the rectal mucosa. The most common types of enemas are cleansing and oil retention. Enemas may also be used in preparing for diagnostic tests or for performing diagnostic tests of the bowel or rectum, such as barium enemas.

Types of Enemas

- Cleansing enemas include tap water, NS, low-volume hypertonic (Fleet), and soap suds.
- Oil retention enemas lubricate the rectum and colon. The feces become softer and easier to pass. The client is advised to hold the enema for 30 minutes to 3 hours.

Nursing Care of Clients Receiving an Enema

- Explain the procedure to the client and ensure privacy.
- Explain how long the client must retain the enema.
- Place the client in the modified left lateral recumbent position position.
- Ensure that the rectal tube attached to the enema bag is lubricated and inserted 7 to 10 cm into the rectum.
- Ensure that the client has access to a bathroom, commode, or bedpan.
- Observe and record the amount and consistency of the return from the enema.

Digital Removal of Stool

Digital removal of stool is used when the client has a fecal impaction. The nurse breaks up the fecal mass with a finger and removes it in sections. This procedure can be painful, can damage the rectal mucosa, and can cause vagal stimulation (resulting in reflex slowing of the heart rate). In some agencies, a physician's order is necessary to remove a fecal impaction. Vital signs should be checked before and after the procedure.

Nasogastric Tubes

Nasogastric (NG) tubes are pliable tubes inserted through the nasopharynx and into the stomach. Commonly used types are Levin or Salem sump NG tubes.

Purposes of NG Tubes

- Decompression: removal of secretions from the gastrointestinal tract for the prevention and relief of abdominal distension
- Feeding or gavage: instillation of liquid nutritional supplements into the stomach for clients unable to swallow
- Compression: internal application of pressure by means of an inflated balloon to prevent internal esophageal or gastro-intestinal hemorrhage
- Lavage: irrigation of the stomach for active bleeding, poisoning, or gastric dilation.

Insertion of an NG Tube

- Place the client in the high Fowler's position.
- Measure from the tip of the nose to the earlobe to the xiphoid process to determine the length of insertion.
- Lubricate 7.5 cm with water-soluble lubricant.
- Instruct the client to bend their head forward to close the epiglottis.
- Insert the tube into the patent nostril and advance it backward into the nasopharynx.
- Have the client dry swallow or sip on water (if allowed) and advance the tube as the client swallows to the predetermined length.
- If the client experiences respiratory distress (coughing or choking), remove the tube and resume the procedure when the client has recovered.
- Tape the tube in place and confirm placement of the tube.

Assessment of Tube Placement

- The initial method to check placement is by radiography.
- Tube placement is assessed every 4 hours and before administering medications or feedings.
- The most reliable method to assess tube placement at the bedside is to monitor the external of the tube and aspirate gastric contents and test the gastric pH. Gastric pH should be less than 4. Intestinal aspirates are greater than 4, and respiratory aspirates are greater than 5.5.
- Auscultation is not considered a reliable method for the identification of tube placement because a tube inadvertently placed in the lungs, pharynx, or esophagus can transmit a sound similar to that of air entering the stomach (Astle & Duggleby, 2024).
- Irrigation of an NG tube is gentle instillation of 30 to 50 mL of water or NS (check agency policy) to check and maintain patency of the NG tube. Check placement of the tube prior to irrigating. A health care provider's order may be required to irrigate the NG tube of gastric surgery clients.
- Obtain repeated radiographic film confirmation if bedside methods create any doubt regarding the location of the tube (Cobbett, 2024).

Medication Administration Via an NG Tube

- Crush medications or open capsules (if allowed) or use liquid forms. Before crushing medications, check for compatibility of medications since not all medications can be crushed together.
- Dissolve medication in 10 to 30 mL of warm water and draw up into a 60-mL syringe.
- Check placement of the NG tube as well as residual volume in the stomach.
- Flush the NG tube with 30 mL of water (check agency policy).
- Instill medication into the tube.
- Flush the NG tube with 30 to 60 mL of water (check agency policy).

Clamp the tube for 30 to 60 minutes if the client is on intermittent suction (check agency policy).

Considerations Relating to Older Persons

- Constipation can be a common complaint among older persons due to a combination of impaired general health, use of medication, decreased motility, and low physical activity.

MOBILITY AND IMMOBILITY

Mobility refers to the ability to move easily and independently. Certain illnesses, surgery, pain, and aging can impair mobility temporarily or permanently. It is important to know the hazards of immobility and how to prevent them as well as how to care for clients who are immobile.

Systemic Effects of Immobility

When there is an alteration in mobility, each body system is at risk for impairment. Some of the changes that can happen—the "hazards of immobility"—are as follows:

- Metabolic changes include a lowered metabolic rate, a negative nitrogen balance, anorexia (loss of appetite), and a negative calcium balance (calcium is lost from bones).
- Respiratory changes include shallow respirations and decreased vital capacity, pooling of respiratory secretions, atelectasis (collapse of alveoli), and hypostatic pneumonia (inflammation of the lung from stasis or pooling of secretions).
- Cardiovascular changes include diminished cardiac reserve, increased use of the Valsalva manoeuvre (such as when the client holds their breath to change position in bed), orthostatic hypotension, and venous dilation and stasis, which can cause edema and deep vein thrombosis (DVT).
- Musculo-skeletal changes include disuse osteoporosis, disuse atrophy, contractures, foot drop (foot permanently fixed in plantar flexion), and external hip rotation.
- Urinary elimination changes include urinary stasis, urinary calculi, urinary retention, and urinary infection.
- Gastro-intestinal system changes include constipation and decreased peristalsis.
- Integumentary changes include less skin turgor (elasticity) and possible skin breakdown, as well as the formation of pressure sores or ulcers (Astle & Duggleby, 2024; Tyerman & Cobbett, 2023).

Positioning and Body Alignment

- Immobile clients need to be repositioned at least every 2 hours or more frequently if there are reddened skin areas. The 30-degree lateral position is best as it does not put direct pressure on the trochanter.
- Clients should be placed in a variety of positions to prevent pressure areas. Different bed positions used include Fowler's; supine (dorsal) recumbent; prone (face down); side-lying (lateral); and semiprone.
- Limbs need to be anatomically aligned in a slightly flexed position. Bony surfaces should not touch; for example, a pillow is often placed between knees. Trochanter rolls can be used to prevent external hip rotation, footboards to prevent foot drop, and hand–wrist or foot–ankle splints to keep the joints anatomically aligned.

Range-of-Motion Exercises

- ROM exercises can be active (the client is able to move all joints through their ROM unassisted) or passive (the client is unable to move some or all of the joints independently, and the nurse assists certain or all joints through their ROM).
- Exercises should begin as soon as possible, as joints begin to stiffen within 24 hours of loss of movement in an extremity or joint. It is best to schedule them at specific times, such as during a bath.
- Each joint movement is repeated five times during each session. No force is exerted.

Moving and Transferring Clients Safely

A thorough assessment must be made prior to moving or positioning a client. The client needs to be assessed for the degree of exertion permitted, capabilities such as mobility and strength, comprehension, pain level, weight, and presence of orthostatic hypotension. The nurse must also assess their own strength and ability to move the client and how much assistance is available from other health care providers or if mechanical lifts are available. Finally, the nurse must assess the environment to make sure the transfer can be done safely.

- Consider the client's abilities and disabilities when deciding appropriate transfer technique and the need for assistive devices; for example, for hemiplegia, place the wheelchair on the side opposite the affected extremities; for paraplegia, the client may use a trapeze, slide board, or wheelchair with a removable arm.
- Use the principles of body mechanics (see Box 7.2).

WOUND CARE

Types of Wounds

- Acute wounds, such as surgical wounds, follow the normal healing process in a predictable and timely fashion.

- Chronic wounds, such as pressure injuries, do not heal easily, and the normal reparative process is interrupted.

Types of Wound Healing

Primary Intention

Wounds that heal by primary intention have little or no tissue loss, have well-approximated wound margins, and heal quickly. Two examples are a clean surgical wound or a paper cut.

Secondary Intention

Wounds that heal by secondary intention have loss of tissue, such as second- or third-degree burns, or pressure injuries, and there is no approximation of the wound edges. Healing and granulation take place from the edges inward and from the base of the wound to the top. The wound is left open and takes longer to heal (Astle & Duggleby, 2024).

Tertiary Intention

Tertiary intention (delayed primary intention) healing occurs with postponing suturing of a wound in which two layers of granulation tissue are sutured together. The wound is left open until the infection is resolved (Tyerman & Cobbett, 2023).

Complications of Wound Healing

- Hemorrhage or bleeding from the wound may occur externally or internally.
- Wound infection is the second most common HAI. Signs of wound infection may include any of the following: pain and tenderness at the site, erythema, edema, inflammation of wound edges, purulent drainage, warmth of tissues at the site, fever or chills, elevated white blood cell (WBC) count, and delayed healing (Astle & Duggleby, 2024).
- Dehiscence is the partial or total separation of the wound layers (Astle & Duggleby, 2024). It usually occurs at 3 to 11 days postinjury or surgery. It most commonly involves surgical wounds of the abdomen and can occur after a vigorous bout of coughing or straining. A strategy to prevent dehiscence is to provide support to the area, such as using a pillow as a splint when the client is coughing.
- Evisceration is protrusion of the abdominal organs through the wound opening. This is a medical emergency and requires surgical intervention. The nurse should cover the organs with sterile saline-soaked towels, keep the client NPO (nil per os, or nothing by mouth), and monitor for signs and symptoms of shock.
- A fistula is an "abnormal passage between two organs or between an organ and the outside of the body" (Astle & Duggleby, 2024, p. 1311). It is the result of infection, poor wound healing, or a complication of diseases such as Crohn's disease.

Types of Wound Drainage

Wound drainage can be serous (clear and watery), purulent (thick green, yellow, or brown and containing pus cells), serosanguineous (thin, watery, and blood-tinged), or sanguineous (bloody).

Wound Assessment

Wound assessment includes observing wound appearance (size, location, stage of healing, approximation, and condition of skin around the wound); the character and amount of drainage; the presence and amount of drainage from drains such as the Penrose, Hemovac, or Jackson-Pratt; and the presence of sutures, staples, or packing. Wound assessment may also involve palpating the wound for warmth, tenderness, hardness, or pain and may require collection of a wound culture if the wound appears infected.

Pressure (Ulcers) Injuries

The term *pressure injury* replaces the term *pressure ulcer*, *decubitus ulcer* or *bedsore* in the National Pressure Ulcer Advisory Panel (NPUAP) Pressure Injury Staging System in 2016 (NPUAP, 2022). The new term is considered to better describe pressure injuries to both intact and ulcerated skin.

A pressure injury is localized damage to the skin and/or underlying soft tissue, usually over a bony prominence or related to a medical or other device. The injury can present as intact skin or an open ulcer and may be painful. The injury occurs as a consequence of intense and/or prolonged pressure or pressure in combination with shear (Astle & Duggleby, 2024). Pressure is the main source of pressure injuries, and they often develop over a bony prominence when tissue is compressed between the bone and a hard surface such as a bed or chair. The following are other factors that work with pressure to cause skin damage and necrosis:

- *Friction* is when two surfaces are rubbed against each other. For example, dragging a client across the sheets can cause an abrasion.
- *Shear* is the parallel force that happens when the skin and underlying subcutaneous tissue are pulled taut, obstructing capillary blood flow and causing tissue necrosis in the deep tissue layers. Shear occurs when the client is moved incorrectly; for example, when they are dragged instead of lifted clear of the mattress, or when the head of the bed is elevated above 30 degrees for long periods of time, causing the client to slide down in bed.
- Moisture caused by wound discharge, excess diaphoresis, or incontinence can be a factor leading to skin breakdown.

Risk Assessment for Pressure Injuries

Identify at-risk clients early by using a validated risk-assessment tool such as the Braden Scale. The Braden Scale measures sensory perception, moisture, activity, mobility, nutrition, and friction and shear. The scale needs to be used preventively (on admission) and consistently (daily in high-risk clients). As soon as a client is identified to be at risk for developing pressure injuries, prevention strategies should be started.

To assess clients with darker skin, the nurse should look for changes in skin colour, such as areas darker (purplish, bluish, brownish) than the surrounding skin. Use natural light or a halogen light source to accurately assess the skin colour. Palpate the skin temperature of the area. The area may feel warm initially and then cooler. Touch the skin to feel its consistency. Boggy or edematous observation may indicate a stage one pressure injury. Inquire if the client feels any itchiness or pain sensation (Tyerman & Cobbett, 2023).

Staging System for Pressure Injuries

Pressure injuries are described according to the following stages:

- Suspected deep tissue injury: A deep red, purple or maroon localized area of discoloured intact skin, nonintact skin or blood-filled blister, caused by damage to the underlying soft tissue from pressure or shear, or both.
- Stage I pressure injury: Intact skin with nonblanchable redness of a localized area, usually over a bony prominence. Darkly pigmented skin may not have visible blanching, but its colour may differ from that of the surrounding skin. The area may be painful, firm, warm, or cooler as compared with adjacent tissue.
- Stage II pressure injury: Partial-thickness loss of dermis presenting as a shallow open ulcer with a red-pink wound bed, without slough. It may also present as an intact, an open, or a ruptured serum-filled blister.
- Stage III pressure injury: Full-thickness tissue loss. Subcutaneous fat may be visible, but bone, tendon, or muscle is not exposed. Slough may be present. It may include undermining or tunnelling. The depth of a stage III pressure injury varies by anatomical location.
- Stage IV pressure injury: Full-thickness skin and tissue loss with exposed bone, tendon, or muscle. Slough or eschar may be present on some parts of the wound bed. Often it includes tunnelling and undermining. The depth of a stage IV pressure injury varies by anatomical location.
- Unstageable pressure injury: Full-thickness skin and tissue loss in which the base of the injury is covered in slough, eschar, or both. *Slough* is a viscous yellow layer that often covers the wound. *Eschar* is thick, dry, black, necrotic tissue covering a wound (Astle & Duggleby, 2024).

Prevention of Pressure Injuries

- Reposition clients every 2 hours or more if they are high risk. Encourage clients with some independent mobility to shift their weight every 15 minutes when sitting.
- Inspect the condition of the client's skin at least daily, and examine bony prominences carefully. Nonblanchable erythema or discoloration of the skin may indicate early signs of tissue injury.
- Keep linens dry to prevent maceration of skin and wrinkle-free to prevent pressure.
- Position the client in a 30-degree lateral position to either side to avoid pressure on the trochanter.
- Do not massage over bony prominences or reddened areas.
- Avoid elevating the head of the bed to more than 30 degrees, as that increases the shearing force.

- Use support surfaces (pressure redistribution devices), such as pressure-reducing and pressure-relieving mattresses, for at-risk clients. A pressure-reducing mattress reduces the interface pressure (the pressure between the body and the support surface) but not below the capillary-closing pressure (Astle & Duggleby, 2024). A pressure-relieving mattress relieves the interface pressure below the capillary-closing pressure, which is 32 mm Hg (Astle & Duggleby, 2024).
- Promote a diet that is high in protein and calories and ensure adequate hydration. Assess teeth or dentures; ensure good mouth care.
- Keep skin clean and well hydrated.

Treatment of Pressure Injuries

- Management of a client with a pressure injuries involves not only care of the wound itself but also support measures for the whole person. Support measures to consider include proper nutrition, pain management, pressure relief, and control of other medical issues. Treatment involves collaboration with many health care professionals like the dietitian, physician, nurse, occupational therapist, and physiotherapist to prevent and manage pressure injuries (Tyerman & Cobbett, 2023).
- Perform a comprehensive assessment of the pressure injury, including staging, measurement of size (depth, width, and length), character and amount of exudate, wound bed characteristics, pain, condition of surrounding skin, and evidence of tunnelling or undermining (Astle & Duggleby, 2024).
- Determine the need for local wound care by assessing the wound bed for debris, infection, and moisture balance. If slough is present, the wound may need to be irrigated, debrided, or both.
- Wound debridement removes necrotic material that interferes with healing. There are different methods of debridement, such as surgical or sharp, autolytic, enzymatic, or mechanical. Mechanical debridement (also called a *wet-to-dry dressing*) is no longer recommended as it is not selective and can damage new granulating tissue (Astle & Duggleby, 2024).
- Moist interactive wound healing involves keeping the wound bed moist and warm and not disturbing it too much by changing the dressing. A moist, interactive wound healing environment results in faster healing, better tissue quality, and reduced pain (Astle & Duggleby, 2024).
- Negative pressure wound therapy (NPWT) is a device that assists in wound closure by applying localized negative pressure to draw the edges of a wound together (Astle & Duggleby, 2024; Tyerman & Cobbett, 2023). It can be used with dehiscence and with acute, traumatic, and chronic wounds. It removes fluid from the area surrounding the wound and can accelerate healing.
- Healing of the wound can be monitored using tools like the NPUAP Pressure Ulcer Scale of Healing (PUSH) tool. Some agencies require pictures of the injury to be taken

initially and at regular intervals during the course of therapy (Tyerman & Cobbett, 2023).

Applying Dry Dressings

- The purpose of dressings is to protect the wound from contamination, aid hemostasis, absorb drainage, and promote a moist healing environment.
- Wounds are commonly cleansed with NS, which is not toxic to cells.
- The wound or incision should be cleansed from the least contaminated area (the wound or incision) to the most contaminated (the surrounding skin).
- Acute wounds usually require aseptic dressing techniques, while chronic wounds may require only clean dressing techniques.
- It is important to observe the character, colour, amount, and odour of drainage on the dressing and the appearance of the wound, as well as the skin around the wound.

Applying an Elastic Bandage

- An elastic bandage is used to create pressure over a body part, to immobilize a body part, to support a wound, to reduce or minimize edema, to secure a splint, or to secure dressings.
- The bandage is applied from distal to proximal to promote venous return.
- Assess distal circulation when the bandage is first applied and every 4 hours afterward. Check the limb distally for colour, warmth, sensation, and movement. Palpate and compare pulses bilaterally and check capillary refill.

SENSORY ALTERATIONS

Sensory deficits are losses in the normal function of sensory reception and perception, such as vision or hearing impairments. Aging most commonly results in a gradual decline of acuity in all senses. Clients who are immobilized or isolated are at risk for sensory alterations.

Sensory Deprivation

Sensory deprivation is the result of inadequate sensory stimuli (either in quality or quantity). Sensory deprivation can be the result of (a) reduced sensory input, as in the case of vision or hearing impairment; (b) the elimination of order or meaning from input, for example, exposure to strange environments; or (c) restriction in the environment, as when a client is confined to bed rest or receives reduced cues or no variation in cues from the environment. When clients are placed in isolation, a decrease in stimuli can occur (Astle & Duggleby, 2024).

Sensory Overload

Sensory overload occurs when clients receive multiple sensory stimuli and cannot disregard or filter out some stimuli. Their tolerance to sensory overload may vary depending on many factors, such as level of fatigue, attitude, or state of well-being (physical, mental, and emotional). It may lead to

delirium, a serious condition experienced by clients with sensory alterations. Providing calendars, clocks, diming lights, family support, and clear communication can help prevent sensory overload and delirium (Astle & Duggleby, 2024).

CARE OF SURGICAL CLIENTS

Preoperative Surgical Phase

Informed Consent

The surgeon is responsible for obtaining the client's informed consent for surgery before sedation is given.

Minors require a parent or guardian to sign the consent.

Three key elements for a consent to be valid include: it must be voluntary; the client must have the mental capacity to consent; and the client must be properly informed (Tyerman & Cobbett, 2023).

Nutrition

When the client is going to have general anaesthesia, solid foods and liquids are usually withheld after midnight the night before surgery to avoid the possibility of vomiting and subsequent aspiration during surgery. Protocols may vary if the client is having local anaesthesia or the surgery is scheduled for late in the day. Varying NPO protocols exist; the NPO protocol of each surgical facility should be followed (Tyerman & Cobbett, 2023). An IV line may be initiated prior to surgery or in the operating room.

Elimination

An enema or laxative may be ordered for clients having intestinal or abdominal surgery. The client should void immediately before surgery, or the insertion of a Foley catheter may be ordered.

Care of Surgical Site

The surgical site may be scrubbed with an antiseptic soap the night before surgery, or the client may be required to take a chlorhexidine shower and scrub the night before and the morning of the surgery. Shaving the skin is no longer recommended because it causes microscopic cuts. Hair is removed only if it interferes with surgery, and clippers instead of razors are used for hair removal.

Preoperative Teaching

The client needs to be informed before surgery about what to expect postoperatively. Teaching involves topics such as pain relief and use of the PCA pump, postoperative breathing exercises and the use of the incentive spirometer, foot and leg exercises, and instructions about invasive lines or devices to be expected after surgery (such as chest tubes, Foley catheter, drains, and NG tubes).

Psychological Preparation

Monitor the client's anxiety level and provide support as needed. Answer any of the client's questions or concerns and those of the client's family.

Preoperative Medication

Most clients will be told to take their routine cardiac, antihypertensive, and asthma medications on the day of surgery, but there is no routine protocol. If the medications are oral, they are taken with a minimal amount of water. Eye drops are often ordered preoperatively for clients undergoing cataract or other eye surgery. IV antibiotics are often given as prophylaxis against infection for orthopaedic, cardiac, and gastrointestinal surgery clients. It is important to clarify the time and amount of the last dose of insulin to be given before surgery. Sedatives are occasionally ordered, and it is important that the consent is signed before the client receives sedatives or narcotics.

Preoperative Checklist

The preoperative checklist needs to be reviewed thoroughly before the client is transferred to surgery. The client needs to be wearing an identification bracelet. The nurse needs to check the chart for recorded allergies, signed consent forms for surgery and blood transfusions, or both; a complete history and physical examination; routine blood work results (including urinalysis, electrolytes, and complete blood count); electrocardiogram and chest X-ray results; and blood cross and type results, if ordered. All jewellery, makeup, nail polish, dentures, and prostheses need to be removed. All valuables should be given to family members or locked away for safekeeping. The nurse needs to document when the client last ate or drank, when the client last voided, if the client was given preoperative medication, and a current set of baseline vital signs.

Intraoperative Surgical Phase

The circulating nurse is an RN. Their responsibilities include verifying the client's identification bracelet with the chart and the client's verbal response, as well as reviewing the chart for completeness and confirming the operative procedure and operative site. The primary focus of the intraoperative phase is to prevent injury and complications related to anaesthesia, surgery, positioning, and equipment used. The circulating nurse acts as the client's advocate during the intraoperative phase. The scrub nurse maintains a sterile field during the procedure, hands the surgeon sterile instruments and supplies, and counts sponges, needles, and instruments during and after the surgery. In many Canadian institutions, a trained practical nurse performs the scrubbing function (Tyerman & Cobbett, 2023). The circulating nurse positions the client on the operating room table, drapes the client, assists the anaesthetist with intubation, assists the surgeon and scrub nurse in donning sterile attire, and maintains complete and accurate written records.

Postoperative Surgical Phase
Immediate Postoperative Stage

The immediate postoperative stage is the period from 1 to 4 hours after surgery in the postanaesthesia care unit (PACU).

Respiratory status. The respiratory status may be depressed as a result of anaesthesia. Maintain a patent airway until the gag reflex returns. Position the client on their side to prevent aspiration and the accumulation of secretions. Monitor heart rate and rhythm, symmetry of chest movement, breath sounds, pulse oximeter readings, and colour. Administer oxygen as ordered and suction as needed to remove secretions.

Circulatory status. The circulatory status may be compromised by anaesthesia and immobility during surgery. Monitor the heart rate and rhythm as well as BP at least every 15 minutes while in the PACU. Monitor peripheral circulation by noting the colour, temperature, capillary refill, and presence of pulses. Monitor for hemorrhage by watching for hypotension and observing and measuring wound drainage.

Neurological status. The client's neurological status may be affected by preoperative and anaesthetic agents that depress the central nervous system. Monitor the client's level of consciousness and responses to stimuli. Monitor blink and gag reflexes. Monitor for loss or return of sensation or movement when specific areas have been surgically treated. Reorient the client to time, place, and situation and call the client by name. Answer questions simply and reassure the client.

Wound care. Note the location of the wound and the colour, odour, amount, and consistency of drainage. Circle drainage on the dressing to assess the extent of bleeding over time. Reinforce postoperative dressings as the first dressing change is often done by the surgeon.

Care of drains and tubes. Maintain the patency of all tubing. Attach to suction when ordered. Monitor drain output to assess for hemorrhage.

Fluid and electrolyte needs. Maintain IV therapy as ordered. Record intake and output accurately.

Comfort needs. Assess the client's level of pain on the 0 to 10 scale. Medicate as ordered to reduce pain and increase postoperative compliance with coughing, deep breathing, and activity. Splinting at the surgical site may decrease discomfort when coughing. Instruct the client in the use of PCA.

Care of clients with regional anaesthesia. Regional anaesthesia causes the loss of sensation to an area of the body. No loss of consciousness occurs, but the client may receive sedation. Examples include nerve blocks and spinal or epidural anaesthesia. For both spinal and epidural anaesthesia, the client must be observed closely for signs of autonomic nervous system blockade, signalled by hypotension, bradycardia, nausea, and vomiting (Tyerman & Cobbett, 2023). If the block or level of anaesthesia rises (in other words, if spinal anaesthesia migrates up the spinal cord), breathing may be affected (Tyerman & Cobbett, 2023). Burns and other trauma can also occur on the parts of the body affected by the anaesthesia without the client feeling it, so it is important to monitor the position of the extremities and the condition of the skin frequently (Astle & Duggleby, 2024).

Postoperative Convalescence Stage

The postoperative convalescence stage varies, again depending on the extent of surgery and client's recovery process. For ambulatory clients, convalescence may occur at home. For hospitalized clients, it may occur in the hospital for one or more days.

Respiratory status. Continue to monitor vital signs every 2 to 4 hours according to agency policy using the same assessments from the immediate postoperative stage. Encourage coughing and deep breathing and incentive spirometer every 1 to 2 hours.

Circulatory status. Continue to monitor circulatory status as described above every 2 to 4 hours, according to agency policy. Use antiembolism or elastic stockings, if prescribed, to promote venous return.

Musculo-skeletal status. Encourage progressive ambulation, starting with leg dangling at the bedside as soon as possible and following health care providers' orders. If the client is unable to ambulate, reposition them in bed every 2 hours.

Gastro-intestinal status. Monitor intake and output. Administer frequent mouth care. Assess for bowel sounds in all four quadrants. When oral fluids are permitted, start with ice chips and water. The client advances from clear fluids to a full diet when bowel sounds are heard. Monitor the client for flatus and encourage ambulation.

Renal status. Monitor urine output, which should be greater than 30 mL per hour (0.5 mL/kg/hr). Clients without Foley catheters should void at least 200 mL within 6 to 8 hours postoperatively.

Wound care. Assess the surgical site and drains and maintain an intact, dry dressing. Monitor the amount of drainage from drains and the incision. Reinforce dressing as needed.

The assessments from the postoperative convalescence stage continue, but less frequently. Continue to encourage ambulation to promote peristalsis and the passage of flatus. Continue to increase ambulation to regain muscle strength. Change the dressing as needed using aseptic technique and assess the incision and drainage. Monitor for signs and symptoms of infection by checking for pain, redness, and swelling at the incision site, fever, or an elevated WBC.

Postoperative Complications

Respiratory complications such as pneumonia and atelectasis are the most common. Other postoperative complications include hypoxia, pulmonary embolism, hemorrhage, shock, thrombophlebitis (inflammation of a vein accompanied by clot formation), urinary retention, constipation, and paralytic ileus (loss of the forward flow of intestinal contents as a result of anaesthetic medications or manipulation of the bowel during surgery, wound infection, wound dehiscence, or wound evisceration).

Postoperative Exercises
Respiratory Exercises

Deep breathing. The client is instructed to take 10 slow deep breaths every hour during the postoperative period until mobile. Diaphragmatic and pursed-lip breathing are examples of different methods of deep breathing.

Use of incentive spirometer. Incentive spirometry (IS) is a way to encourage deep breathing in clients by providing visual feedback about their inspiratory volume. It is used to prevent or treat atelectasis in the postoperative client and should be used hourly while awake. IS is used in many practice settings, but research does not support its benefit over other methods, such as coughing, deep breathing, and ambulation (Astle & Duggleby, 2024).

Controlled coughing. The client is in the upright position and takes two slow, deep breaths, inhaling through the nose and out through the mouth. On the third intake of breath, the client holds to a count of three and gives two to three consecutive coughs without inhaling between coughs.

Leg Exercises

Leg exercises should be performed at least every 2 hours for five successive times while awake. They include foot circles, alternating dorsiflexion and plantar flexion of both feet, quadriceps (thigh) setting, and hip and knee movements.

PRACTICE QUESTIONS

Case 1

A new graduate nurse is working a 12-hour day shift on a complex medicine unit. The nurse has four clients assigned to their care.

Questions 1 to 6 refer to this case.

1. The nurse knows that it is important to take accurate blood pressure measurements because many of their clients are on antihypertensive medications. Which of the following statements is correct about measurement of blood pressure?
   1. All older persons have an auscultatory gap.
   2. Normal pulse pressure, or the difference between systolic and diastolic pressures, is 50 to 60 mm Hg.
   3. Orthostatic hypotension is measured by recording blood pressure and pulse with the client sitting.
   4. An auscultatory gap can cause underestimation of systolic blood pressure or overestimation of diastolic blood pressure.

2. Mrs. Lucas, 88 years old, has been febrile for several days due to a severe kidney infection. The physician asks the nurse to check a core temperature for the next set of vital signs. Which of the following temperature sites can the nurse use to check a core temperature?
   1. Rectal
   2. Oral
   3. Axillary
   4. Skin

3. Mr. Hamas, age 55, requires an elastic wrap applied to his left ankle this morning for a sprained ankle injury. One hour after the nurse applied the elastic wrap around his left foot, he complained of severe discomfort and tingling in the foot. Which action should the nurse take?
   1. Reassure the client that the pain is a direct result of the sprain ankle injury.
   2. Administer an analgesia for the pain in the left foot.

3. Assess the circulation, sensation, and movement in the left foot.
4. Elevate the foot on a pillow to decrease the swelling.

4. The nurse accidentally sustains a needle-stick injury after giving Mr. Hamas his injection. What could have prevented this injury?
   1. Giving the injection quickly and putting the needle directly into the sharps container
   2. Using safety-engineered needles to reduce the risk of needle-stick injuries
   3. Advocating for oral rather than parenteral administration of medications
   4. Wearing gloves when giving the injection

5. Mr. Aboud, 24 years old, has an intravenous (IV) order for 1 000 mL of normal saline to run over 8 hours. The IV is started at 1100 hours, and 600 mL is left in the bag at 1500 hours. What adjustment in the flow rate must the nurse make to ensure that the solution is infused no earlier or later than 1900 hours as ordered?
   1. Regulate the IV flow rate to 75 mL/hr
   2. Regulate the IV flow rate to 100 mL/hr
   3. Regulate the IV flow rate to 125 mL/hr
   4. Regulate the IV flow rate to 150 mL/hr

6. Mrs. Roman, 77, has heart failure and a history of angina. The nurse must apply a transdermal patch of nitroglycerin at 0800 hours. Which of the following statements about transdermal medications is correct?
   1. They may be applied to any area of the body, regardless of hair distribution as this does not interfere with absorption.
   2. Transdermal medications are applied to the skin by patch or disc and stay in place for 7 days.
   3. Removal of the old patch or disc prior to applying the new medication is recommended but not mandatory as all the medication has been absorbed from the old patch.
   4. Transdermal medications can be absorbed through the skin of the nurse's hands in the process of applying the medication to Mrs. Roman.

Case 2

Mrs. Gupta, age 55, has had a total hysterectomy. She has an intravenous drip of normal saline infusing at 100 mL/hr.

Questions 7 to 12 refer to this case.

7. Mrs. Gupta has just returned from surgery. Her vital signs are blood pressure 88/60, pulse 74, respiratory rate 16, and oxygen saturation 95%. What is the first priority for the nurse after taking these vital signs?
   1. Ask Mrs. Gupta how she is feeling and review the health record for baseline vital signs.
   2. Call the doctor to report the vital signs.
   3. Increase the intravenous rate to 125 mL per hour as Mrs. Gupta is probably dehydrated.
   4. Position Mrs. Gupta in a modified Trendelenburg position.

8. After surgery, Mrs. Gupta is started on a clear fluid diet until bowel sounds return. Which of the following foods are permitted on a clear fluid diet?
   1. Porridge, broth, apple juice
   2. Cream soup, ice cream, orange juice
   3. Broth, Popsicles, orange juice
   4. Tea, Jell-O, apple juice

9. Postoperatively, Mrs. Gupta develops a paralytic ileus. What is the most likely reason for this postoperative complication?
   1. She did not ambulate soon enough after surgery.
   2. She should have eaten a full diet after surgery to stimulate peristalsis.
   3. She is experiencing the effects of the anaesthetic and the manipulation of the bowel.
   4. She did not receive a rectal suppository to stimulate peristalsis on the first day after her surgery.

10. The nurse helps Mrs. Gupta wash her legs. She removes the elastic (TED) stockings and notices that one calf is larger than the other. What should the nurse do next?
    1. Examine the calf carefully and ask Mrs. Gupta if she has any pain.
    2. Put the TED stocking back on her leg and elevate her leg.
    3. Measure the calf with a tape measure and call the physician immediately.
    4. Wash her leg and ask her to exercise that leg a bit more to reduce the swelling.

11. Mrs. Gupta vomits 600 mL of bile-coloured fluid. After consulting with the physician, the nurse inserts a nasogastric tube to decompress the stomach. Which of the following is correct with regard to insertion of a nasogastric tube?
    1. Measure from the tip of the nose to the xiphoid process prior to inserting the tube.
    2. Have the client swallow as much water as possible during the insertion to close the epiglottis.
    3. The placement of the nasogastric tube must be confirmed by radiography.
    4. A reliable method of testing the correct placement of the tube is aspirating gastric contents and testing pH.

12. In addition to her primary intravenous (IV) line, an IV infusion of normal saline with 20 mmol KCl is ordered to replace Mrs. Gupta's nasogastric losses. What is the drop rate for her replacement IV if 640 mL must infuse over the next 8 hours and the drop factor is 15?
    1. 80 mL/hr
    2. 100 mL/hr
    3. 20 gtt/min
    4. 25 gtt/min

Case 3

Ms. Abbey, a 20-year-old malnourished woman, requires surgery for her Crohn's disease. The health care team decides to start her on total parenteral nutrition (TPN) prior to surgery. This is the nurse's first time caring for a client with TPN.

Questions 13 to 15 refer to this case.

13. What important nursing consideration does the nurse need to know when managing Ms. Abbey's TPN?
    1. All intravascular delivery system components up to the hub are changed weekly to prevent infection.
    2. Serum glucose levels and weights are checked weekly.

3. TPN requires daily temperatures, as infection is the most common complication of TPN.

4. Speeding up or slowing the infusion rate is contraindicated.

14. Ms. Abbey has a fever of 39°C. The nurse gives her an antipyretic and notifies the physician. What orders might the nurse anticipate?

1. Isolate the client for possible septicemia.

2. Collect blood, urine, and sputum cultures to isolate the cause of infection.

3. Hold the TPN until blood cultures are clear of pathogens.

4. Run dextrose 10% via the central line until the cause of the infection is discovered.

15. Ms. Abbey's dressing for her subclavian central line is changed using strict aseptic technique to prevent infection. Which of the following actions by the nurse would compromise the principles of surgical asepsis during this dressing change?

1. The normal saline cap drops onto the floor after the nurse pours the saline onto her tray.

2. The nurse discards the disposable gloves used to remove the old dressing prior to opening her sterile tray.

3. The nurse uses a hand sanitizer for 15 seconds prior to starting the dressing change.

4. The normal saline was opened previously, and there is no date and time on it.

Case 4

Mr. Roustas, 42 years old, has a spinal cord injury. He is isolated for a methicillin-resistant *Staphylococcus aureus* (MRSA) infection of a decubitus (injury) on his coccyx. He had the pressure injury on admission to the hospital but acquired the infection postadmission. He is in a private room. The sign on his door says "Isolation Precautions."

Questions 16 to 19 refer to this case.

16. Mr. Roustas has a health care–associated infection (HAI). Which of the following would be the most significant factor in his susceptibility to HAI?

1. Administration of antibiotics

2. Diagnosis of spinal cord injury

3. Age

4. Skin breakdown

17. The nurse wears a mask, a gown, and gloves when caring for Mr. Roustas. What is the principal mode of transmission of an antibiotic-resistant organism such as MRSA?

1. A colonized or infected health care worker

2. Transfer from client to client on the hands of hospital personnel

3. Environmental contamination

4. Droplet transmission

18. Mr. Roustas is receiving vancomycin (Vancocin) intravenously for his wound infection. The nurse observes redness around the intravenous site, and Mr. Roustas is complaining that the site is painful. What corrective action should the nurse take?

1. Slow the rate of infusion.

2. Change the site of the infusion.

3. Notify the physician.

4. Stop the infusion for at least 24 hours.

19. Mr. Roustas has his pressure injury debrided by the skin care nurse. His dressing is changed daily after debridement. The nurse irrigates the wound with normal saline and packs it with saline-soaked gauze to promote moist, interactive wound healing. What is the benefit of moist, interactive wound healing?

1. It can be used with iodine, which is an effective antimicrobial agent.

2. It promotes faster healing and better tissue quality.

3. It requires fewer supplies and equipment.

4. There is less incidence of bacterial invasion of the wound.

Independent Questions

Questions 20 to 40 do not refer to a particular case.

20. A nurse enters a client's room and assesses the following. What initial actions should the nurse take?

General assessment:	Client appears very anxious and restless
Respiratory assessment:	Laboured, dyspneic breathing with audible wheezes. Crackles in both lower lobes posteriorly.
Vital signs:	Pulse (beats per minute): 80 Respiratory rate (breaths per minute): 20 Oxygen saturation: 92%

1. Chart the findings and report to the nurse team leader.

2. Encourage the client to deep breathe and cough.

3. Elevate the head of the bed and administer oxygen.

4. Go to the nurses' station and call the health care provider.

21. A postoperative client reports sensations of prickling and itchiness around their abdominal incision site after the initial dressing change. How should the nurse proceed?

1. Administer the client analgesia for the prickling and itchiness sensation.

2. Remove the dressing and assess the skin area around the incision.

3. Inform the client that this is a normal sensation to feel after the surgery.

4. Notify the health care provider of the client's complaints of prickling and itchiness around the incision.

22. What is the most effective method for the nurse to validate the effectiveness of pain relief with most clients?

1. Ask clients to rate their pain verbally from mild to severe.

2. Monitor their facial expressions before and after administration of analgesics.

3. Monitor their vital signs in response to analgesics given.

4. Ask clients to rate pain using a numeric rating scale before and after analgesics.

23. Clients who require special nail and foot care include those with which of the following conditions? **Select all that apply.**
    1. Peripheral neuropathy
    2. Peripheral vascular disease
    3. Pancreatitis
    4. Diabetes
    5. Osteoporosis

24. The nurse is providing care to a client with a tracheostomy tube that has an inner cannula. Which intervention by the nurse follows proper procedure for tracheostomy tube care?
    1. Carefully removes the inner cannula and places it in a basin of 1:10 bleach solution
    2. Scrubs the inner cannula on the inside and outside with a 1:10 bleach solution
    3. After scrubbing the inner cannula, rinses it with normal saline
    4. Uses a wet 4 × 4 gauze and cleans the inside of the outer cannula

25. A client gave birth to their third child 6 hours ago and would like to be discharged. The client has not urinated since the birth. On palpation, the nurse determines a full bladder, and the bladder scanner indicates 1 000 mL of urine in their bladder. What should the nurse do?
    1. Have the client sit in a warm bath to see if they can void in the bathtub.
    2. Insert an intermittent catheter and drain the bladder.
    3. Let the client go home, as the client feels they will be able to void in the privacy of their own home.
    4. Insert an in-dwelling catheter for 24 hours so that the bladder will remain empty and the uterus will involute normally.

26. Which of the following are examples of medical asepsis? **Select all that apply.**
    1. Inserting a urinary catheter for postoperative urinary retention
    2. Changing an abdominal dressing for the first time after surgery
    3. Cleaning the hospital environment and equipment routinely
    4. Giving an intramuscular injection in the ventrogluteal region
    5. Performing hand hygiene prior to entering the client's room

27. A client is prescribed 2 units of packed red blood cells (250 mL/unit). Each unit is to run over 4 hours. The administration set delivers 10 gtt/mL. At what rate should the IV infuse? **Fill in the blank.**
    Answer: _____ gtt/min

28. A 1-month-old infant is receiving ampicillin (Ampicin) every 6 hours. The hospital formulary indicates that a maximum safe dose is 400 mg/kg/day. What is the maximum recommended dosage range for the infant, who weighs 5 kg? **Fill in the blank.**
    Answer: _____ mg/day

29. Which of the following is correct regarding subcutaneous injections? **Select all that apply.**
    1. Pinch the skin at the site of the injection to elevate the subcutaneous tissue.
    2. All subcutaneous injection sites can be massaged, with the exception of those for insulin.
    3. Inject the medication at a 5- to 15-degree angle.
    4. Aspiration is not necessary, as it is rare to inject into a blood vessel.
    5. Give only 0.5 to 1 mL as subcutaneous injections can cause discomfort.

30. An older male client is confused after his hip-replacement surgery and has been trying to get out of bed when the family is not present. His family wants him to be restrained so he does not injure himself. What is the best response by the nurse?
    1. "Restraining your father will only make him more agitated."
    2. "We do not restrain clients anymore, as it is against the law."
    3. "Would it be possible to have a family member stay with him until he is less confused?"
    4. "Would you like me to call the doctor to get an order for restraints for your father?"

31. A client has stomatitis as a result of recent chemotherapy. The nurse knows that the client understands the oral hygiene instructions given by the nurse when the client makes which of the following comments?
    1. "I don't brush my teeth every day, but when I do, I use my ordinary toothbrush."
    2. "I use diluted Listerine mouthwash every 4 hours. It stings, so I know it is working."
    3. "Rinsing my mouth with normal saline every 2 hours has helped me tremendously."
    4. "I never need analgesics. If my mouth is too painful, I just do not brush or rinse for a day or two and the pain passes."

32. A client returns from surgery with chest tubes in place. What should the nurse say to the client concerning their chest tubes?
    1. "You have chest tubes to remove abnormal accumulations of fluid from inside your lungs."
    2. "We will assist you to turn in bed frequently to promote drainage from the pleural space and improve lung expansion."
    3. "Your chest tubes will be clamped every time you get out of bed to prevent a leak from developing in the drainage system."
    4. "The chest tube drainage system should remain at the level of the chest at all times."

33. The client is to receive 1 unit of packed red blood cells (RBCs). The nurse obtains the blood from the blood bank and returns to the unit to find that the client has been taken to radiology for a computed tomography (CT) scan and is expected to return in about an hour. What should the nurse do?

1. Go to radiology and administer the blood.
2. Keep the blood refrigerated until the client returns.
3. Return the blood to the blood bank.
4. Hang the blood in the client's room and start it when the client returns.

34. A nurse gives a client the wrong medication, what is the nurse's first responsibility?
    1. Disclose the incident to the client and their family.
    2. Inform the unit manager and prescriber of the medication error.
    3. Complete an incident report for the agency about the details of the medication error.
    4. Assess the client.

35. What are the responsibilities of a nurse who is caring for a client in wrist restraints? **Select all that apply.**
    1. Remove the restraints and arrange for a paid sitter as soon as possible.
    2. Make sure that the restraints are tied tightly and secured with a knot.
    3. Check skin integrity, pulses, colour, and sensation of the restrained part as often as every 1 to 2 hours.
    4. Ensure that the physician reorders the wrist restraints every 2 weeks.
    5. Ensure that the client and the client's family are involved in the plan of care.

36. Which of the following facts does the nurse need to be aware of when treating older clients? **Select all that apply.**
    1. The older person tends to have a lower body temperature.
    2. The older person might have an advanced infection before it is identified.
    3. The older person has increased sensitivity to pain sensation.
    4. The constipation common in older clients is primarily due to polypharmacy.
    5. The older person will need help in taking medications.

37. What will the nurse teach the family about care of their child during and after a seizure? **Select all that apply.**

1. Restrain the child gently until the seizure passes.
2. Use a padded tongue blade to prevent damage to the tongue during the seizure.
3. Place a pillow or folded blanket under the child's head.
4. Loosen restrictive clothing and clear the area of hazards and articles that might cause harm.
5. Immediately following the seizure, place the child in a side-lying position.

38. An older person is admitted to an acute care hospital from a long-term care facility. The nurse documents the Braden Scale score on the chart shortly after the client arrives on the unit. What is the main purpose of the Braden Scale?
    1. To identify clients at risk for pressure injury early
    2. To identify interventions that can be implemented to treat pressure injuries
    3. To classify the client's stage of pressure injuries on admission to the hospital
    4. To identify preventive measures to reduce the incidence of pressure injuries

39. A client has been diagnosed with lung cancer and is scheduled for resection of their right lung tomorrow. What will the nurse teach the client about what to expect with their postoperative care?
    1. "You will have incentive spirometry at least four times daily to prevent atelectasis."
    2. "Leg exercises will be carried out every 2 hours while you are awake."
    3. "Vigorous coughing will be necessary to expectorate excess sputum."
    4. "There will be a right-sided chest tube, and you will be on bed rest until it is removed."

40. A health care provider orders 1 000 mL of dextrose 5% and sodium chloride 0.45% with 20 mmol KCL to be infused intravenously (IV) over 10 hours. At what rate should the nurse set the drip rate if the intravenous tubing delivers 15 gtt/mL? **Fill in the blank.**
    Answer: _____ gtt/min

REFERENCES

Astle, B., & Duggleby, W. (2024). *Potter and Perry's Canadian fundamentals of nursing* (7th ed.). Elsevier Inc.

Cobbett, S. (2024). *Perry & Potter's Canadian clinical nursing skills and techniques* (2nd ed.). Elsevier Inc.

Dames, S., Luctkar-Flude, M., & Tyerman, J. (2021). *Edelman and Kudzma's Canadian heatlh promotion throughout the life span* (1st ed.). Elsevier.

Government of Canada. (2022). *Canada's food guide.* https://food-guide.canada.ca/en/

Health Quality Ontario. (2018). *Quality standards: Opioid prescribing for chronic pain. Care for people 15 years of age and older.* https://www.hqontario.ca/portals/0/documents/evidence/quality-standards/qs-opioid-chronic-pain-clinician-guide-en.pdf

Hockenberry, M., Rodgers, C., & Wilson, D. (2022). *Wong's essentials of pediatric nursing* (11th ed.). Elsevier.

Ignatavicius, D. D., Workman, M. L., & Rebar, C. (2018). *Medical-surgical nursing: Concepts for interprofessional collaborative care* (9th ed.). Elsevier.

Institute for Safe Medication Practices (ISMP). (2018a). *ISMP high alert medications in acute care settings.* https://www.ismp.org/recommendations/high-alert-medications-acute-list

Institute for Safe Medication Practices Canada (ISMP). (2018b). *ISMP do not use: List of dangerous abbreviations, symbols, and dose designations.* https://ismpcanada.ca/wp-content/uploads/2022/02/ISMPCanadaListOfDangerousAbbreviations.pdf

Institute for Safe Medication Practices (ISMP). (2021). *High-alert medications in long-term care (LTC) settings.* https://www.ismp.org/recommendations/high-alert-medications-long-term-care-list

Institute for Safe Medication Practices (ISMP). (2022). *List of error-prone abbreviations.* https://www.ismp.org/recommendations/error-prone-abbreviations-list

International Association for the Study of Pain (IASP). (2021). *IASP terminology.* http://www.iasp-pain.org/Education/Content. aspx?ItemNumber=1698

Jarvis, C., Browne, A. J., MacDonald-Jenkins, J., & Luctkar-Flude, M. (2024). *Physical examination and health assessment* (4th Cdn ed.). Elsevier Inc.

Mitevska, E., Wong, B., Surewaard, B., & Jenne, C. (2021). The prevalence, risk and management of methicillin-resistant *Staphylococcus aureus* infection in diverse populations across Canada: A systemic review. *Pathogens, 10*(4), 393. https://www. ncbi.nlm.nih.gov/pmc/articles/PMC8064373/

National Pressure Ulcer Advisory Panel. (2022). *Pressure injury stages.* https://npiap.com/page/PressureInjuryStages

Registered Nurses' Association of Ontario (RNAO). (2013). *Clinical best practice guidelines: Assessment and management of pain* (3rd ed.). https://rnao.ca/sites/rnao-ca/files/ AssessAndManagementOfPain2014.pdf.

Registered Nurses' Association of Ontario (RNAO). (2020). *A proactive approach to bladder and bowel management in adults* (4th ed). https://rnao.ca/sites/rnao-ca/files/bpg/Bladder_and_ Bowel_Management_FINAL_WEB.pdf

Sealock, K., Seneviratne, C., Lilley, L., et al. (2021). *Lilley's pharmacology for Canadian health care practice* (4th ed.). Elsevier.

Stephen, T., & Skillen, D. L. (2021). *Canadian nursing health assessment: A best practice approach* (2nd ed.). Wolters Kluwer.

Tyerman, J., & Cobbett, S. (2023). *Lewis's medical-surgical nursing in Canada: Assessment and management of clinical problems* (5th ed.). Elsevier Inc.

World Health Organization. (2021). *WHO issues new guidelines on the management of chronic pain in children.* https://www.who. int/news/item/01-02-2021-who-issues-new-guidelines-on-the-management-of-chronic-pain-in-children

BIBLIOGRAPHY

Centers for Disease Control and Prevention. (2019). *Infection control: Isolation precautions.* https://www.cdc.gov/ infectioncontrol/guidelines/isolation/index.html

College of Nurses of Ontario. (2022). *Practice standard: Medication.* http://www.cno.org/globalassets/docs/prac/41007_medication.pdf

National Pressure Ulcer Advisory Panel. (2016). *Pressure injury prevention points.* https://npiap.com/page/ PreventionPoints#:~:text=Assess%20pressure%20points%2C%20 such%20as,consistency%20compared%20to%20adjacent%20skin

Registered Nurses' Association of Ontario. (2016). *Clinical best practice guidelines: Assessment and management of pressure injuries for the interprofessional team* (3rd ed.). http://rnao.ca/ sites/rnao-ca/files/PI_BPG_FINAL_WEB_June_10_2016.pdf

Registered Nurses' Association of Ontario. (2020). *Best practice guideline: A proactive approach to bladder and bowel management in adults* (4th ed.). https://rnao.ca/sites/rnao-ca/ files/bpg/Bladder_and_Bowel_Management_FINAL_WEB.pdf

Registered Nurses 'Association of Ontario. (2021). *Best practice guideline: Vascular Access* (2nd ed.). https://rnao.ca/sites/rnao-ca/files/bpg/Vascular_Access_FINAL_Web_3.0.pdf

WEBSITES

- **Institute for Safe Medication Practices Canada** (https:// www.ismp.org): This site provides information and research about common medication errors, factors that can potentially lead to medication errors, and methods by which to mitigate these factors.

- **Nova Scotia College of Nursing: Medication Guidelines for Nursing** (https://cdn3.nscn.ca/sites/default/files/doc-uments/resources/MedicationGuidelines.pdf): This site provides practice guidelines for safe medication admin-istration from the College of Licensed Practical Nurses of Nova Scotia (CLPNNS). The guidelines outline the licensed practical nurse's accountability in specific practice contexts. They reflect relevant legislation and are designed to help licensed practical nurses understand their responsibilities and legal obligations so that they can make safe and ethical nursing decisions.

- **Public Health Ontario: Hand Hygiene** (https://www. publichealthontario.ca/en/health-topics/infection-prevention-control/hand-hygiene): This site provides information on hand hygiene. It reviews clinical situations in which hand hygiene is important and links to other educational resources on this subject.

- **Public Health Ontario: Infection Prevention and Con-trol (On-line Learning)** (https://www.publichealthon-tario.ca/en/Education-and-Events/Online-Learning/ IPAC-Courses): This site provides information and on-line learning modules on infection prevention and control for health care providers.

Pharmacology and Nursing Practice

A major component within the scope of practice of nurses practising in Canada is the administration of medications and the care of clients receiving those medications. There is a legal responsibility on the part of the nurse to ensure a sound knowledge base of pharmacology. Nurses must master the physical skill of administering medications to their clients. They are also responsible for the specific nursing interventions required in the administration of medications.

The nursing implications relating to the administration of medications are derived from a thorough understanding of the medications being administered and their actions, therapeutic effects, adverse effects, contraindications, and normal dosage ranges. Only by being aware of the nature of medications, by making the appropriate assessments, and by initiating the appropriate actions prior to, during, and after the administration of medications can the nurse exercise professional responsibility and ensure the safe care of the client.

PHARMACOLOGY

Pharmacology is the study of drugs (chemicals, called "medications" in health care contexts) and how they affect living cells, the nature of those drugs, their biological activity on living cells, and their fate once they are absorbed into the body.

Sources of Drugs

There are many sources of drugs that are natural or synthetic products or a combination of both. Some of these sources are as follows:
- Plants (e.g., heroin and digitalis)
- Soil (e.g., Kaopectate, which includes clay)
- Animals (e.g., insulin and conjugated estrogen [Premarin])
- Minerals (e.g., iron)
- Synthesis in a laboratory provides better standardization of chemical characteristics: more consistency of effects and a reduction in the potential for allergic reactions.
- Semisynthesis: Naturally occurring substances are chemically modified to produce a drug (includes many antibiotics and some human insulins).
- Biotechnology: Drugs are produced through the manipulation of DNA and RNA and cloning (includes human insulin such as Humulin and Novolin, hepatitis B vaccine, and others).

Routes of Administration of Medications

The route of administration depends on the characteristics of the medication, the characteristics of the client, and the desired responses. The route also affects the action, absorption, and distribution of medications.

See Table 8.1 for a comparison of different medication routes and absorption times.

Naming of Drugs
Chemical Name

This name describes the specific molecular structure and chemical composition of a drug and is used mainly by researchers (e.g., 6-chloro-3,4-dihydro-2H-1,2,4-benzothiadiazine-7-sulfonamide 1,1-dioxide).

Generic (Nonproprietary) Name

The generic name is the one commonly used by health professionals that is created when a medication is ready to be marketed, for example, hydrochlorothiazide.

Brand or Trade (Proprietary or Trademark) Name

This name is owned by the manufacturer and can be created as soon as a generic name has been approved. The choice of name is motivated by marketing considerations (e.g., Urozide).

Combination drugs. These are medications made up of a combination of two or more active drugs in a single tablet with complementary modes of action. They provide an additive, therapeutic effect with the possibility of decreasing adverse effects and increasing client adherence, and they reduce the number of prescriptions and administrative costs. For example, atorvastatin–amlodipine is a combination of two drugs, an anticholesterolemic and an antihypertensive agent, and treats two different major risk factors for coronary heart disease.

CANADIAN DRUG LEGISLATION
Food and Drugs Act, 1985

Health Canada administers the *Food and Drugs Act.* In the act, a *drug* is defined as any substance or mixture of substances manufactured, sold, or represented for use in:
(a) the diagnosis, treatment, mitigation, or prevention of disease, disorder, or abnormal physical state, or its symptoms, in human beings or animals,
(b) restoring, correcting, or modifying organic functions in human beings or animals, or
(c) disinfection in premises in which food is manufactured, prepared, or kept.

The purpose of the law is to:
- Govern the distribution and use of drugs in Canada

TABLE 8.1   Drug Administration Routes and Absorption Rates

Drug Administration Route	Absorption Rate
1. Intravenous (IV)	• It has the most rapid and effective absorption and action.
2. Intramuscular (IM)	• Certain preparations can produce drug action in a few minutes, and others have a slower action.
3. Subcutaneous (SC)	• It is slower than IM, but faster than oral.
4. Oral (PO)	• Absorption action is slower than the injectable routes that bypass the digestive system. • Drugs with the fastest absorption rates are liquids, elixirs, and syrups. • Drugs with the slowest absorption rates include enteric-coated tablets. • Drugs undergo "first pass" effects.
5. Topical (Top): skin and mucous membranes)	• Absorption and action vary according to drug form and application site. • It is the slowest route of absorption for systemic applications compared with other parenteral routes.

- Protect the consumer from unsafe drugs
- Investigate discrepancies
- Monitor the advertising and sale of drugs for treatment, prevention, and cure
- Divide drugs into specific categories, depending on the classification of the drug, as follows:

  Schedule I: Prescription drugs (Pr): Require prescription from a practitioner

  Schedule II: Drugs obtained from a pharmacist without a prescription on request, such as Tylenol #1

  Schedule III: Drugs available in a pharmacy

  Unscheduled: Drugs that can be purchased in any store, such as Tylenol or Alka Seltzer

Controlled Drugs and Substances Act, 1996

The *Controlled Drugs and Substances Act* (CDSA) outlines the legal control of addictive and habituating drugs and provides extensive regulation and control over their possession, manufacture, sale, and distribution. Controlled substances require a specific type of prescribing and more stringent recording and record keeping.

The CDSA regulates the following categories of drugs:
- Opiates, fentanyls, and methamphetamine
- Synthetic cannabinoid receptor type 1 agonists
- Amphetamines, LSD
- Barbiturates, anabolic steroids

PHARMACODYNAMICS

The term *pharmacodynamics* describes the action of drugs on target cells and the changes that occur in body fluids as a result of the action of these drugs. The pharmacological effects of a drug on the body can be described as the local or systemic therapeutic effects, or both, as well as any adverse effects and any toxic effects.

Types of Action

Most drugs combine with receptor sites on cells and are characterized by their mechanism of action upon those cells:
- Agonist: A drug that binds to a receptor, producing a biochemical response
- Antagonist: A drug that binds to a receptor, preventing an agonist from binding to that receptor, which results in no agonist-induced biochemical response

Factors That Affect Drug Action

- Drug dosage
- Route of administration
- Individual characteristics (age, sex, race or ethnicity, pathological condition)
- Drug–diet interaction
- Drug interactions
- Use of herbal and dietary supplements
- Genetic makeup

Drug Interactions

- Potentiation (synergism): There is interaction between two drugs with the result that the overall effect is greater than if the drugs are given separately.
- Displacement: The effects of one drug are increased when its normal binding site on plasma protein within the blood is inhibited by another drug, thereby promoting more immediate action of the first drug.
- Antidotal effect: The toxic effects of one drug are reduced by a second drug that takes up the receptor sites of the first drug, thereby preventing a biochemical response.

Nonpharmacological Effects of a Drug on the Body

- Allergic reaction: An undesirable reaction to a drug (of protein origin) that is regarded by the body as an allergen; occurs after the second or subsequent dose of the drug
- Anaphylaxis: A severe, acute, systemic reaction to an allergen, causing massive vasodilation, dyspnea, and shock, that requires immediate emergency care
- Idiosyncratic reaction: An unexpected response to a drug by a specific client; commonly the result of genetic factors that cause the client to respond differently
- Teratogenic reaction: A reaction to a drug that may produce congenital defects if taken by a person who is pregnant, such as thalidomide, which produced deformed limbs
- Drug tolerance: Resistance of the body to the action of a drug because of adaptation to overuse; higher dosages are required to produce the desired effects
- Physical dependence: Dependence on a drug resulting in the body requiring a continuous supply to function

normally; undesirable physical manifestations result if the drug is withdrawn

- Psychological dependence: A psychological dependence on the drug, where there is an overwhelming and uncontrollable desire for the drug that forces continued usage

PHARMACOKINETICS

Pharmacokinetics refers to how the body manages a drug: its absorption, distribution, metabolism (biotransformation), and excretion.

Absorption

Absorption is the process that occurs from the time a drug enters the body until the time it enters the bloodstream. Factors that affect the absorption of a drug include the following:

- Size of the drug molecules
- Properties of the drug (such as being lipophilic)
- Environmental temperature
- Membrane thickness
- Surface area of body
- Blood supply at absorption site
- Route of administration
- Presence of food or other drugs in the gastro-intestinal (GI) tract
- Drug formulation (such as enteric or slow release)
- Bioavailability: How much of the drug actually enters the bloodstream to exert its effects on body cells; the route of administration is a major determinant
- Presence of disease

Distribution

Distribution is the transport of drug molecules within the body. Factors that affect the distribution of a drug include the following:

- Blood circulation
- Plasma protein binding (drug inactivated temporarily while bound to the protein)
- Anatomical barrier (such as the blood–brain or blood–placental barrier)
- Presence of disease (such as peripheral vascular disease)
- Lipid solubility
- Storage in body tissues (the drug is inactive while in the storage site, such as in adipose tissue)

Metabolism

An individual's metabolism determines how drugs are biotransformed by the body into simple, active, or inactive metabolites. For example:

- Lipid-soluble drugs are converted to water-soluble forms to be excreted by the kidney, which is achieved by enzyme systems in the liver, kidney, lungs, GI tract, red blood cells, and plasma mucosa.
- Toxic waste products can be produced if biotransformation is extremely rapid.

- Slow biotransformations result in lower drug dosages to cells.
  - Factors that affect biotransformation include the following:
- Immaturity of organs (infants)
- Degeneration of organs (older persons)
- Reduced circulation
- A diet low in protein
- Drugs that antagonize enzyme action
- Disease (cirrhosis of liver)
- Genetic factors

Excretion

- Elimination of a drug from the body
- Requires an adequately functioning cardiovascular system, kidneys, GI tract, lungs, and skin
- Prior to administering drugs, an assessment of adequate organ functioning needs to be made

DRUGS THAT AFFECT THE CENTRAL NERVOUS SYSTEM

Numerous classifications of drugs affect the nervous system. In general, there are two actions a drug can exert on the nervous system: stimulation or depression. Figure 8.1 shows the drug classifications and their therapeutic actions and effects on either the central nervous system (CNS) or the autonomic nervous system (ANS).

Analgesic Agents

Analgesics are used to relieve pain without causing loss of consciousness. There are two major classifications of analgesics: opioids, prescribed for the treatment of severe pain, and nonopiate preparations, used for milder or more moderate pain. Many nonopioid preparations have both antipyretic and anti-inflammatory effects. The choice of analgesic will depend on the effectiveness of an agent, the route of administration to be used, the duration of action of the drug, the duration of the therapy, potential drug interactions (particularly if the client is receiving other depressant medications), and hypersensitivities that the client may have.

Although opioid analgesics are primarily prescribed for the treatment of pain, other therapeutic uses of specific types of opioid analgesics, such as codeine, include treatment to suppress a dry cough and severe diarrhea.

Opioid Analgesics

These are morphine-like substances that may be natural, derived from opium, or synthesized in the laboratory. These substances:

- Are controlled under the CDSA
- Are associated with a high risk for dependence
- Are prescribed for treatment of moderate to severe pain, such as pain originating from visceral sources, such as surgery, myocardial infarction (MI), colic, and cancer pain

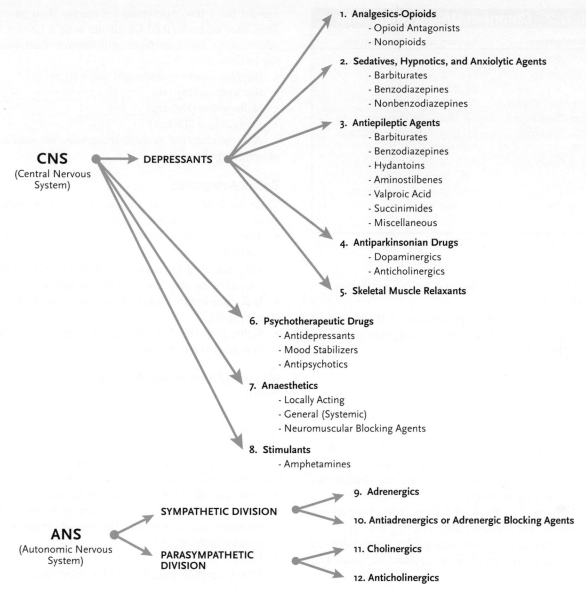

CNS
(Central Nervous
System)

DEPRESSANTS

1. **Analgesics-Opioids**
   - Opioid Antagonists
   - Nonopioids

2. **Sedatives, Hypnotics, and Anxiolytic Agents**
   - Barbiturates
   - Benzodiazepines
   - Nonbenzodiazepines

3. **Antiepileptic Agents**
   - Barbiturates
   - Benzodiazepines
   - Hydantoins
   - Aminostilbenes
   - Valproic Acid
   - Succinimides
   - Miscellaneous

4. **Antiparkinsonian Drugs**
   - Dopaminergics
   - Anticholinergics

5. **Skeletal Muscle Relaxants**

6. **Psychotherapeutic Drugs**
   - Antidepressants
   - Mood Stabilizers
   - Antipsychotics

7. **Anaesthetics**
   - Locally Acting
   - General (Systemic)
   - Neuromuscular Blocking Agents

8. **Stimulants**
   - Amphetamines

ANS
(Autonomic Nervous
System)

SYMPATHETIC DIVISION
9. **Adrenergics**
10. **Antiadrenergics or Adrenergic Blocking Agents**

PARASYMPATHETIC DIVISION
11. **Cholinergics**
12. **Anticholinergics**

Fig. 8.1 Drugs that affect the nervous system.

- Inhibit the release of substance P in the central and peripheral nerves, resulting in interference with the transmission of sensory nerve impulses to the brain from peripheral tissues
- Enhance the release of naturally occurring opioid-type chemicals within the body (enkephalin, dynorphins, and endorphins)
- Include effects such as the suppression of the CNS, preventing the sensation of pain within the CNS (the substantia gelatinosa, spinal cord, brainstem, reticular formation, thalamus, and limbic system)
- Modify the perception of pain
- Include additional actions and effects of opioids, such as the following:
  - Suppression of the cough reflex
  - Suppression of GI motility
  - Stimulation of the vomiting centre

Common opioid analgesics. Common opioid analgesics are listed in Table 8.2.

Analgesic dosages. It is important to refer to a potency chart to ensure the correct dosage when changing the route of administration of an opioid. For example, 10 mg of morphine sulphate by intramuscular (IM) injection equals 30 mg morphine sulphate orally.

Adverse effects of opioid analgesics
- Tolerance, physiological and psychological dependence (addiction)
- Nausea, vomiting, and constipation
- CNS depression, which may lead to respiratory depression
- Weakness, sedation
- Euphoria, disorientation, and hallucinations (particularly in older persons)

Contraindications of opioid analgesics
- Allergy
- Respiratory insufficiency (such as asthma)
- Elevated intracranial pressure
- Pregnancy

TABLE 8.2 Common Opioid Analgesics

Opioid Analgesics	Routes of Administration
Morphine sulphate	PO, IM, epidural, intrathecal, IV
Codeine phosphate	PO, IM, SC
Fentanyl	IM, IV, transdermal
Hydromorphone (Dilaudid)	IM, SC, IV, SUPP
Meperidine (Demerol)	IM, IV, SC, PO
Methadone (Metadol)	PO (not recommended for children)
Oxycodone (Oxyneo, others)	PO (not recommended for children under 12)
Tramadol and acetaminophen (Tramacet)	PO (not recommended for children)

IM, Intramuscular; *IV,* intravenous; *PO,* by mouth; *SC,* subcutaneous; *SUPP,* suppository.

Nursing considerations relating to opioid analgesics

- Assess client need.
- Ask the client about their perception of the degree of pain; medication should be administered prior to the pain becoming too severe.
- Assess the client's history of opioid use.
- Check for the time of the last dosage.
- Assess the previous client response and adverse effects; antiemetics may be administered at the same time to avoid nausea and vomiting.
- Assess respiratory rate, depth, and rhythm prior to administration. Withhold the medication and report if respiration is less than 10 breaths per minute and shallow; an opioid blocker may be required.
- Frequently assess the client's vital signs, level of consciousness, alertness, and cognitive ability during therapy.
- Facilitate the effects of the analgesic administered by promoting an environment of rest, relaxation, peace and quiet, and physical comfort.
- Coughing exercises, deep breathing, and frequent moving help maintain normal functioning.
- Maintain careful documentation of administration of opioids, noting frequency. Observe for signs of dependence; opioids require frequent reordering by a physician or prescriber to minimize overuse and abuse.
- Monitor the client's intake and urine output for possible dehydration and urinary retention.
- Monitor bowel sounds and bowel functioning for signs of constipation.
- When educating clients, include knowledge relating to the nature of the medication and usage, particularly in home use.
- Due to possible drowsiness, caution clients taking opioids at home to avoid situations requiring rapid reactions, including driving a car, the operation of dangerous machinery, and smoking.
- Advise that care should be taken around the concurrent use of other CNS depressants, such as alcohol.

Agonist–Antagonist Agents

Agonist–antagonist combination drugs are narcotics with a narcotic antagonist added. They have the potency of an agonist but a lower potential for misuse than pure agonists. They may be prescribed for clients with a history of opioid addiction or for short-term pain control. Examples include the following:

- Buprenorphine transdermal patch (Butrans)
- Butorphanol tartrate
- Nalbuphine (Nubain)
- Pentazocine (Talwin)

Adverse effects of agonist–antagonists are similar to those of opioid agonists.

Opioid Antagonists

These medications block the receptor sites of opioid analgesics or displace opiates occupying receptor sites.

- They act as an antidote to opioid agonists and agonist–antagonists.
- They are used to relieve CNS and respiratory depression caused by an overdose of opioid analgesics.
- Naloxone hydrochloride is used in the treatment of opioid overdoses.
- Naltrexone (ReVia) maintains an opiate-free state in clients addicted to opiates.

Nonopioid Analgesics (Antipyretic or Anti-Inflammatory Agents)

Nonopioid analgesics relieve mild to moderate pain, fever, and the inflammatory response. Common nonopioid analgesics are listed in Table 8.3.

Uses for nonopioid analgesics (antipyretics, nonsteroidal anti-inflammatory drugs [NSAIDs]) are as follows:

- Pain associated with muscles, joints, and connective tissue
- Treatment of pain and inflammation associated with osteoarthritis (OA) and rheumatoid arthritis (RA) and rheumatic fever
- Fever
- Dysmenorrheal pain (especially ibuprofen)
- Headache

Nursing considerations relating to nonopioid analgesics (antipyretics, NSAIDs)

- Monitor clients for bleeding and petechiae (ASA).
- Administer analgesics with food to reduce gastric irritation.
  Advise self-medicating clients:
- Do not to exceed the recommended dosage and frequency.
- Avoid ASA if there is a history of gastric discomfort or bleeding tendency.
- Avoid activities that require alertness (driving) due to the sedating effects.
- Avoid using other CNS depressants, such as alcohol.
- Seek medical attention if pain or fever persists for greater than 48–72 hours.

Sedative-Hypnotics

Classifications of sedatives and hypnotics include barbiturates, benzodiazepines, and nonbenzodiazepines. Irrespective of the classification of individual drugs, each has a calming, relaxing effect on the body by depressing CNS activity. Many of these drugs are strongly controlled, requiring a

TABLE 8.3   Common Nonopioid Analgesics

Classification	Action	Therapeutic Effects	Adverse Effects
Acetylsalicylic acid (e.g., Aspirin)	• Inhibits prostaglandin synthesis by binding to both forms of cyclo-oxygenase (COX-1 and COX-2)	• Mild analgesia • Antipyretic • Anti-inflammatory • Anticoagulant	• Gastro-intestinal irritation • Tinnitus • Allergic reactions • Bleeding • Drowsiness, weakness, and dizziness
Acetaminophen (e.g., Tylenol)	• Inhibits prostaglandin synthesis in central nervous system	• Mild analgesia • Antipyretic	• Liver and renal damage; not recommended for use in severe liver disease • Drowsiness, weakness, and dizziness
Ibuprofen (e.g., Advil, Motrin)	• Inhibits prostaglandin synthesis by binding to both forms of cyclo-oxygenase (COX-1 and COX-2)	• Mild analgesia • Antipyretic • Anti-inflammatory	• Drowsiness, weakness, and dizziness
Celecoxib (e.g., Celebrex)	• Inhibits prostaglandin synthesis by binding cyclo-oxygenase (COX-2)	• Mild analgesia • Antipyretic • Anti-inflammatory	• Allergic reactions • Drowsiness, weakness, and dizziness
Naproxen (e.g., Naprosyn)	• Inhibits prostaglandin synthesis by binding cyclo-oxygenase (COX-2)	• Mild analgesia • Antipyretic • Anti-inflammatory	• Drowsiness, weakness, and dizziness

prescription; however, mild-acting drugs may be purchased over the counter (OTC). Certain medications may be used for sedation and relief of anxiety in low dosages, and in high doses, they are prescribed to produce sleep.

Sedatives:
- Decrease the functional activity of the brain and response to stimuli without producing sleep
- Produce general CNS depression
- Are used to relax clients prior to procedures and for extreme anxiety

Hypnotics:
- Are used to produce extreme sedation and sleep
- Act on the reticular activation system (RAS) to block the brain's response to incoming stimuli
- Are used to treat insomnia
- May be prescription drugs or OTC

Sedative–hypnotics:
- Produce sedative or hypnotic effects, depending on the dose administered

Classifications of Sedatives-Hypnotics

Benzodiazepines. These drugs act in the limbic and reticular activating systems to make gamma-aminobutyric acid (GABA), an inhibitory neurotransmitter, more effective.

Uses of benzodiazepines:
- To prevent mild to severe anxiety (including panic disorder) and insomnia
- To induce sleep
- For skeletal muscle relaxation
- As preoperative medication

Common benzodiazepines and their uses and dosages are outlined in Table 8.4.

Adverse effects of benzodiazepines:
- Headache
- Drowsiness
- Blurred vision

- Benzodiazepines (contraindicated for pregnancy and lactation and severe respiratory, kidney, or liver disorders)

Common Nonbenzodiazepine Sedatives-Hypnotics

Common uses and dosages of nonbenzodiazepines are outlined in Table 8.5.

Barbiturates

Barbiturates, derivatives of barbituric acid, act by inhibiting the conduction of nerve impulses within the CNS by promoting the inhibitory activity of GABA. They are less commonly used now as sedatives or for insomnia because of their adverse effects and strong addictive properties. The benzodiazepines and nonbenzodiazepines are the treatment of choice for these problems. Phenobarbital, a long-acting barbiturate, is used primarily to treat status epilepticus.

Nursing Considerations Relating to Sedatives-Hypnotics

- Perform a careful assessment prior to administration, including vital signs, level of consciousness, other drugs being taken, health history, and any allergies.
- Instruct clients to avoid the concurrent use of these drugs with other CNS depressants (including alcohol).
- Take all precautions relating to drowsiness, dizziness, reduced awareness, and loss of coordination.
- Ensure that safety measures due to CNS depression are initiated to reduce the risk for injury.
- Assess clients for adverse effects and observations charted and reported.
- Teach and caution clients at home about the following:
  - The risks of overuse, misuse, and dependence
  - The avoidance of dangerous behaviours, such as smoking
  - That these medications should be restricted to short-term use only

TABLE 8.4   Common Benzodiazepines

Medication	Normal Dosage	Common Use
Alprazolam (Xanax)	0.25–0.5 mg tid PO	Anxiety and panic attacks
Diazepam (Valium)	2–10 mg bid PO	Mild anxiety
	2–10 mg IM/IV	Muscle relaxant
Flurazepam	15–30 mg at bedtime, PO	Insomnia
Triazolam	125–500 mcg at bedtime, PO	Insomnia
Chlordiazepoxide HCl	PO/IM/IV 5–25 mg tid/qid	Mild to severe anxiety
Lorazepam (Ativan)	0.5–6 mg per day PO	Anxiety; sedation
Oxazepam	10–30 mg tid/qid PO	Anxiety

bid, Twice a day; IM, intramuscular; IV, intravenous; PO, by mouth; qid, four times a day; tid, three times a day.

TABLE 8.5   Common Nonbenzodiazepines

Drug	Dosage	Uses
Zolpidem tartrate (Sublinox)	5–10 mg at bedtime, SL	Insomnia
Zoplicone (Imovane)	5–7.5 mg at bedtime, PO	Insomnia
Diphenhydramine (Sleep-Eze)	50 mg at bedtime, PO	Antihistamine, mild hypnotic
Hydroxyzine	25–100 mg tid to qid per day 100 mg, IM	Sedative, anxiolytic
Sertraline (Zoloft)	50 mg daily PO	Anxiety and stress disorder

IM, intramuscular; PO, by mouth; tid, three times a day; qid, four times a day; SL, sublingual.

Antiepileptic Drugs

Epilepsy is not a single disorder but a collection of conditions characterized by the sudden discharge of excessive electrical energy by brain cells. The goal of antiepileptic drug (AED) therapy is to effectively limit this uncontrolled firing of neurons and to control the spread of impulses. To achieve this goal, each client's treatment is based on the type of seizure they experience.

The choice of drug therapy is dependent on the proper classification of the type of seizure. This classification is based on the client's clinical symptoms and electroencephalographic (EEG) pattern.

Types of Antiepileptic Drugs

Barbiturates. Barbiturates such as phenobarbital and primidone act to inhibit the conduction of nerve impulses within the CNS by promoting the inhibitory activity of GABA. This reduces the abnormal electrical activity within the brain that is causing seizure activity. Phenobarbital is used for the management of status epilepticus.

Benzodiazepines. Benzodiazepines such as diazepam (Valium) and clonazepam (Rivotril) increase the GABA effect to inhibit neuron firing, thereby reducing abnormal electrical activity.

Hydantoins. The hydantoin class acts on the cell membrane of neurons in the cortex of the brain to stabilize nerve membranes, thus reducing voltage frequency and the spread of electrical discharges. Phenytoin (Dilantin) is the medication of choice for treating adults' tonic–clonic seizures.

Iminostilbenes. Carbamazepine (Tegretol) and oxcarbazepine (Trileptal) block sodium channels which leads to stabilization of nerve membranes. They are used for generalized tonic–clonic and focal seizures.

Valproic acid. Valproic acid (Depakene) increases the GABA effect, resulting in decreased electrical activity. It is used to treat absence, myoclonic, and tonic–clonic seizures.

Succinimides. Ethosuximide (Zarontin) is used for the control of absence seizures.

Miscellaneous AEDs
- Gabapentin (Neurontin)
- Perampanel (Fycompa)
- Pregabalin (Lyrica)
- Lamotrigine (Lamictal)
- Levetiracetam (Keppra)
- Topiramate (Topamax)

Adverse Effects of Antiepileptic Medications
- Epigastric pain
- Nausea and vomiting
- Drowsiness
- Bradycardia
- Hypotension

Nursing Considerations Relating to Antiepileptic Medications
- Prior to administration, perform a complete assessment of past and present health history for allergies, drug interactions, adverse effects experienced, and kidney, liver, and heart disease, and take vital signs.
- Teach clients that the medication should be given at the same time each day.
- Advise clients that food should be eaten to avoid GI irritation, nausea, and vomiting.
- Inform clients of possible drowsiness that may occur initially.

- Caution clients to avoid taking antacids at the same time as medication.
- Caution clients about abruptly stopping medication.
- Advise clients to report any undesirable effects immediately.
- Advise clients to avoid using other CNS depressants, such as alcohol.
- Perform an assessment of therapeutic blood levels for clients on long-term therapy.
- Perform liver function tests on a regular basis.
- Educate clients about the use of a MedicAlert bracelet as a protective measure.

Antiparkinsonian Agents

Antiparkinson's pharmacotherapy is aimed at increasing or enhancing the action of dopamine in the brain (using dopaminergic agents) and inhibiting the action of acetylcholine (Ach, with anticholinergic agents) for the purpose of restoring the balance between dopamine and Ach.

Dopaminergic Agents

These drugs increase the effects of dopamine at receptor sites in the substantia nigra. Since dopamine cannot cross the blood–brain barrier, medications that act like dopamine or increase dopamine concentration are used.

- Levodopa (L-dopa) crosses the blood–brain barrier, where it is converted to dopamine. Large amounts are broken down to dopamine prior to passing through the blood–brain barrier and into the CNS. Levodopa given alone requires a high dosage to produce the desired effects.
- Carbidopa inhibits the breakdown of levodopa outside the CNS, allowing greater amounts of levodopa to enter the CNS. This effect results in a lower dosage requirement. Commonly, a combination of levodopa–carbidopa (Sinemet) is administered.
- Amantadine increases dopamine release and blocks the reuptake of dopamine into the presynaptic neuron.
- Selegiline (Apo-Selegiline) decreases the breakdown of dopamine by monoamine oxidase B (MAO-B) inhibitors. (Monoamine oxidase is an enzyme that breaks down neurotransmitters.)
- Entacapone decreases the breakdown of dopamine by COMT (catechol O-methyltransferase, the enzyme that breaks down levodopa).

Adverse effects of dopaminergic agents

- Nausea and vomiting
- Orthostatic hypotension
- Palpitations
- Dizziness
- Nervousness and agitation
- Muscle irritability

The beneficial effects of dopaminergic medications are not seen until a few weeks after treatment begins. Vitamin B_6 facilitates the breakdown of levodopa, reducing levels outside the CNS and limiting the amount of dopamine reaching the brain.

Anticholinergic Drugs

These drugs oppose the effect of Ach at the receptor sites in the substantia nigra and corpus striatum, thus helping restore chemical balance in the area. They also help alleviate the tremors and rigidity associated with Parkinson's disease. Examples include benztropine and trihexyphenidyl.

Adverse effects of anticholinergic drugs

- Drowsiness
- Confusion
- Constipation
- Dry mouth
- Urinary retention
- Pupillary dilation

Nursing Considerations Relating to Antiparkinsonian Medication

- Prior to administration, perform an assessment of health history for CNS, GI, and urinary functioning and psychological state, such as swallowing, voiding patterns, constipation, peptic ulcer disease, prostate enlargement, depression, and so on, to identify possible contraindications or cautions.
- Administer following meals and at bedtime with a full glass of water.
- Encourage regular mouth care due to drying effects.
- Advise clients to avoid foods high in vitamin B_6 (such as spinach, bananas, liver, and sweet potato).
- Teach the importance of ingesting foods high in fibre to maintain regular GI functioning and avoid constipation.
- Teach clients that entacapone will produce a brownish discoloration of the urine that is normal.
- Observe for and chart desired and adverse effects experienced by clients.
- Encourage clients to report any undesirable effects that are experienced.
- Teach clients that the medications must be taken at the time prescribed. Delaying a dose by even 30 minutes can lead to a return of symptoms that lasts for several hours.

Skeletal Muscle Relaxants

Skeletal muscle relaxants depress the CNS by blocking nerve impulses that cause muscle tone and contraction. The primary use is for the treatment of muscle spasm. Most muscle relaxants act on the CNS by depressing the system and indirectly relaxing the muscles. However, a few act directly by depressing the contraction of muscle fibres (such as dantrolene).

- Baclofen (Lioresal) is used to treat the spasticity of multiple sclerosis (MS) and spinal cord injury.
- Dantrolene (Dantrium) inhibits muscle contraction, relieving muscle spasticity and neuroleptic malignant syndrome.
- Cyclobenzaprine (Novo-Cycloprine) is used for muscle spasm following musculoskeletal injury.

Nursing Considerations Relating to Muscle Relaxants

- Use all safety precautions relating to medications that produce CNS depression.

- Teach clients about avoiding dangerous activities that require alertness and quick reflexes.

Psychotherapeutic Drugs

Psychotherapeutic medications are used to treat clients who have lost the ability to cope with the normal activities of daily living due to changes in their mental state. An inability to cope with normal day-to-day functions can be the result of anxiety, depression, changes in personality and mood, or psychotic behaviour. The four categories of medications used to treat these mental health disorders include anxiolytics, antidepressants, mood stabilizers, and antipsychotics.

Anxiolytics

Anxiolytics are prescribed to produce relief of anxiety and panic disorder by depressing CNS activity. Refer to Table 8.4 on page 7 for common benzodiazepines and their uses and dosages.

Antidepressants

Depression has no known external cause. It is theorized to be the result of decreased levels of the neurotransmitters norepinephrine (NE), dopamine, or serotonin in key areas of the brain. Older medications, such as the tricyclic antidepressants (TCAs) and monoamine oxidase inhibitors (MAOIs), as well as newer medications, such as the selective serotonin reuptake inhibitors (SSRIs), share the following characteristics:

- Relieve depression
- Must be taken for 2 to 4 weeks before depression symptoms improve
- Can be administered by mouth (PO)
- Are metabolized by cytochrome enzyme P-450 in the liver

Classifications of antidepressants

Tricyclic antidepressants (TCAs)

- TCAs reduce the uptake of serotonin and NE into nerves by inhibiting the presynaptic uptake; this, in turn, leads to increased levels in the synaptic cleft. Newer-generation antidepressant classes have largely replaced the use of TCAs for depression.
- Adverse effects of TCAs include the following:
  - Sedation
  - Sleep disturbances
  - Fatigue
  - Hallucination
  - Visual disturbances
  - Tremors
  - GI problems
  - Cardiac dysrhythmias
- Examples include imipramine, used to treat depression and childhood enuresis; amitriptyline (Elavil), used to treat insomnia and neuropathic pain; and clomipramine, used to treat obsessive–compulsive disorder (OCD).

Monoamine oxidase inhibitors (MAOIs)

- They are rarely prescribed today for depression because of the requirement that clients have a specific diet free of tyramine, which produces drug toxicity.
- Examples are phenelzine and tranylcypromine.

Selective serotonin reuptake inhibitors (SSRIs)

- The newest group of antidepressants
- Block the uptake of serotonin with little to no effect on NE; an increase in levels in the synaptic cleft promotes nerve impulse transmission and results in an antidepressant effect
- Examples include the following:
  - Fluoxetine (Prozac): For treatment of depression, obsessive-compulsive disorder (OCD), and bulimia nervosa
  - Fluvoxamine (Luvox): For depression
  - Paroxetine (Paxil): For depression, OCD, and generalized anxiety disorder
  - Sertraline (Zoloft): For depression, OCD, and panic attacks
  - Citalopram (Celexa): For depression
- Adverse effects of SSRIs include the following:
  - Fewer adverse effects are produced than with TCAs; however, because they bind significantly to plasma protein (with a half-life of 24–72 hours), accumulation within the body can occur when taken over a protracted period.
  - Anxiety
  - Dizziness
  - Seizures
  - GI effects
  - Must be used with caution in children and older persons

Mood Stabilizers

Lithium carbonate is used for the treatment and prevention of acute mania and the management of bipolar disorder. Lithium salts appear to alter sodium transport at nerve endings, inhibiting cyclic adenosine monophosphate (AMP) formation in nerve cells and enhancing the uptake of NE and serotonin by nerve cells.

Lithium is not metabolized by the body and is entirely excreted by the kidneys; therefore, renal function assessment is necessary prior to treatment. Cardiac and thyroid status should also be assessed prior to treatment due to the medication's potential adverse effects on these organs.

Sodium levels can affect the reabsorption of lithium; therefore, electrolyte levels should also be monitored. Lithium has a narrow therapeutic index. Early signs of lithium toxicity include gastrointestinal discomfort, drowsiness, muscle weakness, tremors, unsteadiness, and lack of coordination. Examples of other mood stabilizers include the following:

- Olanzapine (Zyprexa): Used to treat mania and schizophrenia
- Oxcarbazepine (Trileptal): Used to treat bipolar disorder (also an antiepileptic)
- Valproic acid (Depakene): Used to treat bipolar disorder (also an antiepileptic)

Nursing Considerations Relating to Antidepressants or Mood-Stabilizing Medications

- Do a careful assessment of the client's history of receiving antidepressant medications.
- Assess for blood dyscrasias (such as leukopenia) and liver functioning.

- Monitor for extrapyramidal symptoms (EPSs) and cardiac dysrhythmias.
- Monitor the behaviour of clients with a history of suicidal attempts.
- Monitor vital signs: blood pressure (BP), pulse, and respiratory rates initially.
  Client teaching points:
- Understand that desirable effects may take several weeks to be established.
- Take the medication as prescribed and avoid missing or doubling dosages.
- Take the medication with food to avoid GI irritation.
- Understand the adverse effects of CNS stimulation.
- Report to a doctor if adverse effects are experienced.
- Do not discontinue prescribed medication independently.
- Avoid taking other CNS-affecting substances, such as alcohol, coffee, or tobacco.
- Avoid exposure to direct sunlight and use sunscreen and protective clothing.

Antipsychotic Drugs

Neuroleptics or major tranquilizers are antipsychotic drugs. They are designed to bind to dopamine receptors and block the action of dopamine. These medications are used primarily in the treatment of psychoses, schizophrenia, and autism but may also be used to treat psychotic symptoms brought about by head injury, tumour, stroke, and other disorders.

Phenothiazines. This is the largest group of antipsychotic drugs and includes chlorpromazine, a prototype medication used in treating adults, older persons, and children.

Major adverse effects include sedation, extrapyramidal reactions, and hypotension.

Thioxanthenes. These drugs cause fewer sedative and hypotensive effects than the phenothiazines but cause extrapyramidal effects. An example is thiothixene (Navane).

Phenylbutylpiperidines. Haloperidol has similar antipsychotic properties to the thioxanthenes and phenothiazines. Use for the long-term treatment of psychosis has largely been replaced by the atypical antipsychotics.

Atypical agents
- These agents block both dopamine and serotonin receptors in the brain and relieve negative and positive symptoms of psychosis.
- Clozapine (Clozaril) is used as a second line of treatment for clients who do not respond well to the typical medications.
- Risperidone (Risperdal) may be used as the first agent in the management of schizophrenia and inappropriate behaviour associated with Alzheimer-type dementia.
  Other examples of atypical agents include olanzapine (Zyprexa) and quetiapine (Seroquel).

Nursing considerations relating to antipsychotic medications
- Perform an assessment of clients' history of receiving antipsychotic medications.
- Monitor for EPSs and cardiac dysrhythmias.

- Monitor the behaviour of clients with a history of suicide attempts.
- Monitor vital signs, including BP, pulse, and respiratory rates (e.g., assess for postural hypotension).
- Monitor blood count and liver function.
  Client teaching points:
- Understand that beneficial effects may take several weeks to become evident.
- Take the medication as prescribed and avoid missing or doubling dosages.
- Understand the adverse effects of CNS stimulation.
- Report to a doctor if adverse effects are experienced and not discontinue prescribed medication independently.
- Avoid taking other CNS-affecting substances, such as alcohol or coffee.
- Wear sunscreen and protective clothing when outdoors or in direct sunlight.
- Take the medications with food or milk to avoid gastric problems.
- Understand the possible sexual irregularities, such as enlargement of the breasts or menstrual irregularities.

Anaesthetics

Anaesthetics depress the CNS, producing loss of sensation. In the case of a local anaesthetic, the loss of sensation is to a particular area of the body; with a general anaesthetic, the result is loss of consciousness. The overall action of an anaesthetic is suppression of nerve impulse conduction, causing loss of sensation. The primary purpose is to desensitize the client to pain.

Local Anaesthetics

Drugs in this classification are primarily used to eliminate sensation to a specific region to prevent discomfort. Dental surgery commonly uses local anaesthesia. It is also used to alleviate the discomfort of certain hospital procedures, such as the suturing of wounds, the insertion of certain therapeutic devices, and during certain diagnostic procedures. Clients need to be cautioned to protect the anaesthetized area until normal sensation returns to avoid injury or damage. A common local anaesthetic is lidocaine (Bactine).

General Anaesthetics

These preparations produce loss of consciousness, skeletal muscle relaxation, and suppression of reflexes. Deep general anaesthetics will depress respirations; thus, the client will require respiratory support. General anaesthetics are used most commonly for the performance of surgical procedures.

Commonly, a combination of anaesthetics is used: an intravenous (IV) short-acting CNS depressant to induce unconsciousness, followed by an anaesthetic gas to maintain unconsciousness for the duration of the surgical procedure. The administration of general anaesthetic medication is carried out by an anaesthesiologist, who is responsible for the client's normal vital functioning during surgical procedures.

Central Nervous System Stimulants

CNS stimulants are used to enhance nervous system activity. CNS stimulants can elevate mood, decrease perception of fatigue, increase alertness, decrease appetite, and improve motor function. Stimulants may be used improperly to maintain alertness in order to avoid sleep. One stimulant commonly used to maintain general alertness is caffeine. However, some CNS stimulants have the potential to produce tolerance and severe physiological and psychological dependence when used continuously. As a result, many are classified as controlled substances.

The main CNS stimulants in use today are the amphetamines, including dextroamphetamine (Dexedrine), amphetamine sulphate (Adderall), and methylphenidate hydrochloride (Ritalin). There are several extended-release (XR) dosage forms of methylphenidate hydrochloride including Ritalin SR, Concerta, and Biphetin. These agents are prescribed primarily for the treatment of narcolepsy and attention-deficit/hyperactivity disorder (ADHD). They act by increasing the amount of norepinephrine and dopamine in the system to promote mood elevation, increase alertness, and prolong wakefulness.

Nursing Considerations Relating to CNS Stimulants

- Perform a careful physical and mental health history, including other medications being taken and any self-medication with herbal remedies, such as ginseng.
- Observe for adverse effects relating to overstimulation of the CNS.
- Check for cardiovascular system effects, mental hyperactivity, and insomnia; report adverse effects immediately to a physician.
- Alert clients to the dangers of overuse and abuse.
- Instruct clients to take only the dosage and frequency prescribed.

DRUGS THAT AFFECT THE AUTONOMIC NERVOUS SYSTEM

The four categories of drugs that affect the functioning of this division of the nervous system can stimulate or suppress the sympathetic and the parasympathetic branches. An easy way to learn the general effects produced by each of the four groups of drugs is to recall the actions of the two systems and the effects they produce on the body. The following drugs will, in general, mimic these effects.

Adrenergic Agonists (Sympathomimetic) Drugs

Drugs belonging to this category stimulate the sympathetic nervous system. Many adrenergic medications are used as emergency agents for treating cardiac arrest and cardiovascular collapse. Adrenergic agonists can stimulate both alpha-adrenergic receptors (alpha agonists) and beta-adrenergic receptors (beta agonists) of the ANS. The action of these agonists mimics the actions of the sympathetic nervous system and the neurotransmitters NE and epinephrine, producing varied effects, including increased cardiac contractions, increased heart rate, bronchodilation, decreased gastric motility, decreased intraocular pressure, and pupil dilation.

Selected vasoactive agents that influence blood vessels
- Dopamine: Used to treat hypotension and shock
- Epinephrine (Adrenalin): Used to treat allergic reactions, cardiac arrest, hypotension and shock, bronchodilation, and cardiac stimulation
- Norepinephrine (Levophed): Used to treat hypotension and shock

Adrenergic agents used to treat asthma and bronchitis
Examples of agents that produce bronchodilation:
- Salbutamol (Ventolin)
- Epinephrine (Adrenalin)
- Isoproterenol HCl

Adrenergic agents used in treating glaucoma. These agents reduce intraocular pressure and dilate the pupil. They include brimonidine (Alphagan P), simbrinza (Lumify), and apraclonidine (Iopidine).

Adrenergic agents used as nasal decongestants. A common decongestant is pseudoephedrine (Sudafed).

Adrenergic Blocking Agents (Sympatholytic) Drugs

Adrenergic blocking agents inhibit or block the responses of adrenergic neurotransmitters at alpha- and beta-adrenergic adrenergic receptor sites. In general, they block the action of the sympathetic nervous system.

Alpha blockers cause a decrease in BP and are commonly used in treating hypertension. These agents promote blood flow to vasoconstricted areas. Examples include doxazosin (Cardura) and prazosin (Minipress). Alpha blockers also relax the smooth muscle within the prostate and bladder and can be used to treat benign prostatic hypertrophy (BPH). Tamsulosin (Flomax) is an example.

Beta blockers also cause a decrease in BP. These agents decrease the heart rate and force of contraction, which decreases the load on the heart. Examples include the following:
- Propranolol (Inderal)
- Metoprolol (Lopressor)
- Atenolol (Tenormin)
- Sotalol (Rylosol)

Cholinergic (Parasympathomimetic) Drugs

In general, cholinergic drugs imitate the parasympathetic nervous system. Cholinergic medications have limited use. Their primary uses are in the treatment of urinary retention and GI disturbances. Their actions mimic the neurotransmitter Ach. Examples include the following:
- Bethanechol chloride (Duvoid): Prescribed for the treatment of urinary retention
- Pyridostigmine (Mestinon) and neostigmine (Prostigmin): Stimulate skeletal muscle contraction and are used in the treatment of myasthenia gravis. These medications

are indirect-acting cholinergic agonists that react chemically with acetylcholinesterase (AchE) in the synaptic cleft to prevent the breakdown of Ach.

- Rivastigmine (Exelon): Alzheimer's disease is associated with decreased Ach levels in the brain, and certain cholinergic agents can be employed to block AchE.

Adverse Effects of Cholinergic Drugs

As previously stated, by recalling the effects of the parasympathetic nervous system, the adverse effects of cholinergic drugs can be identified. Pulmonary secretions, bronchospasm, respiratory depression, and respiratory paralysis are some of the potentially life-threatening adverse effects. Atropine sulphate should be close at hand to reverse the cholinergic effect in the event that a client experiences a cholinergic crisis. Also, prior to administering cholinergic agents, nurses should ensure that intubation equipment is readily available should respiratory depression or arrest occur.

Anticholinergic (Parasympatholytic) Drugs

These agents act by blocking Ach receptors. Their pharmacological action results in pupil dilation, decreased lacrimation, increased heart rate, decreased GI motility, decreased salivation, and suppression of other physiological functions associated with Ach activity. Examples include the following:

- Atropine sulphate: This drug may be used as a preoperative medication to decrease GI and respiratory secretions. It is also used to treat symptomatic bradycardia. Atropine sulphate crosses the blood–brain barrier and in a sufficiently large dose will act as a stimulant. At toxic dose levels, it causes CNS depression.
- Tolterodine (Detrol): This medication is used for the treatment of urinary frequency, urgency, and urge incontinence caused by bladder overactivity.
- Benztropine, procyclidine, trihexyphenidyl, and ethopropazine (Parsitan): These medications are used to treat the cholinergic disorder in Parkinson's disease.
- Oxybutynin (Ditropan): This medication is used in the treatment of overactive bladder.
  Client teaching points:
- Since overdosage of cholinergic-blocking agents may cause life-threatening problems, medications should be administered exactly as prescribed.
- Clients should be warned about undertaking activities that cause perspiration since anticholinergic agents inhibit perspiration, making clients susceptible to heat stroke.
- Clients should also be cautioned to consult with the primary health care provider before taking any other medications, including OTC drugs.

Nursing Considerations Relating to Medications that Affect the ANS

- Maintain awareness of sympathetic and parasympathetic nervous system effects on the body.
- Be aware that observations relating to sympathomimetics include tachycardia, elevation in BP, hyperactivity, sleeplessness, dry mouth, and pupillary dilation.

- Be aware that observations relating to sympatholytics will include bradycardia, decreased BP, sedation, weakness, lethargy, and dizziness.
- Be aware that observations relating to parasympathomimetics will include bradycardia, hypotension, bronchoconstriction, increased salivation, perspiration, abdominal cramps, dizziness, and pupillary constriction.
- Be aware that observations relating to parasympathetic blockers include tachycardia, restlessness, confusion, pupillary dilation, blurred vision, urinary retention, dry mouth, and constipation.
- Monitor vital signs carefully.
- Promote a relaxing environment for clients on stimulant classifications of ANS medications.
- Provide mouth care for dry mouth.
- Teach clients to report adverse effects.
- Caution clients on depressant classifications of ANS medications about safety precautions, particularly to avoid driving or operating dangerous machinery.
- Advise clients taking anticholinergics that these medications may cause sensitivity to light due to pupillary dilation; use of sunglasses and avoidance of bright lights should be encouraged.
- Advise clients taking sympathomimetics and anticholinergics that these medications may cause urinary retention; teach clients to report urination problems.

DRUGS THAT AFFECT THE CARDIOVASCULAR SYSTEM

Drugs that affect the cardiovascular system are outlined in Figure 8.2.

Agents Affecting Blood Coagulation

Two overall classifications of drugs affect blood coagulation: agents that inhibit blood coagulation and those that promote it. Classes of drugs that inhibit abnormal coagulation of blood (clot formation) may be divided into several general classifications: anticoagulants, antiplatelet drugs, hemorheological drugs, and thrombolytics. Agents that promote blood coagulation (to prevent abnormal blood loss) are called *antifibrinolytics*.

Preliminary Tests

Before and during the administration of agents that affect the clotting of blood, several blood tests are used to assess the clotting processes within the body. These include the following (normal values are given in parentheses):

- Platelet count $(150–400 \times 10^9)$
- Hemoglobin (Hgb) (male: 140–180 g/L; female: 120–160 g/L)
- Hematocrit (Hct) (male: 042–0.52 volume fraction; female: 0.37–0.47 volume fraction)
- Prothrombin time (PT) (11–12.5 seconds)
- Partial thromboplastin time (PTT) (60–70 seconds)
- Activated partial thromboplastin time (aPTT) (30–40 seconds)

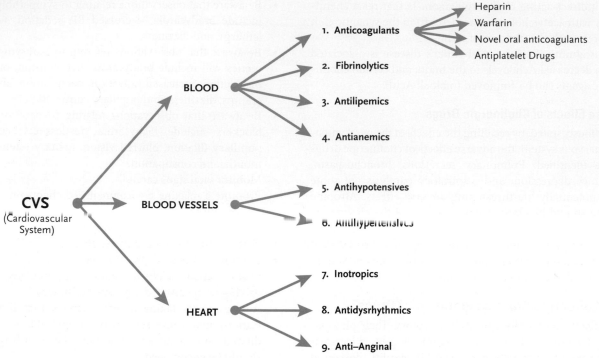

Fig. 8.2 Drugs that affect the cardiovascular system.

- International normalized ratio (INR) (0.81–1.2)

For clients taking heparin, the aPTT or PTT is used to monitor the prescribed therapeutic range. For clients taking oral anticoagulants, PT or INR is used to monitor the prescribed therapeutic range.

Anticoagulants (Coagulation-Modifying Agents)

Anticoagulants prevent the formation of clots by inhibiting certain clotting factors and platelets. They are only given prophylactically as they have no direct effect on a blood clot that has already formed.

Common uses
- Myocardial infarction (MI)
- Unstable angina pectoris
- Atrial fibrillation
- Emboli (pulmonary emboli)
- In-dwelling devices (pacemakers, mechanical valves)
- Pelvic surgeries (prostatectomy)

Anticoagulants drug classes

Heparin
- Heparin is commonly prescribed during the acute stage of a condition requiring anticoagulant therapy.
- Heparin activates antithrombin III, causing neutralization of thrombin and inhibition of clot formation.
- Onset of action following subcutaneous (SC) injection is 20–60 minutes; duration of action is approximately 8–12 hours.
- Dosage is based on PTT or aPTT; therapeutic range is 1.5–2.5 times normal.
- Enoxaparin sodium (Lovenox) and dalterparin sodium (Fragmin) are examples of low molecular weight heparins (LMWHs) which are more specific for activated factor

X). They have a predictable anticoagulant response and frequent laboratory monitoring of bleeding times is not required.

Warfarin (Coumadin)
- Warfarin is commonly prescribed after the acute stage of a condition requiring anticoagulant therapy to maintain therapeutic blood levels of anticoagulation.
- Warfarin interferes with production of vitamin K (necessary for clotting of blood). Vitamin K is necessary for the production of clotting factors II, VII, IX, and X.
- Onset of action is 2 to 7 days.
- Dosage is based on the PT and INR; the desirable therapeutic range is 1.5 to 2.5 times normal.

Novel oral anticoagulants. There are several newer oral anticoagulants including dabigtran (Pradaxa) which is a direct thrombin inhibitor, and rivaroxaban (Xarelto) and apixaban (Eliquis), which are selective factor Xa inhibitor.

Antiplatelet drugs
- These drugs interfere with the ability of platelets to aggregate during the process of blood clotting.
- Antiplatelet medications are commonly prescribed to prevent arterial thrombosis and where a thromboembolism disorder exists, as in the prevention and management of conditions such as MI, cerebrovascular accident, and transient ischemic attacks.
- Bleeding time and PT are used to monitor the therapeutic effects of antiplatelet medications.

Examples include the following:
- Acetylsalicylic acid (Aspirin)
- Clopidogrel bisulphate (Integrilin)
- Clopidogrel (Plavix)

Adverse effects of anticoagulant drugs (coagulation-modifying agents)

- Hemorrhage: Indicated by occult blood in stool, melena stool, petechia, bruising, bleeding from gums
- Gastric ulceration (ASA)

Nursing considerations relating to anticoagulant medications (coagulation-modifying agents)

- Observe for signs of hemorrhage, such as hematuria or black stool, and report.
- Administer oral medications with food to avoid gastric irritation.
- Administer SC heparin to avoid local bruising. Use a 1-cm needle, do not aspirate the plunger, inject into the deep fatty tissue of the abdomen, withdraw carefully, and apply pressure to the site for several minutes; do not massage the site.
- Monitor blood tests for the degree of anticoagulation and report if abnormal for therapeutic dose.
- Use elastic stockings to promote circulation.
- Teach clients to exercise legs to promote circulation and prevent clot formation.
- Teach clients to avoid positions that impede blood circulation, such as dangling or crossing the legs or wearing restricting clothing.
- Maintain proper hydration to avoid hemoconcentration.
- Caution clients to avoid activities that may cause trauma or increase the tendency to bleed, including the following:
  - Contact sports and other potentially risky activities
  - Vigorous teeth brushing or using a coarse-bristled toothbrush
- Remind clients to report abnormal bruising or unusual bleeding.
- Caution clients to avoid food high in vitamin K.
- Caution clients to avoid taking ASA if taking other anticoagulants.
- Instruct clients to take oral medications, particularly ASA, with food.
- Ensure that when a client is changed from heparin to a warfarin preparation, the client will remain on the heparin until the warfarin preparation achieves therapeutic levels in the blood.
- Carefully monitor PPT, aPPT (heparin), and PT and INR (warfarin) during therapy and when the client is changed from a parenteral to an oral preparation.

Fibrinolytic (Thrombolytic) Agents

- These agents act by converting plasminogen to plasmin (an enzyme that breaks down the fibrin in clots that have formed).
- Early initiation of therapy is required immediately after the condition develops to be effective.
- They are prescribed to act on clots that have formed in coronary artery occlusion (MI), pulmonary embolus, cerebral emboli (stroke), and deep vein thrombosis (DVT).
- They are administered by IV infusion.
- Clients receiving fibrinolytic medications require care in the Critical Care Unit during therapy.

Reverse anticoagulant agents. These agents are used when an overdose of anticoagulant has occurred. Examples include the following:

- Protamine sulphate: Used in the case of heparin overdose; neutralizes heparin activity
- Vitamin K: Used for a warfarin overdose

Antilipemics (Agents Used to Treat Dyslipidemia)

Antilipemic medications are used to reduce lipid levels when dietary measures, weight loss, and exercise have been unsuccessful. Indication for treatment includes elevated plasma cholesterol, triglyceride, and low-density lipoprotein (LDL) levels.

Preliminary Tests

The following are the normal ranges for preliminary levels.

- Cholesterol: <5.0 mmol/L
- Triglycerides: Male 0.45–1.81 mmol/L, female 0.40–1.52 mmol/L
- LDL: <2.59 mmol/L

The choice of treatment depends on which type of lipid is elevated.

Bile Acid Sequestrants

These preparations combine with the bile acids in the intestine to form a nonabsorbable complex that is then excreted in the feces. This lack of reabsorption of bile forces the liver cells to metabolize cholesterol to produce more bile acids, thus reducing LDLs and total cholesterol levels. An example is cholestyramine resin (Olestyr).

HMG-CoA Reductase Inhibitors (Statins)

This is the most widely used classification of antilipemics in the treatment of dyslipidemia. Statins block the formation of cellular cholesterol, causing a reduction in blood LDL and total cholesterol within weeks. Examples include the following:

- Rosuvastatin (Crestor)
- Atorvastatin (Lipitor)
- Pravastatin sodium
- Simvastatin (Zocor)
- Lovastatin
- Fluvastatin sodium (Lescol)

Fibric Acids

These acids stimulate the breakdown and reduction in synthesis of very-low-density lipoproteins (VLDLs). Therapeutic effects include the lowering of VLDLs, the reduction of triglycerides, and the increase of high-density lipoprotein (HDL) levels. Examples include fenofibrate and gemfibrozil.

Nicotinic acid (Vitamin B₃)

Nicotinic acid (niacin, vitamin B_3, Niaspan) acts on liver cells to inhibit LDL and triglyceride production. It may be prescribed in combination with other antihyperlipidemic medications.

TABLE 8.6   Nutritional Deficiency Anemia Drug Treatments

Preparation	Uses	Adverse Effects	Nursing Considerations
Iron • Ferrous fumarate • Ferrous gluconate • Ferrous sulphate	• Iron deficiency anemia	• Gastro-intestinal irritation • Discolouration of tooth enamel • Black stool • Drug allergy	• Oral preparations: give with food • Liquid preparations: drink with straw • IM: deep IM, Z-track technique to reduce tissue irritation
Folic Acid • Folate	• Pregnancy • Megaloblastic anemia • Folic acid deficiency • Pernicious anemia	• Rare • Discoloration of urine • Possible allergy	• Take with food
Vitamin B$_{12}$ • Cyanocobalamin		• In large doses: • Diarrhea • Pruritis • Hypokalemia	• Take with food • Usually required for life

IM, intramuscular.

Adverse Effects of Antilipemics

- The reduction of fat-soluble vitamins due to bile salts reducing their absorption
- The formation of gallstones (fibric acid preparations disturb the fat level of the blood)
- The effects of statins are usually mild; however, they should be used with caution in clients with liver and kidney impairment.
- Headache
- GI disturbances: Nausea, vomiting, distension, irritation, diarrhea, or constipation
- Myopathy (muscle aches): Uncommon but significant (with statins)
- Flushing, skin rash, and itchiness (with niacin)
- Jaundice
- Antilipemics are contraindicated in liver and kidney disease.

Nursing Considerations Relating to Antilipemics

Client teaching points:
- Take the medication as prescribed (this point should be stressed).
- Promptly comply with laboratory requests and health care provider appointments.
- Report adverse effects to a health care provider (myopathy with statins, jaundice).
- Change dietary habits; reduce fat intake.
- Supplement fat-soluble vitamins (A, D, E, K).
- Increase dietary fibre and fluid intake.
- Understand the importance of moderate exercise and weight reduction.
- Do not discontinue medications without consulting with a health care provider.
- Understand that mild adverse effects usually dissipate after medication is established within the body.
- Do not take statins with grapefruit juice.
- Ensure that medication is taken with or without meals, according to the preparation.

Anemia Drugs

There are many different classifications of anemia with differing causes, manifestations, and origins. Regardless of the type of anemia, the end result is a decrease in the concentration of circulating red blood cells or a low hemoglobin level.

Anemias result from a deficiency of nutrients necessary for the development of healthy red blood cells and hemoglobin (such as iron deficiency anemia (iron), fetal damage in pregnancy (folic acid deficiency), or pernicious anemia (vitamin B$_{12}$ deficiency), or an abnormality of the bone marrow that produces the cells, such as marrow destruction from radiation, or genetic deviation, such as sickle cell anemia or thalassemia. Refer to Table 8.6, which outlines the medications used to treat nutritional deficiency anemia.

Nutritional Deficiency Anemia

Nursing considerations relating to anemia drugs. When the client takes dietary supplements for the treatment of nutritional deficiency anemia, the nurse should do the following:
- Teach the client to take prescribed medications as required to maintain optimal blood levels.
- Encourage the client not to discontinue medication without consultation with a health care provider.
- Observe the client for adverse effects and measures.
- Encourage the client to take medication in the method prescribed.
- Encourage the client to use natural dietary sources to complement prescribed medication.
- Teach the client not to break or crush preparations into a powder (many are coated to reduce irritation).

Antihypotensive Agents

These agents are used to treat low BP and circulatory shock and to re-establish effective circulation and BP. Sympathomimetic drugs are the most common classification of medications

TABLE 8.7 Classifications of Antihypotensive Agents

Type	Drug	Action
Alpha-adrenergic agents	• Norepinephrine (Levophed) • Phenylephrine (Neosynephrine) • Midodrine (prodrug)	• Causes constriction of vascular smooth muscle, resulting in increased systemic vascular resistance and increased BP
Beta-adrenergic agents	• Dobutamine • Isoproterenol (Isuprel)	• Increases myocardial contractility and heart rate, resulting in increased BP
Alpha- and beta-adrenergic agents	• Dopamine HCl • Epinephrine (Adrenalin)	• Causes constriction of vascular smooth muscle and stimulates cardiac contractility • Increases blood flow to kidneys, preventing renal shutdown (dopamine) • Bronchodilation

BP, Blood pressure; *HCl,* hydrochloric acid.

used for the treatment of the above conditions and are effective in an emergency.

Classifications of Antihypotensive Agents

Table 8.7 summarizes the classifications and actions of antihypotensive agents.

Dopamine and epinephrine are the most commonly used agents for shock and hypotension.

Antihypertensive Agents

Antihypertensive agents are usually prescribed for clients when diet, exercise, and other measures designed to reduce BP have failed to lower BP to a level that does not pose a health risk to the cardiovascular and renal systems. In general, to reduce BP, antihypertensive medications either reduce blood volume (such as diuretics) or cause dilation of blood vessels (i.e., they reduce peripheral resistance).

Treatment for hypertension depends on the severity of the disorder. Antihypertensive therapy for mild to moderate hypertension usually begins with a single medication, such as a thiazide diuretic. In the presence of moderate hypertension, in some clients, it may be necessary to give a combination of two medications (e.g., a thiazide diuretic in addition to one from another antihypertensive drug class). For severe hypertension, a combination of medications designed specifically for the client will be prescribed.

Classifications of Antihypertensive Agents

Table 8.8 summarizes the classifications and actions of antihypertensive agents.

Adverse Effects of Antihypertensive Agents

Adverse effects vary according to the category of drug prescribed. In general, adverse effects most commonly experienced are the result of vasodilation and reduced cardiac action, including the following:
- Hypokalemia (diuretics, such as thiazides)
- Muscle cramps (loop diuretics)
- Lightheadedness, dizziness, weakness, lethargy
- Orthostatic hypotension
- Dehydration (diuretics)
- Urticaria (thiazide and loop)
- Photosensitivity (thiazide and loop)
- Headache (vasodilating effects)
- Gynecomastia (potassium sparing in men)
- Erectile dysfunction (thiazide)
- Menstrual irregularities (potassium sparing in menstruating persons)

Nursing Considerations Relating to Antihypertensive Agents
- Observe for adverse effects related to specific medication prescribed (such as dehydration or electrolyte imbalance).
- Monitor vital signs—BP and pulse, lying and standing—before antihypertensive medication administration.
  Client teaching points:
- Understand the dangers of uncontrolled hypertension.
- Report adverse effects that may occur initially.
- Do not suddenly stop taking the prescribed medication.
- Take the medication as prescribed.
- Do not double up if a dose is missed.
- Take care when ambulating due to postural hypotension.
- Avoid very hot showers or baths due to vasodilating effects and dizziness that could result.
- Ensure proper hydration; avoid becoming dehydrated, monitor fluid intake.
- Avoid excess alcohol use, since it is vasodilating and the effects produced interfere with medication metabolism and cause dehydration.
- Monitor and report signs of swelling of lower extremities.
- Keep health care provider and laboratory appointments for reassessments.
- Understand the importance of the following:
  - Weight reduction
  - Balanced diet (restrict salt intake, potassium supplementation if on diuretics)
  - Stress reduction
  - Adequate rest

Agents Used to Treat Heart Failure

A variety of treatment regimens exist for the management of heart failure. The following classifications of drugs may be prescribed to promote more effective cardiovascular functioning.

TABLE 8.8   Classifications of Antihypertensive Agents

Type	Select Drugs	Action
Diuretics (thiazide and thiazidelike, loop, potassium sparing)	• Hydrochlorothiazide • Furosemide (Lasix) • Spironolactone (Aldactone)	• Reduce circulating and interstitial fluid → reduce peripheral vascular resistance → ↓ BP
ACE inhibitors	• Benazepril (Losentin) • Captopril (Capoten) • Cilazapril (Inhibace) • Enalapril (Vasotec) • Fosinopril sodium • Ramipril (Altace) • Lisinopril (Prinivil) • Perindopril (Coversyl) • Quinapril (Accupril) • Trandolapril (Mavik)	• Block enzyme that converts angiotensin I to angiotensin II → vasodilation → decrease peripheral vascular resistance → ↓ BP
Angiotensin II receptor blockers	• Losartan (Cozaar) • Valsartan (Diovan) • Eprosartan (Teveten) • Irbesartan • Candesartan (Atacand) • Telmisartan (Micardis) • Azilsartan (Edarbi)	• Block binding of angiotensin II to type 1 angiotensin II receptors → blocks vasoconstriction and secretion of aldosterone → vasodilation → decrease peripheral vascular resistance → ↓ BP
Adrenergic drugs: Alpha$_1$-adrenergic blockers	• Doxazosin (Cardura) • Prazosin (Minipress) • Terazosin (Hytrin)	• Block stimulation of alpha-adrenergic receptors in blood → vasodilation → decrease peripheral vascular resistance → ↓ BP
Adrenergic drugs: Beta-adrenergic blockers	• Atenolol (Tenormin) • Metoprolol (Lopressor) • Propranolol	• Block beta-adrenergic receptors within heart muscle → reduce strength and rate of cardiac contraction → decrease peripheral resistance → ↓ BP
Calcium channel blockers	• Amlodipine (Norvasc) • Diltiazem (Cardizem) • Verapamil (Isoptin)	• Prevent the action of calcium at receptor sites, inhibiting smooth muscle contraction → vasodilation → decrease peripheral vascular resistance → ↓ BP
Centrally acting antihypertensives	• Clonidine • Methyldopa	• Stimulate the brain to modify the action of the sympathetic nervous system → reduce strength of cardiac activity and inhibit vasoconstriction → decrease peripheral vascular resistance → ↓ BP
Vasodilators	• Hydralazine (Apresoline) • Minoxidil (Loniten) • Diazoxide (Proglycem) • Sodium nitroprusside (Nipride)	• Produce vasodilation by acting directly on the arterial smooth muscle → decrease peripheral vascular resistance → ↓ BP
Direct renin inhibitors	• Aliskiren (Rasilez)	• Binds directly to the renin enzyme and blocks conversion of angiotensinogen to angiotensin I and angiotensin II → vasodilation → decrease peripheral vascular resistance → ↓ BP

ACE, Angiotensin-converting enzyme; *BP,* blood pressure.

Vasodilators

Vasodilators decrease the workload of the heart and include ACE inhibitors, nitrates, and angiotensin II receptor blockers (used if ACE inhibitors are not tolerated well).

Diuretics

These medications increase urine output and decrease sodium levels in the body. They are commonly used in combination with other medications to treat heart failure and include thiazides and furosemide.

Beta-Adrenergic Blockers

These medications reduce or block the sympathetic nervous system to the heart and the heart's conduction system. This results in decreased contractility of the myocardium, decreased heart rate, and delayed atrioventricular (AV) node conduction and decreased myocardial automaticity. Examples of beta blockers used in the treatment of heart failure include bisoprolol, extended-release metoprolol, and carvedilol.

Beta-Adrenergic Agonists

These agonists stimulate sympathetic nervous system activity to increase calcium flow into the cardiac muscle, resulting in increased contractility. These medications are used for clients who are experiencing acute decompensated heart failure and are hemodynamically unstable. An example is dobutamine hydrochloride.

Cardiac Glycosides

This class of drug was once widely used in the treatment of heart failure, but it has largely been replaced by newer medications. Cardiac glycosides act by increasing the strength of cardiac contraction (positive inotropic effect), which results in increased cardiac output. The drugs also slow the rate of cardiac contraction (negative chronotropic effect), leading to more effective heart action, an increase in renal output, and a decrease in renin release results. An example is digoxin (Lanoxin).

Nursing considerations: Implications relating to digoxin

- They have a narrow therapeutic index.
- They are excreted from the body by the kidney (renal impairment may cause accumulation, leading to toxic levels).
- Dosages should be adjusted to prevent blood levels from becoming toxic.
- Assess for adverse or toxic effects, reporting and charting immediately.
- Do not administer digoxin concurrently with the following medications or substances:
  - Antacids, which reduce absorption.
  - Antimicrobial agents and calcium preparations, which may promote toxicity.
- Monitor digoxin serum levels throughout treatment to detect toxic levels.
- Following each administration of the medication, be aware that charting should include indicating the apical heart rate at the time of administration.
- If the apical pulse rate is erratic, below 60 beats per minute in adults (less than 90 beats per minute in infants), or above 100 to 120 beats per minute, withhold the digoxin and report for additional assessment by the health care provider.
- Monitor clients with hypokalemia, hypothyroidism, and acute MI more frequently for toxic effects.
- Know that the antidote for severe toxicity is digoxin immune fab (Digibind), which inactivates digoxin by drawing the medication from the tissues and binding to it. Client teaching points:
- Monitor for adverse effects, such as visual changes (colour perception).
- Monitor heart rate (teach the client how to do so).
- Report concerns regarding the effects of the medication.
- Eat food high in potassium (due to loss through urine).
- Avoid taking several medications if a drug interaction may occur.
- Do not to take a double dose if a dose is missed.

Symptoms of digitalis toxicity

- Drowsiness, weakness, dizziness
- Confusion
- GI upset: Nausea, vomiting, diarrhea
- Visual disturbances (yellow-green distortion)
- Bradycardia or tachycardia
- Heart block

Digitalization. When a client is initially started on a digitalis preparation, a higher-than-normal dosage of the medication is commonly given to establish therapeutic levels as quickly as possible. The subsequent (maintenance) dosage is established to maintain the therapeutic level in the blood following the initial high dose. Careful monitoring of blood levels is undertaken to avoid possible toxicity and to establish the most effective maintenance dosage.

Phosphodiesterase Inhibitors (PDIs)

- PDIs produce an inotropic effect on the heart as well as dilating arteries and veins.
- They increase the force of contractility of the heart muscles and decrease pre- and afterload on the heart.
- PDIs are administered intravenously.
- An example is milrinone.
- Potential adverse effects of PDI administration include hypotension and dysrhythmias.
- Clients must be evaluated for BP, cardiac rhythm and rate, and cardiac output during and for several hours following administration.

Antidysrhythmic Drugs

Antidysrhythmics are medications used to treat dysrhythmias, to slow conduction of electrical impulses in the heart, to reduce spontaneous depolarization of myocardial cells, or to prolong the effective refractory period.

The Vaughan Williams classification of antidysrhythmic drugs, which is based on the effect that agents produce on action potential in the heart, lists four classes of agents:

Class I: Sodium channel blockers (e.g., quinidine, disopyramide, or procainamide)

Class II: Beta blockers (e.g., sotalol or propranolol)

Class III: Potassium channel blockers (such as amiodarone, bretylium, and ibutilide)

Class IV: Calcium channel blockers (such as diltiazem and verapamil)

Digoxin is used for atrial fibrillation.

Adverse Effects

- Quinidine can result in disturbed hearing, giddiness, and impaired vision (cinchonism).
- Amiodarone can accumulate in tissue, causing photosensitivity rashes and lung problems.
- See the section "Symptoms of Digitalis Toxicity."

Antianginal Drugs

Antiangina medications are prescribed to relieve angina pain and reduce the frequency of angina attacks. They are also prescribed to improve the client's functional capacity and prevent or delay MI. The drugs either help restore oxygen supply to the heart by improving blood supply to the myocardium, reduce myocardial oxygen demand, or both.

Classifications of Drugs Used to Treat Angina Pectoris

Nitrates. Nitrates act by relaxing vascular smooth muscle, which dilates coronary blood vessels and increases blood flow to the myocardium. They also reduce both preload and afterload. Examples are nitroglycerin (Nitrostat) and isosorbide mononitrate.

Calcium channel blockers. These medications act by relaxing vascular smooth muscle, which dilates the coronary blood vessels and increases blood flow to the myocardium. Examples include amlodipine (Norvasc), diltiazem (Cardizem), and extended-release nifedipine (Adalat XL).

Beta-adrenergic blockers. Beta-adrenergic blockers act to help reduce the risk for angina by decreasing the influence of the sympathetic nervous system on stimulating the myocardium, resulting in decreased cardiac output, reduced oxygen demand, and lower BP. Examples are propranolol, atenolol (Tenormin), and metoprolol (Lopresor).

Adverse Effects of Antiangina Pectoris Medications

- Headache
- Flushing of skin
- Dizziness, weakness, and fainting

Nursing Considerations Relating to Antiangina Pectoris Medications

- Oral preparations and patches are used for the prevention of anginal attacks.
- Sprays and sublingual preparations are used for acute attacks.
- For treatment of acute anginal pain, the sublingual dose range for nitrate is 0.3 to 0.6 mg. The dose of nitrate may be repeated twice at 5-minute intervals. If the pain persists after one dose, the client should seek medical attention immediately as the potential for MI exists.
- To avoid developing tolerance, the health care provider may order removal of the nitroglycerin patch for 8 hours overnight.

Clients should be taught the following:

- Techniques for administration
- To recognize adverse effects and report
- To rest while taking medication during an anginal attack
- To avoid swallowing for several minutes when administering sublingual preparations
- To store sublingual medications in a dry, cool, dark place
- To carry medication at all times
- To note and observe expiratory dates and replace
- That sublingual spray preparations should not be frozen, and prior to administration, priming of the pump is required.
- That patches applied to the skin should be stored in a dry environment and applied to an area of skin without hair, the old patch is removed and the skin is cleansed, and the new patch is applied to a different area; apply at the same time each day.
- To take oral preparations on an empty stomach

DRUGS THAT AFFECT THE GASTRO-INTESTINAL SYSTEM

Drugs that affect the GI system are outlined in Figure 8.3.

There are four common disorders of the GI system for which medications are frequently prescribed: constipation, diarrhea, hyperacidity, and nausea and vomiting. Some of these disorders may be treated using OTC preparations, but for clients

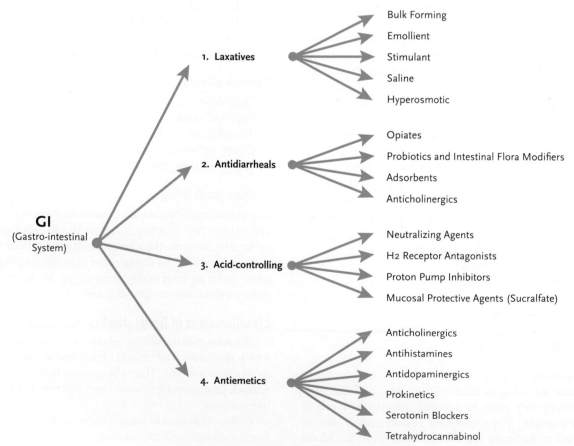

Fig. 8.3 Drugs that affect the gastro-intestinal system.

TABLE 8.9 Classifications of Laxatives

Type of Laxative	Action	Uses
Bulk-Forming Laxative • Psyllium (Metamucil)	• Acts by absorbing water into intestine → increases bulk and distends bowel → reflex bowel activity (peristalsis)	• Slow-acting (12–48 hours) • Long-term therapy for chronic constipation
Stimulant Laxative • Bisacodyl (Dulcolax) • Senna (Senekot)	• Irritates or stimulates the nerve plexus in the mucosa of small intestine and colon → increasing peristalsis	• Rapid evacuation of bowel for diagnostic tests • Acute constipation
Saline Laxative • Magnesium citrate • Magnesium hydroxide (Milk of Magnesia)	• Draws water into the bowel by osmotic action → watery stool and distended bowel → stimulates stretch receptors → stimulates peristalsis	• Bowel cleansing • Acute constipation • Rapid onset
Emollient Laxative (stool softener) • Docusate sodium (Colace) • Mineral oil	• Detergent-like action that lowers surface tension of gastro-intestinal fluids → water and fat absorbed into stool and increased peristalsis • Lubricates bowel for easier passage of stool	• Mild, gentle relief of constipation • Prevention of constipation
Hyperosmotic Laxative • Lactulose (Apo-Lactulose) • Polyethylene glycol (Miralax)	• Produces a hyperosmolar environment in bowel → draws water from intestinal lining into bowel → distension of bowel with added water → stimulation of peristalsis	• Relieves acute constipation • Bowel preparation for diagnostic and surgical procedures • Very cleansing

with serious conditions or those in institutions, the health care provider may prescribe the appropriate medication.

Laxatives

In this group, drugs are used to speed the passage of intestinal contents through the GI tract. They may be administered to prevent or relieve constipation (most common use), to prepare a client for lower GI tract procedures, to reduce the strain of defecation in clients with cardiovascular disease or hemorrhoids, to remove ingested toxic substances, or as treatment for parasitic infestations or other such conditions.

Classifications of Laxatives

Table 8.9 outlines the different classifications of laxatives, their actions, and their uses.

Adverse Effects Relating to the Use of Laxatives

- Diarrhea
- Abdominal cramps (can occur with the rapid-acting stimulant and saline laxatives and irritating stimulant laxative classifications)
- Flatulence
- Tolerance
- Bowel impaction or obstruction (with bulk-forming preparations)
- Electrolyte imbalances (with saline laxatives)

Nursing Considerations Relating to Laxatives

- Assess client need; evaluate record of bowel movements.
- Know that contraindications include bowel surgery and bowel diseases.
- Observe and record therapeutic effects and adverse effects.
- Ambulate client as soon as possible because exercise promotes bowel action.
- Push fluids if not contraindicated.

- Provide a relaxed, unrushed, and private area for defecation. Client teaching points:
- Follow the directions indicated on the medication container (e.g., take with the full glass of water; take before bedtime).
- Increase fluid intake throughout the day if not contraindicated.
- Increase fibre in the diet.
- Reduce constipating foods in the diet.
- Increase exercise.
- Avoid overuse of medications as tolerance can develop.
- If possible, use milder classifications such as stool softeners or bulk-forming laxatives.
- Avoid overuse of bulk-forming laxatives, which can interfere with absorption of other medications and cause distension and possible obstruction.
- Do not take prescribed medication if abdominal pain or nausea and vomiting are present.

Antidiarrheal Agents

Usually, the medication prescribed to treat diarrhea is given to treat the unpleasant symptoms or the underlying cause of the diarrhea. Some medications may be purchased without prescription and are available on pharmacy shelves or OTC, whereas others require a prescription because of the classification of the drug or the severity of the condition to be treated (such as opiate-related medications).

Four general classifications of agents are used for the treatment of diarrhea: opiates, probiotics and intestinal flora modifiers, adsorbents, and anticholinergics. The type of medication prescribed depends on the cause and severity of the diarrhea.

Classifications of Antidiarrheals

Table 8.10 outlines the different classifications of antidiarrheals, their actions, and their uses.

TABLE 8.10 Classifications of Antidiarrheals

Classification	Action	Uses
Opiates • Codeine sulphate • Loperamide (Imodium) • Diphenoxylate + atropine (Lomotil)	• Suppress gastro-intestinal (GI) smooth muscle activity → ↓ GI motility, prolonging transit time → absorption of fluid and nutrients • Analgesic effect	• Acute diarrhea • Not usually recommended for diarrhea caused by infections as infectious agents may be retained within the bowel
Probiotics and Intestinal Flora Modifiers • *Lactobacillus acidophilus*	• Replenish organisms commonly destroyed by antibiotics.	• Treatment of uncomplicated diarrhea associated with antibiotic use.
Adsorbents • Bismuth subsalicylate (Pepto-Bismol)	• Absorb irritants and coat lining of the intestinal tract → inhibit irritation of the lining of intestines and absorb toxic substances for excretion in feces	• Diarrhea associated with intestinal infections and chronic bowel diseases, such as diverticulitis and ulcerative colitis
Anticholinergics • Atropine sulphate	• Suppress parasympathetic nervous system activity of the intestinal tract → suppress peristalsis → reduce spasm and speed of passage of intestinal contents	• Require prescription; administered in conjunction with opioid preparation • Diarrhea associated with irritable and inflammatory bowel conditions

Adverse Effects Related to Antidiarrheal Agents

- Constipation
- Nausea and vomiting
- Dependency (with opiates)
- Sedation, drowsiness, weakness, lethargy (with opiates)
- Urinary retention (with atropine preparations and opiates)
- Clotting disorders (with bismuth preparations)
- Allergic reactions

Nursing Considerations Relating to Antidiarrheal Agents

- Assess the client's history relating to the diarrhea and established bowel patterns.
- Identify possible causes of the diarrhea.
- Adhere to established guidelines for administration of a specific preparation, such as the time to administer.
- Assess for contraindications.
- Increase fluid intake while diarrhea persists to prevent dehydration; monitor for electrolyte imbalances.
- Monitor client's intake and output.
  Client teaching points:
- Follow administration directives, including the correct dosage and when to take the medication.
- Increase fluid intake to replace lost fluids.
- Monitor effects relating to relief of diarrhea.
- Maintain a record of the frequency and consistency of stools until normal bowel patterns resume.
- See a health care provider immediately if diarrhea persists, manifestations increase in severity, or adverse effects develop (child: 24 hours; adult 2–3 days, depending on severity).
- Avoid irritating, gaseous foods that stimulate the bowel, such as cabbage, high-fibre foods, or psyllium fibre.
- Monitor weight for possible fluid deficits.
- Avoid overuse of opioid preparations due to possible development of dependence.
- Try to identify causes of the diarrhea for possible avoidance of a recurrence of the condition.

- Understand that sometimes the diarrhea facilitates removal of undesirable substances from the body and antidiarrheals are not always necessary.
- Understand that bismuth preparations darken the stool and that this is no cause for alarm.

Acid-Controlling Drugs

Acid-controlling drugs form a large group of prescription and OTC medications used to reduce the hyperacidity of the stomach. Antacids can directly neutralize the hydrochloric acid (HCl) secreted into the stomach (such as aluminum, magnesium, and calcium-containing medications). Additives include simethicone, which reduces gaseous buildup and distension, and alginate, which protects the gastric lining and reduces the risk for acid reflux into the esophagus. H_2 receptor antagonists and proton pump inhibitors inhibit the production or release of HCl, which results in a reduction in the amount of HCl in the stomach, thereby relieving gastric irritation.

These medications are used for the treatment of conditions such as mild gastritis, which is caused by indigestion and eating foods that cause "heartburn," gastroesophageal reflux disease (GERD), peptic ulcer disease, and hypersecretion disorders. A prescription for certain preparations may also be used as a preventive of stress ulcers caused by extreme traumatic events, such as extensive burns. The particular type of preparation prescribed is directed toward treating the specific condition.

Classification of Acid-Controlling Drugs

Table 8.11 outlines the different classifications of acid-controlling drugs, their actions, their uses, and adverse effects.

General Adverse Effects of Acid-Controlling Drugs

- Antacids are contraindicated in severe renal failure, GI obstruction
- H_2 receptor antagonists may rarely cause confusion and disorientation in older persons

TABLE 8.11 Classifications of Acid-controlling Drugs

Classification	Action	Uses	Adverse Effects
Neutralizing Agents • Aluminum products (Amphogel) • Calcium products (Tums, Rolaids) • Combination products (Gelucil, Maalox, Diovol, Gaviscon)	• Neutralized HCl in the stomach (e.g., AlOH + HCl → AlCl + H_2O) • Alginic acid-coating action of the stomach • Simethicone is added to some of these agents as an antiflatulent as it inhibits gas formation	• Treatment of acute irritation and inflammation of esophageal and gastric lining due to ingestion of certain foods and gastric reflux • Available in chewable tablets, powders, and liquid preparations • All preparations are available OTC	• Constipation (aluminum and calcium preparations) • Renal calculi (calcium preparations) • Systemic metabolic alkalosis (sodium bicarbonate) • Acid rebound hyperacidity (calcium preparations)
H_2 Receptor Antagonists • Cimetidine (Tagamet) • Ranitidine (Zantac) • Famotidine (Pepcid)	• Inhibit histamine stimulation of H_2 receptors within the parietal cells to produce HCl → reduce HCl secretion → reduce gastric acidity	• Peptic ulcer disease • GERD • Stress ulcers • Zollinger–Ellison syndrome*	• Lethargy, confusion (H_2 receptor antagonists) • Gynecomastia and erectile dysfunction (cimetidine) • Suppression of metabolic activities of the liver (cimetidine)
Proton Pump Inhibitors • Lansoprazole (Prevacid) (for *Helicobacter pylori* infections) • Omeprazole (Losec) • Pantoprazole (Pantoloc)	• Irreversibly bind to H+/K+ ATPase in parietal cells, preventing the movement of H+ out of parietal cells → lowering HCl	• Erosive esophagitis • GERD • Active duodenal ulcers (short-term therapy) • Gastric hypersecretory conditions (Zollinger–Ellison syndrome*)	• GI infections due to decreased acid production (H_2 receptor antagonists, proton pump inhibitors)
Miscellaneous Acid-Controlling Medications Sucralfate • Bismuth • Misoprostol • Metoclopramide	• Sulcrafate combines with HCl and proteins at ulcer site to form a thick paste that covers and sticks to the ulcer site → protect ulcer to allow for healing • Bismuth appears to stimulate prostaglandin and bicarbonate production • Misoprostol is thought to inhibit gastric acid secretion and enhance the local production of mucous. • Metoclopramide increases GI motility	• Active peptic ulcers • Stress ulcers • Esophageal irritation	• Allergic reactions • Urticaria • Nausea • Constipation • Dry mouth • Uterine contractions (misoprostol) • Extrapyramidal effects (metoclopramide)

ATPase, Adenosine triphosphatase; *GERD*, gastroesophageal reflux disease; *H+*, hydrogen ion; *HCl*, hydrochloric acid; *K+*, = potassium ion; *OTC*, over the counter; *NSAIDS*, nonsteroidal anti-inflammatory drugs.

*Zollinger–Ellison syndrome = nonendocrine pancreatic tumours that secrete gastrin, which in turn stimulates parietal cells within the lining of the stomach to secrete HCl and pepsin, resulting in the development of peptic ulcers.

• Proton-pump inhibitors have the potential to cause osteoporosis with long-term use

Nursing Considerations Relating to Acid-Controlling Medications

• Administer at times indicated (such as after meals [pc], at bedtime, with food, for 4–6 weeks, and so on). However, sometimes clients may be prescribed low dosages of medication for extended periods.
• Observe for desired effects and adverse effects (such as constipation or diarrhea).
• Observe for occult blood or melena stool.
Client teaching points:

• Take the medication according to the directions on the label.
• Avoid overuse or long-term use.
• See a health care provider if manifestations continue or if the medication is taken beyond the suggested duration.
• Reduce possible causes of irritation or ulcer formation, such as stress.
• Avoid alcohol and smoking.
• Administer with a full glass of fluid to ensure absorption.
• Take frequent small meals to maintain food within the stomach.
• Avoid irritating foods or foods that stimulate acid production.

TABLE 8.12   Classifications of Antiemetics

Classifications	Action	Uses
Anticholinergics (Ach blockers) • scopalamine	• Block Ach receptors in vestibular region and reticular formation → impulses blocked from stimulating chemoreceptor trigger zone (CTZ) → CTZ prevented from stimulating the vomiting centre	• Prevention and treatment of nausea and vomiting due to motion sickness
Antihistamines • Dimenhydrinate (Gravol) • Diphenhydramine (Benadryl)	• Block H_1 receptors in vestibular region → impulses blocked from stimulating CTZ → CTZ prevented from stimulating the vomiting centre	• Prevention and treatment of nausea and vomiting due to motion sickness
Antidopaminergics • Prochlorperazine (Prochlorazine) • Promethazine (Histantil)	• Block dopamine receptors in CTZ → CTZ prevented from stimulating the vomiting centre	• Prevention and treatment of nausea associated with inner ear disorders
Serotonin Blockers • Granisetron (Apo-Granisetron) • Ondansetron (Zofran)	• Inhibit stimulating effect of serotonin at receptor sites in gastro-intestinal (GI) tract and CTZ → CTZ prevented from stimulating the vomiting centre	• Prevention and treatment of vomiting associated with chemotherapy, postoperative nausea, and vomiting
Prokinetic Agents • Metoclopramide (Metonia)	• Stimulate release of Ach in GI tract → speed gastric emptying → decrease nausea and vomiting relating to gastric retention and distension • Block dopamine in CTZ	• Prevention and treatment of nausea and vomiting relating to gastric distension • Prevention and treatment of vomiting relating to migraine headache, chemotherapy, hiatus hernia
Tetrahydrocannabinol • Marihuana	• Depresses reticular formation, thalamus, and cerebral cortex → reduces sensitivity → reduces nausea and vomiting	• Prevention and treatment of nausea associated with chemotherapy • Prevention and treatment of nausea and anorexia associated with HIV/AIDS

Ach, acetylcholine.

- Remain sitting up for 1 to 2 hours following a meal to reduce the risk for acid reflux.
- Monitor bowel movements for constipation, diarrhea, or black stool.

Antiemetics

Antiemetics are agents used to prevent and treat nausea and vomiting. Conditions that precipitate nausea, vomiting, or both include GI irritation, infections occurring in many parts of the body (such as the brain), metabolic imbalances, severe pain, stress, fear and horror, motion imbalances that originate from the semicircular canals of the ear, or radiation therapy and drug toxicity within the body, such as the vomiting associated with chemotherapeutic agents for cancer.

Antiemetic agents suppress impulses travelling to the vomiting centre within the medulla oblongata of the brain to relieve the manifestation of nausea and vomiting.

Classification of Antiemetics

Table 8.12 outlines the different classifications of antiemetics, their actions, and their uses.

Adverse Effects Relating to Antiemetics

- Drowsiness, dizziness, weakness
- Orthostatic hypotension
- Visual disturbances (blurred vision)
- Dry mouth
- Urinary retention (with antihistamines, anticholinergics)
- Diarrhea (with prokinetics)

Nursing Considerations Relating to Antiemetics

- Administer medication as ordered: dose, route, and time, such as before meals (ac), IV, IM, half an hour prior to nausea-producing treatment or event.
- Monitor and record effects and adverse effects.
- Implement safety precautions due to potential for drowsiness.
- Predict potential for vomiting and administer medication prior to occurrence.
- Withhold fluids until nausea is relieved.
- Offer fluids when nausea has been relieved, initially in small amounts.
- Monitor intake and output to maintain positive balance.
- Promote rest and relaxation when nausea occurs.
- Ensure that tissues and a kidney basin are available when the client is experiencing nausea.
- Provide mouth care during acute episodes of nausea and vomiting.
  Client teaching points:
- Take medications prior to nausea-producing event, such as motion sickness.
- Avoid activities that require constant alertness (such as driving) when taking antiemetics.
- See a health care provider if the nausea and vomiting persists beyond 24 hours.
- Avoid food and situations that cause nausea and vomiting.
- Avoid activity and promote rest when nauseated.
- After nausea has subsided, initially take small amounts of clear fluids to determine tolerance.

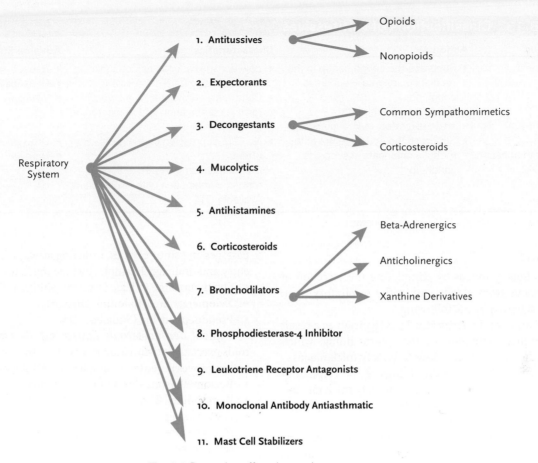

Fig. 8.4 Drugs that affect the respiratory system.

- Recognize specific adverse effects of the classification of medication taken; report adverse effects.

DRUGS THAT AFFECT THE RESPIRATORY SYSTEM

Drugs that affect the respiratory system are outlined in Fig 8.4.

Several classifications of drugs are used to relieve disorders of the respiratory tract. These medications can relieve cough (antitussives), promote the removal of excess secretions from the respiratory passageways (expectorants, decongestants, and mucolytics), or facilitate the dilation of the respiratory passageways (antihistamines, corticosteroids, bronchodilators, phosphodiesterase-4 inhibitor, monoclonal antibody antiasthmatic).

Antitussives

The classification of medications prescribed for the treatment of a cough depends on whether the cough is productive or dry. Productive coughs are usually treated with expectorants and mucolytics, while dry coughs are treated with antitussives.

Antitussives (cough suppressants) are prescribed to decrease the intensity and frequency of the cough without obstructing the elimination of tracheobronchial phlegm. Since the cough reflex is required to clear the upper respiratory tract of obstructive secretions, antitussives are commonly given in combination with expectorants to prevent the congestion of respiratory secretions within the lungs.

Classifications of Antitussives

Table 8.13 outlines the different classifications of antitussives, their actions, their characteristics, and their adverse effects.

Nursing Considerations Relating to Antitussives

- Ensure care regarding dosage and frequency.
- Observe for drowsiness and sedative effects.
- Codeine is not recommended in children under the age of 12 (and children under 18 years posttonsillectomy) due to potential breathing problems.
- Dextromethorphan is unsafe for children under the age of 6.
  Client teaching points:
- Avoid activities that require constant alertness.
- Report excessive drowsiness or sedation, headache, fever, and chest congestion.
- Take only as directed by a prescriber or pharmacist.
- Increase fluid intake to maintain hydration and liquefy respiratory secretions.
- Take syrups undiluted.
- Avoid intake of food or fluid for half an hour after administering the medication to promote local effects of syrup on throat.

TABLE 8.13 Classifications of Antitussives

Classification	Action	Characteristics	Adverse Effects
Opioids • Codeine	• Suppress the cough centre in the medulla oblongata → suppress coughing • Suppress pain receptors → analgesic effect → ↓ cough reflex	• Low dosage reduces risk of addiction and excessive CNS depression • Commonly administered in syrup form in combination with expectorant	• Nausea and vomiting • Constipation • Weakness, dizziness
Nonopioids • Dextromethorphan (Benylin DM)	• Suppress the cough centre in the medulla oblongata → suppress coughing	• No CNS depression or analgesic effects • Commonly administered in syrup form in combination with expectorant • Available OTC	• Drowsiness • Nausea

CNS, Central nervous system; *OTC*, over the counter.

Expectorants

Expectorants liquefy mucus by stimulating the secretion of natural lubricants from glands within the respiratory tract. This effect is achieved by the following:

- Reflex irritation of the respiratory passageways as a result of drug-induced irritation of the gastric lining, which leads to stimulation of secretions to liquefy thick mucus.
- Drug-induced irritation of the linings of the respiratory passageways stimulates secretions to liquefy thick mucus.
- Ciliary action and coughing expel the liquefied phlegm from the pulmonary system.
- Use includes the treatment of productive cough (in combination with an antitussive) and inflammatory conditions of the upper respiratory tract that produce excess secretions, such as pharyngitis and the common cold.

Common Preparation

- Guaifenesin (Robitussin)

Adverse Effects of Expectorant Agents

- Minimal adverse effects
- Nausea and vomiting
- GI irritation

Nursing Considerations Relating to Expectorants

- Increase fluid intake to assist in liquefying mucus.
- Observe for adverse effects, including those relating to antitussives.

Decongestants

Decongestants are medications used to relieve upper airway congestion, primarily nasal, which is caused by swollen mucous membranes irritated by conditions such as allergic rhinitis and the common cold. Many of these preparations may be obtained as OTC medications. Preparations may be oral, inhalation sprays, or nose drops.

Common Decongestant Agents

Common sympathomimetics. These products act by producing local vasoconstriction, which decreases blood flow to irritated and dilated capillaries in the mucous lining of the nasal passages and sinus cavities, widening airways for improved air entry and drainage. Examples include the following:

- Oxymetazoline (Vicks, Drixoral, Sinufrin, Dristan)
- Xylometazoline (Balminil, Otrivin)
- Pseudoephedrine (Sudafed): Oral

Topical corticosteroids (intranasal steroids). Corticosteroids exert an anti-inflammatory action that reduces swelling and improves air entry. Examples are as follows:

- Beclomethasone dipropionate (Beconase AQ)
- Budesonide (Rhinocort)
- Fluticasone propionate (Flonase)

Adverse effects of nasal decongestants. Usually, the dose remains topical; therefore, systemic effects are uncommon. Potential effects of sympathomimetics include the following:

- Headache
- Nervousness
- Dry mouth
- Palpitation
- Increased BP
- Urinary retention (in prostatic hyperplasia)

Potential effects of corticosteroids include the following:

- Nasal irritation
- Nasal itchiness
- Dry mouth
- Oral fungal infections
- Cough

Nursing Considerations Relating to Decongestants

Client teaching points:

- Understand that use of decongestants is cautioned for those who have hypertension, glaucoma, or cardiac disease.
- Increase fluid intake to 2 000 to 3 000 mL per day, unless contraindicated.
- Take them according to label instructions.
- Ensure correct dosage and frequency.
- Avoid prolonged use of OTC medications.
- If manifestations persist for longer than 1 week, consult a health care provider.
- Understand that prolonged use may result in rebound congestion.

- Understand whether they are compatible with other medications.
- Monitor for adverse effects and report to a health care provider.
- Observe for potential adverse effects and, if they arise, discontinue the medication and report the effects to a health care provider.
- Teach correct methods for effectively administering nose drops or sprays:
  - Hyperextend the neck when instilling nose drops.
  - Breathe in while instilling spray.
  - Blow the nose gently prior to administering preparation into the nose.

Mucolytics

Mucolytics are specific preparations prescribed to reduce the stickiness and viscosity of pulmonary secretions.

- Action focuses directly on the thick mucus plugs to liquefy and dissolve them, thereby promoting removal of the secretions by ciliary action, suction, postural drainage, and coughing.
- Mucolytics are prescribed for treatment of chronic bronchitis, emphysema, cystic fibrosis, and pneumonia.
- Examples include acetylcysteine, inhaled by direct instillation or by nebulization, and dornase alfa (Pulmozyme), which exerts an enzyme action on thick mucus (used primarily for cystic fibrosis).

Adverse Effects of Mucolytics

- Drowsiness
- Rhinorrhea
- Bronchospasm (may occur during treatment)
- Nausea and vomiting

Nursing Considerations Relating to Mucolytics

- Assess the effectiveness of air entry prior to and after therapy.
- Follow directions regarding the preparation and administration of the product.
- Encourage increased intake of fluids to 2 000 to 3 000 mL per day.
- Encourage the client to cough deeply following treatment to remove secretions.
- Use suction equipment to remove excess liquefied secretions as necessary.
- Administer mouth care following treatment.

Antihistamines

Antihistamines are used to treat a variety of disorders that result in an increase in capillary permeability, constriction of smooth muscle, and increased respiratory secretions. These effects result in swelling and obstruction of respiratory passageways and can occur with allergies.

These drugs act by opposing the action of histamine at the H_1 receptor sites, which leads to a decrease in capillary permeability, the relaxation of bronchial smooth muscle, and reduced secretions, resulting in more open passageways, reduced swelling, and, therefore, improved air entry.

Common Antihistamine Agents

First-generation preparations include the following:
- Diphenhydramine (Benadryl)
- Chlorpheniramine (Chlor-Tripolon)
- Promethazine (Phenergan)
Second-generation preparations include the following:
- Loratadine (Claritin)
- Cetirizine (Reactine)
- Fexofenadine (Allegra)

Adverse Effects of Antihistamines

Effects vary depending on the preparation; second-generation preparations do not have as sedating an effect as those of the first generation. Possible effects include the following:
- Drowsiness
- Known drug allergies
- Dry mouth
- Urinary retention
- Dizziness, weakness, feeling faint
- Nervousness
- Nausea, vomiting
- Constipation or diarrhea
- Cardiac dysrhythmias, palpitations
- Headache
- Visual disturbances

Nursing Considerations Relating to Antihistamines

- Observe for desired effect and possible adverse effects.
- Note safety precautions relating to preparations with sedating effects and take caution with activities requiring constant attention.
  Client teaching points:
- Follow directions on dosage and frequency.
- Administer with meals to avoid gastric discomfort.
- Suck candies to relieve dryness in the mouth.
- Report to a health care provider if manifestations of the condition persist.
- Understand that weakness and drowsiness may occur.
- Consult with a health care provider before taking sedating products such as alcohol, sleeping pills, analgesics, and so on, which increase drowsiness and weakness.
- Report any unusual adverse effects to a health care provider.

Corticosteroids

Corticosteroids exert their anti-inflammatory action on the respiratory passageways by suppressing airway inflammation, thereby reducing swelling within the bronchioles, as well as by decreasing mucus production, resulting in less airway obstruction.

These desirable effects are produced by inhibiting the production of histamine, which results in reduced capillary permeability and decreased production of tissue chemicals that cause inflammation. This leads to the suppression of the movement of protein, fluid, and blood cells into interstitial spaces, also reducing swelling and inflammation; corticosteroids also facilitate the action of beta$_2$-adrenergic agonists by increasing the sensitivity of their adrenergic receptors. This classification of medication is commonly prescribed for the treatment of asthma and any other conditions that cause bronchoconstriction.

Corticosteroids may be administered by inhalation, orally, or intravenously. They are not generally effective in relieving acute episodes. The medications require several hours to produce their desirable effects.

Common Corticosteroid Agents

- Budesonide (Pulmicort) administered through inhalation
- Fluticasone propionate (Flovent) administered through inhalation
- Methylprednisolone administered intravenously (IV) or orally
- Prednisone administered orally

Adverse Effects of Corticosteroids

- Gastric irritation
- Hypertension
- Dry mouth
- Cough
- Oral fungal infections
- Adrenal failure at high doses (with systemic doses)
- Fluid retention

Nursing Considerations Relating to Corticosteroids

- Administer oral preparations with meals.
- Observe for desirable and adverse effects (optimal effects may take hours to days).
- Caution against prolonged use and abrupt stoppage of medication due to possible adrenal shutdown.
- Instruct clients to use inhalers as directed and only when necessary; they should avoid overuse.
- Have clients rinse their mouths following each treatment to prevent the development of infection.
- Teach clients to administer the corticosteroid inhaler approximately 15 minutes to half an hour following the use of other inhalers, such as bronchodilators.
- Instruct clients to shake the inhaler prior to administration.
  Client teaching points:
- Employ the proper method for use of inhalers.
- Rest until relief of manifestations is achieved.
- Identify and avoid conditions that promote bronchoconstriction.
- Watch for possible adverse effects and report.
- Employ good mouth care to prevent oral infections.
- Drink plenty of fluids if not contraindicated.
- Do not suddenly discontinue a regularly prescribed oral preparation.
- Understand that medications require a slow "weaning" process when discontinuing.

Bronchodilators

Bronchodilators are used in the treatment of airway-obstructive diseases such as asthma. These agents relax the smooth muscles of the tracheobronchial tree, causing dilation of bronchioles and alveolar ducts, thereby decreasing the resistance to airflow.

Preparations are available in inhalation, oral, and IV forms. Inhalation and IV administration are used to treat acute attacks of bronchoconstriction; oral preparations are used for long-term prevention.

Inhalers

Inhalers or puffers release a small dose of medication into the lungs when discharged. They act topically on the lungs and require smaller doses than medications taken enterally.

Nebulizers

These devices pump compressed air through a solution of the medication, producing a fine mist that can be inhaled through a face mask.

Inhaled corticosteroids are used to prevent and treat asthma. This route reduces the need for oral corticosteroids as the inhaled versions have a direct, local effect on the inflammation in the respiratory system, with the result that systemic steroids are not required.

General Classifications of Bronchodilators

Table 8.14 outlines the different classifications of bronchodilators, their actions, their uses, and their adverse effects. Some bronchodilators may be used in combination with corticosteroids for added and more prolonged effects.

Mast Cell Stabilizers

Mast cell stabilizers (sodium cromoglycate and nedocromil) are now rarely used. These drugs act by stabilizing and reducing the response of mast cells to irritating substances, which leads to reduction of the release of substances that stimulate inflammation and smooth muscle constriction.

Leukotrine Receptor Antagonists

Montelukast (Singulair) is a leukotriene receptor antagonist which blocks receptors that control bronchoconstriction, vascular permeability, and mucus secretion. It is used for long-term treatment and prevention of asthma attacks but is ineffective in the treatment of acute asthma attacks. Adverse effects include headache, nausea, diarrhea, and liver dysfunction.

Phosphodiesterase-4 Inhibitor

Roflumilast (Daxas) is a selective inhibitor of the enzyme phosphodiesterase type 4 (PDE4), which leads to decreased inflammation in the lungs. It is effective in reducing the frequency of COPD exacerbations but is not used to treat acute bronchospasm. Adverse effects include nausea, diarrhea, headache, insomnia, dizziness, weight loss, anxiety, and depression.

Monoclonal Antibody Antiasthmatic

Omalizumab (Xolair) is a new medication for asthma. It is a monoclonal antibody that selectively binds to the immunoglobulin IgE and limits the release of mediators of the allergic response. This medication is given subcutaneously and may cause hypersensitivity reactions.

Nursing Considerations Relating to Bronchodilators

- Administer specific medication according to directions (such as dosage, method of administration).

TABLE 8.14 Classifications of Bronchodilators

Classification	Action	Uses	Adverse Effects
Beta-Adrenergics • Salbutamol (Ventolin) • Epinephrine (Adrenalin) • Isoproterenol	• Beta-adrenergic agents (mainly beta$_2$-agonists) stimulate receptors in the muscle → smooth muscle relaxation within the respiratory tract → dilation of bronchial tree	• Acute attacks and long-term treatment of asthma	• Cardiac dysrhythmias, hypertension, and hypotension • Restlessness, nervousness • Hyperactivity, tremors • Dizziness • Insomnia • Headache • Hyperglycemia • Hypokalemia
Anticholinergics • Ipratropium bromide (Atrovent) • Tiotropium bromide monohydrate (Spiriva)	• Anticholinergics block the action of acetylcholine (Ach) in the muscles → smooth muscle relaxation in the respiratory tract → dilation of bronchial tree	• Primarily used to prevent bronchoconstriction • Long-term treatment of asthma	• Hyperactivity • Dry mouth • Dry cough • Dizziness • Insomnia • Anxiety • Gastro-intestinal upset
Xanthine Derivatives • Aminophylline • Theophylline (Theolair)	• Act directly on smooth muscle of bronchi and blood vessels causing relaxation → dilation of bronchial tree • Inhibit release of slow-reacting substances of anaphylaxis (SRSA) and histamine → reduce bronchial swelling and narrowing caused by these two chemicals	• Acute attacks and long-term prevention of bronchoconstriction of asthma attacks	• Cardiac dysrhythmias and hypertension • Tachycardia • Restlessness, nervousness, hyperactivity • Insomnia • Headache • Nausea and vomiting • Gastroesophageal reflux (GERD)

- Observe for desired effects, relief of respiratory distress, and reduced respiratory rate and chart.
- Observe for adverse effects relating to sympathetic nervous system stimulants, including beta-adrenergics, anticholinergics, and xanthines.
- Instruct avoidance of caffeine, smoking, and OTC medications (xanthines).
- Use cautiously with clients who have cardiac, renal, or hepatic disorders.
- Provide a quiet, relaxing environment to reduce stimulation.
- Increase intake of fluids, if not contraindicated.
- When administering medication during an acute attack of bronchoconstriction, institute measures to promote optimal air entry into the lungs, such as a high Fowler's position.
- Ensure the client has basic knowledge about the nature of the condition and the nature of the medications (e.g., dosage, time to be taken, and possible adverse effects). Client teaching points:
- Take the medication as prescribed by the prescriber and pharmacist.
- Identify and reduce possible triggers that produce bronchoconstriction.
- Demonstrate how to administer inhaled preparations correctly.
- Take oral medications with food.
- Try to relax and rest during acute attacks.

- Contact a health care provider immediately if manifestations do not resolve.
- Receive COVID-19, influenza, and pneumococcal vaccinations as eligible to prevent respiratory manifestations.
- Obtain prescriber advice prior to use of OTC medications.

ANTIMICROBIAL AGENTS

Figure 8.5 outlines the major antimicrobial agents.

Antimicrobial agents are used to treat a variety of forms of pathogenic organisms capable of infecting the body. In addition to bacteria and viruses, there are a variety of pathogenic fungi, protozoans, and complex, multicellular organisms, such as worms.

Antimicrobial agents have been developed to destroy organisms or groups of organisms depending on the agent's specific chemical nature and action and the nature of the organism. Diagnosis of a particular infection, and the best antimicrobial agent to prescribe for its treatment, is commonly achieved by gathering a specimen from the client for culture and sensitivity tests. The laboratory identifies the organism and its sensitivity to the various antimicrobial agents.

Antibacterial Agents

Antibiotics is the term commonly used to refer to antibacterial drugs. Agents that destroy living organisms are said to be bactericidal, while those that interfere with their

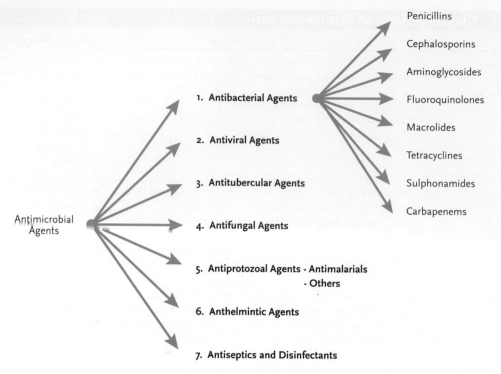

Fig. 8.5 Antimicrobial agents.

development are bacteriostatic. Antibiotics are classified into broad categories based on their chemical structures—sulphonamides, penicillins, cephalosporins, carbapenems, macrolides, quinolones, aminoglycosides, and tetracyclines—in addition to other miscellaneous categories, and their spectrum of activity (broad spectrum or extended spectrum).

The misuse and overprescription of antibiotics have resulted in strains of bacteria resistant to traditional antibiotic therapy. Important current strains include the following:

- Methicillin-resistant *Staphylococcus aureus* (MRSA)
- Vancomycin-resistant *Enterococcus* (VRE)
- Extended-spectrum beta-lactamase-producing *Escherichia coli* (ESBL)

Classification of Antibiotics

Table 8.15 outlines the different classifications of antibiotics, their actions, their characteristics, and their adverse effects.

Antiviral Agents

Viruses can only reproduce within the cells of a host because of their simple cellular structure (they contain only DNA or RNA). Antiviral agents act by inhibiting the entry of the virus into the host cell or by acting on the virus once it has entered the cell.

Antiviral agents most commonly inhibit the virus from replicating, and with the assistance of the body's normal immune system, destruction can then occur. Antiviral agents have been developed to target either DNA-containing viruses (antiviral agents) or viruses containing RNA (antiretroviral agents).

Vaccines and immunoglobulins are probably the best preventive for specific viral diseases. Postexposure prophylaxis (PEP) may protect persons who may have had direct contact with persons with conditions such as influenza A, HIV, or hepatitis B.

Commonly Used Non-HIV Antiviral Agents

- Acyclovir, famciclovir, valacyclovir: Herpes zoster, genital herpes
- Amantadine: Influenza A
- Zanamivir, oseltamivir: Influenza A and B
- Valganciclovir, ganciclovir, cidofovir: Cytomegalovirus infection
- Ribavirin, palivizumab: respiratory syncytial virus (RSV) infection

Commonly Used Antiretroviral Agents in HIV/AIDS

Nucleoside Reverse Transcriptase Inhibitors (NRTI)
- Zidovudine (Retrovir)
- Tenofovir (Viread)

Nonnucleoside Reverse Transcriptase Inhibitors (NNRTI)
- Delaviridine (Rescriptor)
- Efavirenz (Sustiva)

Protease Inhibitors (PI)
- Atazanavir (Reyataz)
- Darunavir (Prezista)

Fusion Inhibitors (FI)
- Enfuvirtide (Fuzeon)

Entry Inhibitor-CCR5 Coreceptor Antagonist
- Maraviroc (Celsentri)

HIV Integrase Strand Transfer Inhibitor (INSTI)
- Raltegravir (Isentress)

TABLE 8.15 Classifications of Antibiotics

Classification	Action	Characteristics	Adverse Effects
Penicillins **Natural Penicillins** • Penicillin G (IV and IM) • Penicillin V (PO) **Aminopenicillins** • Amoxicillin, ampicillin **Extended-Spectrum Penicillins** • Piperacillin, clavulanic potassium/ticarcillin disodium, piperacillin sodium/tazobactam sodium **Penicillinase-Resistant Penicillins** • Cloxacillin sodium	• Interfere with the synthesis of bacterial cell walls	• Bactericidal • Ear, nose, throat, and sexually transmitted infection syphilis • Broad spectrum • Semisynthetic penicillin • Infections of the ear, nose, throat, respiratory tract, urogenital tract, and skin • Broad spectrum • *E. coli* and other pseudomonal organisms • Staphylococcal infections, except for MRSA	• Hypersensitivity (allergic reactions): urticaria, respiratory difficulty, shock • Diarrhea • Thrombophlebitis (in clients receiving IV penicillin) • Superinfections
Cephalosporins • Structurally and pharmacologically related to penicillin • Derivative of cephalosporin C, produced by fungus and synthetically altered to produce an antibiotic • Cephalexin • Cefazolin • cefaclor • Cefoxitin • Cefuroxime • Cefprozil • Cefotaxime • Cefixime • Cefpodoxime • Ceftazidime • Ceftriaxone • cefepime	• Interfere with bacterial cell wall synthesis and bind to penicillin-binding proteins (PBPs) in bacteria cell walls	• Semisynthetic antibiotic • Broad spectrum • Bactericidal • Use with caution as an alternative if client has penicillin allergy • Urinary tract infections (UTIs), respiratory tract infections (RTIs), abdominal infections, septicemia, meningitis, and osteomyelitis	• Diarrhea • Thrombophlebitis • Hyperkalemia • Hypernatremia • Abnormal liver and renal function tests • Secondary infections: oral thrush, genital and anal pruritus, vaginitis, and vaginal discharge • Nephrotoxicity • Antacids, iron, and H_2 receptor antagonists may inhibit absorption
Aminoglycosides **Natural** • Gentamicin • Streptomycin • paromomycin • tobramycin **Semisynthetic** • amikacin	• Bind to ribosomes and thereby prevent protein synthesis within the bacteria	• Bactericidal • Poorly absorbed orally • Commonly used in combination with other antibiotics • Gram-negative bacteria that cause UTIs, wounds, and septicemias • Mainstay treatment of health care–associated infection • Reserved mainly for use in life-threatening infections	• Dizziness • Headache • Skin rash • Fever • Renal failure • Hearing loss (ototoxicity) • Not favourable for long-term use
Quinolones • Norfloxacin (Apo-Norflox) • Ciprofloxacin (Cipro)Levofloxacin (Levaquin) Ofloxacin (Ocuflox) Moxifloxacin (Avelox)	• Inhibit activity of DNA gyrase, an enzyme necessary for replication of bacterial DNA	• Bactericidal • Excellent oral absorption • Used against wide variety of Gram-negative and selective positive bacteria • UTIs, sexually transmitted infections, and respiratory tract infections.	• GI problems • Headache • Dizziness • Fatigue • Insomnia • Depression • Convulsions • Fever • Blurred vision • Tinnitus • Skin problems • Antacids decrease absorption • Contraindicated with cardiac problems

Continued

TABLE 8.15   Classifications of Antibiotics—cont'd

Classification	Action	Characteristics	Adverse Effects
Macrolides • Erythromycin (Erythro-EC) • Azithromycin (Zithromax) • Clarithromycin (Biaxin)	• Inhibit protein synthesis in susceptible bacteria	• Bacteriostatic • Bactericidal in high concentrations • Respiratory and GI tract infections • Sexually transmitted infections when penicillin, cephalosporins, and tetracycline cannot be used	• GI irritation: nausea, heartburn • Palpitations, chest pain • Headache, dizziness, vertigo • Hepatotoxicity • Skin reactions • Tinnitus, hearing loss • Interacts with rifampin and rifabutin to reduce antibiotic effect and may increase adverse GI effects
Tetracyclines **Natural Tetracyclines** • Tetracycline **Semisynthetic Tetracyclines** • Doxycycline	• Inhibit protein synthesis in susceptible bacteria by binding to a portion of the ribosomes and stopping bacterial growth	• Bacteriostatic • Inhibit growth of many Gram-positive and Gram-negative organisms, some protozoa • Treatment of sexually transmitted infections • Lyme disease • Rickettsia • Chlamydia • *Mycoplasma* organisms	• Do not administer with milk, antacids, or iron salts • Contraindicated in pregnancy, allergies • Tooth discoloration in children (younger than 8 years) • Superinfections • Diarrhea, nausea, abdominal cramps, vomiting • Photosensitivity • Enhance the anticoagulant effect of warfarin
Sulphonamides • Trimethoprim-sulphamethoxazole (Co-Trimoxazole)	• Prevent synthesis of folic acid required by the bacteria for proper synthesis of purines and nucleic acid	• Bacteriostatic • Treat both Gram-positive and Gram-negative bacteria • UTIs, respiratory tract infections, pneumonia associated with HIV, outpatient *Staphylococcus* infections.	• GI irritation • Rash • Photosensitivity • Renal calculi
Carbapenems Imipenem/cilastin Meropenem ertapenem	Bacteriocidal Inhibit cell wall synthesis • Broadest antibacterial action	• Reserved for complicated body cavity and connective tissue infections	Drug-induced seizure activity • Cross-sensitivity with penicillin allergies

GI, Gastro-intestinal; *IM,* intramuscular; *IV,* intravenous; *MRSA,* methicillin-resistant *Staphylococcus aureus; PO,* by mouth.

Antitubercular Agents

Tuberculosis is caused by *Mycobacterium tuberculosis,* an aerobic bacterium requiring high concentrations of oxygen to survive and replicate. The bacterium (tubercle bacillus) is very slow-growing and, after infecting the lungs, may become inactivated and encapsulated by fibrous tissue. Because of this slow growth, monotherapy with the usual antibiotics, such as streptomycin, does not provide effective treatment.

The treatment can be either monotherapy or combination therapy using first-line agents or second-line agents. The pre-scribed agent will depend on whether the goal is prevention or active treatment.

Common First-Line Medications for the Treatment of Tuberculosis

• Isoniazid (Isotamine)
• Ethambutol (Etibi)
• Rifampin (Mycobutin)
• Pyrazinamide (Tebrazid)

Common Second-Line Medications for the Treatment of Tuberculosis

• Amikacin sulphate
• Levofloxacin hemihydrate
• Moxifloxacin hydrochloride

Liver damage can result from long-term therapy. Clients should not drink alcohol while on therapy due to alcohol and drug interaction and resultant liver damage.

Antifungal Agents

These medications are used in the treatment of pathogenic fungal diseases, both systemic and local. Fungal diseases vary from superficial (skin, hair, and nail infections) to systemic (histoplasmosis and opportunistic mycotic diseases, such as aspergillosis and candidiasis).

Few mycotic medications are available because most that are effective in treating mycotic infections are toxic to human cells. Human cells are similar to fungal cells.

Common Examples of Antifungal Agents

- Amphotericin B (Fungizone): Used to treat systemic infections (candidiasis and histoplasmosis)
- Fluconazole (Diflucan): Used to treat systemic infections (candidiasis and histoplasmosis), often preferred to amphotericin B as it has a much better adverse effect profile
- Nystatin: Used to treat candidiasis of skin and mucous membranes
- Terbinafine hydrochloride (Lamisil): Used to treat cutaneous mycosis, athlete's foot (*tinea pedis*), jock itch (*tinea cruris*), and ringworm (*tinea corporis*)
- Atovaquone (Mepron): Used to treat *Pneumocystis* pneumonia
- Metronidazole (Flagyl): Used to treat vaginal fungal infections

Antiprotozoal Agents
Antimalarial Agents

These agents are prescribed for the treatment of malaria. The agents are most effective when the malaria parasite is in its nonreproductive stage after entering the human body.

Common antimalarial agents
- Hydroxychloroquine sulphate (Plaquenil): Used to treat an acute infection or as a preventive
- Mefloquine hydrochloride: Used to treat an acute infection or as a preventive
- Primaquine phosphate: Effective against malaria in red blood cells and tissue
- Quinine sulphate: Used to treat chloroquine-resistant strains

Other Antiprotozoal Agents

Other protozoal diseases are common to tropical countries. Protozoal diseases encountered in Canada include trichomoniasis and toxoplasmosis. Metronidazole (Flagyl) is a common treatment used for these conditions.

Anthelmintic Agents

These agents are used for the treatment of infections caused by worms, including pinworms, tapeworms, flatworms, and roundworms. These organisms are large, are sometimes visible to the naked eye, and commonly infest the GI tract. Systemic infections occur with some types of worms, particularly those from the tropics. Medications focus on the specific type of worm infection.

Anthelmintic Agents
- Praziquantel (Biltricide)
- Mebendazole (Vermox)
- Pyrantel pamoate (Combantrin)

Antiseptics and Disinfectants
Antiseptic Agents

Antiseptic agents may be applied locally for cleansing the skin and mucous membranes. Antiseptics inhibit microbial growth and at high concentration may kill microbes (e.g., povidone-iodine is bactericidal).

Common Antiseptics
- Chlorhexidine
- Povidone-iodine
- Benzalkonium chloride

Disinfectant Agents

Disinfectants are agents that are applied to nonanimate objects, usually to destroy microorganism; for example, glutaraldehyde (Cidex) has a bactericidal effect.

Common Disinfectants
- Povidone-iodine
- Hydrogen peroxide
- Formaldehyde

Nursing Considerations Relating to Antimicrobial Agents
- Perform a complete assessment of the client's history of taking antibiotics, including possible allergies, liver or renal disease, culture and sensitivity (C and S) reports, adverse effects previously experienced, and other medications being taken.
- Take C and S specimens prior to administering the first dose of medication.
- Maintain awareness of contraindications and drug interactions with other medications being taken.
- Administer at the times indicated.
- Administer on an empty stomach, if possible, with plenty of liquid.
- Administer for the length of time ordered.
- Monitor the desired effects, such as a reduction in fever or relief of manifestations.
- Monitor the client for possible allergic reactions (skin rash, shortness of breath, etc.) for at least 2 hours following administration.
- Hold medication and report if allergic reactions are observed.
- Monitor for development of superinfections.
- Observe for adverse effects, record, and report.
- Administer IM injections deep intramuscularly to reduce irritation and tissue damage.
- Administer IV preparations according to dilution ordered; monitor the drip rate carefully.
  Client teaching points:
- Report any adverse effects immediately.
- Take medications at the times ordered.
- Ensure that the complete prescription is taken to avoid recurrence of infection.
- Take medication with at least one full glass of liquid.
- Wear a MedicAlert bracelet if any allergies were experienced with past antimicrobial use.

- Take medication with food if gastric manifestations occur.
- Learn about potential adverse effects relating to specific preparations, such as photosensitivity with tetracyclines (avoid exposure to sun).
- Avoid taking tetracyclines with dairy products.
- Drink plenty of liquids when taking sulpha medications to avoid renal calculi.

DRUGS THAT AFFECT THE URINARY SYSTEM

Drugs that affect the urinary system are outlined in Figure 8.6.

Diuretics

Diuretics are drugs or substances that increase the production and excretion of urine by inhibiting the reabsorption of sodium and water from the nephron filtrate. Various diuretics differ in their chemical structure, the region within the kidneys in which they exert their actions, and their potency. Primary uses of diuretics include the following:

- Hypertension: A reduced circulating fluid volume decreases BP.
- Heart failure: A decreased circulating fluid volume decreases the preload and afterload on the heart.
- Kidney failure: Stimulates optimal functioning of the damaged kidney and reduces retained fluid
- Liver failure: Reduces retained fluid and wastes (ascites) by stimulating maximum functioning of the kidney
- Increased intracranial pressure: Removes retained fluids within the brain to relieve pressure
- For hormonal imbalances that result in the retention of fluid, such as during the premenstrual period and with corticosteroid use

Classifications of Diuretics

Table 8.16 outlines the different classifications of diuretics, their actions, their uses, and adverse effects.

Combination Drugs

A combination diuretic is the potassium-sparing drug plus a thiazide type, such as the following:
- Spironolactone + hydrochlorothiazide (Aldactazide)
- Triamterene + hydrochlorothiazide

Nursing Considerations Relating to Diuretics

- Perform a careful assessment of the following:
  - Hydration levels
  - Blood glucose levels
  - Serum electrolyte levels: sodium (Na^+), potassium (K^+), chloride (Cl^-)
  - Vital signs
  - Urine output
  - Relief of fluid overload as manifested by edema and dyspnea
- Ensure that toilet facilities are readily available.
- Be aware that clients may require potassium supplementation based on the class of diuretic and potassium levels.
- Administer with food to avoid gastric irritation.
- Monitor intake and output to assess effects.
  Client teaching points:
- Eat foods high in potassium, such as bananas and orange juice.
- Take potassium supplements as ordered with food.
- Take medication in the morning to reduce the need for nocturnal voiding and loss of sleep.
- Fluid restrictions may be necessary.
- Avoid high-sodium foods.
- Avoid beverages with diuretic effects such as caffeine and alcohol as they may produce excess effects.
- Monitor blood glucose levels carefully if taking thiazide or loop diuretics.
- Use caution when rising from a lying to a sitting position due to possible postural hypotension.
- Keep scheduled health care providers' visits to monitor progress.
- Report adverse effects immediately to a health care provider.
- Monitor weight carefully; increased weight is indicative of fluid retention.

Smooth Muscle Stimulants (Cholinergics)

Specific cholinergic medications may be prescribed to relieve urinary retention that is nonobstructive in nature. Cholinergics act by stimulating cholinergic receptors in the bladder, resulting in the contraction of the bladder smooth muscle and micturition. An example is bethanechol (Urecholine).

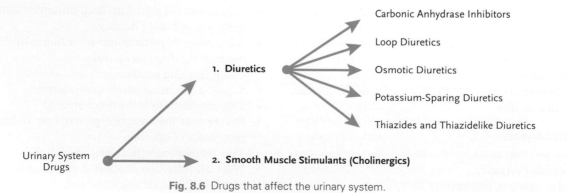

Fig. 8.6 Drugs that affect the urinary system.

TABLE 8.16 Classifications of Diuretics

Classification	Action	Uses	Adverse Effects
Carbonic Anhydrase Inhibitors • Acetazolamide (Acetazolam) • Methazolamide	• Inhibit the enzyme carbonic anhydrate from promoting the reabsorption of Na+ from the proximal tubules → water remains in filtrate and is excreted	• Mild diuretic effect • Reduce intraocular pressure in glaucoma • Altitude sickness • Epilepsy (adjunct with other drugs)	• Drowsiness • Weakness • Visual disturbances • Hyperglycemia • Hypokalemia • Aplastic anemia • Crystalluria
Potent Loop Diuretics • Furosemide (Lasix)	• Block reabsorption of Na+ and Cl– in ascending loop of Henle → water remains in filtrate due to change in concentration gradient	• Provide potent and rapid diuresis • Heart failure • Liver failure • Renal disease • Hypertension	• Hypokalemia • Hypocalcemia • Hyperglycemia • Dizziness, headache, blurred vision • Nausea and vomiting • Abdominal pain
Osmotic Diuretics • Mannitol (Osmitrol)	• Filtered by glomerulus but are not reabsorbed → highly concentrated filtrate produced → inhibits reabsorption of water	• Produce large quantity of urine • Increased intracranial pressure • Acute renal failure • Situations requiring rapid reduction in water content (e.g., intraspinal pressure)	• Lung congestion • Seizures • Thrombophlebitis • Headache • Visual disturbances • Tachycardia
Potassium-Sparing Diuretics • Spironolactone (Aldactone) • Triamterene • Amiloride (Midamor)	• Inhibit the exchange of Na+ and K+ in distal tubules independent of aldosterone → water and Na+ are excreted; K+ is retained	• Produce a mild diuretic effect • Hyperaldosteronism • Hypertension • Heart failure	• Dizziness, headache • Hyperkalemia • Abdominal cramps • Nausea, vomiting, and diarrhea • Gynecomastia in men (with long-term use)
Thiazides and Thiazidelike Diuretics • Hydrochlorothiazide (Urozide) • Chlorothalidone • Metolazone (Zaroxolyn)	• Block reabsorption of Na+, K+, and Cl– in distal tubules → water is retained in tubules and excreted as urine • Arteriole smooth muscle relaxation → ↓ preload and afterload in heart	• Heart failure • Liver failure • Edema due to corticosteroid use or hormonal imbalance	• Hypokalemia • Hypocalcemia • Hyperglycemia • Dizziness, headache • Muscle spasm • Abdominal pain

Cl–, chloride ion; *K+*, potassium ion; *Na+*, sodium ion.

• Clients should be advised of cholinergic effects.
• Adverse effects include abdominal discomfort, bronchospasm, increased salivation, abdominal cramps, hypotension, and bradycardia.
• Clients should be advised to make position changes slowly to avoid postural hypotension.

VITAMINS AND MINERALS

Vitamins and minerals are outlined in Figure 8.7.

Vitamins

Vitamins are complex chemical nutrients present in many foods and required in small amounts by the body to facilitate metabolic processes. Of the 13 major vitamins (A, B complex, C, D, E, and K), only D is made by the body. Vitamins function as coenzymes (except the vitamin B group) and as antioxidants (A, C, and E) to neutralize free radicals in the body.

Vitamin Uses

Vitamins are prescribed as supplements for clients with symptoms of vitamin deficiency or for older persons who may be at risk for deficiencies due to restricted diets. Older persons also may have impaired bowel function and high serum cholesterol levels, both of which can affect vitamin absorption. Vitamin D is prescribed for the treatment of osteoporosis.

Vitamin Deficiencies

Deficiencies may occur if intake is lower than the body's requirement. Shortages of the water-soluble vitamins (B and C) are more likely than of the fat-soluble vitamins (A, D, E, and K) because water-soluble vitamins are not stored in the body. Deficiencies of fat-soluble vitamins may occur in the absence of bile. Vitamin K can be depleted within about 10 days.

The body may also be unable to absorb and utilize nutrients. This malabsorption may be due to diseases, such as celiac disease, which affects the absorption of fat, or a lack of the

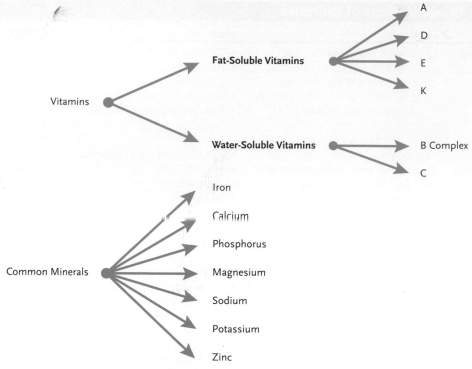

Fig. 8.7 Vitamins and minerals.

intrinsic factor necessary for the absorption of vitamin B_{12}, causing pernicious anemia. A population also may have vitamin deficiencies due to poor food choices and low income.

Table 8.17 outlines the different vitamins and their dosages, effects, and adverse effects.

Natural Sources of Vitamins

- Brewer's yeast is the best source of B-complex vitamins and many minerals and protects against vitamin D toxicity.
- Liver, beans, meat, eggs, wheat germ, yeast, vegetables, and dairy products are sources of vitamins.
- Fresh fruits are rich in vitamin C.

Minerals

Minerals are essential in trace amounts for normal metabolic processes. They are usually obtained from a balanced diet. They function as structural components, helping to form healthy bones, teeth, and nails. In addition, minerals function as components of enzymes.

Other major functions for minerals include regulation of water metabolism, blood volume, cell membrane permeability, generation of nerve fibre action potentials, and maintenance of the acid–base balance. A mineral deficiency may be due to the inability to absorb minerals from the diet or a lack in the diet.

Common Mineral Agents

- Ferrous gluconate, ferrous sulphate, ferrous fumarate and iron dextran and iron sucrose injection may be used to treat iron deficiency anemia.
- Magnesium sulphate is the most common form of magnesium and is used to prevent and treat hypomagnesia,

hypertension, and convulsion associated with toxemia of pregnancy or acute nephritis in children.
- Potassium chloride supplement (Odan K-20, Odan K-8, PMS oral solution) is used to prevent and treat hypokalemia.
- Sodium chloride injections are given to treat hyponatremia.
- Zinc sulphate is used for wound repair.
- Multiple mineral electrolytes such as Pedialyte are used to prevent and treat fluid and electrolyte deficiency.
- Calcium is used to treat deficiency and tetany in newborns.
- Phosphorus may be given to treat a deficiency, although this is rare.

Effects of Deficiency or Excess of Mineral Agents

- Hypernatremia (serum levels >145 mmol/L) causes electrolyte imbalance, nausea, and vomiting.
- Hyponatremia (serum levels <135 mmol/L) may cause nausea and abdominal cramps, as well as cerebral edema (mental deterioration).
- Hyperkalemia (serum levels >5.0 mmol/L) causes hypotension, muscle weakness, nausea, and diarrhea.
- Hypokalemia (serum levels <3.5 mmol/L) causes cardiac arrhythmias, muscle weakness, nausea, vomiting, and delayed gastric emptying.
- Hypercalcemia (serum levels >2.75 mmol/L) may cause muscle weakness and headache, even confusion and coma.
- Hypocalcemia (serum levels <2.25 mmol/L) causes tetany, seizures, mental changes, and delayed ventricular repolarization.
- Excess iron causes diarrhea or constipation, vomiting, and dark stool.
- Iron deficiency causes tachycardia, brittle nails, and glossitis.

TABLE 8.17 Classifications of Vitamins

Vitamin	Therapeutic Dosage	Effects	Adverse Effects
Water-Soluble Vitamins (cannot be stored by the body)			
Vitamin B₁ (thiamine)	5–100 mg/day	• Promotes carbohydrate, aerobic metabolism, transmission of nerve impulses	• Restlessness • Pulmonary edema • Hypersensitivity
Vitamin B₂ (riboflavin)	5–30 mg/day	• Acts as catalyst in oxidation of glucose and amino acid	
Vitamin B₃ (niacin)	300–500 mg/day	• Acts as catalyst in the reactions of cholesterol and fats • Causes vasodilation and treats pellagra	• Nausea, vomiting • Flatulence • Jaundice
Vitamin B₆ (pyridoxine)	2.5–10 mg/day	• Promotes protein, fat, and glucose metabolism and formation of neurotransmitters • Treats neuropathy • Pyridoxine supplements are used to relieve symptoms in women with premenstrual syndrome and neuritis due to treatment with isoniazid for tuberculosis	• Paresthesia • Seizure (these effects are rare)
Vitamin B₉ (folic acid)	0.1–0.4 mg/day	• Helps in protein synthesis and erythropoiesis	• Altered sleep patterns • Irritability • Depression • Anorexia
Vitamin B₁₂ (cyanocobalamin)	50–100 mcg/day	• Essential for cell growth and reproduction • Treatment for pernicious anemia	• Hypersensitivity
Vitamin C (ascorbic acid)	100–250 mg	• Antioxidant • Promotes collagen formation and tissue repair • Treatment for deficiency and used as a dietary supplement.	• Rapid IV administration may lead to fainting • Overdose causes nausea, vomiting, gout attack, and renal stones
Fat-Soluble Vitamins (can be stored by the body)			
Vitamin A (retinol)	50 000–100 000 units/day IM	• Derivates of vitamin A (retinoids) are used to treat severe acne	• Anorexia • Vomiting • Irritability • Muscle pain
Vitamin D (cholecalciferol)	600–800 units/ daily	• Required for absorption and use of calcium and phosphorus by the body • Used to treat calcium deficiencies (e.g., osteoporosis)	• Dehydration • Vomiting • Decreased appetite (anorexia) • Irritability • Constipation • Fatigue
Vitamin E (tocopherol)	60–75 units daily	• Antioxidant	• Fatigue • Nausea • Blurred vision • Diarrhea
Vitamin K (phytonadione)	1-5 mg daily	• Necessary for normal clotting of blood • Used to treat deficiencies resulting in bleeding, petechiae, or bruising	• Can increase coagulation in clients taking warfarin

IM, intramuscular; *IV,* intravenous.

Nursing Considerations Relating to Minerals

- Teach clients that iron should be administered with citrus or fruit juice to enhance absorption.
- When administering liquid iron preparations, have the client use a straw to avoid tooth discoloration.
- Encourage clients to take iron preparations with food to avoid gastric irritation.
- Warn clients that stools may become black and tarry stools when taking iron supplements.
- Teach clients that phosphorus capsules should not be swallowed but broken to dissolve powder in water.
- Monitor clients' sodium and potassium serum levels for desired effects and overdose effects.

ANTIDIABETIC AGENTS

Insulin and oral agents are used in the treatment of diabetes. Insulin is required in clients with type 1 diabetes and it may be required for clients with type 2 diabetes who do not have adequate blood glucose control by other means. Oral antihyperglycemic agents are prescribed for glucose control in clients with type 2 diabetes.

Insulins

Insulin is required to support carbohydrate, protein, and fat metabolism and to facilitate the entry of these substances into cells. Human insulin, synthesized in laboratories, is the most widely used insulin. Insulin can also be derived from pork. Table 8.18 outlines the different types of insulin, their onset, peak, and duration of action.

Oral Antihyperglycemic Agents

Table 8.19 outlines the different types of antihyperglycemic agents, their actions, and adverse effects.

Nursing Considerations Relating to Antidiabetic Medications

- Assess blood glucose levels prior to administration of antidiabetic agents.
- Insulin may be required during times of increased stress, surgery, or infection.
- Roll Neutral Protamine Hagedorn (NPH) or premixed insulin mixtures between the hand before administering.

TABLE 8.18 Types of Insulin, Onset, Peak and Duration

Generic Name	Onset	Peak	Duration
Rapid Acting Insulin lispro Insulin aspart Insulin glulisine	10–15 min	1–2 hour	3.5–6 hr
Short Acting Regular insulin	30 min	2–3 hr	6.5 hr
Intermediate Acting NPH insulin	2–4 hours	4–10 hr	12–18 hr
Long Acting Insulin glargine Insulin detemir		Glargine (none) Detemir (16 to 24 hr)	Glargine (24 hr) Dose dependent

NPH, Neutral Protamine Hagedorn.

TABLE 8.19 Antihyperglycemic Agents for Diabetes Mellitus

Type	Mechanism of Action	Adverse Effects
Insulin secretagogues: Sulphonylureas Gliclazide (Diamicron, DiamicronMR) Glimepiride (Amaryl) Glyburide (Diabeta) (chlorpropamide and tolbutamide are available in Canada but rarely used)	Stimulate release of insulin from β cells; decrease glycogenolysis and gluconeogenesis; glimepiride may improve insensitivity in tissues	Weight gain, hypoglycemia
Meglitinide Repaglinide (GlucoNorm)	Stimulates a rapid and short-lived release of insulin from the pancreas	Less weight gain, decreased incidence of hypoglycemia compared with glyburide
Biguanide Metformin (Glucophage) Metformin ER (Glumetza)	Inhibits hepatic glucose production; increases peripheral and liver sensitivity to insulin	Nausea, upset stomach, diarrhea; less weight gain than sulphonylureas and does not cause hypoglycemia; potential lactic acidosis in renal or hepatic impairment; must be held at the time of or before procedures and held for 48 hr after administration of IV contrast media
α-Glucosidase Inhibitors Acarbose (Glucobay)	Delays absorption of glucose and digestion of CHO in small intestine, lowering after-meal blood glucose levels	Flatulence, abdominal pain, diarrhea
Thiazolidinediones Pioglitazone (Actos) Rosiglitazone (Avandia)	↑ Glucose uptake in muscle and fat; inhibit hepatic glucose production	Edema, weight gain, heart failure; causes ovulation in premenopausal women with PCOS; not recommended for patients with heart failure
Dipeptidyl Peptidase-4 Inhibitors Sitagliptin (Januvia) Saxagliptin (Onglyza) Linagliptin (Trajenta) Alogliptin (Nesina)	Enhance the incretin system, stimulate release of insulin from pancreatic β cells, and inhibit hepatic glucose production	Upper respiratory tract infection, sore throat, headache, diarrhea

TABLE 8.19　Antihyperglycemic Agents for Diabetes Mellitus—cont'd

Type	Mechanism of Action	Adverse Effects
Noninsulin Injectable Agents: GLP-1 Receptor Aagonists Liraglutide (Victoza) Exenatide (Byetta) Dulaglutide (Trulicity) Exenatide QW (Bydureon) Lixesenatide (Adlyxine) Semaglutide (Ozempic)	Stimulate release of insulin; decrease glucagon secretion, increase satiety, decrease gastric emptying	Nausea, vomiting, hypoglycemia, diarrhea, headache
Sodium-Glucose Cotransporter Type 2 (SGLT2) Inhibitors Canagliflozin (Invokana) Dapagliflozin (Forxiga) Empagliflozin (Jardiance) Ertugliflozin (Steglatro)	Enhance urinary glucose excretion	Genital infections, urinary tract infections, hypotension, increased lipids
Combination Therapy Avandamet (rosiglitazone [Avandia] and metformin [Glucophage]) Janumet/Janumet XR (sitagliptin [Januvia] and metformin/metformin XR [Glucophage/Glucophage XR]) Jentadueto (linagliptin [Trajenta] and metformin [Glucophage]) Kazano (alogliptin [Nesina] and metformin [Glucophage]) Komboglyze (metformin [Glucophage] and saxagliptin [Onglyza]) Oseni (alogliptin [Nesina] and pioglitazone [Actos]) Soliqua (glargine [Lantus] U100 and Lixisenatide [Adlyxine]) Xultophy (degludec [Tresiba] and liraglutide [Victoza]) Invokamet (canagliflozin [Invokana] and metformin [Glucophage]) Xigduo (Dapagliflozin [Forxiga] and metformin (Glucophage]) Glyxambi (empagliflozin [Jardiance] and linagliptin [Trajenta]) Synjardy (empagliflozin [Jardiance] and metformin [Glucophage]) Segluromet (ertulgliflozin [Steglatro] and metformin [Glucophage]) Steglujan (ertugliflozin [Steglatro] and sitagliptin [Januvia])	See mechanism of action for individual medications, above	See adverse effects for individual medications, above

CHO, carbohydrates; *GLP-1,* glucagon-like peptide 1; *IV,* intravenous; *PCOS,* polycystic ovarian syndrome.
Source: Tyerman, J., & Cobbett, S. L., (2023). *Lewis's medical-surgical nursing in Canada: Assessment and management of clinical problems* (5th ed., p. 1282, Table 52-7). Elsevier.

- Administer insulins at room temperature.
- Only regular insulin may be administered intravenously.
- In hospital setting, be sure that meal trays have arrived on the unit before giving insulin.
- Glucagon is available as a subcutaneous injection to be given for severe hypoglycemia.
- Instruct client to rotate sites within same general location for about 1 week prior to choosing a new location.
- Instruct client on how to recognize and treat hypoglycemia.
- Encourage the client to avoid smoking and alcohol.
- Provide specific instruction on how and when antidiabetic medication should be taken; for example, some sulfonylureas are to be taken with breakfast.

PRACTICE QUESTIONS

Case 1

Mrs. Mabel Hawkins, 73 years of age, has been admitted to hospital with heart failure (HF). She is prescribed several medications, including digoxin (Lanoxin). Her condition is monitored to assess the effects of the drug therapy.

Questions 1 to 5 refer to this situation.

1. Mrs. Hawkins asks the nurse why her heart rate must be taken prior to giving her the "heart pill" (digoxin). Which of the following statements would be the nurse's best response?
   1. "I will make adjustments in the dosage of the medication depending on what your heart rate is."
   2. "I do not need to give you the medication if your heart rate is normal."
   3. "I will only give you half the dosage if your heart rate is less than 60 beats per minute."
   4. "I will not give the medication and report to the doctor if your heart rate is below the normal rate of 60."

2. Mrs. Hawkins is receiving the diuretic furosemide (Lasix), 40 mg by mouth daily. What is the most appropriate time of day to administer this medication?
   1. Just before bedtime
   2. Any time during the day but always at the same time in order to space the doses
   3. In the morning
   4. With food, preferably the midday meal

3. Mrs. Hawkins is ordered the potassium supplement Slow-K 600 mg twice daily. What is the purpose of administering this medication?
   1. To replace potassium losses produced by the furosemide
   2. To promote the effects of the diuretic
   3. To help facilitate nerve impulse conduction within the heart
   4. To prevent adverse effects produced by digoxin

4. Mrs. Hawkins is scheduled for discharge from the hospital. She has been prescribed nitroglycerin in the form of a dermal patch and sublingual spray. Which of the following should the nurse teach Mrs. Hawkins concerning the correct use of nitroglycerin dermal patches?
   1. Apply a patch once a day for 1 hour to ensure that the medication gets absorbed through the skin.
   2. Apply each patch daily to the same area of skin to maximize absorption.
   3. Remove the old patch and cleanse the area, then apply a new patch to a different area of skin.
   4. Massage the area of skin around the patch to stimulate absorption of the medication.

5. What directions should the nurse provide to Mrs. Hawkins regarding the use of her nitroglycerin sublingual spray when she experiences angina pectoris?
   1. Spray under the tongue at 5-minute intervals. Continue the procedure until the pain subsides.
   2. Spray under the tongue. If pain continues, spray an additional time for better absorption.
   3. Spray under the tongue. If the pain is not relieved, apply a nitroglycerin patch to the skin to help facilitate the action of the spray.
   4. Spray once under the tongue at 5-minute intervals to a maximum of three times. If the pain continues, seek medical attention.

Case 2

Leslie, a nurse educator in the diabetes clinic, is teaching new nurses on a medical unit about type 2 diabetes and the use of insulin. Leslie provides client scenarios for the nurses and asks them to "brainstorm" answers as a group.

Questions 6 and 7 refer to this case.

6. The first client scenario involves Mr. B., a client who is taking regular and NPH insulin. Regular insulin has an onset of 30 to 60 minutes and a peak of 2 to 4 hours. NPH insulin has an onset of 1 to 2 hours, a peak of 6 to 12 hours, and a duration of action of approximately 18 hours. If Mr. B. is given a combination of regular and NPH insulin at 0730 hours, when might he require another injection of insulin?
   1. Noon
   2. Midmorning
   3. Midafternoon
   4. Bedtime

7. Another client scenario concerns Ms. A., who is receiving Novolin 30/70. Novolin 30/70 is a mixture of regular insulin (onset: 0.5–1 hours, peak: 2–4 hours, duration: 5–8 hours) and isophane insulin (onset: 1–3 hours, peak: 5–8 hours, duration: up to 18 hours). The nurse is concerned about hypoglycemia. When would hypoglycemia most likely occur?
   1. Between 0.5 and 1 hour and 2 to 3 hours after administering the insulin
   2. Between 2 and 4 hours and 5 to 8 hours after administering the insulin
   3. Between 5 and 8 hours and 18 hours after administering the insulin
   4. After 18 hours following the administration of the insulin

Case 3

Robert Melnick has been experiencing gastric discomfort for several months. His health care provider prescribes several medications, including H_2 receptor antagonists and simethicone, to alleviate the discomfort. The nurse teaches Mr. Melnick about his medications.

Questions 8 and 9 refer to this case.

8. The nurse is not familiar with H_2 receptor antagonists and asks the pharmacist for information. What would the pharmacist explain about the action of H_2 receptor antagonists?
   1. They neutralize excess hydrochloric acid (HCl) that has been secreted into the stomach.
   2. They compete with histamine for binding sites on the surface of parietal cells and block hydrogen ion (H^+) secretion.

3. They inhibit the secretion of the digestive enzyme pepsin into the stomach.

4. They combine with, and convert, HCl in the stomach to a salt and water.

9. What would the nurse explain to Mr. Melnick about the desirable effect of simethicone for the relief of gastrointestinal distress?

1. It stimulates peristalsis.
2. It reduces gas distension.
3. It prevents diarrhea.
4. It absorbs excess HCl.

Case 4

Francesca, a student nurse, has read about how overprescribing of antibiotics has led to multiple drug-resistant pathogens. Francesca asks the nurse for more information about antibiotics.

Questions 10 and 11 refer to this case.

10. Francesca asks the nurse, "What is meant by the term 'narrow-spectrum antibiotic agent'?" Which of the following would be a correct response by the nurse?

1. An antimicrobial that is effective only against bacteria
2. An antimicrobial that has a narrow therapeutic index
3. An antimicrobial that can only be given in very small doses because of toxicity concerns
4. An antimicrobial that is mainly effective against a few Gram-positive or Gram-negative bacteria

11. Francesca and the nurse discuss the treatment of infections for which antibiotics are not useful. For which of the following conditions is antibiotic treatment not indicated?

1. Chlamydia
2. *E. coli* infection
3. Gonorrhea
4. Influenza A and B

Independent Questions

Questions 12 to 25 do not refer to a particular case.

12. A client has just developed acute renal failure. What is the safest action by the nurse regarding administration of their prescribed medications?

1. Plan to administer lower doses of the medications due to the decreased ability of the kidneys to eliminate the drugs.
2. Consider administering higher doses of the medications to promote more effective elimination of the drugs.
3. Have the prescribed medications and doses reviewed by the prescriber and pharmacist prior to administering the drugs.
4. Do not administer any medications that are known to be eliminated through the kidneys.

13. Which of the following nursing considerations should be addressed prior to the administration of morphine sulphate (morphine) to a client, who is experiencing pain associated with his terminal colorectal cancer?

1. Assess the requirement for an antiemetic to be administered at the same time as the morphine to prevent nausea or vomiting, or both.

2. Administer the lowest dose of the range of morphine that has been prescribed by the physician.

3. Assess the client for any previous history of narcotic abuse prior to administering the medication.

4. Withhold administering the morphine if the client's respiratory rate is less than 15 respirations per minute.

14. A client will be taking oral iron supplements. Which statements should the nurse include when teaching the client? **Select all that apply.**

1. Take the iron tablets with an antacid.
2. Take the iron with meals.
3. Drink 250 mL of milk with each iron dose.
4. Taking iron supplements with orange juice enhances iron absorption.
5. Stools may become black and tarry.
6. Iron tablets may be crushed to enhance iron absorption.

15. Which of the following conditions are an indication for the administration of a central nervous system (CNS) stimulant medication? **Select all that apply.**

1. Insomnia
2. Alzheimer's disease
3. Narcolepsy
4. ADHD
5. Appetite enhancement

16. Nalbuphine (Nubain) is a partial opioid agonist. What characterizes this type of medication? **Select all that apply.**

1. Used for mild pain
2. Used for moderate to severe pain
3. Medication of choice for reversing the effects of opioids in case of overdose
4. Has a lower potential for abuse than a pure agonist
5. Adverse effects are similar to those of opioid agonists.

17. Contraindications to the administration of an opioid analgesic include which of the following? **Select all that apply.**

1. Renal insufficiency
2. Severe chronic obstructive pulmonary disease
3. Liver disease
4. Diabetes mellitus
5. Allergy

18. Which of the following medications are used for acute asthma attack? **Select all that apply.**

1. Salbutamol (Ventolin)
2. Ipratropium bromide (Atrovent)
3. Aminophylline
4. Zafirlukast (Accolate)
5. Fluticasone (Flovent)

19. Which of the following symptoms are indicative of digitalis toxicity? **Select all that apply.**

1. Diarrhea
2. Yellow-green visual distortion
3. Nausea and vomiting
4. Insomnia
5. Urinary retention

20. How would the action and effect of a drug that is metabolized by the liver be affected in a client with severe cirrhosis of the liver?
    1. The rate of the excretion of the drug will increase.
    2. The duration of the action of the drug will decrease.
    3. The action and effects of the drug on body cells will be blocked—hence no effect.
    4. The action and effects of the drug on the body will be prolonged.

21. Which of the following factors will the nurse take into consideration when administering medications to older persons?
    1. Older persons require higher dosages to compensate for degenerative changes in the liver.
    2. Older persons require more frequent dose administration because of high levels of excretion by the kidneys.
    3. Older persons require lower doses due to reduced function of body organs.
    4. With older adults, the parenteral route is preferable because of less efficient absorption from the gastrointestinal system.

22. Which of the following classifications of drugs would be prescribed for the treatment of depression?
    1. Barbiturates
    2. Antianxiolytics
    3. Selective serotonin reuptake inhibitors (SSRIs)
    4. Cholinergic agonists

23. Why do individuals who have been treated with cortisone preparations for an extended period of time have an increased risk of developing infections?
    1. Cortisone attracts microbes into the body.
    2. Cortisone suppresses the body's normal immune response.
    3. Cortisone therapy suppresses the body's natural bacteria.
    4. Cortisone causes increased capillary permeability.

24. A client has just returned to the unit after surgery and requests pain medication. Within 15 minutes of receiving a dose of the prescribed opioid, the nurse completes an assessment on the client. Based on the information provided, which necessary action may the nurse need to perform?

Vital signs	Pulse (beats per minute): 90 Respiratory rate (breaths per minute): 8 (shallow) Temperature: 37.5 C Oxygen saturation 97%
Medications	Morphine sulphate 5 to 10 mg subcutaneously q4H prn Acetaminophen 500 mg 1–2 tabs PO Q6H prn
Neurological assessment	Drowsy

1. Administration of naloxone, an opioid reversal agent
2. Close observation for signs of opioid tolerance
3. Administration of fentanyl, an agonist opioid
4. Immediate intubation and artificial ventilation

25. Which of the following should be taught to a client who is taking isoniazid (INH)?
    1. Urine and saliva may be reddish orange in colour.
    2. Avoid alcohol to limit the danger of hepatic damage.
    3. Clients will need to have weekly chest X-rays.
    4. Take with an antacid to reduce gastric distress.

BIBLIOGRAPHY

Astle, B., & Duggleby, W. (2024). *Potter and Perry's Canadian fundamentals of nursing* (7th ed.). Elsevier.

Canadian Pharmacists Association. (2016, November 1). *Compendium of pharmaceuticals and specialties.*

National Association of Pharmacy Regulatory Authorities. (n.d.) *Outline of the schedules.* https://www.napra.ca/sites/default/files/documents/Schedules-Outline.pdf

Sealock, K., & Seneviratne, C. (2021). *Lilley's pharmacology for Canadian health care practice* (4th ed.). Elsevier.

Skidmore-Roth, L., & Richardson, F. (2021). *Canadian nursing drug reference.* Elsevier.

Tyerman, J., & Cobbett, W. (2023). *Lewis's medical-surgical nursing in Canada: Assessment and management of clinical problems* (5th ed.). Elsevier.

WEBSITES

- **Canadian Pharmacists Association** (http://www.pharmacists.ca): There are many useful medication-related resources on this site, which has sections for health professionals and for the general public.
- **Health Canada: Drug Product Database** (https://www.canada.ca/en/health-canada/services/drugs-health-products/drug-products/drug-product-database.html): This site has updated drug advisories, describes the drug regulation process, and contains other information for health care providers and consumers.
- **Health Canada: Therapeutic Products Directorate** (https://www.canada.ca/en/health-canada/corporate/about-health-canada/branches-agencies/health-products-food-branch/therapeutic-products-directorate.html): The Therapeutic Products Directorate is the government body that regulates therapeutic products, including drugs, in Canada.
- **medSask** (https://medsask.usask.ca): This University of Saskatchewan site has a vast number of resources and links concerning drugs, immunization, and health and pharmaceutical organizations.

Medical-Surgical Nursing

In Canada, our general population is aging, and more people are developing chronic illnesses and disabilities that require skilled nursing intervention. Nursing education requires students to synthesize and critically analyze knowledge in order to provide and promote holistic care to this growing sector of the population. With this point in mind, the following chapter provides a condensed summary of many medical and surgical topics to help students build on the knowledge and skills they will need to promote health, facilitate recovery from injury or illness, and provide support with coping with chronic illness and disability. Please refer to Appendix D (laboratory values) and Appendix E (mathematical calculations) as additional resources for this chapter.

FLUID AND ELECTROLYTE IMBALANCES

Homeostasis

Homeostasis is the state of equilibrium in the internal environment of the body. Body fluids and electrolytes play an important role in homeostasis. Water is the primary component of body fluids and serves many functions:

- Transporting nutrients and oxygen
- Transporting waste
- Providing a medium for metabolic reactions
- Insulating and helping to regulate temperature
- Providing form and substance to body tissues
- Providing lubrication

Water accounts for 60% of body weight in an adult and 70 to 80% of body weight in an infant. Water content will vary with sex, body mass, and age. Fatty tissue has less water content than other tissues. Insensible water loss is unavoidable and immeasurable, such as water loss by evaporation occurring through the skin as perspiration, a nonvisible form of water loss. Another example of insensible water loss is the water lost via respirations. Sensible water loss is observable and measurable, such as water lost in urine.

Electrolytes are substances that dissociate in solutions and are referred to as *ions*. Cations are positively charged electrolytes such as sodium (Na^+). Anions are negatively charged electrolytes such as chloride (Cl^-). Electrolytes help regulate water and the acid–base balance. They contribute to enzyme reactions and are essential to neuromuscular activity.

The following terms relate to the mechanisms controlling fluid and electrolyte movement:

- Diffusion and facilitated diffusion
- Active transport
- Osmosis, filtration, and osmotic pressure
- Tonicity, isotonic, hypertonic, and hypotonic
- Hypovolemia and hypervolemia
- Dehydration and edema

Fluid Shifting

Fluid in the body is divided into different compartments. See Table 9.1 for an explanation of body fluid compartments and fluid spacing.

The amount and direction of fluid movement within the capillaries are determined by the following:

- Capillary hydrostatic pressure
- Plasma osmotic pressure
- Interstitial hydrostatic pressure
- Interstitial osmotic pressure
  Edema occurs when
- Fluid shifts from the plasma to the interstitial fluid.
- There is an elevation of capillary hydrostatic pressure.
- There is a decrease in plasma osmotic pressure.
- There is elevation of interstitial osmotic pressure.
  Fluid is drawn into the plasma space when
- There is an increase in plasma osmotic pressure that causes the fluid to move from the interstitial space to the plasma.
- Osmoreceptors in the hypothalamus sense a fluid deficit or an increase in plasma osmolarity, or both, stimulating the primary regulator, thirst, and the release of antidiuretic hormone (ADH) from the posterior pituitary gland.
- The adrenal cortex releases the mineralocorticoid aldosterone, which has potent sodium-retaining and potassium-excreting capabilities.

The kidneys are the primary organs for regulating fluid and electrolyte balance. The kidneys selectively reabsorb or excrete water and electrolytes. The renal tubules are sites of actions for ADH and aldosterone. Pertaining to cardiac regulation, atrial natriuretic factor (ANF) is released by the cardiac atria in response to increased atrial pressure. ANF causes vasodilation and increased urinary excretion of sodium and water. ANF inhibits the kidneys from releasing the hormone renin.

The gastro-intestinal (GI) tract receives most of the body's water intake, but only small amounts of water are eliminated by the GI tract. About 8 L of fluid is moved in the bowel during an average day; however, only 100 to 200 mL is lost through feces. Insensible water loss, which occurs via vaporization from the lungs and the skin, accounts for about 900 mL per day. No electrolytes are lost with insensible water loss. However, excessive sweating could lead to the loss of both water and electrolytes.

TABLE 9.1 Body Fluid Compartments and Fluid Spacing

Body Compartment and Spacing	Description
Intracellular fluid (ICF)	• ICF fluid is found within the cell. • ICF comprises about 42% of body weight and is about 30 L in total volume. • The most prevalent cation is potassium (K^+). • The most prevalent anion is phosphate (PO_4^-).
Extracellular fluid (ECF)	• ECF fluid is the fluid that is found between cells (called *interstitial fluid*) and in the plasma space (called *intravascular fluid*). • Interstitial fluid bathes the cells and makes up two-thirds of ECF (ECF comprises about 15% of the body's total fluid volume). • The most prevalent anion is chloride (Cl^-). • The most prevalent cation is sodium (Na^+). • Intravascular fluid makes up the last third of the ECF, which is about 5% or 3 L of the body's total fluid volume.
Transcellular fluid	• Transcellular fluid is a small but important fluid compartment and totals about 1 L. • Transcellular fluid includes cerebrospinal fluid, digestive secretions in the gastro-intestinal tract, and fluid in the pleural spaces, synovial spaces, and peritoneal spaces.
First spacing Second spacing Third spacing	• Distribution of fluid in ICF and ECF is within normal limits. • Abnormal accumulation of fluid within the interstitial space, also known as *edema* • Fluid accumulates in a part of the body where it is not easily exchanged with ECF. • Fluid shifts from the vascular space into an area where it is not available for any physiological process. • Fluid is trapped and does not participate in normal functions of the ECF. • Weight does not change as the volume is not lost but is shifted to a nonfunctioning area. • This can lead to a decrease in the volume of the intravascular space. • Damage to tissues may result from the high fluid volume within the nonfunctioning space. • Treatment focuses on treating the underlying cause of the shift of fluid by removing the fluid from the third space, replacing fluid within the intravascular space, and maintaining adequate cardiac output.

Client History and Fluid and Electrolytes

Many conditions affect the fluid and electrolyte balance, such as diabetes or renal failure. The following conditions and topics should be discussed when taking a client history:

• Medications, such as diuretics, steroids, herbs, and total parenteral nutrition
• Abnormal fluid loss, such as vomiting, diarrhea, and polyuria
• Diet, whether prescribed or client initiated
• Present fluid intake history, including the client's ability to obtain fluids, mobility, and actual amount the client drank

Extracellular Fluid Volume Imbalances

Hypovolemia

Hypovolemia can occur with the loss of normal body fluids, such as in the case of diarrhea, hemorrhage, decreased intake, or plasma loss due to interstitial fluid shift. The cause of the hypovolemia must be identified and treated. Once this is done, replacement fluid may be given either orally or intravenously (IV) with balanced solutions, isotonic sodium chloride, or blood, depending on the cause of the hypovolemia.

Hypervolemia

Hypervolemia may result from the excessive intake of fluids, abnormal retention of fluids, or interstitial loss to plasma fluid shift. Treatment for hypervolemia will depend on the cause of the hypervolemia and may include diuretics, fluid restriction, and sodium restriction.

Nursing Management for Hypovolemia and Hypervolemia

Management of both hypovolemia and hypervolemia includes assessment and monitoring of the following:

• Strict intake and output

- Cardiovascular changes
- Respiratory changes
- Daily weights, which is the best way to monitor fluid balance over time
- Skin and mucous membranes
- Neurological status

Nursing Considerations for Older Clients

Older persons are at significant risk for a fluid volume deficit, which can lead to dehydration and heat stroke. The risk is due to the following:

- The decrease in muscle mass in older persons, which leads to a decrease in total body water
- The thirst response, which can be delayed in older persons
- The skin of older persons, which has less elasticity, and sweat gland atrophy
- A decreased ability to concentrate urine and possible kidney function changes
- Changes in the cardiovascular system and GI tract

Many common conditions that affect older persons may also affect fluid balance. These conditions include dehydration, constipation with laxative abuse, and hyperthermia.

Nursing Considerations for the Older Client

Most of the infant's body weight, 70 to 80%, is made up of fluid. Therefore, infants have a larger amount of extracellular fluid (ECF), where water and electrolyte disturbances can occur more frequently and rapidly. Pediatric clients need more fluid intake and output relative to their size due to the large ECF volume and the following:

- Infants exchange more fluid across capillary membranes daily compared with adults.
- Infants have immature renal function and a greater body surface area, which together have an important effect on metabolism, heat production, and heat loss.

Infants exchange half of their body fluids per day, whereas adults exchange one sixth of their fluids per day. Therefore, pediatric clients have smaller fluid reserves, and the balance can be upset more quickly. Note that an infant is less able to handle large quantities of solute-free water than an older child. Therefore, when an infant is being rehydrated, a solution with electrolytes should be used rather than plain water. Rehydration should proceed slowly with infants.

Electrolytes

Sodium

Sodium (the normal, or reference, range is 135–145 mmol/L) plays a major role in electrolyte balance. This role includes its effect on ECF volume and concentration, the generation and transmission of nerve impulses, and acid–base balance. Sodium is readily available in a balanced diet and is normally balanced within a healthy individual by the kidneys.

Hypernatremia. Hypernatremia (>145 mmol/L) is elevated serum sodium occurring with water loss or sodium gain. It is rarely seen in people with intact thirst mechanisms. Hypernatremia is caused by hyperosmolality leading to cellular dehydration. Clinical manifestations of hypernatremia include the following:

- Thirst
- Lethargy or agitation
- Disorientation
- Hallucinations
- Seizures
- Coma

Hypernatremia can be produced by nephrogenic diabetes insipidus. Management includes treating the underlying cause, as well as giving oral fluids or an IV solution of 5% dextrose in water, or hypotonic saline. Note that it is important that sodium levels be reduced gradually to avoid cerebral edema.

Hyponatremia. Hyponatremia (<135 mmol/L), a decreased level of serum sodium, can result from a loss of sodium-containing fluids or from excess water. Clinical manifestations include the following:

- Nausea, vomiting, or both
- Anorexia
- Muscle twitching
- Diminished reflexes
- Respiratory arrest
- Headache
- Confusion
- Seizures
- Coma

If hyponatremia is caused by water excess, fluid restriction is needed. If severe symptoms occur, small amounts of IV hypertonic saline solution (3% NaCl) are given. If hyponatremia is associated with abnormal fluid loss, fluid replacement with sodium-containing solution is required.

Potassium

Potassium (3.5–5 mmol/L) is necessary for the transmission and conduction of nerve impulses, the maintenance of normal cardiac rhythm, skeletal muscle contraction, and acid–base balance. Potassium is critical to the action potential of nerves. Normal renal function is needed for the maintenance of potassium balance because the majority of potassium is excreted from the body by the kidneys. The remaining potassium is lost through the bowel and perspiration. Potassium is plentiful in the normal diet of meats, fruits—particularly citrus fruits—green vegetables, and potatoes.

Hyperkalemia. Hyperkalemia (>5 mmol/L), the condition of an excessive amount of potassium in the body, can result from renal failure, potassium-sparing diuretics, an increased intake of potassium from foods high in potassium, tissue destruction, and acidosis. Clinical manifestations can include the following:

- Muscle weakness or paralysis
- Paraesthesias of the face, tongue, feet, and hands
- Nausea
- Ventricular fibrillation or cardiac standstill
- Impaired cardiac depolarization, resulting in a slow heart rate

Management focuses on elimination of the potassium source and potassium from the body through the use of potassium-wasting diuretics, polystyrene sulfonate (Kayexalate), and dialysis. IV insulin may be administered to force potassium from ECF to intracellular fluid (ICF). IV calcium gluconate may be used to reverse the membrane effects of elevated ECF potassium.

Hypokalemia. Hypokalemia (<3.5 mmol/L) can result from the increased secretion of aldosterone, the use of loop diuretics, severe vomiting, or severe diarrhea and is associated with magnesium deficiency. Clinical manifestations include the following:

- Ventricular dysrhythmias and impaired repolarization
- Muscle fatigue and weakness
- Cramps
- Decreased GI motility
- Altered airway responsiveness
- Impaired regulation of arterial blood flow
- Hyperglycemia

Management of hypokalemia focuses on replacement of the potassium, either orally or intravenously. In addition, it is important to teach preventive measures, such as eating foods containing adequate amounts of potassium or ingesting potassium supplements when dietary intake is not adequate.

Calcium

Calcium (2.25–2.75 mmol/L) is obtained through food sources. Calcium has an inverse relationship with phosphorus. The majority of calcium is stored in bones. Calcium blocks sodium transport and stabilizes cell membranes. Calcium functions include the transmission of nerve impulses, myocardial contractions, blood clotting, muscle contractions, and the formation of teeth and bones. Calcium is controlled by parathyroid hormone (PTH). When this hormone is released, it stimulates calcium resorption from the bones. Calcitonin, secreted by the thyroid gland, inhibits the resorption of calcium from the bones. Vitamin D is needed to increase the intestinal absorption of calcium, which is excreted by the intestinal and urinary tracts.

Hypercalcemia. Hypercalcemia (>2.75 mmol/L) can result from hyperparathyroidism, malignancy, vitamin D overdose, and prolonged immobilization. Clinical manifestations of hypercalcemia include the following:

- Confusion, disorientation, and decreased memory
- Fatigue
- Decreased neuromuscular excitability, weakness, and decreased deep tendon reflexes

Management of hypercalcemia includes loop diuretics, hydration with isotonic saline, synthetic calcitonin, and client mobilization.

Hypocalcemia. Hypocalcemia (<2.25 mmol/L) can result from the decreased production of PTH, acute pancreatitis, multiple blood transfusions, alkalosis, and the decreased intake of calcium. Deficiency of vitamin D or insufficient exposure to the sun can cause reduced calcium absorption from the gut. Clinical manifestations include the following:

- Positive Trousseau's sign, which indicates neuro-excitability; a positive sign is indicated if twitching of the

hands and fingers occurs when a blood pressure (BP) cuff is inflated 10 mm Hg above the systolic pressure
- A positive Chvostek's sign, which indicates neuro-excitability as well; it is indicated if tapping over the facial nerve (the area below the temple) with a finger causes muscle spasms of the mouth and cheek
- Increased neuromuscular activity; tetany
- Laryngeal stridor, dysphagia, numbness, tingling around the mouth or extremities
- Decreased myocardial contractility

Management of hypocalcemia focuses on treating the cause, replacing the calcium, and ensuring that the intake of vitamin D is adequate.

Phosphate

Phosphate (0.97–1.45 mmol/L) is the primary anion in ICF and is essential for muscle and nerve function, as well as red blood cell (RBC) formation. Along with calcium, phosphate is important in the formation of bones and teeth. It is involved in the acid–base buffering system, adenosine triphosphate (ATP) production, and cellular uptake of glucose. A normal diet, including red meat, fish, poultry, eggs, milk products, and legumes, usually is sufficient for adequate phosphate absorption. However, vitamin D is needed in the absorption of phosphate. The kidneys are the major route of excretion for phosphate.

Hyperphosphatemia. Hyperphosphatemia (>1.45 mmol/L) can result from acute or chronic renal failure, chemotherapy, excessive ingestion of milk or phosphate-containing laxatives, and large doses of vitamin D. Clinical manifestations include the following:

- Hypocalcemia
- Muscle tetany
- Deposition of calcium–phosphate crystals in skin, soft tissue, cornea, viscera, and blood vessels
- Tingling of mouth and fingertips and numbness

Management focuses on identifying and treating the underlying cause, restricting foods and fluids containing phosphorus, and ensuring adequate hydration.

Hypophosphatemia. Hypophosphatemia (<0.97 mmol/L) can result from malnourishment or malabsorption, alcohol withdrawal, and the use of phosphate-binding antacids. Clinical manifestations include the following:

- Central nervous system (CNS) depression, confusion, delirium, and seizures
- Muscle weakness and pain
- Dysrhythmias, cardiomyopathy
- Acute respiratory failure (ARF)

Management includes phosphate replacement.

Magnesium

Magnesium (0.65–1.05 mmol/L) acts directly on the myoneural junction. It is also important for normal cardiac function. About two thirds of the body's magnesium is stored in the bones, with the remaining one third in the ICF. The kidneys are the primary route of excretion of magnesium, helping maintain a normal balance of magnesium within the body.

Hypermagnesemia. Hypermagnesemia (>1.05 mmol/L) can result from an increased intake or ingestion of products containing magnesium when renal insufficiency or failure is present. Clinical manifestations include the following:

- Lethargy, drowsiness, somnolence
- Peripheral vasodilation, causing flushing, warm skin, decreased BP, and rhythm disturbances with possible cardiac arrest
- Impaired reflexes
- Possible respiratory arrest

Management focuses on prevention, increased fluids, and IV calcium chloride or calcium gluconate.

Hypomagnesemia. Hypomagnesemia (<0.65 mmol/L) can result from prolonged fasting or starvation, chronic alcoholism, fluid loss, prolonged parenteral nutrition without supplementation, diuretics, osmotic diuretics, or high glucose levels. Hypomagnesemia is a common clinical condition. Clinical manifestations include the following:

- Hyperactive deep tendon reflexes, tremors, and seizures
- Cardiac dysrhythmias, increased heart rate and BP
- Confusion, convulsions, and disorientation

Management focuses on replacement of magnesium orally or intravenously. To prevent hypomagnesemia from occurring, adequate dietary intake of magnesium, including green vegetables, seafood, nuts, and grains, should be encouraged. Table 9.2 summarizes the major serum electrolyte concentrations and the significance of abnormal values.

Intravenous Fluids

IV fluids are used to maintain fluid balance when oral intake is not adequate and to replace fluids and electrolytes when fluid losses have occurred and electrolytes are out of balance. The amount and type of fluid replacement depend on the client's daily maintenance requirements and on any imbalances identified through laboratory work.

IV solutions can be hypotonic, isotonic, or hypertonic. These types of IV solutions are described in Table 9.3.

Acid–Base Balance and Arterial Blood Gases
Regulating Mechanisms to Balance Acids and Bases

The proper balance between the acids and bases in the human body is called *acid–base homeostasis*, in other words, the body's pH, which must be maintained within a very narrow range. Arterial blood gases (ABGs) provide information about the various concentrations of the gases dissolved in the blood before the blood is distributed to the tissues. pH is the indirect measure of hydrogen (H^+) ion concentration and measures the ratio of base bicarbonate (HCO_3^-) to acid carbon dioxide (CO_2). This ratio is normally 20:1. Acids give up (donate) H^+ ions, and bases pick up H^+ ions. The body maintains a slightly alkaline pH of 7.34 to 7.45 in arterial blood.

The three regulating mechanisms to maintain acid–base homeostasis are as follows:

- Chemical buffer regulators
- Respiratory regulators
- Renal regulators

Buffer regulator system. The buffer system comprises the primary chemical regulators that act immediately. They are found in the blood and tissues and include bicarbonate, proteins, and hemoglobin.

Respiratory regulator system. The respiratory system eliminates CO_2 and water (H_2O), which, when joined, are carbonic

TABLE 9.2   Major Serum Electrolyte Concentrations and Significance of Abnormal Values

Electrolyte	Reference Range	Significance of Abnormal Values
Sodium (Na^+)	136–145 mmol/L	*Elevated:* Hypernatremia; dehydration; kidney disease; hypercortisolism *Low:* Hyponatremia; fluid overload; liver disease; adrenal insufficiency
Potassium (K^+)	3.5–5.0 mmol/L	*Elevated:* Hyperkalemia; dehydration; kidney disease; acidosis; adrenal insufficiency; crush injuries *Low:* Hypokalemia; fluid overload; diuretic therapy; alkalosis; insulin administration; hyperaldosteronism
Calcium (Ca^{2+})	2.25–2.75 mmol/L	*Elevated:* Hypercalcemia; hyperthyroidism; hyperparathyroidism *Low:* Hypocalcemia; vitamin D deficiency; hypothyroidism; hypoparathyroidism; kidney disease; excessive intake of phosphorous-containing foods and drinks
Chloride (Cl^-)	98–106 mmol/L	*Elevated:* Hyperchloremia; metabolic acidosis; respiratory alkalosis; hypercortisolism *Low:* Hypochloremia; fluid overload; excessive vomiting or diarrhea; adrenal insufficiency; diuretic therapy
Magnesium (Mg^{2+})	0.65–1.05 mmol/L	*Elevated:* Hypermagnesemia; kidney disease; hypothyroidism; adrenal insufficiency *Low:* Hypomagnesemia; malnutrition; alcoholism; ketoacidosis

Adapted from Astle, B., & Duggleby, W. (2024). *Potter and Perry's. Canadian fundamentals of nursing* (7th ed., Table 41.4, p. 1022). Elsevier. Data from Tyerman, J., & Cobbett, S. (2023). *Lewis's medical-surgical nursing in Canada: Assessment and management of clinical problems* (5th Cdn, ed., p. 349, Table 19.2). Elsevier.

TABLE 9.3 Intravenous Fluids

Type of Solution	Description
Hypotonic intravenous solution	• It has fewer electrolytes and solutes than plasma and therefore dilute the extracellular fluid (ECF). • Osmosis moves the fluid from ECF to intracellular fluid (ICF), hydrating the cells. • An example of a hypotonic solution is 0.45% NaCl (sodium chloride).
Isotonic intravenous solution	• It has the same tonicity as plasma. • It is given to expand ECF only. • It does not change ICF volume. • Examples of an isotonic solution are 0.9% normal saline (NS) and Ringer's lactate.
Hypertonic intravenous solution	• It contains more electrolytes or solutes than are normally found in plasma. • When intravenous (IV) hypertonic fluid is given, the osmotic pressure within the vessel increases, drawing fluid from the tissues into the vascular system, thereby decreasing fluid within the tissues and increasing fluid in the IV space. • An example of a hypertonic solution is 10% dextrose in water.

TABLE 9.4 Interpreting Blood Gases

Normal ABG values are as follows:

pH	7.35–7.45
$PaCO_2$	35–45 mm Hg (respiratory component)
HCO_3^-	21–28 mmol/L (metabolic component)
PaO_2	80–100 mm Hg
SaO_2	95–100% arterial O_2 saturation

HCO_3^-, Bicarbonate; $PaCO_2$, partial pressure of carbon dioxide in arterial blood; PaO_2, partial pressure of oxygen in arterial blood; SaO_2, oxygen saturation.

acid (H_2CO_3), thus eliminating acid from the body through respiration. The respiratory centre within the medulla controls breathing. When the blood has too much carbonic acid in it, the respiratory centre will instruct the lungs to increase the respiratory rate in order to "blow off" the acid.

If the carbonic acid levels are low, the centre will instruct the lungs to decrease the respiratory rate in an effort to conserve carbonic acid. The respiratory regulating system works within minutes to hours to balance acid–base levels.

Renal regulator system. The renal regulator system is the most powerful of the three systems. The kidneys secrete hydrogen ions and reabsorb bicarbonate ions. This activity is increased when the pH is acidotic and decreases when the pH is alkalotic. The renal system responds within hours to days to restore acid–base homeostasis.

When interpreting ABGs, the nurse must evaluate the pH and determine whether it is acidotic or alkalotic. A value under 7.35 indicates acidosis; a value above 7.45 indicates alkalosis (See Table 9.4).

If there is an abnormality in the pH, the cause must be determined. Next, the respiratory component must be evaluated. If there is a high level of CO_2, above 45 mm Hg, this indicates an elevated level of carbonic acid ($H_2O + CO_2 = H_2CO_3$), and acidosis. If the level is low, below 35 mm Hg, this indicates a low level of carbonic acid (H_2CO_3) and therefore alkalosis.

The metabolic component is determined by looking at the amount of base HCO_3^-. If there is a lot of base, indicated by a reading above 28 mmol/L, then the blood is alkalotic. If there is insufficient base, indicated by a reading below 21 mmol/L, the blood would be acidotic. See the blood gas summary using the mnemonic ROME in Box 9.1.

BOX 9.1 Blood Gas Summary Using the Mnemonic ROME

For acid-base imbalances, the mnemonic ROME can be used.

In **R**espiratory conditions, the pH and $PaCO_2$ are in **O**pposite directions.

• In respiratory alkalosis, the pH is increased and the $PaCO_2$ is decreased.
• In respiratory acidosis, the pH is decreased and the $PaCO_2$ is increased

In **M**etabolic conditions, the pH and the HCO_3 go in the same direction (**E**qual or **E**quivalent). The $PaCO_2$ may also go in the same direction.

• In metabolic alkalosis, pH and HCO_3 are increased and the $PaCO_2$ is increased or normal.
• In metabolic acidosis, pH and HCO_3 are decreased and the $PaCO_2$ is decreased or normal.

Adapted from Tyerman, J., & Cobbett, S. (2023). *Lewis's medical-surgical nursing in Canada: Assessment and management of clinical problems* (5th Cdn. ed., p. 364, Table 19.17). Elsevier.
HCO_3^- = bicarbonate; $PaCO_2$ = partial pressure of carbon dioxide in arterial blood.

If both respiratory and metabolic components match the pH, a mixed complicated disorder may be present.

The body must maintain the correct pH. The body's regulatory systems will attempt to compensate for respiratory or metabolic conditions by adjusting the levels of acid or base to bring the pH back to the normal range. Compensation is evident in ABGs if the pH is normal or near normal and the partial pressure of carbon dioxide (PCO_2) or HCO_3^- is not within normal limits.

TABLE 9.5 Acid–Base Imbalances

Common Causes	Pathophysiology	Laboratory Findings
Respiratory Acidosis		
Chronic obstructive pulmonary disease	CO_2 retention from hypoventilation	↓ Plasma pH
Barbiturate or sedative overdose	Compensatory response to HCO_3^-	↑ Pco_2
Chest wall abnormality (e.g., obesity)	retention by kidney	HCO_3^- normal (uncompensated)
Severe pneumonia		↑ HCO_3^- (compensated)
Atelectasis		Urine pH <6 (compensated)
Respiratory muscle weakness (e.g., Guillain-Barré syndrome)		
Mechanical hypoventilation		
Respiratory Alkalosis		
Hyperventilation (caused by hypoxia, pulmonary emboli, anxiety, fear, pain, exercise, fever)	Increased CO_2 excretion from hyperventilation	↑ Plasma pH
	Compensatory response of HCO_3^-	↓ Pco_2
Stimulated respiratory centre caused by septicemia, encephalitis, brain injury, salicylate poisoning	excretion by kidney	HCO_3^- normal (uncompensated)
		↓ HCO_3^- (compensated)
Mechanical hyperventilation		Urine pH >6 (compensated)
Metabolic Acidosis		
Diabetic ketoacidosis	Gain of fixed acid, inability to excrete acid, or loss of base	↓ Plasma pH
Lactic acidosis		Pco_2 normal (uncompensated)
Starvation	Compensatory response of CO_2 excretion	↓ Pco_2 (compensated)
Severe diarrhea	by lungs	↓ HCO_3^-
Renal tubular acidosis		Urine pH <6 (compensated)
Renal failure		
Gastro-intestinal fistulas		
Shock		
Metabolic Alkalosis		
Severe vomiting	Loss of strong acid or gain of base	↑ Plasma pH
Excess gastric suctioning	Compensatory response of CO_2 retention	Pco_2 normal (uncompensated)
Diuretic therapy*	by lungs	↑ Pco_2 (compensated)
Potassium deficit		↑ HCO_3^-
Excess $NaHCO_3$ intake		Urine pH >6 (compensated)
Excessive mineralocorticoids		

*Commonly used diuretics such as thiazides and furosemide are known to produce mild alkalosis by affecting tubular excretion of electrolytes and bicarbonate.
CO_2, carbon dioxide; HCO_3^-, bicarbonate; Pco_2, partial pressure of carbon dioxide.
From Tyerman, J., & Cobbett, S. (2023). *Lewis's medical-surgical nursing in Canada: Assessment and management of clinical problems* (5th Cdn. ed., p. 361, Table 19.12). Elsevier.

Respiratory acidosis occurs when the CO_2 is too high, causing the pH to be low (acidotic). This can be caused by hypoventilation, respiratory failure, pneumonia, pulmonary emboli, or long-standing chronic obstructive pulmonary disease (COPD).

Respiratory alkalosis occurs when the CO_2 is too low, causing the pH to rise above 7.45. It can be caused by the following:

- Hyperventilation
- Extreme anxiety
- High fever
- Sepsis
- Hypoxemia

Metabolic acidosis occurs when the HCO_3^- is low, causing the pH to fall below 7.35. It can be caused by the following:

- Anaerobic metabolism
- Lactic acidosis
- Diabetic ketoacidosis
- Anoxia
- Poisoning
- Overdose

Metabolic alkalosis occurs when the HCO_3^- is high, causing the pH to rise above 7.45. It can be caused by the following:

- Excessive vomiting
- Poisoning or overdose
- Antacid ingestion (most common)

Mixed diagnoses do occur. This mixed picture occurs when the client has multiple system conditions and experiences both respiratory and metabolic imbalances.

Hyperkalemia may occur in an acidotic state as the hydrogen ion drives the potassium ion out of the cell into the ECF. Once the acidosis is resolved, the hyperkalemia resolves. Acid–base imbalances are listed in Table 9.5.

IMMUNE SYSTEM DYSFUNCTION

Overview of the Immune System

The immune system has three lines of defence. Chemical and mechanical barriers such as the skin, GI tract, and mucous membranes are the first line of defence. The second line is the inflammatory response, and the third line is the immune response. The immune response is slower to develop as it is more specific and can result in permanent protection.

Central lymphoid organs include the thymus gland and bone marrow. Peripheral lymphoid organs include the tonsils; gut-, genital-, bronchial-, and skin-associated lymphoid tissues; lymph nodes; and spleen (Tyerman & Cobbett, 2023). The two immunity classifications are innate (natural) and acquired. Innate immunity is present in a person who has not been in contact with an antigen (a substance that elicits an immune response). Active acquired immunity is the consequence of an invasion of the body by foreign substances, such as microbes, and the subsequent development of antibodies and sensitized lymphocytes. Passive acquired immunity is one in which the host receives antibodies to an antigen, rather than synthesizing them, as with the immunoglobulins passed from mother to fetus.

Humoral immunity is made up of antibody-mediated immunity. This type of immunity is from antibodies that are produced in plasma (differentiated B lymphocytes [B cells]). B lymphocytes, formed in the bone marrow, will differentiate into plasma cells when activated. These plasma cells will produce antibodies (immunoglobulins IgA, IgG, IgM, IgD, IgE) that will recognize and attack antigens. The primary immune response is seen 4 to 8 days after the first contact with the antigen. When the individual is exposed to the antigen a second time, a secondary antibody response occurs. This response will occur faster, is stronger, and will last longer than the primary response (Tyerman & Cobbett, 2023).

Cell-mediated immunity is initiated through specific antigen recognition by T lymphocytes, or T cells. T lymphocytes develop from cells that migrate from the bone marrow to the thymus, where they differentiate. These T cells respond directly to specific targets (antigens). T cytotoxic cells attack antigens on the cell membrane of the foreign pathogens, releasing cytolytic substances that destroy the pathogen. T helper lymphocytes (CD4s) and T suppressor lymphocytes (CD8s) play a role in the regulation of cell-mediated immunity and the humoral antibody response. Natural killer cells (NK cells) are not T or B cells but are large lymphocytes that do not require prior sensitization. NK cells recognize and kill virus-infected cells, tumour cells, and transplanted grafts. Cell-mediated immunity plays an important role against pathogens that survive inside cells, as well as in tumour immunity, fungal infections, the rejection of transplanted tissues, and contact hypersensitivity reactions.

Cells involved in the immune response include mononuclear phagocytes, lymphocytes, including B lymphocytes and all forms of T lymphocytes (T cytotoxic cells, T helper cells, and T suppressor cells), and NK cells. Cytokines are soluble factors secreted by white blood cells (WBCs) and a variety of other cells in the body that act as messengers between the immune cell types.

Inflammation

Inflammation provides protection against the effects of cell injury. Regardless of the injury, the response is the same. The inflammatory agent will be diluted and neutralized, necrotic materials will be removed, and an environment will be established that supports healing and repair. The inflammatory response can be caused by heat, radiation, trauma, chemical injury, microbial injury, ischemic injury, allergens, and normal body fluids. The intensity of the response depends on the extent and severity of the injury and the health of the injured or ill person. The inflammatory response comprises a vascular response and a cellular response.

Vascular Response

After cell injury, the following vascular changes occur:

- Arterioles in the area briefly undergo transient vasoconstriction.
- Histamines and other chemicals are released from the injured cells, resulting in vasodilation.
- Vasodilation and chemical mediators increase capillary permeability, allowing fluid to move from the capillaries to the tissues.
- Initially, fluid is serous but later contains plasma proteins, primarily albumin, which exert oncotic pressure that draws additional fluid from the blood vessels.
- As the plasma protein fibrinogen leaves the blood, it is activated to form fibrin by-products of the injured cells. This fibrin strengthens a blood clot formed by platelets. The purpose of the clot is to ensnare bacteria and prevent them from spreading. The clot also serves as a frame for the healing process (Tyerman & Cobbett, 2023).

Cellular Response

In the cellular response to an injury, the following events occur:

- Blood flow through capillaries in the injured area slows.
- Neutrophils are first to arrive at the injury site (at 6–12 hours), and they phagocytize (engulf) foreign material and damaged cells.
- Monocytes arrive within 3 to 7 days after the onset of inflammation. They transform into macrophages, which are necessary for cleaning the area so that healing can occur. Unlike neutrophils, which have a short lifespan, macrophages have a long lifespan, can multiply, and may stay in the damaged tissues for weeks.
- Lymphocytes have a primary role related to humoral and cell-mediated immunity.
- Eosinophils are active during an allergic reaction, releasing chemicals that act to control the effects of histamine and serotonin, as well as phagocytizing allergen–antibody complexes.
- Basophils carry histamine and heparin, which are released during inflammation.
- Chemical mediators include histamine, serotonin, kinins, complement components, fibrinopeptides, prostaglandins, and leukotrienes, as well as cytokines.

Understanding Inflammation and Its Treatment

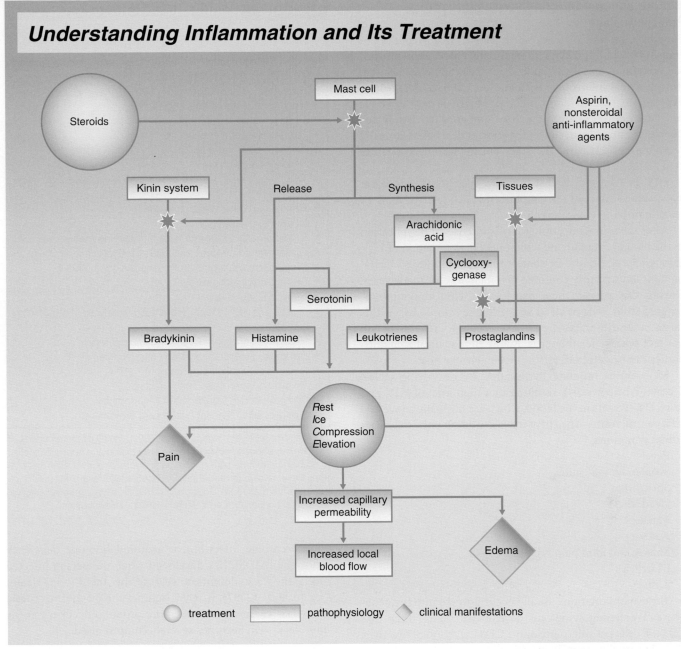

Fig. 9.1 Understanding inflammation and its treatments. (From Black, J. M., & Hawks, J. H. [2009]. *Medical-surgical nursing: Clinical management for positive outcomes* [8th ed., p. 306]. Saunders.)

The complement system is the primary mediator of the inflammatory response. The most important functions of this system are increased phagocytosis, increased vascular permeability, cellular lysis, and chemotaxis.

Prostaglandins are substances that can be produced from the phospholipids of the cell membranes of most body tissues, including blood cells. Prostaglandins are powerful vasodilators that cause increased permeability. Exudates made up of fluid and leukocytes move from the circulation to the site of injury. The nature and quantity of exudates depend on the type and severity of the injury and the tissues involved (Tyerman & Cobbett, 2023).

Local clinical manifestations of inflammation include the following:

- Redness
- Heat
- Pain
- Swelling
- Loss of function
  Systemic clinical manifestations include the following:
- Leukocytosis with a shift to the left
- Malaise
- Nausea
- Anorexia
- Increased heart rate and respiratory rate
- Fever
  See Figure 9.1 for more on inflammation and its treatment.

Human Immunodeficiency Virus Infection

Pathophysiology

Human immunodeficiency virus (HIV) is a fragile virus transmitted only through contact with blood, semen, vaginal secretions, and breast milk. The virus can be transmitted during sexual intercourse with an infected partner; through exposure to infected blood, blood products, or needles; or via pregnancy and breastfeeding. The number of newly infected people continue to decline each year and people with HIV receiving antiretroviral therapies are living longer (Dames et al., 2021).

HIV is a retrovirus that binds to specific CD4 receptor sites on the surface of the lymphocytes (also referred to as *T4 cells*) in order to enter the cell.

After the initial infection, there is intense viral replication in the blood (viremia) and widespread dissemination of HIV throughout the body. In some situations, the level of HIV remains low and may continue to remain low for many years. During this period, there may be few clinical symptoms, ranging from none at all to severe flulike symptoms. At this stage, antibodies are not being developed yet, so the client will not test positive for the virus. By the time neutralizing antibodies can be detected, HIV is thriving in the host.

HIV causes immune dysfunction by destroying CD4+ T-cells (T helper cells), resulting in a high level of HIV and low CD4+ counts in the blood, which are normally above 800 cells per microlitre. The client may now develop the following flulike symptoms:

- Fever
- Swollen lymph glands
- Sore throat
- Headaches
- Malaise
- Nausea
- Muscle and joint pain
- Diarrhea
- Rash

These manifestations usually occur 3 weeks into the acute phase. Worsening symptoms develop with fewer than 200 CD4+ T cells per microlitre and a CD4+ fraction of less than 15%. Eventually in HIV infection, so many CD4+ T cells are destroyed that not enough remain to regulate immune response (Tyerman & Cobbett, 2023).

Clinical Manifestations

Early chronic infection can last about 10 years and is defined as the stage at which the CD4+ T-cell counts remain above 500 cells per microlitre. In this stage, the clients often feel relatively well, with symptoms ranging from none to headache, low-grade fever, and night sweats.

Intermediate chronic infection is marked by a drop in the CD4+ T-cell count to 200 to 500 cells per microlitre. Earlier symptoms become worse. Fever is persistent, night sweats are excessive, diarrhea may be constant, and fatigue is severe. With the CD4+ count dropping, opportunistic diseases such as oral hairy leukoplakia, *Candida* infections, and Kaposi's sarcoma may develop.

BOX 9.2   Diagnostic Criteria for AIDS

AIDS is diagnosed when an individual with HIV develops at least one of these conditions:

- HIV wasting syndrome (*wasting* is defined as a loss of 10% or more of ideal body mass)
- *Pneumocystis* pneumonia
- Recurrent bacterial pneumonia
- Chronic herpes simplex virus infection
- Esophageal candidiasis
- Extrapulmonary tuberculosis
- Kaposi's sarcoma
- Cytomegalovirus disease (other than liver, spleen, or lymph nodes)
- Central nervous system toxoplasmosis
- HIV encephalopathy
- Extrapulmonary cryptococcosis (including meningitis)
- Disseminated nontuberculous mycobacteria infection
- Progressive multifocal leukoencephalopathy (PML)
- Chronic cryptosporidiosis
- Chronic isosporiasis
- Disseminated mycosis (coccidiomycosis or histoplasmosis)
- Recurrent nontyphoid *Salmonella* bacteremia
- Lymphoma (cerebral or B-cell non-Hodgkin's)
- Invasive cervical carcinoma
- Atypical disseminated leishmaniasis
- Symptomatic HIV-associated nephropathy
- Symptomatic HIV-associated cardiomyopathy

Source: World Health Organization. (2007). *WHO case definitions of HIV for surveillance and revised clinical staging and immunological classification of HIV-related disease in adults and children.* https://apps.who.int/iris/bitstream/handle/10665/43699/9789241595629_eng.pdf; Tyerman, J., & Cobbett, S. (2023). *Lewis's medical surgical nursing in Canada* (5th ed.), Table 17.10, p. 290. Elsevier.

Late chronic infection, or acquired immune deficiency syndrome (AIDS), has developed when the person infected meets the case definition set out by the World Health Organization (2007). Box 9.2 outlines the diagnostic criteria for AIDS. These criteria are more prone to occur when the immune system becomes severely compromised.

Diagnostics

Several screening tests are used to diagnose HIV infection, while other tests are used to assess the stage and severity of the infection. Screening tests for HIV-specific antibodies include the following:

- Enzyme immunoassay (EIA), formerly called *enzyme-linked immunosorbent assay*, is undertaken.
- If the blood is found to be positive for antibodies, the test is repeated.
- If the blood continues to test positive for antibodies, the Western blot or immunofluorescence assay test is done to confirm seropositivity from the EIA test.
- If the blood proves positive in all tests, the individual is considered to be HIV positive.

However, there is a period of up to 2 months during which antibodies may not be detected.

To monitor the stage, severity, and effectiveness of treatment of the HIV infection, CD4+ T-cell counts as well as laboratory tests measuring viral activity are done throughout the course of the infection. Viral load testing counts the number of viral particles in a sample of blood. New "rapid" HIV-antibody tests are now available that provide results in 20 minutes (Tyerman & Cobbett, 2023).

Therapeutics

Protocols of care change often as new knowledge about both the infection and the treatment develop. However, collaborative management of the HIV-infected person still focuses on monitoring the following:

- HIV disease progression
- Immune function
- Acute retroviral treatment
- Development of opportunistic diseases
- Symptoms
- Preventing or decreasing the complications of treatment

There is no cure for HIV. Therefore, HIV continues for the rest of the client's life, causing increasing physical disability, impaired health, and eventual death. Although there is no cure, signs and symptoms can be managed with treatment.

Primary therapy for HIV infection includes six different types of antiretroviral medications:

- Protease inhibitors, such as tipranavir (Aptivus), indinavir (Crixivan), nelfinavir (Viracept), and atazanavir (Reyataz).
- Nucleoside reverse transcriptase inhibitors, such as zidovudine (AZT), didanosine (Videx-EC), abacavir (Ziagen), emtricitabine (Emtriva), and lamivudine (3TC)
- Nonnucleoside reverse transcriptase inhibitors, such as nevirapine (Viramune) and delavirdine (Rescriptor)
- Nucleotide reverse transcriptase inhibitors such as tenofovir disoproxil fumarate (Viread)
- Integrase inhibitors, such as dolutegravir (Tivicay) and raltegravir (Isentress)
- Fusion inhibitors, such as enfuvirtide (Fuzeon) and maraviroc (Celsentri)

These medications are used in various combinations and are designed to suppress the viral replication process. The medications can be toxic, and the client must be monitored for these toxicities. Other drug therapies used in AIDS include immunomodulatory medications that are designed to boost the weakened immune system and antimicrobial and antineoplastic agents that are used to combat opportunistic infections and associated cancers.

Health promotion focuses on prevention of HIV by decreasing the risks related to sexual practices, drug use, and perinatal transmission, and by encouraging abstinence or safer-sex practices.

The risk of a client with HIV/AIDS transmitting HIV to a sexual contact is reduced if the individual:

- Is engaged in treatment and regularly taking antiretrovirals
- Has a suppressed viral load (meaning that high levels of the virus are not detected in that person's blood) for 6 months or more
- Has no other sexually transmitted infection
- Is undergoing regular monitoring of the HIV infection (Fournier & Karachiwalla, 2021).

The client with HIV/AIDS is likely to develop infections and cancers that will have an effect on their ability to cope psychosocially and economically. As with most chronic diseases, most of the nursing care will take place in the client's home. Family members and those people caring for a client with HIV/AIDS need to understand that the client will be anxious, fearful, and depressed at times and may develop a variety of symptoms, such as diarrhea, pain, nausea, vomiting, and fatigue, throughout the course of their disease. Symptom management is important.

Some clients may develop metabolic disorders, such as dyslipidemia, insulin resistance, and bone disease. The caregiver must be knowledgeable in assessing the client so that early detection and treatment can take place. Dementia often is present in the final stages of HIV.

Nursing Considerations

Assessment is important in order to identify persons at risk for HIV. Individuals should be asked if they received blood products before 1985 or shared needles, syringes, or other injection equipment with another person. They need to be asked whether they have had sexual experience with their penis, vagina, rectum, or mouth in contact with these areas of another person. Information regarding the client's history of diagnosed sexually transmitted infection is important.

Ongoing health and psychosocial assessment is paramount. Education about HIV should include what the infection is, how it is transmitted, treatment, preventing transmission, improving health, and family planning. Initially, the client may be in denial or shock, so the information needs to be repeated.

Assessment is dependent on the stage of the disease; focuses on prevention, treatment, or terminal-phase care; and must include social factors such as self-esteem, sexuality, family interactions, and finances.

The client should be encouraged to adhere to the medication regimens, to maintain a healthy lifestyle, to prevent opportunistic infections, and, most importantly, to prevent transmission to others. This plan requires developing supportive relationships, encouraging the client to maintain activity, and eventually to come to terms with issues related to living with HIV/AIDS and death and spirituality. Health care professionals should incorporate "treatment as prevention" practices which is advocating for people to get tested and treated, as well as following up with people who are potentially exposed (Fournier & Karachiwalla, 2021).

In the terminal stages of HIV, palliative care is important to provide comfort and support to the client and the family. See Chapter 13, "End-of-Life Care" for further nursing considerations.

CANCER OVERVIEW

Pathophysiology

Cancer is an umbrella term for a group of disorders in which certain cells grow and multiply uncontrollably. Cancer cells

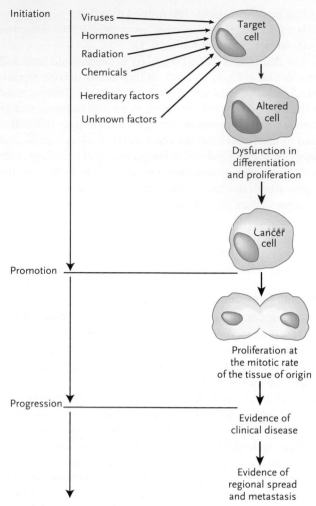

Fig. 9.2 Process of cancer development. (From Tyerman, J., & Cobbett, S. [2023]. *Lewis's medical-surgical nursing in Canada: Assessment and management of clinical problems* [5th Cdn. ed., p. 310, Figure 18-3]. Elsevier.)

are characterized by the loss of contact inhibition. They have altered recognition and adhesion and altered anchorage-dependent growth, have lost their restrictive point control, and keep on dividing. These cells do not stay put but invade other cells and are viable in blood and lymph fluid.

Cellular differentiation is normally an orderly process in which the cell progresses from a state of immaturity to a state of maturity. Malignant cells do not resemble their parent cells; they take on more of the appearance and some of the behaviours of fetal cells. The appearance of the cell and the degree of differentiation of the cell help classify the cancer. The less differentiated the cell is from the normal cell, the worse the grade of classification is. Normal cellular differentiation is illustrated in Figure 9.2.

Proto-oncogenes are normal cellular genes that are important regulators of normal cellular processes. Mutations that alter their expression can activate them to act as oncogenes, tumour-inducing genes that promote the development of cancer. Tumour-suppressor genes help suppress the growth of tumours, and render mutation inactive. Malignant tumours

are able to metastasize, infiltrate, and expand; they frequently recur and have moderate to marked vascularity.

In many cases, the exact cause of cancer is unknown; however, specific factors have been implicated as causing genetic mutations. External stimuli include the following:
- Chemical carcinogens, such as tobacco smoke, arsenic, vinyl chloride benzene, exposure to viruses, and exposure to ultraviolet light
- A diet high in fat and low in fibre, which encourages the development of colon cancer
- Genetic abnormalities that affect the presence of oncogenes, proto-oncogenes, and tumour-suppressor genes
- Chromosomal abnormalities, such as increased number (as in Down syndrome), deletion, translocation, and breakage of chromosomes, have been found to be present with cancer development.

Stages of Cancer Development

Cancer development follows a three-stage pattern: initiation, promotion, and progression.

First stage: Initiation. The first stage begins with the "initiation," when the mutation of the cell's genetic structure first occurs. Carcinogens can initiate this mutation. This is the event that causes the change in the cell. The cell is still functioning normally but has the potential to develop into a clone of a neoplastic cell (Tyerman & Cobbett, 2023).

Second stage: Promotion. The promotion stage is characterized by the reversible proliferation of altered cells. A cancer cell is not a health threat unless it can divide. Lifestyle choices such as obesity, diet, and smoking can enhance promotion. If these behaviours improve, the promotion may be reversible. If not, the initial genetic alteration proceeds to clinical cancer (Tyerman & Cobbett, 2023).

Third stage: Progression. The progression stage is characterized by the increased growth rate of the tumour, as well as its invasiveness and metastasis. As progression continues, the malignant tumour will develop its own blood supply (angiogenesis). Figure 9.2 illustrates the process of this development.

The body's immune system will attempt to reject or destroy cancer cells if they are perceived as nonself. This attempt may be inadequate, however, as the cancer cells arise from normal human cells that the immune system may perceive as self. Some cancers cells have changes on their surface, called *tumour-associated antigens* (TAAs). The response to TAAs is termed *immunological surveillance.* Lymphocytes continually check cell surfaces and detect and destroy cells with abnormalities. T cytotoxic cells, NK cells, macrophages, and B lymphocytes are involved. However, there are mechanisms by which cancer cells evade the immune system by suppressing factors that stimulate the T cells. Sometimes weak surface antigens allow cancer cells to "sneak through" surveillance. The cancer cells may develop a tolerance to the immune system. There may be a suppression of the immune response to products secreted by cancer cells, and antibodies that bind with TAAs may be blocked (Tyerman & Cobbett, 2023).

Children develop different cancers than adults. Pediatric cancers are usually embryonic in origin or due to oncogenes.

The child's immune system is less mature, and treatment protocols tend to be much longer than adult treatment protocols. See the section "Cancer" in Chapter 11, page 386.

Clinical Manifestations

Clinical manifestations are dependent on the type of cancer, the stage of its development, and its metastatic progression.

Diagnostics

Diagnosis involves the following:
- History and physical examination
- Blood work
- Biopsy
- Tumour markers (oncofetal antigens)
- X-ray, computed tomography (CT), and magnetic resonance imaging (MRI)
- Ultrasonography and nuclear medicine
- Visualization via scopes
- Definitive diagnosis is done by biopsy. A biopsy of the suspected tumour is helpful only if the cancer is going to be treated.

Cancers are classified according to the following:
- Tissue of origin
- Anatomical site
- Degree of differentiation
- How closely the cancer cell resembles its parent cell

Some cancers are classified according to their receptor status, such as breast cancer; chromosomal abnormalities, including chronic myelogenous leukemia (CML), characterized by the Philadelphia chromosome; and tumour markers, such as those present in testicular cancer.

Therapeutics and Nursing Considerations

Cancer treatment goals include cure, in which the cancer is eradicated; control, in which containment of the tumour is attempted to prolong and improve quality of life; and palliation, which focuses on comfort and the relief of symptoms. Factors that determine treatment modality depend on cell type, location and size of the tumour, and extent of the disease. The physiological and psychological status of the client and their expressed needs must also determine treatment. Cancer treatment can involve one or more of the following:
- Surgery
- Radiation
- Chemotherapy
- Biological therapy

Surgical therapy is used to cure or control the disease process or for palliative reasons. When surgery is done, a margin of normal tissue surrounding the tumour will be removed, as well as the tumour itself. Preventive measures are used to reduce the risk of surgical seeding of the cancer cells. The usual sites of regional spread may also be removed.

Radiation therapy involves the use of high-energy particles or waves to treat the cancer. When radiation is used, many factors must be considered. The type of cell determines whether radiation will be beneficial. Malignant melanomas are not sensitive to radiation, whereas Hodgkin's disease is highly sensitive to radiation. The cycle of cell division also must be considered. Cells in the mitosis (M) and RNA synthesis (G_2) cycles are more sensitive to radiation than at other times within the cell division process. Well-oxygenated cells, as well as rapidly dividing cells, are more sensitive to radiation. The radiation breaks the chemical bonds in DNA, causing loss of the proliferative capacity. The radiologist will decide on a tumoricidal dose that can be delivered within the limits of tolerance of the surrounding tissues. Radiation is considered local therapy and will affect tissues directly radiated. Radiation can be delivered by external beam (teletherapy) or internal radiation (brachytherapy). Radiolabelled antibodies may also be used. The number of treatments will depend on the type of cancer, extent of the disease, area to be treated, dose, and fractionation, which is the administration of a course of therapeutic treatments planned as a series of fractions of the total prescribed dose. Side effects are related to damage to the normal cells in and around the treatment field. Factors affecting the development of side effects include the following:
- Tumour location
- Dose of radiation needed
- Method of delivery
- Individual factors

The destruction of the cells and the body's attempt to rid itself of the dead cells will cause fatigue. Anorexia may develop. Skin reactions may occur, and precautions should be taken in the proper care of the skin, such as using warm water, mild soap, and no antiperspirant or perfume.

The goal of chemotherapy is to reduce the number of cancer cells in the tumour site(s). Cancer cells are not sensitive to some chemotherapeutic agents when the cell is in the resting phase. Chemotherapy attacks rapidly dividing cells systemically. Because chemotherapy is systemic therapy, the adverse effects are different from the adverse effects of radiation. Some chemotherapeutic agents have known adverse effects, and these should be managed aggressively. Chemotherapeutic agents also have less common, unexpected toxicities, and the client should be carefully assessed to allow for early identification. Refer to Table 9.6 for details of nursing management of adverse effects of radiation therapy and chemotherapy.

Complications of cancer include the following:
- Malnutrition
- Altered taste sensation
- Infection
- Superior vena cava syndrome
- Spinal cord compression
- Third space syndrome
- Syndrome of inappropriate antidiuretic hormone (SIADH)
- Hypercalcemia
- Tumour lysis syndrome
- Cardiac tamponade
- Carotid artery rupture

Leukemia

Pathophysiology

Leukemia is a generalized term used to describe complex cancers of the blood that affect the blood and blood-forming

TABLE 9.6   Nursing Management of Conditions Caused by Radiation Therapy and Chemotherapy.

Condition	Cause	Nursing Management
Gastrointestinal System		
Stomatitis, mucositis, esophagitis	Destruction of cells in radiation treatment field. Destruction of epithelial cells by chemotherapy. Inflammation and ulceration, which result from rapid cell destruction.	Be aware that eating, swallowing, and talking may be difficult and necessitate changes in diet and fluid intake. Encourage client to use artificial saliva. Assess the mucosa daily. Teach the client to do this and encourage the client to practice good oral hygiene. Use evidence informed guidelines and protocols to minimize the occurrence or reduce the severity or oral mucositis. Discourage use of irritants such as tobacco and alcohol, spicy foods, and drinks. Apply topical anaesthetics such as lidocaine (Xylocaine Viscous) or oxethazaine.
Nausea and vomiting	Cellular breakdown, which stimulates vomiting centre in the brain. Drugs that stimulate vomiting centre. Destruction of GI lining by radiation and chemotherapy.	Counsel the patient to eat and drink when not nauseated. Administer antiemetics and teach the patient and family caregiver when to use antiemetic therapy to maximize symptom control.
Anorexia	Release of TNF and IL-1 from macrophages, which has appetite-suppressant effect. General reaction to therapy.	Use diversional activities (if appropriate). Monitor the client's weight. Encourage the client to eat small, frequent meals of high-protein, high-calorie foods (e.g., Ensure or supplements). Reassure family caregivers and teach them to provide gentle encouragement to the patient.
Diarrhea	Denuding of epithelial lining of intestines	Suggest low-fibre diet, low residue diet. Increase fluids. Provide antidiarrheal agents as required.
Constipation	Autonomic nervous system dysfunction. Neurotoxic effects of plant alkaloids (vincristine, vinblastine). Use of opioids.	Encourage the client to keep a record to monitor bowel movements and report to the health care team as needed. Provide stool softeners and laxatives as needed. Encourage intake of high-fibre foods.
Hepatotoxicity	Toxic effects from chemotherapy drugs	Monitor liver function lab values.
Hematological System		
Anemia	Bone marrow depressed due to therapy. Malignant infiltration of bone marrow by cancer	Monitor hemoglobin and hematocrit levels. Encourage intake of foods that promote RBC production (e.g., green leafy vegetables, okra, meat, liver, fish, legumes, whole grains, orange juice, peanuts, lentils, avocado).
Leukopenia	Depression of bone marrow due to chemotherapy or radiation therapy. Febrile neutropenia. Infection resulting from immune suppression (main cause of morbidity or death in clients with cancer. Infection mainly in the genitourinary or respiratory systems	Monitor WBC count, especially the neutrophils. Educate and counsel clients and family caregivers to do the following: • Monitor changes in temperature and report any elevation to the health care providers immediately. • Advise the client to maintain good personal hygiene, including frequent handwashing. • Recommend that the client report any signs of infection (swelling, unusual cough, vomiting, severe headache, redness) immediately to the nearest hospital. • Advise the client to avoid large crowds and people with infections and encourage masking.

TABLE 9.6   Nursing Management of Conditions Caused by Radiation Therapy and Chemotherapy.—cont'd

Condition	Cause	Nursing Management
Thrombo-cytopenia	Bone marrow depression secondary to chemotherapy. Malignant infiltration of bone marrow, Spontaneous bleeding, which can occur with platelet counts at or below 20 x 10^9/L	Observe for signs of bleeding (e.g., petechiae, ecchymosis). Monitor hemoglobin, hematocrit, and platelet counts. Recommend use of a soft-bristle toothbrush and electric razor.
Integumentary System		
Alopecia (usually temporary with chemotherapy and usually permanent in response to radiation.	Destruction of hair follicles by chemotherapy or radiation to scalp.	Offer supports to help to cope with hair loss (e.g., hairpieces, scarves, wigs). Discuss effects of hair loss on body image. Recommend cutting long hair before therapy. Advise the client to avoid excessive shampooing, brushing and combing of hair. Recommend avoiding use of electronic hair dryers, curlers, and curling irons.
Skin reactions	Extravasation of vesicant chemotherapeutic drugs. Radiation therapy damage to skin.	Protect the client from extravasation through careful attention to delivery of chemotherapeutic drugs and assess of venous access. Recommend lubricating dry skin with non irritating creams. Recommend avoid use of harsh soaps. Advise client to wear loose clothing and cotton underwear and to avoid tight garments. Inform client of possible photosensitivity reactions.
Genitourinary System		
Cystitis	Destruction of cells lining the bladder by chemotherapy Adverse effects of radiation when located in the treatment region	Monitor manifestations such as urgency, frequency, and hematuria. Discuss these changes with the client.
Reproductive dysfunction	Damage of cells of ova or testes by therapy	Provide health teaching about the effects on fertility and referral to fertility resources (e.g., sperm banking) before delivery of radiation to the pelvis, high-dose chemotherapy, or bone marrow transplantation.
Nephrotoxicity	Accumulation of drugs in the kidney, and tumour lysis, which cause necrosis of proximal renal tubules.	Monitor BUN and serum creatine lab values.
Nervous System		
Increased intracranial pressure	Radiation related edema in the central nervous system	Administer steroids and pain medication. Monitor neurological status.
Peripheral neuropathy	Paresthesias, areflexia, skeletal muscle weakness, and smooth muscle dysfunction, which can occur as adverse effects of plant alkaloids and cisplatin	Monitor for such symptoms in clients receiving these medications.
Respiratory System		
Pneumonitis (develops 2-3 months after the start of treatment). Fibrosis (develops after 6-12 months and is evident on X-rays).	Radiation. Adverse effects of some chemotherapeutic drugs.	Monitor for dry, hacking cough, fever, and exertional dyspnea.
Cardiovascular System		
Pericarditis and myocarditis (complication when chest wall is irradiated; may occur up to 1 year after treatment).	Inflammation secondary to radiation injury. Adverse effects of some chemotherapeutic drugs.	Monitor for clinical symptoms of these disorders. Monitor heart function with ECG studies and cardiac ejection fractions.

Continued

TABLE 9.6   Nursing Management of Conditions Caused by Radiation Therapy and Chemotherapy.—cont'd

Condition	Cause	Nursing Management
Cardiotoxicity	Some chemotherapeutic drugs (e.g., doxorubicin, daunorubicin) can cause ECG changes and rapidly progressive heart failure.	Medication therapy may have to be modified.
Biochemical		
Hyperuricemia, secondary gout, and obstructive uropathy.	Cell destruction by chemotherapy	Monitor uric acid levels in bloodwork. Allopurinol (Zyloprim) may be given as a prophylactic measure. Encourage high fluid intake.
Multidimensional Effects		
Fatigue	Increased metabolic rate. Anabolic processes that result in accumulation of metabolites from cell breakdown.	Provide health teaching to client that fatigue is an expected adverse effect of therapy, but that there are ways to manage fatigue such as sleep hygiene, moderate exercise, and pacing activities. Encourage the client to rest when fatigued, to maintain usual lifestyle patterns as closely as possible, and to pace activities in accordance with energy levels.
Pain	Compression or infiltration of tumour involving nerves. Inflammation, ulceration, or necrosis of tissues.	Refer to the analgesic ladder to provide basis for pain medication administration. Encourage health teaching on various alternative therapies like use of imagery, relaxation therapy, deep breathing exercise, etc.

BUN, Blood urea nitrogen (Serum urea (nitrogen); *ECG*, electrocardiographic; *GI*, gastro-intestinal; *IL-1*, interleukin 1; *RBC*, red blood cell; *TNF*, tumour necrosis factor; *WBC*, white blood cell.

Adapted from Tyerman, J., & Cobbett, S. (2023). *Lewis's medical-surgical nursing in Canada: Assessment and management of clinical problems* (5th Cdn. ed., p. 326, Table 18.14). Elsevier.

tissues of the bone marrow, lymph system, and spleen. Leukemia results in an accumulation of dysfunctional cells because of loss of regulation in cell division. Most leukemias result as a combination of several genetic and environmental factors, including chromosomal factors, immunological factors, viruses, and exposure to radiation or certain chemicals.

The classification of leukemia is based on the type of WBCs involved and on whether the condition is acute or chronic. Acute leukemia is characterized by the proliferation of immature cells. Chronic leukemia involves more mature forms of WBCs, and the disease onset is more gradual. Acute and chronic leukemias are classified as lymphocytic or myelogenous according to the predominant cell type (Tyerman & Cobbett, 2023). The four major types of leukemia are as follows:

- Acute myelogenous leukemia (AML)
- Acute lymphocytic leukemia (ALL)
- Chronic myelogenous leukemia (CML)
- Chronic lymphocytic leukemia (CLL)

Clinical Manifestations

The clinical manifestations of leukemia will vary. Essentially, symptoms relate to bone marrow failure and the formation of leukemic infiltrates. The leukemic cells will crowd out normal WBCs, RBCs, and platelets, causing anemia with associated fatigue, dyspnea, pallor, frequent infections and flulike

symptoms, and bleeding tendencies. As the abnormal WBCs continue to accumulate, they infiltrate the client's organs, leading to splenomegaly, hepatomegaly, lymphadenopathy, bone pain, meningeal irritation, and oral lesions (Tyerman & Cobbett, 2023).

Diagnostics

The definitive test for leukemia is bone marrow aspiration and biopsy, which will determine the cell type, the type of erythropoiesis, and the maturity of the leukopoietic and erythropoietic cells.

A complete blood count (CBC) will show decreased hemoglobin and hematocrit, a low platelet count, and an abnormal WBC count. A physical examination may reveal lymph node enlargement.

Therapeutics and Nursing Considerations

Treatment of the leukemia is dependent on the type. When possible, treatment will focus on achieving remission. Systemic chemotherapy is used to eradicate leukemic cells and induce remission, restoring normal bone marrow function. The type of chemotherapy will vary with the type of leukemia present. Other treatments may include the following:

- Antibiotics, antifungals, and antivirals to control infections
- Platelet transfusions to prevent bleeding

- Blood or RBC transfusions to treat the anemia
- For some clients, bone marrow transplantation

Hodgkin's Lymphoma

Pathophysiology

Hodgkin's lymphoma is a malignant lymphoma characterized by abnormal gigantic tumour cells called *Reed-Sternberg cells*, which are morphologically unique and thought to develop from immature lymphoid tissue. This lymphatic cancer initially develops in a single lymph node or chain of nodes. The disease then spreads in a predictable manner to nearby lymph tissue. If left unchecked, it will then spread to nonlymph tissue. All organs are susceptible to invasion as the disease progresses. The exact cause of Hodgkin's lymphoma is unclear, although key factors, such as infection with the Epstein–Barr virus, genetic predisposition, and exposure to occupational toxins, could be possible causes (Tyerman & Cobbett, 2023).

Clinical Manifestations

The onset of Hodgkin's lymphoma is usually insidious. The initial development is most often painless enlargement of one or more lymph nodes. As the disease progresses, the client may experience the following symptoms:

- Pruritus
- Persistent fever
- Night sweats
- Fatigue
- Weight loss
- Malaise
- Headaches
- Changes in mentation
- Seizures (Tyerman & Cobbett, 2023)

Diagnostics

Biopsy of the enlarged lymph nodes showing the presence of the Reed-Sternberg cell confirms the diagnosis. Other diagnostic tests should be done to rule out any infectious origin for the disease. A bone marrow biopsy will be done to identify the stage of the disease. Other tests will include a chest X-ray and a CT scan of the head, neck, chest, abdomen, and pelvis to look for possible spread of the disease.

Therapeutics and Nursing Considerations

Treatment will depend on the disease stage rather than the histological type and may include chemotherapy, radiation, or both.

Non-Hodgkin's Lymphoma

Pathophysiology

Non-Hodgkin's lymphoma (NHL) a group of malignant neoplasms of primarily B-, T- or natural-killer (NK)-cell origin that can affect people of all ages. The exact cause is unknown. It may result from chromosomal translocations, infections, environmental factors, or immunodeficiency states (Tyerman & Cobbett, 2023). NHLs usually develop in the lymph nodes or lymphatic tissue. NHLs involve lymphocytes arrested in various stages of development.

Clinical Manifestations

NHLs can origin outside the lymph nodes, the way it spreads is unpredictable, and the majority of clients have widely disseminated disease at the time of the diagnosis. The main symptom is painless enlarged lymph nodes. Other symptoms will present depending on where the disease has spread. Clients with high-grade lymphomas may have night sweats, fever, and weight loss. The peripheral blood is usually normal but some lymphoma manifest in a leukemic phase (Tyerman & Cobbett, 2023).

Diagnostics

The diagnostic testing is similar to that for Hodgkin's disease but the client may require more diagnostic tests due to the potential to spread to other areas of the body. Tests may involve: MRI scan to rule out CNS or bone marrow infiltration; barium enema or CT scan to rule out potential GI involvement. Clinical staging will help determine the course of treatment, but the establishment of the precise histological subtype is extremely important. Lymph node biopsy will determine cell type and the pattern (Tyerman & Cobbett, 2023).

Treatment and Nursing Considerations

Treatment is determined by the cell type, cytogenetic studies, and clinical behaviour: indolent (low grade), aggressive (high grade), or highly aggressive (very high grade). The International Prognostic Index (IPI) may be considered for each subtype to help determine the appropriate treatment for each client. Treatment involves chemotherapy and sometimes radiation. More aggressive lymphomas tend to be responsive to treatment whereas indolent lymphomas generally have a naturally long course but are difficult to treat effectively. Clients with indolent lymphoma may live for 10 years or more without treatment. Nursing care is similar to that for Hodgkin's lymphoma. The nursing care is centred on managing conditions related to the disease (for example pain caused by a tumour or spinal cord compression) and other adverse effects of therapy.

RESPIRATORY SYSTEM DYSFUNCTION

Asthma

Pathophysiology

Asthma is a chronic reactive airway disorder that is characterized by chronic inflammation, bronchoconstriction, and bronchial hyper-responsiveness, causing increased mucus production. There is often a family history of asthma, and symptoms can occur seasonally. Asthma is commonly accompanied by nocturnal flare-ups.

Extrinsic asthma results from exposure to sensitizing agents such as pollen, animal dander, house dust, or mould. Intrinsic asthma may result from the following causes:

- Irritants
- Emotional stress
- Fatigue
- Endocrine changes

- Cold temperatures
- Exposure to noxious fumes

Other triggers of asthma include but are not limited to the following:

- Exercise
- Nonsteroidal anti-inflammatory drugs (NSAIDs)
- Upper airway infections
- Food dye

The triggers initiate the inflammatory response that contributes to the airway inflammation, mucus production, and bronchoconstriction, all of which cause airway obstruction.

Clinical Manifestations

Symptoms of asthma may include the following:

- Intermittent attacks of dyspnea and wheezing
- Tightness of the chest
- Coughing that is productive of thick, clear, or yellow sputum
- Tachypnea, with the result that the client needs to use the accessory respiratory muscles to breathe
- Orthopnea, with clients sitting upright with shoulders hunched forward

Clients in severe distress may experience diaphoresis, cyanosis, pallor, and diminished breath sounds. Between attacks, the client will breathe normally.

Diagnostics

A history and physical examination revealing dyspnea, wheezing, and coughing are highly suggestive of asthma. Two main areas that must be looked at when considering a diagnosis of asthma are the client's symptoms and variable airflow.

Pulmonary function tests are helpful in determining the extent of the client's asthma. Other tests used in diagnosing asthma are spirometry testing, alternative lung testing and bronchoprovocation challenge testing. Chest X-rays are used to reveal complications of asthma such as pneumothorax, mucoid impaction, and atelectasis (Tyerman & Cobbett, 2023).

Therapeutics and Nursing Considerations

Treatment is usually tailored to each client and focuses on identifying and avoiding precipitating allergens and irritants. Primary drug therapy generally includes inhaled bronchodilators and steroids, either individually or in combination.

During an acute attack, respiratory function needs to be monitored closely while attempts are made to relieve the bronchoconstriction and expulsion of mucoid plugs. The client needs close supervision as they are likely to be frightened and need to have constant reassurance. The nursing considerations are as follows:

- Encourage the client to sit in a semi- or high Fowler's position.
- Encourage the client to breathe using the diaphragm.
- Inhaled salbutamol should be administered immediately. Inhaled beta$_2$-adrenergic agonists are preferably administered through a metered-dose inhaler with a spacer (a holding chamber that holds the medication for a few seconds

after it has been released from the inhaler) at a frequency of 4 to 8 puffs every 15 to 20 minutes, usually repeated three times. Ipratropium bromide may be added (4–8 puffs inhaled every 15–20 minutes, repeated three times) to salbutamol during moderate and severe acute asthma episodes. In emergency departments, bronchodilators may be administered via a nebulizer. Oral corticosteroids are required for treatment of an acute exacerbation that requires a visit to the emergency department. IV corticosteroids are usually administered to clients with difficulty swallowing (Tyerman & Cobbett, 2023).

- Deliver supplemental oxygen to keep arterial oxygen saturation above 92%.
- Monitor for "silent chest," an indication that the client may be progressing to status asthmaticus.
- Perform a chest assessment before and after bronchodilator inhalations.

If an asthma attack is severe and unresponsive to treatment the client may require mechanical ventilation (Tyerman & Cobbett, 2023).

Chronic Obstructive Pulmonary Disease
Pathophysiology

COPD is an umbrella term that refers to emphysema and chronic bronchitis, conditions characterized by airflow obstruction. COPD clients may have asthma as well. Exposure to tobacco smoke is the primary cause of COPD. Other risk factors include recurrent or chronic respiratory tract infections, allergies, and familial or hereditary factors, such as alpha-antitrypsin deficiency.

Smoking causes the following complications:

- Nicotine acts as a sympathetic nervous system (SNS) stimulant, causing vasoconstriction and increased heart rate, BP, and cardiac workload.
- Smoking decreases ciliary activity and increases proteolytic enzymes that destroy elastin and collagen and cause cellular hyperplasia. This increases the production of mucus, reduces the airway diameter, and increases the difficulty in clearing secretions.

Emphysema is an abnormal permanent enlargement of the air space distal to the terminal bronchioles accompanied by destruction of alveolar walls without obvious fibrosis. Emphysema pathology includes the following:

- Hyperinflation of the alveoli
- Destruction of alveolar walls (bullae development)
- Destruction of alveolar capillary walls
- Small airway collapse (air trapping)
- Loss of lung elasticity

Chronic bronchitis is diagnosed when an individual has had a productive cough for three or more months in each of two successive years. Figure 9.3 illustrates chronic bronchitis. Chronic bronchitis pathology includes the following:

- Hyperplasia of mucus-secreting glands in the trachea and bronchi
- An increase in the goblet cells
- Disappearance of cilia
- Chronic inflammatory changes

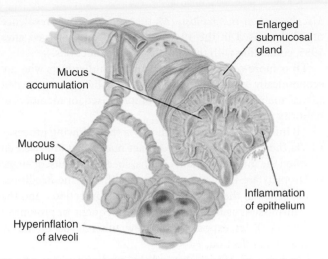

Fig. 9.3 Chronic bronchitis. (Modified from Des Jardins, T., & Burton, G. G. [1995]. Clinical manifestations and assessment of respiratory disease [3rd ed.]. Mosby.)

- Altered alveolar macrophage function
- Normal alveolar structures and capillaries

Clinical Manifestations

Clinical findings may be absent in the early stages of COPD. As the disease progresses, various symptoms develop depending on the underlying disease entity. Regardless of this underlying entity, progressive airflow obstruction will eventually lead to poor ventilation–perfusion, resulting in hypoxia. The client may experience barrel chest, cyanosis, and clubbing of the fingers and nails. Dyspnea is usually the first symptom to develop. In chronic bronchitis, cough is usually the first symptom to develop, and it may be either productive or nonproductive. The typical posture of persons with COPD is illustrated in Figure 9.4. Complications may include the following:

- Polycythemia
- Acidosis
- Pulmonary hypertension
- Cor pulmonale
- Acute respiratory failure

Diagnostics

Diagnosis is based on client history and physical examination. Pulmonary function tests may show an increase in residual volume, total lung capacity, and adherence, with decreased vital capacity, diffusing capacity, and forced expiratory volumes. Blood work may show polycythemia due to the hypoxia. A chest X-ray is not diagnostic for COPD or chronic bronchitis but is often necessary to rule out other conditions.

Therapeutics and Nursing Considerations

Treatment focuses on airway expansion and airway clearance with improved gas exchange. The treatments are as follows:

- Oxygen is administered at low-flow settings to ensure not to suppress the respiratory drive and to treat hypoxia These clients rely on low oxygen levels as their stimulus to breathe. Long term oxygen therapy (15 hours per day or

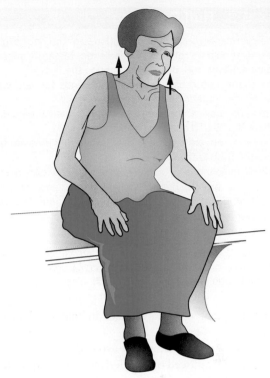

Fig 9.4 Typical posture of person with chronic obstructive pulmonary disease, primarily emphysema. The person tends to lean forward and uses the accessory muscles of respiration to breathe, forcing the shoulder girdle upward and causing the supraclavicular fossae to retract on inspiration.

more to achieve an oxygen saturation of 90% or greater) prolongs life in clients with hypoxemia.

- Antibiotics are prescribed to treat infections.
- Avoidance of smoking or air pollutants is encouraged.
- Bronchodilators are prescribed to relieve bronchospasm and facilitate mucociliary clearance. As with asthma, the preferred route of administration is inhalation because it targets the lungs directly.
- Steroids may be prescribed to reduce inflammation.
- Breathing techniques, such as pursed-lip breathing, are taught to control dyspnea and reduce air trapping.
- Diaphragmatic breathing, breathing using the muscles of the diaphragm rather than the accessory muscles, is also encouraged.
- Often huff coughing is taught to overcome ineffective cough patterns. Huff coughing is summarized in Box 9.3.

Nursing Considerations

Clients with severe COPD expend an increasing amount of energy doing the work of breathing. They can expend 30 to 50% more energy on breathing than the average person. Eating becomes an effort as a result of dyspnea. A full stomach presses up on the flattened diaphragm, causing increased dyspnea and discomfort. It is difficult for the client to eat and breathe at the same time (Tyerman & Cobbett, 2023).

- The client will need to be encouraged to rest prior to eating and again after eating.

BOX 9.3   Huff Coughing

1. The client assumes a sitting position with the neck slightly flexed, shoulders relaxed, knees flexed, forearms supported by a pillow, and, if possible, feet on the floor.
2. The client then drops the head and bends forward while using slow, pursed-lip breathing to exhale.
3. Sitting up again, the client uses diaphragmatic breathing to inhale slowly and deeply.
4. The client repeats steps 2 and 3 three to four times to facilitate the mobilization of secretions.
5. Before initiating a cough, the client should take a deep abdominal breath, bend slightly forward, and then huff cough (cough three to four times on exhalation). The client may need to support or splint their thorax or abdomen to achieve maximum effect.

Adapted from Tyerman, J., & Cobbett, S. L. (2023). *Lewis's medical-surgical nursing in Canada: Assessment and management of clinical problems* (5th Cdn. ed., p. 665, Table 31-17). Elsevier.

- Small, frequent meals are easier to tolerate than larger meals.
- Food that causes gas should be avoided.
- In some cases, pureed or blenderized food is easier for the client to tolerate.
- If there are no other medical conditions, the client should be encouraged to drink 3 L of fluid each day. Fluids should be offered between meals so that the client will eat a nutritious meal and then take the fluids.

COPD education focuses on the client maintaining the following:
- Effective airway clearance
- Effective gas exchange
- A balanced diet
- Adequate sleep
- Prevention of infection

To accomplish these goals, the client needs to be encouraged to be as physically active as their condition permits: walking each day, practising the breathing exercises, and practising energy-conserving strategies, such as assuming the tripod position (elbows supported on table and chest flexed) when tired. Relaxation techniques can be very beneficial to relieve dyspnea. Appropriate use of medications prior to an activity is helpful. Long-acting theophylline (Theolair) or a long-acting bronchodilator medication may be needed to assist the client during sleep. Oxygen therapy at low settings is frequently required for hypoxemia. Long-standing home oxygen settings are often needed for these clients.

Many lifestyle changes may occur during the progression of COPD. Clients may go through the stages of grief as more and more of their normal activities may be lost (Tyerman & Cobbett, 2023).

Tuberculosis
Pathophysiology

Tuberculosis (TB) is an acute or chronic infection characterized by pulmonary infiltrates and formation of granulomas with caseation, fibrosis, and cavitation. TB is caused by *Mycobacterium-tuberculosis (M. tuberculosis)*. The prevalence of TB decreased in the 1940s and 1950s but resurged after 1985, coinciding with the spread of HIV infections.

TB is more commonly found among individuals who are economically disadvantaged, homeless, living in crowded spaces, malnourished, immunocompromised, or members of minority groups.

TB infection is spread to others via the following process:
- Via the airborne route by droplet nuclei that are released when the infected person coughs, sneezes, speaks, or sings.
- Droplets are inhaled by the recipient, and the bacilli are deposited in the lung. TB is not highly infectious, and the transmission usually requires close, frequent, or prolonged contact. Brief exposure to a few tubercle bacilli rarely causes an infection.
- The immune system responds by sending leukocytes and macrophages to the area, ultimately resulting in encapsulation of the bacilli in the Ghon tubercle.
- At this stage, the client will demonstrate exposure to the TB bacilli via skin testing but does not have an active TB infection.
- If the tubercle and inflamed nodes rupture, the infection contaminates the surrounding tissue and may spread through the blood and lymphatic circulation to distant sites such as the kidneys, epiphyses of bone, cerebral cortex, or adrenal glands.
- Increase incidence of TB risk factors may be found in poor living conditions, homelessness and overcrowded spaces. "Populations most at risk in Canada are the Indigenous and immigrant populations" (Tyerman & Cobbett, 2023, p. 595).

Clinical Manifestations
- Clients in the early stages of TB are usually asymptomatic.
- Nonspecific symptoms such as fatigue, weakness, anorexia, weight loss, night sweats, and low-grade fever may develop as TB progresses.
- The client may experience cough, productive mucopurulent sputum, and chest pain.
- Hemoptysis develops in advanced cases.

Diagnostics
Definitive diagnosis is made by the following:
- Sputum cultures and stains
- Skin testing, which detects exposure to TB but does not distinguish between exposure and infection
- Chest X-rays, which may show nodular lesions, patchy infiltrates, cavity formation, scar tissue, and calcium deposits but which cannot distinguish between active or inactive TB
- Nucleic acid amplification, a new test that gives results within hours. However, this test does not replace smears and sputum cultures.
- Interferon gamma release assays is a blood test that provides rapid results in 24 hours and is an effective diagnostic tool in certain client populations.

Purified protein derivative (PPD) of tuberculin is used primarily to detect the delayed hypersensitivity immune response of the individual. Two-step testing (the Mantoux test) is recommended for initial testing for health care workers. Once a two-step test has been done, follow-up testing requires only the one-step test (Tyerman & Cobbett, 2023).

Therapeutics and Nursing Considerations

Prevention of TB is very important. If the living conditions of the client cannot be changed, immunization with Bacillus Calmette-Guérin (BCG) may be given to prevent TB. This is commonly done in the Northwest Territories and Nunavut.

Treatment for TB includes the following:

- Antitubercular therapy usually consists of a combination of at least four drugs that are administered for at least 6 months. The five primary medications used are isoniazid (INH), rifampin (RMP), pyrazinamide, streptomycin, and ethambutol.
- Combination therapy is used to increase the therapeutic effectiveness and decrease the development of resistant strains of *M. tuberculosis*.
- Newer medications that are sometimes used include ciprofloxacin (Cipro), ofloxacin (Floxin), sparfloxacin (Zagam), and rifapentine (Priftin), particularly when the client develops complications from one of the earlier antitubercular agents.

The client is taught health practices such as using tissues when coughing or sneezing, discarding the tissues in appropriate garbage containers, and washing hands after each cough and sneeze. Directly observed therapy (DOT) is now being used in many overcrowded areas to help ensure that the client takes the medications as instructed for the length of time they are needed. Nonadherence is a major factor in the emergence of multidrug resistance and treatment failures (Tyerman & Cobbett, 2023). Latent TB infection occurs when an individual becomes infected with *M. tuberculosis* but does not become acutely ill. INH is generally used to prevent a TB infection from developing into a clinical disease.

Acute Respiratory Distress Syndrome
Pathophysiology

Acute respiratory distress syndrome (ARDS) is a form of pulmonary edema that can lead to acute respiratory failure. ARDS results from the following:

- Increased permeability of alveolocapillary membrane, causing the alveoli to fill with fluid and resulting in severe dyspnea
- Hypoxemia refractory to supplemental oxygen
- Reduced lung compliance
- Diffuse pulmonary infiltrates
- Aspiration
- Infection or sepsis
- Lung trauma
- Head injury
- Embolism
- Oxygen toxicity
- Drug overdose of barbiturates
- Blood transfusion
- Smoke or chemical inhalation
- Pancreatitis uremia
- Near-drowning

Clinical Manifestations

With ARDS, the client will have rapid, shallow breathing, dyspnea, hypoxemia that does not respond to supplemental oxygen, tachycardia, intercostal and suprasternal retractions, crackles, and wheezing. The client will be restless, apprehensive, and then mentally sluggish, with motor dysfunction. As ARDS progresses, it is associated with profound respiratory distress requiring endotracheal intubation and positive pressure ventilation.

Diagnostics

The history and physical examination are important where risk factors can be ascertained. The following symptoms indicate ARDS:

- Acute onset of the distress
- Bilateral pulmonary infiltrates
- Clinical absence of heart failure

Therapeutics and Nursing Considerations

Treatment focuses on correcting the underlying cause of ARDS. Aggressive supportive care is usually required. Clients with ARDS are critically ill and require close monitoring and support.

Atelectasis
Pathophysiology

Atelectasis is a condition of the lungs that may be acute or chronic and that is characterized by collapse of the alveoli. In atelectasis, a blockage impedes the passage of air to and from the alveoli. The trapped alveolar air becomes absorbed into the bloodstream, and without any replacement air, that area of the lung becomes airless and collapses.

The prognosis depends on prompt treatment, including removal of the airway obstruction, relief of hypoxia, and re-expansion of the collapsed area of the lung. Possible causes of atelectasis include the following:

- Bronchial obstruction by excessive secretions, a mucus plug, or a foreign object. This is the most common cause.
- Cancer
- Oxygen toxicity, pulmonary edema, and conditions that inhibit full lung expansion

Clinical Manifestations

Signs and symptoms are variable and may include the following:

- Cough, sputum production, and fever
- In acute atelectasis, respiratory distress is evident, and dyspnea, tachypnea, pleural pain, and central cyanosis may also be present.

Diagnostics

Decreased breath sounds and crackles during auscultation are indicators of atelectasis. A chest X-ray may be done. Pulse oximetry is usually found to be below 90%.

Therapeutics and Nursing Considerations

Strategies to prevent the development of atelectasis and to minimize or treat it by improving ventilation include the following:

- Frequent turning in bed, early ambulation, and deep-breathing exercises
- Coughing or suctioning may be needed to remove secretions that could be causing obstruction.
- Bronchodilators may be ordered to assist with removal of the secretions.
- If a pleural effusion is present, a thoracentesis may be needed to remove fluid from the lung.

Pulmonary Embolism

Pathophysiology

A pulmonary embolism (PE) is an obstruction of a pulmonary artery or a branch of the artery by a thrombus that has developed in the venous circulation or right side of the heart from blood, amniotic fluid, air, fat, bone marrow, or foreign IV material.

- The most common source of the thrombus is the deep veins of the legs.
- The thrombus breaks loose and travels as an embolus until it lodges in the pulmonary vasculature.
- This thrombus can result in complete or partial occlusion of the pulmonary arterial blood flow.
- The lung tissue distal to the embolus is ventilated but not perfused.
- This ventilation–perfusion imbalance leads to an increase in pulmonary arterial pressure. This increases the work of the heart's right ventricle to maintain pulmonary blood flow, which could lead to right-sided heart failure.

Clinical Manifestations

The severity of clinical manifestations of PE depends on the size of the emboli and the size and number of blood vessels occluded. The most common manifestations of PE are as follows:

- Anxiety and the sudden onset of unexplained dyspnea and tachypnea
- Pleuritic chest pain that often mimics angina pain
- Cough, hemoptysis, and crackles
- Fever
- Changes in mentation

A massive embolus may produce sudden collapse of the client, with shock, pallor, severe dyspnea, and crushing chest pain. The pulse is likely to be rapid and weak, and the BP will be low. Death occurs in 60% of clients with massive PE, frequently within the first hour of symptom development.

Diagnostics

Diagnosis is based on the client's history and physical examination. The following tests are done to diagnose the embolism:

- Ventilation–perfusion scan
- Pulmonary angiography
- Chest X-ray
- Electrocardiography (ECG)
- Peripheral and arterial blood studies
- Plethysmography, depending on the amount of time available
- D-dimer level
- spiral (helical) CT scan

Therapeutics and Nursing Considerations

Treatment for PE should be instituted immediately. The objectives of treatment are to prevent further growth or multiplication of thrombi in the lower extremities, to prevent embolization from the upper or lower extremities to the pulmonary vascular system, and to provide cardiopulmonary support if indicated. The following treatments may be needed:

- Oxygen by mask or nasal cannula
- Mechanical ventilation
- Thrombolytic therapy may be used to dissolve clots.
- IV anticoagulant therapy will be initiated to prevent further clots from forming.
- Pulmonary embolectomy may be done in life-threatening situations.
  Nursing care will focus on the following considerations:
- Minimizing the risk for more thrombi development
- Monitoring anticoagulation therapy and thrombolytic therapy
- Managing pain
- Managing oxygen therapy
- Relieving anxiety
- Monitoring for complications
- Educating the client and family regarding ways to prevent further thrombi formation

Pneumothorax

Pathophysiology

A *pneumothorax* is air in the pleural space. There is a resultant complete or partial collapse of a lung due to the accumulation of this air. Pneumothorax may be closed or open and, when associated with trauma, may be accompanied by hemothorax, a condition called *hemopneumothorax*. A closed pneumothorax has no associated external wound. The most common form is a spontaneous pneumothorax, which is accumulation of air in the pleural space without an apparent reason. It is caused by the following conditions:

- Rupture of small blebs on the visceral pleural space
- Trauma
- TB
- COPD

Spontaneous pneumothorax may occasionally occur in lean adolescents and young clients with no apparent precipitating cause.

An open pneumothorax occurs when air enters the pleural space through an opening in the chest wall, such as a stab or gunshot wound. A penetrating chest wound is often referred to as a *sucking chest wound*. A *tension pneumothorax* is a pneumothorax with rapid accumulation of air in the pleural space causing severely high intrapleural pressures with resultant tension on the heart and great vessels. In tension pneumothorax, air that enters the pleural space during expiration does not exit during inspiration.

Clinical Manifestations

Pneumothorax may not produce symptoms in mild cases, but in moderate to severe cases, it may produce the following symptoms:

- Profound respiratory distress
- Weak rapid pulse, pallor, jugular vein distension
- Anxiety
- Severe chest pain accompanied by tachypnea
- Asymmetrical chest wall movement
- Dyspnea, cyanosis, decreased or absent chest sounds, or hyper-resonance on the affected side

Diagnostics

Diagnosis is made from a chest X-ray revealing air in the pleural space and a possible mediastinal shift. ABGs reveal hypoxemia and respiratory alkalosis. ECG changes may be present.

Therapeutics and Nursing Considerations

Treatment depends on the cause and severity of the pneumothorax.

- In mild cases, re-expansion can be achieved using a conservative approach, with bed rest, oxygen therapy, and close monitoring of the client's vital signs.
- In more severe cases, needle aspiration of the pleural space with a large-bore needle may be required.
- The most definitive and common form of treatment is to insert a chest tube and connect it to suction (usually 20 mm Hg suction). Repeated spontaneous pneumothorax may need to be treated surgically by a partial pleurectomy, stapling, or pleurodesis to promote adherence of the pleurae to one another.

Pneumonia

Pathophysiology

Pneumonia is an acute inflammation of the lungs that commonly impairs gas exchange. The inflammatory response causes fluid or blood to fill the lung tissue, creating an excellent environment for pathogens. The invading pathogen starts changing epithelial lung cells to allow it to adhere to the cell wall. The pathogen then destroys the macrophages that travel to the site, resulting in further congestion with decreased lung ventilation.

Pneumonia is more likely to result when

- Defence mechanisms are incompetent or become overwhelmed. Pneumonia is the leading cause of death in debilitated clients.
- There are infecting pathogens, either bacterial or viral, or chemical or other irritants, such as aspirated material.
- There are predisposing factors that increase the risk for pneumonia, including chronic illness, cancer, abdominal and thoracic surgery, atelectasis, aspiration, colds, COPD, smoking, alcoholism, malnutrition, chemotherapy, radiation, and immunosuppressive therapy.

- If there is onset in the community or within the first 2 days of hospitalization, it is referred to as *community-acquired pneumonia.*
- Hospital-acquired pneumonia is that which occurs 48 hours or longer after admission.
- The abnormal entry of secretions into the lower airway causes aspiration pneumonia. There is usually a history of unconsciousness in which the gag and cough reflexes are suppressed. Gastrostomy tube feeding also carries a risk for aspiration pneumonia.

A less severe form of pneumonia is often termed "walking pneumonia." These clients often respond well to treatment at home.

Complications of pneumonia may include the following:
- Pleurisy
- Pleural effusion
- Atelectasis
- Delayed resolution
- Lung abscess
- Empyema
- Pericarditis
- Arthritis
- Meningitis
- Endocarditis

Clinical Manifestations

Clinical manifestations vary depending on the cause of the pneumonia. Symptoms may include fever, chills, tachypnea, tachycardia, dyspnea, cough with production of purulent sputum, hypoxemia, possible pleuritic chest pain, and possible confusion or stupor.

Diagnostics

Diagnosis is suspected by the history and physical examination and confirmed with a chest X-ray showing infiltrates. Blood cultures and sputum smears will define the causative agent.

Therapeutics and Nursing Considerations

Treatment focuses on clearing the infection and improving gas exchange and may include the following:
- Antibiotic therapy
- Oxygen for hypoxemia
- Analgesics for chest pain
- Antipyretics
- Influenza drugs
- Inhaled bronchodilator and corticosteroid therapies
- Increased fluid intake
- Adequate caloric intake

Lung Cancer

Pathophysiology

Lung cancer is the leading cause of cancer-related deaths in Canada. It most commonly occurs in individuals over age 50 with a history of cigarette smoking. Smoking is responsible for 85% of all lung cancers in Canada (Tyerman & Cobbett, 2023). Other risk factors for the development of lung cancer include genetic predisposition and exposure to carcinogenic industrial or air pollutants, such as asbestos, uranium arsenic, chromates, radon, nickel, iron, iron oxides, second-hand smoke, and personal history of lung disease.

Ninety percent of lung cancers originate from the epithelium of the bronchus, developing squamous cell carcinoma. It takes 8 to 10 years for a tumour to reach 1 cm, the smallest lesion detectable on X-ray. The lesions usually occur on segmental bronchi and the upper lobes of the lung. Pathological changes in the bronchial system result in hypersecretion of mucus, desquamation of cells, reactive hyperplasia of basal cells, and metaplasia of normal respiratory epithelium to stratified squamous cells.

Lung cancers metastasize by direct extension, blood circulation, and the lymph system. Common sites for metastatic growth include the following:

- Liver
- Brain
- Bones
- Lymph nodes
- Adrenal glands (Tyerman & Cobbett, 2023)

Clinical Manifestations

Clinical manifestations appear late in the disease and depend on the type of primary lung cancer, location, degree of obstruction, and metastatic spread. The manifestations may include the following:

- Pneumonitis, persistent cough with sputum, and hemoptysis
- Chest pain
- Dyspnea
- Anorexia
- Fatigue
- Nausea and vomiting
- Hoarse voice
- Unilateral paralysis of diaphragm
- Dysphagia
- Palpable nodes in in the neck and axilla area

Diagnostics

Diagnostic studies include a chest X-ray, which can detect a tumour 2 years before it becomes symptomatic, as well as the following:

- CT scans, MRI, and positron emission tomography (PET) to help find metastatic tumours
- Sputum specimens obtained from fibre-optic bronchoscopy, mediastinoscopy, and video-assisted thoracoscopy for cytological studies
- Biopsy of the tumour, to provide the definitive diagnosis and allow for staging of the cancer

Therapeutics and Nursing Considerations

Treatment involves combinations of surgery, radiation, and chemotherapy. However, surgery is contraindicated for small cell carcinomas. Squamous cell carcinomas, adenocarcinoma, and large cell cancer are likely treated with surgery. Radiation may be used prior to surgery to reduce the tumour size. If the tumour is nonresectable or other conditions exist, such as cardiac disease, surgery is not an option. Radiation therapy is usually recommended for stage 1 and stage 2 lesions if surgery is contraindicated. Radiation can be used as an adjunct to surgery postoperatively.

Chemotherapy is the primary treatment for small cell lung cancer. Other therapies include biological therapy, prophylactic cranial therapy, bronchoscopic laser therapy, phototherapy, airway stenting, and cryotherapy. Treatment focuses on providing comprehensive supportive care and client teaching to minimize complications and promote recovery from surgery, radiation, chemotherapy, or all of these. Overall goals include the following:

- Effective breathing patterns
- Adequate airway clearance
- Adequate oxygenation of tissues
- Minimal or no pain
- Providing psychological support and developing realistic attitudes toward treatment and prognosis

HEMATOLOGICAL HEALTH CHALLENGES

Anemia

Pathophysiology

Anemia is a decrease in the number of erythrocytes (RBCs), the amount of hemoglobin, or the volume of packed RBCs (hematocrit), all of which will result in a decreased amount of oxygen being delivered to the cells. Anemia is not itself a disease but rather is a clinical sign of an underlying disorder. Anemia can result from blood loss, impaired production of erythrocytes, or increased destruction of erythrocytes. The various types of anemia can be grouped according to a morphological (cellular characteristics) or an etiological (underlying cause) classification. A morphological classification gives information about the size and colour of the RBCs. Etiological classification is related to the underlying cause of the anemia.

Clinical Manifestations

Symptoms of anemia are caused by the body's response to the level of tissue hypoxia, which will depend on the severity of the anemia. When present, clinical symptoms may include the following:

- Palpitations
- Dyspnea
- Diaphoresis
- Pallor, due to reduced hemoglobin and reduced blood flow to the skin
- Jaundice, due to the increased hemolysis of RBCs, leading to increased concentrations of bilirubin
- Pruritus, due to an increased serum and skin bile salt concentration
- Cardiovascular manifestations of severe anemia result from additional attempts by the heart and lungs to provide adequate amounts of oxygen to the tissues
- Heart rate is increased in an attempt to maintain adequate cardiac output. Murmurs and bruits may develop due to the low viscosity of the blood.

- Angina, myocardial infarction (MI), and heart failure may develop due to the extreme increase in workload of the heart.
- Fatigue is common due to the increased heart rate and ineffective transportation of oxygen to the tissues.

Diagnostics

Laboratory assessment is needed to detect the type and size of RBCs as well as possible causes of the anemia. The following laboratory tests are used in the diagnosis:

- Hemoglobin, hematocrit, and reticulocyte counts
- Serum iron levels
- RBC indexes, particularly the mean corpuscular volume

Therapeutics and Nursing Considerations

Treatment of anemia is directed at correcting the cause of the anemia and maintaining adequate tissue perfusion. Oral or occasionally parenteral iron supplementation is used to replace iron. Acute interventions may include the following:

- Transfusion of blood or blood products
- Drug therapy, such as erythropoietin, vitamins, and supplements
- Oxygen therapy

Nursing considerations will be specific to the client's needs; however, all clients with anemia should be encouraged to balance rest with activity, eat a balanced diet rich in iron and folate, and be adherent to their drug therapy.

Aplastic Anemia

Pathophysiology

Aplastic anemia is a deficiency of circulating RBCs due to failure of the bone marrow to produce these cells. Stem cells in the bone marrow, or the bone marrow matrix itself, are either injured or destroyed, resulting in pancytopenia (decrease in all blood cell types). The damaged marrow is replaced by fat, resulting in bone marrow hypoplasia (decreased hematopoiesis).

Aplastic anemia may be congenital, acquired, or idiopathic. Some causes of aplastic anemia may include the following:

- Adverse drug reactions to certain medications
- Exposure to toxic agents, such as benzene, inorganic arsenic, insecticides, and radiation
- Viral or bacterial infections, such as hepatitis

Clinical Manifestations

Clinical manifestations of aplastic anemia vary with the severity of the pancytopenia. Infection, bleeding tendencies, fatigue, pallor, and dyspnea are common.

Diagnostics

Diagnosis is confirmed by laboratory studies. RBCs, WBCs, and platelets will be decreased. Morphologically, aplastic anemia is considered normocytic, normochromic anemia. A bone-marrow biopsy may show hypoplasia or aplasia, with cells being replaced by fat.

Therapeutics and Nursing Considerations

Management of aplastic anemia is based on identifying and removing the causative agent (when possible) and providing supportive care. The following treatments are used:

- Blood transfusions are the mainstay of treatment. Transfusions are discontinued once the bone marrow starts producing RBCs.
- Bone marrow transplantation is the preferred treatment of aplastic anemia for clients needing constant blood transfusions.
- A splenectomy may be performed when the spleen is destroying normal RBCs.

The prognosis for aplastic anemia is poor, with a mortality rate as high as 70%. Death may result from bleeding or infection.

Sickle Cell Anemia

Sickle cell anemia is an inherited childhood disorder of autosomal recessive defects, characterized by the presence of an abnormal form of hemoglobin (called *sickle cell hemoglobin*, or HgbS) in the erythrocyte. This abnormal hemoglobin causes erythrocytes to become rigid and to take on a crescent shape in response to low oxygen levels, causing vaso-occlusive crises, and, over time, tissue hypoxia and necrosis. For more information on sickle cell anemia, see Chapter 11.

Thrombocytopenia

Pathophysiology

Thrombocytopenia is characterized by a deficiency of circulating platelets. Platelet disorders can be inherited or acquired due to decreased platelet production, increased sequestration in the spleen, or increased platelet destruction. Types of thrombocytopenia are as follows:

- Acquired thrombocytopenia may result from medications such as NSAIDs or antibiotic chemotherapeutic agents.
- In children, idiopathic thrombocytopenia is common.
- Transient thrombocytopenia may follow a viral infection such as Epstein–Barr virus or other infections.
- Immune (idiopathic) thrombocytopenic purpura (ITP) is an autoimmune disorder with platelet destruction.
- Thrombotic thrombocytopenic purpura (TTP) is a rare disease in which thrombi occlude small vessels.

The key factor with all types of thrombocytopenia is the low platelet level: below 150×10^9/L of blood.

Clinical Manifestations

Many clients with thrombocytopenia are asymptomatic. When manifestations are present, the most common symptom is bleeding, usually noticeable only when the platelet count drops below 20000/mL of blood. The major complication of thrombocytopenia is hemorrhage.

Diagnostics

Diagnosis is made by a laboratory test of platelets. The platelet count will be decreased. Any reduction below 150×10^9/L is termed *thrombocytopenia*.

Therapeutics and Nursing Considerations

Treatment of thrombocytopenia depends on the etiology of the decreased platelet count. The underlying cause must be treated, and treatment may include the following:

- Splenectomy for hypersplenism
- Chemotherapy for acute or chronic leukemia
- Corticosteroids to enhance vascular integrity
- Steroids, danazol (Cyclomen), or IV immune globulin for idiopathic thrombocytopenia
- Platelet transfusions for a count below 20×10^9/L
- Plasmapheresis (plasma is removed from the client and replaced with fresh frozen plasma) is the primary treatment for acute thrombocytopenia.

INGESTION, DIGESTION, ABSORPTION, AND ELIMINATION CHALLENGES

Nausea and Vomiting

Nausea is a feeling of discomfort in the epigastrium with a conscious desire to vomit. Vomiting is the forceful ejection of partially digested food and secretions (emesis) from the upper GI tract. Nausea and vomiting can occur independently but usually are closely related and treated as one condition. A client can feel nauseated and vomit in response to many conditions. Some of these conditions include the following:

- Pregnancy
- GI disorders
- Infectious diseases
- Food poisoning
- CNS disorders (meningitis, traumatic brain injury, concussion, CNS tumour)
- Cardiovascular disorders (myocardial infarction, heart failure)
- Metabolic disorders (Addison's disease, uremia) and adverse effects of medications
- Other triggers of nausea may include odours, intense activity or emotional stress, or certain types of food (Tyerman & Cobbett, 2023).

Clinical Manifestations

Nausea is a subjective, unpleasant, wavelike sensation the client experiences in the back of the throat, epigastrium, or abdomen. This feeling may or may not lead to the urge to vomit.

Diagnostics

Diagnosis is arrived at via a client history and physical assessment.

Therapeutics and Nursing Considerations

The goals of management are to determine and treat the underlying cause of the vomiting, remove the cause, and provide symptomatic relief. Differentiation between vomiting, regurgitation, and projectile vomiting is important. The colour and odour of the emesis can supply important information. Fecal odour and bile indicate a lower obstruction of the bowel. The colour of the emesis aids in determining whether bleeding is taking place. Vomiting with "coffee-ground" appearance is associated with bleeding in the stomach, and bright red blood is associated with active bleeding (Tyerman & Cobbett, 2023). Many different medications can be used to treat nausea and vomiting. The exact medication therapy will depend on the cause. IV fluids may be needed to replace fluids and electrolytes. If vomiting is continuous, a nasogastric (NG) tube may be inserted to decompress the stomach. The client will be started on clear fluids when tolerated. The client will be encouraged to drink fluids between meals rather than with meals.

Hiatus Hernia

Pathophysiology

Hiatus hernia is a protrusion of the stomach into the esophagus through an opening in the diaphragm. A sliding hiatus hernia occurs when the stomach slides through the gastro-esophageal junction. A paraesophageal, or rolling, hiatus hernia occurs when the fundus or greater curvature of the stomach rolls up through the esophageal hiatus.

Many different factors may cause the development of a hiatus hernia. These include the following:

- A weakness in the muscles of the diaphragm
- Increased intra-abdominal pressure
- Obesity
- Pregnancy
- Ascites
- Tumour
- Heavy lifting
- Increasing age
- Trauma
- Poor nutrition
- Prolonged recumbent position

Potential complications of hiatus hernia are hemorrhage, obstruction, and strangulation of the hernia.

Clinical Manifestations

Clinical manifestations are similar to those of gastroesophageal reflux disease (GERD) and are as follows:

- Pyrosis, dysphagia, reflux, and discomfort are associated with position.
- Bending over may cause pain.
- Large meals may cause pain.
- Smoking and alcohol may cause pain.
- Nocturnal symptoms of heartburn are common.
- Reflux symptoms are more common with a sliding hiatus hernia, and fullness is more typical in the paraesophageal hernia.

Complications that may occur with hiatus hernia include GERD, hemorrhage from erosion, stenosis of the esophagus, ulcerations of the herniated portion of the stomach, strangulation of the hernia, and regurgitation with tracheal aspiration (Tyerman & Cobbett, 2023).

Diagnostics

Diagnosis of hiatus hernia begins with the history and a physical examination as well as barium swallow X-ray, endoscopic examination, or both, looking for any protrusion of the gastric mucosa through the esophageal hiatus or abnormalities in the mucosa.

Therapeutics and Nursing Considerations

Conservative care is attempted first and may include the following:

- Lifestyle modifications similar to those for GERD
- Elevation of the head of the bed to 30 degrees
- Use of antacids and antisecretory agents such as H_2 receptor blockers
- Weight reduction if the client is overweight

Surgical treatments attempt to reduce reflux by enhancing the integrity of the lower esophageal sphincter (LES). Different types of surgery all involve "wrapping" the fundus of the stomach around the lower portion of the esophagus in order to reduce the hernia, provide acceptable LES pressure, and prevent movement of the gastroesophageal junction. Postoperative care involves the following:

- Monitoring vital signs and airway and chest sounds
- Monitoring any chest tubes and possible respiratory distress
- Monitoring an abdominal incision for infection
- Monitoring the NG tube for patency and checking the abdomen for distension
- Always assessing clients for venous thrombus following these types of surgery

Education of the client will revolve around preventing respiratory complications by deep breathing and coughing frequently. Clients should be taught to prevent gas-bloat syndrome by slowing and progressively advancing their diet. Small, frequent meals will prevent overloading of the stomach. Carbonated drinks and gas-producing foods should be avoided (Ignatavicius et al., 2018).

Esophageal Cancer

Pathophysiology

Factors predisposing to the development of esophageal cancer include the following:

- Smoking and excessive alcohol use
- A diet low in fruits, vegetables, and certain vitamins and minerals, which increases the risk
- Achalasia (peristalsis is absent in the lower two thirds of the esophagus), which results in delayed emptying of the lower esophagus; exposure to asbestos and metal; and a history of swallowing lye

Cancer of the esophagus is caused by malignant advancement into the esophageal area. If the malignancy spreads into the submucosa, the risk for metastasis and death increases drastically. The major types of esophageal cancers are adenocarcinoma and squamous cell cancers.

Complications with esophageal cancers include the following:

- Hemorrhage that may occur if cancer erodes through the esophagus and into the aorta
- Esophageal perforation with fistula formation into the lung or trachea
- Obstruction of the esophagus
- Spread of the cancer through the lymph system; the liver and lungs are common sites of metastasis

Clinical Manifestations

Symptoms appear late in the development, usually when the esophagus is 50 to 60% occluded, and include progressive dysphagia, pain in the epigastric area, substernally, or in the back, which may radiate to the neck and jaw. Other common symptoms may include a sore throat, choking and hoarseness, and weight loss.

Diagnostics

Diagnostic tests used to find esophageal cancer include barium swallow with fluoroscopy, which may show a narrowing of the esophagus at the site of the tumour. Endoscopy and biopsy are needed to make a definitive diagnosis and identify the malignant cells. A CT scan and MRI may be needed to assess the extent of the disease.

Therapeutics and Nursing Considerations

Since the disease is often not diagnosed until late in its development, the prognosis is poor. Treatments include the following:

- Surgery, which may include esophagectomy, removal of part or all of the esophagus
- Esophagogastrostomy, resection of a portion of the esophagus and anastomosis of the remaining portion to the stomach
- Esophagoenterostomy, resection of a portion of the esophagus and anastomosis of a segment of colon to the remaining portion
- Chemotherapy and radiation before or after the surgery
- After surgery, parenteral fluids are given. When allowed to drink orally, 30 to 60 mL of water is given hourly and gradually increased to small, frequent bland diet. Position the client in a high Fowler's position to prevent regurgitation of the fluid. Monitor the client for signs of leakage into mediastinum such as pain, increased temperature and dyspnea. Also monitor the client for signs of intolerance to feeding (Tyerman & Cobbett, 2023).

Palliative therapy consists of restoration of the swallowing function and maintenance of nutrition and hydration. Further palliative care focuses on pain management and maintaining as normal a lifestyle as possible.

Peptic Ulcer Disease

Pathophysiology

Peptic ulcer disease includes conditions characterized by erosion of the GI mucosa in the lower esophagus, stomach and duodenum, and jejunum. The ulcer may be acute with either superficial or minimal erosion. It can be of short duration and resolve quickly when the cause is identified and removed. A chronic ulcer is of long duration, eroding through the muscular wall with the formation of fibrous tissue. Peptic ulcers develop only in the presence of an acid environment. The stomach is normally protected from autodigestion and damage by the gastric mucosal barrier. When that barrier is damaged, acid–pepsin freely enters the mucosa, and cellular inflammation and destruction occur. The precise cause of peptic ulcers is not known; however, common risk factors include the following:

- *Helicobacter pylori* infection
- The use of NSAIDs, salicylates, or steroids
- Exposure to irritants, such as alcohol, coffee, and tobacco, increases the risk for peptic ulcer development.
- Other predisposing factors include emotional stress, physical trauma, and aging.

The major complications of peptic ulcers include hemorrhage, perforation, and gastric outlet obstruction. All three complications are considered emergencies requiring prompt medical treatment.

Clinical Manifestations

Clinical manifestations are variable. Those with gastric or duodenal ulcers often do not have any pain. When pain is present, it is described as burning or cramplike and most often is located in the midepigastric region. Eating or ingesting antacids often relieves the pain.

Diagnostics

Diagnostic testing includes the following:

- An upper GI tract X-ray will show abnormalities in the mucosa.
- A barium swallow examination can diagnose gastric outlet obstruction.
- Gastric secretory studies will show hyperchlorhydria.
- An upper GI endoscopy will confirm the presence of an ulcer.
- A biopsy will help rule out cancer.
- A serological or breath urea test is done to test for the presence of *H. pylori*.
- Stool may need to be tested for occult blood.
- Laboratory studies (CBC, liver enzymes, serum amylase, and urinalysis).

Therapeutics and Nursing Considerations

Treatment is essentially symptomatic, with an emphasis on medication therapy and rest. The following treatments are used:

- Antacids reduce gastric acidity. Histamine-2 receptor blockers and proton pump inhibitors reduce gastric secretions in short-term therapy.
- Anticholinergics inhibit the vagus nerve effect on the parietal cells and reduce gastrin production and excessive gastric activity in duodenal ulcers.
- Sucralfate (Sulcrate), a cytoprotective drug, is used in short-term therapy and is cytoprotective of the esophagus, stomach, and duodenum.
- Antibiotic treatment may be used to reduce *H. pylori*.
- Physical rest promotes healing.
- Gastroscopy can facilitate coagulation of the bleeding site by cautery or laser therapy.
- If hemorrhage occurs, saline lavage, sclerotherapy, and angiography with vasopressin may postpone the need for surgery until the client stabilizes.

Surgery is indicated for clients with perforation or those unresponsive to conservative measures. Surgical procedures include vagotomy and pyloroplasty or distal subtotal gastrectomy.

Nutritional therapy identifies foods that cause distress, such as the following:

- Hot, spicy foods, and pepper
- Alcohol
- Carbonated drinks
- Tea and coffee
- Foods high in roughage, which may irritate an inflamed mucosa

Protein is considered the best neutralizing food, but it does stimulate gastric secretions. Milk can neutralize gastric activity and contains prostaglandins and growth factors.

Diet should consist of small, dry feedings daily that are low in carbohydrates and that include a moderate amount of protein and fat. Fluids should not be taken during the meal. Clients are encouraged to rest for 30 minutes following every meal.

With an acute exacerbation when bleeding is occurring, the client often has increased pain with nausea and vomiting. The following treatment is required in this situation:

- An NG tube will be placed in the stomach with intermittent suction for 24 to 48 hours.
- Fluids and electrolytes will be replaced by IV infusion until the client is able to tolerate oral feedings without distress.

Management will be similar to that for upper GI bleeding. Blood, blood products, or both may be needed. The client will require the following nursing considerations:

- Careful monitoring of vital signs
- Monitoring of intake and output
- Laboratory studies
- Monitoring for signs of impending shock
- Endoscopic evaluation will reveal the degree of inflammation or bleeding as well as the location of the ulcer.

Perforation of the ulcer requires immediate action to stop spillage of gastric or duodenal contents into the peritoneal cavity and to restore blood volume. The following interventions are essential:

- An NG tube will be placed into the stomach as close to the perforation as possible.
- Circulating blood volume must be replaced.
- Packed RBCs may be needed.
- A central venous pressure line may be needed.
- An in-dwelling urinary catheter should be inserted and monitored every hour.

Surgery is not the usual method of treatment; however, it is indicated for such conditions as an intractable ulcer, history of hemorrhage, perforation, or obstruction. Surgical procedures done to treat ulcers include gastroduodenostomy (Billroth I), gastrojejunostomy (Billroth II), vagotomy, and pyloroplasty.

Postoperative complications include dumping syndrome, postprandial hypoglycemia, and bile reflux gastritis. The dumping syndrome is a direct result of surgical removal of a large portion of the stomach and pyloric sphincter. The syndrome results from the rapid emptying of gastric contents into the small bowel, which creates a fluid shift into the gut, resulting in abdominal distension. The client will feel dizzy and weak and complain of abdominal cramps.

Gastritis
Pathophysiology
Gastritis is not a disease but rather a condition of inflammation of the gastric mucosa.

- Acute gastritis is often due to eating foods contaminated with microorganisms or food that is highly seasoned.
- Chronic gastritis is sometimes associated with autoimmune disease, such as pernicious anemia. It can also be due to benign or malignant ulcers caused by *H. pylori* bacteria.

Gastritis occurs as a result of a breakdown in the gastric mucosal barrier. In gastritis, the mucous membrane becomes edematous and hyperemic and undergoes superficial erosion. This erosion may lead to hemorrhage.

Clinical Manifestations
Acute and chronic symptoms are the same and include anorexia, nausea and vomiting, epigastric tenderness, and a feeling of fullness. Hemorrhage is particularly common with alcohol abuse.

Diagnostics
Diagnosis is often suspected with a thorough history and physical examination where ingestion of drugs and alcohol may be discussed. Definitive diagnosis is made with an endoscopic examination and biopsy of the gastric mucosa from which a histological examination will occur. Upper GI radiographic studies may be ordered.

Therapeutics and Nursing Considerations
Treatment and management revolve around removal of the precipitating cause. Initially, the client will be nothing by mouth (NPO), with possible NG insertion to remove the causative agent. The client must be monitored for dehydration, which can occur quickly. Medication therapy focuses on reducing irritation of the gastric mucosa and providing symptomatic relief. Antacids and H_2 receptor blockers such as ranitidine (Zantac) are helpful in reducing HCl secretion and in raising the pH to a more alkaline level. Nursing considerations will focus on promoting optimal nutrition, promoting fluid balance, relieving pain, and promoting self-care.

Gastroesophageal Reflux Disease (GERD)
Pathophysiology
GERD refers to any clinically significant symptomatic condition of reflux of the gastric contents into the lower esophagus. There is no single cause for GERD. Predisposing factors include the following:

- Hiatus hernia
- Incompetent LES
- Decreased gastric emptying
- Pyloric stenosis

The acidic gastric secretions that reflux up into the lower esophagus result in esophageal irritation, inflammation, and corrosion.

Clinical Manifestations
Clinical manifestations include heartburn, described as a burning or tight sensation radiating to the neck. Clients with heartburn (pyrosis) that occurs more than once a week, becomes more severe, or occurs at night and wakes the client from sleep should be investigated for GERD. Regurgitation is common and is frequently described as hot, bitter, or sour liquid coming into the mouth or throat.

Gastric symptoms may also include the following, which are related to delayed gastric emptying:
- Early satiety
- Postmeal bloating
- Nausea, vomiting

Diagnostics
Diagnosis of GERD is made by barium swallow or endoscopy to evaluate damage to the esophageal mucosa. Other tests may include biopsy with histological examination, esophageal manometric studies to monitor pH, and radionuclide tests to detect reflux and the rate of esophageal clearance.

Therapeutics and Nursing Considerations
Management focuses on lifestyle modifications and avoidance of situations that decrease LES pressure or that cause esophageal irritation. Nutritionally, clients are encouraged to avoid high-fat foods, avoid milk products at night, and avoid late-night snacking.

Medication therapy may include the following:
- H_2 receptor blockers
- Proton pump inhibitors
- Antacids
- Sucralfate
- Prokinetic drugs

If medical management is unsuccessful, fundoplication surgery (wrapping a portion of the gastric fundus around the sphincter of the esophagus) is performed. Nurses need to educate clients to
- Avoid factors causing reflux, such as smoking and acid-producing foods.
- Have the head of the bed elevated to about 30 degrees.
- Not lie down for 2 to 3 hours after eating. Not to wear tight clothing around the waist and not to bend over (especially after eating).
- To eat small, frequent meals to prevent gastric distension.
- Take medications correctly.

Gastroenteritis
Pathophysiology
Gastroenteritis is an inflammation of the mucosa of the stomach and small intestine, resulting in vomiting and diarrhea. The condition usually is caused by infectious agents, such as the noroviruses and *Escherichia coli*. Most cases are self-limiting and do not require hospitalization. However, older

persons and chronically ill clients may be unable to consume adequate fluids orally to compensate for fluid loss.

If the symptoms are severe, or if the client is experiencing frequent watery stools, a culture for *Clostridium difficile* should be performed.

Clinical Manifestations

Clinical manifestations include the following:
- Nausea and vomiting
- Diarrhea
- Possible fever
- Abdominal cramping and distension
- Depending on the amount of fluid that is lost, the client may experience symptoms of hypovolemia.

Diagnostics

The history and physical examination of the client are usually diagnostic. However, Gram stain of stool specimens will confirm the causative agent.

Therapeutics and Nursing Considerations

Until vomiting stops, the client should be NPO. Thereafter, the client should have bland food and fluids as tolerated. Most gastroenteritis is managed at home. If the symptoms are severe, the following treatments may be needed:
- IV replacement therapy for dehydration
- Accurate monitoring of intake and output
- Potassium supplements
- Antibiotic, antimicrobial therapy, if the causative organism is identified
- Enteric precautions

Symptomatic nursing care is given for nausea, vomiting, and diarrhea. The nurse should assess complaints of pain, vomiting, and diarrhea as gastroenteritis is often confused with appendicitis.

Appendicitis
Pathophysiology

Appendicitis is an inflammation of the vermiform appendix, a narrow, fingerlike appendage found just below the ileocecal valve. Inflammation of the appendix usually occurs when the lumen is obstructed by fecal material, foreign bodies, or a tumour of the cecum. This obstruction can lead to distension, venous engorgement, and the accumulation of mucus and bacteria, which can, in turn, lead to gangrene and perforation of the appendix. If the appendix ruptures or perforates, the infected contents can spill into the abdominal cavity, causing peritonitis.

Clinical Manifestations

Appendicitis typically begins with periumbilical pain, followed by anorexia, nausea, and vomiting. The pain eventually will shift to the right lower quadrant and localize at McBurney's point, with rebound tenderness (Blumberg sign) and muscle guarding. The client will probably want to lie still with knees flexed. Coughing aggravates the pain.

Diagnostics

Diagnosis of appendicitis can be difficult, so although the history and physical examination are important, further tests should be done, including the following:
- Rovsing's sign may be elicited by palpating the left lower quadrant.
- WBCs will be elevated, but this is not considered diagnostic.
- An ultrasonogram or CT scan of the abdomen is often needed to confirm the diagnosis.

Therapeutics and Nursing Considerations

Appendectomy is the only effective treatment for appendicitis. If the appendix has ruptured, treatment will also include insertion of an NG tube, IV fluids and electrolytes, and administration of antibiotics. Nursing care will focus on the following:
- Pain relief
- Maintaining fluid balance
- Support to reduce anxiety
- Maintaining skin integrity
- Monitoring and managing complications that may arise

Diverticulitis
Pathophysiology

The diverticulum is a saccular outpouching of the mucosa through the muscular intestinal wall. Diverticulitis is an inflammation of the diverticular sacs, most commonly due to obstruction with fecal matter. Diverticula may occur at any point within the GI tract but are more commonly found in the sigmoid colon.

Diverticula in the sigmoid colon are thought to be associated with high luminal pressure from a deficiency in dietary fibre perhaps combined with a loss of muscle mass and collagen with the aging process. When diverticula form, the smooth muscle of the colon wall becomes thickened. Lack of dietary fibre slows transit time, and more water is absorbed from the stool, making it more difficult for it to pass through the lumen. Decreased stool size raises intraluminal pressure, thus promoting diverticula formation.

Clinical Manifestations

The majority of people with diverticulitis are asymptomatic. When symptoms are present, they usually include the following:
- Abdominal pain localized over the involved area of the colon
- Fever, chills, nausea
- Anorexia
- Leukocytosis
- Sometimes a palpable mass

Complications of diverticulitis include perforation with peritonitis, abscess and fistula formation, bowel obstructions, ureteral obstruction, and bleeding.

Diagnostics

Diagnostic tests include CBC, urinalysis, and fecal occult blood test, as well as X-ray of the abdomen or ultrasound and

CT scan to confirm diagnosis and evaluate the severity of the condition.

Therapeutics and Nursing Considerations

In acute diverticulitis, the goal of treatment is to allow the colon to rest and the inflammation to subside. Treatments include the following:

- Ensuring the client is NPO with IV therapy to maintain fluid and electrolyte balance
- Initiating broad-spectrum antibiotic therapy
- Monitoring the client for signs of peritonitis
- Surgery is reserved for clients with complications such as abscess or obstruction.

Nursing considerations focus on maintaining normal elimination patterns, relief of pain, maintaining fluid balance, and monitoring and managing potential complications. Teaching the client that diverticular disease can be prevented by a diet high in fibre and low in fats is important.

Inflammatory Bowel Disease

Inflammatory bowel disease consists of the immunologically related disorders of Crohn's disease and ulcerative colitis. Inflammatory bowel disease is characterized by chronic, recurrent inflammation of the intestinal tract. Clinical manifestations are varied for both conditions, but these often include long periods of remission interspersed with episodes of acute inflammation. Both diseases can be debilitating. The cause of inflammatory bowel disease is unknown; however, causes may include the following:

- Infectious agents
- Autoimmune reaction
- Food allergies
- Heredity

Ulcerative Colitis

Pathophysiology

Ulcerative colitis is characterized by inflammation and ulceration of the colon and rectum. It may occur at any age but tends to peak between the ages of 15 and 25 years. It is equally prevalent in both sexes. The inflammation of ulcerative colitis usually starts in the rectum and moves in a continuous pattern toward the cecum. Ulcerative colitis is characterized by multiple ulcerations, inflammations, and shedding of the epithelium. The affected mucosa is hyperemic and edematous. The ulcerations destroy the mucosal epithelium, causing bleeding and diarrhea. This can lead to fluid and electrolyte losses, protein losses, and the development of pseudopolyps. Granulation tissue develops, and the mucosa musculature becomes thickened, shortening the colon. Intestinal complications include the following:

- Hemorrhage
- Abscess formation
- Perforation
- Toxic megacolon and colonic dilation
- Cancer

Clinical Manifestations

Clients with ulcerative colitis usually present with mild to severe acute exacerbations that occur at unpredictable intervals over many years. The major symptoms are bloody diarrhea and abdominal pain.

Diagnostics

Diagnosis of ulcerative colitis includes ruling out other diseases with similar symptoms and determining whether the client has ulcerative colitis or Crohn's disease. The following tests are done:

- CBC, serum electrolytes, and serum protein levels
- Stool will be examined for blood, pus, and mucus.
- Sigmoidoscopy and colonoscopy examination of the mucosa to look for inflammation, ulcerations, pseudopolyps, and strictures
- A double-contrast barium enema for areas of granular inflammation with ulceration

Therapeutics and Nursing Considerations

Goals of treatment include the following:

- Resting the bowel
- Control of inflammation
- Combatting infection
- Correcting malnutrition
- Alleviating stress
- Symptomatic relief and improving quality of life
- Sulfasalazines are the principal drugs of choice. They are effective in the maintenance of remission.
- Other medications that may be used are corticosteroids, 5-ASA and 4-ASA, and immunosuppressants such as azathioprine (Imuran).

Surgery is indicated if the client does not respond to medical treatment, has frequent or debilitating exacerbations, has massive bleeding or obstruction, or develops dysplasia or carcinoma. Surgical procedures include total proctocolectomy with permanent ileostomy, total proctocolectomy with continent ileostomy (Kock pouch), or total colectomy with rectal mucosal stripping and ileoanal reservoir.

Postoperatively, the nurse must monitor for the following:

- Stoma viability, mucocutaneous juncture, and peristomal skin integrity
- Signs of hemorrhage, abdominal abscess, small bowel obstruction, dehydration, and other complications

Diet is an important component in the treatment of ulcerative colitis. The goal is to provide adequate nutrition without exacerbating symptoms. This diet must correct and prevent malnutrition, replace fluid and electrolyte losses, and prevent weight loss. The diet should be

- High calorie
- High protein
- Low residue with vitamin and mineral supplements

Other nursing considerations include the following:

- Maintaining normal elimination patterns
- Relieving pain
- Promoting rest
- Reducing anxiety

- Preventing skin breakdown
- Enhancing coping mechanisms

Crohn's Disease

Pathophysiology

Crohn's disease is a chronic nonspecific inflammatory bowel disorder of unknown origin that can affect any part of the GI tract from mouth to anus. Crohn's disease can occur at any age but usually presents between the ages of 15 and 30 years and affects both sexes equally.

Crohn's disease is characterized by inflammation of segments of the GI tract, and although the disease can affect any section, it is most often found in the terminal ileum. The inflammation of Crohn's disease affects all layers of the bowel wall. Eventually, deep ulcerations develop. There are also "skip lesions," in which segments of normal bowel occur between diseased portions. As the disease continues, the wall of the bowel thickens, and as strictures develop, the lumen of the bowel narrows. Severe diarrhea and malabsorption of nutrients result from the damaged bowel. Complications of Crohn's disease are similar to those of ulcerative colitis.

Clinical Manifestations

The onset of Crohn's disease is usually insidious, with nonspecific complaints of the following:

- Diarrhea
- Fatigue
- Abdominal pain
- Weight loss
- Fever

Diarrhea (non-bloody) and abdominal pain are usually the symptoms that cause the client to seek medical attention. As the disease progresses, the pain may increase in severity, abdominal distension may develop, and the client may develop arthritis and finger clubbing.

Diagnostics

Diagnostic studies are similar to those needed for ulcerative colitis, including barium studies, endoscopy with biopsy, blood work, and upper GI barium swallow.

Therapeutics and Nursing Considerations

The goals of treatment revolve around controlling the inflammatory process, relieving symptoms, correcting metabolic and nutritional conditions, and promoting healing of the affected area.

Treatments include the following:

- Medication therapy similar to that used with ulcerative colitis. Sulfasalazines, corticosteroids, immunosuppressive agents, metronidazole, and infliximab may be used.
- Nutritional therapy, including elemental diets; parenteral nutrition when needed; and low-residue, low-roughage, low-fat, high-calorie, and high-protein diets are recommended.

The majority of clients will eventually require surgery at least once in the course of their disease. The disease is not cured by surgery, and the recurrence rate following surgery is high.

Nursing management is similar to that required for ulcerative colitis, with frequent rest periods and skin care. Client education is very important. Teaching includes the following:

- The importance of rest and diet management
- Teaching about the medications, what they are, why they are needed, and what they will do for the client helps clients be compliant with their medications. Clients should also be taught about possible adverse effects of their medications and symptoms of disease recurrence.
- When to seek medical care
- The use of diversional activities to reduce stress

Colorectal Cancer

Pathophysiology

Colorectal cancer (CRC) is equally common in males and females. Nearly all CRCs are adenocarcinomas, most arising from adenomatous polyps. Tumours spread through the walls of the intestine and into the lymphatic system. Tumours commonly spread to the liver because venous blood flow from the colorectal tumour is through the portal vein.

CRC is the second leading cause of death from cancer in Canada. However, if diagnosed early, the cure rate is very high. Screening via *fecal occult blood test* (FOBT) or *fecal immunochemical test* (FIT) once a year and flexible sigmoidoscopy every 5 years beginning at age 50 are important aspects of the examination (Tyerman & Cobbett, 2023). People with an increased risk for colorectal cancer (family history with one or more first degree relatives with the disease) need to be tested more often. They require colonoscopy 10 years earlier than the age the relative was diagnosed or age 50, whichever every comes first (Colorectal Cancer Canada, 2021).

The cause of CRC is unclear. However, risk factors for the development of CRC include the following:

- Familial tendencies
- Increasing age
- A diet high in fat and calories
- A history of inflammatory bowel disease

Clinical Manifestations

Clinical manifestations are nonspecific and may not appear until the disease is advanced. Most people with CRC have hematochezia (passage of blood through the rectum) or melena (black, tarry stools) and abdominal pain or changes in bowel habits, or both. Occult bleeding and iron deficiency anemia lead to weakness and fatigue. The signs of CRC depend on the location of the tumour.

- Left-sided lesions tend to bleed. Clients tend to alternate between constipation and diarrhea, and they tend to have narrow, ribbonlike stools.
- Right-sided lesions are usually asymptomatic or cause vague abdominal discomfort.

In later stages, findings result from extension of the cancer to adjacent organs and reflect the symptoms of advanced cancer.

Diagnostics

Diagnostic studies include family history and physical examination, distal rectal examination, colonoscopy, endorectal ultrasonography, CT scan, fecal occult blood tests, and carcinoembryonic antigen. Only a biopsy will verify the presence of CRC.

Therapeutics and Nursing Considerations

Prognosis and treatment correlate with the pathological staging of the disease. Surgery seeks to remove the cancerous tumour and adjacent tissues, as well as lymph nodes that may contain cancer cells. Chemotherapy and radiation therapy are recommended for clients with positive lymph node involvement at the time of surgery or those who have metastatic disease. Chemotherapy and radiation may be the primary treatment when the CRC is nonresectable.

- A right hemicolectomy for advanced tumours of the cecum or ascending colon may include resection of the terminal segment of the ileum, cecum, ascending colon, and right half of the transverse colon with corresponding mesentery.
- A right colectomy may be done for tumours of the proximal and middle transverse colon, which includes the resection of the transverse colon and mesentery corresponding to midcolonic vessels.
- Alternatively, the surgeon may perform segmental resection of the transverse colon and associated midcolonic vessels.
- For sigmoid colon tumours, surgery is usually limited to the sigmoid colon and mesentery.
- Upper rectum tumours usually call for anterior or low anterior resection. A newer method using a stapler allows resection much lower than previously possible.
- For tumours in the lower rectum, abdominoperineal resection and permanent sigmoid colostomy are usually performed.

The overall goals for the client being treated for CRC are to attain normal bowel elimination patterns, maintain quality of life appropriate for the disease progression, be free of pain, and maintain feelings of comfort and well-being.

Other nursing considerations include the following:

- Providing emotional support
- Maintaining optimal nutrition
- Providing pain relief
- Providing wound care following a surgical procedure
- Educating about colostomy care, if applicable
- Supporting a positive image

Jaundice

Pathophysiology

Jaundice results from bilirubin diffusing into tissues and giving them a yellow or greenish-yellow tinge. In the spleen, during RBC destruction, the heme is separated from the globulin. The heme further breaks down to iron and bilirubin. In the blood, bilirubin joins with albumin and travels via the blood to the liver, where it is processed and excreted in bile, urine, and feces.

Jaundice is often the first and sometimes the only symptom of liver disease. In hepatitis, it is evident in the icteric phase as hyperbilirubinemia.

The three major types of jaundice are hemolytic, hepatocellular, and obstructive jaundice.

Hemolytic jaundice. Hemolytic jaundice occurs when there is an increase in the number of RBCs destroyed, which increases the amount of bilirubin in the blood. The liver cannot handle the increased load, and the increased bilirubin remains in the blood and is not excreted in the urine or feces. Predisposing factors that may cause hemolytic jaundice are the following:

- Blood transfusions
- Anemia, especially sickle cell
- Reabsorption of extravascular blood found postoperatively or in hematomas
- Certain medications, such as chlorpromazine and penicillin

Hepatocellular jaundice. Hepatocellular jaundice develops from damaged liver cells that are unable to clear bilirubin from the blood. There is impairment of uptake, conjugation, and excretion of bilirubin. Bile salts will deposit on the skin, and the client will have yellow discoloration. Predisposing factors for hepatocellular jaundice include hepatitis, cirrhosis, and liver cancer.

Obstructive jaundice. Obstructive jaundice results from an obstruction to bile flow. Bile will back up into the liver and then into the blood. Urine will take on a deep orange colour. Stool will be light or clay coloured. Pruritus will be evident. Intrahepatic predisposing factors include the following:

- Swelling or fibrosis of the canaliculi and bile ducts in the liver
- Hepatitis
- Cirrhosis
- Tumours
- Medications

Predisposing extrahepatic factors include bile duct obstruction.

Clinical Manifestations

Body tissues including the sclera and skin become yellow or greenish-yellow tinged. The urine may be dark brown or brownish-red due to the presence of bilirubin. Depending on the cause of the jaundice, the client may experience the following symptoms:

- Loss of appetite
- Nausea
- Malaise
- Fatigue
- Weakness
- Pruritus
- Dyspepsia
- Intolerance to fatty foods

Diagnostics

The history and physical examination are important in diagnosing jaundice. Blood work including serum bilirubin, both direct and indirect, will assist in finding the cause of the jaundice. Liver function tests will give information regarding conditions in the liver. Viral hepatitis testing may be needed.

Therapeutics and Nursing Considerations

Nursing management involves promoting the following:

- Acceptance of altered body image
- Control of pruritus
- Preventing skin irritation or injury
- Administering medications
- Monitoring clinical findings and laboratory data
- Providing distraction and rest

Adequate nutrition can be a challenge as the clients are often anorexic. Offering small, frequent meals of foods that the client enjoys can be beneficial. Measures to stimulate the appetite, such as mouth care and antiemetics, should be included in the nursing plan. Rest is an important factor in promoting liver cell regeneration (Tyerman & Cobbett, 2023). To treat the irritating pruritus, lanolin oil or oatmeal may be added to the bath. Skin irritation and injury can be prevented by keeping nails short or wearing mitts. Antihistamines may be prescribed in some situations.

Psychological and emotional rest is as essential as physical rest. Strict bed rest may produce anxiety and extreme restlessness in some clients, which may be more damaging than reasonable ambulation (Tyerman & Cobbett, 2023). Educating the family is important so they understand what is happening to the client. Family can be instrumental in supplying diversional activities.

Cholelithiasis

Pathophysiology

Cholelithiasis refers to stones in the gallbladder. *Cholecystitis*, or inflammation of the gallbladder, is usually associated with cholelithiasis. The stones vary in size, shape, and composition and may be lodged in the neck of the gallbladder or in the cystic duct and common bile duct. Cholelithiasis may be acute or chronic. The incidence is higher in multiparous persons over the age of 40 years. Sedentary lifestyle, obesity, and family tendency also are risk factors.

The actual cause of the stone is unknown. The most common gallstones are formed from cholesterol, a major component of bile. The stones may remain in the gallbladder or migrate to the cystic duct or common bile duct. They cause pain as they pass through the ducts and may lodge in the ducts and produce an obstruction. Stasis of bile in the gallbladder can lead to cholecystitis.

Clinical Manifestations

Cholelithiasis may produce severe symptoms or none at all. Severity of symptoms depends on whether the stones are stationary or mobile and whether obstruction is present. When the stones are lodged in the cystic duct, the obstruction prevents the movement of bile, so the gallbladder becomes distended, inflamed, and possibly infected. This results in biliary colic with severe upper right abdominal pain that radiates to the back or right shoulder. Other symptoms may include the following:

- Tachycardia
- Diaphoresis
- Nausea and vomiting

Pain may last up to an hour, and when it subsides, a residual tenderness in the right upper quadrant is usually felt. The attacks frequently occur 3 to 6 hours after a heavy meal or when the client lies down. When total obstruction occurs, symptoms related to bile blockage are manifested, including steatorrhea, pruritus, dark amber urine, a tendency to bleed, and jaundice.

Diagnostics

The following tests are used in the diagnosis:

- Ultrasonography to diagnose gallstones
- CT scan to identify ductal stones
- Endoscopic retrograde cholangiopancreatography (ERCP) allows for visualization of the gallbladder, cystic duct, common hepatic duct, and common bile duct. Bile taken during the procedure is sent for analysis to identify any possible infecting organism.
- Percutaneous transhepatic cholangiography may be used to diagnose obstructive jaundice and to locate stones within the bile ducts.
- Laboratory studies may demonstrate liver function test abnormalities, elevated serum enzymes, pancreatic enzymes, increased WBCs, elevated direct and indirect bilirubin levels, and urinary bilirubin.

Therapeutics and Nursing Considerations

Cholelithiasis is most commonly treated by means of ERCP, which will clear the stones from the biliary tree. In some cases, surgical intervention is needed. Cholecystectomy is often the preferred surgical procedure. This can be done through laparoscopic surgery, in which the gallbladder is removed through one of four tiny punctures in the abdominal wall. Clients experience minimal postoperative pain and are usually discharged home the day of surgery or the day after surgery. Nonsurgical removal of gallstones involves dissolving the gallstones, using extracorporeal shock wave lithotripsy or intracorporeal lithotripsy, but these methods have proven to be only temporary solutions. Medication therapy for gallbladder disease includes the following:

- Analgesics
- Anticholinergics
- Fat-soluble vitamins
- Bile salts
- Pharmacological therapy to dissolve small stones; this method of treatment is beneficial for clients unable to undergo surgery

Nurses need to focus on the following considerations:

- Pain relief
- Improving respiratory status
- Promoting skin care
- Promoting biliary drainage
- Improving nutritional status
- Monitoring for potential complications
- Low-fat diet, and if the client is obese, also a low-calorie diet

Hepatitis

Pathophysiology

Hepatitis is an inflammation of the liver marked by liver cell destruction, necrosis, and autolysis. In most clients, hepatic cells eventually regenerate, with little or no residual damage. However, advanced age and serious underlying disorders make complications more likely. Prognosis is poorer if edema and hepatic encephalopathy develop. The most common cause of hepatitis is viral infection.

Viral hepatitis may be caused by one of six viruses:

- Hepatitis type A (HAV) is transmitted almost exclusively by the fecal–oral route, and outbreaks are common in areas of overcrowding and poor sanitation. Child care centres and other institutional settings are common sources of outbreaks. The incidence is also increasing in homosexuals and in people with HIV. HAV is the most common type of hepatitis worldwide.
- Hepatitis type B (HBV) is transmitted by blood and blood products, by sexual intercourse, and through perinatal transmission.
- Hepatitis type C (HCV) is transmitted by blood and blood products as well as sexual activity with an infected partner. HCV accounts for 45% of all cases of hepatitis and is the most common liver disease in Canada. Many people infected with HIV also have HCV.
- Hepatitis type D (HDV) can cause an infection only if HBV is present; therefore, the routes of transmission are blood and blood products, as well as sexual intercourse with an infected partner.
- Hepatitis type E (HEV) is transmitted by the fecal–oral route.
- Hepatitis type G (HGV), also known as GB virus C, is transmitted parenterally and sexually.

Infection with HAV or HBV provides immunity to that virus, but the client may still develop another type of viral hepatitis. Clients with HCV can be infected with another strain of hepatitis C.

Hepatitis may also be caused by cytomegalovirus (CMV), Epstein–Barr virus, the herpes virus, coxsackievirus, and the rubella virus. Despite the different causative viruses, changes in the liver are usually similar in each type of viral hepatitis.

Liver damage is mediated by cytotoxic cytokines and NK cells that cause lysis of infected hepatocytes. In hepatitis, liver cell damage results in hepatic cell necrosis. This necrosis occurs in a spotty fashion, resulting in a piecemeal appearance. Many of the cells swell and rupture, while others shrink. Inflammation then occurs with proliferation and enlargement of the Kupffer cells. Inflammation of the periportal areas may interrupt bile flow, causing jaundice. Cholestasis may occur, as well as hepatomegaly and splenomegaly. Regeneration of liver tissue normally occurs alongside the death of liver cells. The ongoing necrosis, inflammation, and regeneration distort the normal structure and may interfere with blood and bile flow. If there are no complications, the liver cells will resume their normal appearance and function. Along with the hepatic changes, there may be some systemic effects, which may include rash, angioedema, arthritis, fever, and malaise.

Many clients with chronic HBV and HCV are asymptomatic. Most clients with hepatitis recover completely, with no complications. The mortality rate is less than 1%. Complications due to hepatitis include fulminant hepatic failure, chronic hepatitis, cirrhosis, and hepatocellular carcinoma. The characteristics of hepatitis viruses are summarized in Table 9.7.

Clinical Manifestations

The three phases of hepatitis are the preicteric phase, the icteric phase, and the posticteric phase. The preicteric phase is sometimes called the *intestinal phase* and may last from 1 to 21 days.

The *preicteric phase* is the period of maximal infectivity for HAV. This phase precedes the development of jaundice. The symptoms of this phase are as follows:

- Anorexia, nausea, and sometimes vomiting
- Abdominal discomfort, particularly the right upper quadrant
- Constipation or diarrhea
- Malaise and weight loss
  Other symptoms may include the following:
- Headache
- Low-grade fever
- Arthralgias
- Skin rashes
- A distaste for dietary protein and cigarette smoke

The *icteric phase* can last from 2 to 4 weeks and is characterized by jaundice. Symptoms in the icteric phase include pruritus and dark urine with light-coloured stools.

As the *posticteric phase* begins, the jaundice begins to disappear. This phase may last weeks to months, with the average being 2 to 4 months. Symptoms found in this phase include malaise and easy fatiguability. The disappearance of jaundice does not indicate recovery. Not all clients with viral hepatitis have jaundice; anicteric hepatitis does occur.

- In HAV, the onset of symptoms is acute, but the actual symptoms are a mild flulike manifestation.
- In HBV, the onset is insidious, and the symptoms tend to be more severe, with fewer GI symptoms.
- In HCV, the majority of clients are asymptomatic. HCV has a high rate of persistence and can induce chronic liver disease.

Diagnostics

Diagnosis of HBV will be confirmed by testing for the presence of hepatitis surface antigens and hepatitis B antibodies. These tests are as follows:

- Detection of an antibody to type A hepatitis confirms past or present infection with HAV.
- Detection of an antibody to type C hepatitis confirms a diagnosis of HCV.
- Viral load is measured by quantitative polymerase chain reaction assay and is useful in determining the need for treatment and monitoring therapy.
- The prothrombin time (PT) will be prolonged, indicating liver damage.

TABLE 9.7   Characteristics of Hepatitis Viruses

Incubation Period and Mode of Transmission	Sources of Infection	Infectivity
Hepatitis A Virus (HAV)		
15–50 days (average 28) Fecal–oral route (primarily fecal contamination and oral ingestion)	Crowded conditions (e.g., day care, long-term care facility). Poor personal hygiene. Poor sanitation. Contaminated food, water, shellfish. Persons with subclinical infections, infected food handlers. Sexual contact with infected partner. IV drug users.	Most infectious during 2 wk before onset of symptoms. Infectious until 1–2 wk after the start of symptoms.
Hepatitis B Virus (HBV)		
45–180 days (average 56–96) Percutaneous (parenteral) or permucosal exposure to blood or blood products Sexual contact Perinatal transmission	Contaminated needles, syringes, and blood products. Sexual activity with infected partner. Contact with asymptomatic carrier. Tattoos or body piercing with contaminated needles.	Before and after symptoms appear. Infectious for 4–6 mo. Carriers continue to be infectious for life.
Hepatitis C Virus (HCV)		
14–180 days (average 56) Percutaneous (parenteral) or mucosal exposure to blood or blood products High-risk sexual contact Perinatal contact	Blood and blood products. Needles and syringes. Sexual activity with infected partners.	1–2 wk before symptoms appear. Continues during clinical course. 75%–85% go on to develop chronic hepatitis C and remain infectious.
Hepatitis D Virus (HDV)		
2–26 wk HBV must precede HDV Chronic carriers of HBV always at risk	Same as HBV. Can cause infection only when HBV is present. Routes of transmission same as for HBV.	Blood infectious at all stages of HDV infection.
Hepatitis E Virus (HEV)		
15–64 days (average 26–42 days) Fecal–oral route Outbreaks associated with contaminated water supply in developing countries	Contaminated water, poor sanitation. Found in Asia, Africa, and Mexico. Not common in United States.	Not known. May be similar to HAV.

IV, Intravenous.

From Tyerman, J., & Cobbett, S. (2023). *Lewis's medical-surgical nursing in Canada: Assessment and management of clinical problems* (5th Cdn. ed., p. 1081, Table 46.1). Elsevier.

- Serum transaminase levels (alanine aminotransferase [ALT] and aspartate aminotransferase [AST]) will be elevated.
- Serum alkaline phosphatase will be slightly elevated.
- Serum and urine bilirubin levels are elevated.
- Serum albumin levels are low, and serum globulin levels are high.
- A liver biopsy and scan will show patchy necrosis.

Therapeutics and Nursing Considerations

There is no specific treatment for acute viral hepatitis. The following interventions are used:

- Most clients can be managed at home. Emphasis is on measures to rest the body and assist the liver in regenerating. Rest will help decrease the metabolic demands on the body and liver.
- Adequate nutrients and rest seem to be most beneficial for healing and liver cell regeneration. Dietary emphasis is on a well-balanced diet that the client can tolerate.

There is no specific drug therapy for viral hepatitis. Supportive medication therapy may include antiemetics, antihistamines, and sedatives, if needed.

Medication therapy for chronic hepatitis B is focused on decreasing the viral load, serum levels of AST and ALT, and the rate of disease progression. Alpha-interferons (Pegasys, PegIntron) and nucleoside analogues (Epovor, Hepsera) help suppress viral activity and decrease viral loads.

Medication therapy for chronic hepatitis C is directed at reducing the viral load, decreasing the progression of disease, and promoting seroconversion. Treatment includes direct-acting antiviral agents (DAAs), which have fewer adverse effects (headache and fatigue) compared to previous IFN therapies. The most common DAAs used in Canada include sofosbuvir (Sovaldi), sofosbuvir/ledipasvir (Harvoni), ombitasvir/paritaprevir/ritonavir/dasabuvir (Holkira, pak), daclatasvir (Daklinza) and elbasvir/grazoprevir (Zepatier) (Tyerman & Cobbett, 2023).

Both hepatitis A vaccine and immune globulin are used for prevention of hepatitis A. The vaccine is used for pre-exposure prophylaxis, and the immune globulin can be used either before or after exposure. Immunization with hepatitis B vaccine is the most effective method of preventing HBV infection. Health care workers are vaccinated for hepatitis B. For postexposure prophylaxis, the vaccine and hepatitis B immune globulin (HBIG) are used.

The diet needs to be adequate to assist hepatocytes to regenerate. The diet should be high in carbohydrates and calories. Protein may be limited if the liver is failing. Fat and sodium should be limited. Vitamin K supplements may be needed, and the client is encouraged to avoid drinking alcohol.

Cirrhosis

Pathophysiology

Cirrhosis of the liver refers to the chronic, progressive, irreversible, and widespread destruction of hepatic cells, with scar tissue (fibrosis) replacing healthy tissue. Cirrhosis can occur at any age but is more common in males between the ages of 40 and 60. Cirrhosis is the tenth leading cause of death in Canada, with alcohol ingestion being the most common cause. There are four major forms of cirrhosis:

- Alcoholic (Laennec's or portal/nutritional) cirrhosis results from malnutrition, especially protein deficiency and chronic alcohol intake. Alcohol alone has a direct hepatotoxic effect; it can produce necrosis of cells and fatty infiltrates.
- Postnecrotic cirrhosis is a complication of viral, toxic, or idiopathic hepatitis. Hepatitis C and alcohol are the two major causes of liver disease in Canada.
- Biliary cirrhosis results from bile duct disease.
- Cardiac cirrhosis is due to severe right-sided heart failure with cor pulmonale, prolonged constrictive pericarditis, and tricuspid insufficiency.
- Other forms of cirrhosis include nonspecific metabolic cirrhosis from infiltrating infections and cirrhosis due to inherited diseases such as hemochromatosis or Wilson's disease. Cirrhosis can be caused by drugs, toxins, and parasites. Nonalcoholic steatohepatitis (NASH) is found when fat builds up in the liver and eventually causes scar formation.

The pathophysiology of cirrhosis involves the destruction of hepatocytes. This hepatocyte necrosis leads to the development of scar tissue, which, in turn, disrupts blood and bile flow. This disruption then leads to an increase in pressure in the portal circulatory system, which causes portal hypertension. This hypertension damages more hepatocytes, resulting in loss of function and liver death.

Clinical Manifestations

Early manifestations of cirrhosis may be absent or minimal and then develop insidiously. These manifestations are as follows:

- Fatigue and weakness
- Decreased appetite and weight loss
- Nausea and vomiting
- Flatus
- Dull right upper quadrant discomfort due to swelling and stretching of the liver
- Possibly fever and pruritus
  Later manifestations may include the following:
- Jaundice
- Skin lesions

- Hematological conditions (thrombocytopenia, anemia, leukopenia)
- Endocrine disturbances (testicular atrophy, menstrual irregularities)
- Peripheral neuropathies
- Peripheral edema
- Infections

As the liver begins to fail, the normal functions of the liver also fail.

Diagnostics

Cirrhosis is typically advanced before it is diagnosed. The following tests are done to diagnose cirrhosis:

- A liver biopsy is the definitive test to diagnose cirrhosis.
- Blood work will show abnormal liver function, impaired clotting factors, thrombocytopenia, leukopenia, and anemia, as well as electrolyte imbalances due to an increase in aldosterone and ADH.
- A liver scan will show abnormal thickening and mass.

Therapeutics and Nursing Considerations

Treatment is aimed at removing or alleviating the underlying cause of the cirrhosis, preventing further liver damage, and preventing or treating complications. Complications that may result from cirrhosis are as follows:

- Portal hypertension
- Peripheral edema
- Ascites
- Varices
- Hepatic encephalopathy
- Hepatorenal syndrome
- Fetor hepaticus

Portal hypertension can result in retention and pooling of visceral blood, which, in turn, causes congestion of adjacent viscera. The high portal venous pressure will shunt blood into the systemic circulation, causing esophageal, gastric, spleen, and rectal varices. These vessels are fragile and may rupture. Treatment for ruptured varices begins with finding the source of the bleeding and stopping it. Esophagoscopy may be done if possible to find and treat the bleeding. Gastric lavage, sclerotherapy, vasopressin injection, and an esophagogastric tamponade (Minnesota or Blakemore tube) may be used to stop the bleeding. Once stabilized, a portacaval shunt or a transjugular intrahepatic portosystemic shunt may be put in place. Fluid volume must be replaced. Vital signs must be monitored, assessing for any signs of shock.

The failing liver impairs the synthesis of albumin. With the decrease in albumin, vascular oncotic pressure decreases, resulting in peripheral edema. Ascites develop due to the decreased hepatic synthesis of albumin, increased portal vein pressure, obstructed hepatic lymph flow, and increased serum aldosterone level. Ascites may be treated with sodium restriction, diuretics, and albumin. A paracentesis may be done to remove the excess fluid. A peritoneal venous shunt (LeVeen or Denver) may be inserted to remove fluid from the peritoneum to the superior vena cava. With the removal of fluid, the BP may drop, so the nurse must monitor the vital signs closely. Fluid replacement may be needed.

Hepatic encephalopathy is frequently a terminal complication. It is caused by increased levels of ammonia. Classic symptoms of hepatic encephalopathy include impaired attention span, irritability and restlessness, apathy, loss of interest, lethargy, somnolence, and coma. Hepatic encephalopathy is treated by identifying the precipitating cause and treating it with antibiotics, enemas, and lactulose. Lactulose will bind with the ammonia and help evacuate it via the bowel.

Hepatorenal syndrome results from functional renal failure with advancing azotemia, oliguria, and intractable ascites. The kidneys fail due to the redistribution of blood flow from the kidneys to the periphery and visceral circulation, or as a result of hypovolemia due to ascites. Vital signs need to be monitored closely.

Fetor hepaticus is a musty, sweetish odour detected on the client's breath. The odour is due to the accumulation of digested by-products. Additional complications of cirrhosis may include exhaustion, gallstones, complications with pharmacological therapy, and pruritus.

An important role of the nurse is educating the client about the general management of cirrhosis, which includes rest, avoidance of alcohol and anticoagulants, managing the possible complications, and ensuring adequate and appropriate nutrition.

Pancreatitis
Pathophysiology
Pancreatitis is an inflammation of the pancreas that can be acute or chronic. The degree of inflammation varies from mild edema to severe necrosis. Pancreatitis can affect both males and females, but it is more commonly found in males. The prognosis is good when pancreatitis follows biliary disease but poor when it is a complication of alcoholism. The causes of pancreatitis are as follows:

- Alcohol is the number one cause of pancreatitis in Canada.
- Gallbladder disease is the next most common cause of pancreatitis.
- Other causes include viral infections, duodenal or peptic ulcers, pancreatic cancer, medications such as glucocorticoids, metabolic disorders such as hyperparathyroidism and dyslipidemia, and postsurgical trauma from ERCP.

In acute pancreatitis, the inflammation that occurs is caused by premature activation of digestive enzymes, which leads to autodigestion of the surrounding tissue. The pancreatic enzymes are activated while they are still in the pancreas rather than in the small intestine, so they digest pancreatic cells, causing severe edema, interstitial hemorrhage, and necrosis, which can lead to hypotension, shock, and disseminated intravascular coagulation (DIC).

Two major complications of pancreatitis are pseudocyst and pancreatic abscess. The pseudocyst is a cavity that develops around the pancreas that is filled with necrotic products and liquid secretions. If the cyst perforates, exudate inflames the surrounding tissues, causing peritonitis, followed by scar tissue. The pseudocyst may heal by itself or require draining. A pancreatic abscess is a large fluid-containing cavity within the pancreas that results from extensive necrosis of the pancreatic cells. This abscess may become infected and perforate.

Other complications of pancreatitis include pulmonary conditions such as pleural effusion, atelectasis, and pneumonia. Cardiovascular conditions such as hypotension and tachycardia may occur, and the client may develop tetany due to the low calcium levels in the blood.

Clinical Manifestations
Abdominal pain unrelieved by vomiting may be the first and only symptom of mild pancreatitis. A severe attack may cause a sudden onset of extreme pain in the left upper quadrant with possible radiation to the back. The pain is often described as severe, deep, piercing, and steady. The pain is aggravated by eating or drinking alcohol and does not subside with vomiting. Other manifestations may include flushing, cyanosis, edema, nausea, vomiting, low-grade fever, leukocytosis, jaundice, hypotension, and tachycardia.

Diagnostics
Diagnosis is made through the history and physical examination. Blood work may show elevated serum amylase levels, which rules out appendicitis, acute cholecystitis, perforated ulcer, and bowel infarction. Serum lipase, glucose, and WBC levels are likely to increase, while serum calcium levels are likely to decrease. An abdominal CT scan can help distinguish between cholelithiasis and pancreatitis.

Therapeutics and Nursing Considerations
Management of pancreatitis focuses on the following:
- Pain relief
- Maintenance of circulation and fluid volume
- Decreasing pancreatic enzymes
- Analgesics, vasodilators, and antispasmodics may be given. Dopamine may be needed for hypotension.
- The client will be NPO. An NG tube will be in place to remove secretions. IV therapy will be needed to maintain fluid volume. The client will be monitored for complications. Once the client is allowed food, small, frequent meals are offered. The diet should be high in carbohydrates and protein and low in fat.

Nursing considerations will focus on the following:
- Pain relief (e.g., with hydromorphone, morphine)
- Improving breathing patterns
- Improving nutritional status
- Improving skin integrity
- Monitoring and managing any complications

The nurse will also be involved in client teaching about discontinuing alcohol consumption, proper nutrition and rest, and ways to improve the client's general health.

Pathophysiology of chronic pancreatitis. Chronic pancreatitis develops from repeated attacks of pancreatitis. These repeated attacks cause scarring and calcification of the pancreatic cells, which leads to the permanent and progressive destruction of the pancreas. Both exocrine and endocrine functions of the pancreas are affected. Chronic obstructive pancreatitis results from inflammation of the sphincter of Oddi and is associated with cholelithiasis. Chronic calcifying pancreatitis is alcohol-induced pancreatitis.

Clinical manifestations of chronic pancreatitis. Chronic pancreatitis manifestations include abdominal pain, usually described as a severe, heavy, gnawing feeling, burning, or cramplike pain. The client will experience malabsorption, constipation, steatorrhea, mild jaundice, and diabetes mellitus (DM).

Diagnostics for chronic pancreatitis. Diagnosis is the same as for acute pancreatitis.

Therapeutics and nursing considerations for chronic pancreatitis. Management of chronic pancreatitis focuses on prevention of attacks. During an attack, treatment is similar to that of acute pancreatitis. With chronic pancreatitis, the client needs to be taught about diet, pancreatic enzyme replacement, exogenous insulin, antacids, and cessation of alcohol intake. The client cannot tolerate fatty or rich foods. The DM is often "brittle" in response to insulin; therefore, the client may require frequent injections to control blood sugars. Client education is very important.

REGULATORY MECHANISM HEALTH CHALLENGES

Addison's Disease

Pathophysiology

Addison's disease is the most common form of adrenal insufficiency. Although Addison's disease usually results from an autoimmune disorder, it can be caused by TB, histoplasmosis, adrenal hemorrhage, cancer, lymphoma, and certain drugs. Surgical removal of the adrenal glands and abruptly stopping long-term corticosteroid therapy can also cause Addison's disease. When the cause is autoimmune, antibodies against the client's own adrenal cortex destroy the adrenal gland's ability to secrete hormones.

Clinical Manifestations

Manifestations do not tend to become apparent until about 90% of the cortex has been destroyed. Manifestations that do develop do so insidiously and may include the following:
- Progressive weakness and fatigue
- Weight loss and anorexia
- Skin hyperpigmentation (bronze colouring) is a striking feature.
- The client also may have orthostatic hypotension, a weak irregular pulse, decreased tolerance for even minor stress, poor coordination, fasting hypoglycemia, a craving for salty foods, and amenorrhea.

Diagnostics

Diagnosis is made based on clinical features and decreased serum cortisol and sodium levels. Corticotrophin, serum potassium, and blood urea nitrogen (BUN) levels are all increased. A failure of serum cortisol to rise following adrenocorticotropic hormone (ACTH) stimulation indicates primary adrenal disease.

Therapeutics and Nursing Considerations

Treatment of Addison's disease is focused on management of the underlying cause and replacement therapy.
- Hydrocortisone has both glucocorticoid and mineralocorticoid properties and is frequently used as replacement therapy.
- During periods of stress, the replacement therapy may need to be increased.
- In an adrenal crisis, the client may need prompt administration of dexamethasone, hydrocortisone, or both, and doses continue until they stabilize.
- Vital signs must be monitored for signs of volume depletion and hypotension.
- Blood work needs to be monitored for altered electrolytes both before and during treatment.
- Blood glucose needs to be monitored as steroid replacement may alter insulin requirements.

Client education regarding medication adherence is essential.

Cushing's Syndrome

Pathophysiology

Cushing's syndrome is a spectrum of clinical abnormalities caused by excess corticosteroids, particularly glucocorticoids. This adrenal hyperfunction can be caused by prolonged administration of high doses of corticosteroids, an ACTH-secreting pituitary tumour, or a cortisol-secreting neoplasm within the adrenal cortex that can be either carcinoma or adenoma.

Clinical Manifestations

Unmistakable manifestations of Cushing's syndrome include the following:
- Adiposity of the face (moon face) and neck (buffalo hump)
- Purple striae on the skin of the trunk, especially the abdomen
- Weight gain
- Muscle weakness and fatigue
- Thinning of the extremities with muscle wasting and fat mobilization
- Thin, fragile skin, ruddy complexion, hirsutism, acne, bruising, and impaired wound healing
- Mood disturbances such as irritability, euphoria, anxiety, insomnia, irrationality and occasionally psychosis may occur.

Diagnostics

When Cushing's syndrome is suspected, a 24-hour urine collection test for free cortisol and a low-dose dexamethasone suppression test are done. If these tests are inconclusive, then a high-dose dexamethasone suppression test is done. Ultrasonography, CT scan, and angiography localize adrenal tumours. CT scan and MRI of the head help localize pituitary tumours.

Therapeutics and Nursing Considerations

The primary goal of treatment is to normalize hormone secretion. Radiation, drug therapy, or surgery may be needed to

restore hormone balance and reverse Cushing's syndrome. Some examples of treatments are as follows:
- Trans-sphenoidal resection and radiation may be used for pituitary adenomas.
- Surgical removal or radiation may be used for an ectopic ACTH-secreting tumour.
- Nonendocrine corticotropin-secreting tumours require excision.
- Medication therapy with ketoconazole (Nizoral), or mitotane (Lysodren) decreases cortisol levels if symptoms persist or if the tumour is inoperable.

Before surgery, the client will require special monitoring and control of hypertension, edema, diabetes, and cardiovascular manifestations and to prevent infection. Glucocorticoid administration the morning of surgery can help prevent acute adrenal insufficiency during surgery. Nursing considerations will focus on the following:
- Decreasing risk for injury
- Decreasing risk for infection
- Encouraging rest and activity
- Promoting skin integrity
- Improving body image
- Improving thought processes
- Monitoring and managing complications

Clients with Cushing's syndrome require thorough ongoing assessment and supportive care, including emotional support, as the syndrome produces emotional lability. In some cases, sedation may be needed to help the client rest.

Hyperthyroidism
Pathophysiology
Hyperthyroidism is a clinical syndrome in which there is a sustained increase in synthesis and release of thyroid hormones by the thyroid gland. The most common form of hyperthyroidism is Graves' disease (diffuse toxic goitre), an autoimmune disease that increases T_4 (thyroxine) production, enlarges the thyroid gland (goitre), and causes multisystem changes. In Graves' disease, a thyroid-stimulating hormone (TSH) receptor autoantibody stimulates the thyroid gland to produce high concentrations of T_3 (tri-iodothyronine) and T_4. Graves' disease has also been associated with the production of several autoantibodies formed because of a defect in suppressor T-lymphocyte function.

Thyrotoxic crisis (thyroid storm) is an acute, rare condition in which all hyperthyroid manifestations are heightened. This is a life-threatening condition for which aggressive measures must be taken to prevent death.

Clinical Manifestations
Classic manifestations of Graves' disease include the following:
- A diffusely enlarged thyroid
- Nervousness and insomnia
- Hair loss
- Fatigue and muscle weakness
- Edema
- Heat intolerance

- Weight loss and increased appetite
- Splenomegaly
- Hepatomegaly
- Sweating
- Diarrhea
- Tremor
- Palpitations
- Systolic hypertension
- Arrhythmias and atrial fibrillation
- Reproductive abnormalities
- Possible exophthalmos

Treatment is aimed at reducing circulating thyroid hormone levels and treating manifestations such as high fever with antipyretics, IV therapy for fluid replacement, and elimination of stressors.

Diagnostics
Graves' disease is diagnosed by the history and physical examination and laboratory tests finding decreased TSH and increased free T_4 levels. Radioactive iodine uptake test is needed to differentiate Graves' disease from other forms of thyroiditis. A thyroid sonogram helps distinguish cystic and solid lesions. A CT scan or an MRI helps identify deep thyroid nodules.

Therapeutics and Nursing Considerations
The overall goal in the treatment of hyperthyroidism is to block the adverse effects of the thyroid hormones and stop their oversecretion. The primary forms of treatment for hyperthyroidism are as follows:
- Antithyroid medications
- Radioactive iodine therapy
- Subtotal thyroidectomy

Choice of treatment will depend on the client's age, severity of the disease, client's present physical condition, and the client's preference.
- Propylthiouracil (Propyl-Thyracil) and methimazole (Tapazole) block thyroid hormone synthesis.
- The administration of iodine in large doses rapidly inhibits synthesis of T_3 and T_4 and blocks the release of these hormones into the circulatory system.
- Beta-adrenergic blockers are used for symptomatic relief of thyrotoxicosis that results from increased beta-adrenergic receptor stimulation caused by excess thyroid hormone.
- Radioactive iodine damages or destroys thyroid tissue, thus limiting thyroid hormone secretion. This treatment is effective but leaves the client with hypothyroidism, requiring thyroid hormone replacement therapy.
- A subtotal thyroidectomy removes a significant portion (90%) of the thyroid gland and is needed for clients who do not respond to antithyroid therapy.
- Endoscopic thyroidectomy is a minimally invasive procedure that involves making several small incisions in which the endoscope and other instruments can be passed to remove thyroid tissue or nodules. This procedure is appropriate for clients with small nodules (less than 3 cm in diameter) and have no evidence of malignancy.

Nursing considerations focus on improving nutritional status, enhancing coping measures, improving self-esteem, maintaining normal body temperatures, and monitoring and managing any complications.

Hypothyroidism
Pathophysiology

Hypothyroidism is a state of low levels of serum thyroid hormones. Hypothyroidism may result from a number of causes but is mainly caused by the following:

- A thyroidectomy
- Radiation therapy
- Chronic autoimmune thyroiditis (Hashimoto's disease)
- Inflammatory diseases, such as amyloidosis

In primary hypothyroidism, thyroid hormone production is decreased due to decreased thyroid tissue. The pituitary gland will still secrete TSH, and a goitre may develop. In secondary hypothyroidism, the pituitary fails to synthesize or secrete adequate amounts of TSH, or target tissues fail to respond to normal blood levels of the thyroid hormone. Either type may progress to myxedema (an advanced form of hypothyroidism). This condition is considered a medical emergency.

Clinical Manifestations

Clinical manifestations of hypothyroidism will vary with the severity of the condition regardless of the cause. Symptoms develop insidiously and may include the following:

- Fatigue and lethargy
- Forgetfulness
- Slow speech
- Low exercise tolerance
- Weight gain
- Bradycardia
- Anemia
- Constipation
- Cool, dry, flaky skin; dry, sparse hair; and thick, brittle nails.

Symptoms of the life-threatening myxedema include progressive personality and mental changes moving toward stupor, hypoventilation, hypoglycemia, hyponatremia, hypotension, and hypothermia.

Diagnostics

The most common and reliable laboratory tests used to evaluate thyroid function are those that measure TSH and free T_4. When TSH levels are high, the defect is in the thyroid, and when the levels are low, the defect is in the pituitary or hypothalamus.

Therapeutics and Nursing Considerations

The goal of treatment for clients with hypothyroidism is replacement of the hormones by administering synthetic levothyroxine (Synthroid, Eltroxin). The nurse provides the following care:

- Routinely assesses the client to see whether the medication is adequate or not

- Encourages weight loss with a high-bulk, low-calorie diet
- Encourages activity balanced with rest
- Administers laxatives and stool softeners when needed

Teach the client to watch for signs of hyperthyroidism, such as sweating, tachycardia, or rapid weight loss, and to always wear a MedicAlert bracelet or carry a MedicAlert card.

Syndrome of Inappropriate Antidiuretic Hormone
Pathophysiology

Syndrome of inappropriate antidiuretic hormone (SIADH) occurs when ADH is released despite normal or low plasma osmolarity. SIADH results from an abnormal production or sustained secretion of ADH and is characterized by fluid retention. The hyponatremia that can occur with SIADH can lead to cerebral edema. SIADH can occur due to malignant lung disease, infections, trauma, or medications that stimulate ADH release.

Clinical Manifestations

One of the chief clinical manifestations of SIADH is fluid retention; therefore, the client will gain weight and have a decreased urine output. The serum hyponatremia may cause the client to have the following symptoms as well:

- Muscle cramps, weakness, and muscle twitching
- Vomiting
- Seizures

If the hyponatremia progresses and sodium levels continue to decline, the client may experience cerebral edema, leading to lethargy, anorexia, confusion, headaches, seizure, and coma.

Diagnostics

The diagnosis of SIADH is made by simultaneous measurements of urine and serum osmolality. A serum osmolality of less than 280 mmol/kg and a urine specific gravity greater than 1.005 are indicative of SIADH.

Therapeutics and Nursing Considerations

Once SIADH is identified, the care is directed at the underlying cause of the condition. The immediate treatment is aimed at restoring normal fluid volume and osmolality. Fluid restriction may be all that is needed. If the hyponatremia is severe, hypertonic saline solutions may be administered cautiously as rapid administration could overload the heart.

Diabetes Insipidus
Pathophysiology

Diabetes insipidus (DI) is a group of conditions associated with a deficiency of production or secretion of ADH (vasopressin) or a decreased renal response to ADH. DI may be familial, acquired, or idiopathic.

- It can be acquired as the result of intracranial neoplastic or metastatic lesions.
- Other causes may include hypophysectomy or other neurosurgery, head trauma, infection, granulomatous disease, vascular lesions, or autoimmune disorders.

Normally, the ADH is synthesized in the hypothalamus and stored in the posterior pituitary gland. When released, ADH works on the distal and collecting tubules of the kidneys, causing water to be reabsorbed. If ADH is absent or not released, the water is excreted in the urine. As a result, the client will void copious amounts of urine.

Clinical Manifestations

The classic sign of DI is polyuria, or the passage of a large volume of urine, with amounts from 5 to 20 L and possibly up to 30 L a day. Polydipsia, or excessive thirst, may be present. Nocturia and fatigue are common, as well as dehydration with weight loss, poor tissue turgor, dry mucous membranes, constipation, muscle weakness, dizziness, tachycardia, and hypotension.

Diagnostics

A complete history and physical examination are needed to diagnose DI. Baseline vital signs and weight are taken, and urine and plasma osmolalities and specific gravity of the urine tests are usually performed. A urinalysis may reveal almost colourless urine with a low osmolality and low specific gravity. A water deprivation test confirms the diagnosis. The client will be denied water for 8 to 16 hours. The client will be anxious and thirsty and will require reassurance and support. Vital signs will be monitored closely, and the test will be stopped if the client develops orthostatic hypotension or body weight drops by 3% and until the urine osmolality stabilizes (hourly increase <30 mmol/kg in 3 consecutive hours).

Therapeutics and Nursing Considerations

Determining the cause of DI is critical to its treatment. Hormone replacement of ADH is needed. Care of a client with DI resulting from nephrogenic conditions includes a low-sodium diet and utilizing thiazide diuretics. The thiazides are able to slow the glomerular filtration rate (GFR), allowing the kidneys to reabsorb more water in the loop of Henle and distal tubules. If this does not work, indomethacin (an anti-inflammatory) may be prescribed.

Nursing management revolves around early detection, maintenance of adequate hydration, client teaching for long-term management, and encouragement and support while the client is undergoing diagnostic studies and treatment.

Diabetes Mellitus
Pathophysiology

DM is a multisystem disease related to abnormal insulin production, impaired insulin utilization, or both. It is the leading cause of heart disease, stroke, adult blindness, and nontraumatic lower limb amputation.

Normally, insulin is produced by the beta cells in the islets of Langerhans of the pancreas. Insulin facilitates the normal glucose range of approximately 4 to 6 mmol/L. Insulin is a storage hormone that promotes glucose transport from the bloodstream across the cell membrane into the cytoplasm of the cell. Ingesting food stimulates the release of insulin from the pancreas into the blood. Insulin stimulates the storage of glucose as glycogen and inhibits gluconeogenesis. Insulin also enhances fat deposition in adipose tissue and increases protein synthesis. Glucagon is a hormone produced in the alpha cells of the pancreas and functions by increasing blood glucose levels.

Type 1 diabetes was formerly known as *juvenile-onset* or *insulin-dependent* diabetes. Type 1 diabetes usually affects people under the age of 30, peaking at 11 to 13 years, but it can affect people older than 30 years of age. Type 1 diabetes involves the progressive destruction of pancreatic beta cells. Autoantibodies cause a reduction of 80 to 90% of normal beta-cell function before manifestations occur. The causes of type 1 diabetes may be due to genetic predisposition or exposure to a virus. Manifestations develop when the pancreas can no longer produce insulin. Symptoms tend to be rapid in onset, and the client often presents to the emergency department with ketoacidosis. Other classic symptoms include weight loss, polyuria, polydipsia, and polyphagia. Diabetic ketoacidosis (DKA) occurs in the absence of exogenous insulin. It is a life-threatening condition that results in metabolic acidosis.

Type 2 diabetes accounts for over 90% of clients with diabetes. It usually occurs in people over the age of 35; however, children are now being diagnosed with type 2 diabetes, usually due to obesity and a sedentary lifestyle. With type 2 diabetes, the pancreas continues to produce some endogenous insulin; however, the amount produced is either insufficient or is poorly utilized by the tissues. Insulin resistance is the key to type 2 diabetes, a situation in which the body does not respond to the insulin and hyperglycemia results. Some people experience glucose intolerance, in which the alteration in the beta cells is mild. In these situations, the blood glucose levels are higher than normal but are not high enough for a diagnosis of diabetes. Inappropriate glucose production by the liver is not considered a primary factor in the development of type 2 diabetes. Insulin resistance syndrome (syndrome X) is a cluster of abnormalities that act synergistically to increase the risk for cardiovascular disease. Type 2 diabetes typically has a gradual onset; the person may go many years with undetected hyperglycemia. See Table 9.8 for further characteristics of type 1 and 2 diabetes.

Diabetes can also develop during pregnancy, when it is usually detected at 24 to 28 weeks of gestation. With gestational diabetes, there is an increased risk for a caesarean delivery, perinatal deaths, and neonatal complications.

Diabetes can also develop secondary to another medical condition or the treatment of a medical condition. For example, there can be abnormal blood values in a client experiencing Cushing's syndrome or as a result of the use of parenteral nutrition.

Clinical Manifestations

Manifestations of type 1 diabetes include classic polyuria, polydipsia, and polyphagia. The client will also experience weight loss, weakness and fatigue, and ketoacidosis. Nonspecific symptoms include fatigue, recurrent infections, prolonged wound healing, and visual changes.

TABLE 9.8   Characteristics of Type 1 and Type 2 Diabetes Mellitus

Factor	Type 1 Diabetes Mellitus	Type 2 Diabetes Mellitus	Factor	Type 1 Diabetes Mellitus	Type 2 Diabetes Mellitus
Age at onset	More common in young people but can occur at any age	Usually ≥35 yr but can occur at any age Incidence is increasing in children	Endogenous insulin	Minimal or absent	Possibly excessive; adequate but delayed secretion or reduced utilization; secretions diminish over time
Type of onset	Signs and symptoms abrupt, but disease process may be present for several years	Insidious; may go undiagnosed for years	Nutritional status	Thin, normal, or obese	Obese or normal
Prevalence	Accounts for 5%–10% of all types of diabetes	Accounts for 90% of all types of diabetes	Symptoms	Thirst, polyuria, polyphagia, fatigue, weight loss	Frequently none, fatigue, recurrent infections
Environmental factors	Viruses, toxins	Obesity, lack of exercise	Ketosis	Prone at onset or during insulin deficiency	Resistant except during infection or stress
Primary defect	Absent or minimal insulin production due to an autoimmune process	Insulin resistance, decreased insulin production over time, and alterations in production of adipokines	Nutritional therapy	Essential	Essential
Islet-cell antibodies	Often present at onset	Absent	Insulin	Required for all	Required for some
			Oral antihyperglycemic agents	Not indicated	Usually beneficial
			Vascular and neurological complications	Frequent	Frequent

From Tyerman, J., & Cobbett, S. (2023). *Lewis's medical-surgical nursing in Canada: Assessment and management of clinical problems* (5th Cdn. ed., p. 1271, Table 52.1). Elsevier.

Diagnostics

Diagnosis of DM is made when glycosylated hemoglobin (hemoglobin A1c) is greater than 6.5%, fasting plasma glucose is greater than 7 mmol/L, a random plasma glucose measurement is greater than 11.1 mmol/L, or a 2-hour oral glucose tolerance test (OGTT) is greater than 11.1 mmol/L when using a glucose load of 75 g. Tests used to evaluate glucose control and monitor for complications of diabetes include hemoglobin A1c, lipid profile, BUN, serum creatinine, electrolytes, and TSH. Urine can be checked for glucose and ketones.

Therapeutics and Nursing Considerations

Goals for the treatment of DM include the following:
- Reducing symptoms
- Promoting well-being
- Preventing acute complications
- Delaying the onset and progression of long-term complications

Collaborative care includes five components: education, nutrition, medications, exercise, and self-monitoring of blood glucose.

Exogenous insulin is required for type 1 diabetes. It may be prescribed for clients with type 2 diabetes who cannot control their blood glucose by other means or when the client is under stress. Human insulin is the most widely used insulin; it is cost-effective, and there is less chance of the client developing an allergic reaction. Insulin can also be derived from pork.

Insulin types differ in regard to onset, peak action, and duration. Different types of insulin may be used for combination therapy. Some common types of insulin are as follows:
- Lispro (Humalog), Lispro U200 (Humalog), Aspart (NovoRapid), Glulisine (Apidra) are rapid-acting insulins.
- Regular (Novolin ge) Toronto, Humulin R) are short-acting insulins.
- NPH (Humulin N, Novolinge ge NPH) are intermediate-acting insulins.

- Detemir (Levemir), Glaragine U300 (Toujeo) and Glargine (Lantus) are long-acting insulins.
- Premixed (cloudy): (Regular/NPH 30/70+, regular/NPH 50/50 and 40/60, Lispro/lispro protamine 25/75 Humalog Mix 25, 50/50(Humalog mix 50), Aspart/ aspart protamine 30/70 (NovaMix 30).

Insulin may be administered subcutaneously. At present, insulin cannot be taken orally; however, new research is finding alternative delivery methods, including aerosol, skin patches, oral spray, and pills. Difficulties with insulin therapy include hypoglycemia, allergic reactions, lipodystrophy, and the Somogyi effect.

Oral agents are not insulin. These medications work to improve the mechanisms through which insulin and glucose are produced and used by the body. These medications include the following:

- Sulfonylureas, meglitinides, biguanides
- Alpha-glucosidase inhibitors
- Thiazolidinediones
- Dipeptidyl peptidase-4 inhibitors
- Sodium-glucose cotransporter type 2 (SGLT) inhibitors
- Glucagon-like peptide (GLP)-1 receptor agonists (incretin mimetrics). These drugs stimulate GLP-1 (one of the incretin hormones), which is found to be decreased in people with type 2 DM.
- Many combination therapy medications are available. These drugs combine two different classes of medication to treat DM. One advantage of combined therapy is improved clients compliance.
- Other drugs affecting blood glucose levels are beta-adrenergic blockers, thiazide diuretics, and loop diuretics.

Nutrition and exercise in DM management. Research has shown that within the context of an overall healthy eating plan, a person with diabetes can eat the same foods as a person who does not have diabetes. The overall goal of nutrition therapy is to assist people in making changes in nutrition and exercise habits that will lead to improved metabolic control.

- A type 1 DM meal plan is based on the individual's usual food intake and is balanced with insulin and exercise patterns.
- In type 2 DM, emphasis is placed on achieving glucose, lipid, and BP goals. Calorie reduction is often needed.

Individual meal plans are developed with the assistance of a dietitian. The plan promotes a nutritional balance and does not prohibit the consumption of any one type of food. Alcohol can be included within the plan with the full understanding that alcohol is high in calories, promotes hypertriglyceridemia, and can cause severe hypoglycemia. The dietitian should provide instructions to the client and family or significant other. It is important for the nurse to consider the food preferences of a cultural group when giving dietary instructions. Diabetes Canada has nutritional resources specifically designed for members of different cultural groups (Tyerman & Cobbett, 2023).

Exercise is an essential part of diabetes management as it increases insulin sensitivity, lowers blood glucose levels, and decreases insulin resistance. Exercise also improves circulation and muscle tone, increases the resting metabolic rate, and alters blood lipids. The body considers exercise to be stress. In type 1 diabetes, the physiological decrease in circulating insulin that normally occurs with exercise cannot occur; therefore, clients with DM need to have small carbohydrate snacks every 30 minutes during exercise to prevent hypoglycemia. Exercise is best done after meals and should be individualized for every client. Blood glucose levels should be monitored before, during, and after exercise.

Self-monitoring of blood glucose (SMBG) enables clients to make self-management decisions regarding diet, exercise, and medications. SMBG is important for detecting episodic hyperglycemia and hypoglycemia. Client teaching is crucial. SMBG requires good visual acuity, fine motor coordination, cognitive ability, comfort with technology, willingness, and sufficient finances to pay for it.

Urine testing for glucose was a technique used before the development of SMBG. It is a less expensive technique, but it does not represent an accurate reading as the urine tested could have been in the bladder for a matter of hours. However, urine testing for ketones is essential when the client is ill.

Overall goals for the management of DM should include active participation of the client, no episodes of hypoglycemia or hyperglycemia, maintenance of normal blood glucose levels, prevention of complications, and lifestyle adjustments with minimal stress.

Acute complications of DM. Acute complications pertaining to DM are hypoglycemia, DKA, and hyperosmolar hyperglycemic nonketotic syndrome (HHNK).

Hypoglycemia. Hypoglycemia is found in clients whose blood glucose level is abnormally below 4 mmol/L. Hypoglycemia may be caused by too little food or too much insulin. Symptoms of hypoglycemia include the following:

- Sweating
- Trembling
- Blurred vision
- Extreme tiredness and paleness
- Headache
- Hunger
- Mood changes
- Dizziness

To treat hypoglycemia, give 10 to 15 g of a fast-acting simple carbohydrate, such as 3 to 4 commercially prepared glucose tabs, 175 mL of fruit juice or a regular soft drink, or 6 to 8 Life Saver candies; for a client taking acarbose: 15 mL (1 tbsp) syrup or honey, 125 to 150 mL low-fat milk, or dextrose tabs because the absorption of glucose itself is not affected (Tyerman & Cobbett, 2023). The blood should be retested after 15 minutes. If the blood glucose remains low, the carbohydrate intake should be repeated. When the level goes up, the client should be given a protein with a starch. An unconscious client can be injected with 1 mg of glucagon, either subcutaneously or intramuscularly. If this is not available, a source of glucose, such as corn syrup, honey, or icing, may be placed in the client's buccal pouch. After consciousness returns, the client should be given a protein or starch snack. Hypoglycemia is preventable. Clients with diabetes should always carry a simple sugar with them and have identification confirming their diagnosis. Family and friends need to know the signs and symptoms of hypoglycemia and what they can do to assist the client. In an acute care setting, clients with hypoglycemia are treated with 20 to 50 mL of 50% dextrose IV push.

Diabetic ketoacidosis. DKA is caused by an absence or a markedly inadequate amount of insulin. Clinical features of DKA include hyperglycemia, dehydration, and acidosis. DKA can be caused by a decreased or missed dose of insulin, an illness or infection, or undiagnosed and untreated diabetes. Clinical manifestations include the following:

- Blurred vision
- Weakness
- Headache
- Orthostatic hypotension
- Anorexia, nausea and vomiting, and abdominal pain
- Acetone breath
- Hyperventilation
- Possible mental changes

Laboratory findings include an elevated blood glucose above 14 mmol/L, arterial blood pH below 7.35, serum bicarbonate level less than 15 mmol/L, and an anion gap greater than 12 mmol/L. The severity of DKA is not necessarily related to the actual blood glucose level. Ketones will be found in the blood and urine, and the electrolytes may be low, normal, or high, depending on the level of dehydration.

Prevention of DKA is based on understanding the importance of food replacement during illness. A typical sick-day routine is as follows: take insulin or oral antidiabetic agents as usual. Test blood glucose and urine for ketones every 3 to 4 hours. Report elevated blood glucose levels of 16 mmol/L or more or the presence of ketones in the urine to the health care provider. Treatment of DKA focuses on rehydration and balancing the electrolytes and pH. Clients receive potassium in the IV solution as long as they remain polyuric and hypokalemic. The acidosis is reversed by administering insulin via an IV pump. Nursing management focuses on the following:

- Monitoring fluid and electrolyte balance
- Monitoring blood glucose levels
- Giving fluids, insulin, and other medications as ordered
- Ensuring renal function
- Monitoring for arrhythmias
- Monitoring vital signs
- Reassessing factors leading to the development of DKA

Hyperosmolar hyperglycemic nonketotic syndrome. HHNK includes hyperglycemia, dehydration, and hyperosmolality of the plasma, with the absence of ketones in the urine. HHNK differs from DKA in that HHNK does not cause fat tissue to break down; thus, ketones will not be released. Clinical manifestations include hypotension, profound dehydration, and tachycardia, with variable neurological signs. Medical and nursing management focuses on fluid replacement, correction of electrolyte imbalances, administering IV insulin, and monitoring fluid and electrolyte balance. Insulin is not used to treat acidosis in HHNK, but it is used to treat the hyperglycemia.

Chronic complications of DM. Chronic complications of DM include microvascular and macrovascular complications and neuropathic complications. DM can cause macrovascular damage to the large blood vessels providing circulation to the brain, heart, and extremities. Dyslipidemia, hypertension, and impaired fibrinolysis have been found in uncontrolled DM.

Microvascular complications create abnormal thickening of the basement membrane in the capillaries by hyperglycemia. Hyperglycemia also disrupts platelet function.

- Retinopathy starts with small hemorrhages in the retinal capillaries. Neovascularization occurs, which can lead to proliferative retinopathy. People with DM have an increased risk of developing cataracts and open-angle glaucoma.
- Nephropathy is the leading cause of end-stage renal disease (ESRD), with the characteristic lesion being glomerulosclerosis.
- Neuropathic complications can be found in 40 to 50% of those with diabetes; paraesthesia, autonomic complications, and sensory disturbances are common.
- Peripheral polyneuropathy involves both neuropathy and vascular conditions. The real danger for the client with this condition is that the client cannot feel pain.
- Individuals with diabetes need to watch for any signs of infection. There is a defect in the mobilization of inflammatory cells and an impairment of WBCs in phagocytosis. Persistent glycosuria encourages bladder infections. There is a delay in healing due to decreased circulation as well as protein waste leading to poor wound healing.

Pancreas transplantation is done for clients with type 1 DM who have ESRD and have had or plan to have a kidney transplantation. The pancreas transplantation eliminates the need for exogenous insulin and eliminates hypoglycemia and hyperglycemia.

REPRODUCTIVE HEALTH CHALLENGES

Breast Cancer

Pathophysiology

Breast cancer is the most diagnosed cancer in Canadian females, excluding nonmelanoma skin cancer. Genetic abnormalities account for 5 to 10% of breast cancers. *BRCA* gene carriers are also at risk of developing ovarian cancer. Having a first-degree relative with breast cancer increases the risk of developing breast cancer by 1.5 to 3 times. Secondary risk factors include never giving birth, giving birth to a first child after the age of 30, prolonged hormonal stimulation, exposure to excessive ionizing radiation, and a history of endometrial, ovarian, or colon cancer.

Types of breast cancer are based on histological characteristics and growth patterns. Infiltrating ductal carcinoma is considered to be the most common form of breast cancer. The cancers generally arise from the epithelial lining of the ducts or from the epithelium of lobules. Breast cancer may be invasive or in situ. Most cancers that arise from the ducts are invasive. Factors affecting prognosis include the size of the tumour, axillary node involvement, tumour differentiation, DNA content, and estrogen and progesterone receptor status.

Ductal carcinoma in situ (DCIS) tends to be unilateral and progresses to invasive if untreated. Lobular carcinoma in situ (LCIS) appears to be more of a premalignant cancer. Individuals with LCIS have a greater risk of developing invasive breast cancer in the same or opposite breast.

Clinical Manifestations

Symptoms of breast cancer include the following:

- Detecting a lump or mass in the breast
- Changes in breast symmetry or size
- Changes in breast skin, such as dimpling
- Edema
- Skin ulcers
- Changes in nipples causing itching, burning, erosion, or retraction
- Skin temperature changes

The cancer often occurs in the upper outer quadrant; will present as hard, irregularly shaped, poorly delineated, and nonmobile; and will feel nontender when palpated. A serious complication of breast cancer is recurrence. Metastasis occurs primarily through lymphatic chains but can spread without invading axillary nodes.

Diagnostics

Diagnosis of breast cancer is based on biopsy and pathological evaluation of suspected tissue. Diagnostic studies used are lymph node dissection, axillary lymph node status, estrogen and progesterone receptor status, DNA content analysis, and cell proliferative indices.

Therapeutics and Nursing Considerations

Common surgical therapy involves breast conservation surgery (lumpectomy) with radiation therapy or modified radical mastectomy with or without reconstruction. Axillary node dissection is often performed regardless of treatment as it provides excellent prognostic data and helps develop further treatment.

Breast conservation surgery removes the entire tumour along with a margin of normal tissue. Radiation is delivered to the entire breast following surgery. Attempts are made to preserve as much of the breast as possible, including the nipple. A modified radical mastectomy removes the entire breast along with the axillary lymph nodes. The pectoral major muscle is preserved. This is done when the tumour is too large to excise with good margins. The client has the option of breast reconstruction.

Lymphedema, swelling caused by the localized retention of lymphatic fluid, can result from the excision or radiation of lymph nodes. This fluid can cause obstructive pressure. Lymphedema can be prevented by frequent and sustained elevation of the arms, performing arm exercises, and avoiding constrictive clothing.

The client will experience postmastectomy pain in the chest and upper arm. Tingling down the arm, numbness, and shooting or prickling pain are felt. Unbearable itching may

also be present. This pain is treated with NSAIDs, antidepressants, topical lidocaine patches, eutectic mixture of local anaesthetics (EMLA) cream, and antiseizure medications.

Radiation is employed to destroy a cancerous tumour or as a companion to surgery. The radiation will shrink the tumour to an operable size. Radiation can be used for palliative care as well.

Chemotherapy is systemic therapy designed to destroy cells that have spread undetected to distant sites, as well as to decrease the primary tumour and suppress tumour growth.

Hormonal therapy will block and destroy estrogen receptors and suppress estrogen synthesis.

Biological therapy attempts to stimulate the body's natural defences to recognize and attack cancer cells.

Mammoplasty surgically changes the size and shape of the breast for cosmetic or reconstructive reasons. Possible complications include hematoma, hemorrhage, and infection. It is often done simultaneously with or after a mastectomy. When done simultaneously, reconstruction avoids surgery after scar tissue or adhesions develop. Mammoplasty can include breast implants and tissue expansions, or a musculocutaneous flap procedure may be done. This procedure involves using the client's own tissue, usually from the back or abdomen, to repair soft tissue defects if there is insufficient muscle after a mastectomy. Nipple and areolar reconstruction can also be done.

Ovarian Cancer

Pathophysiology

Ovarian cancer, malignant neoplasm of the ovaries, has the highest mortality rate of all gynecological cancers because most clients have advanced disease at diagnosis. It occurs most frequently in females between the ages of 55 and 65 years. Risk factors are as follows:

- Family history of ovarian, breast, or colon cancer
- Nulliparity; persons who have never been pregnant are at greater risk
- High-fat diet
- Increased number of ovulatory cycles
- Hormone replacement therapy (HRT)
- Use of infertility drugs

Oral contraceptives, breastfeeding, multiple pregnancies, and early age at birth of a first child are associated with lower risk.

Ninety percent of ovarian cancers are epithelial carcinomas. Germ cell tumours account for 10% of ovarian cancers. Ovarian cancer can metastasize directly by shedding malignant cells that often implant in the uterus, bladder, bowel, and omentum. The cancer can also spread via the lymph system.

Clinical Manifestations

Manifestations include general abdominal discomfort, a sense of pelvic heaviness, loss of appetite, feeling of fullness, and a change in bowel habits. As the malignancy grows, there can be an increase in the abdominal girth, bowel and bladder dysfunction, persistent pelvic or abdominal pain, menstrual irregularities, and ascites.

Diagnostics

There are no screening tests at present. A yearly bimanual pelvic examination should be done. Postmenopausal persons should not have palpable ovaries. An abdominal or vaginal ultrasonogram can be used to detect ovarian masses. A combination of testing for the tumour marker CA-125 (ovarian antibody) and ultrasonography is recommended in addition to the pelvic examination. CA-125 is also used to monitor the course of the disease.

Therapeutics and Nursing Considerations

Treatment usually is a total hysterectomy and bilateral salpingo-ophorectomy. Abdominal and pelvic radiation, intraperitoneal radiation, and systemic combination chemotherapy may be done after tumour-reducing surgery has been completed. Other surgical procedures include subtotal hysterectomy, panhysterectomy, simple and radical vulvectomy, vaginectomy, and radical hysterectomy. It is very important that the client and family participate in treatment decisions. Psychological support both preoperatively and postoperatively is necessary. The client will be encouraged to continue to practise cancer detection strategies postoperatively. A "second-look" procedure (laparoscopy or laparotomy) is performed a year after completion of primary treatment to confirm the absence or presence of the tumour.

Cervical Cancer
Pathophysiology

Cervical cancer is the second most common cancer affecting females in the world. Noninvasive cervical cancer is approximately four times more common than invasive cervical cancer. The development of cervical cells to dysplasia occurs slowly over time. A strong connection exists between dysplasia and HPV infections. Cancers rates expected to decline further with vaccines against HPV (e.g. Gardasil, Cervarix) now being used. Cervical cancers deaths have declined among persons who undergo regular Papanicolaou (Pap) tests.

Clinical Manifestations

Early cervical cancer is generally asymptomatic, but leukorrhea and intermenstrual bleeding eventually occurs. The discharge is usually thin and watery, eventually becoming dark with a foul odour as the disease progresses. Vaginal bleeding begins as spotting but as the tumour enlarges, the bleeding becomes more frequent and heavier. Pain is a late symptom, followed by weight loss, anemia, and cachexia (Tyerman & Cobbett, 2023).

Diagnostics

Cervical cancer screening is recommended in all sexually active females between the ages of 21 and 69 years of age. The Canadian Cancer Society recommends that females have a Pap test every 1 to 3 years, depending on guidelines in their province or territory and depending on their previous test results. Clients with abnormal previous test results may be screened more often. Clients with more prominent changes will receive additional procedures such as a colposcopy and biopsy. Colposcopy and biopsy have improved diagnosis and treatment plans (Tyerman & Cobbett, 2023).

Therapeutics and Nursing Care

Treatment will depend on the staging of the tumour, clients age and health status. (e.g., conization, laser therapy, cautery, and cryosurgery). Invasive cancer of the cervix will be treated with surgery, irradiation, and chemotherapy as single treatments or in combination. Surgical procedures include hysterectomy, radical hysterectomy and rarely pelvic exenteration. Radiation can be external or internal implants may be used. Cisplatin-based chemotherapy regimens benefits clients with cancer that has metastasis beyond the cervix (Tyerman & Cobbett, 2023).

Benign Prostatic Hyperplasia
Pathophysiology

Benign prostatic hyperplasia (BPH) is an enlargement of the prostate gland resulting from an increase in the number of epithelial cells and stomal tissue. It is the most common condition of the male reproductive system. It occurs in 50% of men over the age of 50. BPH does not predispose the client to the development of prostate cancer. The etiology is not really understood, but it is thought to result from endocrine changes as part of the aging process. Other theories suggest that BPH is due to the effect of chronic inflammation of the prostate gland. Research supports the theory that BPH results from a systemic hormonal (testicular androgen) alteration. As the prostate gland grows, it extends upward into the bladder and inward, narrowing the prostatic urethral channel. This obstructs urine flow.

Risk factors include family history, environment, lack of physical activity, smoking, and diabetes.

Clinical Manifestations

Symptoms usually appear gradually and include the following:
- Voiding symptoms, including a decrease in the calibre or force of the urinary stream, difficulty in initiating urination, intermittency, dribbling at the end of voiding, and incomplete bladder emptying
- Urinary frequency and urgency, dysuria, bladder pain, nocturia, and incontinence

Diagnostics

Diagnostic tests include a history and physical examination, urinalysis with culture, a prostate-specific antigen (PSA) level, serum creatinine levels, transrectal ultrasound scan (TRUS), uroflowmetry, and cystourethroscopy. A digital rectal examination should be done yearly.

Therapeutics and Nursing Considerations

The goal of treatment is to restore bladder drainage, relieve symptoms, and prevent complications. Pharmacological therapy includes finasteride (Proscar), which reduces the size of the prostate gland. Alpha-blocking agents such as terazosin, doxazosin, and tamsulosin are given to constrict the prostate gland, reducing urethral pressure and improving urine flow. Improvement can be seen in 2 to 3 weeks. The adverse effects of these medications are orthostatic hypotension and dizziness. Some clients benefit from herbal therapy such as saw palmetto extract.

Invasive therapy is indicated when there is persistent residual urine in the bladder, acute urinary retention, or hydronephrosis causing decreased urine flow and discomfort. Urinary retention leaves residual urine in the bladder and creates a favourable environment for bacterial growth. Calculi may develop in the bladder due to alkalinization of residual urine. Hydronephrosis can cause renal failure. Pyelonephritis may develop, or the bladder could be damaged. Acute urinary retention is an indication for surgical removal in 25 to 30% of clients with BPH. Long-term catheter use is contraindicated because of the risk for infection. The choice of treatment depends on the size and location of the prostatic enlargement and the age of the client.

Transurethral resection of the prostate (TURP) removes the prostate tissue using a resectoscope inserted through the urethra. The enlarged portion of the prostate gland is then resected in small pieces.

Transurethral microwave thermotherapy (TUMT) delivers microwaves directly to the prostate in order to raise the temperature to 45°C, causing tissue death and relief of the obstruction. Postoperative urinary retention is common following the procedures. Transurethral needle ablation (TUNA) increases the temperature of the prostate tissue for localized necrosis. A low-wave frequency is used, and only the tissues that the needle touches are affected. Urinary retention, urinary tract infection (UTI), and irritative voiding symptoms may result. Laser prostatectomy delivers a beam that is used for cutting, coagulation, and vaporization of the prostatic tissue. Intraprostatic urethral stents are used for clients who are poor surgical candidates with symptoms from obstruction. The stents are placed directly into the prostatic tissue.

Goals for postoperative care include the following:
- The client is free of complications.
- The client has restored urinary control and complete bladder emptying.
- The client has satisfying sexual expression.

Clients will require teaching for adequate fluid intake, aseptic technique if using a catheter at home, medication information, and providing an opportunity to express concerns of alteration in sexual function.

Prostate Cancer
Pathophysiology
Prostate cancer is the most common cause of cancer in males, excluding skin cancer. Prostate cancers are androgen-dependent adenocarcinomas that usually develop in the outer aspect of the gland. The cancer is usually slow-growing and metastasizes in a predictable pattern. Common sites of metastasis include the lymph nodes, bone marrow, pelvis, sacrum, and lumbar spine. Risk factors include the following:
- Increasing age
- Family history
- Being of African descent
- High-fat diet
- Exposure to certain chemicals
  A history of BPH is not considered a risk factor.

Clinical Manifestations
The client is usually asymptomatic in the early stages. Eventually, symptoms similar to those with BPH develop, such as dysuria, hesitancy, dribbling, frequency, and urgency. Gross painless hematuria is the most common presenting symptom. The client may experience lumbosacral pain that radiates to the hips or legs. When these symptoms are coupled with urinary symptoms, metastasis should be considered.

Diagnostics
Diagnostic studies include a physical examination and history. A PSA blood test is likely to show elevated levels of PSA with prostatic pathology. Elevated levels of prostatic acid phosphatase (PAP) indicate prostate cancer. A direct rectal examination may find the prostate hard and enlarged with areas of indurations or nodules. A biopsy of the prostate gland is the only definitive diagnostic tool. A bone scan, CT, MRI, and TRUS are used to determine the location and extent of the spread of the cancer. Single-photon emission computed tomography (SPECT) can detect the spread of the cancer to pelvic lymph nodes.

Therapeutics and Nursing Considerations
Conservative treatment is recommended when life expectancy is less than 10 years, there is significant comorbid disease, or the cancer is a low-grade, low-stage tumour. Surgical treatment is a radical prostatectomy, in which the entire gland, seminal vesicles, and part of the bladder neck are removed. Retroperitoneal lymph node dissection is usually done for the most effective long-term survival. Complications of a radical prostatectomy include the following:
- Hemorrhage
- Urinary retention
- Infection and wound dehiscence
- Deep vein thrombosis (DVT)
- Pulmonary emboli

Sometimes nerve-sparing procedures are done to spare the nerves responsible for an erection. This type of surgery is done only when the cancer is contained in the prostate. Cryosurgery destroys cancer cells by freezing them and can be used as an initial or second-line treatment. Other surgical approaches may be a laparoscopic prostatectomy or robotic-assisted prostatectomy. Radiation therapy can be done by external and internal beam. External radiation is used to treat cancer confined to the prostate or the surrounding tissue. Brachytherapy includes implantation of radioactive seeds into the prostate gland. This spares the surrounding tissue and is best suited for stage A or B prostate cancers. Hormonal therapy focuses on androgen deprivation and can be used before surgery or radiation to reduce the tumour. The hormones commonly used are luteinizing hormone–releasing agonists, androgen receptor blockers, and estrogen. An orchiectomy (surgical removal of the testes) may be done in the advanced stages of prostate cancer. Chemotherapy is primarily limited to treatment for those with hormone-resistant tumours and prostate cancer in the late stages. The goal of chemotherapy is palliative.

The client is encouraged to actively participate in the therapeutic plan, which includes thorough discussion about possible sexual dysfunction.

Testicular Cancer

Testicular cancer is the most common cancer in men 15 to 29 years of age. It is a highly treatable and usually curable cancer (Tyerman & Cobbett, 2023).

Pathophysiology

The testicles can develop both germinal and nongerminal tumours. Germinal tumours are the most common form of testicular cancer. About half of germinal tumours are seminomas (tumours developing from sperm-producing cells of the testes). Seminomas tend to remain localized and therefore have a more favourable prognosis. Nonseminoma germinal cell tumours tend to develop earlier in the lifespan and grow quickly. Nonseminomas tend to metastasize quickly. A small percentage of testicular tumours develop in the supportive and hormone-producing tissues or stroma. Secondary testicular tumours have metastasized from other organs.

Clinical Manifestations

A painless mass or lump gradually appears on the testicle. Testicular cancer is rarely bilateral. The client may experience heaviness in his scrotum, inguinal area, or lower abdomen. Back pain, abdominal pain, weight loss, and general weakness suggest that metastasis has already occurred.

Diagnostics

Palpation of the scrotal contents is the first step in diagnosing testicular cancer. Ultrasonography of the testes is indicated whenever testicular cancer is suspected or when persistent or painful mass testicular swelling is present. Tumour markers are substances synthesized by the tumour cells and released into the circulation in abnormal amounts. Human chorionic gonadotropin and alpha-fetoprotein are tumour markers for testicular cancer. Benign testicular tumours do not elevate the levels of these markers. The markers can also be used to evaluate the responses to therapy for testicular cancer. Effective treatment drops the level of the markers. The persistence of elevated levels of markers after orchiectomy is evidence the client has metastatic disease. Other diagnostic tests could include CT of the abdomen and chest to assess for metastasis. Lymphangiography may be ordered to assess possible spread to the lymph system. Microscopic analysis is the definitive way to determine the presence of cancer.

Therapeutics and Nursing Considerations

Treatment selection is based on cell type and the extent of the disease. An orchiectomy is performed surgically to remove the cancerous testis. The client may also undergo a radical retroperitoneal lymph node dissection. Chemotherapy and radiation therapy may be indicated for clients who are at high-risk for metastasis.

Issues related to body image and sexuality need to be addressed. The client will require encouragement to maintain a positive attitude during the course of their treatment. Unilateral orchiectomy and radiation will not necessarily prevent the client from fathering children. The client will be encouraged to perform testicular self-examinations (TSE).

GENITOURINARY HEALTH CHALLENGES

Urinary Tract Infections

Pathophysiology

UTIs are the second most common bacterial disease in females. Usually, the bladder and its contents are free of bacteria in the majority of healthy clients. A small minority of healthy individuals have colonizing bacteria in their bladder. This is called *asymptomatic bacteriuria* and does not justify treatment. *E. coli* is the most common pathogen causing UTIs. Clients who are immunosuppressed, have diabetes, or have undergone multiple courses of antibiotics are vulnerable to developing UTIs.

UTIs may be classified as upper and lower, depending on their location within the urinary system:
- Infections of the upper tract involve the renal parenchyma, pelvis, and ureters.
- Lower tract infections involve the lower urinary tract, bladder, and urethra.

Pyelonephritis refers to infection of the renal parenchyma and collecting system, *cystitis* indicates inflammation of the bladder wall, and *urethritis* is inflammation of the urethra. *Urosepsis* is a UTI that has spread into the systemic circulation and is a life-threatening condition requiring emergency treatment.

UTIs may also be classified as uncomplicated and complicated infections. Uncomplicated infections occur in an otherwise normal urinary tract. Complicated infections occur with coexisting conditions, such as obstruction, stones, catheters, diabetes, or neurological disease, or are recurrent infections.

The physiological and mechanical defence mechanisms that help maintain the normally sterile condition of the bladder include the actual emptying of the bladder, normal antibacterial ability of the mucosa and the urine, the ureterovesical junction competence, and the peristaltic activity of the urinary tract. Alterations in any of these factors increase the risk of contracting a UTI. Organisms causing UTIs are usually introduced via the ascending route from the urethra. Less commonly, organisms can be introduced via the bloodstream or the lymphatic system. Gram-negative bacilli from the GI tract are the most common cause. Contributing factors that enhance development include urological instrumentation that allows bacteria present in the opening of the urethra to enter the urethra or bladder. Sexual intercourse promotes the "milking" of bacteria from the perineum and vagina. UTIs rarely result from the hematogenous route.

Clinical Manifestations

Symptoms of UTIs include the following:

- Dysuria, frequent urination, urgency, and suprapubic discomfort or pressure
- Urine itself may contain visible blood or sediment, giving it a cloudy appearance.
- Flank pain, chills, and fever are indicative of an upper UTI.
- Older persons may not experience these classic symptoms of a UTI. Older persons tend to experience nonlocalized abdominal discomfort rather than dysuria and suprapubic pain. Older persons are less likely to have a fever with an infection from a UTI. Adults aged 80 years and older may see a decline in temperature. There may also be cognitive impairment, delirium, and falls

Diagnostics

Diagnostic studies include a urinalysis and urine for culture and sensitivity (C and S), following a complete history and physical examination of the client. Urine cultures may be obtained by clean-catch technique, catheterization, or suprapubic needle aspiration. Sensitivity testing determines susceptibility to antibiotics.

Therapeutics and Nursing Considerations

Uncomplicated cystitis is treated by a short-term course of antibiotics. A complicated UTI requires a long-term treatment. Trimethoprim-sulfamethoxazole (TMP-SMX) and nitrofurantoin (Macrobid) are frequently used to treat uncomplicated or initial infections. Local application of heat to the suprapubic area or lower back region may help to relieve discomfort associated with an acute UTI. Teach clients to avoid caffeine, alcohol, citrus juices, chocolate, and highly spiced foods or beverages as they are potential bladder irritants.

Prophylactic or suppressive antibiotics are sometimes administered to clients with repeated UTIs. Suppressive therapy is effective on a short-term basis, but the strategy is limited because of the risk for antibiotic resistance, leading to breakthrough infections with increasingly virulent pathogens (Tyerman & Cobbett, 2023).

Client teaching is important to help prevent UTIs, and includes the following:

- Emptying the bladder on a regular basis and wiping the perineal area from front to back
- Avoiding constipation
- Maintaining good fluid intake

Pyelonephritis
Pathophysiology

Acute pyelonephritis is a bacterial infection of the renal pelvis, tubules, and interstitial tissue of the kidney. It usually begins with colonization and infection of the lower tract via the ascending urethral route and is frequently caused by *E. coli*, *Proteus*, *Klebsiella*, or *Enterobacter* agents. Often preexisting factors are present, such as vesicoureteral reflux or a dysfunction of the urinary tract by obstruction, stricture, or stones. Recurring episodes lead to scarred, poorly functioning kidneys and chronic pyelonephritis.

Clinical Manifestations

Symptoms will vary from mild fatigue to sudden onset of chills, fever, vomiting, malaise, flank pain, and lower urinary tract symptoms characteristic of cystitis. Costovertebral tenderness is usually present on the affected side.

Diagnostics

Diagnostic studies such as a urinalysis will show pyuria, bacteriuria, and varying degrees of hematuria. WBC casts indicate involvement of renal parenchyma. CBC will show leukocytosis with an increase in immature bands. Ultrasonography of the urinary system helps identify anatomical abnormalities or the presence of obstructing stones. Imaging studies also are helpful to assess for impaired renal function, scarring, chronic pyelonephritis, and abscesses.

Therapeutics and Nursing Considerations

Clients with severe infections may need hospitalization for control of nausea, vomiting, and dehydration. At home, clients are encouraged to drink an adequate amount of fluids, rest to increase comfort, and take their antibiotics until the prescription has been finished.

Nephrotic Syndrome
Pathophysiology

Nephrotic syndrome is a condition characterized by marked proteinuria, hypoalbuminemia, dyslipidemia, and edema. Although nephrotic syndrome is not a disease itself, it results from a specific defect that makes the glomeruli more permeable to plasma proteins. Nephrotic syndrome usually is caused by an immune or inflammatory process. The increased glomerular permeability is responsible for a massive excretion of protein in the urine, especially albumin and immunoglobulin. This results in decreased serum protein, leading to decreased oncotic pressure with subsequent edema formation, which may include ascites and anasarca. The diminished plasma oncotic pressure also stimulates hepatic lipoprotein synthesis, which results in dyslipidemia. Fat bodies commonly appear in the urine. Because of the loss of immunoglobulins, the immune response is affected, and infections can be serious complications. Hypercoagulability with thromboembolism is potentially the most serious complication of nephrotic syndrome. The renal vein is the most common site for thrombus formation. Pulmonary emboli are also a risk.

Clinical Manifestations

Characteristic manifestations may include massive proteinuria, dyslipidemia and hypoalbuminemia, peripheral edema, possible third space shifting, foamy urine, orthostatic hypotension, malaise, and irritability.

Diagnostics

Diagnosis is made with a thorough history and physical examination. Urinalysis will reveal large quantities of protein and an increased number of hyaline, granular, and waxy, fatty casts.

Blood work shows the following:

- Increased cholesterol, phospholipid, and triglyceride levels
- Decreased albumin

Protein electrophoresis may be done to identify the type of protein lost in the urine.

Therapeutics and Nursing Considerations

Treatment aims at correction of the underlying cause if possible. Supportive treatment is aimed at protein replacement and relief of edema. Diuretics and a restricted sodium diet are ordered, with low to moderate protein in the diet (0.5–1 g of protein per kilogram of body weight per day). Antibiotics may be given for infection. Some clients may need steroid medication; others may need lipid-lowering medications.

The nurse will pay particular attention to the relief of edema. Weigh the client daily. Accurate intake and output measurements are necessary. Abdominal girths may need to be measured. Edematous skin needs careful cleaning and care to protect it from trauma. Education regarding diet and fluid management is important.

Glomerulonephritis
Pathophysiology

Glomerulonephritis is an inflammation of glomerular capillaries caused by an immunological process. It affects both kidneys equally and can lead to renal failure. The antigen–antibody complexes can be deposited in the glomeruli, causing obstruction. The kidney tissue itself may also serve as the antigen. Inflammation occurs within the glomeruli, followed by thickening and scarring of the glomerular membrane, which decreases glomerular filtration.

Clinical Manifestations

Clinical manifestations of glomerulonephritis include varying degrees of hematuria, proteinuria, and elevated serum creatinine and BUN. Other manifestations may include some degree of hypertension and edema.

Diagnostics

Diagnosis is based on the history and physical examination along with a urinalysis, CBC, BUN, creatinine, serum albumin, complement levels, and an antistreptolysin O (ASO) titre. Renal biopsy may be used to confirm the presence of the disease.

Therapeutics and Nursing Considerations

In most cases, recovery is complete following rest and symptomatic treatment. This includes diuretics for fluid retention and antihypertensives if the client is hypertensive. If progressive involvement occurs, the result is destruction of renal tissue and marked renal insufficiency.

Renal Cancer
Pathophysiology

Renal cell carcinoma, also called *adenocarcinoma*, is the most common type of malignant kidney tumour. It usually starts in the proximal renal tubules. Local extension of kidney cancer into the renal vein and vena cava is common. The most common sites of metastases include the lungs, liver, and long bones. Some forms of renal carcinoma are inherited.

Clinical Manifestations

There are no characteristic early symptoms. The most common symptoms are hematuria, flank pain, and a palpable mass in the flank or abdomen. Other symptoms may be weight loss, fever, hypertension, and anemia.

Diagnostics

Diagnosis is made through the history and physical examination. An intravenous pyelogram (IVP) with nephrography or sonography is used to detect renal masses. Ultrasound helps differentiate between a tumour and a cyst. Angiography, percutaneous needle aspiration, CT scan, and MRI can also be used for diagnosis.

Therapeutics and Nursing Considerations

The treatment of renal cancer involves destruction or removal of the cancer. Radiofrequency ablation is a minimally invasive procedure that can be done to destroy the tumour. Nephrectomy (removal of a kidney) or radical nephrectomy, which is removal of the kidney, adrenal gland, surrounding fascia, part of the ureter, and draining lymph nodes, may be needed. Radiation therapy is used palliatively in inoperable cases and when there are metastases to the bone or lungs. Postoperative care focuses on the following:

- Monitoring for hemorrhage and adrenal insufficiency, which may cause hypotension
- Loss of urine output
- Changes in the level of consciousness (LOC)
- Pain management
- Fluid assessment
- Possible antibiotics and steroid replacement

The nurse needs to support the client and the family and share available resources with them.

Polycystic Kidney Disease
Pathophysiology

Polycystic kidney disease (PKD) is a common genetic disease. Cysts form in the renal tubules, and as they advance and increase in size, they fill the cortex and the medulla and destroy surrounding tissue by compression. The cysts are various sizes, involve both kidneys, and are filled with fluid, including blood or pus.

Clinical Manifestations

Symptoms appear when the cysts begin to enlarge. Often the first symptoms to appear are hypertension, hematuria, and feelings of heaviness in the back, side, or abdomen. On physical examination, palpable bilateral enlarged kidneys are often found. UTIs, urinary calculi, or both may be found, and chronic pain is common. The disease usually progresses to ESRD.

Diagnostics

Diagnosis is based on clinical manifestations, family history, IVP, ultrasonogram, and CT scan.

Therapeutics and Nursing Considerations

There is no specific treatment for PKD. A major aim of treatment is to prevent infections and to treat them promptly and effectively if they occur. Nephrectomy may be necessary if pain, bleeding, or infection becomes chronic. A kidney transplant may be the only cure.

Nursing management is the same as that used for the treatment and management of renal failure, namely diet modification, fluid restriction, medications, and helping the client accept the chronic disease process.

Urinary Tract Calculi
Pathophysiology

Nephrolithiasis refers to kidney stone disease. Urolithiasis (calculi) is stones in the urinary tract. Except for struvite stones, which are associated with UTI, stone disorders are more common in males than in females. The majority of clients are 20–55 years of age. Renal calculi may result from the following:

- Dehydration
- Infection
- Changes in urine pH
- Diet
- Immobilization
- Metabolic factors, such as hyperparathyroidism, cancers, and granulomatous disease

Calcium is the most common type of urolithiasis. Struvite stones are composed of magnesium, phosphate, and ammonium. Cystine and xanthine stones are associated with hereditary factors. Uric acid can also form stones. Different theories attempt to explain the development of stones in the urinary tract. One theory is that urinary constituents exceed their solubility. Keeping urine dilute reduces the risk for recurrent stone formation. Another theory is that the urinary pH affects the formation of stones. A higher pH is an environment that supports the development of calcium and phosphate stones. A lower pH supports the development of uric acid and cystine stones. Struvite stones usually form in the presence of a UTI with urea-splitting bacteria such as *Proteus* or *Klebsiella*.

Clinical Manifestations

Clinical manifestations of urinary stones occur because of the obstruction of urinary flow. Symptoms include a sudden onset of unilateral abdominal or flank pain. The type of pain is determined by the location of the stone. If the stone is not obstructing, there will not be any pain. Other symptoms include the presence of hematuria, urinary infections accompanied by fever, vomiting, nausea, and chills.

Diagnostics

Diagnosis is determined by an accurate history and physical examination. Urine pH will be checked. An X-ray of the abdomen and renal ultrasonography will reveal larger radiopaque stones. Ultrasonography can be used to identify radiopaque or radiolucent calculi in the renal pelvis, calyx, or proximal ureter. A CT scan will differentiate between a nonopaque stone and a tumour. IVP or a retrograde pyelogram localizes the degree and site of obstruction or confirms the presence of nonradiopaque stones (from cystine and uric acid). When stones are recovered, chemical analysis will be done to provide an indication of the underlying disorder.

Therapeutics and Nursing Considerations

The history and physical examination will reveal a family history of stone formation, nutritional assessment, activity pattern, a history of any prolonged illness with immobilization or dehydration, and a history of any condition or surgery involving the genitourinary or GI tract or endocrine disturbances.

Various medications are prescribed that prevent stone formation by altering urine pH, preventing excessive urinary excretion of a substance, or correcting a primary disease such as hyperparathyroidism.

Treatment for struvite stones requires control of infection. If the infection cannot be controlled, the stone will have to be surgically removed. Indications for surgical therapy include stones that are too large to pass through ureters, a client who cannot be treated medically, and a client with one kidney.

Calculi that are too large for natural passage may require surgical removal, percutaneous ultrasonic lithotripsy, or extracorporeal shock wave lithotripsy (ESWL), or chemolysis.

Hematuria is common following lithotripsy procedures. Adequate fluid intake to prevent dehydration is encouraged prior to stone removal as an increase in fluids may exacerbate the colic associated with the episode. After the stone has passed, the client is encouraged to drink enough to ensure at least a 2 L output, as this will dilute concentrations of minerals. Diet modifications may be needed to help prevent further stone formation.

Nursing considerations are as follows:

- Pain management and client comfort are primary nursing responsibilities when managing a person with an obstructing stone and renal colic.
- All urine voided by the client should be strained so it can be inspected for the stone.
- Ambulation with support is encouraged to promote movement of the stone.
- Client and family teaching is necessary regarding diet and fluid intake.
- Follow-up care should be discussed with both client and family.

Renal Failure
Pathophysiology and Clinical Manifestations

Renal failure is a partial or complete impairment of renal function and is classified as acute or chronic. Acute renal failure has a rapid onset. Chronic renal failure (CRF) usually develops slowly over months or years.

Acute renal failure. ARF is a clinical syndrome characterized by a rapid loss of renal function with progressive azotemia (accumulation of nitrogenous wastes). Causes of ARF include conditions that reduce the blood flow to the kidneys, renal parenchymatous disease, and obstruction. Prerenal ARF is due to factors external to the kidney that reduce renal blood flow and lead to decreased glomerular perfusion and filtration. Prerenal causes are the most common cause of ARF and include the following:

- Hypovolemia
- Decreased cardiac output
- Decreased peripheral vascular resistance
- Vascular obstruction

Prerenal disease can lead to intrarenal disease (acute tubular necrosis) if renal ischemia is prolonged.

Intrarenal causes include the conditions that cause direct damage to the renal tissue (parenchyma), resulting in impaired nephron function. Intrarenal ARF is usually due to the following:

- Prolonged ischemia
- Nephrotoxins
- Rhabdomyolysis
- Glomerulonephritis
- Complications of diabetes on the glomerular basement membrane

Causes of postrenal ARF involve obstruction of urinary outflow. The most common causes are as follows:

- Prostate cancer and BPH
- Urinary tract calculi
- Extrarenal tumours

ARF progresses through four phases: initiation, oliguric, diuretic, and recovery.

The *initiation phase* begins at the time of the insult. This phase continues until symptoms become evident.

The *oliguric phase* reflects a reduction in the GFR that causes oliguria.

- The oliguric phase usually starts 1 to 7 days after the initiating event and lasts about 10–14 days.
- The longer the oliguric phase lasts, the poorer the prognosis is for complete recovery of renal function.
- Due to the decrease in urine in the oliguric phase, the client will have fluid retention.
- Fluid overload can lead to heart failure, pulmonary edema, and pericardial and pleural effusions.
- Metabolic acidosis results when the kidneys cannot synthesize ammonia, which is needed for the excretion of hydrogen ions.
- The client may exhibit Kussmaul breathing (rapid and deep) as the respiratory tract attempts to compensate and blow off carbon dioxide.
- Waste products are not eliminated and remain in the blood.
- Potassium levels rise in the blood as the kidneys are unable to eliminate potassium.
- The kidneys are unable to eliminate phosphate, so the calcium levels within the blood will drop.
- As the waste products build in the blood, the client may become anorexic and experience nausea and vomiting with bowel disturbances.

- Uremic breath may develop.
- The kidneys are unable to produce the active form of vitamin D, so absorption of calcium from the intestine is limited.
- Anemia occurs due to the kidneys' inability to produce erythropoietin.
- Hematological changes may result in GI bleeds and the development of stomatitis as the waste products damage the leukocytes, immunoglobulins, and platelets.
- Neurological changes can occur as nitrogenous waste products accumulate in the brain and other nervous tissue. Symptoms can be as mild as fatigue and difficulty concentrating or can escalate to seizures, stupor, and coma.

The *diuretic phase* begins with the gradual increase in urine output. As this phase continues, the output may be as high as 3 to 5 L per day or more. The diuretic phase may last 1 to 3 weeks or more.

- The kidneys are starting to recover their ability to excrete waste and fluid.
- During this period, the client's acid–base, electrolyte, and waste product values are beginning to normalize.
- Because of the large volume of fluid and electrolytes lost during this phase, the client must be monitored closely for hypovolemia, hypotension, hyponatremia, and hypokalemia.

The *recovery phase* begins when the GFR increases and the BUN and creatinine levels plateau.

- Although major improvements occur in the first 2 weeks of this phase, renal function may take up to 12 months to stabilize.
- Many clients who survive ARF never regain a normal GFR.

Chronic renal failure. CRF refers to the progressive, irreversible destruction of nephrons, resulting in systemic damage to all organs. The causes are as follows:

- The most common cause of CRF is uncontrolled diabetes, followed closely by uncontrolled hypertension.
- Other causes may include glomerulonephritis, renal vascular disease, pyelonephritis, and polycystic disease.

CRF is insidious; symptoms do not become evident until the GFR has dropped to 20% of its norm.

A client with CRF exhibits the following changes:

- A severely decreased GFR, with azotemia (high levels of BUN and creatinine)
- Metabolic acidosis
- Fluid retention
- Increased serum potassium, phosphate, and possibly sodium
- Decreased calcium
- Severe anemia
- Oliguria

Figure 9.5 illustrates the manifestations of this condition. The term *uremia* refers to the entire signs and symptoms of CRF.

The final stage of CRF is ESRD. The client experiences uremic syndrome with severe metabolic acidosis and severe fluid and electrolyte imbalance. ESRD is fatal if clients do not receive dialysis or a kidney transplant.

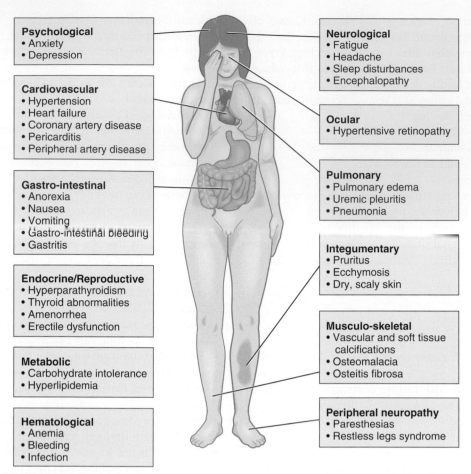

Psychological
• Anxiety
• Depression

Cardiovascular
• Hypertension
• Heart failure
• Coronary artery disease
• Pericarditis
• Peripheral artery disease

Gastro-intestinal
• Anorexia
• Nausea
• Vomiting
• Gastro-intestinal bleeding
• Gastritis

Endocrine/Reproductive
• Hyperparathyroidism
• Thyroid abnormalities
• Amenorrhea
• Erectile dysfunction

Metabolic
• Carbohydrate intolerance
• Hyperlipidemia

Hematological
• Anemia
• Bleeding
• Infection

Neurological
• Fatigue
• Headache
• Sleep disturbances
• Encephalopathy

Ocular
• Hypertensive retinopathy

Pulmonary
• Pulmonary edema
• Uremic pleuritis
• Pneumonia

Integumentary
• Pruritus
• Ecchymosis
• Dry, scaly skin

Musculo-skeletal
• Vascular and soft tissue calcifications
• Osteomalacia
• Osteitis fibrosa

Peripheral neuropathy
• Paresthesias
• Restless legs syndrome

Fig. 9.5 Clinical manifestations of chronic uremia. (From Tyerman, J., & Cobbett, S. [2023]. *Lewis's medical-surgical nursing in Canada: Assessment and management of clinical problems* [5th Cdn. ed., p. 1189, Figure 49-3]. Elsevier.)

Diagnostics

Diagnostic studies include a thorough history to determine the etiology of the failure.

Blood work shows the following:
• Elevated BUN and creatinine levels
• Elevated potassium and phosphate levels
• Acidic pH, with low levels of bicarbonate
• Hemoglobin and hematocrit
  Urine specimens show the following:
• Casts, cellular debris, and decreased specific gravity, and in glomerular disease, proteinuria and urine osmolality close to serum osmolality
• The creatinine clearance test measures the GFR and is used to estimate the number of remaining functioning nephrons.
• Other studies include ultrasonography of the kidneys, renal scan, CT scan, retrograde pyelography, MRI, and plain X-ray films of the abdomen, kidneys, ureters, and bladder (KUB).

Therapeutics and Nursing Considerations

The primary goal of treatment is to find the underlying cause of the ARF and eliminate it. Management of signs and symptoms and prevention of complications are also high priorities. Assessing for adequate cardiac output is mandatory. Diuretic therapy along with volume expanders may be used to prevent fluid overload. If ARF has already been established, conservative measures may be necessary until renal function improves. Fluid intake is closely monitored. Blood work is closely monitored for changes in potassium, sodium, bicarbonates, phosphates, blood gases, BUN, creatinine, and calcium.

The diet will be high in carbohydrates and low in protein until the diuretic phase begins. Restriction of potassium- and sodium-containing foods will be regulated according to the levels of these electrolytes in the blood. If potassium levels rise too high, the client may be given polystyrene sulfonate (Kayexalate) to rid the body of potassium, glucose, and insulin to help move the potassium into the cells or calcium gluconate to decrease the excitability of the cell membrane. In some situations, dialysis will be initiated.

Treatment of CRF is to find the precipitating cause and treat or manage it as well as treat the consequences of the progressive condition. Once CRF has progressed to ESRD, dialysis and renal transplantation are the only options. See Figure 9.6.

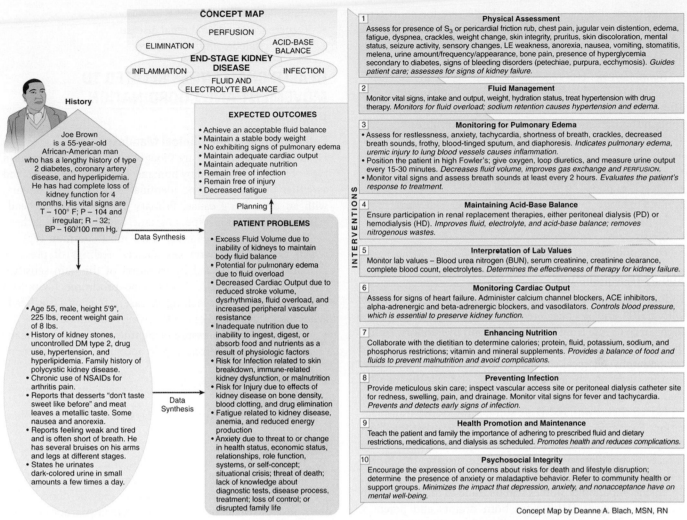

Fig. 9.6 Concept map: End-stage renal disease. (From Ignatavicius, D. D., Workman, M. L., & Rebar, C. [2018]. *Medical-surgical nursing: Concepts for interprofessional collaborative care* [9th ed.]. Elsevier. Concept map by Deanne A. Blach, MSN, RN.)

Dialysis

Dialysis is a technique in which substances move from the blood through a semipermeable membrane and into a dialysis solution (dialysate). Dialysis is used to correct fluid and electrolyte and acid–base imbalances and to remove excess waste products. The two main methods of dialysis include hemodialysis (HD) and peritoneal dialysis (PD). In PD, the peritoneal membrane acts as a semipermeable membrane. In HD, an artificial membrane is used as the semipermeable membrane and is in contact with the client's blood. Generally, dialysis is initiated when the GFR or creatinine clearance of the client is less than 15 mL/min (normal is 100–125 mL/min); however, these criteria can vary widely in different clinical situations. Certain uremic complications indicate an immediate need for dialysis and are as follows:

- Encephalopathy
- Neuropathies
- Uncompensated metabolic acidosis
- Uncontrollable hyperkalemia
- Pericarditis
- Accelerated hypertension

The general principles of diffusion, osmosis, and ultrafiltration are involved in both forms of dialysis.

Peritoneal dialysis. With PD, a catheter is surgically placed through the anterior wall of the abdomen into the peritoneum. The catheter is sutured in place. Dialysis solutions are available commercially in 2-L to 3-L plastic bags with glucose concentrations of 0.5%, 1.5%, 2.5%, or 4.25%. The electrolyte concentration is similar to plasma. There are two forms of PD: automated peritoneal dialysis (APD) and continuous ambulatory peritoneal dialysis (CAPD), as well as three phases: the inflow, the dwell, and the drainage.

Complications pertaining to PD include the following:

- Exit site infection, peritonitis, and abdominal pain
- Outflow conditions and hernias
- Lower back pain
- Bleeding
- Pulmonary complications
- Protein loss
- Carbohydrate and lipid abnormalities
- Encapsulating sclerosing peritonitis
- Loss of ultrafiltration

Peritoneal dialysis is considered effective for short-term dialysis, allowing the client more independence and ease of travelling. There are fewer dietary restrictions for clients using PD compared to those having HD.

Hemodialysis. HD requires vascular access and incorporates shunts and internal arteriovenous fistulas and grafts. The HD dialyzers are basically long plastic cartridges that contain thousands of parallel hollow tubes or fibres.

Complications to monitor for with HD include the following:

- Hypotension
- Muscle cramps
- Loss of blood
- Hepatitis
- Sepsis
- Disequilibrium syndrome

Kidney Transplantation

Kidney transplantation is the treatment of choice for clients with ESRD and is considered extremely successful, with a high survivor rate from both cadaver and live donors. Unlike dialysis, the transplanted kidney is able to reverse many of the pathophysiological changes associated with renal failure, eliminates the dependence on dialysis, and is less expensive than dialysis after the first year following surgery.

Not all clients with ESRD are suitable for kidney transplantation. Each transplant team will have criteria that the client must meet in order to be a transplant recipient. Clients with spreading malignancies, severe cardiac disease, or chronic respiratory failure are not suitable recipients.

Histocompatibility studies will be done to identify human leukocyte antigens (HLAs) for both donors and potential recipients. Donor sources include compatible blood type cadaver donors, blood relatives, and living donors. The donor kidney will be removed (nephrectomy) either conventionally or by laparoscope. The transplanted kidney is usually placed extraperitoneally in the iliac fossa.

Emotional and psychological supports are important for both clients. Immunosuppressive medications will be given to the recipient to prevent rejection of the new kidney. The goal of immunosuppressive therapy is to adequately suppress the immune response to prevent rejection while maintaining sufficient immunity to prevent overwhelming infection. Postoperative care for the donor is similar to care for laparoscopic nephrectomy, with close monitoring of remaining renal function. The recipient will be monitored closely for fluid and electrolyte balances.

Rejection of the kidney by the recipient is the antibody-mediated humoral reaction to the new organ. Hyperacute rejection may occur within minutes to hours of the transplant. Acute rejection can occur days to months after the transplant. Chronic rejection is a process that occurs over months to years and is irreversible.

Complications following transplantation include the following:

- Infection
- Cardiovascular disease
- Malignancies
- Recurrence of original renal disease
- Steroid-related complications

HEALTH CHALLENGES RELATED TO MOVEMENT AND COORDINATION

Headache

Pathophysiology and Clinical Manifestations

Headaches (cephalalgia) are thought to be the most common type of pain experienced by humans. Headaches are classified as either primary, with no identifiable cause, or secondary, with an underlying cause. Primary classifications of headaches include tension-type, migraine, and cluster headaches.

The tension-type headache is the most common type, in which the client experiences bilateral feelings of pressure around the head caused by irritation of the pain-sensitive structures of the brain. There is no prodrome (symptom indicative of an approaching disease). Tension-type headaches have at least two of the following characteristics:

- The sensation of pressure or tightness or band-like headache associated with neck pain and increased muscle tension
- Mild to moderate severity
- Bilateral location
- Sensitivity to light (photophobia) or sound (phonophobia)

Diagnostics

To diagnose tension-type headaches, a careful history and physical examination, including a neurological examination, are needed. Routine laboratory studies may be done. CT of the sinuses, MRI, angiography, and electromyography (EMG) may be performed.

Migraine Headaches

Pathophysiology and Clinical Manifestations

Migraine headaches are characterized by unilateral or bilateral throbbing pain caused by vasodilation of the dural blood vessels that then stimulate the trigeminal nerve pain pathway. Neuropeptides are released, which make the vasodilation worse. There is usually a family history of migraine headaches. The onset is usually in childhood or adolescence.

Migraine headaches may be preceded by an aura (sensation occurring before a disorder) and prodrome by days or hours. The prodrome can include psychic disturbances, GI upset, and changes in fluid balance.

The headache itself may be triggered by the following:

- Stress
- Physical exertion
- Weather
- Bright lights
- Menstruation
- Alcohol
- Certain foods
- Fatigue
- Head trauma
- Drugs

Migraine headaches are subdivided into migraine with aura and migraine without aura. A classic symptom of an aura is flashing lights in one quadrant of the visual field (scintillating scotomata). Other auras could be tingling or burning sensations, paresthesia's, motor dysfunctions, dizziness, confusion, or even loss of consciousness that precede the onset of the migraine headache.

Migraine without aura involves at least one of the following: nausea and vomiting, photophobia, and phonophobia. Migraine without aura is the most common type of migraine.

Symptoms of a migraine with or without an aura are as follows:

- Generalized edema
- Irritability
- Pallor
- Nausea and vomiting
- Sweating

Clients may seek shelter from noise, light, odours, people, or other stressors. They feel a steady, throbbing pain synchronous with the pulse.

Diagnostics

Diagnostic tests are the same as those for tension headaches.

Cluster Headaches

Pathophysiology and Clinical Manifestations

Cluster headaches are thought to be variants of migraine headaches and are characterized by repeated headaches that occur for weeks or months at a time, followed by periods of remission. Cluster headaches are considered one of the most severe forms of head pain. The etiology of cluster headaches is unknown. The pathophysiology of cluster headaches is similar to that of migraine headaches. Common triggers for cluster headaches include beer, caffeine, nicotine, bright lights, and histamines.

Clinical manifestations of cluster headaches include the following:

- Severe unilateral orbital, supraorbital, or temporal pain
- Associated symptoms, including nasal congestion, lacrimation, rhinorrhea, constriction of the pupil, facial flushing or pallor, and forehead and facial swelling

Cluster headaches do not cause nausea and vomiting. The onset of the headache is usually abrupt, without prodrome. It commonly occurs at night and may recur several times a day for several days. Cluster headaches typically last 2 weeks to 3 months and then go into remission for months or years (Tyerman & Cobbett, 2023). The pain is described as deep, steady, and penetrating but not throbbing. Clients with cluster headaches often pace the floor, cry out, and avoid being touched by others.

Diagnostics

Diagnostic tests are the same as those for tension headaches.

Therapeutics and Nursing Considerations

Drug treatments for headaches are as follows:

- Tension-type headache medications may include nonnarcotic analgesics used alone or in combination with a sedative, muscle relaxant, tranquilizer, or codeine.
- Migraine headache medications focus on terminating or decreasing the symptoms.
- ASA (Aspirin) or acetaminophen (Tylenol) may be effective for mild forms of the headache.
- Other medications may include serotonin receptor agonists, alpha- and beta-adrenergic blockers, tricyclic antidepressants, ergot derivatives, calcium channel blockers, and antiseizure medications.
- Cluster headaches are treated with alpha-adrenergic blockers and vasoconstrictors. An acute treatment for cluster headaches is inhalation of 100% oxygen delivered at a rate of 8 to 12 L per minute for 15 minutes.

Overuse of analgesics can lead to chronic daily headache or drug-induced headache.

Client and family teaching regarding the medication regimen, nonpharmacological management, and stress-reduction techniques can be very helpful. Alternative therapy such as heat or cold applications, acupuncture, or hypnosis has been found to be beneficial for many clients.

Head Injury
Pathophysiology

Head injury is any trauma to the scalp, skull, or brain. Head trauma includes an alteration in consciousness, no matter how brief. There are many causes of head injury, such as firearm-related injuries, motor vehicle accidents, falls, assaults, sports-related injuries, and recreational accidents. There is a high potential for a poor outcome when the head is injured. Not all brain damage is evident at the time of the event.

Scalp lacerations are the most minor type of head trauma. The scalp is very vascular and therefore can bleed profusely. Trauma can result in an abrasion, contusion, laceration, or hematoma. The major complication from a scalp laceration is infection.

Skull fractures may be linear, comminuted, depressed or compound, closed or open. The type and severity of a skull fracture depends on the velocity, momentum, and direction of the injuring agent and the site of impact. The force of the damaging impact could be due to the mechanism of acceleration or deceleration. Specific manifestations of a skull fracture are generally associated with the location of the injury. The major potential complications of skull fractures are as follows:

- Intracranial infections
- Hematomas
- Meningeal and brain tissue damage

Minor head trauma includes concussions and postconcussion syndrome. A concussion involves a change in the LOC. Major head traumas are contusions and lacerations that involve severe brain trauma. Contusions are bruising of brain tissue most commonly found at the site of impact (coup injury) or in the line opposite the site of impact (contrecoup injury). Lacerations involve the actual tearing of the cortical surface vessels, which may lead to secondary hemorrhage and cerebral edema and inflammation. Intracerebral hemorrhage can be associated with cerebral laceration. The prognosis is generally poor for the person with a large intracerebral hemorrhage. Chronic traumatic encephalopathy (CTE) is the term used to describe degeneration in the brain after repeated concussions, including those sustained during sports. Research continues to examine the link between repeated concussions and brain degeneration (Tyerman & Cobbett, 2023).

When major head trauma occurs, many delayed or secondary responses can be seen, including the following:
- Hemorrhage and hematoma formation
- Seizures
- Cerebral edema

Complications of head trauma include an epidural, subdural, or intracerebral hematoma. An epidural hematoma results from bleeding between the dura and the inner surface of the skull. Laceration of the middle meningeal artery is the usual cause, and as such, the hematoma develops rapidly and requires immediate control of the bleeding and evacuation of the blood in the epidural space.

Subdural hematomas occur from bleeding between the dura mater and arachnoid layer of the meningeal covering of the brain and are usually venous in origin and much slower to develop into a mass large enough to produce symptoms. The accumulation of clots puts pressure on the brain surface and eventually displaces brain tissue.

An intracerebral hematoma can be due to a hemorrhagic stroke or ruptured aneurysm.

Clinical Manifestations

Signs of a concussion may include a brief disruption in LOC, amnesia, and headache. Symptoms are generally of short duration. The postconcussion syndrome can occur anywhere from 2 weeks to 2 months after the head injury and involves the following:
- A persistent headache
- Lethargy
- Personality and behaviour changes
- Shortened attention span
- Decreased short term memory
- Changes in intellectual ability

With acute subdural hematoma, the client exhibits the following signs within 48 hours of the injury:
- Appears drowsy and confused
- Ipsilateral pupil dilates and becomes fixed

With a subacute subdural hematoma, symptoms take longer to appear, between 2 to 14 days after the injury.
- Failure to regain consciousness may be an indicator.

Chronic subdural hematomas develop over weeks or months after a seemingly minor head injury. The damaged area is filled with fluid rather than blood clots, and symptoms tend to be less acute.

Diagnostics

Diagnosis of a head injury includes the history and physical examination. A CT scan is considered the best diagnostic test to determine craniocerebral trauma. MRI, PET, cervical spine and skull X-ray series, and the Glasgow Coma Scale (GCS) are also used.

Therapeutics and Nursing Considerations

Care for the client with head trauma focuses on the following:
- Monitoring the neurological status and using the GCS
- Observing for cerebrospinal fluid (CSF) leak

The overall goals are to maintain adequate cerebral perfusion; to keep the client normothermic and free from pain, discomfort, and infection; and to attain maximal cognitive, motor, and sensory function. In some situations, craniotomy, craniectomy, cranioplasty, or burr-hole surgery is done to remove the hematoma.

Nursing considerations will focus on the following:
- Promoting good air entry
- Controlling intracranial pressure (ICP)
- Maintaining temperature control
- Monitoring fluid and electrolyte balance
- Preventing infection
- Assisting the client to resume normal activities
- Providing emotional support to the client and the family

Inflammatory Brain Disorders

Bacteria, viruses, fungi, and chemicals can cause inflammatory brain disorders. Meningitis, encephalitis, and brain abscesses are among the most frequently occurring CNS infections. During an infection, infectious agents can enter the bloodstream. Once the organisms reach the brain, the CSF in the subarachnoid spaces and the pia-arachnoid membrane may become infected. The infection spreads quickly through the meninges and can invade the ventricles. This infectious process can cause serious long-term neurological deficits.

Bacterial Meningitis

Pathophysiology, clinical manifestations, and diagnostics. Bacterial meningitis is a medical emergency with a high mortality rate. The inflammatory response increases CSF production and ICP. The major bacteria associated with bacterial meningitis are *Streptococcus pneumoniae* and *Neisseria meningitidis*.

Symptoms include fever, severe headache, nausea and vomiting, nuchal rigidity (resistance to flexion of the neck), positive Kernig sign, positive Brudzinski sign, photophobia, decreased LOC, and signs of increased ICP. Seizures occur in 20% of all cases. The headache becomes progressively worse. Vomiting and irritability may accompany the worsening headache. Delirium and complete disorientation may develop quickly.

Rapid diagnosis is done by history and physical examination. A blood culture, lumbar puncture, and analysis of CSF are done. A head X-ray, CT scanning, and MRI may be done.

Therapeutics and nursing considerations. Antibiotic therapy is initiated after all necessary specimens are collected. The antibiotic needs to be able to cross the blood–brain barrier to be effective. The client is cared for while in a comfortable position in a darkened room to help prevent hallucinations. Pain medication is administered as needed. The client must be observed and treated for any neurological conditions, such as seizures. Antipyretics should be given as needed. Hydration must be monitored and small, frequent meals offered. Aseptic technique must be utilized at all times. Progressive range-of-motion (ROM) exercises are required, and client activity should be increased as tolerated. The nursing considerations for all of the following inflammatory brain disorders are similar to those for bacterial meningitis.

Viral Meningitis

Pathophysiology, clinical manifestations, and diagnostics. Viral meningitis is most commonly caused by enterovirus, arbovirus, HIV, or herpes simplex virus (HSV). Viral meningitis, also known as *aseptic meningitis*, usually presents with a headache, fever, photophobia, myalgias, and a stiff neck. Diagnosis is done by the history and physical examination and a lumbar puncture with cultures done on CSF. In viral meningitis, the CSF will show lymphocytosis, but no organisms will be present in Gram stains or acid-fast smears.

Therapeutics and nursing considerations. Symptomatic management with full recovery should be expected. The nursing considerations for viral meningitis are similar to those for bacterial meningitis.

Encephalitis

Pathophysiology, clinical manifestations, and diagnostics. Encephalitis is an acute inflammation of the brain that can be fatal. It can be caused by a number of viruses, including West Nile virus. Ticks or mosquitoes can transmit epidemic encephalitis. Advanced age is a risk factor for developing encephalitis. Most cases have mild flulike symptoms in addition to nonspecific symptoms, such as the following:
- Fever and headache
- Nausea and vomiting
- Stiff neck
- Declining LOC

Signs appear 2 to 3 days postinfection and may vary from minimal alterations to coma. Abnormalities in brain function are common in encephalitis. Diagnosis is done by the history and physical examination, MRI, PET, and tests for the IgM antibody to West Nile virus in CSF. Polymerase chain reaction tests for HSV, DNA, RNA levels in CSF allow for early detection of HSV viral encephalitis. Diagnosis between meningitis and encephalitis is based on brain function.

Therapeutics and nursing considerations. The treatment for encephalitis may include diuretics, corticosteroids, acyclovir (Zovirax), vidarabine (Vira-A) for HSV infection, and antiseizure medications. Mosquito control may be used as a preventive measure. The nursing considerations for encephalitis are similar to those for bacterial meningitis.

Brain Abscess

Pathophysiology, clinical manifestations, and diagnostics. Brain abscess is a purulent infection of the brain with an accumulation of pus within brain tissue. The infection may be due to an ear, tooth, mastoid, or sinus infection; skull fracture; brain trauma or surgery; or a complication of meningitis. *Streptococcus* and *Staphylococcus aureus* are the causative agents. The client will present with headache, fever, and nausea and vomiting and may show signs of increased ICP. The symptoms will reflect the local area of abscess. CT and MRI will be used for diagnosis.

Therapeutics and nursing considerations. Antimicrobial therapy is the primary treatment, as well as symptomatic treatment for any manifestation. The abscess may need to be drained or removed. If the abscess is left untreated, the client will not survive. The nursing considerations for brain abscesses are similar to those for bacterial meningitis.

Multiple Sclerosis
Pathophysiology
Multiple sclerosis (MS) is a chronic, progressive, degenerative neuromuscular disease that is characterized by inflammation of the white matter of the CNS. The disease usually affects young to middle-aged adults, with onset 30 years of age. Females are affected more than males. The cause is unknown; however, it may be related to infectious, immunological, and genetic factors. Other autoimmune theories include the possibility that autosensitization occurring in response to an antigen on the myelin membrane or a cell-mediated immune reaction triggers the demyelination process. There is no cause-and-effect relationship between a pathogenetic agent and MS. Possible precipitating factors include the following:
- Infection
- Physical injury
- Emotional stress
- Excessive fatigue
- Pregnancy
- Poor state of health

The disease process consists of loss of myelin, disappearance of oligodendrocytes, and proliferation of astrocytes. Changes result in plaque formation, with plaques scattered throughout the CNS. Initially, the myelin sheaths of the neurons in the brain and spinal cord are attacked, but the nerve fibre is not affected. Clients may complain of noticeable impairment of function. Myelin can regenerate and symptoms disappear, resulting in remission, or myelin can be replaced by glial scar tissue. Nerve impulses slow down without myelin. With the destruction of axons, impulses are totally blocked, resulting in permanent loss of nerve function.

Clinical Manifestations
Vague symptoms can occur intermittently over months and years. The disease may not be diagnosed until long after the onset of the first symptom. Symptoms of MS are characterized by chronic, progressive deterioration in some clients, with remissions and exacerbations in others. Common signs and symptoms of MS include the following:
- Motor manifestations, which may include weakness or feelings of heaviness in the legs, paralysis of limbs, diplopia, hyper-reflexia and spasticity of muscles, and sensory, cerebellar, and neurobehavioural conditions.
- Sensory manifestations can include numbness and tingling, blurred vision, vertigo, and tinnitus.

- Cerebellar manifestations include nystagmus, ataxia, dysarthria, and dysphagia.
- Neurobehavioural manifestations may include emotional lability.
- Other symptoms may include bowel and bladder dysfunction, optic neuritis, and fatigue. Sexual dysfunction can also occur with MS.

Diagnostics

Diagnosis is based primarily on the history, clinical manifestations, and the presence of multiple lesions over time as measured by an MRI. Laboratory tests will show an increase in activated T4 lymphocytes and IgG content.

Therapeutics and Nursing Considerations

The goal of treatment is to maintain the client's independence for as long as possible. Medication therapy for the treatment of MS includes the following:

- Corticosteroids, which are used to treat acute exacerbations by reducing edema and inflammation at the site of demyelination
- Immunosuppressive therapy is beneficial in clients with progressive relapsing, secondary-progressive, and primary-progressive types of MS.
- Immunomodulators include interferon-beta 1b (Betaseron), interferon-beta-1a (Avonex), glatiramer (Copaxone), teriflunomide (Aubagio) and mitoxantrone (Novantrone).
- Antispasmodics, CNS stimulants, anticholinergics, tricyclic antidepressants, and antiseizure medications may also be prescribed. Dopamine agonists my be effective in treatment of erectile dysfunction, while hormone therapy has shown efficacy in increasing libido. Cannabinoids have been used to treat both spasticity and pain with mild adverse effects (Tyerman & Cobbett, 2023).

Surgical interventions, such as a neurectomy, rhizotomy, or cordotomy, or dorsal column electrical stimulation, or use of an intrathecal baclofen pump may be required if spasticity is not controlled with antispasmodics. Neurological dysfunction sometimes improves with physical therapy and speech therapy. Nutritional therapy prescribes a high-protein diet with supplementary vitamins. Clients will be encouraged to balance rest with activities and maintain optimal nutrition.

As the condition progresses, symptomatic treatment and assistance will be needed. Support groups for MS have been very beneficial for clients and their families.

Parkinson's Disease
Pathophysiology

Parkinson's disease is a disease of the basal ganglia characterized by slowing down in the initiation and execution of movement (bradykinesia), increased muscle tone (rigidity), tremor at rest, and impaired postural reflexes. The diagnosis of Parkinson's increases with age, with the peak onset being in the sixth decade. Parkinson's is more common in males than in females and is caused by the following conditions:

- Onset of Parkinson's before age 50 is usually due to a genetic defect.

- In many cases, the cause of Parkinson's is unknown.
- Some cases are caused by exposure to toxins from drugs and chemicals that destroy the cells in the substantia nigra of the brain.
- Other causes of Parkinson's include hydrocephalus, hypoxia, dementia with Lewy bodies, infections, stroke, tumour, and trauma.

Parkinson's affects the extrapyramidal system, which influences movement. A dopamine deficiency occurs in the basal ganglia. Reduction of dopamine in the corpus striatum upsets the normal balance between the dopamine (inhibitor) and acetylcholine (excitatory) neurotransmitters. Symptoms occur when affected brain cells can no longer perform their normal inhibitory function within the CNS.

Clinical Manifestations

Symptoms of the disease do not occur until 80% of neurons in the substantia nigra are lost. The classic triad of manifestations includes tremor, rigidity, and bradykinesia.

- Insidious tremor begins in the fingers (unilateral pill-roll tremor). The tremor is more prominent at rest and is aggravated by emotional stress or increased concentration.
- Rigidity is caused by sustained muscle contraction and consequently elicits complaints of soreness and feeling tired and achy. Rigidity inhibits the alternating contraction and relaxation in opposing muscle groups, slowing movement. The rigidity may be uniform or jerky (cogwheel rigidity). The client may have difficulty walking, with the gait lacking normal parallel motion. Bradykinesia (slow and delayed movement) is particularly evident.
- Other symptoms include a high-pitched, monotone voice, drooling, a masklike facial expression, slow, slurred speech, and dysphagia.

Complications of Parkinson's are caused by progressive deterioration and the negative impact this deterioration may have on the client. For example, dysphagia can lead to malnutrition. As the disease advances, it often results in severe dementia which is associated with an increase in mortality. (Tyerman & Cobbett, 2023).

Diagnostics

There are no specific tests for diagnosing Parkinson's. Diagnosis is based solely on the history and clinical features. A firm diagnosis can be made when at least two of the three classic symptoms are present. The ultimate confirmation of the disease is a positive response to antiparkinsonian medications.

Therapeutics and Nursing Considerations

The medication therapy is aimed at correcting imbalances of neurotransmitters within the CNS. These medications either enhance the release or supply of dopamine or antagonize or block the effects of acetylcholine. The treatments are as follows:

- Levodopa with carbidopa (Sinemet) is often the first medication used. Levodopa is a precursor of dopamine and can cross the blood–brain barrier. It is converted to dopamine in the basal ganglia. Carbidopa inhibits an enzyme that breaks down levodopa before it reaches the brain. The effect of Sinemet could wear off after a few years of therapy.

- Anticholinergics may be used in the management of Parkinson's.
- Antihistamines, monoamine oxidase inhibitors and catechol-O-methyltransferase (COMT) inhibitors are also used.
- As Parkinson's progresses, a combination therapy is often required.

Surgical procedures are aimed at relieving symptoms in clients who are usually unresponsive to medication therapy or who have developed severe motor complications. Ablation therapy has largely been replaced by deep brain stimulation, which involves placing electrodes in the thalamus, globus pallidus, or subthalamic nucleus. Both ablation and deep brain stimulation procedures work by reducing the increased neuronal activity produced by the dopamine depletion.

Transplantation of fetal neural tissue into the basal ganglia provides dopamine-producing cells in the brains of clients with Parkinson's. This type of therapy is still experimental.

Since malnutrition and constipation can cause serious consequences, adequate nutrition is essential. Clients with dysphagia and bradykinesia need food that is easily chewed and swallowed. The client needs adequate roughage. Small, frequent meals are best to prevent fatigue. Ample time must be allowed for the client to eat and not become frustrated. Levodopa can be impaired by protein ingestion.

The goals of treatment focus on maximizing neurological function and maintaining independence in activities of daily living for as long as possible. Optimizing psychosocial well-being is very important.

Spinal Cord Injury

Pathophysiology

Spinal cord injuries (SCIs) are most common in young people between the ages of 20–30 years and occur much more frequently in males. The causes of this injury include motor vehicle accidents, falls, violence, and sports injuries. Types of SCI include cord concussion, in which the cord is severely jarred, as in a sports injury. There may be cord contusion, in which compression of the cord results in bleeding into the cord, causing bruising and edema. The extent of the damage will depend on the severity of the inflammatory response. Cord laceration, in which there is an actual tear in the cord, results in permanent injury as the neurons of the CNS do not regenerate. Cord transection, either complete or incomplete, results in loss of neurological function below the site of the injury.

The extent of the neurological damage caused by an SCI results from the primary injury, which is the actual physical disruption of an axon, and the secondary injury damage due to ischemia, hypoxia, microhemorrhage, and edema. Secondary injury occurs over time; therefore, a prognosis of recovery is more accurate 72 hours after the initial injury. The secondary injury refers to the ongoing progressive damage that occurs after the initial injury. This ongoing injury can be due to free radical formation, uncontrolled calcium influx, ischemia, lipid peroxidation, or some combination of these.

Spinal shock can last days to months and is characterized by the following:
- Decreased reflexes
- Loss of sensation
- Flaccid paralysis below the level of injury, which is experienced by 50% of people with acute SCI (Tyerman & Cobbett, 2023)

The six syndromes associated with incomplete cord lesions are summarized in Table 9.9.

Spinal shock is manifested by the following:
- Decreased reflexes
- Loss of sensation
- Flaccid paralysis below the level of injury

These symptoms may last days to months and may mask postneurological function. In clients with spinal injuries at T6 or higher, return of the reflexes once spinal shock has been resolved may trigger the development of autonomic

TABLE 9.9 Incomplete Cord Lesion Syndromes

Syndrome	Cause and Results
Central cord syndrome	• Damage is to the central spinal cord, with the client experiencing motor weakness and sensory loss in both upper and lower extremities.
Anterior cord syndrome	• Damage is to the anterior spinal artery, resulting in motor paralysis and loss of pain and temperature sensation below the level of injury. • Position, vibration, and touch sensations remain intact.
Brown-Seguard syndrome	• Typically, it results from a penetrating injury involving half of the spinal cord. • Loss of motor function, position, and vibratory sense occur on the same side as the injury, with contralateral loss of pain and temperature sensation.
Posterior cord syndrome	• This syndrome is the least common of the six spinal cord lesions; it involves damage to the posterior spinal artery, resulting in loss of proprioception. • Pain, temperature sensation, and motor function below the site of the lesion will be intact.
Conus medullaris syndrome and Cauda equina syndrome	• Damage is to the very lowest portion of the spinal cord (conus) and lumbar and sacral roots (cauda equina). • These types of syndromes result in lower motor neuron injury with flaccid paralysis of the bowel and bladder and loss of sexual function.

dysreflexia, which is a massive uncompensated cardiovascular reaction mediated by the SNS. Autonomic dysreflexia is life-threatening and usually occurs in response to visceral stimulation once the spinal shock is resolved. A distended bladder or rectum is the most common precipitating cause of autonomic dysreflexia. Manifestations of autonomic dysreflexia include the following:

- Extreme hypertension
- Blurred vision
- Throbbing headache
- Marked diaphoresis and flushed skin
- Piloerection
- Nasal congestion
- Nausea
- Anxiety (Tyerman & Cobbett, 2023)

Clinical Manifestations

Clinical manifestations are generally a direct result of trauma. The manifestations are related to the level and degree of injury. With the incomplete lesion, there will be a mixture of symptoms.

A higher injury will have more serious manifestations. Sensory function closely parallels motor function at all levels. Disturbances of respiratory function in injuries below T6 are minimal. The following manifestations are common for upper-level injuries:

- Hypoventilation can be a serious complication with a cervical spine injury. Mechanical ventilation is required. Atelectasis and pneumonia can easily develop, and the client may require an artificial airway.
- An injury above the T6 level greatly decreases the influence of the SNS, resulting in bradycardia, peripheral vasodilation, and hypotension.
- With spinal cord lesions, the client may experience urinary retention and bladder distension and may need an in-dwelling catheter.

When lesions involve lower motor neurons, flaccid muscle weakness or paralysis, loss of reflex activity, and atrophy of the involved muscles are usually evident. Any lesion that destroys or interferes with upper motor neurons initially results in muscle flaccidity and hyporeflexia. Gradually, the reflex arcs become reactive. Voluntary muscle function is lost, but hyperreflexia of all cord segments occurs, with increased muscle tone and spasticity. Pressure sores can develop. Temperature regulation can be problematic as the client will have a decreased ability to sweat or shiver. Loss of body weight is common. DVT is common, with pulmonary embolism being one of the leading causes of death in clients with SCIs.

Diagnostics

SCIs are initially diagnosed on the basis of the presenting clinical manifestations. Diagnostic studies include complete spine films, CT scans, and MRIs.

Therapeutics and Nursing Considerations

The initial goals focus on sustaining life and preventing further cord damage. As the client's condition stabilizes, retraining takes place. The client:

- Will require a balanced diet with adequate calories and dietary fibre.
- May require an in-dwelling catheter or intermittent catheterization to regularly and completely empty the bladder to avoid UTIs.
- Will require a bowel training program.
- Will require monitoring of the environment to maintain proper body temperature.
- Will require respiratory rehabilitation, which may include a diaphragmatic pacemaker, ventilator care, assisted coughing, incentive spirometry, and deep-breathing exercises.

Sexuality is an important issue for all individuals who experience SCI. Reflexogenic erection is possible with upper motor neuron lesions. Drugs, vacuum devices or surgery for erectile dysfunction may be used. Affected females usually remain fertile; however, uterine contractions are not felt, and menses may cease for up to 6 months following injury. Open discussion with the client and their partner is essential.

Surgical interventions for SCI may help to stabilize, realign, and decompress the spinal column. It depends on health care provider preference and availability of surgical services. Research has shown early surgical intervention is safe and feasible and may improve clinical and neurological outcomes and reduce health care costs (Tyerman & Cobbett, 2023).

Grief and depression should be anticipated. The client may regress at different stages of recovery. Wide fluctuations of emotion should be expected. Mourning is normal and must be allowed. Assistance to obtain control during the anger phase is difficult but helpful. Above all, promotion of independence is critical.

Osteomyelitis

Pathophysiology

Osteomyelitis is a severe infection of the bone, bone marrow, and surrounding soft tissue. The most common infection microorganisms are *S. aureus*, *Staphylococcus epidermis*, *E. coli*, and *M. tuberculosis*. Osteomyelitis is usually a bloodborne disease that affects rapidly growing children.

Common sites of infection include the lower end of the femur and the upper ends of the tibia, humerus, and radius. In adults, the most common sites are the pelvis and vertebrae. The infection causes tissue necrosis, breakdown of bone structure, and decalcification.

Acute osteomyelitis refers to an infection of less than 1 month in duration. Chronic osteomyelitis is rare and is characterized by multiple draining sinus tracts and metastatic lesions.

Clinical Manifestations

Clinical manifestations are both systemic and local and include the following:

- Fever
- Night sweats
- Chills
- Restlessness

- Nausea
- Malaise
- Constant bone pain that is unrelieved by rest and worsens with activity
- Swelling, tenderness, and warmth at the infection site
- Restricted movement of the affected part and possible drainage from the sinus tracts (later sign) with chronic osteomyelitis

Long-term and rare complications of osteomyelitis include septicemia, septic arthritis, pathological fractures, and amyloidosis.

Diagnostics

Diagnostic studies include a bone or soft tissue biopsy, blood or wound cultures, or both; elevated WBC and erythrocyte sedimentation rate (ESR); bone scans; MRI; and CT.

Therapeutics and Nursing Considerations

Vigorous and prolonged IV antibiotic therapy is the treatment of choice for acute osteomyelitis as long as bone ischemia has not yet occurred. Cultures or bone biopsy should be done prior to medication therapy. If antibiotic therapy is delayed, surgical debridement and decompression are often needed. Clients are discharged to home care with IV antibiotics delivered via a central venous catheter or peripherally inserted central catheter (PICC).

Surgical treatment includes the removal of the poorly vascularized tissue and dead bone. Antibiotic-impregnated polymethylmethacrylate bead chains may be implanted at this time to aid in combatting the infection. After debridement, the wound may be closed and a suction irrigation system is inserted. Intermittent or constant irrigation of the affected bone with antibiotics may also be initiated. Protection of the limb or surgical site with casts or braces is frequently done.

Hyperbaric oxygen therapy of 100% oxygen may be administered in chronic osteomyelitis. Amputation of the extremity may be necessary to preserve life and improve quality of life.

Upon discharge, family members need to know their role in monitoring the client's health. Key points of client and family education include the following:

- Family members should be aware that symptoms of bone pain, fever, swelling, and restricted limb movement should be reported immediately.
- Immobilization may be indicated to decrease pain, and excessive manipulation should be avoided.
- Pain assessment and interventions need to be taught.
- Instructions concerning wound care with sterile management and frequent changes of open wound dressings, if present, are needed.
- The family needs to understand the infection is not contagious.
- Heat application and activities such as exercise should be avoided.
- Uninvolved joints and muscles should continue to be exercised.

- Care and management of the venous access device are needed, as well as instruction about antibiotic administration.
- The importance of continuing to take the antibiotics even after the symptoms have subsided needs to be strongly impressed upon the family.

The family should be advised that periodic home nursing visits will provide support and help reduce anxiety.

Osteoporosis
Pathophysiology

Osteoporosis is a chronic, progressive, metabolic bone disease characterized by low bone mass and structural deterioration of bone tissue. The rate of bone resorption accelerates as the rate of bone formation decelerates, resulting in decreased bone mass and the bones becoming porous and brittle. Osteoporosis occurs more frequently in the spine, hips, and wrists. Risk factors for developing osteoporosis include the following:

- Being female
- Family history
- Being of European or Asian descent
- Being of small stature
- Excess alcohol intake
- Cigarette smoking
- Early menopause
- Anorexia
- Liver disease
- Oophorectomy
- Sedentary lifestyle
- Insufficient calcium intake
- Long-term use of corticosteroids

Clinical Manifestations

Osteoporosis is often referred to as the "silent disease" because there are no symptoms. Later manifestations include fractures, back pain, kyphosis, and loss of height.

Diagnostics

Diagnosis includes a history and physical examination as well as a bone mineral density test, quantitative ultrasonography, and dual-energy X-ray absorptiometry.

Therapeutics and Nursing Considerations

Treatment focuses on proper nutrition, with calcium supplements, exercise, medications, and prevention of fractures. The following treatments are recommended:

- Taking supplemental vitamin D
- Increasing nutritional intake of good sources of calcium, including milk and milk products, green leafy vegetables, seafood, almonds, and hazelnuts
- Encouraging exercise to build up and maintain bone mass
- Advising quitting smoking and cutting down on alcohol intake to decrease bone loss
- Medication therapy may include the following:
  - HRT and calcitonin to inhibit osteoclastic activity
  - Bisphosphonates to inhibit osteoclast-mediated bone resorption

- Selective estrogen receptor modulators, such as Evista, may be ordered, as well as Forteo, which contains recombinant PTH.

Nursing plays an important role in health promotion and teaching how to optimize bone health and prevent osteoporosis.

Fibromyalgia Syndrome

Pathophysiology

Fibromyalgia syndrome (FMS) is a widespread, nonarticular, musculo-skeletal pain condition that causes fatigue and multiple tender points. The etiology is unknown, but there is a link between sleep disturbances, lack of exercise, and fibromyalgia, and multiple theories exist. Some include possible CNS involvement with serotonin and substance P, abnormal levels of norepinephrine, hyperfunctioning of the hypothalamic–pituitary–adrenal axis, an increase in cortisol, a decrease in ACTH, a dysfunction in the autonomic nervous system (ANS), viral illness or Lyme disease, a decreased amount of growth hormone, or simply a low pain threshold with increased muscle tenderness.

Clinical Manifestations

Clinical manifestations include widespread burning or gnawing pain that worsens and improves throughout the day. It is difficult to discriminate the origin of the pain.

- Head or facial pain may develop from a stiff neck and shoulder muscles and can accompany temporomandibular joint dysfunction.
- There is joint tenderness at 11 or more of the 18 specific tender point sites.
- The client has difficulty concentrating, has memory lapses, and often feels overwhelmed by multiple tasks.
- Depression, anxiety, numbness or tingling in hands or feet, restless legs syndrome, and irritable bowel syndrome frequently develop.
- The client often has difficulty swallowing, perhaps due to abnormalities in esophageal smooth muscle function.
- The client experiences urinary frequency and urgency and may experience dysmenorrhea with worsening of symptoms.

Diagnostics

Laboratory tests can rule out other suspected disorders. A muscle biopsy may have a nonspecific moth-eaten appearance or show fibre atrophy. Rheumatology classifies a client as having FMS when the following criteria are met: pain is experienced in 11 of 18 tender points on palpation and there is a history of widespread pain for at least 3 months.

Therapeutics and Nursing Considerations

Treatment focuses on restoring sleep and relieving pain. This consists of the following:

- Balancing rest with activity
- Using analgesics for pain relief
- Drug treatment for widespread pain associated with the disease includes pregabalin (Lyrica) and duloxetine (Cymbalta).

Administering low-dose tricyclic antidepressants or skeletal muscle relaxants for stress, fatigue, and sleep disturbances. Selective serotonin reuptake inhibitors (SSRIs) may be used for depression and benzodiazepines for anxiety.

- Massage combined with ultrasound or application of alternating heat and cold to sore muscles is often beneficial.
- Practising gentle stretching, yoga, Tai Chi, or low-impact aerobics is encouraged.
- Limiting the intake of sugar, caffeine, and alcohol is recommended.
- Vitamin and mineral supplements are suggested to assist the immune system.
- Relaxation strategies are discussed.

Chronic Fatigue Syndrome

Pathophysiology

Chronic fatigue syndrome (CFS) also known as *systemic exertion intolerance disease or myalgic encephalomyelitis,* is characterized by unexplained debilitating fatigue in which any type of exertion (physical, emotional, cognitive) can affect multiple organs in a person. Immune abnormalities are also present.

The precise cause is unknown, but viral infections such as herpes, Epstein–Barr virus, CMV, and retroviruses are suspected to be involved.

CFS often follows a cyclical course, alternating between illness and relatively symptom-free intervals. An abnormal immune function appears to be the central event, which leads to decreased immunoglobulin production, reduced NK cell activity, and altered cytokine production. CFS is sometimes referred to as a mental illness due to the mild to moderate depression that develops in these clients. CFS is often difficult to distinguish from FMS.

Clinical Manifestations

Clinical manifestations include sleep disturbances, low-grade fever, generalized musculo-skeletal pain, fatigue, sore throat, cervical or axillary adenopathy, multijoint pain without swelling, and headaches.

Diagnostics

Ruling out other possible causes assists in the diagnosis. No specific laboratory test is used for diagnosis. According to Tyerman & Cobbett, 2023, the diagnosis requires that the client have three of the following symptoms:

- Profound fatigue lasting at least 6 months
- Postexertional malaise: total exhaustion after even minor or physical exertion that clients sometimes described as a "crash"
- Unrefreshing sleep
  At least on of the following two symptoms is also required:
- Cognitive impairment ("brain fog")
- Worsening of symptom when standing (orthostatic intolerance)

Therapeutics and Nursing Considerations

Treatment is aimed at controlling the symptoms. Education of the client with CFS focuses on managing the fatigue while improving functioning and quality of life. Management consists of informing the client about what is known about the disease and recognizing the fears and concerns of the clients as real. The treatments are as follows:

- NSAIDs for relief of pain and fever
- Treatment for any allergic symptoms
- Tricyclic antidepressants and SSRIs for mood and sleep difficulties
- Clonazepam (Rivotril) for sleep disturbances or panic disorders
- Exercise to improve conditioning and restore energy, with gradual increases in intensity and duration
- Total rest is not advised as it can potentiate the client's self-image of being an invalid; rather, a carefully graduated exercise program is encouraged.
- Clients are taught to maintain a balanced diet, as good nutrition is essential to producing adequate energy stores. Referrals to agencies and CFS groups are very helpful for the client.

Osteoarthritis

Pathophysiology

Osteoarthritis (OA) is a noninflammatory disorder of the diarthrodial (synovial) joints. It is slowly progressive, with the majority of adults being affected by age 40. After menopause, more females than males are affected by OA. OA is usually caused by a known event or condition that directly damages the cartilage or causes joint instability. It may occur from previous infection, trauma, or skeletal deformity. Estrogen reduction at menopause, as well as genetic factors, seems to play a significant role. Modifiable risk factors include obesity, sedentary lifestyle, and occupations that require frequent kneeling and stooping.

OA causes deterioration of the joint cartilage and reactive new bone formation at the margins and subchondral areas. The progression of OA causes cartilage to gradually become softer, less elastic, and less able to resist wear with heavy use. Continued changes in the cartilage collagen lead to erosion of the articular surface. Uneven joint surfaces create an unequal distribution of stress across the joint, resulting in limited joint movement. Although inflammation is not characteristic of OA, a secondary synovitis may result when phagocytic cells try to rid the joint of small pieces of cartilage torn from the joint surface. These inflammatory changes contribute to the early pain and stiffness of OA. In later stages of OA, contact can occur between exposed bony joint surfaces after cartilage has completely deteriorated.

Clinical Manifestations

Clinical manifestations do not include systemic symptoms. The symptoms are as follows:

- Joint pain is the most common symptom and occurs particularly after exercise or weight-bearing.
- Joint pain may worsen as barometric pressures fall before inclement weather.
- Sometimes crepitation, a grating sensation caused by loose particles of cartilage, can be felt in the joint cavity.

- The joint pain is asymmetrical, and the client may experience early-morning stiffness, but this stiffness is usually resolved within 30 minutes.
- Joints that are commonly involved include the distal interphalangeal, proximal interphalangeal, and carpometacarpal joint of the thumb. Weight-bearing joints such as the hips and knees are commonly affected, as well as the metatarsophalangeal and the cervical and lower lumbar vertebrae.
- Heberden's nodes are deformities of the distal interphalangeal joint and indicate osteophyte formation. Bouchard's nodes are deformities found on the proximal interphalangeal joint. These deformities often appear red, swollen, and tender.

Diagnostics

Diagnosis is based on a history and physical examination. Bone scans, CT scans, MRIs, and X-rays are used to look for joint changes. Blood work would include ESR showing minimal elevated levels in acute synovitis. CBC and kidney and liver function tests are useful for screening for related conditions or establishing baseline values prior to the initiation of treatments. Synovial fluid analysis will rule out an inflammatory arthritis.

Therapeutics and Nursing Considerations

There is no cure for OA; therefore, treatment is focused on the following:

- Management of symptoms of pain and inflammation
- Prevention of deformity and maintenance of joint function
- Rest and joint protection
- Heat and cold applications, which may help reduce pain and stiffness
- Nutritional therapy
- Exercise
- Complementary and alternative therapies
- Supportive devices such as braces, which can be used to protect the joint

Medication therapy is based on the severity of the symptoms. Clients with mild to moderate joint pain may receive relief from acetaminophen. Salicylates or NSAIDs may provide greater relief for moderate to severe OA pain. Corticosteroids, disease-modifying antirheumatic drugs (DMARDs), immunosuppressants, biological therapy, and antibiotics may be added, depending on the client.

Education is a necessary element for the client. The client needs to know about medications and the treatment plan and be a full participant in their own care.

Arthroscopic surgery (reconstruction or replacement of a joint to relieve pain, improve or maintain ROM, and correct deformity) may be recommended for clients less than 55 years of age for knee OA. This may delay the need for more serious surgery such as a knee replacement. A total hip arthroplasty is a surgical procedure to relieve pain and improve function for clients with advanced hip OA (Tyerman & Cobbett, 2023).

Rheumatoid Arthritis

Pathophysiology

Rheumatoid arthritis (RA) is a chronic, systemic disease characterized by inflammation of the connective tissue in the diarthrodial (synovial) joints and surrounding tissues. Systemic manifestations include pulmonary, cardiac, vascular, ophthalmological, dermatological, and hematological effects. RA typically has periods of remission and exacerbation. It affects all ethnic groups and can occur at any time of life; however, the incidence increases with age. Females are affected more than males. Smoking appears to play a role in the development of RA.

The cause of RA is unknown, although an autoimmune etiology is currently the most widely accepted theory. The unknown antigen triggers the formation of an abnormal IgG. RA is characterized by the presence of autoantibody, rheumatoid factor (RF). RF and IgG form immune complexes that initially deposit on synovial membranes or superficial articular cartilages in the joints, which leads to activation of complement and an inflammatory response. Joint changes from inflammation begin when the hypertrophied synovial membrane invades the surround cartilage, ligaments, tendons, and joint capsule. Pannus forms with the joint and eventually covers and erodes the entire surface of the articular cartilage. Inflammatory cytokines further contribute to cartilage destruction. The pannus scars and shortens supporting structures, causing joint laxity, subluxation, and contracture. A genetic predisposition appears to be important in the development of RA.

Anatomical changes of RA follow four stages:

- Stage 1—early: There are no destructive changes on X-ray, although there may be evidence of osteoporosis.
- Stage 2—moderate: X-rays reveal evidence of osteoporosis with or without slight bone or cartilage destruction. There is no joint deformity. Adjacent muscle will atrophy, and extra-articular soft tissue lesions may be present.
- Stage 3—severe: X-rays reveal cartilage and bone destruction in addition to osteoporosis. There will be joint deformity with extensive muscle atrophy, and extra-articular soft tissue lesions may be present.
- Stage 4—terminal: Fibrosis, bony ankylosis, or both are present, as well as all the criteria for stage 3.

Clinical Manifestations

The onset of RA is typically insidious. Nonspecific manifestations may precede the onset of arthritic complaints. These may include the following:

- Fatigue
- Anorexia and weight loss
- Generalized morning stiffness

Specific articular involvement of pain, stiffness, limitation of motion, and signs of inflammation develop. The joint symptoms occur symmetrically and frequently. The joints most frequently affected include the small joints of the hands and feet and the larger peripheral joints of the wrists, elbows, shoulders, knees, hips, ankles, and jaw.

The cervical spine may also be involved. The client with RA will often experience joint stiffness after periods of inactivity. Morning stiffness may last from 60 minutes to several hours or more. Joints become tender, painful, and warm to the touch. Joint pain increases with movement, varies in intensity, may not be proportional to the degree of inflammation, and may make it difficult for the client to grasp things (tenosynovitis). The inflammation and fibrosis of the joint capsule and supporting structures may lead to deformity and disability.

RA can affect nearly every system of the body. The three most common complications include rheumatoid nodules, Sjögren's syndrome, and Felty's syndrome. Rheumatoid nodules develop in 25% of all clients with RA who have high titres of RF. Sjögren's syndrome affects 10–15% of clients with RA and can occur as a disease by itself or in conjunction with other arthritic disorders. Felty's syndrome occurs most commonly in clients with severe nodule-forming RA.

Diagnostics

Diagnosis depends on an accurate history and physical examination. RF can be found in 75–80% of clients with RA. ESR and C-reactive protein are indicators of active inflammation. Antinuclear antibody (ANA) titres may also be present in some clients with RA. Testing for anticitrullinated protein antibody (ACPA) is another important diagnostic test for RA. X-rays are not specifically diagnostic in the early stages. A bone scan may detect early changes and confirm the diagnosis. Synovial fluid analysis will show increased volume and turbidity but decreased viscosity. The client might be slightly anemic with slight leukocytosis.

Therapeutics and Nursing Considerations

Treatment focuses on medication therapy, education, physical therapy, and occupational therapy. Medication therapy is the cornerstone of RA treatment and is as follows:

- DMARDs such as methotrexate, sulphasalazine (Salazopyrin), leflunomides (Arava) have the potential to lessen the permanent effects of RA. Tofacitinib (Xeljanz) is used to treat moderate to severe active RA.
- Biological or targeted therapy are also used to slow disease progression in RA.
- NSAIDs, salicylates, and steroids are also used.
- In some situations, immunosuppressants, gold sodium thiomalate, or antibiotics may be used.

The choice of medication depends on the disease activity, the client's level of function, and lifestyle considerations.

Other important treatments include the following:

- Balanced nutrition can control weight loss, which may result from loss of appetite and inability to shop for and prepare food.
- Corticosteroids or immobility may result in unwanted weight gain.
- Exercise reduces stress on arthritic joints. The client is encouraged to alternate rest and activity.

- Lightweight splints help rest inflamed joints and prevent deformity.
- Occupational therapists are helpful in teaching the client about work simplification techniques and time-saving joint protection devices.
- Nonpharmacological management may include the use of therapeutic heat and cold, relaxation techniques, biofeedback, transcutaneous electrical nerve stimulation (TENS) and hypnosis.

Psychological support is important as clients are constantly threatened by limited function and fatigue, loss of self-esteem, altered body image, fear of disability and deformity, and loss of sexuality.

The major goals of therapy for clients with RA include the following:
- Promoting comfort and satisfactory pain relief
- Promoting independence and self-care with minimal loss of functional ability of affected joints
- Reducing fatigue
- Maintenance of a positive self-image
- Preventing injury and promoting mobility and maintenance of activities of daily living

Systemic Lupus Erythematosus
Pathophysiology
Systemic lupus erythematosus (SLE) is a chronic multisystem inflammatory disorder of the connective tissue. SLE affects multiple organ systems, including the skin, and can be fatal. It mostly affects young females of African, Asian, or Indigenous descent, although it does affect people of European descent as well. The etiology is unknown; however, genetic influences, hormones, environmental factors, and certain medications have been known to precipitate the disease. The onset of SLE usually occurs following menarche. The autoimmune reactions are directed at the body producing antibodies against components of its own cells, resulting in immune complex disease. Clients with SLE may produce antibodies against RBCs, neutrophils, platelets, lymphocytes, or any organ or tissue in the body.

Clinical Manifestations
Since SLE has multisystem involvement and characteristics of remission and exacerbation, the clinical manifestations can be many. These may include the following:
- Characteristic facial butterfly rash
- Photosensitivity
- Oral ulcers
- Alopecia
- Arthritis
- Pleuritis
- Pericarditis
- Renal disorders (proteinuria)
- Neurological disorders (seizures, psychosis)
- Hematological disorders (hemolytic anemia, leukopenia, lymphopenia, thrombocytopenia)
- Immunological disorders and development of antinuclear antibodies

Diagnostics
There is no specific diagnostic test for SLE, which is primarily diagnosed on examination of criteria relating to client history, physical findings, and laboratory findings. Antinuclear antibodies are positive for most clients with SLE.

Therapeutics and Nursing Considerations
Management of SLE revolves around medication therapy. The following medications are used:
- NSAIDs
- Antimalarial drugs
- Steroid-sparing drugs
- Corticosteroids
- Immunosuppressive drugs

Since SLE is a chronic condition, the client's physical, psychological, and sociocultural conditions should be assessed and managed. Pain and fatigue need to be monitored daily. The client needs to be educated regarding management of these ongoing issues. The overall goals for managing clients with SLE include satisfactory pain relief and adherence to the therapeutic regimen to achieve maximum symptom management. Other goals are to demonstrate awareness of and avoid activities that cause disease exacerbation and to maintain optimal function and a positive self-image.

With an acute exacerbation, it is important to record the severity of symptoms and the client's response to therapy. The client needs to be observed for the following:
- Fever pattern
- Joint inflammation
- Limitation of motion
- Location and degree of discomfort
- Fatigue
- Signs of bleeding
- Weight, fluid, and electrolyte anomalies need to be monitored if on corticosteroid therapy.
- Neurological disorders

The client will require support with explanations through the exacerbation. Once the exacerbation has ended, further client teaching needs to focus on adherence to the treatment plan and minimizing exposure to precipitating factors.

Low Back Pain
Pathophysiology
Low back pain is a prevalent population issue and is a common workplace condition resulting in lost of productivity that can result in significant economic and social costs. The lumbar region is susceptible to injury as this area bears most of the weight of the body and is the most flexible region of the spinal column. This region has poor biomechanical structure, and the nerve roots in the area are vulnerable to injury. Risk factors for developing low back pain are as follows:
- A lack of muscle tone
- Excess weight
- Poor posture
- Cigarette smoking
- Stress
- Repetitive heavy lifting

- Vibrations
- Prolonged periods of sitting

Low back pain is most often due to musculo-skeletal conditions, such as acute lumbosacral strain, instability of the lumbosacral bony mechanism, and OA of the lumbosacral vertebrae. Low back pain can also be due to intervertebral disc degeneration or herniation of the intervertebral disc.

Chronic back pain lasts for more than 3 months or is manifested in repeated incapacitating episodes. The causes of chronic back pain include the following:

- Degenerative disc disease
- Lack of physical exercise or prior injury
- Obesity
- Structural and postural abnormalities
- Systemic disease; OA of the lumbar spine is found in clients over the age of 50 years
- Cold, damp weather, which can aggravate back pain

Clinical Manifestations

Acute low back pain lasts 6 weeks or less and is usually associated with some activity that causes undue stress on the tissues of the lower back. The actual lower back pain with or without spasms will often appear later. Straight-leg raises will increase the pain.

Diagnostics

A thorough history and physical examination are needed to rule out serious conditions that may present as low back pain. MRI and CT scanning are not usually done unless trauma or systemic disease is suspected.

Therapeutics and Nursing Considerations

The client is cared for on an outpatient basis with the following treatments:

- Analgesics
- Muscle relaxants
- Massage
- Possible use of a corset to prevent rotation, flexion, and extension
- Rest may also be beneficial.

The client will be encouraged to avoid lifting, bending, twisting, and prolonged sitting. Most cases improve within 2 weeks.

Once an acute episode has resolved, health promotion is very important. Suggestions such as maintaining an appropriate weight, avoiding sleeping in the prone position, and using a firm mattress are beneficial. The client will be instructed not to lean forward without bending the knees, lift anything above the level of the elbows, stand in one position for a prolonged time, or exercise without consulting a health care provider. Treatment of chronic low back pain is similar to that for acute low back pain.

Herniated Intervertebral Disc
Pathophysiology

A herniated intervertebral disc is often referred to as a "slipped disc." It is a protrusion of the nucleus pulposus between adjacent surfaces of vertebral bodies and may occur anywhere along the spine. It can result from trauma, a sharp or sudden movement, or natural degeneration due to age. The gelatinous centre of the disc may rupture, causing acute injury and back pain. Common sites of rupture include L4–L5, L5–S1, C5–C6, and C6–C7. Herniation of thoracic discs is less common.

Clinical Manifestations

Clinical manifestations of a herniated disc are dependent on the location and size of the herniation. Manifestations may include low back pain that radiates down the leg in dermatomal distribution. Lying down often relieves pain. Reflexes may be depressed or absent. Muscle weakness is found in the legs, feet, and toes. There may be incontinence and erectile dysfunction.

Diagnostics

Diagnostic studies include X-ray, myelography, MRI, CT, epidural venography, discography, and EMG to determine the severity of nerve irritation and to rule out other pathological conditions.

Therapeutics and Nursing Considerations

Treatment involves limitation of extremes of spinal involvement; the local application of heat, ice, or both; ultrasound and massage; and traction and transcutaneous electrical nerve stimulation (TENS).

Medication therapy can include analgesics such as NSAIDs, and muscle relaxants. Once symptoms subside, back-strengthening exercises are encouraged. The client should be taught the principles of good body mechanics. Surgical therapy is needed when the client is unresponsive to conservative treatment or experiences consistent pain or there is a persistent neurological deficit. Several surgical procedures can be used to treat a herniated disc, which are as follows:

- Laminectomy, removal of a portion of the lamina, is the most common surgery for a herniated disc.
- A discectomy, removal of all or part of the herniated disc.
- A spinal fusion is done to stabilize two or more vertebrae by the insertion of bone grafts with or without the addition of rods, plates, screws, or other hardware.

After surgery, the client will be on a flat bed for 1–2 days, depending on the extent of the surgery. The client will be turned by log-rolling. Pillows will be placed under the thighs of each leg when the client is supine and between the legs when the client is in the side-lying position. The client is often fearful of any movement; therefore, explanation and reassurance are essential. IV narcotics will manage pain. Muscle relaxants may be prescribed. The client should be monitored for CSF leakage, which would manifest by a severe headache or the appearance of clear or slightly yellow fluid at the surgical site. Neurological assessment is ongoing, comparing the movement of the arms and the legs with preoperative movement. The client should be assessed for paraesthesia in all appropriate dermatomes. Movement and muscle strength of all extremities should be monitored. Wound care is done when needed. The donor site for a bone graft must be regularly assessed. The posterior iliac crest is the most common donor site. The donor site often produces more pain than the fused area. A pressure dressing may be needed to prevent excessive bleeding at the site.

Complications following surgery may include the following:
- Paralytic ileus and interference with bowel function may arise.
- Nausea, abdominal distension, and constipation; stool softeners may be ordered.
- Bladder emptying may be altered due to limited activity, the use of narcotics, or anaesthesia.
- Loss of sphincter tone or bladder tone may indicate nerve damage.

The client will have to adjust to a permanent immobility at the graft or fusion site. The client and family will need education regarding proper body mechanics, avoiding standing or sitting for long periods of time, balancing rest with activity, and that bending, lifting, and stooping could be injurious. Walking should be encouraged. Twisting movements of the spine are contraindicated.

Fractures
Pathophysiology
A fracture is a disruption or a break in the continuity of the structure of a bone, usually due to a blow to the body, a fall, or another accident. Fractures are described and classified according to their type and anatomical location and whether there is communication or noncommunication with the external environment. Other classification categories include appearance, position, alignment of the fragments, classic names, and whether they are stable or unstable. Figure 9.7 illustrates various types of fractures.

Typical complete fractures include the following:
- Closed (simple) fractures are noncommunicating wounds between bone and skin.
- Open (compound) fractures are communicating wounds between bone and skin.

- **Complete fracture** is when a bone breaks into two parts that are completely separated.

- An **incomplete fracture** is when a bone breaks into two parts that are not completely separated.

- A **comminuted fracture** is one in which the bone is broken and shattered into more than two fragments.

- A **closed (simple) fracture** is one in which there is no break in the skin.

- An **open (compound) fracture** is one in which there is a break in the skin through which the fragments of broken bone protrude.

- A **greenstick fracture**, common in children, is one in which the bone is partially bent and partially broken.

Fig. 9.7 Types of fractures. (From deWit, S. C., Stromberg, H., & Dallred, C. [2017]. *Medical-surgical nursing: Concepts and Practices* [3rd ed., p. 739, Box 32-1]. Elsevier.)

- Other types include comminuted, linear, oblique, spiral, transverse, impacted, pathological, avulsion, extracapsular, and intracapsular fractures.

Typical incomplete fractures include greenstick, torus, bowing, stress, and transchondral fractures.

Clinical Manifestations
Clinical manifestations of fractures include the client reporting a mechanism of injury resulting in immediate localized pain, loss of function, and obvious deformity. Other symptoms could include excessive motion at the site, crepitus, soft tissue edema in the area of injury, warmth over the injured area, ecchymosis of skin surrounding the injured area, paralysis, impairment or loss of sensation distal to the site of injury, signs of shock, and inability to bear weight on or use the affected part.

Therapeutics and Nursing Considerations
Fracture healing is a reparative process of self-healing (union) that occurs in the following stages:
1. Fracture hematoma
2. Granulation tissue
3. Callus formation
4. Ossification
5. Consolidation
6. Remodelling

Treatment focuses on anatomical realignment of fragments (reduction), immobilization to maintain alignment, and restoration of normal function or near-normal function of the injured part. A closed reduction involves nonsurgical manual realignment. An open reduction is the correction of bone alignment through a surgical incision. Forms of immobilization include skin traction for short-term immobilization and skeletal traction for long-term immobilization.

Traction is the mechanism by which a steady pull is exerted on a part or parts of the body while countertraction pulls in the opposite direction. Traction is used to prevent or reduce muscle spasm, immobilize the limb, reduce the fracture, stretch adhesions, and correct deformities. Suspension is the use of traction equipment, such as frames, splints, pulleys, and weights, to suspend but not exert pull on a body part. Balanced suspension is often used with traction to allow the client more freedom. A Buck traction boot is a form of skin traction used to immobilize a fracture, prevent hip flexion contractures and reduce muscle spasms.

Casts are considered temporary circumferential immobilization devices and are commonly used with closed reductions. There are many different types of casts.

External fixation uses metallic devices composed of pins that are inserted into the bone and attached to external rods. Internal fixation uses pins, plates, rods, and screws that are surgically inserted at the time of realignment.

Medication therapy for the treatment of fractures may include the following:
- Muscle relaxants
- Tetanus–diphtheria toxoid or immunoglobulins

- Bone-penetrating antibiotics, such as cephalosporin and analgesics as needed

The overall goals for treatment of the fracture include physiological healing with no associated complications, pain relief, and achievement of maximal rehabilitation potential. The following considerations are important:

- Neurovascular assessment of colour, temperature, capillary refill, peripheral pulses, edema, sensation, motor function, and pain should be ongoing. Both extremities are compared for an accurate assessment.
- Fractures pose a risk for peripheral neurovascular dysfunction, pain, and infection.
- A high fluid intake and a diet high in fibre are important due to the immobility of the client
- Traction equipment should be checked for proper functioning, and pin site care must be done.
- Too tight a cast can result in neurovascular complications; extremities must be checked frequently.
- If a cast is applied, the limb should be elevated above the level of the heart if possible when the client is resting.
- The client should be encouraged to exercise the joints above and below the cast to decrease muscle atrophy.
- Assistive devices such as canes, walkers, or crutches may be needed to help mobilize the client.

Complications of fractures include infections. Open fractures and soft tissue injuries have an increased risk of developing infections. Osteomyelitis may become chronic. If infection is present in an open fracture, surgical debridement may be necessary. Antibiotic therapy will be initiated.

Compartment syndrome is a condition in which elevated intracompartmental pressure within a confined myofascial compartment compromises the neurovascular function of the tissues within the space. This causes capillary perfusion to be reduced below a level necessary for tissue viability and is classified as acute, chronic or exertional, or crush. Two basic etiologies create compartment syndrome. There may be a decreased compartment size due to restrictive dressings, splints, or casts, or there may be increased compartment content due to bleeding or edema. Clinical manifestations of compartment syndrome include the following "six P's":

- Paraesthesia
- Pain
- Pressure
- Pallor
- Paralysis
- Pulselessness

Clients may present with one or all of the six Ps. Absence of a peripheral pulse is considered an ominous late sign. Treatment requires prompt, accurate diagnosis. Early recognition is key. The bandage or cast should be removed and traction weight reduced, and the limb should not be placed above the heart, nor should it receive hot or cold applications. Surgical decompression (fasciotomy) may be needed.

Venous thrombus is another potential complication of fractures. Precipitating factors include venous stasis, caused by incorrectly applied casts or traction, local pressure on the vein, and immobility.

Fat embolism syndrome (FES) is characterized by the presence of fat globules in tissues and organs after a traumatic skeletal injury. The fractures that most often cause FES include fractures of the long bones, ribs, tibia, and pelvis. Tissues that are most affected are the lungs, brain, heart, kidneys, and skin. Symptoms will occur within 24–48 hours after injury and may manifest as interstitial pneumonitis, which may produce symptoms of ARDS (chest pain, tachypnea, cyanosis, decreased PaO_2, dyspnea, apprehension, and tachycardia). The course of FES is rapid, with an acute onset and feelings of impending doom, and the client may be comatose for a short while. Treatment is directed at prevention; careful immobilization of the bone fracture is the most important preventive factor.

Stroke (Brain Attack or Cerebrovascular Accident)
Pathophysiology

A cerebrovascular accident (CVA) occurs when there is a sudden interruption of circulation in one or more of the cerebral blood vessels, resulting in the death of brain cells. Functions such as movement, sensation, and emotion that were controlled by the affected area of the brain are impaired or lost. The severity of the loss of function varies according to the location and extent of involvement.

Nonmodifiable risk factors for developing a stroke include increasing age, being male, being female postmenopause, heredity, low birth weight, and being of African, Latin American, or South Asian descent or Indigenous. Modifiable risk factors include the following:

- Poorly controlled DM
- Heart disease, arrhythmias, hypertension, hypercoagulability, and dyslipidemia
- Obesity, sedentary lifestyle, smoking, and heavy alcohol use
- Sickle cell disease (if sickling episodes can be prevented)
- Oral contraceptives
- Sleep apnea

Blood is supplied to the brain by two major pairs of arteries, the internal carotid arteries and the vertebral arteries. The brain requires a continuous supply of blood to provide the oxygen and glucose that neurons need to function. If blood flow to the brain is totally interrupted, neurological metabolism is altered in 30 seconds. Metabolism stops within 2 minutes, and cellular death occurs in 5 minutes. Arteriovenous malformation (AVM) is an abnormal group of tangled arteries and veins in the brain which are more likely to bleed.

Atherosclerosis is the major cause of stroke. It can lead to thrombus formation and contribute to emboli development. In response to ischemia, a series of metabolic events (ischemic cascade) occur, which include inadequate ATP production, loss of ion homeostasis, release of excitatory amino acids, free radical formation, and cell death. Around the core area of ischemia is a border zone of reduced blood flow where ischemia may be reversed. If adequate blood supply can be restored (in less than 3 hours), the ischemic cascade can be interrupted, with the result that there is less brain damage and less neurological function is lost.

Transient ischemic attack (TIA) is a temporary focal loss of neurological function caused by ischemia. TIAs usually resolve within 3 hours but may last as long as 24 hours. TIAs may be due to microemboli that temporarily block the blood flow and are warning signs of progressive cerebrovascular disease.

Strokes are classified based on the underlying pathophysiological findings and are either ischemic or hemorrhagic in nature. Ischemic strokes result from inadequate blood flow to the brain from partial or complete occlusion of an artery. Ischemic strokes constitute 87% of all strokes and are due to either thrombus or emboli damage. Thrombotic stroke occurs in relation to injury to a blood vessel wall and subsequent formation of a blood clot that narrows the blood vessel, resulting in a decreased amount of blood delivered to the tissue. This is the most common type of stroke and is usually associated with hypertension, DM, or both. Thrombotic stroke is often preceded by a TIA.

Embolic stroke occurs when an embolus lodges in and occludes a cerebral artery. This results in no blood to the distal tissues, leading to infarction and edema. This is the second most common cause of a stroke. The majority of emboli originate in the inside layer of the heart, with plaque breaking off from the endocardium and entering the circulation. Clients with an embolic stroke commonly have a rapid occurrence of severe clinical symptoms that may or may not be related to activity. Clients experiencing an embolic stroke usually remain conscious, although they often have a headache. Recurrence is common unless the underlying cause is aggressively treated.

Hemorrhagic strokes account for about 15% of all strokes. They result from bleeding into the brain tissue itself or into the subarachnoid space or ventricles. Intracerebral hemorrhage is bleeding within the brain caused by a rupture of a vessel, usually during activity. Hypertension is the most common cause. The onset is sudden, with a progression of symptoms over minutes to hours due to ongoing bleeding. Manifestations include neurological deficits, headache, nausea, vomiting, hypertension, and decreased levels of consciousness.

Subarachnoid hemorrhage occurs when there is intracranial bleeding into the CSF-filled space between the arachnoid and pia mater. This bleeding is commonly caused by rupture of a cerebral saccular or berry aneurysm. The majority of aneurysms are in the circle of Willis. Clients often describe the pain as "the worst headache in my life."

Clinical Manifestations

Motor impairment is the most obvious effect of stroke and can involve the following:
- Mobility
- Respiratory function
- Swallowing, speech, and gag reflex may be affected. Client may experience dysphagia; therefore a swallowing assessment by dietitian, speech language pathologist or OT should be performed.

- Self-care abilities
- Skilled voluntary movement
- The integration of movements, and alteration in muscle tone
- Alterations in reflexes
- An initial period of flaccidity, which may last from days to several weeks and is related to nerve damage
- Spasticity of the muscles, which follows the flaccid stage and is related to interruption of upper motor neuron influence

Stroke can also have the following neurological effects:
- The client may experience aphasia (total loss of comprehension and language) when a stroke damages the dominant hemisphere of the brain.
- Many clients also experience dysarthria (impairments with pronunciation, articulation, and phonation). Dysarthria does not affect the meaning of communication or the comprehension of language, but it does affect the mechanics of speech

For various neurological deficits of stroke and their nursing considerations, see Table 9.10.

Clients who suffer a stroke may have difficulty controlling their emotions, with the result that their emotional responses may be exaggerated or unpredictable. Depression and feelings associated with changes in body image and loss of function can make this worse. Clients may also be frustrated with immobility and communication difficulties.

Both memory and judgement may be impaired as a result of stroke. A left-brain stroke is more likely to result in memory impairment related to language. Stroke on the right side of the brain is more likely to cause impairments in spatial perceptual orientation, although this can also occur with left-brain stroke. The client may neglect all input from the affected side. This may be worsened by homonymous hemianopia, in which blindness occurs in the same half of the visual fields of both eyes. The client may also have difficulty judging distances (Tyerman & Cobbett, 2023). Most difficulties with urinary and bowel elimination occur initially and are temporary. Manifestations for right-brain and left-brain stroke are summarized in Figure 9.8.

Diagnostics

A CT scan is the primary diagnostic test used when stroke is suspected. The CT scan or MRI brain imaging diagnoses either hemorrhage or ischemic stroke and thus assists in appropriate treatment. Brain scans reveal ischemia but may not be positive for up to 2 weeks after a stroke. Carotid ultrasonography may detect a blockage, stenosis, or reduced blood flow of the carotid arteries. Ophthalmoscopy may detect signs of hypertension and atherosclerosis in retinal arteries. Angiography can help pinpoint the site of occlusion or rupture. An electroencephalogram (EEG) may help localize the area of damage. Laboratory tests include CBC, platelets, PT, partial thromboplastin time (PTT), electrolytes, glucose, renal and hepatic studies, and lipid profile.

TABLE 9.10   Neurological Impairments of Stroke

Neurological Impairment	Manifestation	Nursing Considerations and Client Teaching Applications
Visual Field Deficits		
Homonymous hemianopsia (loss of half of the visual field)	• Unaware of persons or objects on side of visual loss • Neglect of one side of the body • Difficulty judging distances	• Place objects within intact field of vision. • Approach the client from side of intact field of vision. • Instruct/remind the client to turn their head in the direction of visual loss to compensate for loss of visual field. • Encourage the use of eyeglasses if available. • When teaching the client, do so within the client's intact visual field.
Loss of peripheral vision	• Difficulty seeing at night • Unaware of objects or the borders of objects	• Avoid night driving or other risky activities in the darkness. • Place objects in centre of client's intact visual field. • Encourage the use of a cane or other object to identify objects in the periphery of the visual field.
Diplopia	• Double vision	• Explain to the client the location of an object when placing it near the client. • Consistently place client care items in the same location.
Motor Impairments		
Hemiparesis	• Weakness of the face, arm, and leg on the same side (due to a lesion in the opposite hemisphere)	• Place objects within the client's reach on the nonaffected side. • Instruct the client to exercise and increase the strength on the unaffected side.
Hemiplegia	• Paralysis of the face, arm, and leg on the same side (due to a lesion in the opposite hemisphere)	• Encourage the client to perform range-of-motion exercises to the affected side. • Provide immobilization as needed to the affected side. • Maintain body alignment in functional position. • Exercise unaffected limb to increase mobility, strength, and use.
Ataxia	• Staggering, unsteady gait • Unable to keep feet together; needs a broad base to stand	• Support client during the initial ambulation phase. • Provide supportive device for ambulation (walker, cane). • Instruct the client not to walk without assistance or supportive device.
Dysarthria	• Difficulty forming words	• Provide the client with alternative methods of communicating. • Allow the client sufficient time to respond to verbal communication. • Support the client and family to alleviate frustration related to difficulty in communicating.
Dysphagia	• Difficulty swallowing	• Test the client's pharyngeal reflexes before offering food or fluids. May have a depressed gag reflex. • May be a risk for aspiration and require a swallowing assessment. Offer thickened fluids as required • Assist the client with meals. • Place food on the unaffected side of the mouth. • Allow ample time to eat

TABLE 9.10   Neurological Impairments of Stroke—cont'd

Neurological Impairment	Manifestation	Nursing Considerations and Client Teaching Applications
Sensory Impairments Paraesthesia (occurs on the side opposite the lesion)	• Numbness and tingling of extremity • Difficulty with proprioception	• Instruct the client to avoid using this extremity as the dominant limb due to altered sensation. • Perform range-of-motion exercises on affected areas and apply corrective devices as needed.
Verbal Impairments Expressive aphasia	• Unable to form words that are understandable; may be able to speak in single-word responses	• Encourage the client to repeat sounds of the alphabet.
Receptive aphasia	• Unable to comprehend the spoken word; can speak but may not make sense	• Speak slowly and clearly to assist the client by modelling sounds.
Global (mixed) aphasia	• Combination of both receptive and expressive aphasia	• Speak clearly and in simple sentences; use gestures or pictures when possible. • Establish alternative means of communication.
Cognitive Impairments	• Short- and long-term memory loss • Decreased attention span • Impaired ability to concentrate • Poor abstract reasoning • Altered judgement	• Reorient the client to time, place, and situation frequently. • Use verbal and auditory cues to orient the client. • Provide familiar objects (family photographs, favourite objects). • Use simple language. • Match visual tasks with a verbal cue; holding a toothbrush, simulate brushing of teeth while saying, "I would like you to brush your teeth now." • Minimize distracting noises and views when teaching the client. • Repeat and reinforce instructions frequently.
Emotional Impairments	• Loss of self-control • Emotional lability • Decreased tolerance to stressful situations • Depression • Withdrawal • Fear, hostility, and anger • Feelings of isolation	• Support the client during uncontrollable outbursts. • Discuss with the client and the family that the outbursts are due to the disease process. • Encourage the client to participate in group activity. • Provide stimulation for the client. • Control stressful situations, if possible. • Provide a safe environment. • Encourage the client to express feelings and frustrations related to the disease process.

From Day, R. A., Paul, P., Williams, B., et al. (2016). *Brunner & Suddarth's textbook of medical-surgical nursing* (3rd Cdn. ed., p. 2047, Table 63.2). Williams & Wilkins. Reprinted with permission.

Therapeutics and Nursing Considerations

Goals for collaborative care during the acute phase of a stroke are to preserve life, prevent further brain damage, and reduce disability. The nurse monitors and reports vital signs and neurological assessments, including LOC, motor and sensory function, pupil size and reactivity, oxygen saturation, and cardiac rhythm.

Rehabilitation care begins after the stroke has been stable for 12 to 72 hours. Collaborative care shifts from preserving life to lessening disability and attaining optimal function. Goals at this time include maintaining a stable or improved LOC, attaining maximum physical functioning, attaining maximum self-care abilities and skills, and maximizing communication abilities. A plan to prevent recurrence of stroke is developed with the client and family.

Management of the following systems is very important. Nursing considerations:
• The respiratory system is a priority as the client may be at risk for aspiration pneumonia and airway obstruction.
• The neurological system requires close monitoring for changes that might suggest an extension of a stroke.

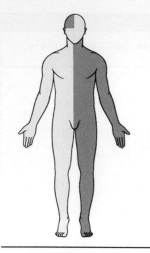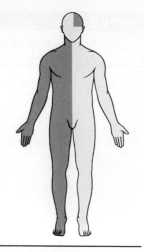

Right-brain damage
(stroke on right side of the brain)

- Paralyzed left side: hemiplegia
- Left-sided neglect
- Spatial–perceptual deficits
- Tends to deny or minimize problems
- Rapid performance, short attention span
- Impulsive; safety problems
- Impaired judgement
- Impaired time concepts

Left-brain damage
(stroke on left side of the brain)

- Paralyzed right side: hemiplegia
- Impaired speech–language (aphasias)
- Impaired right–left discrimination
- Slow performance, cautious
- Aware of deficits: depression, anxiety
- Impaired comprehension related to language, math

Fig. 9.8 Manifestations of right-brain and left-brain stroke. (From Tyerman, J., & Cobbett, S. [2023]. *Lewis's medical-surgical nursing in Canada: Assessment and management of clinical problems* [5th Cdn. ed., p. 1491, Figure 60-5]. Elsevier.)

- The cardiac system (vital signs and cardiac rhythm) also requires close monitoring due to the potential for a decreased cardiac reserve.
- Monitoring the lungs for sounds of fluid and the heart for the sound of murmurs is important for early detection of heart failure.
- Fluid and electrolyte balance is important.
- Proper positioning with appropriate supports and ROM exercises are needed to help prevent joint contracture and muscle atrophy.
- The skin of a client with stroke is susceptible to breakdown related to loss of sensation, decreased circulation, and immobility. This can be compounded by the client's age, poor nutrition, dehydration, edema, and incontinence. Pressure relief by proper turning and positioning is needed, along with good skin hygiene.
- Early mobility is helpful.
- Stress of the illness contributes to a catabolic state that can interfere with recovery. Good nutrition is essential, but the client must be checked for an active gag reflex before oral feedings are initiated. Feedings should be followed by thorough oral hygiene.
- Constipation is a common bowel condition for clients with stroke. Physical activity will promote bowel function.

Stool softeners and suppositories may be needed. Urinary incontinence is more common in the acute stage of the illness. Efforts should be made to promote normal bladder function and avoid the use of in-dwelling catheters.

It is imperative to meet the psychological needs of the client. The client will be assessed for the ability to speak and understand. Speaking slowly and calmly with simple words and sentences assists the client in speech improvement. Blindness in the same half of each visual field is a common condition after a stroke. Other visual conditions may be diplopia, loss of the corneal reflex, and ptosis.

Explanations about what has happened to the client and about diagnostic and therapeutic procedures should be clear and understandable to the client and family.

HEALTH CHALLENGES RELATED TO ALTERED SENSORY INPUT

Otitis Media

Pathophysiology

Inflammation or infection of the middle ear is considered the most common cause of conductive hearing loss. It can be caused by viruses or bacteria, with *Streptococcus* infections being the most common causative factor in bacterial otitis media. An accumulation of fluid can build up behind the tympanic membrane, resulting in loss of movement of the membrane, which can prevent the ossicles from moving and result in temporary hearing loss.

Clinical Manifestations

Symptoms of otitis media vary according to the severity of the infection. They may include tugging at the ears, pain and irritability, poor sleeping, diarrhea, vomiting and fever, inability to hear soft sounds, fluid draining from the ear, and possibly loss of balance *Chronic otitis media* is characterized by purulent exudate and inflammation that can involve the ossicles, eustachian tube and mastoid bone. It often presents as painless and may be accompanied by hearing loss, nausea, and episodes of dizziness. See Chapter 11 for more information on otitis media.

Diagnostics

Diagnosis is made based on otoscopic examination, which reveals that the tympanic membrane is red and bulging (Tyerman & Cobbett, 2023). Audiography may demonstrate a hearing loss if the ossicles have been damaged or separated. Sinus radiographic studies, MRI or CT of the temporal bone may show bone destruction, absence of ossicles, or a presence of a mass.

Therapeutics and Nursing Considerations

Treatment for this condition includes acetaminophen for pain and fever control and antibiotics specific to the infectious organism.

The nurse should monitor the effectiveness of the antibiotic and acetaminophen. Educating the client regarding adherence to the medication regimen, awareness of complications such as a perforated tympanic membrane, and when to seek medical assistance is important.

Chronic tympanic membrane perforation may require surgical interventions such as a tympanoplasty or mastoidectomy.

Cataracts
Pathophysiology

Cataracts are a common cause of vision loss. Vision is lost gradually due to the developing opacity of the lens or lens capsule of the eye. Cataracts commonly occur bilaterally but progress independently. They can be due to the following:

- Blunt force trauma
- Congenital factors
- Radiation and ultraviolet exposure
- Systemic corticosteroids
- Ocular inflammation

Most cataracts occur due to age-related changes in the lens and are called "senile cataracts." Frequent exposure to ultraviolet light may cause cataracts to occur earlier in life.

Clinical Manifestations

The client presents with a decrease in vision and abnormal colour perception. There may be whitening of the pupil, and the client may complain of halos around lights and a blinding glare from headlights at night. The client also is likely to experience glare and poor vision in bright sunlight.

Diagnostics

Diagnostic testing includes a detailed history and physical examination along with a visual acuity measurement. Ophthalmoscopy, slit lamp microscopy, and glare testing will confirm the diagnosis.

Therapeutics and Nursing Considerations

Nonsurgical treatment includes visual aids to compensate for the decreased ability to see. Surgical treatment consists of removal of the opaque lens and insertion of a prosthetic intraocular lens. The procedure is usually done on an outpatient basis. Postoperatively, the client requires antibiotic and anti-inflammatory eye drops and possibly an eye patch and may be advised against activities that increase intraocular eye pressure. Clients with an eye patch should be informed they will not have depth perception until the patch is removed (usually within 24 hours). Client is to restrain from any strenuous activities, avoid lifting (anything over 4.5 kilograms and bending for the first two weeks after surgery or as recommended by health care provider).

Glaucoma
Pathophysiology

Glaucoma refers to a group of disorders characterized by abnormally high intraocular pressure (IOP, fluid pressure in the eye), which can damage the optic nerve. Glaucoma occurs in three primary forms: open-angle (primary), acute angle-closure, and secondary to other causes. Risk factors for chronic open-angle glaucoma include genetics, hypertension, diabetes, aging, being of African descent, and severe myopia.

Acute angle-closure glaucoma (also called *narrow-angle glaucoma*) results from obstruction to the outflow of aqueous humour from anatomically narrow angles between the anterior iris and posterior corneal surface. It also results from shallow anterior chambers, a thickened iris that causes angle closure on pupil dilation, or a bulging iris that presses on the trabecular meshwork, closing the angle. Precipitating risk factors for acute angle-closure glaucoma include drug-induced mydriasis (extreme dilation of the pupil) and excitement or stress, which can lead to hypertension.

Secondary glaucoma may result from uveitis, trauma, steroids, diabetes, infections, or surgery.

Diagnostics

Ophthalmoscopic examination will show cupping and atrophy of the optic disc. Diagnostic studies include tonometry measurements of IOP, slit-lamp microscopy, gonioscopy to examine the angle between the iris and the cornea, and peripheral and central vision tests.

Therapeutics and Nursing Considerations

Chronic open-angle glaucoma can be treated by medication therapy, cyclocryotherapy, argon laser trabeculoplasty, or trabeculectomy. Acute angle-closure glaucoma can be treated with miotics, hyperosmotic solutions, laser peripheral iridotomy, or surgical iridectomy. Secondary glaucoma is managed by treating the underlying condition and with antiglaucoma medications.

It is very important that the client is able to understand and comply with the treatment. The client's ability to react to sight-threatening disorders needs to be assessed. The expected goals of treatment are no progression of vision loss, the client and family understanding the disease process and treatment, the client's adherence to the treatment, and no postoperative complications.

Macular Degeneration
Pathophysiology

Age-related macular degeneration (AMD) is a degeneration of the macula, the central area of the retina, which results in varying degrees of central vision loss. AMD is divided into two classic forms: dry (nonexudative), which is the most common, and wet (exudative), which is more severe. AMD is the most common cause of irreversible central vision loss in people over the age of 60.

AMD is related to retinal aging. Risk factors include the following:

- Family history is a major risk factor, and a gene responsible for some cases of AMD has been identified.
- Long-term exposure to ultraviolet light
- Hyperopia (farsightedness)
- Cigarette smoking
- Light-coloured eyes

In dry AMD, the client notices reading and other close vision tasks becoming more difficult. This form starts with the abnormal accumulation of yellowish coloured extracellular deposits called *drusen* in the retinal pigment epithelium. Atrophy and degeneration of macular cells then result, leading to a slowly progressive and painless vision loss.

Wet AMD is characterized by the growth of new blood vessels from their normal location in the choroids to an abnormal location in the retinal epithelium. As the new blood vessels leak, scar tissue gradually forms. Acute vision loss may occur in some cases due to this bleeding.

Clinical Manifestations

Symptoms include blurred and darkened vision, the presence of scotomata (blind spots), or metamorphopsia (distortion of vision).

Diagnostics

Diagnosis is based on the history and physical examination, visual acuity measurements, ophthalmoscopic examinations, an Amsler grid test, fundus photography, and IV fluorescent angiography.

Therapeutics and Nursing Considerations

When visual acuity is compromised, laser photocoagulation of abnormal blood vessels has been the therapy of choice, but it can also destroy the retinal pigment epithelium and photoreceptor cells. Photodynamic therapy is a newer therapy that results in fewer complications.

The permanent loss of central vision associated with AMD has serious psychological implications for nursing care. Uncorrectable vision impairment needs specific care and consideration.

HEALTH CHALLENGES RELATED TO OXYGEN PERFUSION

Hypertension

Pathophysiology

Hypertension refers to an intermittent or sustained elevation in the diastolic or systolic BP. Primary (also known as *essential* or *idiopathic*) hypertension is the most common form. Secondary hypertension results from a number of disorders, such as coarctation of the aorta or renal disease.

There is no single cause of hypertension, but there are numerous risk factors, including the following:

Nonmodifiable risk factors include the following:
- Family history
- Being of African or South Asian descent
- Males are more at risk than females, but the risk level reverses postmenopause
- Aging

Modifiable risk factors include the following:
- Stress
- Obesity
- High dietary fat and sodium intake
- Cigarette smoking
- Hormonal contraception
- Sedentary lifestyle

- DM

Complications of hypertension target the heart, brain, kidneys, arterial vessels of the lower extremities, and eyes. Individuals with poorly controlled hypertension have an increased risk for developing the following diseases:
- Coronary artery disease, left ventricular hypertrophy, and heart failure
- Cerebrovascular disease and peripheral vascular disease
- Nephrosclerosis
- Retinal damage
- Intermittent claudication, arterial thrombosis, gangrene

Clinical Manifestations

Primary hypertension usually begins insidiously and progresses slowly. If left untreated, even mild cases can lead to major complications. Initially, the client is asymptomatic. As the disease progresses, the client may experience the following symptoms:
- Fatigue and reduced activity tolerance
- Palpitations, angina, and dyspnea
- Epistaxis headache, or dizziness occurs only if blood pressure is extremely high or low

Diagnostics

Along with the client's history and physical examination, the following tests may identify underlying causes: urinalysis, blood glucose, CBC, lipid profile, BUN and creatinine, electrolyte levels, and ECG.

Therapeutics and Nursing Considerations

Treatment of primary hypertension focuses on lifestyle changes and medication therapy. Secondary hypertension is treated by treating the underlying cause. The goal of therapy is to reduce the overall cardiovascular risk factors and control the BP by the least intrusive means possible. Follow-up monitoring is very important, as is gaining the client's trust to help enhance adherence to therapy. Lifestyle modifications may include the following:

Dietary changes to low-fat, low-sodium products
- Weight reduction
- Limitation of alcohol intake and avoidance of tobacco use are important.
- Regular physical exercise and stress management are encouraged.

If lifestyle modifications are not enough or the BP remains high, drug therapy will be initiated. Medication therapy is directed at reduction of systemic vascular resistance (SVR) and a decreased volume of circulating blood. The types of medications used include the following:
- Diuretics
- Adrenergic inhibitors
- Direct vasodilators
- Angiotensin inhibitors
- Calcium channel blockers

See Chapter 8, page 145, for more specific information on antihypertensive drugs. The client will require regular follow-up to monitor BP. Explanation and encouragement are necessary with every visit to encourage adherence to treatment.

In rare situations, a client may go into a hypertensive crisis, in which there is a severe, abrupt elevation in BP. This more commonly affects a client who is not compliant with the treatment or who have been undermedicated. A hypertensive crisis puts the client at risk for developing renal insufficiency, heart failure, pulmonary edema, severe diaphoresis, and, in extreme cases, hypertensive encephalopathy. This is an emergency, and the client requires immediate medical assistance.

Coronary Artery Disease
Pathophysiology

Coronary artery disease (CAD) refers to any narrowing or obstruction of arterial lumina that interferes with cardiac perfusion. Deprived of sufficient blood, the myocardium can develop angina pectoris, infarction, arrhythmias, heart failure, and sudden death. The vessels involved are the right coronary artery, the left coronary artery, and the left anterior descending artery.

The right coronary artery supplies blood to the right atrium, right ventricle, inferior portion of the left ventricle, and posterior walls of the septum. The left coronary artery branches off to form the left circumflex artery, which supplies blood to the left atrium, lateral and posterior walls of the left ventricle, and posterior intraventricular septum. The left anterior descending artery supplies blood to the anterior wall of the left ventricle. The majority of blood passes into the coronary arteries when the heart muscle is at rest (diastole).

Every myocardial cell has four unique properties: automaticity, excitability, conductivity, and contractility. When a blockage occurs in an artery, the cells distal to the blockage will suffer, and these unique properties will be damaged or destroyed. The ejection fraction (EF), the percentage of blood ejected from the ventricle per beat, will be affected when any property is compromised.

Risk factors for the development of CAD include the following:

Nonmodifiable risk factors:
- Family history and genetic predisposition
- Increasing age
- Sex (males at greater risk than females until age 65 years)
- Ethnicity (White people at greater risk than Black people)
Modifiable risk factors:
- Obesity
- Smoking
- A high-fat diet
- A sedentary lifestyle
- Stress
- Diabetes
- Hypertension
- Dyslipidemia
- Elevated homocysteine levels

Atherosclerosis begins as soft deposits of fat accumulate along the inner wall of an artery. As the atherosclerosis progresses, luminal narrowing is accompanied by vascular changes that impair the diseased vessel's ability to dilate.

When oxygen demand exceeds what the diseased vessels can supply, localized myocardial ischemia develops. Transient ischemia can cause angina pectoris, a reversible change that can depress myocardial function. If untreated, actual tissue injury or necrosis (infarction) may result. Oxygen deprivation causes a shift to anaerobic metabolism in the myocardium, resulting in the formation of lactic acid. The accumulation of lactic acid—with a subsequent drop in pH—further impairs cardiac function and results in decreased cardiac output (CO). When occlusion of the coronary arteries occurs over a long period of time, there is a greater chance that collateral circulation will develop. Some clients have an inherited predisposition to developing new vessels.

Angina pectoris has four main forms. Chronic stable angina refers to cardiac pain that is predictable in frequency and duration and can be relieved with rest and nitrates. (Refer to Chapter 8, page 147, Anti-Angina Pectoris drugs). Unstable angina is unpredictable, with increasing cardiac pain. Prinzmetal's angina also called (variant angina) is a variant of unpredictable angina that is caused by vasospasm. Microvascular angina results from myocardial ischemia that affects the small, distal branches of the walls and inner lining of the coronary artery blood vessel.

Myocardial infarction (MI) occurs as a result of sustained ischemia causing irreversible cellular death. The degree of altered function depends on the area of the heart involved and the size of the infarct. Within 24 hours of the infarct, leukocytes infiltrate the area of cell death. Enzymes are released from the dead cells, and proteolytic enzymes of neutrophils and macrophages remove all necrotic tissue by the second or third day. Collateral circulation improves areas of poor perfusion. The necrotic zone can be identified on the ECG and by nuclear scanning. Ten to 14 days following an infarct, scar tissue is developing but is still very weak. By 6 weeks, the scar tissue has replaced the necrotic tissue and the area is said to be healed. Ventricular remodelling is an attempt by the heart to compensate for the infarcted muscle and includes hypertrophy and dilation.

Complications of a MI include the following:
- Dysrhythmias
- Heart failure (most common)
- Cardiogenic shock
- Papillary muscle dysfunction
- Ventricular aneurysm
- Pericarditis
- Dressler syndrome, which is pericarditis with effusion and fever that can develop 4–6 weeks post-MI
- Pulmonary embolism

Clinical Manifestations

Clinical manifestations of MI include the following:
- Pain in the chest, neck, jaw, arms, or epigastric region
- Dyspnea
- Nausea and vomiting
- Cool, clammy, pale skin
- Low-grade fever within the first 24 hours
- Initially an increase in BP and heart rate, which may later drop due to decreased CO

- Decreased urine output
- Crackles
- Peripheral edema
- Fear with feelings of impending doom

Recent research has shown that females present differently than men. In females, severe fatigue prior to the MI is the most common complaint. Sleep disturbances, shortness of breath, and anxiety are also symptoms of CAD in females. They can experience chest discomfort, but they are more likely to express discomfort in the diaphragm, neck, or jaw.

Diagnostics

Diagnosis will be based on the client's history and physical examination. Pain is the chief complaint and can be described as a heavy pressure on the chest, up the neck, along the arms, and in the back or as epigastric discomfort. The cardiac pain usually does not change with respiration or position change. An ECG can show ischemia or an infarct. Laboratory work will show elevation in the following blood work:

- Cardiac enzymes (troponin I and T)
- Creatine kinase (CK)
- Cardiac isoenzyme (CK-MB)

Coronary angiography can reveal coronary stenosis or obstruction. A stress ECG may provoke chest pain and signs of myocardial ischemia.

Therapeutics and Nursing Considerations

Treatment for angina consists of the following considerations:

- Rest to decrease the oxygen demand
- Nitrates
- Acetylsalicylic acid (ASA)
- Possible stent placement
- With some clients with angina, beta blockers or calcium channel blockers may be needed.

Invasive interventions may include percutaneous coronary interventions, atherectomy, laser angioplasty and myocardial revascularization with coronary artery bypass graft (CABG), or minimally invasive direct coronary artery bypass grafting (MIDCABG). The same management may be used for treating a client with an infarct, with the addition of thrombolytics to dissolve the clot and allow blood to pass. The main complications following thrombolytic therapy are bleeding arrhythmias and reocclusion. Medications used in the acute management of an infarct include the following:

- Oxygen
- Nitrates
- Morphine
- Antiarrhythmic drugs
- Beta-adrenergic blockers
- Angiotensin-converting enzyme inhibitors
- Stool softeners may also be used.

Once the acute phase has ended, the client will need cardiac rehabilitation to help them return to as normal a lifestyle as possible. This rehabilitation includes physical, emotional, and psychological assistance.

Sudden Cardiac Death

Sudden cardiac death is unexpected death from cardiac causes. There is a disruption in cardiac function causing an abrupt loss of cerebral blood flow. Death usually occurs within an hour of the onset of symptoms and is mostly caused by ventricular arrhythmia.

Dysrhythmias
Pathophysiology

The normal electrical pattern of the heart begins at the sinoatrial (SA) node, which is considered the pacemaker of the heart. It is found in the right atrium and usually sets a rate of 60 to 100 beats per minute (bpm). The electrical signal spreads through the atria and then travels to the atrioventricular (AV) node, where it is held for a short period of time to allow the atria to contract. If there is interference with the SA electrical impulse, the secondary pacemaker nodes (AV and Purkinje fibres) will automatically activate to keep the heart contracting. The AV node is normally the only avenue of connection with the ventricles. If an impulse starts at the AV node, the rate is usually around 40 to 60 bpm. The impulse then travels down the bundle of His and spreads to the ventricles via the Purkinje fibres. Once all cells in the ventricle are stimulated, the ventricles contract. If the impulse is formed in the ventricle, the normal rate is around 20–40 bpm. Refer to Figure 9.9 Electrocardiogram showing a normal sinus rhythm.

A dysrhythmia is an abnormal heartbeat. It is very important to assess how this abnormal rhythm is affecting the CO. Refer to Figure 9.10 demonstrating examples of two dysrhythmic ECG tracings.

The ECG is a display of electrical activity of the heart. The ECG can detect rate, rhythm, and conduction abnormalities; left ventricular hypertrophy; electrolyte imbalance; and digoxin (Lanoxin) toxicity.

The ECG also shows the voltage and duration of waves. The voltage gives information regarding the thickness of the

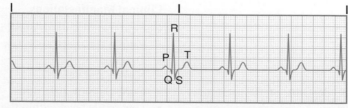

Fig. 9.9 Electrocardiogram depicting normal sinus rhythm in Lead II. (From Tyerman, J., & Cobbett, S. [2023]. *Lewis's medical-surgical nursing in Canada: Assessment and management of clinical problems* [5th Cdn. ed., p. 853, Figure 38-7]. Elsevier.)

chamber walls, and the duration gives information about the formation and conduction.

The action potential is the impulse generated by the movement of ions across a cell membrane. A cell is resting in a polarized state. A change in the electrical charge across the membrane causes an action potential, or cell depolarization. Once the heart is completely depolarized, it will attempt to return to its resting state via cell repolarization. The cycle of depolarizing and repolarizing includes the following five phases:

- Phase 0: Is the upstroke of rapid depolarization. The cell receives the impulse and is depolarized. Sodium moves rapidly into the cell, and calcium moves slowly into the cell.
- Phase 1: Early or rapid repolarization occurs, and the sodium channel closes.
- Phase 2: A plateau phase, slow repolarization occurs. Calcium is still slowly moving into the cell, and now potassium flows out of the cell.
- Phase 3: Rapid repolarization returns as the calcium channels are closed, and potassium flows out of the cell rapidly.
- Phase 4: Is the complete repolarization state. The resting phase (polarized state), active transport through the sodium–potassium pump returns potassium to the inside of the cell and sodium to the outside of the cell. The cell is now impermeable to sodium. Potassium can still move out of the cell. This is the end of the cycle, and the cell is ready for a new impulse. The phases of the cardiac action potential on an ECG are shown in Figure 9.11.

Refractory periods refer to the stage of resistance to stimulation. In the absolute refractory period, no depolarization can occur. In the relative refractory period, a strong stimulus is needed to initiate an impulse. In the supernormal refractory period, only a mild stimulus is needed to initiate an impulse. Many dysrhythmias are triggered in the relative and supernormal refractory periods, with the T wave being the most vulnerable.

Antidysrhythmic drugs are classified according to the phase they affect. The classes of antidysrhythmic drugs are as follows:

- Class I drugs block the influx of sodium into the cell in phase 0. These are sodium channel blockers.
- Class II drugs block the betareceptors; therefore, they block the SNS, depress depolarization, slow the SA node impulses, and increase the AV nodal refractory period. They are considered general myocardial depressants.
- Class III drugs block the potassium movement in phase 3, thereby prolonging the repolarization and refractory periods.
- Class IV drugs block calcium in phase 2 and so are calcium channel blockers or slow channel blockers. They act to prolong conductivity and increase the refractory period and time at the AV node.

Other medications do not fit into these classifications and are as follows:

- Adenosine (Adenocard) decreases conduction at the AV node.
- Atropine sulfate is an anticholinergic that blocks the vagal effect on the SA and AV nodes, thereby increasing the heart rate.
- Digoxin (Lanoxin) is an inotropic medication that strengthens the myocardial contraction and slows conduction at the AV node.
- Epinephrine (Adrenalin) acts on alpha- and beta-adrenergic receptor sites of the SNS, helping to restore normal sinus rhythm in a cardiac arrest.
- Magnesium sulfate decreases excitability and conduction.

Dysrhythmias are triggered by internal forces such as acid–base imbalances, electrolyte imbalances, and hypoxia, and by external forces such as illness, medication, and stress. Dysrhythmias are characterized by an alteration in impulse formation affecting the rate, rhythm, and development of entopic beats (those outside the normal pathway) or by alterations in conductivity, where failure or delay of impulse transmission may occur. The rhythms are classified according to

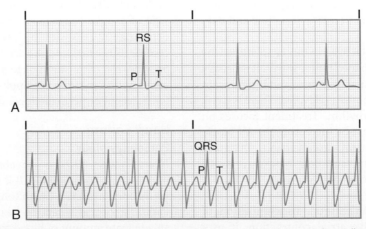

Fig. 9.10 A, ECG demonstrating sinus bradycardia. B, ECG demonstrating sinus tachycardia. (From Tyerman, J., & Cobbett, S. [2023]. *Lewis's medical-surgical nursing in Canada: Assessment and management of clinical problems* [5th Cdn. ed., p. 855, Figure 38-10]. Elsevier.)

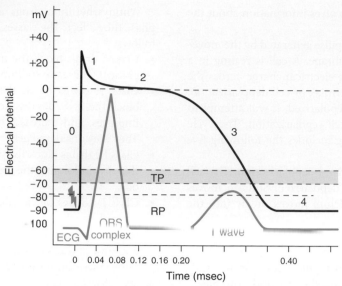

Fig. 9.11 Phases of the cardiac action potential on an electrocardiogram (ECG). The electrical potential, measured in millivolts, is indicated along the vertical axis of the graph, Time, measured in milliseconds, is indicated along the horizontal axis. The action potential (*black line*) has five phases, labelled 0 through 4. Each phase represents a particular electrical event or combination of electrical events. Phase 0 is the upstroke of rapid depolarization and corresponds with ventricular contraction. Phases 1, 2, 3 represent repolarization. Phases 4 is known as *complete repolarization* (*or the polarized state*) and corresponds to diastole. *RP*, resting membrane potential; *TP*, threshold membrane potential. (From Lewis, S., Bucher, L., McLean Heitkemper, M., et al. [2019]. *Medical-surgical nursing in Canada: Assessment and management of clinical problems* [4th ed., p. 867, Figure 38-1]. Elsevier Canada.)

the site of impulse formation and the degree of conduction block.

Sinus bradycardia is a slow sinus rhythm with a rate below 60 bpm. This rhythm can be normal in trained athletes. It becomes significant when CO is decreased and hypotension develops. Sinus bradycardia can predispose a client with an acute MI to develop escape arrhythmias and premature ectopic beats. If the bradycardia is compromising the CO, it can be treated with atropine.

Sinus tachycardia is a sinus rhythm with a rate over 100 bpm. It can cause dizziness and hypotension. The increased rate increases the oxygen consumption of the heart. It can create angina and extend the size of an infarct. Treatment depends on determining the underlying cause. Beta-adrenergic blockers are used to decrease heart rate and oxygen consumption.

Atrial flutter is an atrial tachyarrhythmia identified by recurring, regular, sawtooth-shaped flutter waves. It is usually associated with slower ventricular responses and is significant only when the ventricular response is elevated. There is a risk for clot formation with this rhythm. Treatment focuses on slowing the ventricular response by increasing the AV block. The client may require electrical cardioversion. Diltiazem (Cardizem), digoxin (Lanoxin), and beta blockers may be used. Anticoagulant therapy is needed to prevent the formation of clots.

Atrial fibrillation (AF) is the total disorganization of atrial activity without effective atrial contraction. It may be chronic or intermittent, can result in decreased CO, and carries a risk for stroke. AF is sometimes found in clients

experiencing heart failure. Treatment is the same as for atrial flutter.

Premature ventricular contractions (PVCs) are contractions originating in an ectopic focus in the ventricles. Ventricular tachycardia is a run of three or more PVCs. It is considered life-threatening because of decreased CO and the possibility of deterioration to ventricular fibrillation. Ventricular fibrillation is a severe derangement of the heart rhythm. This is an emergency, and the client needs cardiopulmonary resuscitation (CPR) and advanced cardiac life support (ACLS) with medication therapy and defibrillation.

Defibrillation is the most effective method of terminating ventricular fibrillation. Ideally, it is performed 15 to 20 seconds after the onset of the arrhythmia. It involves the passage of a direct current of electricity through the heart to depolarize all cells with the intent of allowing the SA node to resume its normal role. A pacemaker is a pulse generator that provides electrical stimulus to a heart that cannot conduct its own impulse in order to supply adequate CO. It can be used for transient or permanent conduction defects.

Heart Failure

Pathophysiology

Heart failure (HF) is an abnormal condition involving impaired cardiac pumping. It is not a disease but a syndrome. HF is often associated with long-standing hypertension and CAD. HF occurs when the heart is no longer able to pump an adequate amount of blood to meet the metabolic needs of the client. It is the most common reason for hospitalization in adults over age 65 years.

Risk factors for developing HF include the following:
- CAD
- Advanced age
- Hypertension
- Obesity
- Cigarette smoking
- DM
- High cholesterol
- Being of African descent

Conditions that can precipitate or exacerbate HF include the following:
- Stress
- Dysrhythmias
- Infection
- Anemia
- Thyroid disorders
- Pregnancy
- Paget's disease
- Nutritional deficiency of B vitamins
- Pulmonary disease
- Hypervolemia

HF may be caused by any interference with normal mechanisms regulating cardiac output. CO depends on preload, afterload, myocardial contractility, heart rate, and metabolic rate.

Heart failure with reduced ejection fraction (HF-REF) (systolic failure) is the most common cause of HF. The left ventricle loses its ability to generate enough pressure to eject blood into the body. The hallmark of systolic failure is a decrease in the left ventricular ejection fraction.

Heart failure with preserved ejection fraction (HF-PEF) (diastolic failure) is the impaired ability of the ventricles to fill during diastole and usually is the result of left ventricular hypertrophy. Pulmonary congestion results from diastolic failure, and there will be a normal ejection fraction until systolic failure develops.

There can also be mixed systolic and diastolic failure, as seen in dilated cardiomyopathy. This is known as *biventricular failure*. The ejection fraction in this case is extremely poor.

The four basic factors that cause HF are as follows:
- An increase in the volume of blood to be pumped
- An increase in the resistance against which the blood must be pumped
- A decrease in contractility
- A decrease in the filling of the cardiac chambers

Cardiac reserve refers to the heart's ability to increase CO in response to stress. A failing heart has limited ability to respond to increased demand.

There are four cardiac compensatory mechanisms: Sympathetic nervous system (SNS) activation, neurohormonal responses, ventricular dilation, and ventricular hypertrophy. Systemic compensatory mechanisms involve the SNS, kidneys, and liver.

Clinical Manifestations

Clinical manifestations of HF depend on the specific ventricle involved, precipitating causes of the failure, the duration of the failure, and any underlying condition the client may have. One-sided failure eventually leads to biventricular failure.

Left-sided (left ventricular) heart failure is the most common classification of HF. With this type of HF, blood backs up through the left atrium into the pulmonary veins, causing congestion and edema. Hypertension is the most common cause of left-sided HF, followed by cardiomyopathies, rheumatic heart disease, and CAD.

Right-sided (right ventricular) heart failure results in the backward flow of blood to the right atrium and venous circulation, which creates venous congestion, peripheral edema, hepatomegaly, splenomegaly, and jugular venous distension. The primary cause of right-sided HF is cor pulmonale.

Complications of HF are pleural effusions, arrhythmias, left ventricular thrombus, and hepatomegaly.

Classifications of HF are based on the person's tolerance to physical activity. Classifications are as follows:
- Class 1 is no limitation of physical ability.
- Class 2 is slight limitation to physical ability.
- Class 3 is a marked limitation.
- Class 4 is the inability to carry on any physical activity without discomfort.

Manifestations of acute HF include the following symptoms:
- Agitation
- Pale and cyanotic skin, and cold and clammy extremities
- Severe dyspnea and tachypnea

If untreated, the client may develop pulmonary edema. Chronic symptoms of HF include the following:
- Fatigue
- Dyspnea, orthopnea, and cough
- Tachycardia, pulse alterans, and AF
- Edema and nocturia
- Restlessness and confusion
- Chest pain
- Weight changes
- Skin with a dusky appearance
- Heart enlargement
- Cheyne-Stokes respirations

Death usually results from asphyxiation, pulmonary acidosis, shock, or dysrhythmias.

Diagnostics

Diagnostic studies are done to determine the underlying cause and extent of present failure, and they include the history and physical examination of the client. Chest X-ray, ECG, electrolytes, liver function tests, CBC, BUN and creatinine, and cardiac enzyme tests are performed. An echocardiogram with measurement of the ejection fraction may be done, along with stress testing and cardiac catheterization.

Therapeutics and Nursing Considerations

Treatment is focused on the following:
- Decreasing intravascular volume
- Decreasing venous return (preload)
- Decreasing the afterload
- Improving the gas exchange and oxygenation

- Improving cardiac function
- Reducing anxiety

Medications that are frequently prescribed for HF include diuretics, ACE inhibitors, beta-blockers, nitrates, calcium channel blockers, mineralocorticoid receptor antagonists and angiotensin-converting enzyme inhibitors.

The client will be encouraged to be in a high Fowler's position with the legs down to help decrease blood return to the heart. Oxygen therapy is usually needed as the condition deteriorates. Symptom management is important. Teaching regarding the activity–exercise balance, nutrition with a low-sodium diet, medications, weight management, support systems, and possible psychological changes will be helpful for the client with HF. Monitoring client's weight daily for fluid retention is important. A weight gain of 2 kg (4 lb) over a 2-day period or 2.5 kg (5 lb) gain over a 5-day period requires intervention.

Abdominal Aortic Aneurysm

Pathophysiology

An abdominal aortic aneurysm is an abnormal dilation in an arterial wall, commonly in the aorta between the renal arteries and iliac branches. Aneurysms commonly result from atherosclerosis, which weakens the aortic wall and gradually distends the lumen. Other causes include fungal infections, congenital disorders, trauma, syphilis, and hypertension.

Degenerative changes in the tunica media create a focal weakness, allowing the tunica intima and tunica adventitia to stretch outward. BP within the aorta progressively weakens the vessel walls and enlarges the aneurysm.

The most serious complication of an aneurysm is rupture. If it is a posterior rupture into the retroperitoneal space, bleeding may tamponade by surrounding structures, preventing exsanguination. If the rupture occurs anteriorly into the abdominal cavity, mortality is very high due to uncontained massive hemorrhage.

Clinical Manifestations

Clients are often asymptomatic. On physical examination, a pulsating mass is found in the periumbilical area. There may be a systolic bruit over the aorta, and the client may experience tenderness on deep palpation. Lumbar pain that radiates to the flank and groin can occur. If the aneurysm ruptures, there is severe, persistent, abdominal and back pain, often mimicking renal colic. Tachycardia, profuse diaphoresis, decreased urine output, altered level of consciousness and hypotension can occur.

Diagnostics

Diagnosis is made by history and physical examination, chest X-ray, echocardiography, ECG, CT scan, angiography, and MRI.

Therapeutics and Nursing Considerations

The goal of management is to prevent rupture of the aneurysm and extension of dissection. Early detection and prompt treatment are imperative. The aneurysm will be surgically removed and replaced with a Dacron graft. If the aneurysm is small and the client is asymptomatic, surgery may be delayed. Endovascular grafting may be used to repair an abdominal aneurysm. This is a minimally invasive procedure, in which a catheter with an attached graft is inserted through the femoral or iliac artery and advanced over a guide wire into the aorta. The graft is then positioned across the aneurysm. A balloon on the catheter expands, affixing the graft to the vessel wall.

Peripheral Vascular Diseases

Pathophysiology

Peripheral vascular disease (PVD) is an imbalance between the supply and demand of blood and nutrients that results from the degeneration of the peripheral vascular system. PVD includes arterial insufficiency and occlusion and venous insufficiency and occlusion.

Peripheral arterial diseases (PADs) can affect any artery but tend to affect the aorta, iliac, femoral, popliteal, tibial, and peritoneal arteries. Risk factors for developing PAD include the following:

- Increasing age, smoking, diabetes, obesity, sedentary lifestyle, and stress
- Heredity
- Being male
- Hyperhomocysteinemia
- CVD

There are two forms of PAD: organic and functional. Organic disease is caused by structural damage to the blood vessel with plaque or inflammation blocking blood flow. Functional disease is a reversible disturbance in the SNS. The vasospasm of Raynaud's disease is an example of functional disease.

Clinical Manifestations

The classic symptom of organic PAD is intermittent claudication, in which ischemic muscle ache or pain is precipitated by a constant level of exercise. The pain usually resolves within 10 minutes or less of rest. The pain is reproducible. Other manifestations may be as follows:

- Paraesthesia
- Thin, shiny, and taut skin on lower legs
- Loss of hair on lower legs
- Diminished or absent pedal, popliteal, or femoral pulses
- Pallor
- Reactive hyperemia

Complications of PAD include the following:

- Atrophy of the skin and underlying muscles
- Delayed wound healing
- Wound infections
- Tissue necrosis
- Arterial ulcers

Diagnostics

Diagnostic studies include Doppler ultrasonography, ankle–brachial index, duplex imaging, angiogram, or magnetic resonance angiography.

Therapeutics and Nursing Considerations

Treatment focuses on preventing further damage to the vessel. The client is encouraged to do the following:

- Stop smoking
- Treat the dyslipidemia, hypertension, and diabetes
- Exercise, as this improves oxygen delivery to the legs
  Pharmacological therapy may include the following:
- ASA (Aspirin)
- Ticlopidine (Ticlid)
- Clopidogrel (Plavix)
- Pentoxifylline (Trental) may be prescribed for intermittent claudication.

If PAD progresses and the intermittent claudication becomes incapacitating, the client has pain at rest, or ulceration and gangrene develop, surgical intervention will be needed.

A percutaneous transluminal balloon angioplasty could be done. The most common surgical procedure is a peripheral arterial bypass operation with autogenous vein or synthetic graft material to bypass the lesion.

An endarterectomy may need a patch graft. A sympathectomy may be done. When gangrene is present, amputation is needed.

Peripheral Venous Disease

Pathophysiology

The most common peripheral disorder of the veins is venous thrombus, which is the formation of a clot in association with inflammation of the vein. Three important factors, known as *Virchow's triad*, are involved in the etiology of the clot formation. These factors are venous stasis, damage to the endothelium lining, and hypercoagulability of the blood. Some of the risk factors for developing either superficial or DVT include the following:

- Major abdominal surgery
- Pelvic or orthopaedic surgery
- Oral contraceptives and hormone replacement therapy
- Obesity
- Pregnancy and postpartum period
- Heart disease
- Advanced cancer
- Coagulation disorders

Blood cells, platelets, and fibrin accumulate together to form the thrombus. A common site of clot formation is the cusps of the veins. An enlarged clot may occlude the lumen of the vein. Emboli can break away from the clot and lodge anywhere else in the body. The most serious complications of venous conditions include pulmonary emboli and phlegmasia cerulea dolens (swollen, blue, painful legs).

Varicose veins are dilated tortuous subcutaneous veins that usually affect the saphenous system. Risk factors for developing varicosities include the following:

- Congenital defective valves
- Prolonged standing
- Obesity
- Systemic conditions such as pregnancy, ascites, heart disease, and abdominal masses

Clinical Manifestations

Clients with superficial thrombophlebitis may present with the following:

- A palpable, firm, cordlike vein
- Surrounding area may be red and tender and warm to touch
- A slight fever
  Many clients with a DVT are asymptomatic. Those clients who are symptomatic experience the following:
- Unilateral leg edema
- Pain
- Warm, red skin
  Varicosities present as prominent, superficial, discoloured, tortuous veins. The client usually complains of the following:
- A dull ache or heaviness
- Fatigue
- Leg cramps and edema
- Some varicosities have nodular protrusions.

Diagnostics

Diagnoses can be made from the client's history and physical examination, blood work such as platelet count, bleeding time and international normalized ratio (INR), venous Doppler evaluation, duplex scanning, and venogram.

Therapeutics and Nursing Considerations

Treatment of superficial thrombophlebitis involves elevating the affected limb and applying warm moist heat to the area. ASA and acetaminophen may be used to relieve discomfort. NSAIDs may be used to treat the inflammation.

To prevent DVT development, early mobilization following surgery is encouraged. If the client is to remain in bed, frequent position changes are encouraged, as well as dorsiflexing the feet and rotating the ankles. Preventive measures such as compression stockings or support hose should be employed.

People with venous disorders should be encouraged not to cross their legs or ankles, not to stand in one place for long periods of time, and not to wear constrictive clothing.

If a DVT does develop, the client is usually started on anticoagulants to prevent the growth of the present clot and the development of any new clots. Unfractionated heparin, low-molecular-weight heparin, and warfarin (Coumadin) derivatives are the most commonly used anticoagulants. Coumadin requires 48 to 72 hours to have an effect on the PT; therefore, Coumadin is started before the heparin infusion is completed. A venous thrombectomy or insertion of a vena cava interruption device may be done to prevent pulmonary emboli. The client usually remains on prophylactic Coumadin.

Varicose vein management involves education concerning prevention, including lifestyle modifications, exercise, use of support hose, not standing for long periods, and reducing obesity. Surgical therapy for varicose veins may include sclerotherapy, ligation and stripping, or laser therapy for smaller varicosities.

CRITICAL HEALTH CHALLENGES

Burns

Pathophysiology

Burns occur when there is injury to the tissue of the body caused by heat, chemicals, electrical current, or radiation and can lead to many local and systemic conditions. Burns are classified according to the depth, extent, and location of the burn, as well as the client's own risk factors. The depth of the burn is now categorized as a partial- or full-thickness burn, as follows:

- A superficial partial-thickness burn involves the epidermis.
- A deep partial thickness burn involves the dermis.
- A full-thickness burn involves, fat, muscle, and bone.

The location of the burn is related to the severity of the injury. Face, neck, and chest burns can result in respiratory complications. Circumferential burns of the extremities can cause circulatory conditions and compartment syndrome. Older clients or clients who have pre-existing cardiovascular conditions, respiratory conditions, renal disease, diabetes, alcoholism, a history of drug use, or malnutrition are slower at healing from a burn.

Clinical Manifestations

Manifestations of burns are as follows:

- Shock
- Blisters
- Adynamic ileus
- Shivering
- Altered mental status
  Many complications can result from burns:
- Cardiovascular complications include arrhythmias, hypovolemic shock, edema, ischemia, necrosis, gangrene, and increased blood viscosity.
- Respiratory complications can be mechanical obstruction and asphyxia, interstitial edema, pneumonia, and pulmonary edema.
- Renal complications because of acute tubular necrosis can result in kidney damage.
- GI changes that can occur from burns include impairment of gastric mucosal integrity and motility. Paralytic ileus may develop. Abdominal distension can occur, and curling ulcer (acute ulcerative gastroduodenal disease) can develop.
  Metabolic complications can include hypermetabolism, increasing body temperature, and increasing catabolic rates.
  Skin complications occur due to the burn injury's disruption of the protective barrier of the skin, which increases the risk for infection.

Therapeutics and Nursing Considerations

Care begins at the time of the burn. The client must first be removed from the source of the burn. For smaller burns, cover the burn with a clean, cool, tap water–dampened towel. For larger burns, remove burned clothing and wrap the client in a clean sheet, without using any cool water or ice.

Emergent phase. The emergent (resuscitative) phase is from the onset to 2 to 5 or more days following the burn. In the first 24–48 hours, the client will lose fluid and form edema until fluid mobilization and diuresis occur. At this time, the client is at risk for the following complications:

- Hypovolemic shock
- Edema, decreased BP, and increased pulse
- Increased insensible water loss
- Thrombosis
- Potassium and sodium shifts
- The immune system is compromised.
  Initial management focuses on survival. Goals of management include the following:
- Securing the airway
- Supporting circulation by fluid replacement
- Keeping the client as comfortable as possible with analgesics
- Preventing infection
- Maintaining body temperature
- Providing emotional support
- Airway management
- Fluid management
  Wound care is delayed until a patent airway, adequate circulation, and adequate fluid replacement have been established. When time permits, the wound should be cleansed by using a hydrotherapy tub, shower, or bed. Debridement is the removal of loose, necrotic skin and may require sedation. An open wound is covered with a topical antibiotic without a dressing. The closed method or multiple-dressing change involves sterile gauze dressing impregnated with or laid over a topical antimicrobial. Dressings are changed at various intervals, from every 12–24 hours to once every 14 days, depending on the product.
  Be aware of the following:
- Allograft or homograft skin grafts are commonly used, along with newer biosynthetic options.
- Routine blood work is important to monitor for electrolyte imbalance and homeostasis.
- Early ROM exercises help prevent contractures.
- Analgesics and sedatives are given, as well as a tetanus immunization.
- Antimicrobial agents, both topical and systemic, are used.
- Fluid replacement takes priority over nutritional requirements. Oral intake can be started once the bowel sounds return. Due to the increased metabolic state, the client will need high-calorie meals with vitamin and mineral supplements.

Acute phase. The acute phase begins with the mobilization of ECF and subsequent diuresis and ends when the burned area is completely covered by skin grafts or when the wounds are healed. Necrotic tissue will begin to slough off, and granulation tissue will form. A partial-thickness wound will heal from the edges. Full-thickness wounds must be covered by skin grafts. Partial-thickness wounds form eschar initially, and then epithelialization begins once the eschar is removed. Full-thickness wounds require debridement. The interventions required are as follows:

- Wound care in the acute phase includes daily observation, cleansing, and debridement.
- Appropriate coverage of the graft is needed. A fine mesh gauze is placed on the graft, followed by a middle and outer dressing. Sheet skin grafts must be kept free of blebs. Eschar is removed down to the subcutaneous tissue of fascia. Cultured epithelial autographs, grown from biopsies of the client's own skin, or artificial grafts may be used.
- Analgesics and sedation are needed.
- Passive and active ROM exercises should be performed.
- Splints help prevent deformities.
- A high-protein, high-carbohydrate diet helps meet the client's increased metabolic needs.

Rehabilitation phase. The rehabilitation phase begins when the client's burn wounds are covered with skin or healed, and the client is able to resume a level of self-care activity. The burn wound will heal either by primary intention or by grafting. Layers of epithelialization begin rebuilding the tissue structure. Collagen fibres add strength to weakened areas. In about 4–6 weeks, the burn area becomes raised and hyperemic. Mature healing is reached in 6 months to 2 years. The skin will never completely regain its original colour. The following are nursing considerations:

- Skin and joint contractures are the most common complication in the rehabilitation phase.
- Both the client and the family become active learners regarding wound care.
- An emollient water-based cream is recommended.
- Cosmetic surgery may be needed.
- The client will require constant encouragement and reassurances. The family will need to understand the importance of re-establishing the client's independence while participating in client care. It is important to assess for psychoemotional cues and understand that psychiatric intervention may be needed.

Shock

Pathophysiology

Shock is a syndrome characterized by decreased tissue perfusion and impaired cellular metabolism. Shock may be classified as *low flow*: cardiogenic and hypovolemic shock or *distributive*: neurogenic, anaphylactic, or septic shock. Cardiogenic shock or low-blood-flow shock involves systolic and diastolic dysfunction and compromised CO. The causes are as follows:

- MI, cardiomyopathies, and blunt cardiac injury
- Severe systemic or pulmonary hypertension
- Severe sepsis can cause cardiogenic shock.

Diastolic dysfunction results from the impaired ability of the ventricle to fill during diastole and a decrease in stroke volume. Early signs of cardiogenic shock include the following:

- Tachycardia
- Hypotension and narrowed pulse pressure
- Increased SVR
- Increased myocardial oxygen consumption, tachypnea, pulmonary congestion, and crackles

- Since the CO is low, renal blood flow, and urine output decrease.
- Lack of oxygen to the tissues can result in anxiety.

Hypovolemic shock. Hypovolemic shock is loss of intravascular fluid, either an absolute or relative volume loss. Absolute hypovolemia can be due to the following:

- Hemorrhage
- GI loss
- Fistula drainage
- Diuresis

Relative hypovolemia occurs when fluid moves out of the intravascular space into an extravascular space (third spacing). With hypovolemic shock, the size of the vascular compartment is unchanged, and there is a decreased venous return to the heart, decreased preload, and decreased CO, which results in impaired cellular metabolism. If the loss of blood is more than 30% of total volume, blood replacement is needed.

Neurogenic shock. Neurogenic shock occurs after SCI, at T5 or above. Neurogenic shock results in massive vasodilation, leading to pooling of blood in the vessels. Clinical signs include hypotension and bradycardia. Hypothalamic dysfunction is characteristic, with temperature dysregulation.

Spinal shock. Spinal shock is manifested by decreased reflexes, loss of sensation, and flaccid paralysis below the level of injury. These symptoms may last days to months and may mask postneurological function. Once spinal shock has been resolved in clients with spinal injuries at T6 or higher, return of the reflexes may trigger the development of autonomic dysreflexia, which is a massive uncompensated cardiovascular reaction mediated by the SNS. Autonomic dysreflexia is life-threatening and usually occurs in response to visceral stimulation once the spinal shock is resolved. A distended bladder or rectum is the most common precipitating cause of autonomic dysreflexia. Manifestations of autonomic dysreflexia include extreme hypertension, blurred vision, throbbing headache, marked diaphoresis, piloerection, flushed skin, nasal congestion, nausea, and anxiety (Tyerman & Cobbett, 2023).

Anaphylactic shock. Anaphylactic shock is an acute life-threatening hypersensitivity reaction that causes massive vasodilation, increased capillary permeability, and release of mediators. This can lead to respiratory distress and circulatory failure. Sudden symptoms are anxiety, confusion, and a sense of impending doom.

Septic shock. Septic shock is a systemic inflammatory response to infection. It is the leading cause of death in noncoronary critical care units (CCUs). The primary causative agents are Gram-negative and Gram-positive bacteria. With septic shock, there is increased coagulation and inflammation. The decreased fibrinolysis results in the formation of microthrombi that can obstruct microvasculature. SVR will decrease, leading to hypotension. The client will be tachypneic and have temperature dysregulation, decreased urinary output, altered neurological status, GI dysfunction, and respiratory failure (Tyerman & Cobbett, 2023).

Clinical Manifestations

Initial stage of shock. The initial stage of shock may not be clinically apparent. Metabolism changes from aerobic to anaerobic with lactic acid accumulation. Lactic acid must be removed by the blood and broken down in the liver, which requires oxygen that is not available.

Compensatory stage. During the compensatory stage, the body attempts to re-establish homeostasis. Baroreceptors in the carotid and aortic bodies activate SNS in response to the decreased BP. The following actions happen as listed:

- Peripheral vasoconstriction occurs to maintain blood to the visceral organs. The client's extremities will be cool and clammy. However, the septic client will be warm and flushed.
- The decreased renal blood flow activates the renin–angiotensin system in an attempt to increase venous return to the heart and increase CO and BP.
- The impaired GI motility can lead to paralytic ileus.
- The decreased arterial oxygen levels cause increased respirations. SNS stimulation increases myocardial oxygen demand.

Progressive stage. If the perfusion deficit is corrected, the client will recover with no residual sequelae; if the deficit is not corrected, the client enters the progressive stage, which begins when the compensatory mechanisms fail.

Aggressive intervention is needed to prevent multiorgan dysfunction syndrome. Decreased cellular perfusion and altered capillary permeability are hallmarks for the progressive stage of shock.

Refractory stage. The refractory stage involves the exacerbation of anaerobic metabolism, accumulation of lactic acid, and increased capillary permeability. The client may be hypotensive and tachycardic and may experience both cardiac and cerebral ischemia, as well as hypoxia. In the refractory stage, failure of one organ will affect the other organs. Recovery at this stage is unlikely.

Diagnostics

There is no single diagnostic test to determine shock. Integration of the physical examination and medical history is key.

Therapeutics and Nursing Considerations

Treatment focuses on interventions to control or eliminate the cause of decreased perfusion and to protect the organs from dysfunction. Multisystem care is needed, including the following:

- Ensuring a patent airway and optimizing oxygen delivery
- Possible blood transfusions or other fluid replacement therapy
- An in-dwelling catheter allows for frequent checks of output.
- Vital signs and ABGs must be monitored frequently.
- Vasopressor agents may be given for hypotension.
- Vasodilators may be given.
- Cardiac monitoring may be done.
- A pulmonary catheter may be used to monitor venous pressures.

- Chest and bowel sounds should be assessed frequently.

The goals of treatment are to provide adequate tissue perfusion, to restore normal BP, to recover organ function, and to have no complications.

Treatment for life-threatening autonomic dysreflexia includes the following:

- Raising the head of the bed to 45 degrees
- Immediate urinary catheterization if the bladder is distended
- A digital rectal examination with topical anaesthesia may be needed if the client is constipated.
- Constrictive clothing and tight shoes need to be removed to prevent excessive skin stimulation.
- BP must be closely monitored and treated with an alpha-adrenergic blocker or an arteriolar vasodilator (Tyerman & Cobbett, 2023).

CONCEPTS IN NURSING PRACTICE

Preoperative Care

Surgery can be described as the art and science of treating diseases, injuries, and deformities by operation and instrumentation. Surgery can be performed for purposes of diagnosis, cure, palliation, prevention, exploration, and cosmetic improvement. A surgery may be a planned event (elective surgery) or arise unexpectedly (emergency surgery).

Part of preoperative care includes interviewing the surgical client. The purpose of this interview is to obtain health information, determine client expectations, provide and clarify information about the surgery, and assess the emotional state and readiness of the client. During the interview and any other interactions, the use of a common language is important; therefore, translators may be needed.

Preoperative care also includes nursing assessment of the client undergoing surgery. The goals of the nursing assessment should include the following:

- Determining the client's psychological status in order to reinforce coping strategies
- Determining any psychological factors of the procedure that may contribute to risks
- Establishing baseline data
- Identifying medications and herbs taken that may affect surgical outcomes
- Identifying, documenting, and communicating results of laboratory and diagnostic tests
- Identifying cultural and ethnic factors that may affect the surgical experience
- Determining whether the client has signed the informed consent for surgery

Psychosocial assessment is important as a magnified stress response can affect recovery. During this assessment, the nurse can identify any emotional reactions to hospitalization, allay anxieties or fears, assess coping mechanisms, and help restore self-esteem. The nursing assessment includes obtaining information on the following:

- The client's health history
- Medical conditions

- Previous surgeries
- Menstrual and obstetric history
- Familial diseases
- Reaction to anaesthesia
- Current prescribed medications and over-the-counter medications
- Herbs or homeopathic preparations used
- Vitamins
- Recreational drugs
- Alcohol
- Tobacco
- Allergies

There are different methods of performing the physical assessment; however, they should contain a review of the systems of the body: the cardiovascular, respiratory, nervous, urinary, GI, integumentary, musculo-skeletal, endocrine, and immune systems. Other assessments include fluid and electrolyte status and nutritional status.

Preoperative teaching is very important. The client has the right to know what to expect during and after surgery. By having this knowledge, the client will have decreased anxiety and an increased sense of control. Instruction on postoperative deep breathing, coughing, and ambulation, and giving the client the rationale for these actions, increases the client's success and adherence in performing them. Methods of pain control should be discussed. The client and family should be informed about any tubes, drains, monitoring devices, or special equipment that might be present postoperatively. This knowledge will decrease client and family fears and anxiety. Information should be provided to the client and the family about fluid or food restrictions, the need for certain treatments prior to surgery, the need for a shower prior to surgery, and the need to remove jewellery and prosthetics prior to surgery.

Legal preparation is important. Ensure that all forms have been correctly signed and witnessed. These forms could include the informed consent form, a blood refusal form, if needed, an advance directive, a living will, and a power of attorney. With voluntary consent, the client must have a clear understanding and comprehension of what is going to happen prior to signing the consent form. An anaesthesiologist will assess the client for anaesthetic risk and discuss the type of anaesthetic that will be used. The surgeon is responsible for obtaining the client's consent on the agency consent form after the surgical procedure and risks have been clearly explained. The nurse may witness the signature if required. The client has the right to withdraw consent at any time. Legally appointed representatives of the family may give consent if the client is a child, unconscious, or mentally incompetent. Medical emergencies may override the need for consent. If no next of kin is available, the surgeon may document the necessity of the surgery.

On the day of surgery, the following nursing interventions are essential for any type of surgery:
- Preoperative teaching should be reinforced.
- Consent should be verified.
- Preoperative charting of baseline data and vital signs should be complete.
- Clients cannot wear any cosmetics.
- Dentures should be removed.
- Correct client identification and allergy bands must be in place.
- Valuables are given to the family or locked in a safe.
- The client is encouraged to void prior to surgery.
- Preoperative medication is given.

Intraoperative Care

The surgical suite is a controlled environment designed to minimize the spread of infection and to allow for the smooth flow of clients, personnel, and instruments or equipment. The operating room is geographically, environmentally, and bacteriologically controlled.

The basic surgical team includes the perioperative nurse, the circulating nurse, the scrub nurse, the surgeon, and the anaesthetist. The perioperative nurse ensures that the client is fully prepared for the surgery. The circulating nurse is not scrubbed, gowned, or gloved. The circulating nurse assists the scrub nurse with the surgical count, provides supplies as needed to the scrub team, assists the anaesthesiologist as needed, and documents the procedure. The scrub nurse follows a designated scrub procedure, participates in the surgical count, monitors blood loss and medications used during surgery, requests sterile supplies as needed, passes instruments and implements to the surgeon, and remains within the sterile field. Practical nurses with advanced training perform the scrubbing function in many Canadian institutions. The surgeon is the physician who performs the procedure. Registered Nurse First Assistant (RNFA) is a registered nurse with formal surgical education, skills, and knowledge who facilitates and supports the health care needs of the client. RNFAs handle instruments, provide exposure, manipulate tissue, assist with hemostasis, and suture under direct supervision of the surgeon (Tyerman & Cobbett, 2023). The anaesthesiologist administers the anaesthesia, maintains the client's physiological homeostasis, and monitors their physical status throughout the surgery. A registered nurse anaesthesia assistant is an RN with advance education, knowledge and skill in anaesthesia who work in collaboration with and under the supervision of the anaesthesiologist (Tyerman & Cobbett, 2023).

Proper positioning of the client is important to provide accessibility of the operative site and for the administration of anaesthetic agents, the maintenance of the airway, and the correct skeletal alignment. The client should be protected from pressure on nerves and skin over bony prominences. The eyes should be protected. Adequate thoracic excursion should be provided. Arteries and veins should not be occluded. Modesty in exposure of the body should be respected. Any painful area or deformity should be recognized and respected. Client safety is a priority.

Anaesthetics are classified as general, local, conscious sedation, and regional. General anaesthetics provide loss of sensation with loss of consciousness, skeletal muscle relaxation, and analgesia. General anaesthetics can affect somatic, autonomic, and endocrine responses. General anaesthetics are usually given to clients who require significant skeletal muscle relaxation, must be placed in awkward positions, or require extended surgical time. These anaesthetics are also given to clients who are extremely anxious or refuse or have contraindications for a local or regional anaesthetic. General anaesthetics may be inhaled or administered by IV line. IV administration is rapid, quickly inducing a pleasant sleep. Inhalation agents enter the body through the alveoli and are excreted rapidly by ventilation. Complications of inhalation agents include coughing, laryngospasm, bronchospasm, increased secretions, and respiratory depression. Adjuncts to general anaesthetics include opioids, benzodiazepines, and neuromuscular blocking agents.

Local anaesthesia results in a loss of sensation without loss of consciousness. Local anaesthetics can be administered topically, intracutaneously, and subcutaneously. Local anaesthesia produces ANS blockage and skeletal muscle paralysis in the area of the affected nerve. There is little systemic absorption, and recovery tends to be rapid, with little residual "hangover." Possible complications include discomfort, hypotension, and seizures.

Conscious sedation results in a minimally depressed LOC with maintenance of the client's protective airway reflexes. The goal with conscious sedation is to reduce the client's anxiety and discomfort and facilitate co-operation. A sedative–hypnotic and opioid are frequently used with conscious sedation. The client can maintain their own airway and respond to appropriate commands.

Regional anaesthesia results in loss of sensation in a body region without loss of consciousness, when the administration of a local anaesthetic blocks a specific nerve or group of nerves. Spinal anaesthesia and epidural blocks are a form of regional anaesthesia. The client will need to be monitored for ANS blockage, bradycardia, hypotension, nausea, and vomiting.

Other management techniques that may be done during surgery include controlled hypotension, in which the BP is decreased during the administration of the anaesthetic to decrease blood loss during surgery. Hypothermia results from the deliberate lowering of the client's body temperature in order to reduce the demand for oxygen and anaesthesia. Cryoanaesthesia freezes a localized area to block pain impulses. Hypoanaesthesia is hypnosis to alter pain consciousness. Acupuncture decreases sensation to specific areas.

Catastrophic events that may happen in the operating room include anaphylactic reactions, which may be masked by the anaesthesia. Malignant hyperthermia is a rare metabolic disease that can be fatal. Hyperthermia with skeletal muscle rigidity can also occur. This is possibly due to exposure to succinylcholines. Other factors such as trauma, heat, and stress may be triggers of malignant hyperthermia. Some clients have inherited hypermetabolism of the skeletal muscles, resulting in altered control of intracellular calcium.

Manifestations of malignant hyperthermia include the following:

- Tachypnea
- Hypercarbia
- Hyperthermia
- Tachycardia
- Ventricular dysrhythmias, which can result in cardiac arrest and death

Postoperative Care

Care of the client in the postoperative (anaesthesia) care unit (PACU) includes monitoring and managing the following:

- Respiratory and circulatory function
- Pain
- Temperature
- Surgical site
- Airway patency, rate, and quality of respiration, and auscultation of breath sounds in all fields will be assessed.
- Oxygen therapy may be established.
- Cardiac monitoring, including the rate and rhythm of the client's heartbeat, will be compared with preoperative findings.
- BP and temperature will also be compared with the previous baseline.
- Neurological assessment will include LOC, orientation, sensory and motor status, and size and equality of pupils.
- Intake and output will be monitored.
- Surgical sites and the condition of dressings will be noted, with the amount and type of drainage.

Figure 9.12 outlines potential problems in the postoperative period. See Figure 9.13 for an example of airway obstruction.

In order for the client to be discharged from the PACU, the client must be mobile, alert, and able to provide a degree of self-care. Pain, nausea, and vomiting should be controlled. The PACU nurse will give a report to the receiving nurse on the ward that summarizes the operative and postoperative periods. The client will be transferred to the bed, and then an in-depth assessment must be done, postoperative orders will be initiated, and ambulation may be encouraged.

Atelectasis and pneumonia are complications that may occur after abdominal and thoracic surgery (see Figure 9.14 There may be postoperative development of mucous plugs and decreased surfactant related to hypoventilation, a recumbent position, ineffective coughing, or smoking.

To help prevent the development of atelectasis and pneumonia, the nurse will encourage the client to breathe deeply and cough. Other techniques to encourage full lung expansion include the use of incentive spirometry, splints, diaphragmatic breathing, and changing position every 2 hours.

Fluid and electrolyte imbalances may contribute to cardiovascular alterations. Fluid retention in the first 2 to 5 days could occur due to the stress response. Fluid overload may occur when IV fluids are administered too quickly, if chronic disease exists, or if the client is an older person. Fluid deficits may result from inadequate fluid replacement, causing a decreased CO and tissue perfusion. Hypokalemia can result from urinary or GI losses.

The stress response can contribute to an increase in clotting factors, causing DVT or pulmonary emboli. Symptoms of a pulmonary embolus include the following:

- Tachypnea
- Dyspnea

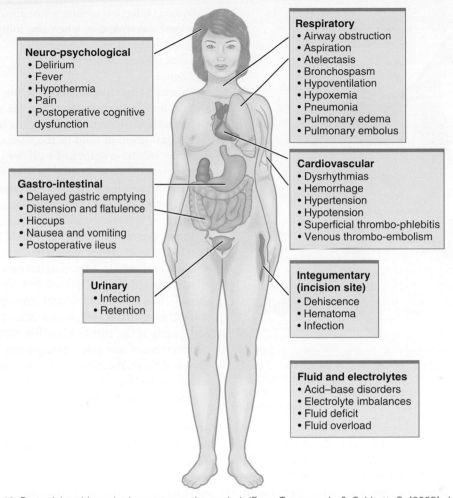

Neuro-psychological
- Delirium
- Fever
- Hypothermia
- Pain
- Postoperative cognitive dysfunction

Respiratory
- Airway obstruction
- Aspiration
- Atelectasis
- Bronchospasm
- Hypoventilation
- Hypoxemia
- Pneumonia
- Pulmonary edema
- Pulmonary embolus

Cardiovascular
- Dysrhythmias
- Hemorrhage
- Hypertension
- Hypotension
- Superficial thrombo-phlebitis
- Venous thrombo-embolism

Gastro-intestinal
- Delayed gastric emptying
- Distension and flatulence
- Hiccups
- Nausea and vomiting
- Postoperative ileus

Urinary
- Infection
- Retention

Integumentary (incision site)
- Dehiscence
- Hematoma
- Infection

Fluid and electrolytes
- Acid–base disorders
- Electrolyte imbalances
- Fluid deficit
- Fluid overload

Fig. 9.12 Potential problems in the postoperative period. (From Tyerman, J., & Cobbett, S. [2023]. *Lewis's medical-surgical nursing in Canada: Assessment and management of clinical problems* [5th Cdn. ed., p. 410, Figure 22-1]. Elsevier.)

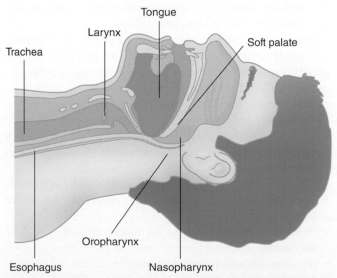

Fig. 9.13 Obstruction of airway by tongue. (From Rothrock, J., & McEwen, D. [2019]. *Alexander's care of the patient in surgery* [16th ed., p. 265, Figure 10.3]. Elsevier.)

- Tachycardia
- Chest pain
- Hypotension
- Dysrhythmias
- Heart failure
- Hemoptysis

Syncope can indicate decreased CO, fluid deficits, or deficits in cerebral perfusion.

Vital signs need to be monitored and compared with the preoperative status. Intake and output need to be assessed accurately. Laboratory work, especially electrolytes, needs to be monitored. Mouth care and leg exercises are also part of postoperative care of the client.

A low urinary output can be expected for the first 24 hours due to an increase in aldosterone and ADH levels in the client's body due to the stress response of surgery, fluid losses during surgery, drainage, and diaphoresis. The anaesthesia may depress the nervous system, allowing the bladder to fill to a greater than normal extent before the urge to void is felt. Anticholinergic and narcotic medications may also interfere with the ability to initiate voiding. Fluid retention is more likely to develop with abdominal or pelvic surgery where pain may alter the perception of a full bladder. The recumbent

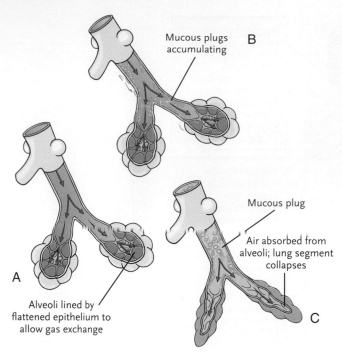

Fig. 9.14 Postoperative atelectasis. **A,** Normal bronchiole and alveoli. **B,** Mucus plug in bronchiole. **C,** Collapse of alveoli due to atelectasis following absorption of air. (From Tyerman, J., & Cobbett, S. [2023]. *Lewis's medical-surgical nursing in Canada: Assessment and management of clinical problems* [5th Cdn. ed., p. 413, Figure 22-4]. Elsevier.)

position may also impair the ability to void. The normal urine output should be at least 0.5 millilitres per kg body weight per hour. This would mean about 30 millilitres per hour for an adult. If the client does not have a catheter, they should be able to void about 200 mL following surgery. To assist the client to void, place the client in the normal voiding position. Use techniques such as running water, pouring water over the perineum, or ambulation or use the bedside commode.

Nausea and vomiting may be caused by anaesthetic agents or narcotics, delayed gastric emptying, slowed peristalsis, or resumption of oral intake too soon after surgery. Abdominal distension results from a decreased peristalsis caused from the handling of the bowel during surgery or by the client swallowing air. Hiccups occur due to irritation of the phrenic nerve. The client will remain NPO until the gag reflex has returned and the client has bowel sounds. Bowel sounds indicate that peristalsis has resumed. Clear fluids are introduced first and advanced fluids added as tolerated. Regular mouth care is essential when the client is NPO. An NG tube may be inserted if the vomiting persists and to help decompress the abdomen. Early ambulation is helpful to prevent abdominal distension.

The surgical incision disrupts the skin barrier, and healing is a major concern during the postoperative period. Adequate nutrition is important to help fight the catabolic effect of the stress response and assist in wound healing. Wound infections may be caused by oral flora, intestinal flora, or exogenous flora on the skin or in the environment. The incidence of wound sepsis is higher in clients who are malnourished, immunosuppressed, older persons, or experiencing a prolonged hospital stay.

Wound infection usually is not apparent until the third to fifth postoperative day, when the following symptoms may appear:

- Local manifestations of redness
- Edema
- Pain and tenderness around the site
- Purulent drainage leaking from the surgical incision
- Systemic manifestations, including leukocytosis and fever

Accumulation of fluid in the wound may impair healing and may require a drain to be placed in the area. The nurse should note the type, amount, colour, and consistency of the drainage. Assessment of position changes on the drainage should also be noted. The physician should be notified of excessive or abnormal drainage.

Postoperative pain may be caused by traumatization of skin and tissues, reflex muscle spasms, and anxiety or fear. Analgesics should be administered on a timely basis to ensure effectiveness during activities and for comfort. The nurse should observe for behavioural clues of pain and ask clients about their pain, as well as assess for the location, intensity, and quality of the client's pain. The nurse should evaluate the effectiveness of any pain management technique that is utilized and notify the physician if alternative pain management orders are needed.

Anxiety and depression may be more pronounced with clients experiencing a poor prognosis. Attention to a history of neurotic or psychotic disorders is important. The client's response may be part of the grief process. Confusion and delirium may result from psychological or physiological sources, including the following:

- Fluid and electrolyte imbalances
- Hypoxemia
- Drug effects
- Sleep deprivation
- Sensory alteration or overload

Delirium tremors may result from alcohol withdrawal. The nurse must provide adequate support for the client. Listen and talk with the client, offer explanations, reassure, and encourage involvement of the significant other.

Planning for discharge begins in the preoperative period. The client is informed and prepared to gradually assume greater responsibility for self-care. The following client teaching topics should be covered:

- Information should be provided regarding care of the wound site and dressing.
- Information should be provided about the action and adverse effects of medications as well as when and how to take medications.
- Dietary restrictions or modifications should be explained.
- Any symptoms that should be reported should be described.
- Where and when to return for follow-up care should be explained.
- Written instructions to help in reinforcement and remembering should be provided to the client.

The nurse should always allow plenty of time for the client to ask questions regarding postoperative care at home.

PRACTICE QUESTIONS

Case 1

Fred Kingsley, a 52-year-old country and western singer, has been diagnosed with vocal cord polyps, requiring surgical laser removal.

Questions 1 to 3 refer to this case.

1. What is the nurse's priority assessment in Mr. Kingsley's immediate postoperative period?
   1. Hemorrhage
   2. Pain
   3. Difficulty swallowing
   4. Oral pharyngeal edema

2. What is the recommended postoperative position for Mr. Kingsley?
   1. Prone with his head on a pillow
   2. Reverse Trendelenburg with the neck extended
   3. Semi-Fowler's with the neck flexed
   4. Supine with his neck hyperextended and supported with a pillow

3. What nursing action can best alleviate Mr. Kingsley's throat discomfort?
   1. Having him drink warm fluids
   2. Giving him ASA (Aspirin)
   3. Giving him acetaminophen (Tylenol) elixir or pills
   4. Placing a heating pad around his throat

Case 2

Consuela Gomez, age 58, moved to Canada from Mexico 10 years ago. For the past few months, she has been experiencing fatigue, cough, and occasional blood-tinged sputum. The nurse administers a Mantoux tuberculin skin test, and Mrs. Gomez returns to the clinic for the test to be read.

Questions 4 to 7 refer to this case.

4. Mrs. Gomez's Mantoux test yields an induration area of 10 mm. What is the most accurate interpretation of a 10-mm result?
   1. Active disease is present.
   2. She has been exposed to *M. tuberculosis* or has been vaccinated with bacille Calmette-Guérin.
   3. The disease is not active, but preventive treatment should be initiated.
   4. The reaction is questionable and should be repeated.

5. Which of the following tests is most reliable to confirm a diagnosis of tuberculosis (TB) for Mrs. Gomez?
   1. A chest X-ray
   2. Acid-fast bacilli in a sputum smear
   3. A nucleic acid amplification test
   4. Second-step Mantoux test with induration of 10 mm or greater

6. Mrs. Gomez is started on a multiple-drug regimen. The nurse teaches Mrs. Gomez about the medications. Which of the following drugs have adverse effects of ototoxicity and nephrotoxicity?
   1. Ethambutol (Myambutol)
   2. Isoniazid (INH)
   3. Rifampin (Rifadin)
   4. Streptomycin (Streptomycin)

7. The nurse discusses with Mrs. Gomez the importance of adherence to her medication regimen. How long will Mrs. Gomez be required to take the pharmacological treatment for TB?
   1. 1–2 months
   2. 3–4 months
   3. 5–6 months
   4. 6–9 months

Case 3

Ms. Juliet Mathias, age 34, has been overweight most of her life. Because she began feeling light-headed and dizzy, she came to the health clinic for a checkup. She was diagnosed with primary hypertension following serial blood pressures of 150/100 mm Hg. The community nurse visits her in her home.

Questions 8 to 10 refer to this case.

8. Which of the following statements about primary hypertension is true?
   1. It requires management by medication therapy.
   2. It has no identifiable cause.
   3. It is related to another underlying condition.
   4. Obesity is not a factor.

9. Ms. Mathias is started on hydrochlorothiazide (HydroDIURIL) by the physician for her hypertension. Which dietary modification, related to the HydroDIURIL, would the nurse teach Ms. Mathias in order to prevent an electrolyte imbalance?
   1. Increase potassium-containing foods.
   2. Decrease sodium-containing foods.
   3. Increase sodium-containing foods.
   4. Decrease potassium-containing foods.

10. The nurse determines that Ms. Mathias's hypertension is not well controlled on the diuretic. She is referred back to the physician, who prescribes a calcium channel blocker. What would be priority teaching for her regarding this medication?
    1. She should watch for decreased urine output.
    2. She may develop hair loss.
    3. She may develop high blood pressure.
    4. She may feel dizzy when she stands quickly.

Case 4

Linda Hynes, age 52, is admitted to the hospital in preparation for surgery for an adrenal tumour that has caused Cushing's syndrome. A health assessment reveals Ms. Hynes to be manifesting truncal obesity, thin arms and legs, a round face, and a "buffalo hump" on her upper back. She is irritable during the assessment and says she just wants to be left alone.

Questions 11 and 12 refer to this case.

11. In addition to the manifestations noted in the initial health assessment, which of the following, observed by the nurse, may be additional manifestations of Cushing's syndrome?
    1. Petechiae and abdominal purplish red striae on the abdomen
    2. Decreased axilla and pubic hair

    3. Tachycardia and bulging eyes
    4. Hypotension and hypoglycemia

12. Later in the day, Ms. Hynes apologizes for her irritability and tells the nurse she just does not like anyone examining her because she looks so bad. Which response by the nurse is most appropriate?
    1. "You really shouldn't worry about how you look. It's what you are on the inside that counts."
    2. "There are some really good ways to dress so that the changes wouldn't seem so noticeable."
    3. "You are going to look much better right after your surgery."
    4. "Most of the physical and mental changes caused by the disease will gradually improve after your surgery."

Case 5

Brian Wilson, a 17-year-old student, sustains a mandibular fracture while playing rugby. There was no loss of teeth. His treatment includes intermaxillary fixation surgery.

Questions 13 to 15 refer to this case.

13. Postoperatively, how should the nurse position Brian?
    1. Prone to facilitate lung expansion
    2. On his side with his head slightly elevated to prevent aspiration
    3. Supine with his head to the side to promote the drainage of secretions
    4. Slight Trendelenburg to prevent aspiration of fluids

14. What is the most important postoperative goal for Brian?
    1. Adequate nutrition
    2. Jaw immobilization
    3. Oral hygiene
    4. Patent airway

15. Which of the following is the most important to be available at Brian's bedside?
    1. Nasogastric suction tube
    2. Nasopharyngeal suction catheter
    3. Wire cutter
    4. Oxygen cannula

Case 6

Mrs. Cheng, age 78 years, fell on the ice and injured her hip. She was transported to the nearest emergency department, where a fractured hip was diagnosed.

Questions 16 and 17 refer to this case.

16. Mrs. Cheng is on bed rest with immobilization of her hip while she is waiting for an operating room to be available for surgery later in the day. What assistive device will the nurse provide for Mrs. Cheng?
    1. A urinary catheter, as a bedpan may not be used
    2. A trapeze to facilitate lifting movement
    3. Side rails in the "up" position for Mrs. Cheng to use for moving herself
    4. A "geri-chair" so Mrs. Cheng may sit up for meals

17. It is determined that Mrs. Cheng has osteoporosis. Prior to discharge from rehabilitation, the nurse discusses measures to prevent further fractures. Which of the following would be important to discuss with Mrs. Cheng?

    1. Calcium supplements and prescribed bisphosphonate medication
    2. Incorporating non–weight-bearing exercise into her daily routine when allowed by the physician
    3. Vitamin D, 200 international units (IU)
    4. Planning for a move from her residential home to an assisted living facility

Case 7

The nurse in a walk-in, ambulatory clinic assesses Sandra Procinski, 33 years old. Ms. Procinski states she experienced a sore throat about a week ago but has not had any problems until today. This morning she awoke to find her face swollen, particularly around her eyes. She also has noted that her urine appears foamy.

Questions 18 and 19 refer to this case.

18. The nurse suspects that Ms. Procinski is manifesting symptoms of which of the following?
    1. Urinary tract infection
    2. Pyelonephritis
    3. Nephrotic syndrome
    4. Acute glomerulonephritis

19. What is the likely initial treatment for Ms. Procinski?
    1. A diet low in potassium
    2. Rest
    3. Antihypertensives
    4. Antibiotics

Case 8

Bernard Cowler, 36, was admitted to hospital with a diagnosis of pulmonary embolism.

Questions 20 and 21 refer to this case.

20. Mr. Cowler is started on heparin (Hepalean) therapy. What blood test result does the nurse need to monitor closely?
    1. International normalized ratio (INR)
    2. Partial thromboplastin time (PTT)
    3. Platelet function assay (PFA)
    4. Prothrombin time (PT)

21. Several days later, the nurse transcribes a physician order for Mr. Cowler: "Discontinue heparin, start warfarin (Coumadin) at 5 mg OD each morning." What action should the nurse take?
    1. Stop the heparin and notify the pharmacy to prepare Coumadin for Mr. Cowler.
    2. Stop the heparin and give Mr. Cowler his first dose of Coumadin.
    3. Question the doctor regarding the dose of Coumadin.
    4. Question the doctor about discontinuing heparin before therapeutic levels of Coumadin are reached.

Case 9

The nurse interviews Arnold Hampton, age 69 years, at the clinic. He states he has been experiencing muscle cramps in his legs that are getting worse, and he is not able to walk as much as he once did. He tells the nurse the pain gets better when he sits but starts again shortly after he gets up and begins walking.

Questions 22 to 24 refer to this case.

22. When performing the physical assessment on Mr. Hampton, the nurse instructs him to abduct his leg. What does *abduction* mean?
    1. Movement of part toward midline of body
    2. Movement of part away from midline of body
    3. Rotating the joint outward
    4. Rotating the joint inward

23. The nurse and physician suspect Mr. Hampton may have peripheral arterial disease (PAD). What assessment would the nurse perform with a client with presumed PAD?
    1. Assess for diminished or absent pulses in the extremities.
    2. Assess for pallor or blanching of the foot when in a dependent position.
    3. Assess for lower leg edema.
    4. Assess blood pressure in both thighs.

24. What self-care activities would the nurse suggest to Mr. Hampton?
    1. Use a heating pad to help him become comfortable while resting.
    2. Purchase support stockings to wear daily.
    3. Walk at least 30 minutes a day.
    4. Inspect his feet for redness once a week.

Case 10

Sarah Sawchuk is an 18-year-old female who is admitted to the hospital with severe diarrhea, anorexia, weight loss, and abdominal cramps. She is diagnosed with ulcerative colitis.

Questions 25–27 refer to this case.

25. What symptoms of fluid and electrolyte imbalance caused by ulcerative colitis should the nurse report immediately?
    1. Thirst and dry, sticky mucous membranes
    2. Extreme muscle weakness and tachycardia
    3. Development of tetany and muscle spasms
    4. Numbness and tingling of fingers, mouth, and toes

26. Ms. Sawchuk's condition deteriorates, and she requires an ileostomy. What would her postoperative care include?
    1. Removing rectal packing 4 hours after surgery
    2. Continuous, slow feedings via nasogastric tube
    3. Monitoring intake and output accurately
    4. Removing the nasogastric tube on arrival at the unit

27. The nurse teaches Ms. Sawchuk about nutrition related to her ileostomy. Which of the following foods may cause an obstruction and should be avoided by Ms. Sawchuk?
    1. Raw fruits and vegetables
    2. Beans and legumes
    3. Eggs
    4. Cheese

Case 11

Mrs. Edna O'Brien, age 90 years, lives in a retirement home. Although she is generally healthy, she has bilateral cataracts that she has been reluctant to have treated. Mrs. O'Brien is presently almost totally blind.

Questions 28–29 refer to this case.

28. The nurse instructs the dietary aide in assisting Mrs. O'Brien with her meals. What direction might the nurse give to the aide?
    1. Do not give Mrs. O'Brien sharp utensils.
    2. Provide Mrs. O'Brien with finger foods that she can feel and pick up easily.
    3. Help Mrs. O'Brien locate the food on her plate by comparing it to a clock; for example, say, "The toast is at nine o'clock."
    4. Stay with Mrs. O'Brien throughout the meal and feed her when necessary.

29. Mrs. O'Brien consents to have her cataracts treated. At a local clinic, she has an initial right cataract extraction with intraocular lens implant and is discharged the same day. What discharge instructions would the nurse provide to Mrs. O'Brien?
    1. "I will give you a stool softener to prevent constipation."
    2. "You need to drink at least six glasses of water or fluids this evening."
    3. "You will not be allowed to bathe until you return to see the doctor in 2 days."
    4. "You are allowed to watch TV, but you should not read for the next 48 hours."

Case 12

Mrs. Gardner, age 84, was diagnosed with heart failure 2 years ago. She has been a pack-a-day cigarette smoker for over 50 years. She has never had a myocardial infarction. Mrs. Gardner has been admitted to her local hospital with severe shortness of breath and only able to speak in one-word sentences. She is pale, diaphoretic, and cool to the touch. Her pulse is rapid and irregular.

Questions 30 to 33 refer to this case.

30. What position should the nurse encourage Mrs. Gardner to assume while being treated for the shortness of breath?
    1. Prone, to allow her to rest more effectively
    2. Semi-Fowler's, to allow her to breathe more easily
    3. Trendelenburg, to encourage drainage of fluids from the upper respiratory airway
    4. High Fowler's with legs down, to decrease preload

31. Mrs. Gardner is given furosemide (Lasix) to initiate urinary output. When she starts to void, what is the priority assessment?
    1. Electrolyte levels
    2. Blood pressure
    3. Hourly output
    4. Respiratory rate

32. It is determined that Mrs. Gardner has left-sided heart failure. Which of the following would the nurse assess for in Mrs. Gardner?
    1. Pitting edema
    2. Jugular venous distension
    3. Hepatomegaly
    4. Lung crackles

33. During Mrs. Gardner's hospitalization, blood work showed elevated BUN and creatinine levels, with reduced creatinine clearance. Chronic renal failure was diagnosed, and she was placed on a renal diet. The nurse should teach Mrs. Gardner to avoid which of the following foods?
    1. Red meat and shellfish
    2. Potatoes and citrus fruit
    3. Cookies and cake
    4. Lean meat and chicken

Independent Questions

Questions 34 to 60 do not refer to a particular case.

34. Positioning of clients to maintain correct body alignment is essential to prevent which of the following complications? **Select all that apply.**
    1. Thrombus
    2. Pressure injury
    3. Kyphosis
    4. Contractures
    5. Incontinence

35. A client has a history of hypertension and has been admitted to hospital with a myocardial infarction (MI). What laboratory tests will confirm the diagnosis of MI?
    1. PT, PTT, INR
    2. Troponin, CK-MB, LDH
    3. Na$^+$, K$^+$, CK-BB
    4. BUN, Cr, CK-MM

36. A nurse is at a pool where a swimmer dives into the shallow end of the pool and sustains a high neck fracture and spinal cord injury. The nurse suspects a C2-level injury. What priority first aid measure will the nurse likely need to provide until paramedics arrive?
    1. Immobilize the client on a firm board, such as a Styrofoam "flutter board."
    2. Fashion a roll out of clothes to stabilize the neck.
    3. Maintain the client in the pool without attempting to lift them out.
    4. Provide rescue breathing.

37. A 16-year-old client diagnosed with asthma has been prescribed salbutamol (Ventolin) and beclomethasone (Beclovent) metered-dose inhalers. The client asks the nurse why they need to take these medications. What is the nurse's most appropriate response?
    1. "The Beclovent is a steroid, and the Ventolin is a bronchodilator."
    2. "You take both of these so that you don't have another asthma attack."
    3. "The Ventolin opens your airways, and the Beclovent decreases the swelling, so together they stabilize your asthma."
    4. "You must be careful to take both of these inhalers exactly as they are prescribed to prevent another attack."

38. What would be the most helpful approach by the nurse when meeting with a client who has just received a diagnosis of Parkinson's disease from the physician?
    1. "I am really sorry about your diagnosis, but the medications can keep you stable for a long time."
    2. "What did the physician explain to you about your diagnosis of Parkinson's disease?"
    3. "There is a lot of research about Parkinson's disease these days, so many new treatments may be available."
    4. "I understand that you are upset by this very bad diagnosis. I will sit here with you for a while."

39. A client has a hemoglobin of 100 gl/L. What will be the most likely manifestations of their condition? **Select all that apply.**
    1. Fatigue
    2. Bradycardia
    3. Yellow sclera
    4. Palpitations
    5. Headache

40. A client has experienced several weeks of diarrhea as a result of a viral gastroenteritis. The client is at risk of being deficient in which of the following due to the diarrhea?
    1. Magnesium
    2. Calcium
    3. Potassium
    4. Sodium

41. Which of the following information should the nurse include when teaching a client with a newly diagnosed gastroesophageal reflux disease (GERD)? **Select all that apply.**
    1. "Peppermint tea may be helpful in reducing your symptoms."
    2. "You should avoid eating between meals to reduce acid secretion."
    3. "You might try an antacid preparation to soothe the heartburn."
    4. "It will be helpful to keep the head of your bed elevated on blocks."
    5. "Vigorous physical activities may increase the incidence of reflux."

42. A client with a history of peptic ulcer disease is unable to be discharged from the surgical unit after a hip replacement because of a sudden onset of frank gastric bleeding. What priority intervention should the nurse anticipate?
    1. Sengesten-Blakemore tube insertion
    2. An intravenous bolus of normal saline
    3. Insertion of a nasogastric tube and saline lavage
    4. Administration of oxygen

43. Which of the following actions should the nurse implement when initiating the initial plan of care for a client admitted with acute diverticulitis? **Select all that apply.**
    1. Give stool softeners.
    2. Administer IV fluids.
    3. Order a diet high in fibre and fluids.
    4. Place the client on NPO status.
    5. Prepare the client for colonoscopy.

44. The nurse is admitting a client for evaluation of right lower quadrant abdominal pain with nausea and vomiting and an O_2 saturation of 90%. Which of the following actions should the nurse take? **Select all that apply.**
    1. Place the client on NPO status.
    2. Assist the client to cough and deep breathe.
    3. Administer oxygen via nasal cannula.
    4. Encourage the client to take sips of clear liquids.
    5. Check for rebound tenderness.

45. In a client with viral hepatitis, the nurse should closely monitor for indications of which of the following abnormal laboratory values? **Select all that apply.**
    1. Decreased vitamins C and E
    2. Decreased serum albumin
    3. Prolonged prothrombin time
    4. Decreased calcium
    5. Elevated serum potassium

46. During recovery from hepatic coma, a high-fibre diet is recommended. What is the primary rationale for recommending this diet?
    1. To prevent dyslipidemia
    2. To prevent diarrhea
    3. To decrease hypokalemia
    4. To decrease serum ammonia

47. A client has radical neck surgery for cancer of the larynx. Which of the following is the most important assessment postsurgery?
    1. Pain
    2. Temperature of 38°C
    3. Stridor
    4. Serosanguinous oozing from the operative site

48. A client has primary adrenal insufficiency (Addison's disease). The nurse assessing the client should anticipate which of the following manifestations? **Select all that apply.**
    1. Bronze pigmentation
    2. Moon face
    3. Hypotension
    4. Buffalo hump
    5. Exophthalmos

49. Which of the following is descriptive of cluster headaches?
    1. Constant, squeezing tightness at the base of the skull
    2. A severe throbbing headache often associated with photophobia, nausea and vomiting
    3. Palpable neck and shoulder muscles, stiff neck, and tenderness
    4. Severe "bone-crushing" pain radiating up and down from one eye

50. The nurse is helping the client prepare for surgery. The client has removed their jewellery and glasses. Which action should the nurse take to keep the jewellery safe?
    1. Put these items in the client's bedside stand.
    2. Inventory the items and give them to the family or caregiver.
    3. Place the items in a plastic bag and send them to the operating room with the client.
    4. Keep these items at the nursing station until the client returns.

51. The nurse is teaching a client about avoiding the recurrence of a urinary tract infection. Which of the following information should be included in the teaching plan? **Select all that apply.**
    1. Teach the client to wipe from back to front after voiding.
    2. Suggest the use of a diaphragm during intercourse.
    3. Advise the client to report cloudy urine.
    4. Advise the client to include high-fibre foods in their diet to avoid constipation.
    5. Advise the client to urinate every 2-4 hours during the day.

52. The nurse is providing foot care instructions to a client. Based on the information provided, what will the nurse include in the client teaching?

Client profile	Type 2 diabetes mellitus Peripheral arterial disease
Neurological assessment	Absent pain and touch sensation soles of feet Decreased touch sensation lower legs
Vision assessment	Vision both eyes 20/200

    1. Choose flat-soled leather shoes.
    2. Soak the feet in warm water for an hour every day.
    3. Examine feet daily in well-lit room owing to poor eyesight.
    4. Buy callus remover for corns or calluses.

53. The clinic nurse performs a physical examination on an older person. What assessment data would support the diagnosis of abdominal aortic aneurysm (AAA)? **Select all that apply.**
    1. Epigastric discomfort
    2. Pyrosis
    3. Abdominal bruit
    4. Tearing abdominal pain
    5. Periumbilical pulsating mass

54. An older person is admitted to hospital from a long-term care facility because of extreme lethargy. The client's hematocrit is 54% and sodium is 120 mmol/L. Which intervention should the nurse anticipate?
    1. Pushing oral fluids
    2. Establishing an intravenous (IV) line of 10% dextrose solution
    3. Starting an IV line of normal saline (0.9% NaCl)
    4. Inserting a nasogastric tube for enteral feeding

55. The client spends most of their working day in the sun. The nurse performs a skin assessment. What type of skin cancer is the client most at risk for?
    1. Adenocarcinoma
    2. Basal cell carcinoma
    3. Malignant melanoma
    4. Spongioblastoma

56. Which of the following are characteristics of delirium? **Select all that apply.**
    1. Develops over a short period of time
    2. Presence of apraxia

3. Memory impairment or deficits
4. Occurs as a result of a medical condition, such as systemic infection
5. Presence of agnosia

57. The client, age 92, has osteoporosis. The client is generally well but uses a walker frame to assist with mobility. What activity would the nurse recommend to improve the osteoporosis?
    1. Swimming
    2. Walking
    3. Aerobics
    4. Range-of-motion exercises

58. A client is diagnosed with multiple sclerosis. What manifestations is the client likely to have initially experienced?
    1. Sensory disturbances that include blurred vision and tinnitus
    2. Bradykinesia, rigid muscle tone, tremors, and impaired postural reflexes

3. Fluctuating weakness of certain skeletal muscle groups
4. Unpleasant motor and sensory abnormalities (paraesthesias)

59. Six hours following a transurethral resection of the prostate (TURP), a client experiences abdominal pain and bladder distension. What action will the nurse implement?
    1. Pain assessment
    2. Flushing of the continuous bladder irrigation catheter
    3. Decreasing the flow rate in the bladder irrigation
    4. Notifying the physician

60. Which of the following are high potassium-containing foods? **Select all that apply.**
    1. Oranges
    2. Potatoes
    3. Spinach
    4. Pasta
    5. Corn

REFERENCES

Astle, B., & Duggleby, W. (2024). *Potter and Perry's Canadian fundamentals of nursing* (7th ed.). Elsevier.

Black, J. M., & Hawks, J. H. (2009). *Medical-surgical nursing: Clinical management for positive outcomes* (8th ed.). Saunders.

Colorectal Cancer Canada. (2021). *Cancer prevention: Colorectal cancer screening.* https://www.colorectalcancercanada.com/prevention/screening/

Dames, S., Luctkar-Flude, M., & Tyerman, J. (2021). *Edelman and Kudzma's Canadian health promotion throughout the life span* (1st ed.). Elsevier.

Day, R. A., Paul, P., Williams, B., et al. (2016). *Brunner & Suddarth's textbook of medical-surgical nursing* (3rd ed.). Williams & Wilkins.

deWit, S. C., Stromberg, H., & Dallred, C. (2017). *Medical-surgical nursing: Concepts and practices* (3rd ed.). Elsevier.

Fournier, B., & Karachiwalla, F. (2021). *Shah's public health and preventive health care in Canada* (6th ed.). Elsevier Inc.

Huether, S., Power-Kean, K., El-Hussein, M. T., et al. (2018). *Understanding pathophysiology* (Cdn. ed.). Elsevier.

Ignatavicius, D. D., Workman, M. L., & Rebar, C. (2018). *Medical-surgical nursing: Concepts for interprofessional collaborative care* (9th ed.). Elsevier.

Lewis, S. M., Bucher, L., Heitkemper, M. M., et al. (2019). *Medical-surgical nursing in Canada: Assessment and management of clinical problems* (4th ed.). Elsevier Canada.

Rothrock, J., & McEwen, D. (2019). *Alexander's care of the patient in surgery* (16th ed.). Elsevier.

Tyerman, J., & Cobbett, S. (2023). *Lewis's medical-surgical nursing in Canada: Assessment and management of clinical problems* (5th ed.). Elsevier.

World Health Organization. (2007). *WHO case definitions of HIV for surveillance and revised clinical staging and immunological classification of HIV-related disease in adults and children.* https://apps.who.int/iris/bitstream/handle/10665/43699/9789241595629_eng.pdf

BIBLIOGRAPHY

Hockenberry, M., Rodgers, C., & Wilson, D. (2022). *Wong's essentials of pediatric nursing* (11th ed.). Elsevier.

Sealock, K., Seneviratne, C., Lillye, L. L., & Snyder, J. S. (2021). *Lilley's pharmacology for Canadian health care practice* (4th ed.). Elsevier.

WEBSITES

- **Health Finder.gov** (https://www.healthfinder.gov/): This US Department of Health and Human Services site includes a health library that has information on a wide variety of topics and a search engine on health topics. It also provides access to DrugDigest, a medication database that provides a wealth of information (including interactions) on medications, vitamins, and herbs.

- **National Center for Complementary and Integrative Medicine**(https://nccih.nih.gov/health/integrative-health): This US National Institutes of Health site offers comprehensive health information on a variety of herbs and other dietary supplements. It also includes information on alternative treatment modalities, such as acupuncture and relaxation techniques.

- **Public Health Agency of Canada** (https://www.canada.ca/en/public-health.html): This federal government site provides many resources on health promotion and health prevention. It includes information on diseases and conditions, immunization and vaccines, and drug and health products.

Maternal–Newborn Nursing

Pregnancy and childbirth are profound, life-changing events. Factors influencing the client's health and well-being include life experiences, beliefs, and culture; and the diverse Canadian society in which they live. Family-centred maternal–newborn nursing reflects an evidence-informed practice that respects pregnancy and childbirth as a normal physiological event unique to each client and their family.

This approach also acknowledges the complexity of the childbirth experience and the potential for health and social complications. Nurses respond by providing care through a collaborative relationship that is founded on respect and adaptation to the varied and changing needs of the family.

WELL-CLIENT CARE: HEALTH IN THE CHILD-BEARING YEARS

Although the child-bearing years begin with the onset of puberty and sexual maturation, a female's lifetime supply of immature eggs is present in the ovaries at the time of their own birth. Puberty and menarche represent not only a time of rapid and multiple physical changes but also psychological and social development. Throughout the child-bearing years, many health, societal, and personal issues will influence the person's decisions regarding sexual and reproductive choices and the lifestyle they choose to live.

Puberty

Physical sexual maturity and reproductive potential begin when the primary and secondary sexual characteristics develop during puberty in response to neuroendocrine hormonal changes. The timing of puberty varies widely, beginning about 2 years earlier for girls than for boys. For both, puberty is usually completed by the mid- to late teens. The psychological and cognitive developmental stages of adolescence also greatly affect an individual's identity and relationships with peers and family.

Female Manifestations

Between the ages of 8 and 14, the maturing brain begins to produce and secrete hormones that stimulate the ovaries and uterus of the young female to mature in preparation for potential pregnancy. Growth hormones are also produced, which, over 3 to 4 years, bring about the characteristic physical changes in appearance and size that announce the transition from childhood into adolescence and early adulthood. These changes include the following:

- Reproductive changes: The uterus, ovaries, and vagina increase in size and blood supply, and hormones stimulate maturation of an ovum each month at the time of menarche. Menstruation may be irregular for the first year or two, and the first few menstrual cycles may be anovulatory (infertile). Ovulation marks the onset of fertility.
- The development of secondary sexual characteristics: Growth of pubic, leg, and axillae hair; breast development and growth; subcutaneous fat stores with characteristic curves and softness to body shape; sweat gland activity increases; and facial acne may develop.
- Skeletal changes: The pelvis widens, and there is sudden skeletal growth, with adult height typically reached at 2 to 2½ years after menarche.

Male Manifestations

Between the ages of 9.5 and 14, the maturing brain stimulates a marked increase in the production of androgens, the male sex hormones, especially testosterone. In males, this stimulates the following changes:

- Reproductive changes: Testosterone stimulates sexual interest, the production of sperm, and the growth and maturation of the penis, scrotum, testes, prostate gland, and seminal vesicles. Onset of fertility begins with ejaculation of mature sperm and continues throughout life, with new sperm formed about every 10 weeks.
- The development of secondary sex characteristics: Increased body hair on the face, chest, axillae, and pubic area; thickening of the vocal cords and deepening of the voice; enlargement and thickening of the muscles; and increased sebaceous gland activity and acne formation take place.
- Skeletal and other physical changes: Rapid growth takes place in skeletal bones, including length and density, that continues until almost 18 or 20 years of age; widening of the shoulders, increased cellular metabolism, and increased red blood cell (RBC) production also takes place.

Nursing Considerations

There are many important nursing considerations regarding these developmental stages. These considerations include the following:

- Provide factual, nonjudgemental information.
- Be aware that teenagers may obtain inaccurate information from peers and be reluctant to discuss their concerns with adults.

- Recognize that both females and males may have body-image conflicts as they naturally gain weight and experience body changes.
- Offer reassurance and clarification of normal variations in puberty changes.

Chapter 11 has more detailed information on adolescent growth and development.

The Menstrual Cycle

The menstruating person's reproductive cycle begins at puberty and ends at menopause. It is composed of the ovarian and endometrial cycles or phases, which are influenced by hormones released by the brain. All work in unison in preparation for a potential pregnancy. If pregnancy does not occur, hormone levels decrease, menstruation occurs, and the cycle repeats. A cycle typically lasts 28 days, plus or minus 5 days, but may vary and last as long as 38 days. See Figure 10.1 for an illustration of the menstrual cycle.

The Ovarian Cycle

Follicular phase. The follicular phase of the cycle occurs in the following sequence:
- The follicular phase occurs in the first half of the cycle, approximately 14 days prior to ovulation. In menstruating persons who experience irregular menstrual cycles, the follicular phase varies in length.
- The anterior pituitary gland in the brain releases follicle-stimulating hormone (FSH) and luteinizing hormone (LH). FSH stimulates the ovarian follicle, and the immature oocyte grows. As the follicle matures, it releases estrogen. LH stimulates the final maturation of the follicle just prior to ovulation. A mature graafian follicle develops by the midpoint of the cycle under the influence of both FSH and LH.
- Under the influence of progesterone, body temperature increases 0.3°C to 0.6°C for 24 to 48 hours after the time of ovulation and remains elevated until menstruation begins.
- Ovulation usually occurs on day 14, or the midpoint, of the cycle; the follicle ruptures, and the mature ovum is released.

Luteal phase. The luteal phase of the cycle occurs in the following sequence:
- The luteal phase begins when the ovum leaves the follicle, which occurs between day 15 and day 28 of a 28-day cycle.
- LH influences the development of the corpus luteum from the ruptured follicle. As it reaches a peak, estrogen levels drop, and progesterone secretion begins.
- When fertilization occurs, the corpus luteum is maintained until weeks 10 to 12 of the pregnancy; it secretes human chorionic gonadotropin (HCG), estrogen, and progesterone to maintain the pregnancy until the placenta is mature.
- If fertilization does not occur, the corpus luteum degenerates, causing a decrease in estrogen and progesterone hormone levels, and menstruation follows by day 28 of the cycle.

The Endometrial Cycle

Menstrual phase. The menstrual phase of the cycle occurs in the following sequence:
- The menstrual phase occurs during days 1 to 5, when estrogen and progesterone levels are low.
- Menstrual discharge or uterine blood loss is dark red and may contain small clots.

Proliferative phase. The proliferative phase of the cycle occurs in the following sequence:
- On days 7 to 14, the proliferative phase of the endometrium corresponds to the follicular phase of the ovary.
- Estrogen causes the endometrial lining of the uterus to thicken in anticipation of the implantation of a fertilized ovum, and the cervical mucus becomes more hospitable to sperm: clear, thin, elastic, and alkaline.
- Mittelschmerz (midcycle abdominal pain), midcycle spotting, or both may occur as the ovum is released from the follicle at the time of ovulation.

Secretory phase. The secretory phase of the cycle occurs in the following sequence:
- The secretory phase occurs on days 15 to 26, corresponding to the luteal phase of the ovary.
- Estrogen decreases as progesterone levels remain high and the vascularity of the endometrium and uterus increases. If fertilization and implantation occur, the endometrium remains thickened and continues to develop.

Ischemic phase. The ischemic phase of the cycle occurs in the following sequence:
- On days 27 to 28, if fertilization does not occur, the corpus luteum degenerates, and estrogen and progesterone levels fall. The endometrium becomes ischemic and pale as the vasculature constricts.

Nursing Considerations

It is important to be aware of and sensitive to religious and cultural beliefs that may affect practices and behaviours at the time of menstruation.

Client teaching points about the menstrual cycle include the following:
- Basal body temperature and cervical mucus changes may be used to predict ovulation.
- Super-absorbent tampons should be used with caution; they are associated with the rare but serious condition of toxic shock syndrome.
- The best time for performing (and teaching) breast self-examination is following the menstrual phase, when hormonal levels are lowest.

CANADIAN FAMILIES

Maternal–newborn nursing focuses on a family-centred approach. It is important for nurses to recognize and respect the diversity of family structures found within their communities and professional practices. The Vanier Institute (2022) defines the concept of *family* as a combination of two or more persons who are bound together over time by ties of

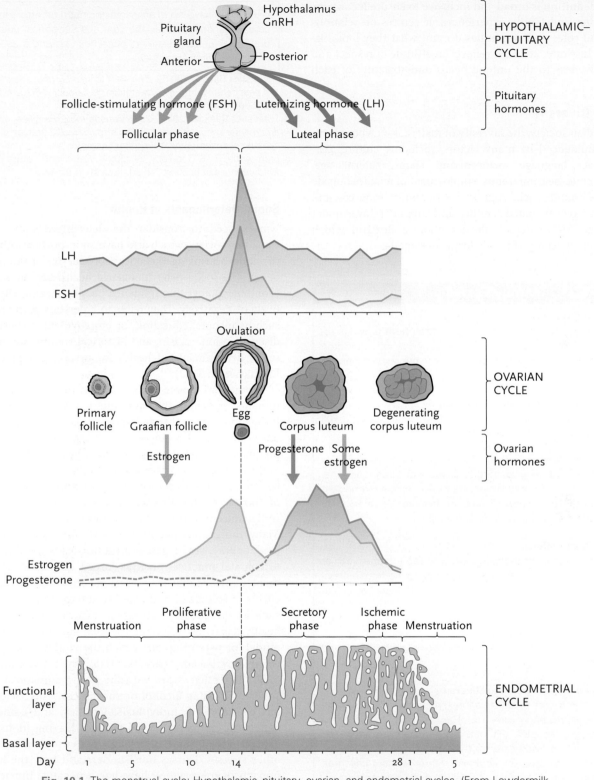

Fig. 10.1 The menstrual cycle: Hypothalamic–pituitary, ovarian, and endometrial cycles. (From Lowdermilk, D. L., Perry, S. E., Cashion, K., et al. [2020]. *Maternity & women's health care* [12th ed., p. 54, Figure 4-7]. Elsevier.)

mutual consent, birth, adoption, or placement and who, together, deliver some of the following:

- Physical care and maintenance of group members
- Addition of new members through procreation or adoption

- Socialization of children
- Social control of members
- Production, consumption, and distribution of goods and services
- Affective nurturance—love

The definition is broad and inclusive to ensure it contains all families and family experiences. It centres on relationships and roles—what families do, not what they look like (Vanier Institute, 2022). It reflects an attitude of respect and responsiveness to the unique needs and structure of each family.

Family Diversity

In Canadian society, the diversity of maternal–newborn families is influenced by many factors, including culture, ethnicity, race, language, socioeconomic status, maternal age, delayed child-bearing trends, employment of females outside the family home, social supports, community resources, and isolation from extended families and support (Government of Canada, 2021a). Refer to the definitions in Box 10.1, which capture the diversity of family forms in Canada.

BOX 10.1　Family Forms

Blended Family
Formed when both parents bring children from previous relationships into a new, joint living situation or when children from the current union and children from previous unions are living together.

Extended or Multigenerational Family
Includes the nuclear family and other relatives (perhaps grandparents, aunts, uncles, cousins).

Lone-Parent Family
Consists of one parent and one or more children. The lone-parent family is formed when one parent leaves the nuclear family because of death, divorce, or desertion or when a single person decides to have or adopt a child.

Same-Sex Family
Consist of people of the same sex who live together with or without children. The children may be offspring from a previous heterosexual marriage or through therapeutic insemination or be adopted children.

Traditional Nuclear Family
Consists of a mother and father (married or common-law) and their children.

Family Forms—Increasing Diversity
Family forms and family relationships within Canada have become increasingly diverse. They include married and common-law couples without children, families in which grandparents provide care for their grandchildren, adults living alone, and same-sex couples (with or without children). The proportion of traditional families (two married parents and children living together) in Canada is declining, while the proportion of common-law and lone-parent families is increasing. Today, the average Canadian household consists of 2.5 people, and for the first time in 2011, there were more one-person households (27.6%) (a number now totaling 28.2%, based on the 2016 Census*) than couple households with children (26.5%).[†] These changes hold significant societal implications. For instance, smaller families and more people living alone have led to an increasing need for affordable child care in Canada. Further, the care and support of young children or older Canadians is now spread among a decreasing number of family members.

* Statistics Canada. (2018). *The shift to smaller households over the past century.* http://www.statcan.gc.ca/pub/11-630-x/11-630-x2015008-eng.htm
[†] Statistics Canada. (2017). *2016 Census topic: Families, households and marital status* (Revised 2021). http://www12.statcan.gc.ca/census-recensement/2016/rt-td/fam-eng.cfm
From Astle, B., & Duggleby, W. (2024). *Potter and Perry's Canadian fundamentals of nursing*, 7th ed., Box 20.1. Elsevier.

Social Determinants of Health

Nurses need to consider the determinants of health in Canadian society, which also have an important influence on the child-bearing aged client's reproductive health and well-being. The social determinants of health are the social and economic factors that influence people's health, either positively or negatively. They relate to a person's place in society, such as income, education, or employment. Experiences of discrimination, racism, and historical trauma are important social determinants of health for certain groups (Keenan-Lindsay et al., 2022).

Indigenous people in Canada may be impacted by determinants of health that are different from those of non-Indigenous people. Indigenous families living in poverty have poorer health outcomes and a greater risk of adverse pregnancy and poor infant and child health outcomes. Some of these health disparities are due to lack of access to quality health care resulting from living in remote areas and lack of Indigenous health care providers who understand the Indigenous traditions that promote health and wellness. Many Indigenous people have lost their identity to their land, culture, languages, and traditional ways of life, owing to colonial practices such as forced relocation and placement in residential schools (Keenan-Lindsay, 2020). The effects of colonization that led to intergenerational trauma, such as the abuse of children, creates a vicious cycle in health disparities. The abuse by their caregivers was the role model for parenting, one which the victims often repeated when they became parents. Also, when the children got older, they often coped with the post-traumatic stress they suffered by using alcohol or substances. This vicious cycle has continued as individuals, families, and communities cope with intergenerational trauma, leaving its impact on generations of families through parenting difficulties and other stresses. Nurses must understand how the historical impacts of colonization have had a negative impact on the health of Indigenous peoples. Health care providers must be knowledgeable of Indigenous health, Indigenous views of health and illness, and Indigenous healing practices in order to provide care in a culturally safe manner (Keenan-Lindsay et al., 2022).

With the availability of alternate methods of conception, nurses need to have a strong perception of lesbian, gay, bisexual, transgender, queer, two-spirited (2SLGBTQI+)

couples' needs and explore ways to make the birthing experience more positive throughout the pregnancy (preconception, pregnancy, and postpartum) (Dames et al., 2021). It is important that nurses provide care in a culturally safe manner for 2SLGBTQI+ clients and their partners. Health care can be seen as heteronormative, a view holding that the normal expression of sexuality is only between individuals of the opposite sex. This attitude does not facilitate appropriate care for 2SLGBTQI+ clients. Asking about clients' partners and not assuming heterosexuality are important in this context. Some 2SLGBTQI+ people may be reluctant to access and use the health care system because they feel they may experience discrimination (Keenan-Lindsay, 2020).

Principles of Providing Family-Centred Maternity and Newborn Care in Canada

The family-centred maternity and newborn care (FCMNC) guiding principles provide direction to ensure safe, skilled, and individualized care. FCMNC addresses the physical, emotional, psychosocial, and spiritual needs of child-bearing parents, the newborn, and the family. FCMNC considers pregnancy and birth to be normal, healthy life events and recognizes the significance of family support, participation, and informed choice.

The Public Health Agency of Canada's principles of FCMNC (Government of Canada, 2021a) include the following:

- A family-centred approach to maternal and newborn care is optimal.
- Pregnancy and birth are normal, healthy processes.
- Early parent-infant attachment is critical for newborn and child development and the growth of healthy families.
- Family-centred maternal and newborn care applies to all care environments.
- Family-centred maternal and newborn care is informed by research evidence.
- Family-centred maternal and newborn care requires a holistic approach.
- Family-centred maternal and newborn care involves collaboration among care providers.
- Culturally appropriate care is important in a multicultural society.
- Indigenous peoples have distinctive needs during pregnancy and birth.
- Care as close to home as possible is ideal.
- Individualized maternal and newborn care is recommended.
- To make informed choices, the child-bearing person and their families require knowledge about their care.
- Child-bearing clients and their families play an integral role in decision-making.
- The attitudes and language of health care providers have an impact on a family's experience of maternal and newborn care.
- Family-centred maternal and newborn care respects reproductive rights.

FAMILY COMPOSITION AND CHILDBIRTH TRENDS

National and regional trends in family composition and childbirth practices are relevant to maternal–newborn nursing as they influence the required resources, choices, needs, and even expectations of the client and their families. The health care system and nurses who provide direct care must recognize and respond to the many significant changes taking place in Canadian families.

Changes in Canadian Families
Factors Influencing Canadian Families

- A lower birth rate across the country: The annual number of births continues to decline (Fostik & Galbraith, 2021).
- Delayed motherhood: In 2019, the average age of first-time mothers was 30 to 34 (Statistics Canada, 2020). Moreover, the number of persons giving birth after the age of 40 has continued to increase each year. Live births for individuals between 40 and 44 years of age in 2016 were 13 506, and in 2019 the number was 15 077 (Statistics Canada, 2021a). An exception to this trend is Indigenous persons, who often have their children at a younger age (Keenan-Lindsay et al., 2022).
- Smaller families: Large families are now rare; the number of families with three or more children has decreased. Families have, on average, 1.4 children (Battams, 2021).
- A decrease in married couples: Married couples remain the predominant family structure, although their proportion has declined over time (Statistics Canada, 2019).
- A rise in common-law families: The proportion of common-law families has increased (Statistics Canada, 2019).
- A rise in same-sex families: The proportion of same-sex married and common-law families has risen significantly (Statistics Canada, 2021b). Many same-sex families have children through adoption, through donor insemination, or from previous heterosexual relationships.
- A rise in 2SLGBTQI+ family building using assisted reproductive technologies (ART): There has been a significant increase within the 2SLGBTQI+ community of those seeking out ART at infertility clinics to have children.
- A rise in step and blended families: Step and blended families have also increased over the past decade (Battams, 2018).
- A rise in the number of lone parents raising children: In 2016, 16% of all Canadian families were lone-parent families, compared with 11% in 1981. Women head 78% of these families. Male lone-parent families are also increasing (Battams, 2018).
- Changes in the Indigenous population and Indigenous families: The Indigenous population is projected to continue to remain younger than the non-Indigenous population. In 2016, the median age of the Indigenous population was 29.1 years and is projected to range from 38.2 to 38.4 years by 2041. The median age of the non-Indigenous population is

projected to increase from 41.4 to 44.7 years over the same period (Statistics Canada, 2021c). The Indigenous population is experiencing rapid growth: from 2006 to 2016, the First Nations population grew by 39.3%, the Métis population grew by 51.2%, and the Inuit population grew by 29.1% (Statistics Canada, 2018). The size of the Indigenous youth population living in urban areas, especially in Western Canada, has more than doubled in the last 20 years.

- COVID-19 pandemic: In 2020, 14% of persons of child-bearing age indicated they want to have children later than before due to the pandemic. In 2020, the average age of child-bearing clients at the time of delivery was 31.3 years old. This postponement in childbirth could lead to some families not obtaining their desired family size due to biological limits. In 2021, persons aged 15 to 49 changed their fertility plans because of the COVID-19 pandemic. Based on the pandemic, 19% reported they want to have fewer children than previously planned, or to have a baby later than previously planned (Fostik & Galbraith, 2021).

Childbirth Choices and Trends

Within the philosophy of family-centred care, families have many options and decisions to make when planning for prenatal care, the birth of the baby, and the family's postpartum transition. These plans include the following:

- Prenatal education and birth preferences: Community or private classes and programs, specialized programs such as Lamaze, breathing techniques, hypnosis, therapeutic touch, acupuncture, medication and pain control options and preferences
- Family participation: Identifying participants and their roles at each stage of the birth experience, attendance of the partner or other support persons at childbirth classes and during labour and birth, the involvement of siblings and extended family members
- Health care setting: Deciding on home birth, a birthing centre, a community hospital, or a high-risk pregnancy hospital
- Health care providers and support: Doula, registered or nonregistered midwife, family general practitioner, obstetrician, nurses, lactation consultant
- Postpartum: Breastfeeding or bottlefeeding, circumcision, early discharge programs, in-home support and community follow-up, newborn and maternal assessment, family involvement

Nursing Considerations

Nursing considerations are many and include the following:
- Provide information on available pregnancy and birth choices in the community.
- Refer as appropriate to community and hospital resources.
- Consider and respect cultural beliefs and preferences when discussing choices with families.
- Recognize that when families are provided with current, accurate information regarding choices, they are the experts at understanding which options will best fit their beliefs, preferences, and needs.

- Provide support to families whose personal birth plans may require adaptation due to the need for specialized care or medical intervention.

Midwifery

Historically, midwifery has a long and respected role as a childbirth option for families. Midwives, often working in teams of two, provide holistic care for the client and family throughout the pregnancy and birth process. Birth options may include hospital, birth centre, health clinic, or home-birth settings. Postpartum care and support are integral parts of midwifery practice.

Access to regulated midwifery care varies across Canada. Most provinces now offer publicly funded, legislated midwifery services. Midwives must be registered with the regulatory body or college in their province to legally practise as midwives (Canadian Midwifery Regulators Council, 2022). The Canadian Association of Midwives (CAM) and various provincial groups continue to be active in raising public awareness and lobbying governments to provide this option to all Canadian families.

- Midwives collaborate with other health care providers, including nurses, as appropriate and as indicated by the needs of the child-bearing parents and families they care for.
- In 1994, Ontario became the first province to regulate and publicly fund midwives. Midwives are legislated under the *Regulated Health Professions Act* (RHPA).
- Midwifery as a legislated and regulated profession is currently available to families in British Columbia, Alberta, Saskatchewan, Manitoba, Ontario, Quebec, Nova Scotia, Newfoundland and Labrador, New Brunswick, and the Northwest Territories (Canadian Association of Midwives, 2022).
- The National Aboriginal Council of Midwives (NACM) are active members under the umbrella of CAM. Indigenous midwifery care provides a diverse model of care for Indigenous peoples respecting their historical, cultural, and spiritual needs of each community (NACM, 2020).
- In some parts of Canada, Indigenous midwives trained in community-based programs are exempt from midwifery regulations (NACM, 2020).

DOULAS

A specially trained labour attendant is called a doula. They provide a continuous, one-on-one caring presence throughout the labour and birth process of the client they are attending. The primary role of the doula is to focus on the labouring client and their partner and provide physical and emotional support by using soft, reassuring words and physical touch. The doula administers comfort techniques to reduce pain and enhance relaxation, walks with the client, helps with position changes, and provides encouragement during the bearing-down efforts. They provide information and explain procedures and events. These forms of caring help to reduce a person's level of anxiety and fear, making the labouring client more confident and calm, and reduce the stress response that could inhibit the progress of labour (Keenan-Lindsay et al., 2022). Some hospitals employ doulas to work in the labour and birth unit, others have volunteer doula programs, although most labouring persons who use a doula pay for the service privately (Keenan-Lindsay et al., 2022).

ACCESS TO CARE: REGIONALIZATION

Regionalization of care refers to the coordination of the many facilities and professional services needed to provide optimal maternal–newborn care to families. Regions are catchment areas within defined geographical boundaries that are structured to provide all the necessary maternal–newborn services required for both uncomplicated and high-risk births. The provision of comprehensive services may be affected by challenges such as geography, funding constraints, and the availability of health care providers. Despite these challenges, advantages to regionalization include lower maternal and newborn morbidity and mortality rates, improved reproductive outcomes, and more efficient, economical utilization of facilities and personnel. Regionalization uses the principles of risk assessment and referral to provide access to the care that is appropriate to the needs of the child-bearing client, baby, and family at a location that is as close to their home as possible.

The Goals of Regionalization

The goals of regionalization are as follows:
- The provision of quality care for all clients, newborns, and their families (preconception, pregnancy, birth, postpartum, newborn) and the provision of referral mechanisms
- The coordination of services, the appropriate use of personnel and facilities, the provision of professional education, and the incorporation of research and evaluation (Canadian Institute of Health Research, 2020)

FERTILITY CONTROL AND INFERTILITY HEALTH CHALLENGES

Fertility Control

More than any other time in history, people today have many options by which they can exercise control over the planning and prevention of pregnancies. Despite this, Canadian statistics show that even in stable relationships, 45 to 50% of pregnancies are unplanned.

In Canada, under the *Health Information Act*, minors can refuse to consent to the disclosure of information to their parent, including information on their use of birth control, as long as they have the mental capacity to understand this decision (Information and Privacy Commissioner of Ontario, 2015).

Each contraceptive method has associated advantages and disadvantages, and its success at preventing pregnancy varies. Birth control methods are most effective when used consistently and correctly all the time. Only total sexual abstinence is 100% effective in preventing pregnancy and the transmission of sexually transmitted infections (STIs).

When educating clients in making a choice of the best contraceptive method, several considerations must be taken into account:
- The client's overall health status, sexual patterns and frequency, the number of sexual partners, if children are desired in the future, effectiveness, potential side effects and risks, and financial costs and availability
- Ease of use and comfort level with using the method
- Cultural beliefs and religious practices that may limit acceptable birth control options
Client teaching points on contraception:
- Most birth control methods *do not* offer protection from STIs such as human immunodeficiency virus (HIV), chlamydia, herpes, or gonorrhea. The use of a male condom is recommended in addition to a primary method of birth control—this is known as *dual protection.*
- Two types of emergency contraceptive are available in Canada: hormonal contraception pills and the placement of a copper intrauterine device. Emergency contraception is not intended as a regular method of birth control.
- Breastfeeding is *not* a reliable method of birth control unless the client accurately uses the lactational amenorrhea method (LAM). LAM is not recommended in North America because most breastfeeding clients do not maintain the required feeding patterns.

Common Methods of Contraception and Nursing Considerations

Fertility Awareness-Based Methods
- Sexual intercourse is avoided on the seventh day of the cycle or later, when a client with regular menstrual cycles is fertile.
- Awareness, knowledge, and careful monitoring of menstrual patterns, cervical mucus changes, and basal body temperature changes are required. Effectiveness can be 80% when used with considerable knowledge, motivation, and consistency.

Male Condoms
- Male condoms can be purchased without a prescription; this is a barrier method that blocks the sperm from reaching the ovum and protects against HIV and STIs.
- Effectiveness is 85 to 98%, depending on correct use and early application during sexual activity. Condoms are most effective when used with a vaginal spermicide.
- Oil- and petroleum-based lubricants can cause latex to break down, resulting in the condom tearing or breaking. Only water-soluble lubricants should be used if needed. Condoms should be made from latex or polyurethane; animal- or natural-product condoms have micro-openings that can allow HIV to be transmitted.

Female Condoms
- Effectiveness is 80 to 90% with this barrier method.
- Female condoms can be inserted up to 24 hours in advance of sexual intercourse; they offer protection against HIV and STIs.

Oral Contraceptives

- Oral contraceptives are commonly known as "the pill" and are taken daily. The pill contains the hormones estrogen and progestin, which suppress the release of the ovum. Effectiveness is 95 to 99%. The pill does not protect against HIV and STIs.
- Extended-cycle pills containing levonorgestrel/ethinyl-estradiol were approved in July 2007 by Health Canada and are taken for 12 consecutive weeks followed by 1 week of nonhormonal pills. This limits menstruation to four cycles per year, which can help manage endometriosis.
- Some antibiotics may interfere with effectiveness or oral contraceptives. Clients who are prescribed antibiotics should be advised to use an additional method of birth control.
- Clients over 35 years of age or who smoke may be advised to choose an alternative method of birth control to minimize the known risks of high blood pressure, blood clots, and arterial blockage. The pill may be contraindicated in clients with a history of blood clots, cerebrovascular accident, heart disease or breast, liver, or endometrial cancers.

Transdermal Contraceptive Patch

- A transdermal contraceptive patch containing the hormones estrogen and progestin is a small patch applied once a week for 3 weeks on the skin. During the fourth week, the client does not wear a patch. This allows menstruation to occur.
- The patch may be less effective for a client with a weight greater than 90 kg (Keenan-Lindsay, 2020).
- The patch provides safe and effective birth control similar to oral contraceptives if used correctly (Keenan-Lindsay, 2020).

Contraceptive Vaginal Ring

- The contraceptive vaginal ring is a flexible, soft, transparent ring made of copolymer ethylene vinyl that delivers continuous levels of progesterone and ethynyl estradiol, which are absorbed through the vaginal epithelium.
- One ring is worn for 3 weeks, followed by a week without the ring. Withdrawal bleeding occurs during the "no ring" week.
- The ring can be inserted by the client and does not have to be fitted (Keenan-Lindsay et al., 2022).

The "Mini" Oral Contraceptive

- The "mini pill" contains only the hormone progestin and acts by thickening the cervical mucus so that sperm cannot reach the egg. In addition, if an egg does become fertilized, it is prevented from implanting in the uterine wall.
- The mini pill may be an option for those clients who cannot take estrogen-based contraceptives.
- Effectiveness is 92 to 99%, but only if taken at the same time each day.

Intrauterine Devices (IUDs)

- The device is placed inside the uterus, preventing sperm from reaching the egg, the implantation of the fertilized egg, or both. The device may use copper or the hormone progesterone as an active ingredient to prevent pregnancy.

- Effectiveness is 98 to 99%. The device can offer up to 5 years of protection.

Depo-Provera

- This is an injection of the hormone progestin given every 3 months. Its effectiveness is 97%.
- Use of depot medroxyprogesterone acetate (Depo-Provera) has been associated with loss of bone mineral density that may not be completely reversible. It is to be used for the shortest time period possible (Pfizer, 2021).

Diaphragm, Cervical Cap

- These are barrier methods, used with spermicidal gel or foam prior to sexual intercourse. Both must be properly fitted to cover the cervix; if used correctly, they can be 83 to 91% effective.
- They must be left in place 6 to 8 hours after intercourse to prevent pregnancy and be removed no later than 24 hours after intercourse.

Surgical Sterilization

- Tubal ligation prevents the egg from reaching the fallopian tube and uterus and is a permanent method of birth control with 99.9% effectiveness.
- Vasectomy, with 99% permanent effectiveness, involves ligation, the removal of a piece of the vas deferens, or both, thereby eliminating sperm from the semen.

Emergency Contraception (EC)

- Emergency contraception is a method used to prevent pregnancy after having unprotected sexual intercourse. It can be used in situations when a condom slips off or breaks or a diaphragm or cervical cap slips out of place. It can also be used in sexual assault cases or any other case of unprotected intercourse.
- There are two types:
  1. Hormonal EC methods:
     a) A special formulation containing progestin only (Plan B, NorLevo, Option 2, Next Choice). Hormones interfere with ovulation, and possibly implantation, preventing pregnancy from occurring. This pill can be used up to 72 hours after unprotected intercourse or contraceptive failure such as a broken condom, providing 75% effectiveness.
     - This contraception is sold in Canada under the name "Plan B" and is available from pharmacists without a medical prescription.
     - This pill does not prevent the transmission of HIV or STIs.
     b) A series of four pills containing high doses of estrogen and progestin (called the Yuzpe method). Adverse effects for both hormonal EC methods include nausea and vomiting, irregular bleeding, fatigue, headache, and dizziness. Clients report less nausea with the progestin-only regimens (Keenan-Lindsay et al., 2022).
  2. Copper intrauterine device (IUD)

- The copper IUD should be inserted within 5 days of unprotected sexual intercourse. It is the most effective method of EC. The IUD is inserted by a heath care professional and available only by prescription (Keenan-Lindsay et al., 2022).

Pregnancy Termination Through Induced Abortion

Induced abortion is the purposeful interruption of pregnancy before 20 weeks' gestation. The term elective abortion is used for the client requesting an abortion and therapeutic abortion refers to abortions performed for maternal health, fetal health, or disease reasons (Keenan-Lindsay et al., 2022).

While induced abortions are legal in Canada and many countries in the world, they continue to be a source of controversy among those with strongly opposing views based on moral, religious, and ethical beliefs. Pregnancies may be ended by medical or surgical means depending on the gestational age, with the majority occurring in the first trimester of pregnancy. Factors influencing a client's decision to choose to have an abortion may include the following:

- Contraceptive failure
- Diseases or a life-threatening medical condition affecting the client or fetus
- Psychosocial factors, including distress due to the timing and circumstances of the pregnancy

Medical Abortion

Medical abortions are available up to 9 weeks' gestation using methotrexate and misoprostol (Cytotec).

Surgical (Aspiration) Abortion

- The most common procedure done in the first trimester is an aspiration (vacuum or suction curettage).
- Second-trimester surgical methods include dilatation and evacuation, systemic or intrauterine prostaglandins, and intrauterine hypertonic saline administration.
  Risks and side effects of surgical abortion include cramping, bleeding, infection, perforation of the uterus, and laceration to the cervix.

Nursing Considerations

- Be aware of your own beliefs regarding elective induced abortion.
- Know the applicable and relevant rules and guidelines of the nursing regulatory body for your province or territory regarding providing nursing care for clients seeking or undergoing elective abortions.
- Provide accurate information regarding side effects to be expected following the abortion, including cramping, bleeding, and pain.
- Provide emotional support throughout and possibly request a referral by a physician or nurse practitioner for follow-up psychological support and possible contraceptive planning.

Infertility

Infertility, which affects 10 to 20% of couples trying to conceive, is diagnosed when pregnancy does not occur following a year without contraception. *Primary infertility* refers to a couple who has never conceived. *Secondary infertility* describes a couple who experiences infertility after having at least one previous conception. Sterility is an absolute inability to conceive. Many infertility issues may respond to interventions. The psychological impact on the couple dealing with infertility must not be underestimated and can be extremely challenging.

Female Infertility Factors

Female infertility factors include the following:

- Age: Delaying child-bearing until age 30 and beyond may lead to corresponding lowered fertility.
- Weight: Excessive weight gain or loss can decrease fertility levels.
- Reproductive organs: Tubal obstructions, cervical stenosis, infections, especially with pelvic inflammatory disease, scarring of the uterus, congenital anomalies, uterine fibroids, inhospitable cervical mucus, in utero exposure to diethylstilbestrol (DES), polycystic ovarian syndrome, antibodies to partner's sperm, and endometriosis can contribute to infertility.
- Endocrine disorders: Abnormal hormone production in the hypothalamus, anterior pituitary, ovary, thyroid, or adrenal glands can contribute to infertility.
- Unknown causes: Ten to 15 percent of female infertility is due to unknown causes.

Male Infertility Factors

Male factors account for 35 to 40% of infertility causes. Male infertility factors include the following:

- Social factors: Prolonged bicycling, hot tubs, malnutrition, or trauma can decrease fertility levels.
- Environmental factors: Testicular radiation or heavy marijuana, cocaine, or alcohol use can contribute to infertility.
- Reproductive organs: Congenital anomalies, hypospadias, varicocele, cryptorchidism, infections, STIs, retrograde ejaculation, ejaculatory failure, impaired circulation, diabetes, obstructions, and faulty spermatogenesis can contribute to infertility.
- Endocrine disorders: Cushing's syndrome, pituitary tumour, or acromegaly can contribute to infertility.
- Unknown causes: Ten percent of male infertility is due to unknown causes.

Diagnostic Assessment

Diagnostic assessments include the following:

- Complete health and reproductive history, respecting individual confidentiality issues
- Physical examination, which may also include tests for anatomical abnormalities, tubal patency, endometrial biopsy, transvaginal ultrasonography, laparoscopy to evaluate peritoneal factors, a postcoital examination of cervical mucus and the quantity and quality of sperm present, and basal body temperature monitoring
- Analysis of semen: Volume, sperm count, motility
- Laboratory assessment for STIs and infections, hormonal analysis of endocrine and ovarian function, ovulation predictor kits or LH surge kits to detect ovulation

Therapeutics

Therapeutic interventions for infertility are directed at the underlying cause or causes.

Male factors
- Sperm washing and assisted intrauterine insemination, use of donor sperm, antibiotic treatment for infections, androgen (testosterone) hormone therapy
- Referral to a urologist for treatment of reparable structural disorders

Female factors
- Surgery for tubal occlusions, pelvic adhesions, fibroids, or reparable structural abnormalities
- Pharmacological therapy is often directed toward treating ovulatory dysfunction

Assisted reproductive technologies (ARTs). These are also known as *assisted human reproduction* (AHR). These technologies include any therapeutic intervention in which the sperm, eggs, or both are managed outside the body. There are several techniques, and the use of donor sperm and eggs may be part of the intervention. National guidelines have been established to regulate the process. There has been an increase in the use of assisted reproduction services by the 2SLGBTQI+ community (Keenan-Lindsay et al., 2022). Often multiple steps are required to prepare the body for ART interventions. The medications used may have several adverse effects.

The most effective form of ART is in vitro fertilization (IVF). This is a complex procedure that allows fertilization to occur outside the client's body. The client's eggs are collected from their ovaries, fertilized in a laboratory with sperm, and transferred to their uterus after normal embryo development has occurred. IVF can use a client's own eggs or sperm, or eggs, sperm, and embryos donated (Lowdermilk et al., 2020).

IVF is an expensive procedure that can cost about $10, 000 to $15,000 for one cycle of treatment. Provinces vary in their financial assistance for the procedure (Burman, 2019).

Nursing Considerations
- Psychological support and counselling are essential when managing fertility because infertility issues are often accompanied by feelings of helplessness, frustration, and grief.
- Clients need to be informed of and closely monitored for adverse effects and risks when undergoing hormonal therapies and ART interventions. Maternal and fetal morbidity and mortality rates in pregnancy, birth, and postpartum are higher for ART interventions.
- It is important to be sensitive to the language used during the ART process when working with 2SLGBTQI+ clients.

NORMAL PREGNANCY

A client's body undergoes tremendous physiological changes as it adapts to the demands of supporting a pregnancy. This major life event inevitably also brings many developmental and psychosocial adjustments as roles and relationships change within a family. Nurses play a significant role in educating and supporting a client and their family during this profoundly important event.

Conception, Fertilization, and Implantation

The sequencing of these stages includes the following:
- At the time of ovulation, the ovum is released and swept up by cilia in the ampulla of the fallopian tube. The ovum is fertile and viable for about 24 hours after ovulation.
- Spermatozoa are viable and optimally fertile for 24 hours postejaculation, although they may survive and remain mobile in the cervical mucus for 2 to 3 days but may survive as long as 7 days (Keenan-Lindsay et al., 2022). Although 200 to 500 million sperm may be contained in the ejaculate, only one will penetrate and fertilize the ovum. Prostaglandins in the semen stimulate uterine smooth muscle contractions and help propel the sperm to the fallopian tube, where fertilization commonly takes place.
- Capacitation: Enzymes in the sperms' heads are released, changing the outer coating of the ovum to allow one sperm to penetrate the ovum.
- Zonal reaction: Once a sperm has penetrated the ovum, cellular changes occur on the ovum's surface membrane, preventing other sperm from entering.
- At the time of fertilization, the nuclei of the sperm and ovum fuse, and the 23 chromosomes from each combine to restore the diploid number of 46. Sex is determined by the 23rd pair of chromosomes, the male contributing either an X chromosome for an XX (female) or a Y chromosome for an XY (male) chromosome pair.

Chromosomal disorders may or may not be linked to hereditary causes. Hazards such as radiation or chemical exposure may also cause chromosomal defects.

Multifetal Pregnancy

A multiple pregnancy occurs naturally in about 1 in 43 pregnancies. It arises from two different processes:
- Monozygotic or identical twins occur due to the spontaneous division of one fertilized ovum early in development.
- Dizygotic or fraternal twins occur when two or more separate ova are fertilized by two or more different spermatozoa. Fetuses have separate placentas and individual chromosomal genotypes.

ART fertility treatments may produce multiple fertilized ova. The Society of Obstetricians and Gynaecologists of Canada (SOGC) currently recommends implantation of no more than one embryo, depending on maternal age and reproductive status, due to the increased maternal–fetal morbidity and mortality risks (SOGC, 2022a).

Embryonic and Fetal Development

Development is divided into three stages: the ovum, embryonic, and fetal stages. The amniotic cavity provides a climate-controlled environment for the developing fetus. The placenta is a key structure with multiple functions. As the uterus receives 10% of the maternal cardiac output, anything that impairs uteroplacental circulation will adversely affect the fetus. Knowledge of this relationship is crucial for nurses when assessing risk factors for maternal–fetal well-being.

Ovum Stage

The ovum stage lasts from conception to day 14. It is characterized by cellular division, formation of the blastocyst and beginnings of the embryonic membranes, and differentiation of the primary germ layers.

- The two-celled zygote continues to undergo mitotic cellular division (also known as *cleavage*) while travelling through the fallopian tube toward the uterine cavity.
- With each mitotic division, two-, four-, and eight-celled groups called *blastomeres* form until a solid ball of 16 cells called a *morula* reaches the uterus and prepares to implant into the uterine wall.
- Inside the morula, development continues as a solid inner mass of cells called the *blastocyst* forms. This marks the first important differentiation from which specific structures will develop, including the embryo, which will develop into a fetus.
- Implantation occurs 7 to 10 days after fertilization, as chorionic villi on the blastocyst implant into the top one-third of the fundus of the uterine wall.
- Following implantation, the endometrium is called the *decidua.*
- The chorionic villi then secrete the hormone HCG, maintaining the corpus luteum until the placenta develops enough to take over hormone production. HCG is the hormone detected in pregnancy testing.
- The primary layers form (ectoderm, mesoderm, and endoderm), from which all tissues and organs will develop.
- The ectoderm is the source of the central and peripheral nervous systems, sensory epithelium, tooth enamel, nails and hair, and lens of the eye.
- The mesoderm produces the skeletal bones and cartilage, muscles, connective tissue, cardiovascular and reproductive systems, kidneys, and spleen.
- The endoderm's lower layer forms the pancreas, liver, bladder, epithelial lining of the respiratory tract, and vagina.

Embryonic Stage

The embryonic stage lasts from gestational day 15 until the embryo reaches a crown-to-rump length of 3 cm, or approximately to the end of the eighth week. This is a critical time of development of all organ systems and external body features and a high-risk time for teratogenic substances to interfere with and harm organ and tissue development.

- From the blastocyst, the amnion (innermost layer) and chorion (outermost layer) membranes form to protect the developing embryo.
- The amnion continues to grow, enclosing the developing embryo in a protective, fluid-filled cavity.
- The chorion becomes the fetal side of the placenta and contains the umbilical blood vessels—two arteries and one vein—surrounded by Wharton's jelly connective tissue.

Fetal Stage

This stage begins at week 9 and lasts until birth or the end of the pregnancy. Major developmental milestones are outlined in Table 10.1.

Amniotic Fluid

- Amniotic fluid is derived initially from maternal blood filtrates and eventually consists mostly of fetal urine. Normal volume is 500 mL to a maximum of 1 000 mL.
- Oligohydramnios is a volume of less than 300 mL, which impairs fetal movement and symmetrical growth and may be associated with fetal abnormalities, and if prolonged, does not allow for normal alveoli development.
- Polyhydramnios is a volume greater than 1.5 to 2 L and is also associated with fetal abnormalities.
- The amniotic fluid functions to control temperature, protect the fetus from trauma, and allow symmetrical growth, fetal breathing, and motor movements.

The Placenta

- The placenta is structurally complete by week 12 gestation; it continues to grow and expand until 20 weeks.
- Fetal and maternal blood are independent, although separated only by a thin layer of cells.
- Placental functions include gas exchange, heat transfer, antibody transfer, transportation of nutrients, excretion of metabolic wastes, and hormone production essential for maintaining the pregnancy.
- Most substances are of a molecular size that allows for transfer across the maternal circulation and into the fetal circulation. This can include protective maternal immunoglobulins but also harmful antibodies, viruses, most drugs, and other external teratogenic substances, including alcohol, nicotine, caffeine, and cocaine.

Hormone production

- Estrogen is a steroid that stimulates growth of the uterus and breast tissue, increases in amount as the pregnancy reaches term, and helps stimulate uterine muscle contractility, thereby helping to stimulate the onset of labour.
- Progesterone is a protective hormone that may help maintain the pregnancy by decreasing uterine contractility. It also decreases smooth muscle contractions in maternal circulation and helps maintain the endometrium.
- Human chorionic gonadotropin (hCG) is detected by pregnancy tests, found in maternal serum and urine 8 to 10 days postconception, and maintains the function of the corpus luteum until the placenta is fully developed.
- Human placental lactogen (HPL) is a growth-type hormone that supports fetal growth by stimulating maternal metabolism and increasing the transport of glucose to the fetus. It also prepares the breasts for milk production and lactation.

Uteroplacental Circulation

- The uterus receives 10% of maternal cardiac output by the end of the pregnancy.
- Anything that adversely affects maternal circulation will impair placental function and put the fetus at risk.

TABLE 10.1	**Essentials of Fetal Development by Pregnancy Trimester**	
First Trimester	**Second Trimester**	**Third Trimester**
Up to 12 Weeks' Gestation	**13–24 Weeks' Gestation**	**25–40 Weeks' Gestation**
Weight: 45 g Heart beats at 28 days; fetal circulation complete; fetal heartbeat (FHB) heard by Doppler; all body organs are formed; differentiation of sex glands; sex determination possible; fingers and toes are distinct; face appears human; eyelids closed; tooth buds appear; skin pink and smooth; palate has developed and closed; outlines of bones visible on ultrasonogram; lungs acquire shape; kidneys produce urine, contribute to amniotic fluid; able to move limbs.	Weight: 60–780 g By 16 weeks, there is rapid growth; transparent skin; blood vessels visible; active movements present; sucking motions; meconium produced; sweat glands developing; skeletal system obvious. At 20 weeks, the mother feels fetal movement ("quickening"); lung alveoli appear; surfactant begins production; respiratory movements occur, called *fetal breathing movements* (FBM); eyes are closed; there is rapid growth. By 24 weeks, eyebrows and lashes are formed; skin is red, wrinkled; there is little subcutaneous fat; fingerprints, footprints are present; vernix covers the body; lanugo is abundant; myelination of the spinal cord begins; fetal suck and swallow reflexes are present; peristalsis begins; teeth form; grasp reflex is present.	Weight: 900–3 500 g By 28 weeks, weight 1 200 g; eyes open and close; gas exchange possible; two thirds of final size; testes descend; nervous system begins some regulation; germinal matrix of brain rich in blood, increasing risk of bleeding if born now. By 32 weeks, weight 2 000 g; central nervous system regulation rapidly developing; bones fully developed; iron stores begin; subcutaneous fat stores develop; skin less wrinkled and red; pupils react to light. By 35 weeks, lung surfactant peaks, signalling lung maturity; lanugo and vernix decrease. By 38 to 40 weeks, the pregnancy is considered full term.

Uterine blood flow

- Uterine blood flow is decreased by maternal hypotension, supine hypotensive disorder, prolonged labour contractions, and vigorous or prolonged cardio exercises.
- Uterine blood flow is increased by maternal positioning to a left or right lateral position.

Nursing Considerations

- Key considerations:
  - Normal placental function depends almost entirely on normal maternal circulation. Any health conditions that decrease maternal circulation may adversely affect placental function.
  - Blood flow is decreased by maternal vasoconstriction related to diabetes, hypertension, either chronic or pregnancy induced (PIH), vasopressor medications, nicotine, and cocaine.
- Assess the learning needs of families and provide resources for understanding fetal growth and development. Assess the need for genetic counselling based on family history or teratogenic exposure and refer as appropriate.
- Teach the client measures by which to maximize uteroplacental circulation throughout their pregnancy: avoiding unsupported supine position, following treatment plans for medical and circulatory conditions, using a left or right lateral sleeping and resting position, and avoiding excessive or prolonged cardio exercise practices.
- Be aware that maternal elevated core body temperature or a fever of 38.5°C or higher may increase the risk of harm in embryological development. Teach the client the balance

between benefits and risks regarding avoiding excessive body temperature overheating. For example, to protect the embryo, hot tubs and saunas should be avoided, especially during the sensitive embryonic development stage. Reducing fever with medications such as acetaminophen (Tylenol) is a safe practice in pregnancy.

Calculating Length of Pregnancy

- The length of a pregnancy is calculated from the first day of the last menstrual period (or cycle, LMP). It can be described as approximately 280 days, 40 weeks, 9 calendar months, or 10 lunar months. Nine calendar months are divided into three trimesters of 3 months each.
- *Term* refers to the normal length of a pregnancy, with labour and birth occurring between 38 and 42 weeks' gestation. *Preterm* refers to labour and birth between 20 and 37 weeks' gestation. *Post-term* is labour and birth after 42 weeks' gestation.
- Naegle's rule: The estimated date of confinement (EDC, that is, labour and birth) is calculated as follows: EDC = LMP + 7 days – 3 months + 1 year.

Key Terms Related to Pregnancy

- *Gravida* is a person who is pregnant.
- *Nulligravida* is a person who has never been pregnant.
- *Primigravida* is a person who is pregnant for the first time.
- *Multigravida* is a person who has been pregnant more than once.
- *Viability* refers to an infant sufficiently developed enough to live outside the womb, with no clear limits on gestational

age or weight. True viability is realistic after 22 to 25 weeks' gestation, but would still require neonatal intensive care support.

- *Para* is a person who has given birth after 20 weeks' gestation. The outcome or number of infants born is not taken into account.
- *Nullipara* is a person who has not given birth to an infant of viable age. Note that the person may have been pregnant but may have had a spontaneous abortion (miscarriage) or induced abortion.
- *Primipara* is a person who has given birth at more than 20 weeks' gestation, regardless of outcome and regardless of how many infants were born (e.g., twins count as one para event).
- *Multipara* is a person who has had two or more viable births.
- *GTPAL* (*g*ravidity, *t*erm, *p*reterm, *a*bortions, *l*iving) is a more accurate way of describing parity and outcome.

See the section "Labour and Birth Processes" for additional key terms.

PRECONCEPTION

Ideally, individuals of child-bearing age should have preconception access to information and health practices that will increase the likelihood of a healthy pregnancy. To improve healthy outcomes and lower risk factors, pregnancy health promotion should take place in the classroom, the public media, and any health care setting before a pregnancy is planned or occurs. Nurses, by virtue of their wide range of professional practice settings, are ideally situated to assess and support individuals in all stages of pregnancy planning and care.

Antenatal Health Assessment

This assessment includes nursing assessment, teaching, support, and referral in the following areas:

- Social support: Factors include life stressors, economic status, stability of housing and accommodations, employment, community resources, quality and nature of relationships and available support, and family support.
- Abuse and violence: Incidence of violence in intimate relationships increases during pregnancy.
- Female genital mutilation (FGM): The diversity of the Canadian population and the worldwide prevalence of this cultural practice mean that nurses may provide counselling and care to clients who have undergone FGM, despite the practice being banned in Canada.
- Lifestyle practices: The type and amount of exercise and activity, as well as tobacco, alcohol, and medicinal and non-medicinal drug use, are identified as potentially adverse lifestyle practices; support, education, and resources are provided.
- Exposure to environmental chemicals and toxic hazards: Previous and current exposure is identified, including exposure in home, recreational settings, and the workplace.

Hazardous substances include anaesthetic gases, radiation, lead, and pesticides.

- Health history: Factors include past medical and family history, especially cardiovascular disease, diabetes, congenital disorders, genetic family history, STIs, past illnesses and hospitalizations, chronic conditions, mental health, bleeding disorders, surgeries, partner's health history, and family mortality and causes.
- Current health status: Factors include weight, age, occupation, current medications and herbal supplements, allergies, teratogenic exposure or risks, chronic conditions, nutrition and dietary patterns, and immunizations.
- Sociocultural factors: They include spiritual or religious, and ethnic considerations and practices and language barriers.
- Pregnancy plans: Factors include pregnancy and birth plan preferences, education, and family involvement and roles.
- Psychological factors: They include psychological readiness for pregnancy and attitudes toward this pregnancy (e.g., excitement, ambivalence, anxiety, emotionally labile).
- Gynecological and reproductive history: Factors include age at menarche, STIs or other infections, menstrual cycle, last Pap smear, contraceptive history, infertility, past pregnancies, postpartum depression, GTPAL, breastfeeding history, complications of past pregnancies or births, prenatal education, blood type, and Rh factor.
- Current pregnancy: This includes calculating the first day of LMP; pregnancy test results, if known; weight gain; discomforts of pregnancy or complications such as spotting, cramping, or bleeding; any medications, vitamins, or supplements; attitude regarding this pregnancy; and family and support system.

High-Risk Pregnancy Screening

High-risk pregnancy screening identifies health and social issues that may adversely affect the pregnant client or fetus during the pregnancy, labour, and birth. Early identification of these factors provides an opportunity to monitor, intervene, or make referrals promptly, thereby providing the best chance for a healthy pregnancy outcome.

Many provincial and territorial health systems use standardized antenatal risk screening assessment profiles to identify those at risk and in need of referral for specialized monitoring or care. The assessment tool is completed at the first prenatal visit and updated at each visit. For example, pregnancy risk levels may be differentiated and defined as a healthy pregnancy with no predictable risk, a pregnancy at risk, or a pregnancy at high risk.

COVID-19 vaccination is recommended during pregnancy in any trimester and while breastfeeding (Centers for Disease Control and Prevention, 2022). SOGC (2021b) recommends the child-bearing client follows their provincial and territorial guidelines on the type of vaccine to receive.

Social risk factors. There are many social risk factors, including the following:

- Low socioeconomic status and education level, housing instability, and social isolation
- Living in a high-altitude geographical location
- Extremes in weight: Obesity (greater than 90 kg) or extreme underweight (less than 46 kg)
- Extremes in age: Adolescent (younger than 16 years) or mature (older than 35 years)
- Lifestyle: Alcohol, tobacco, or recreational drug use
- Culture: Infant mortality rates are higher among Indigenous peoples. Indigenous clients describe past negative experiences with health care providers such as racism, judgement of their lifestyle choices, and discrimination. Some clients have stated they will seek health care for their children but are hesitant to see a health care provider for their own needs because of previous negative encounters. Other factors affecting whether they will attend prenatal care visits include complex life situations, lack of transportation, and whether they had experiences with child protection services (Keenan-Lindsay et al., 2022).
- Exposure to occupational or environmental hazards or toxin exposure, past or present (Keenan-Lindsay et al., 2022)

Reproductive health risk factors
- Past or pre-existing conditions: Cardiovascular disease, diabetes, thyroid disorders, blood or bleeding disorders, blood incompatibility or Rh sensitization, renal disease, mental health disorders, and congenital or genetic disorders
- Past and current obstetrical complications with pregnancy or birth: DES exposure; ectopic pregnancy; cervical insufficiency (premature dilation of cervix); surgeries; stillbirths; Caesarean births; premature or prolonged rupture of membranes; multiple gestation; STIs or other infections, especially rubella, cytomegalovirus (CMV), herpes, and syphilis; abruption or placenta previa; PIH; or gestational diabetes
- Fetal or past neonatal complications of morbidity or mortality: Prematurity or postmaturity, teratogen exposure, small for gestational age (SGA) or large for gestational age (LGA), or fetal compromise

Initial Prenatal Physical Examination

In addition to a detailed history, the physical examination will include vital signs, height, weight, weight gain, pelvic examination, including assessment of pelvic type and adequacy, and breast examination.

Initial Laboratory Assessment

- Blood work entails a complete blood count (CBC); ABO and Rh typing; screening for syphilis, HIV, gonorrhea, and CMV; rubella titre; hepatitis B screening; glucose; screening for sickle cell disease if parent is of African descent; and screening for thalassemia trait if parent is of Mediterranean descent
- Urinalysis
- Pap smear

Danger Signs of Pregnancy

At any time during the pregnancy, the following signs and symptoms should be reported at once:
- Cramping and uterine contractions, vaginal spotting or bleeding
- Persistent vomiting
- Painful, frequent urination or oliguria
- Temperature above 38°C
- Persistent or severe headache, edema of hands or face, dizziness, muscle irritability, epigastric pain related to PIH
- Unusual pain, especially abdominal or uterine pain, absence of fetal movement
- Signs of preterm or impending labour: Rupture of membranes, bloody show, uterine contractions that are regular and increasing in intensity and duration, expulsion of mucus plug

Nursing Considerations

- Key client teaching point:
  - Teach the client the danger signs and symptoms of pregnancy that should be reported immediately. Provide health teaching for immediate interventions.
- Create an interview atmosphere that ensures privacy, safety, and sensitivity to encourage honest, open communication and responses. Ask direct questions, especially regarding abuse and risk factors for abuse.
- Provide information and refer to community and professional services for any identified preconception and antenatal risks, including information about antenatal screening procedures and rationales for testing.
- Advise that moderate exercise appears advantageous if already part of the client's prepregnancy lifestyle. Emphasize the avoidance of hot tubs, saunas, or strenuous, prolonged activity, which may cause overheating.

PERINATAL ASSESSMENT AND CARE

Health Assessment in Normal Pregnancy

Routine health assessment for a normal pregnancy is performed according to the following schedule:
- First visit within the first trimester (12 weeks)
- Every 4 weeks until 28 weeks' gestation
- Every 2 weeks until 36 weeks' gestation
- Thereafter, every week until birth of the infant

Routine assessment includes physical assessment, maternal weight and weight gain patterns, adjustment to pregnancy, discomforts of pregnancy, presence of edema, nutritional assessment, family life and psychosocial status, vital signs, urine testing, fundal height and uterine growth, fetal heart rate (FHR), and a pelvic examination at 36 weeks' gestation to assess for signs of impending labour. For biophysical profile scoring, see Table 10.2.

Laboratory and Maternal Screening

- Urinalysis for protein, glucose, ketones; trace glucose may reflect normal alterations to renal function in pregnancy

TABLE 10.2 Biophysical Profile

Biophysical Variable	Adequate Score (Score = 2)	Inadequate Score (Score = 0)
Nonstress test may or may not be done	2 accelerations in 20 minutes, 15 beats above baseline lasting 15 seconds (normal)	<2 accelerations in 20 minutes Abnormal - atypical
Fetal breathing movements	≥1 episodes of rhythmic fetal breathing of ≥30 seconds within 30 minutes	Episodes absent or no episode ≥30 seconds of sustained fetal breathing movements in 30 minutes
Fetal movements	≥3 discrete body/limb movements in 30 minutes of observation*	<3 episodes of fetal movement
Fetal tone	≥1 episode of active extension with rapid return to flexion of fetal limb(s), trunk, or opening and closing of hand considered normal tone	Either slow extension with return to partial flexion or movement of limb in full extension or absent fetal movement
Amniotic fluid volume	Single pocket of fluid present measuring ≥2 cm in a vertical axis†	Evidence of decreased amniotic fluid or oligohydramnios† No single pocket of fluid that is 2 cm by 2 cm

*Simultaneous limb and trunk movements are considered one movement.
†Some protocols use a single-pocket measurement, and some use the amniotic fluid index: ≤5.0 = oligohydramnios; 5.1–8 = low normal; 8.1–24 = normal; >24 = polyhydramnios.
From Blackburn, S. T. (2017). *Maternal, fetal, and neonatal physiology: A clinical perspective* (5th ed.). Saunders.

- Glucose tolerance testing at 24 to 28 weeks' gestation if there is excessive glucose in urine or a history of diabetes or gestational diabetes
- Indirect Coombs test on Rh-negative individuals at 28 weeks to assess for Rh sensitization
- Fetal ultrasonogram at 18 to 22 weeks
- Group B *Streptococcus* (GBS) at 35 to 37 weeks' gestation
- Maternal CBC at 28 weeks' gestation to assess for anemia

Expected Physical Assessment Findings in Normal Pregnancy
Vital Signs
- Temperature: 36.5 to 37.5°C
- Heart rate: 60 to 90 bpm; heart rate may increase by 10 bpm due to cardiovascular adaptations
- Blood pressure: 90–120/60–80 mm Hg, with a decrease in the second trimester due to smooth muscle relaxation of blood vessels

Fetal Heart Rate and Movement
- 110 to 160 bpm
- Detected at 8 to 17 weeks by Doppler ultrasonography, 16 to 20 weeks by stethoscope

Fundal Height
After 20 to 22 weeks' gestation, fundal height in centimetres for a client of average weight corresponds approximately to the gestational age in weeks. Individual differences in growth make this inaccurate after 36 weeks' gestation.

Weight Gain
Clients of normal prepregnancy weight (body mass index [BMI] 18.5–24.9) can expect to gain an average of 11.5 to 16 kg (25–35 lb.) during a 40-week pregnancy. According to Health Canada's *Prenatal Nutrition Guidelines for Health Professionals*, gestational weight gain is based on preconception BMI (Government of Canada, 2014). In addition to the fetal weight, expected increases in weight are due to increased blood volume, reproductive tissue growth (especially uterine growth), as well as the placenta, amniotic fluid, and products of conception.

The weight gain for the average BMI weight is as follows:
- First trimester: Approximately 1 to 2 kg (2–4 lb.), almost all of which is due to maternal physiological changes and growth
- Second and third trimester: On average, 0.4 kg (1.0 lb.) per week

Nursing Considerations
- Key consideration:
  - Weight gain of more than 1 kg (2 lb.) in 1 week may be a sign of excess fluid retention or hypertension and should be assessed further.
- *Canada's Food Guide* (Government of Canada, 2022) can be used as a guide to make daily food choices during pregnancy and lactation.
- Quickening or maternal awareness of fetal movement occurs at around 20 weeks' gestation, earlier in multiparas.
- Higher than expected fundal height may be related to polyhydramnios, or multiple gestation.
- Lower than expected fundal height may be due to oligohydramnios, a fetus that is SGA, or intrauterine growth restriction.

- Clients may need to be reassured regarding body image and weight gain fears and be made aware of the risks of excessive weight gain or being underweight.
- Clients should be aware that the varied and changing emotional responses to pregnancy are normal and expected. Encourage discussion between partners regarding feelings of ambivalence, uncertainty, and insecurities regarding changing roles and body image. These feelings are an expected part of adapting to a major life change. If feelings continue beyond the first trimester to be a source of distress or conflict, encourage and offer resources and referral to appropriate counselling services. Also promote childbirth preparation classes in a group setting for health information and peer support.

Physical and Physiological Adaptations to Pregnancy

For the client's body to accommodate the demands of a pregnancy, all body systems undergo normal changes. While the reproductive system undergoes the most significant and noticeable changes, all body systems adapt as necessary.

Reproductive System Changes

Reproductive body system changes are as follows:

- Uterus: There is increased growth, elasticity, and enlargement of pre-existing muscles; and increased vascularity and blood supply (10% of cardiac output by term). Irregular Braxton Hicks contractions (involuntary uterine tightening) provide regulatory blood flow to placenta and are felt after the second trimester.
- Cervix: It becomes softer (Goodell's sign), shorter (especially as term approaches), and closed by a protective mucus plug; increased vascularity makes it appear cyanotic on a prenatal examination (Chadwick's sign).
- Ovaries: They may be enlarged on palpation in the first trimester due to hormone-producing corpus luteum.
- Vagina: There is an increase in vascularity, elasticity, and secretions, and the pH changes to alkaline with added risk of infections.
- Perineum: There is increased vascularity (Chadwick's sign) and hypertrophy of tissues.
- Breasts: There is greater sensitivity, increased vascularity with more prominent veins, increased size of periareolar glands and areola, and increased pigmentation in response to increased melanin production.

Cardiovascular System Changes

Significant changes occur in the cardiovascular system as the body supports the added blood volume, flow, and transportation demands:

- Blood volume and flow: Blood volume increases 40 to 50% as plasma volume peaks at 28 to 34 weeks, with a marked increase in flow to the uterus and kidneys.
- Blood constituents: RBCs increase by 20 to 30%, but not in proportion to the increase in plasma volume, creating the condition known as *physiological anemia*. Hemoglobin should remain at or above 120 mmol/L, or the client

should be assessed for true anemia. Fibrinogen increases by 50% (to help prevent excess bleeding at birth and postpartum), and the erythrocyte sedimentation rate (ESR) increases.
- Cardiac output: It increases by 30 to 50%, peaking at 20 to 24 weeks' gestation.
- Heart rate: It increases by 10 to 15 bpm. A systolic murmur may be heard.
- Blood pressure: It decreases slightly in the second trimester due to progesterone; low blood pressure may lead to postural hypotension or fainting.

Respiratory System Changes

Respiratory system changes during pregnancy include the following:

- Respiratory rate and tidal volume increase due to progesterone and slight respiratory alkalosis, 30 to 40% increased volume. Oxygen requirements increase 20 to 40%.
- The diaphragm is displaced upward, leading to shortness of breath as the pregnancy progresses; there is lateral expansion of the ribs and chest wall with increased elasticity and dilation of airways.
- Increased vascularity is secondary to estrogen; resulting nasal congestion and nosebleeds are common.

Gastro-Intestinal System Changes

Gastro-intestinal system changes during pregnancy include the following:

- Carbohydrate metabolism with insulin secretion increases, although its effectiveness is impaired by the action of hormones, and demand may exceed the pancreas's ability, resulting in symptoms of gestational diabetes. Fasting blood sugar decreases secondary to the accelerated utilization of glucose to meet fetal demands, and hypoglycemia may lead to fainting and dizziness.
- Gastric motility decreases with prolonged gastric emptying, slower peristalsis secondary to progesterone, and increased risk of constipation and hemorrhoids.
- Esophageal smooth muscle relaxation is secondary to progesterone and regurgitation.
- The gallbladder has decreased tone, distension, and slower emptying, and there is increased risk for gallstone formation.
- The liver has increased alkaline phosphatase and cholesterol and decreased albumin.
- Gingivitis is secondary to increased estrogen.

Renal System Changes

Renal system changes during pregnancy include the following:

- Bladder has decreased tone, increased capacity, and urinary stasis with increased risk of urinary tract infections.
- Renal blood volume and flow changes the glomerular filtration rate, which increases by 50%; kidneys receive one fifth of cardiac output.
- There is impaired reabsorption of glucose and nitrogen with excretion into urine.

Integumentary System Changes

Skin system changes during pregnancy include the following:

- Increased melanin from the anterior pituitary leads to linea nigra darkening down the midabdomen, facial chloasma (mask of pregnancy) with brown patchy pigmentation over cheeks and forehead, darkening of areola, and development of secondary areola.
- Pruritis (itching) is due to increased estrogen and liver changes.
- Increased sweat and sebaceous gland stimulation can lead to acne, perspiration, and night sweats.
- Striae gravidarum, or stretch marks, are due to underlying connective tissue weakening and breakage; they are dark red or bluish during pregnancy and fade to silver.
- Spider nevi, which are fine red dilated arterioles over the face, neck, and thorax, are secondary to increased estrogen.

Musculo-Skeletal System Changes

Musculo-skeletal system changes during pregnancy including the following:

- Joints become hypermobile secondary to the hormones relaxin and progesterone with increased risk for injury.
- Postural changes consist of an accentuated lumbar spinal curvature and a waddling gait.

Metabolic System Changes

Metabolic system changes during pregnancy are as follows:

- Basal metabolic rate increases by 15 to 20%.
- In carbohydrate metabolism, insulin production increases and fasting blood sugar decreases.

Endocrine System Changes

The endocrine system is affected by pregnancy as follows:

- Increased hormone production by the hypothalamus–pituitary–ovarian axis: Menstruation ceases, and estrogen and progesterone increase.
- Adrenal cortex: There is increased antidiuretic hormone (ADH), aldosterone, and cortisol.
- Pancreas: There is increased insulin demand and production but increased maternal resistance to insulin.
- Thyroid: The thyroid experiences a slight enlargement, and thyroxine (T_4) increases.
  Light-headedness and fainting in early pregnancy are secondary to hypoglycemia or postural changes.

Common Discomforts of Pregnancy

Some of these changes will lead to what are commonly referred to as minor or normal discomforts of pregnancy. Although minor from a health viewpoint, many pregnant clients view these discomforts as a source of concern and distress. Nurses can use prenatal visits to educate their clients concerning what to expect and to help plan interventions for relieving these discomforts.

First-Trimester Discomforts and Nursing Considerations

Discomforts of early pregnancy can include the following:

- Nausea and vomiting: 70 to 80% of clients complain of nausea, with or without vomiting. Nausea and vomiting of pregnancy appear at approximately 4 to 6 weeks' gestation and usually subside by the end of the first trimester. The severity ranges from mild distaste to certain foods to severe vomiting (Keenan-Lindsay et al., 2022).
- Urinary frequency: Related to uterine pressure on the bladder until the uterus expands out of the pelvis
- Fatigue
- Breast tenderness: Secondary to progesterone and estrogen hormone changes
- Vaginal discharge: Leukorrhea
- Nasal congestion and nosebleeds: Secondary to increased estrogen
  Recommend that pregnant clients do the following:
- Eat small, frequent meals, eat dry foods separate from liquids, and eat dry crackers early in the morning to help relieve nausea.
- Avoid large fluid intakes prior to sleep and void frequently during the day.
- Try to plan times for increased rest and naps.
- Wear a supportive bra, adjust it for increased breast size, and even wear a bra to bed if helpful.
- Shower daily and avoid douching.

Second- and Third-Trimester Discomforts and Nursing Considerations

Common discomforts of the second and third trimesters include the following:

- Heartburn and regurgitation of gastric contents
- Leg cramping due to imbalance in the phosphorus–calcium ratio and postural changes
- Varicose veins
- Hemorrhoids and constipation
- Backache
- Ankle edema: Related to poor venous return and increased sodium levels
- Carpal tunnel syndrome related to medial nerve compression, especially in the dominant hand
- Shortness of breath
- Sleep disturbances
  Recommend the following to clients:
- Continue to eat small, frequent meals, avoid spicy, high-fat meals, and use extra pillows to elevate the head.
- Evaluate dietary intake and increase calcium intake, eat fewer phosphorus-rich foods, and increase fluids and fibre for constipation and hemorrhoids.
- Elevate legs, take frequent breaks when driving long distances or sitting for prolonged periods, and wear supportive stockings and dorsiflex ankles to relieve cramping.
- When lightening (the perceived sensation that the fetus is lower in the pelvis) occurs as the uterus moves lower in the pelvis in the primigravida, shortness of breath will be relieved; in bed, elevate the head with pillows.

Psychological Tasks of Pregnancy

Pregnancy involves a myriad of emotional responses and psychological adjustments as a new developmental role is undertaken and family members adjust to accepting a new member into their lives. In addition to the pregnant client, all family members, including involved extended family such as grandparents, must adjust to the changes in their roles and responsibilities. This can be a time of both happiness and anticipation but also of ambivalence and stress. Nurses can help families in understanding the feelings and role changes and can provide support and reassurance.

Many steps are important to attachment between the child-bearing client and baby.

1. Planning the pregnancy
2. Confirming the pregnancy through testing and medical confirmation
3. Accepting the pregnancy; even planned pregnancies are associated with feelings of ambivalence and conflict
4. Perception of fetal movements
5. Accepting the fetus as an individual, role-playing, and fantasizing
6. After birth, reconciling the imagined infant with reality
7. Sensory interactions, such as seeing, touching, and giving care to the baby (Keenan-Lindsay, 2020)

All family members, especially the child-bearing client and their partner, need the opportunity to discuss their emotions and adaptations to the pregnancy. Pregnancy, even when carefully planned for, represents a major developmental change for the child-bearing client and their partner. The challenges of integrating all the practical, physical, financial, and role changes into a relationship and family can threaten the stability a family may or may not have. The adaptations, conflicts, and changing roles need to be acknowledged. Community childbirth classes, prenatal programs, and prenatal visits provide an opportunity for open discussion, support, and, when needed, referral to counselling services. Many community programs also offer classes to prepare siblings for the changes that happen when a new family member arrives.

Sexuality in Pregnancy

Body image, sensuality, and sexuality are all affected by the demands and changes pregnancy brings on both individual and relationship levels. Concerns may include fear of harming the developing fetus, fear of miscarriage, and cultural beliefs and practices. Physical changes may also influence desire and comfort with sexual practices.

Contraindications

There are few absolute contraindications to sexual activity or intercourse during pregnancy. They include vaginal spotting or bleeding, premature rupture of membranes, active vaginal infection, uterine cramping, and a history of spontaneous abortions.

Nursing Considerations

- Assess for beliefs, fears, and concerns and offer reassurance and factual information.
- Assess for contraindications and offer support and alternative suggestions.
- First trimester: Sexual desire may be decreased due to nausea, fatigue, breast tenderness, psychological ambivalence, and fear of harming the fetus. Suggest alternatives to sexual intercourse if desire is decreased; reassure that unless risk factors are present, there is no risk of harming the fetus during sexual intercourse.
- Second trimester: Increased interest and satisfaction take place due to increased vaginal and perineal vascularity; the discomforts of the first trimester decrease.
- Third trimester: Increased size and discomfort may affect comfort level. Suggest changes in positions or alternatives to sexual intercourse that will offer closeness and intimacy.

PERINATAL NUTRITION

The anatomical and physiological changes of pregnancy result in increased daily requirements for energy, nutrients, and vitamins. Ideally, optimal nutrition is part of preconception planning for pregnancy. Meeting nutritional needs during pregnancy is an important factor in promoting healthy outcomes for both the child-bearing client and the infant. For many clients, due to inadequate preconception dietary intake, special attention should be paid to ensuring that there is an adequate intake of calcium, vitamin D, folate, iron, and essential fatty acids. *Canada's Food Guide* recommends eating a varied, nutrient-dense diet during pregnancy, adding a little more food each day during the second and third trimesters (Government of Canada, 2021b). SOGC suggests that, in general, adding two or three *Canada's Food Guide* servings each day during the second and third trimester will meet the needs of pregnancy.

Nutritional Supplements

- Prenatal multivitamin: A prenatal daily multivitamin is recommended because it contains the additional minerals, vitamins, and folic acid necessary to support the pregnant person and fetus during pregnancy. A multivitamin with folic acid is recommended for persons who could become pregnant or are planning a pregnancy.
- Calcium and vitamin D: Calcium is essential for the development and maintenance of bone mass, both prior to and during pregnancy. Adequate intake is also needed for fetal skeletal development. The body needs vitamin D to enhance the intestinal absorption of calcium. The recommended daily intake for calcium during pregnancy is between 1 000 and 1 300 mg, depending on age. Vitamin D daily recommended intake is 600 IU (15 mcg) for pregnant and lactating clients (Canadian Paediatric Society [CPS], 2022; Government of Canada, 2020).
- Iron: Additional iron is needed to support the increase in maternal RBC production The Government of Canada recommends that all pregnant clients take a daily multivitamin with 16 to 20 mg of iron (Keenan-Lindsay et al., 2022).

- Folate: Folate (folic acid) supplementation significantly reduces the risk of neural tube defects (NTDs), which affect about one in 1 000 babies born in Canada (live births and stillbirths). A supplement of 0.4 mg daily in addition to dietary intake is recommended for all child–bearing-aged clients, as well as during pregnancy and when breast-feeding. Clients who have a high risk of having a fetus with an NTD (e.g., diabetes, epilepsy, obesity or a family history of NTD) should take 1.0 mg of folic acid for at least 3 months prior to conception and for the first 3 months of the pregnancy, at which time this can be decreased to 0.4 mg.
- Essential fatty acids: They are important during pregnancy for proper fetal neural and visual development. The fetus is dependent on maternal sources, especially during the rapid growth period of the last trimester of pregnancy. Clients are encouraged to increase dietary intake of foods rich in essential fatty acids, including nonhydrogenated vegetable oils, nuts, eggs, meat, and fatty fish such as wild salmon.

Nursing Considerations

- Assess and work to develop a plan toward optimal pre-conception and perinatal nutrition practices, including adequate caloric intake of nutrient-dense foods that meet the requirements of pregnancy and follow *Canada's Food Guide*.
- Be aware of and sensitive to the reality that dietary habits and practices are influenced by socioeconomic status, cultural diversity, and religious dietary practices and beliefs.
- When considering individual differences for caloric energy increases, suggest that clients use appetite as a guide to satisfying hunger. Review strategies for managing nausea in the first trimester.
- Refer clients to dietary supplement programs sponsored by the Government of Canada and administered by local community agencies, such as the Canada Prenatal Nutrition Program (CPNP, Government of Canada, 2021c).
- Provide suggestions for dietary sources of foods rich in folate, calcium, and iron.
- Increase awareness and understanding of potential adverse effects of excessive use of some vitamins, especially vitamin A, and over-the-counter herbal supplements.
- Ensure that vegetarians understand sources for increased protein and iron dietary intake.
- Assess for risk factors for inadequate iron stores and including a diet deficient in meat, fish, poultry, or vitamin C, as well as frequent consumption of tea or coffee (more than two cups of coffee or equivalent), multiple gestations, and parity of three or more (Keenan-Lindsay, 2020).
- Include in teaching that there is increased absorption of iron from heme sources such as meat, poultry, and fish. Particularly for vegetarians, nonheme iron is found in vegetables, fruit, grains, nuts, eggs, iron-enriched cereals, and pastas. Vitamin C and meat, poultry, and fish enhance the absorption of nonheme iron. Iron absorption is inhibited when consumed with tea, coffee, whole grains, and calcium.
- Assess for risk factors of low calcium intake, including low socioeconomic status, pregnant adolescents, and vegetarians who do not consume milk products.
- Assess for risk factors for inadequate vitamin D production, including dark-pigmented skin, inadequate exposure to sunlight due to northern geographical location during the winter months, which includes most of Canada (Government of Canada, 2020).
- Promote the consumption of healthy essential fatty acids through increased dietary intake. Reassure clients who may have misconceptions that all dietary fats are harmful.

MATERNAL HEALTH CONDITIONS AND PREGNANCY

With advances in technology, research, high-risk referral, and professional expertise, clients with health concerns and their infants are experiencing better outcomes. It is essential, however, to recognize the very real risks and complications that are associated with many maternal health issues. Clients need to be informed of the potential risks for increased maternal and fetal morbidity and mortality and educated on the early monitoring and intervention provided.

Cardiac and Blood Disorders

As previously discussed, the cardiovascular system is challenged during pregnancy to accommodate a 50% increase in circulating volume and an increase in cardiac output. For clients with a pre-existing heart condition, the needed cardiac reserve to accommodate those changes may not be sufficient. Heart disease is a significant cause of maternal morbidity and mortality, and it puts a client into a high-risk pregnancy classification.

- If the condition is associated with cyanosis and decreased systemic circulation, regardless of treatment, pregnancy should be avoided.
- If maternal oxygenation and systemic circulation are impaired, the fetus will suffer the effects of decreased uterine blood flow and hypoxia. This can result in fetal compromise, fetal death, SGA, or spontaneous abortion.
- Routine intrapartum antibiotic prophylaxis for the prevention of endocarditis is not recommended as the risk for bacteremia is low (Keenan-Lindsay et al., 2022).

Nursing Considerations

- Emphasize a preventive approach to minimizing complications of known conditions.
- Provide realistic information about the risks and a plan of care, which will enable the client to participate in their care and reduce anxiety.
- Be aware that throughout pregnancy, labour, and birth, care is directed at minimizing cardiac workload for those clients at high risk for hypoxemia. Bed rest or restricted activity may be recommended. Cardiology referral and high-risk care will be required.

- Know that the first hours following birth present a high-risk time as the body begins to remobilize the extra circulating blood volume acquired during pregnancy. This adds to the workload of the heart. Assess the client for signs of respiratory distress and pulmonary edema.

Infections

During pregnancy, the client's immune system is suppressed, leading to an increased risk of acquiring infections. TORCH infections (toxoplasmosis, other [such as syphilis, varicella zoster, parvovirus B19], rubella, CMV, and herpes) are those caused by a group of organisms that can cross the placenta. In the client, symptoms may be flulike but can cause significant developmental issues in the fetus that increase the risk of illness and death

Toxoplasmosis

- Detected in maternal serum antibodies, this infection can be acquired by handling cat feces or garden soil or through raw meat consumption. Abortion is common; surviving newborns may present with severe neurological conditions, seizures, hepatic splenomegaly, jaundice, and developmental delay.
- Pregnant clients should be advised to wear gloves while gardening and to avoid handling cat litter and eating raw meat products.

Rubella

- Exposure in the first trimester has a high incidence of spontaneous abortion and congenital anomalies, including heart, eye, ear, and brain defects.
- Preconception titre testing is recommended and vaccination with 3 months of contraception. Vaccination is often offered during the postpartum period.

Cytomegalovirus (CMV)

Pregnant clients may be asymptomatic, but the fetal effects of CMV can be severe. CMV is easily transmitted in all body fluids and crosses the placenta to infect the fetus. Fetal effects include microcephaly and severe intellectual and developmental delays, seizures, hydrocephaly, SGA, cerebral calcifications, and deafness.

Herpes Simplex Virus (HSV)

Type 1 infections cause cold sores; type 2 infections are sexually transmitted. Transmission is via the birth canal; however, Caesarean birth is recommended only when active lesions are present.

Fetal and newborn effects include microcephaly, severe intellectual and developmental impairment, patent ductus arteriosus, and eye defects.

Human Papilloma Virus (HPV)

- HPV is the most common sexually transmitted virus, and certain strains are correlated with precancerous lesions, which can lead to cervical cancer. Transmission to the fetus is unknown, but infection can result in respiratory tract papillomatosis.
- An HPV vaccine is available and recommended for all persons prior to becoming sexually active (Government of Canada, 2021d).

HIV and AIDS

- All pregnant clients should be offered voluntary HIV screening and counselling at their first prenatal visit.
- Pregnant clients can be treated with antiretroviral prophylaxis to effectively help prevent HIV transmission to the fetus, and treating the pregnant client decreases risk from 25 to 2%.
- Caesarean birth is preferred.

Group B Streptococcus (GBS)

- GBS is a bacterial infection vertically transmitted from the pregnant client to infant.
- Pregnancy complications include preterm labour and preterm rupture of membranes.
- Fetal neonatal conditions, including blindness, deafness, developmental delay, neonatal sepsis, and meningitis, may appear within 72 hours of birth with significant morbidity and mortality.
- Prenatal assessment and treatment intrapartum with penicillin is recommended.

Varicella (Chicken Pox)

- Varicella infections during pregnancy can cause serious complications to the fetus or neonate.
- In first-trimester exposure, fetal defects include microcephaly, skin, eye, and limb anomalies, and low birth weight.
- Third-trimester infection may rarely result in neonatal complications. A varicella zoster immune globulin (VZIG) is available to exposed pregnant clients.
- Varicella vaccine is recommended to all susceptible child–bearing-aged clients (those lacking immunity). It cannot be given during pregnancy. Pregnant clients who are not immune should have the vaccination offered postpartum (Government of Canada, 2021e).

Chlamydia

- This epidemic infection is the result of a parasitic transmission that occurs by direct sexual contact or exposure at birth. Infection, often asymptomatic in the child-bearing client, is associated with increasing infertility rates in Canada.
- Fetal and newborn effects are common and include prematurity, low birth weight, and stillbirth.
- Prophylaxis erythromycin or azithroymycin eye treatment is a recommended practice and is mandatory by law in most provinces and territories to prevent conjunctivitis and potential eye sequelae (Keenan-Lindsay et al., 2022).

Gonorrhea

- This bacterial infection is spread by direct contact in the lower genital tract, causing only maternal symptoms but potentially serious infections.

- Fetal effects include preterm birth and the premature rupture of membranes. Newborns are at risk for pneumonia and eye infections. Prophylaxis erythromycin eye treatment is administered to prevent conjunctivitis and potential eye sequelae.

Nursing Considerations

- Know that routine screening for STIs should be part of all initial prenatal assessments. Nurses need to know reportable STIs.
- Know that thorough history-taking in a private setting with a nonjudgemental approach is important for honest disclosure of high-risk behaviours.
- Stress the importance of consistency and adherence to treatment protocols for infections.
- Refer to appropriate community resources for information and follow-up care.
- Administer prophylactic treatment to all newborns as indicated.

Respiratory Disorders
Asthma
- The severity of asthma during pregnancy is unpredictable; symptoms may improve or worsen.
- Poorly controlled asthma can increase the risk of preterm births, preeclampsia, low birth weight, perinatal mortality and fetal growth restrictions.

Infections
- Most upper respiratory tract infections are self-limiting and pose no added risk to the fetus.
- Bacterial pneumonia should be treated with antibiotics that are considered safe in pregnancy, including those in the penicillin family.

Nursing Considerations
- For all respiratory conditions, the approach to care centres around the prevention of hypoxemia in the pregnant client. This includes promoting effective control of asthma attacks.
- Systemic steroids when used in the treatment of asthma in the first trimester may be teratogenic.
- Over-the-counter cold and cough remedies cause vasoconstriction of blood vessels, which may elevate blood pressure and therefore should be avoided. Herbal treatments may have unknown adverse effects, including potential harm to the fetus, and should be avoided.
- Hypoxemia associated with acute respiratory distress or pneumonia may cause fetal compromise, and chronic hypoxia may increase the risk for SGA.

Connective Tissue Disorders

These disorders are characterized by an autoimmune-mediated abnormality and include rheumatoid arthritis, multiple sclerosis, scleroderma, myasthenia gravis, and systemic lupus erythematosus (SLE). SLE has the most significant and serious consequences for the pregnant client, fetus, and infant.

Nursing Considerations
- When health teaching, emphasize the importance of adequate rest, especially with the increased metabolic demands of pregnancy. Teach the client to recognize the signs of preterm labour.
- Educate the client about antenatal fetal well-being monitoring techniques.

Cancers

The occurrence of pregnancy and cancer together during the child-bearing years represents a devastating time of fear and crisis for the client and their family. Although relatively rare, the incidence is rising because individuals are postponing pregnancy until later in life. Pregnancy is a growth event as the hormones of pregnancy work to prepare and sustain the client's body to support the pregnancy and developing fetus. Hormone-responsive cancers may also experience accelerated growth as a result (SOGC, 2022c).

Nursing Considerations
- A multidisciplinary approach in collaboration with the family is essential in all stages of treatment and care.
- Decisions regarding treatment options and continuing with the pregnancy are deeply personal and need to be supported and informed by the best available research.

Hypertension

Hypertension in pregnancy can be a pre-existing chronic condition or can be associated with the pregnancy itself. PIH, also known as *pre-eclampsia* and *eclampsia*, poses a more significant risk for the client and the fetus.

Chronic Hypertension Disorders
Chronic Hypertension
- Chronic hypertension is present before birth or evident prior to 20 weeks of gestation.

  Clients with chronic hypertension (or prepregnancy) hypertension may also be at risk for developing superimposed pre-eclampsia.
- Increases the risk for intrauterine growth delay, fetal still birth
- Preconception counseling recommended (Keenan-Lindsay et al., 2022)

Chronic Hypertension With Superimposed Pre-eclampsia:
- Chronic hypertension associated with pre-eclampsia
- Onset after 20 weeks' gestation
- Increase risk for severe maternal and fetal complications (Keenan-Lindsay et al., 2022)

Gestational Hypertension
- Hypertension develops as a complication of the pregnancy.
- Onset of hypertension without proteinuria and without changes in bloodwork occurs after 20 weeks of pregnancy.
- Gestational hypertension is not usually associated with fetal growth restriction.

- Most clients with gestational hypertension will develop few pregnancy complications, although up to 25% of clients will go on to develop pre-eclampsia (Keenan-Lindsay et al., 2022).

Pre-eclampsia

- Increase in blood pressure after 20 weeks of pregnancy with proteinuria in a pregnant client who had normal blood pressure prior to pregnancy or a client with pre-existing hypertension
- It may also be hypertension with a new onset of any of the following: thrombocytopenia, impaired liver function, renal insufficiency, pulmonary edema, or cerebral or visual issues (Lowdermilk et al., 2020).
- Increased risk for uteroplacental insufficiency and placental abruption and maternal complications

Eclampsia

- Development of seizures or coma not identifiable to other causes in a client with pre-eclampsia
- Seizures can occur antepartum, intrapartum, or postpartum
- Increase in maternal risk factors
- Increased complications for the fetus including placental abruption, preterm birth, acute hypoxia, and intrauterine growth restriction (IUGR) (Keenan-Lindsay et al., 2022).

Hypertensive Disorders of Pregnancy

Predisposing Factors

- Primigravida
- Adolescent or advanced client age: Younger than 18 years or older than 40 years
- Diabetes mellitus
- Chronic hypertension or chronic renal disease
- Multifetal pregnancy
- Previous or family history of hypertensive disorders of pregnancy (HDP)

Pathophysiology

Placental arteries do not widen as needed to increase placental perfusion, and the resulting ischemia leads to damage of all blood vessel walls. This damage results in generalized vasoconstriction, which leads to poor tissue perfusion, elevated blood pressure and damage to cell wall permeability, and fluid leakage and loss. Other consequential changes include the following:

- A decrease in placental perfusion (placental vascular insufficiency), renal blood flow, glomerular filtration rate, and oliguria
- Central nervous system (CNS) effects such as edema, cerebral hemorrhage, hyper-reflexia, and severe headache with progression to seizure activity

Clinical Manifestations

- Cardinal signs are hypertension, proteinuria, and obvious generalized edema after 20 weeks' gestation.
- Subjective signs are complaints of headache, photophobia, blurred or double vision, oliguria, nausea, and vomiting,

epigastric or right upper quadrant pain, hematuria, and severe headache.
- Pulmonary edema
  Manifestations quickly resolve following the birth of the infant within 48 hours.

Maternal and Fetal Risks

- Maternal risks: Placental abruption leading to hemorrhage or disseminated intravascular coagulation (DIC), maternal seizures, pulmonary edema, stroke, renal failure, and ruptured liver
- Fetal risks: SGA, prematurity, fetal hypoxia or demise, neonatal hypocalcemia

Diagnostics and Therapeutics

Diagnostics

- Nonsevere pre-eclampsia: Hypertension and proteinuria—If diastolic blood pressure is greater than 90 mm Hg and systolic blood pressure is greater than 140 mm Hg, monitor closely for diastolic hypertension; monitor for generalized edema of the face or hands, 1+ proteinuria, 1–2+ deep tendon reflexes, and adequate urine output.
- Severe pre-eclampsia: Monitor for blood pressure greater than 160–180/110 mm Hg, oliguria (less than 400 mL/24 hr), 2+ proteinuria, 3+ to 4+ deep tendon reflexes, visual disturbances, retinal detachment, severe headache, epigastric pain, pulmonary edema, generalized edema, and weight gain of more than 1 kg in 1 week.
- Eclampsia: Seizures or coma are preceded by severe headache, visual disturbances, epigastric pain, or right upper quadrant abdominal pain (Keenan-Lindsay et al., 2022).

Therapeutics for nonsevere pre-eclampsia

- Therapeutics include rest; fetal antenatal monitoring, including ultrasonography, nonstress testing (NST), and intrapartum monitoring; laboratory work-up for liver, blood, clotting factors, and renal function. Magnesium sulphate may be administered.

Therapeutics for severe pre-eclampsia

- Hospitalization includes advanced hemodynamic monitoring; an early birth is planned if symptoms worsen or the fetus is compromised; the fetus should be monitored.
- Antihypertensive therapy and magnesium sulphate ($MgSO_4$) are recommended.

Therapeutics for eclampsia

- A patent airway is maintained, head is turned to one side, and oxygen support is provided. Monitor time and duration of seizure as well as any urinary or fecal incontinence.
- A bolus amount of $MgSO_4$ is given, as well as diazepam (Valium), if needed. Vital signs, fetal monitoring, intake and output, and uterine activities are closely monitored-every 5 minutes while loading dose is being administered IV and then every hour during the infusion and until the client's condition stabilizes (Keenan-Lindsay et al., 2022). Vaginal birth is preferred when the child-bearing client has been stabilized.

Nursing Considerations

- Assess for worsening cardinal and other manifestations through careful monitoring and teach the pregnant client, if still at home, to assess blood pressure and urine protein.
- Diet should be high in protein and moderate in salt.
- Assess weight daily and carefully monitor fluid intake and output.
- Promote and teach methods to maximize uteroplacental circulation, including lying in the left or right lateral position.
- Monitor fetal well-being with FHR monitoring and NST.
- Promote rest and a quiet environment to minimize distress from cerebral manifestations.
- Observe for signs of placental abruption and be prepared for an emergency birth.
- Provide psychological support to all family members.

Diabetes Mellitus and Gestational Diabetes

Pregnancy is a diabetogenic event. The normal carbohydrate and hormonal changes that occur in the body during pregnancy create a situation that challenges the pancreas to produce more insulin while some of the hormones of pregnancy make the cells more resistant to the effects of insulin. For a client with pre-existing diabetes mellitus, pregnancy is a high-risk event requiring careful ongoing management. For other clients, the manifestations of diabetes will become apparent only during the pregnancy. In this situation, a diagnosis of gestational diabetes is made. For the client with gestational diabetes, the disease process stops after the birth of the infant, although they will carry a higher risk of developing type 2 diabetes later in life. In both types of diabetes, maternal risks are present, and the fetus and newborn are also at risk for complications and must be carefully monitored.

Pathophysiology

- Placental hormones cause an anti-insulin effect, allowing the fetus to receive the increased amounts of glucose in the first half of the pregnancy that it needs for growth and development. Maternal glucose crosses the placenta; maternal insulin does not.
- At around 20 weeks' gestation, the maternal pancreas is challenged to produce increasing amounts of insulin, which it normally does. A client with pre-existing diabetes cannot meet this challenge, and their symptoms of diabetes will worsen. In other clients, if the pancreas fails to match the increased demand for insulin, signs and symptoms of diabetes will appear.
- If the resulting hyperglycemia is not diagnosed or well controlled, the fetus will continue to receive high amounts of glucose, resulting in excessive growth. This creates added risk during labour and at the time of birth.
- The fetal pancreas produces increased amounts of insulin to match the high levels of glucose it is receiving. Following birth, the infant no longer receives high amounts of glucose, but the pancreas needs time to adjust and continues to produce large amounts of insulin. This can quickly lead to moderate to severe hypoglycemia in the newborn.

Clinical Manifestations

Maternal:
- In the first trimester, hypoglycemia is present.
- At around 20 weeks' gestation, the development of hyperglycemia and glucosuria, ketonuria, increased risk for urinary tract infections due to glucosuria, increased risk of PIH and spontaneous abortion if there is pre-existing diabetes, risk of polyhydramnios, risk of postpartum hemorrhage due to increased macrosomia.

Fetal:
- Risks include increased growth, LGA (over 4 kg), risk of congenital anomalies, preterm birth, birth trauma, and hypoglycemia.

Diagnostics and Therapeutics

- Monitor for glucosuria and ketonuria at all prenatal visits. Normal values are a fasting glucose level of 5.8 mmol/L or less. If the result is abnormally high, a three-hour oral glucose tolerance test is done with an oral load of glucose. Blood glucose levels are taken hourly for 3 hours, which exceeds normal limits; a diagnosis of impaired glucose tolerance (IGT) is made.
- Management includes consultation between the pregnant client, dietitian, endocrinologist, obstetrician, pediatrician, and nurse.
- Frequent monitoring of blood glucose levels, up to four times daily, and administration of insulin injections to maintain a normal glucose level. A dietary plan is developed with the dietitian.
- Additional, frequent prenatal visits and possible planned earlier delivery at 37 to 38 weeks' gestation, depending on NST results and maternal well-being. Morbidity and mortality are lowest if the birth takes place as close to term as possible.
- Fetal monitoring may include additional ultrasonograms, NST, biophysical profile, amniocentesis, an alpha-fetoprotein test, and electronic fetal monitoring during labour.
- During labour and birth, the labouring person is kept nothing by mouth (NPO), and an intravenous (IV) with 5% glucose is used to maintain normal serum glucose levels. Insulin is given as needed. Postpartum, insulin requirements decrease, especially for the first 48 hours.
- Breastfeeding is encouraged as it lowers the amount of insulin required.
- The newborn is monitored closely for respiratory distress and hypoglycemia. Care in a level 2 or 3 nursery may be required.

Nursing Considerations

- Know that because oral hypoglycemics cross the placenta, they are considered teratogenic and are not used in the first trimester. Glyburides are used in later trimesters. Injectable insulin is the preferred medication to decrease blood glucose levels during pregnancy since oral hypoglycemics require supplemental insulin injections to maintain blood glucose control (Keenan-Lindsay, 2020).

- Teach the pregnant client the manifestations of hyperglycemia and insulin reaction and measures to take for each.
- Support and encourage adherence to and diligence in glucose testing, insulin self-administration, dietary control, balancing rest and activity levels, accurate record-keeping, and follow-up visits to specialists.
- Provide information and support for additional tests monitoring fetal well-being.
- Prepare the client and family for a possible earlier planned birth and the potential need for Caesarean birth.
- Observe for signs of hypoglycemia in the newborn, including lethargy, jitteriness, poor sucking reflex, and a blood glucose level of less than 2 to 2.5 mmol/L.
- Observe the newborn for signs of respiratory distress, birth trauma, hypothermia, and possible congenital anomalies.
- Promote and support breastfeeding as the ideal feeding option for clients with diabetes.

PREGNANCY COMPLICATIONS

Adolescent Pregnancy

The teen pregnancy rate continues to decline in Canada (Lowdermilk et al., 2020). Pregnancy during the teen years presents many life challenges and interrupts the normal developmental tasks of adolescence. Pregnant adolescents and their newborns are at an increased risk for complications; the younger the teen, the higher the risk. All the determinants of health need to be addressed during and after the pregnancy, and if the young parent chooses to raise their child, community support is essential.

Risk Factors

- Obstetrical: Premature birth; high risk of PIH, anemia, and poor nutrition; lack of knowledge about the harm of using tobacco and alcohol; poor prenatal care if the pregnancy is hidden; cephalopelvic disproportion; SGA infants; postpartum hemorrhage
- Psychosocial: Lack of partner and family support, interruption to education, feelings of isolation and fear, lack of knowledge and life experience to manage changes and transitions, risk of poor coping strategies, lack of community support in isolated areas with minimal resources, negative attitudes and judgement from others
- Socioeconomic: Unless community support through services directed at adolescent parents is available and accessible, teen parents are at risk for not completing high school or progressing to postsecondary education, low earning potential, lack of affordable housing, continued social isolation, chronic stress and poor self-esteem, and increased risk of inadequate nutrition for themselves and their child.

Nursing Considerations

- Provide collaborative, early intervention and prenatal care that focuses on the young client's strengths in a trusting and supportive environment of care. Assess the adolescent's maturity, coping strategies, health history, and support systems, both available and needed. Use a collaborative approach to decision making and planning for the birth of the baby and understanding the demands of the pregnancy.
- Identify the needs of the adolescent and their obstetrical risk factors.
- Arrange referral to community resources and programs for teen parents, including those sponsored by Health Canada. Needs may include programs for prenatal nutrition; healthy-baby programs; parenting programs; social services for housing, child care, and employment; and educational opportunities to finish high school.
- Provide counselling and nonjudgemental support to assist the new parent with postpartum decisions regarding appropriate birth control options.

Advanced Maternal Age

Clients who become pregnant after 35 years of age have increased risks for complications during pregnancy and labour. There is an increased risk of ectopic pregnancy, miscarriage, placenta previa, pregestational diabetes, eclampsia, gestational hypertension, Caesarean birth, and induction of labour. If fertility medications were used, potential risk for multiple pregnancies is increased, which increase fetal risks. Special tests during pregnancy may be ordered such as chorionic villi sampling and amniocentesis if there is a greater risk for congenital anomaly (Keenan-Lindsay, 2020).

Miscarriage (Spontaneous Abortion)

A miscarriage is the natural termination of the pregnancy before viability is established, which is usually at 20 weeks' gestation or a fetal weight of less than 500 g. Early miscarriage occurs in the first 12 weeks of pregnancy. The term *miscarriage* is a more therapeutic term to use than *spontaneous abortion* especially for grieving parents and families (Lowdermilk et al., 2020).

Pathophysiology

- Maternal factors: Infection, cervical insufficiency, failure of the placenta to develop or implant normally, trauma, teratogenic exposure
- Fetal factors: Genetic or developmental abnormality, faulty implantation into endometrium

Clinical Manifestations

- Threatened: No cervical dilatation, cramping, vaginal spotting or bleeding; the pregnancy may or may not terminate
- Imminent or inevitable: Bleeding, cramping, with cervical dilatation
- Incomplete: Bleeding, expulsion of only some of the products of conception
- Complete: All products of conception expelled
- Missed abortion: Embryo or fetal death without cervical dilatation, cramping, or bleeding; no FHR detected; a negative pregnancy test
- Recurrent pregnancy loss: Three or more consecutive miscarriages

Diagnostics and Therapeutics

- Threatened: Rest, avoidance of sexual intercourse, restricted activities
- Incomplete: Outpatient day surgery for dilation and evacuation (D&E) or vacuum extraction.
- Missed abortion: Vaginal or abdominal ultrasound, hCG hormone test, D&E to remove products of conception; if the missed abortion is between 16 and 20 weeks, induction of labour may be required with prostaglandins
- Complete: No medical treatment is necessary; emotional support and follow-up provided
- Recurrent pregnancy loss: Referral for infertility investigation, possible surgical intervention for incompetent cervix

Grief reactions to the loss of the pregnancy include shock, disbelief, sadness, anger, depression, and fear for fertility and the future ability to carry a pregnancy.

Nursing Considerations

- Provide an injection of Rh-immune globulin (Rhogam) to any pregnant client who is Rh-negative to prevent a maternal immune antibody response.
- Know that for each client, a pregnancy has very individual meaning and significance. Support the client's emotional reaction and response; dispel any feelings of blame or guilt.
- Teach what to expect with either natural completion of the miscarriage process or operative D&E or vacuum extraction procedures.
- Assess vital signs and vaginal bleeding; provide pain relief and emotional support.

- Refer as appropriate to community resources for follow-up counselling, including local grief support and infertility groups.

Placenta Previa
Pathophysiology

- The placenta implants in the lower uterus, at or near the internal os at the cervix, instead of the top one-third of the uterine fundus. The cause is unknown. This condition affects about 1 in 200 pregnancies, and the following risk factors have been identified: multiparity, previous Caesarean birth or uterine surgery, previous placenta previa, tobacco use, and maternal age greater than 35 years. Figure 10.2A depicts placentia previa.
- Close to term, around 30 weeks' gestation or later, placental villi become separated from the uterine wall as the uterus contracts and the cervix thins and dilates.
- Placenta previa is classified by the position of the placenta:
  - Total or complete: The placenta completely covers the internal os.
  - Partial or incomplete: The placenta covers some of the internal os.
  - Low-lying or marginal: The placenta reaches but does not cover the internal os.

Clinical Manifestations

Placenta previa manifests as painless, bright red vaginal bleeding with a uterus that is soft and relaxed or relaxes between contractions.

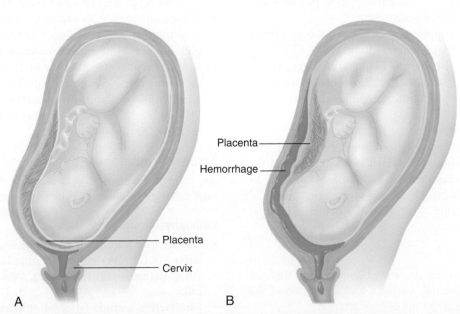

Placenta

Hemorrhage

Placenta

Cervix

A   B

Fig. 10.2 Placenta previa and placental abruption. A. Placenta previa: The placenta is situated in a lower position within the uterus. Separation of the placenta from the uterine wall takes place when the cervix dilates, leading to bleeding. B. Placenta abruption: The placenta is initially implanted in its usual position within the uterus but then detaches from the uterine wall. If the fetal head is engaged, bleeding may accumulate within the uterus rather then being discharged externally. (From Patton, K. T., & Thibodeau, G. A. [2015]. Anatomy & physiology [9th ed.]. St. Louis: Mosby.)

Diagnostics and Therapeutics

- Many low-lying placenta previas are commonly detected on early antenatal ultrasonograms and resolve by term as the uterus elongates. Repeat ultrasonography in the third trimester is needed for confirmation of true placenta previa. The need for Caesarean birth is determined by the classification of the previa, the amount of vaginal bleeding, and fetal well-being.
- In unconfirmed placenta previa, vaginal examination may be deferred until emergency operative interventions are in place.
- The decision to allow a vaginal birth is based on ultrasound findings, which locate the placenta.
- Outpatient management may be used if the client is stable, home support is available, bed rest is an option, and there is proximity to the hospital with readily available transportation and telephone access (Lowdermilk et al., 2020).
- If blood loss is significant or worsens, interventions must include maternal resuscitation for blood loss and shock. Immediate delivery must be done to treat fetal distress due to hypoxia.
- Blood typing, cross-match, and available blood products for maternal resuscitation are needed.

Nursing Considerations

- Reinforce the need for bed rest and accurate pad counts to monitor bleeding. Teach the client to report immediately any changes in condition.
- Ensure that clients who are discharged home prior to labour and birth understand and are able to adhere to outpatient management. Sexual intercourse is contraindicated.
- Observe for signs of shock and be prepared to insert a large-bore IV catheter to administer blood products and proceed to emergency operative birth.
- Provide emotional support and an opportunity to discuss fears and anticipatory grieving response.
- Monitor for fetal well-being and FHR and conduct an NST; birth will be delayed, if possible, to allow for fetal lung maturity. Steroids may be given to advance lung maturity.

Placental Abruption

Placental abruption occurs when a normally implanted placenta prematurely separates or partially separates in the second half of pregnancy or during labour. Abruption is an emergency situation with a high risk of maternal and fetal morbidity and mortality. Figure 10.2B. depicts placental abruption.

Pathophysiology

- The exact cause or causes are unknown, but theories include the degeneration, necrosis, and separation of the placental arterioles at the site of implantation.
- The bleeding can be concealed (no vaginal bleeding) due to formation of retroplacental clot.
- Risk factors include primary hypertension or PIH, multiparity, abdominal trauma short umbilical cord, previous

Caesarean birth, large placenta, smoking, vasoconstrictive drugs, decompression of overdistended uterus, delivery of first twin, and older pregnant clients.
- Complete abruption with massive hemorrhage can lead to complications including fetal demise, maternal shock, DIC, and death.

Clinical Manifestations

- Sudden, intense pain with or without bright red vaginal bleeding
- Concealed bleeding within the uterus
- A hard uterus that does not relax between contractions
- Sudden onset of acute, severe fetal compromise
- Signs of maternal shock with tachycardia, hypotension, cold clammy skin, pallor, loss of consciousness

Diagnostics and Therapeutics

- Often this is an obstetrical emergency, and interventions may be initiated based on clinical findings without confirmation by ultrasound, especially if maternal and fetal compromise is present. If maternal and fetal vital signs are stable, an ultrasound may be used to confirm bleeding but not to diagnose concealed abruption.
- Immediate birth is planned for, vaginal or Caesarean, depending on the stage and progression of labour.
- Nursing staff need to be prepared for the possible resuscitation of the pregnant person and infant.

Nursing Considerations

- Key consideration:
  - Note the distinguishing difference between placenta previa (painless) and placental abruption (painful) bleeding in your immediate assessment.
- Initiate emergency measures to assist in prompt resuscitation efforts and emergency birth: establish an IV and administer volume expansion fluids, administer oxygen 6 to 8 L/min at 100%, monitor FHR continuously, perform ultrasonography if time and condition allow, cross-match and administer blood when necessary (prn).
- Provide information and support to the client and family members.

Ectopic Pregnancy

An ectopic pregnancy occurs when the fertilized ovum implants itself in a location outside the uterine endometrium.

Pathophysiology

- Implantation can occur anywhere, including the abdominal cavity, but, overwhelmingly, implantation occurs in the fallopian tube, mainly on the right side, for reasons that are unknown.
- Risk factors include fallopian tube damage secondary to pelvic inflammatory disease, STIs, structural abnormalities, tumours, scarring and partial obstruction, IUD contraceptive, endometriosis, history of ectopic pregnancy, tobacco use, maternal age greater than 35 years.

Clinical Manifestations

- Early rupture: The client experiences a missed menstrual period or a delayed or abnormal period, signs and symptoms of early pregnancy and positive pregnancy test, abdominal tenderness over lower abdomen.
- Rupture: If the fallopian tube ruptures, acute lower quadrant abdominal pain occurs, often on the right side, along with referred shoulder pain, low-grade fever, and possible shock due to blood loss.

Diagnostics and Therapeutics

- Careful history-taking is important, as manifestations mimic other conditions, including appendicitis, ovarian cyst, and urinary tract infection.
- Pelvic examination and ultrasonography confirm the ectopic pregnancy; laparoscopic surgery is used to remove the products of conception, possibly repair or remove the fallopian tube, and control bleeding.
- Medical management: Systemic methotrexate may be considered for unruptured or chronic ectopic pregnancies as it destroys the pregnancy over several weeks while preserving the fallopian tube.
- Surgical management: depends on tissue involvement, cause and location of the ectopic implantation and childbearing client's plans for future fertility. Various surgical options include salpingectomy or salpingostomy.

Nursing Considerations

- Be sure to take menstrual history carefully; in particular, take note of missed or unusual menstrual periods, use of IUD, or history of STIs or infections.
- Observe for signs of shock and prepare for surgery.
- Offer support and counselling, as often the client may not have been aware a pregnancy had occurred. Encourage the client to share their feelings and concerns related to the loss. The client may require a referral to a grief or infertility support group.
- Be aware that a pregnant client with an Rh-negative blood type must have Rh-immune globulin administered to prevent blood incompatibility antibody formation.

Hyperemesis Gravidarum

This condition of severe, unrelenting nausea and vomiting occurs in about 0.3–3% of pregnancies and greatly impacts the quality of life of the client affected.

Pathophysiology

This condition is poorly understood and likely related to many factors. Theories have included high levels of circulating hCG. It is also associated with multifetal gestation and hydatidiform molar pregnancy.

Clinical Manifestations

- Physiological aspects: Symptoms include persistent vomiting that leads to a 5% prepregnancy weight loss with associated electrolyte balance and ketonuria. The client may show symptoms of dehydration such as decreased blood pressure, increased pulse, and poor skin turgor (Keenan-Lindsay et al., 2022).
- Psychosocial aspects: Anxiety, worry, exhaustion, and depression related to quality-of-life issues, including absence from employment and relationship and family stress. The severity of the personal impact has led some clients to consider or undertake elective termination of the pregnancy.

Diagnostics and Therapeutics

- Diagnosis is made on the basis of history-taking and presenting manifestations, including confirmation by blood electrolytes, urinalysis and weight loss confirmation.
- Oral pharmacological interventions considered safe for use in pregnancy include doxylamine–pyridoxine combination as the standard of care. Other medications may be used for breakthrough episodes or as adjunct therapy.
- Corticosteroids are avoided, if possible, in the first trimester due to their teratogenic effect.

Nursing Considerations

- Provide information and reassurance regarding current pharmacological interventions.
- Know that supportive therapies may include ginger, acupuncture, acupressure, and meditation.
- Encourage dietary and lifestyle changes that support the client's choices in choosing foods that are appealing.
- Know that early recognition and prompt treatment can restore metabolic balance and quality of life.
- Provide accurate intake and output; monitor weight, assess for fetal well-being.
- Offer reassurance and counselling to address psychosocial distress, fears, and concerns.
- Refer to social services as appropriate if hospitalization is prolonged.

Teratogens and Substance Use

A *teratogen* is any agent, drug, toxin, chemical, or infection that can harm the developing embryo or fetus. Depending on molecular size and fat solubility, many, if not most, substances cross the placenta. During the embryonic stage of development in the first trimester, exposure to teratogens can have devastating consequences for the developing embryo, resulting in spontaneous abortion, congenital defects, or death. Even with over-the-counter and prescription medications, teratogenic effects are still poorly understood, and decisions to use medications must be made balancing the risks and benefits to maternal and fetal well-being. A few commonly used teratogenic substances and their effects are described next.

Alcohol

- The severity of fetal effects is influenced by development at the time of exposure, genetic sensitivity, and quantity of alcohol exposure. No safe amount of alcohol consumption is known.

- Adverse effects of fetal alcohol spectrum disorder (FASD) and fetal alcohol syndrome (FAS) include congenital defects, including craniofacial deformities, skeletal abnormalities, cardiac anomalies, moderate to severe intellectual and development delays, recurrent ear infections, neurodevelopmental disorders including impulsivity, attention-deficit/hyperactivity disorder (ADHD), and short-term memory impairment. These anomalies persist into adulthood with ongoing negative outcomes and adverse effects on quality of life.
- The newborn may exhibit irritability, a high-pitched cry, inconsolability, jitteriness, and poor suckling and feeding.
- Other consequences include increased risk for miscarriage, still birth, sudden infant death syndrome (SIDS), and preterm birth.
- Nursing considerations include careful antenatal assessment and teaching that no amount of alcohol is safe. Screen for alcohol use. Referral to community agencies and ongoing support to stop drinking should be provided. Referral should be made to FAS follow-up programs and provision made for long-term support for newborn effects.

Tobacco

- Nicotine in tobacco products, inhaled via smoking or exposure to second-hand smoke, is a powerful alkaloid vasoconstrictor that can affect uteroplacental blood flow.
- Fetal effects include prematurity, SGA, increased incidence of childhood asthma, ADHD, neurodevelopmental disorders and increased risk of SIDS.

Cocaine

- Cocaine is a powerful vasoconstrictor that leads to decreased cardiac output, uteroplacental insufficiency, and an increased level of fetal neurotransmitters.
- Maternal effects include onset of premature labour, risk of spontaneous abortion, cardiovascular failure, hypertensive crisis, seizures, and placental abruption.
- Fetal complications include prematurity, SGA, IUGR, brain damage, cardiac anomalies, CNS abnormalities including cerebral infarcts, and fetal compromise.
- Neonatal complications include neurobehavioural abnormalities at birth, including hyper-reflexia, high-pitched cry, extreme sensitivity to environmental stimuli, poor feeding, diarrhea, and an increased risk for SIDS.

Marijuana

- Derived from the cannabis plant and can be either smoked or eaten. Considered more harmful if smoked. Cannabis crosses the placenta and causes increased maternal carbon monoxide blood levels, which decreases the fetal oxygen supply.
- Cannabis is considered one of the most commonly used substances during pregnancy.
- Fetal complications include preterm birth, SGA, hyperactivity in childhood, IUGR.

- Since the legalization of cannabis in 2018, further research is required to determine the newborn and long-term effects on child development (Keenan-Lindsay et al., 2022).

Prescription Medications

SOGC (2022b) recommends that pregnant persons should not take medications during pregnancy, ideally. If medication is prescribed for a diagnosed medical condition, the decision to continue needs to be made on an individual basis.

FETAL EVALUATION AND MONITORING

Essentials of Fetal Evaluation

Some of the most frequently used tests to assess for fetal well-being in the antenatal and intrapartum periods are described next. Daily monitoring of fetal movements starting at 26 to 32 weeks should be done in clients at risk for adverse outcomes. The contraction stress test is used when biophysical profile is not accessible.

Nonstress Test (NST)

The fetal brain is extremely sensitive to the amount of oxygen it receives. Any maternal condition that adversely affects blood and oxygen supply to the placenta can lead to fetal hypoxia and distress. A sign that the fetus is receiving enough oxygen for the CNS to respond normally is seen when the FHR increases in response to fetal activity. This is considered a reassuring sign of fetal well-being. This ability to respond is assessed during an NST. When the fetus does not respond as expected, it may be an indication of acute or chronic conditions of hypoxia.

An NST is indicated for any high-risk maternal condition that may cause uteroplacental insufficiency, including hypertension, hypertension in pregnancy (HDP), renal disease, diabetes, cardiac disease, or multiple gestation. Also, if the pregnant client reports decreased fetal activity, an NST may be used along with ultrasound to assess well-being. This test is also part of the biophysical profile test.

Nursing considerations

- Educate the client about the purpose and procedure; the test is completed in 30 to 45 minutes and is noninvasive and not painful.
- Be aware that occasionally, the fetus will be sleeping and nonactive. In that case, the test may have to be repeated. The client should be reassured that this is not uncommon.

Ultrasonography

High-frequency sound waves are painlessly transmitted via a vaginal or abdominal transducer. Sound waves reflect different body tissue densities and are displayed on a monitor. This diagnostic tool is widely used to assess the status of the pregnancy and fetal growth and well-being.

- First-trimester indications: If used before 20 weeks' gestation, fetal gestational age can be calculated within 3 days' accuracy by measuring crown–rump length and biparietal skull diameters. Ultrasound at 8 to 12 weeks is most accurate.

- Second- and third-trimester indications: Ultrasound is used to assess placental location, source of vaginal bleeding, polyhydramnios, congenital anomalies, fetal presentation and position.
- Procedure: Before 20 weeks' gestation, the pregnant person drinks enough fluids (1–2 litres) to have a full bladder to lift the uterus up out of the pelvis for better visualization. Gel is applied to the abdomen with the client lying on their back. It takes about 20 minutes to complete the test. Ultrasonography is widely used because to date no harmful effects have been found. It is considered inappropriate to use ultrasound to view the fetus to only determine the gender (Government of Canada, 2019).

Amniocentesis

This is a test used to obtain a sample of amniotic fluid for biochemical and genetic analysis. It is performed at 15 to 17 weeks' gestation when enough amniotic fluid is available to sample. Clinical trials using early amniocentesis before 12 weeks' gestation showed increased risk of complications and spontaneous abortion. In Canada, the test is not performed before 15 weeks' gestation.

- Indications: Amniocentesis is indicated for pregnant clients over 35, karyotyping assessment for chromosomal abnormalities, assessing bilirubin levels, assessing alpha-fetoprotein levels, and assessing fetal lung maturity.
- Procedure: The client is prepped and empties their bladder, and abdominal ultrasonography is used to locate a pocket of amniotic fluid and avoid fetal and placental structures. By needle aspiration, 15 to 20 mL of amniotic fluid is removed. The pregnant client and fetus are monitored throughout the procedure.
- Complications: They are less than 1% but may include spontaneous abortion, hemorrhage, Rh isoimmunization, infection, fetal injury, leaking of amniotic fluid, and premature rupture of membranes. The client may experience mild cramping postprocedure.
  - Rh-immune globulin is administered to Rh-negative clients to prevent antibody formation.

LABOUR AND BIRTH PROCESSES

The intrapartum period, composed of four stages, begins with the onset of regular, true contractions that result in cervical dilatation and end with the recovery and stabilization of the client and infant following the birth.

Factors That Affect the Labour Process

The five factors, also known as the *five P's*, are the passageway, the passenger, the powers, position of labouring client, and the psychological response of the client.

The Passageway

The passageway is made up of the maternal structures of the pelvis and soft tissues that the fetus must navigate through in the process of being born.

- Bony pelvis: Of the four types of pelvis (android, anthropoid, platypelloid, and gynecoid), the gynecoid pelvis is the most common (50%) and is ideally suited in its shape and dimensions to accommodate the movements of the fetus toward birth.
- Soft tissues: The lower uterus, cervix, vaginal canal, and introitus (opening) must all thin, stretch, and open to allow the fetus to pass through.

The Passenger

The fetus, or passenger, travels through the passage with an ease or degree of difficulty that is influenced by several factors:

- Fetal head size: The skull of the fetus is made up of bony plates connected by unfused suture lines and two fontanelles. The anterior and posterior fontanelles can be palpated vaginally to help determine the position and presentation of the fetus. The fetal skull can fit through the bony pelvis with the help of a slight overlapping of the bones, called *moulding*, during labour. Following birth, the head resumes its normal shape within a few days.
- Fetal lie: This describes the relationship between the long axis of the pregnant client and the long axis of the fetus. Normal lie for a vaginal birth is longitudinal.
- Fetal presentation: The bony part of the fetus that presents or enters the pelvic inlet first. A cephalic, or head, presentation occurs in 97% of births. A breech presentation occurs in about 3%.
- Fetal attitude: The relationship of fetal body parts to each other. A normal attitude is one of moderate flexion, with the fetal chin tucked in toward the chest. A flexed attitude ideally allows for the smallest diameter of the head, the suboccipito-bregmatic diameter, to enter the true pelvis. The biparietal diameter of the fetal head is the widest diameter.
- Fetal position: The relationship of the bony presenting part of the fetus to the four quadrants of the maternal pelvis. Using three letters, the position indicates if the presenting part (occiput, sacrum) is to the right or left of and anterior or posterior to the pelvis. *ROA* (right occipitoanterior) means that the occiput is facing toward the front and right of the pelvis. Posterior positions may result in persistent back pain during labour and a more prolonged labour.
- Engagement: This occurs when the largest transverse diameter (usually the biparietal) of the presenting part has passed through the pelvic inlet and into the true pelvis. Engagement can be determined by vaginal examination. For the primipara, engagement may occur a few weeks before the onset of labour.
- Station: Station is the relationship of the presenting part to the ischial spines of the maternal pelvis. The ischial spines are designated as station zero; above the spines is noted as a negative number from 1 to 5 cm and below is plus 1 to 5 cm. Station is assessed during a vaginal examination. Birth is imminent at +4 or +5 cm.

The Powers

Primary powers. These are the involuntary uterine contractions, measured by their frequency, duration, and intensity as they thin and dilate the cervix. Contractions are initiated by pacemaker points at the top of the fundus and radiate down over the uterus in rhythmic waves.

- The relaxation phase (minimum 60 seconds) between contractions is essential for restoring blood flow to the uterus and placenta.
- Frequency is measured as the time from the beginning of one contraction to the beginning of the next contraction. For example, contractions can be 3 minutes apart in frequency.
- Duration is the length a contraction lasts in seconds. Normal contractions last a maximum of 90 seconds in duration. After 90 seconds, there is a risk of fetal compromise and hypoxia.
- Intensity indicates the strength of the contraction, assessed by palpating the firmness of the uterus, and is recorded as mild, moderate, or strong.
- Effacement is measured as a percentage from 0 to 100%. During a contraction, the upper half of the uterus shortens and pulls up the lower uterine segment, stretching and thinning the cervix until only a thin edge can be palpated. In primiparas, effacement is quite advanced by the time contractions begin. In multiparas, effacement and dilatation occur together.
- Dilatation is the opening of the cervix and cervical canal from less than 1 cm to full dilatation, about 10 cm. Full dilatation marks the end of stage 1 of labour.

    Secondary powers. When the cervix is completely dilated, the secondary powers are an important aid in assisting with the descent of the fetus through the birth canal. When the presenting part of the fetus descends to the pelvic floor, the contractions become expulsive. The client experiences the urge to "bear down," which is the secondary power and is additional help in expelling the fetus.
- Uterine contractions continue.
- The client feels an overwhelming urge to bear down and push, contracting their abdominal muscles and diaphragm with each contraction.
- Maternal position can aid the secondary powers. Being in an upright or squatting position improves uterine blood flow and uses gravity to help with the descent and birth of the fetus.

Position of the Labouring Client

- Position affects the child-bearing client's anatomical and physiological adaptions to labour.
- Frequent position changes decrease discomfort, fatigue, and improves circulation. It is important for the labouring client to be encouraged to find positions that are most comfortable for them.
- An upright position (walking, sitting, kneeling, or squatting) may be beneficial in assisting the descent of the fetus. Uterine contractions are generally stronger and more efficient in effacing and dilating the cervix when in an upright position, resulting in a shorter labour (Keenan-Lindsay et al., 2022).
- Positioning for second-stage labour may be choosing the position that the client would like but choices are limited

by their condition, the fetus, the environment, and the health care provider's confidence in assisting in a birth in a specific position (Lowdermilk et al., 2020).

Psychological Response

This important factor encompasses all the psychosocial influences, past experiences, preparation, hopes, and beliefs the client brings to the labour and birth experience. This event and the support they receive will impact the memories and beliefs they will integrate into their life after the experience. Supporting, educating, and collaborating with the client and family during all stages of the labour and birth process are essential parts of the nursing role.

Pain Management During Labour and Birth

Intrapartum pain is complex and has both physiological and psychological components. Uterine contractions cause visceral hypoxic pain, while traction, pressure, and stretching can also cause various pain sensations to be felt. The client's previous experience with pain and their coping strategies, fears, support systems, and beliefs about their control over the pain will also influence their perception of pain. The goal of pain management is to collaborate with the client in finding measures that provide comfort and superior pain relief that is safe and appropriate to the stage of labour. The need for pharmacological agents is often reduced when timely information is provided about the progress of labour and supportive comfort measures are used.

Alternatives to pharmacological pain relief can include breathing techniques, walking or rocking motions, warm showers, hypnosis, meditation, effleurage, transcutaneous electrical nerve stimulation (TENS), therapeutic touch, and acupuncture.

It is important for nurses to understand how the child-bearing client's and, their partner and family's cultural background may affect the child-bearing client's response to pain. Understanding their beliefs, values, practices, and expectations may help the nurse understand how they perceive, interpret, manage, and respond to pain. This will help the nurse provide appropriate pain relief measures that support the child-bearing client's sense of control and self-confidence. The client's respond to pain may not reflect the intensity of pain being experienced, so the nurse must continue to assess the physiological aspects of pain and their verbal responses to describe the sensory and affective qualities of pain. It is important for the nurse to remember that pain is individualized and subjective for each client (Keenan-Lindsay et al., 2022).

Pharmacological Interventions

- Systemic opioids such as morphine sulphate provide pain relief and mild sedation; however, they cross the placenta, causing fetal CNS depression. They are avoided if birth is anticipated within 2 to 3 hours.
- Barbiturates and tranquilizers are not recommended for use in labour as they cross the placenta, cannot be reversed, and have a long half-life that may lead to respiratory and CNS depression in the client and newborn.

- General anaesthesia is used less often for emergency Caesarean births. Maternal aspiration is a risk. Fetal CNS depression (including bradycardia, respiratory depression) may result from the drugs used and can be reversed with a narcotic antagonist.
- Regional anaesthesia usually provides very effective pain relief without affecting the client's level of consciousness. Narcotic and anaesthetic agents are injected into a localized area and block the transmission of sensory nerve impulses to the brain. Limitations include only achieving partial pain relief, nerve damage (rare), and the need for skilled administration and careful monitoring for potential adverse effects.
- Regional anaesthesia methods include local infiltration of perineal tissues, pudendal block of perineal pain via local injection near the nerve plexus beside the ischial spines of the pelvis, and epidural block. In 2018–19 in Canada, the percentage of births using epidural anaesthesia varied among the provinces. About 73.5% of vaginal births in Quebec and Ontario (61.7%) were preceded by an epidural, as compared to rates of 44.1% in British Columbia and in Manitoba (38.8%) (Keenan-Lindsay et al., 2022).

Epidural Regional Anaesthesia

The anaesthetic agent is usually administered when the client is in active labour. Injection is performed by a skilled anaesthetist into the lumbar epidural space between L2 and L3 or L3 and L4. Dermatome testing is done to assess for pain and respiratory distress. Epidural anaesthesia can be used for vaginal or Caesarean births.

- Preparation: Consent is obtained, an IV is established, and vital signs are recorded. A bolus of fluid is often given to increase maternal circulating volume and prevent hypotension. The client is positioned in a curled side-lying or upright position leaning over to open the epidural spaces for maximum exposure. The nurse supports the client in holding still during the needle insertion and alerts the physician to the onset of any contractions. If the catheter is left in place, it is securely taped to the client's back.
- Monitoring: Pain relief is often obtained within 5 to 10 minutes, and the client will experience a heaviness and numbness of the abdomen and legs. Turning the client from one side to the other may help with even distribution of pain relief. Maternal vital signs and FHR are monitored frequently (every 2–5 minutes initially) for hypotension and adverse effects.
- Complications: Although very rare, they may include inadvertent puncture of the dura with leakage of cerebrospinal fluid and respiratory distress. Injection into a vein rarely occurs but may result in seizures, loss of consciousness, cardiovascular collapse, and even death.
- Current recommendations for child-bearing clients with low back tattoos are that they should not be denied an epidural, although direct tattoo puncture should be avoided, if possible, as there is a potential for the epidural to be ineffective (Keenan-Lindsay et al., 2022).

Nursing Considerations

- Discuss and plan for comfort and pain management strategies early in the labour process based on assessment findings and the wishes of the client.
- Be aware that effective support includes promoting open communication, providing anticipatory teaching, offering praise and encouragement, and providing information about the progress of labour.
- Prepare the client for the administration of any pharmacological agents and continuously monitor the client and fetus for any potential adverse effects. Document all findings.
- Assist with epidural block by positioning the client during the procedure, securing a continuous epidural line, establishing IV access, administering fluids, monitoring volumetric solution changes, especially hypotension, monitoring contractions and FHR, assessing the effectiveness of pain relief, assessing for bladder distension, and monitoring the progress of labour.
- Have emergency equipment and narcotic antagonists such as naloxone (Narcan) available to reduce the effects of CNS depression if narcotic analgesics have been used.
- Evaluate the effectiveness of the pain management plan and modify strategies as needed.

Intrapartum Fetal Monitoring

Assessment of the FHR is the accepted standard of care to assess for fetal well-being and detect fetal compromise during active labour (Keenan-Lindsay, 2020). FHR can be assessed using noninvasive periodic auscultation with a stethoscope or electronic transducer or via continuous electronic FHR monitoring devices. All have their advantages and disadvantages. The most appropriate and least invasive means is used to provide the information needed for optimal care of the client and the fetus during labour.

Intermittent Auscultation of FHR

This is the preferred method of FHR monitoring for persons in active labour with no identified fetal or maternal risks (Lowdermilk et al., 2020).

- The FHR is heard best over the fetal back via Leopold's manoeuvres (abdominal palpation). These manoeuvres help to identify the number of fetuses; the presenting part, fetal lie, and fetal attitude; the degree of descent of the presenting part into the pelvis; and expected location of the point of maximal intensity of the FHR on the client's abdomen. Take the maternal pulse at the same time to ensure the fetal pulse is not the pregnant client's.
- Fetoscope or Doppler transducer: Listen for 1 full minute; apply gel to the client's abdomen when using a transducer to improve sound wave transmission.

Continuous Electronic FHR Monitoring

This method is used to monitor the response of and relationship between the FHR and the uterine contractions.

- Indications: It is used in high-risk pregnancies with a risk of uteroplacental insufficiency, apparent signs of fetal compromise, or oxytocin induction in labour.

- External monitoring: A flexible disc attached to an elastic belt, called a *tocotransducer*, is strapped over the fundus to detect and monitor contractions, but does not accurately measure uterine intensity or resting tone. An intrauterine pressure catheter measures uterine pressure. A second transducer is placed over the fetal back to assess FHR.
- Internal monitoring (scalp clip): This method is used when electronic fetal monitoring patterns are not reassuring. The scalp clip can only be applied to the fetal scalp if the amniotic membranes are ruptured, the cervix is at least 2 cm dilated, and the fetal position and presentation are known.
  - Advantages: Allows ongoing assessment and early intervention for signs of fetal distress during active labour; potential decrease in fetal morbidity and mortality
  - Disadvantages: Potential interference with the labour process due to restriction on the client's activity, inaccurate interpretation and increased risk for medical and surgical interventions, including Caesarean birth, increased risk of infection with scalp clip monitoring, false reassurance, or increased fears and anxiety regarding fetal well-being

Baseline FHR Patterns

- Baseline FHR is 110 to 160 bpm over 10 minutes.
- Fetal tachycardia is a rate greater than 160 bpm over a 10-minute period. The tachycardia may be related to maternal anxiety, infection, or prematurity or may indicate distress if accompanied by other changes in FHR patterns, such as poor variability.
- Fetal bradycardia is an FHR of less than 110 bpm for 10 minutes. The bradycardia may be related to maternal hypotension, fetal hypoxia, placental separation, or cord compression. Bradycardia associated with poor variability and late deceleration patterns requires clinical assessment. It may be necessary to prepare for an early delivery.

Variability

FHR variability is the term used to describe the normal small fluctuations in heartbeat rate observed over 1 minute. The average FHR variability is 6 to 25 bpm. Count maternal and fetus pulse. Variability that is absent or minimal (≤5 bpm) for 40 minutes is atypical and requires ongoing close monitoring. If this pattern continues for greater than 80 minutes, immediate intervention is needed.

Periodic Changes in FHR

The following periodic changes in FHR last less than 2 minutes and are in response to uterine contractions. They occur early, late, or variably during the course of the contractions.

- Accelerations: FHR normally increases with fetal activity 15 bpm for 15 seconds for the term infant and is a sign of normal sympathetic nervous system response.
- Early decelerations: They occur early in the contraction with a return to normal baseline by the time the contraction is over. They are repetitious. They are associated

with head compression as labour progresses. They do not require intervention.
- Variable decelerations: They vary in duration, degree of severity, length of time, and timing during the contractions. They are associated with umbilical cord compression, and as the cord becomes compressed during or between contractions, the FHR drops and then recovers. These decelerations are considered ominous, with an immediate need for intervention if variability is also depressed and the decelerations are 60 bpm below normal baseline and last longer than 60 seconds in duration. Reduce maternal anxiety and coach to change breathing or pushing.
- Late decelerations: They occur late in the contraction, with recovery during the resting phase between contractions. They are associated with uteroplacental insufficiency as seen with maternal hypertension disorders, diabetes, or obstetrical emergencies such as placental abruption. Persistent, late decelerations are ominous, even if the FHR does not decrease dramatically, since they represent fetal compromise and hypoxia. If there is also poor variability, intrauterine resuscitation measures should be initiated promptly.

Nursing Considerations for FHR Monitoring

- Assess the most appropriate means of monitoring FHR. Provide explanations and answer questions regarding the use of electronic monitoring.
- Document electronic fetal monitoring patterns with uterine contractions; they are every 15 minutes in the active phase of labour and every 5 minutes in the second stage of labour once pushing.
- Respond to changing situations in FHR patterns by providing the client with information and ongoing rationales for actions.
- Initiate intrauterine resuscitation measures to correct early distress by increasing uterine blood flow and perfusion, decreasing umbilical cord compression, improving fetal oxygen supply, and allowing time for preparing for an emergency Caesarean birth if needed.

Premonitory Signs of Labour

There are many theories concerning what triggers labour, including decreasing progesterone levels, increasing oxytocin and prostaglandins that stimulate contractions, and placental aging and uterine distension that irritate the uterus and stimulate contractions. The following list includes some of the most significant indicators that labour is imminent:

- Lightening occurs anytime in the last 4 weeks of pregnancy for the primipara and closer to or at the time of labour for the multipara.
- Braxton Hicks contractions become stronger and more frequent.
- A nesting instinct or a burst of energy may result from lowered progesterone levels.
- Gastro-intestinal symptoms such as nausea, vomiting, indigestion, diarrhea or loose stools may occur.
- Weight loss of just over 1 kg occurs a few days before onset of labour.

- Increased vaginal secretions or bloody show may indicate that the mucus plug has been expelled.
- Spontaneous rupture of membranes is confirmed with nitrazine paper; amniotic fluid is alkaline and will fern on a glass slide; it should be clear and odourless.

Stages and Mechanisms of Labour and Birth

First Stage of Labour

The first stage of labour is from the onset of regular uterine contractions to the full effacement and dilatation of the cervix. It is divided into two phases: latent and active. Primiparas tend to labour longer than multiparas (20 hours versus 14 hours, on average). Research has shown that childbearing clients who are older and heavier progress more slowly through the active phase of labour than previously believed and experience longer labours (Lowdermilk et al., 2020).

- Latent phase: Up to 3 cm dilatation, extends from the onset of labour, with regular, painful contractions that causes effacement cervical change and little increase in descent
- Active phase: 4 to 10 cm dilatation, there is more rapid dilation of the cervix and increased rate of descent of the presenting part (Lowdermilk et al., 2020)

Second Stage of Labour

- From 10 cm dilation and effacement to the birth of the infant, up to 2 hours for a primipara, often much less time for a multipara
- Divided into two phases: latent phase (passive fetal descent) and active pushing phase
- The term *crowning* means that the widest diameter of the head is encircled by the introitus. Pushing is stopped to allow for controlled delivery of the head and to prevent perineal trauma.

Third Stage of Labour

- From the birth of the infant to the expulsion of the placenta, lasting up to 60 minutes
- The uterus maintains a contracted state, constricting the blood vessels and controlling bleeding.

Fourth Stage of Labour

The fourth stage is the immediate recovery and stabilization time, from the delivery of the placenta to at least 2 to 4 hours after the birth. In this stage, parent–child bonding and attachment begins, along with initiating of breastfeeding.

Mechanisms of Labour

Also known as the *cardinal movements*, these are the various positions the fetus assumes in a cephalic presentation as it moves through the confines of the pelvis and birth canal. See Figure 10.3.

1. Engagement and descent: The fetus moves downward into the pelvic passageway.
2. Flexion: The head flexes downward, chin to chest.
3. Internal rotation: The head rotates 45 degrees.
4. Extension: The head passes under the symphysis pubis and reaches the perineum.
5. External rotation: The head rotates back to its original position (restitution), followed by shoulder rotation.
6. Expulsion: The shoulders pass under the pubic arch and perineum; the body is delivered.

Nursing Considerations During Labour and Birth

In a hospital birth, the nurse spends a great deal of time with the client and their family during the labour and birth process. This presents a significant responsibility to provide safe, effective care while enjoying a place of privilege in welcoming a new family member and person into the world.

Labour Nursing Considerations for the First Stage of Labour

- Undertake initial maternal and fetal assessment: This includes history, length of pregnancy, onset of labour and progression, spontaneous rupture of membranes, contractions, bloody show, preparation and plans for pain management and childbirth, family support, vital signs, FHR, gestational age, risk factors or complications, plans for infant feeding, vaginal examination for cervical dilatation, effacement, station, and fetal presentation and position.
- Provide ongoing support: It is recommended that clients in active labour receive ongoing support with 1:1 nursing care (Keenan-Lindsay et al., 2022).
- Monitor labour: Observe and check the progress of labour and the maternal and fetal responses to labour according to unit protocols or more frequently as indicated by assessment findings. The minimum should be vital signs, vaginal show each hour, contractions and FHR every 15 to 30 minutes during active labour and more frequent assessment of bloody show, contractions, FHR monitoring (every 5–10 minutes) during transition.
- Monitor for bladder fullness: Do so especially if an epidural block is used.
- Monitor for spontaneous or artificial rupture of membranes (AROM): Assess FHR for distress due to possible cord prolapse or compression; fluid should be clear and odourless, with no meconium.
- Assess for complications of labour: They include duration of contractions longer than 90 seconds, resting phase shorter than 60 seconds, FHR outside normal limits or periodic changes, maternal temperature above 38°C, rupture of membranes more than 24 hours before, foul-smelling amniotic fluid or maternal show, persistent dark or bright red vaginal bleeding, or sustained abdominal pain with rigid abdomen.
- Vaginal examinations should be kept to a minimum to reduce the risk of infection: After the initial examination, a repeat examination may be done prior to giving additional pain medication or when the client feels increased perineal pressure and the urge to bear down.
- Prepare for the birth: Birth is imminent for the multiparous client or client who had delivered vaginally previously, since they tend to demonstrate more rapid dilation

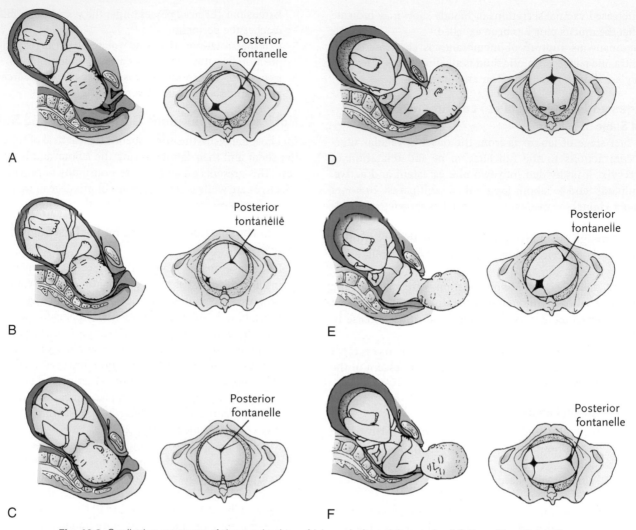

Fig. 10.3 Cardinal movements of the mechanism of labour. Left occipitoanterior (LOA) position. Pelvic figures show the position of the fetal head, as seen by the birth attendant. **A,** Engagement and descent. **B,** Flexion. **C,** Internal rotation to occipitoanterior (OA) position. **D,** Extension. **E,** External rotation beginning (restitution). **F,** External rotation. (From Lowdermilk, D. L., Perry, S. E., Cashion, K., et al. [2021]. *Maternity & women's health care* [12th ed., p. 329, Fig. 16.12]. Elsevier.)

and may only require a brief period in the in the active phase of the first stage of labour. The active phase may take longer for the nulliparous client to become fully dilated (Keenan-Lindsay et al., 2022).

Nursing Considerations for the Second and Third Stages of Labour

- Prepare the child-bearing client: Ensure that their bladder is empty prior to pushing, assist them into a birthing position, give support for relaxing between contractions and pushing effectively during contractions, and monitor contractions and FHR.
- Prepare for the infant: Have warm and dry blankets, a preheated radiant overhead warmer, and resuscitation equipment available.
- Provide immediate newborn care: Assess and maintain a patent infant airway, use maternal–fetal skin-to-skin contact and immediately dry the infant to minimize hypothermia, note the time of birth, assess Apgar scores

at 1 and 5 minutes, document first voiding or passing of meconium, assess for gestational age and obvious defects, provide resuscitation as needed, administer vitamin K (1.0 mg intramuscular [IM] if birth weight is greater than 1 500 g) and eye prophylaxis as ordered, verify and apply identification, weigh and measure the infant, and promote attachment with the client and family through early breastfeeding, holding the infant, and interacting.

- Apgar scores are used to assess adaptation to extrauterine transitions. Parameters are heart rate, respiratory effort, muscle tone, reflex irritability, and colour. A score of 0 to 3 indicates severe distress, scores of 4 to 6 indicates moderate difficulty, scores of 7 to 10 indicate the newborn is having minimal or no difficulty adjusting to extrauterine life. The Apgar score is reassessed in 10 minutes if the score was less than 7 at 5 minutes (Keenan-Lindsay et al., 2022).
- Provide maternal care: Assist with placental delivery; obtain cord blood samples if required; monitor vital signs,

perineal trauma, vaginal bleeding, lochia, and uterine contractility; administer oxytocin for uterine contractility; assess the bladder; and provide pain medication and a perineal ice pack.

Nursing Considerations for the Fourth Stage of Labour

- Assess for uterine contractility. Check fundal height (midway between the umbilicus and symphysis). The uterus rises to just below the umbilical height after several hours. Assess the position (midline) and tone (firm).
- Assess the perineum and lochia. Check the amount of lochia, its character, and whether there are clots or hemorrhage. Hemorrhage (blood loss greater than 500 mL) is suspected if uterine tone is soft and a perineal pad is saturated within 15 minutes. Assess the perineum for hematomas, swelling, and hemorrhoids; offer ice packs.
- Assess maternal vital signs, bladder tone, and ability to void.
- Promote early parental attachment and provide support for breastfeeding choice.
- Assess fetus for ongoing ease of transition to extrauterine life, monitor vital signs and responsiveness, and prevent heat loss.

Essentials of Labour and Birth Complications
Dystocia

Dystocia is a prolonged, abnormal labour related to maternal factors (uterus or pelvis) or fetal factors (size, presentation, position, number of fetuses):

- Abnormal uterine contractions: Hypertonic contractions in the latent phase are abnormally painful and irregular but ineffective in effacing or dilating the cervix. Narcotic analgesia may allow the client to rest and uterine patterns to revert to normal. Hypotonic contractions become ineffective or stop at the active phase. Oxytocin may be used to augment labour once fetal pelvic relationship problems have been ruled out.
- Precipitous labour: It lasts less than 3 hours, with increased risk of uterine rupture, amniotic fluid embolism, and postpartum hemorrhage. Fetal complications include distress and hypoxia.
- Pelvic dystocia: This relates to a pelvic shape that does not allow for descent of the fetus, leading to prolonged labour, increased risk of assisted birth with forceps or vacuum, risk of birth trauma, or Caesarean birth.
- Cephalopelvic disproportion: Excessive fetal size causes problems with descent through the pelvis or under the pubic arch. Assisted birth with forceps, vacuum suction, or Caesarean birth may be needed.
- Breech position: The breech position occurs in 3% of presentations, with the sacrum (buttocks) most commonly presenting to the pelvis. There is an increased risk of birth trauma, prolonged labour, asphyxia, cord prolapse, and the need for Caesarean birth.
- Multiple fetuses: More than one fetus increases the risk of preterm labour, breech or shoulder presentation of one or more fetuses, cord prolapse, fetal compromise, and operative birth.

Episiotomy and Lacerations

- An *episiotomy* is a surgical incision made into the perineum to enlarge the vaginal outlet.
- Episiotomies are seen less often in Canada because of the side-lying position used for birth. This position places less tension on the perineum, making it possible for gradual stretching with fewer indications for episiotomy. Improved outcomes occur with an intact perineum (less blood loss, less postpartum pain, and decreased risk for infection) (Lowdermilk et al., 2020). Indicated episiotomy may be performed in specific considerations such as the need to hasten birth when FHR abnormalities are present (Lowdermilk et al., 2020).
- Episiotomies are sutured afterward with dissolvable stitches to promote healing, prevent residual damage, and decrease the possibility of infection. There are two types: midline (extends from lower vaginal border to the anus) and mediolateral (extends from the lower vaginal border toward the child-bearing client's right side).
- Vaginal lacerations are a tear of the tissues that results in a jagged wound.
- Perineal lacerations and often episiotomies are described by the amount of tissue involved:
  - First degree involves the superficial vaginal mucosa or perineal skin.
  - Second degree involves the vaginal mucosa, perineal skin, and deeper tissues of the perineum.
  - Third degree involves the same as second degree and the anal sphincter.
  - Fourth degree extends through the anal sphincter into the rectal mucosa.

Nursing considerations

- Clients with third-degree and fourth-degree lacerations are often prescribed stool softeners to prevent discomfort with constipation after childbirth. Instruct the client to increase water and fibre in their diet.
- A covered ice packs (20 minutes on and off) applied to the client's perineum for the first 24 hours may help to reduce pain, edema, and bruising. A warm (sitz) bath deep enough to cover the client's buttock and hips for 5 minutes three times a day may help with pain.
- Encourage the client to pour or spray warm water over the perineum after voiding. Spraying from front to back will help to keep the area clean.
- Teach the client that after a bowel movement they should wipe front to back and pat dry the perineum. Perineum pads are applied and removed front to back to prevent fecal contamination of the perineum and vagina.
- The client may apply topical or systemic medications for the perineal pain as ordered by health care provider. Topical anaesthetic ointments or sprays reduce inflammation and numb the perineum. Persons with first- and second-degree lacerations have less pain than a person with an episiotomy (Keenan-Lindsay, 2020).
- Assess the perineum for redness, edema, ecchymosis, discharge, and approximation (REEDA). Explain the signs and symptoms of infection and explain when to see a health care provider. The following may all indicate an infection:

if they have severe, persistent, or increasing pain, chills or fever, foul-smelling vaginal discharge, or red, swollen skin around the incision or tear.

- To reduce pain when sitting, the child-bearing client should to squeeze the buttock together as they lower themselves to a sitting position and then relax their buttock (Keenan-Lindsay, 2020).

Induction or Augmentation of Labour

Methods, including (artificial rupture of membrane) AROM or medications, are used to initiate labour prior to the onset of spontaneous contractions.

- AROM usually stimulates contractions within 12 hours. Amniotic fluid is slowly released. The fetal head should be engaged to prevent cord prolapse. Nursing considerations include noting the time of rupture and the colour, amount, and presence of meconium and monitoring maternal temperature every 2 hours as the risk of infection increases 24 hours after rupture of membranes.
- Cervical ripening methods include Foley catheter insertion into the cervix, cervical prostaglandin gel, and augmentation 24 hours later with oxytocin infusion.
- Oxytocin infusion requires following a careful protocol for administering IV oxytocin with an infusion pump. The dosage should be increased no more frequently than every 30 minutes followed by frequent maternal and fetal monitoring. Fetal monitoring is used, and contractions are closely monitored for excessive uterine activity or tetanic contractions (greater than 90 seconds). At any sign of maternal or fetal compromise, the oxytocin infusion is stopped until further assessment can be made (Keenan-Lindsay, 2020).

Caesarean Birth

- Indications for a Caesarean birth are often related to preventing or intervening in situations of fetal compromise or maternal medical emergencies that require an immediate response or operative birth.
- Surgical incision is most commonly low segment transverse (bikini line) with improved healing and lower risk of hemorrhage or subsequent rupture. The classic and longitudinal incision increases the risks of hemorrhage, pain, healing time, and future uterine rupture is related to location of incision.
- Regional anaesthesia is the preferred method for pain management as the client is awake and there are fewer complications than with general anaesthesia. General anaesthesia is primarily used when rapid birth is necessary in emergency situations.
- Maternal risks and complications include aspiration, infection, hemorrhage, anaesthesia complications, prolonged postpartum recovery, thrombophlebitis, pain, and immobility.
- Fetal risks include transient tachypnea with "wetter lungs" as fetal lung fluid was not removed during passage through the birth canal, as well as CNS depression from the general anaesthetic.

- Additional nursing considerations include postoperative vital sign monitoring, assessment of incision, pain management, extra assistance with infant care and feeding, monitoring for complications, and encouraging early ambulation.

Vaginal Birth After Caesarean (VBAC)

Following a Caesarean birth, it may be possible for the child-bearing client to attempt to give birth vaginally in subsequent pregnancies. Recommended parameters for VBAC are the desire to have a vaginal birth, the absence of previous indications for Caesarean birth, uncomplicated pregnancy, fetal vertex presentation, normal labour, and a previous incision that was low segment transverse (Trojano et al., 2019).

Preterm Labour and Birth

- Labour between 20 and 37 weeks' gestation with uterine contractions and cervical dilatation is considered preterm and presents the risk of premature birth of an immature fetus.
- Maternal risk factors include underweight (less than 45 kg), smoker, strenuous physical activity, physical abuse, no antenatal care, chronic illness, premature rupture of membranes, infection, multifetal pregnancy (50% of twin gestations are premature), history of preterm labour, maternal age less than 18 years, advanced maternal age, polyhydramnios, cervical insufficiency, cardiovascular disease, placental disorders, and unknown causes (Keenan-Lindsay et al., 2022).
- Therapeutic interventions include early risk screening, early detection of onset, stopping uterine contractions, and preparing for care of the premature infant. High-risk clients should be knowledgeable of preterm labour and know how to immediately report all signs of preterm labour; activities may be restricted or admission to hospital indicated.
- If birth is inevitable, an episiotomy may be used to reduce the risk of intraventricular hemorrhage from pressure on the fragile premature skull. A pediatrician or neonatologist should be present to assist in the resuscitation and transportation of the newborn. Nursing considerations, in addition to assisting with the birth, include supporting the parents with factual information, avoiding false hope, acknowledging their concerns, taking photos if the infant is to be admitted to a neonatal intensive care unit, and providing ongoing psychological support and information.

Perinatal Loss and Bereavement

When perinatal loss occurs during a pregnancy, it is a tragedy and crisis for the parents and family. For many young families, it may be their first encounter with the death of a family member. Maternal newborn nurses and staff are also affected by the death of a fetus or newborn. Perinatal loss is unique in that it often occurs suddenly, with little warning, and interrupts the normal developmental processes of pregnancy and parenthood. Nurses need to understand the grief process as it applies to perinatal loss and provide skilful, sensitive care during this highly vulnerable time.

Losses include stillbirths, prematurity, newborns with anomalies, and neonatal deaths.

Grief is a personal experience of deeply felt sorrow at the loss of something highly valued. Grief occurs in stages, slowly over a period of time, allowing the individuals to work their way through the various defences the psyche uses to protect itself from the full impact of the loss. Grief does not follow a linear path—it is a dynamic process.

Stages of Grief

- Parents experience disbelief and shock as they cannot take in the reality of the news. In being overwhelmed, parents may appear not able to hear or understand what is being said to them; they may be immobile or emotionally numb in their initial reactions.
- Anger may be expressed as the reality of the situation is absorbed. Women often have more difficulty than men in expressing anger; this may result in depression and feelings of guilt. Anger may be directed at staff.
- Bargaining occurs when there is an understanding of the reality of the situation but hope that something can change it.
- Depression, overwhelming sadness, and withdrawal represent a greater level of acceptance of the impact of the loss.
- Acceptance is the process of integrating the experience and its meaning into one's life. Normal activities slowly resume, and memories of both sorrow and joy can be recounted.
- Acute grief reactions are intensely felt for 6 to 10 weeks, but the full process of grieving usually takes time, frequently over 1 to 2 years.

Behavioural and Physical Symptoms of Grief

- Somatic manifestations include weight gain or loss, nausea, hyperventilating, sighing respirations, tightening of the throat, heavy feeling in the chest, palpitations, headaches, loss of muscle strength, and extreme fatigue.
- Behavioural manifestations include preoccupation; nightmares; feelings of guilt, shame, apathy, loneliness, isolation, anger, sorrow, and irritability; decreased sexual interest; social withdrawal; crying; exhaustion; loss of concentration and motivation; and restlessness.

Nursing Considerations

- Promote an empathetic environment that openly acknowledges the death of the newborn and supports the reactions of the client and family. Provide time for the parents to see, touch, and be with the infant. Take photos and collect as many mementos as possible: locks of hair (requires parental permission), footprints, ID band, and weight and length information.
- Provide information about community resources on grief counselling and bereavement, and follow-up in the postpartum period.
- Be sensitive to and accommodate cultural and religious practices.
- Grieving parents are vulnerable to well-meaning but harmful comments and clichés that minimize their loss.

Educate others as to why these comments are harmful. Offer suggestions for helping the family acknowledge and cope with the loss.
- Understand that immediate and extended family members are all affected by the loss. Sibling responses will be dependent on their age and stage of development. Simple language that is honest and clear in its meaning and uses words such as "death" lessens confusion and fears.
- Nurses need to take the time to understand their own beliefs and reactions to loss and death in order to be emotionally available to others who are grieving. Finding ways to nurture oneself following these painful experiences is beneficial and important.

THE POSTPARTUM STAGE

Sometimes referred to as the *fourth trimester*, this 6-week puerperium is when the mother's body returns to its prepregnant state, the newborn adapts to an extrauterine life, and family members begin to adjust to the many changes a newborn brings into their lives.

Maternal Adaptations
Physiological Changes

- Reproductive changes: The uterus remains firmly contracted and undergoes involution, descending from the height of the umbilicus by about one fingerbreadth per day until it can no longer be palpated by days 10 to 14. By 6 weeks postpartum, the uterus has returned to its nonpregnant state. The cervix becomes thicker and firmer and contracts over several weeks to an elongated rather than a circular opening. The perineum remains swollen, perhaps bruised for a few days, and the vaginal rugae and tone return within 6 to 10 weeks.
- Sexual intercourse: Assuming that there is no infection or complications, intercourse may resume when the client feels physically and emotionally comfortable and ready. Appropriate methods of birth control should be discussed and planned for as part of postpartum teaching prior to discharge home.
- Lochia, or uterine discharge: It changes over the course of about 3 weeks from lochia rubra (dark red, with small clots) for 3 to 4 days, to lochia serosa (pinkish, serosanguinous) from days 3 to 10, to lochia alba (whitish to clear, no odour) from day 10 to week 3.
- Breast changes: Colostrum is present at the time of birth, and breast milk is produced by the third or fourth day postpartum. Engorgement is common when milk production starts and lasts 24 hours. Newborn suckling and feeding stimulates prolactin, which stimulates more milk production. See the Newborn Nutrition section.
- Cardiovascular changes: They are significant as the circulating blood volume decreases rapidly and is lost through diuresis and diaphoresis (perspiration). Blood pressure remains stable; transient bradycardia (as low as 50 bpm) lasts up to 3 months.
- Renal changes: The glomerular filtration rate is elevated to help mobilize excess vascular volume; overdistension of

the bladder and difficulty voiding in the first 24 hours are fairly common. A full bladder may displace the uterus in the early postpartum stages.

- Endocrine changes: Estrogen and progesterone drop rapidly following birth, and prolactin rises, reaching a peak at day 3, when breast milk production begins. Menstruation is often delayed with breastfeeding until 12 to 24 weeks postpartum. Menstruation returns for nonbreastfeeding mothers by 6 to 12 weeks postpartum.

Psychological Adaptations and Attachment

- The disruption to normal sleep patterns, the increased need for rest and recovery, the needs of a newborn, and changing roles and relationships all add to the stress of adapting to parenting in the postpartum period.
- The transition to parenting is aided by family and community support, positive past experiences, cultural beliefs and practices that promote attachment, and learned adaptive behaviours for coping with change.
- The term *attachment* is preferred to the older term *bonding* when describing the process by which the parents interact and form a relationship with their newborn. The newborn is more awake and sensitive to their surroundings in the first hour of life than they will be for the next 2 weeks, so it is an ideal time for interaction. While this time is ideal, parents should not feel guilty if circumstances do not allow for this first intimate contact to happen. Attachment is the reciprocal relationship that develops over time as parents and newborn interact with each other, using cues and responses to learn to understand each other and to connect on an emotional level.
- Most clients experience postpartum blues, often on days 3 to 5, when milk production begins and prolactin levels surge. This condition is characterized by feelings of inexplicable sadness, letdown, and increased crying and usually resolves within 10 days.

Maternal Complications
Postpartum Hemorrhage

- Risk factors include polyhydramnios, multiple gestation, rapid labour, prolonged rupture of membrane, placenta previa, high parity, a history of coagulation disorder, uterine atony, retained placenta, and trauma.
- Early postpartum hemorrhage is a blood loss of 500 mL or more that occurs in the first 24 hours after giving birth. It is usually related to the uterus not contracting or staying contracted following delivery of the placenta, lacerations of the cervix or vagina, parts of the placenta being retained, or clotting disorders. It presents a greater risk of morbidity and mortality to the client than does a late hemorrhage.
- Late postpartum hemorrhage occurs after 24 hours following birth and is most often related to retained placental fragments.
  Nursing considerations
- Assess uterine involution and teach the client what to expect with vaginal discharge and what signs of complications to report, including fever greater than 38°C, lochia

that changes back to rubra or bright red bleeding, a pad that soaks through in 15 minutes, foul-smelling lochia or urine, or feelings of inability to cope and sadness that last more than 1 or 2 weeks.

- Know that an inability to void and a full bladder may displace the uterus from its midline position, impairing the normal contractility and increasing the risk of hemorrhage. Assess the bladder frequently early in the postpartum period and encourage frequent voiding.
- Monitor the uterus tone and vaginal blood loss every 15 minutes following birth for the first hour and as per unit protocol for the next 24 hours. Gentle massage of the uterus may stimulate uterine contractility, as will breastfeeding. Know the policy and procedure for responding to a postpartum hemorrhage.
- Following birth, it is recommended to administer oxytocin to promote uterine contractility and prevent postpartum hemorrhage.
- Report findings of a bleeding laceration. A continuous trickle of blood may develop more blood loss than from hemorrhage associated with uterine atony. Keep the client nothing by mouth (NPO) until orders received as the client may require surgery for the repair of the laceration (Keenan-Lindsay, 2020).

Hypertensive Disorders

- Hypertension disorders may persist postpartum, and the client should be monitored 3 to 6 days after delivery of the infant.
  Nursing considerations
- Monitor intake and output, reflexes, and level of consciousness.
- Closely monitor uterine tone and lochia flow. There is an increased risk for a boggy uterus and large lochia flow due to the magnesium sulphate therapy muscle relaxant effects. Administration of oxytocin infusion is recommended (Keenan-Lindsay et al., 2022).
- Educate the client to seek health care if increased blurred vision or headache increases in severity after discharge (Keenan-Lindsay, 2020).
- Providing family-centred care is important, especially if the baby is being cared for in the neonatal intensive care unit (NICU). Keep the family informed of the infant's condition and encourage the partner to visit the NICU and the child-bearing client to visit the NICU via wheelchair as soon as their condition stabilizes (Lowdermilk et al., 2020).

Infection

Infection is a significant cause of maternal morbidity and may include the uterus, post–Caesarean birth incision, urinary tract, or breasts (mastitis).
  Nursing considerations.
- Assess the client for signs of infection, including a temperature of 38°C or higher, tachycardia, pain and tenderness, redness or swelling, nausea and feeling unwell, foul-smelling discharge, and excessive fatigue.

- Teach the client how to recognize and report any signs of fever and infection. Teach the importance of taking all doses of antibiotics as prescribed.

Mastitis

Mastitis is inflammation and infection of the breast. It can occur at any time but most commonly occurs in the first 2 to 4 weeks postpartum.

- Signs and symptoms include sudden onset of flulike symptoms, including fever, malaise, chills, body aches, headaches, nausea, and vomiting. The child-bearing person has localized breast pain and tenderness and hot, reddened area on the breast. Most commonly it occurs in the upper outer quadrant of the breast; one or both breasts may be affected. Purulent discharge may or may not be present.
- Risk factors predisposing a child-bearing person to mastitis are inadequate emptying of the breasts related to engorgement, plugged ducts, abrupt weaning, sudden decrease in the number of feeding, or wearing underwire bras. Stress, fatigue, maternal illness, breast trauma, and poor maternal nutrition are other factors that increase the probability for mastitis. Sore, cracked nipples can lead to mastitis, allowing for a portal of entry for the causative organism. *Staphylococcus, Streptococcus,* and *Escherichia* are the most common organisms.

Nursing considerations

- Provide health teaching on taking antibiotics for the prescribed length of time to treat the infection—usually 10 to 14 days. If an abscess forms, the child-bearing client may require IV administration of antibiotics and may need an incision to drain the infected area.
- Reinforce to the child-bearing client to frequently breastfeed or pump from the affected breast and empty the milk from the affected breast adequately.
- Mild analgesics may be given to help promote the child-bearing client's comfort.
- Infection cannot be transmitted to the newborn.
- Apply warm compresses to the affected region to promote blood flow to the area and comfort before feeding and pumping.
- Encourage taking a warm shower before breastfeeding to help stimulate milk flow and provide cleanliness and warmth.
- Encourage the child-bearing client to rest as much as possible.
- Encourage the child-bearing client to drink plenty of fluids to achieve adequate fluid intake.
- Teach the child-bearing client to wear a good, supportive bra (Lowdermilk et al., 2020).

Perinatal Depression—Postpartum Period (PPD)

Unlike those of the postpartum blues, the manifestations of depression continue and worsen over time. They include feelings of despair, hopelessness, inadequacy, ambivalence or apathy toward the newborn, inability to feel joy, and somatic symptoms of headache, appetite changes, sighing, excessive fatigue, or hyperactivity. This disorder is the most common complication of childbirth and must be part of health teaching and follow-up care.

Nursing considerations. It is essential that nurses teach the parents to be aware of the manifestations of depression and to seek support and medical help promptly. Depression is a disease process of neurochemical imbalance; it is not a personal failure or weakness. It is crucial to seek help, follow the treatment plan, and involve others who may provide support, including extended family and community programs. Untreated postpartum depression can result in a client feeling a lack of attachment, gratification, or fulfillment in their role as a parent, or miss cues for their infant, such as hunger, changing diapers, and other needs. For children of parents with untreated depression there is an increased risk for delayed motor, language, cognitive and social developmental and neurodevelopmental disorders (RNAO, 2018a).

Nursing considerations

- The nurse should observe for signs and symptoms during prenatal and postpartum clinic visits and screen with a valid perinatal depression screening tool.
- Provide health teaching that the treatment may involve antidepressant medications and psychotherapy as an outpatient and that breastfeeding clients should consult with their health care provider regarding medications that are safe to take.
- Provide health teaching measures to help clients decrease PPD, such as exercise, relaxation techniques, promoting adequate sleep, and time for themselves.
- Encourage social support from the client's partner, family, community support, and friends.
- Provide counselling for the partner and family (Keenan-Lindsay, 2020).
- Provide referral for additional support services in mental health (refer to Chapter 12 Mental Health Nursing).

Newborn Adaptations

Beginning with the process of labour, the fetus undergoes many changes on a physiological and developmental level. These transitional changes allow the newborn to adapt to life outside the uterine environment. While remaining dependent on others for nutrition, warmth, and a nurturing environment, the newborn is remarkably well equipped to interpret, respond to, and make known their needs.

Transition to Extrauterine Life

Transition is a critical time in the first 6 to 24 hours of life, when many newborn anatomical and physiological changes occur, especially in the cardiovascular and respiratory systems. The fetus has three unique cardiac features that change during transition, beginning with the stimulation of labour and the newborn's first breath. External and internal stimuli initiate these changes. Nurses assess the newborn's ability to adapt during the different transitional periods of reactivity.

Respiratory adaptations

- By 35 to 37 weeks, the fetal lungs are structurally developed enough to do the work of breathing. Surfactant, a phospholipid that lubricates the lungs and helps keep them partially inflated after each breath, peaks, with an L:S ratio of 2:1.
- Fetal anatomical structures that change during transition as the newborn initiates breathing are the ductus venosus, ductus arteriosus, and foramen ovale.
- Stimuli that initiate respirations include chemical, mechanical, and sensory factors:
  - Chemical stimuli: Uterine contractions temporarily decrease fetal oxygen supply, causing a mild acidosis that stimulates the respiratory centre of the brain to initiate breathing.
  - Mechanical stimuli: Most of the lung fluid is squeezed out as the fetal chest is compressed in the birth canal. There is a passive intake of breath once the chest is past the birth canal.
  - Sensory stimuli: The abrupt change in environmental temperature at birth is a major stimulus to breathe, in addition to touch, light, sound, noise, and pain.
- After the first breath, pressure changes occur in the lungs and circulation. The lungs open and pulmonary vessels dilate, changing from a closed high-pressure system to an open low-pressure system.

Circulatory adaptations

- The fetal circulatory system changes from a low-pressure to a higher-pressure system, causing the fetal circulatory structures to close.
- The foramen ovale, located between the right and left atrium, closes as blood flow and pressure on the left side of the heart become greater than on the right side of the heart.
- The ductus venosus, located between the inferior vena cava and the umbilical vein, closes when the umbilical cord is clamped.
- The ductus arteriosus, located between the pulmonary artery and the aorta, closes when pulmonary blood flow and pressures increase. Rising oxygen levels are detected by chemoreceptor sites on the ductus, which also helps stimulate the ductus arteriosus to close.
- **Note:** These anatomical structures functionally close within 15 to 20 minutes of birth, but a murmur may be heard for 6 to 12 hours in the newborn. If the infant is hypoxic or asphyxiated, the ductus arteriosus may open again. Refer to Figure 10.4, which illustrates fetal circulation.

Temperature adaptation

- All newborns are at increased risk for heat loss (via convection, radiation, evaporation, and conduction) due to their large body surface compared with body mass, blood vessels close to the skin surface, an inability to shiver, and immature CNS temperature-control mechanisms. Newborns can also easily overheat if wrapped in too many layers of clothes.
- Maintaining a neutral thermal environment means that the newborn must use only minimum amounts of oxygen, glucose, and metabolic energy to keep warm.

- Newborns use nonshivering thermogenesis to metabolize their unique brown fat stores to generate body heat.

Renal adaptations

- Full-term infants normally void in the first 24 hours of life. They have a limited ability to concentrate urine and may lose 10% of their body weight in the first 3 days of life due to fluid shifts and losses. They will regain the weight within 1 week with normal feeding.
- **Note:** In the first week, a newborn who is receiving adequate hydration through feeding should have one heavy wet diaper for each day of life.

Gastro-intestinal adaptations

- Bowel sounds begin within the first few hours, the first meconium stool passes within 24 hours, and the newborn requires frequent feedings of 30 to 90 mL—or until satisfied at the breast—every few hours.
- There is an increased risk of bleeding in the first week of life since the gut is sterile at birth and newborns do not have the intestinal flora to synthesize vitamin K in the first week of life. Therefore, vitamin K IM is routinely administered as it promotes the creation of clotting factors (II, VII, IX, and X) in the liver. The formation of bacteria begins with the first feedings, and by day 7, healthy newborns can produce their own vitamin K (Keenan-Lindsay et al., 2022).
- The cardiac sphincter between the esophagus and stomach is immature, and regurgitation of feeding is common. Burping following feeding will help.
- Stool characteristics change from meconium (thick, sticky, black, passed in the first 24 hours) to transitional stools (thin, brownish green). Breastfed stools are bright mustard yellow, loose, and frequent. Formula-fed stools are pasty, pale yellow, and less frequent. Elimination patterns may vary, from 1 to 5 or 6 per day in the first few weeks.
- The fetal liver is immature and unable to conjugate bilirubin well at term. Most preterm and 50% of full-term infants will experience physiological jaundice in the first week of life.
- **Note:** Physiological jaundice or hyperbilirubinemia (indicated by yellowed skin, mucous membranes, and eye sclera) appears after 24 hours of life in infants who are otherwise well, peaks at 3 days, and resolves itself by 10 days. Phototherapy may be used as ultraviolet light aids in conjugating bilirubin into a water-soluble form that can be excreted in urine and stools. Frequent feedings help resolve physiological jaundice. Newborns should breastfeed early (usually one hour after birth) and often. Colostrum acts as a laxative to promote stooling, which helps rid the body of bilirubin. Formula fed newborns should be fed after birth, when physiological status is stabilized and then on demand feedings every 3 to 4 hours (Keenan- Lindsay et al., 2022).

Nursing Considerations for the Newborn

- Be aware that adequately hydrated newborns should wet six to eight diapers each day.
- Monitor for physiological jaundice, encourage early and frequent feedings, and implement phototherapy as needed, covering eyes while exposing skin to ultraviolet

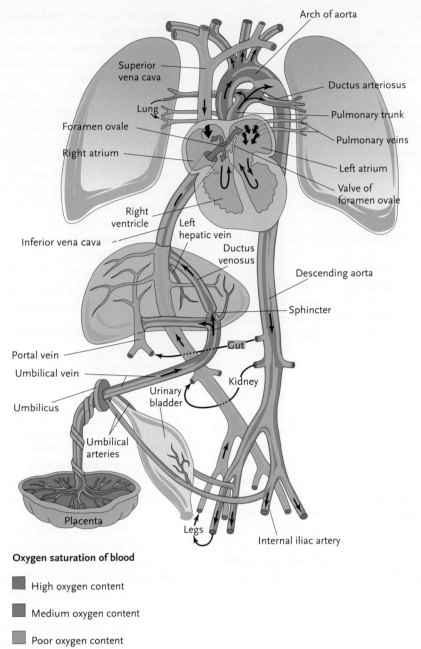

Oxygen saturation of blood

■ High oxygen content

■ Medium oxygen content

■ Poor oxygen content

Fig. 10.4 Schematic illustration of the fetal circulation. The organs are not drawn to scale. The arrows show the course of the blood from the placenta to the heart. A small amount of highly oxygenated blood from the inferior vena cava remains in the right atrium and mixes with poorly oxygenated blood from the superior vena cava. The medium-oxygenated blood then passes into the right ventricle. Observe that three shunts permit most of the blood to bypass the liver and lungs: (1) ductus venosus, (2) oval foramen, (3) ductus arteriosus. The poorly oxygenated blood returns to the placenta for oxygen and nutrients through the umbilical arteries. (From Lowdermilk, D., Perry, S., Cashion, K., Rhodes Alden, K., & Olshansky, E. [2020]. *Schematic illustration of the fetal circulation* [12th ed., p. 239, Fig. 12-13]. Elsevier.)

lights. Phototherapy side effects include a sleepy newborn, loose stools, and an increased need for fluids of 10%.

- As newborns are obligate nose breathers from birth up until 3 months of age, ensure that nasal passages are clear.
- Closely monitor for expected vital signs and physical and behavioural adaptations.
- First period of reactivity:
  - Immediately after birth, tachypnea up to 80 breaths per minute with nasal flaring

- Tachycardia up to 180 bpm
- Murmur may be heard; hands and feet may appear blue (acrocyanosis) as peripheral circulation is sluggish
- Neurologically awake and alert
- Period of relative inactivity:
  - Heart and respiratory rate and effort decrease to normal range of heart rate 120 to 160 bpm
  - Respiratory rate of 30 to 50
  - Newborn falls asleep

- Second period of reactivity:
  - Very responsive and awake
  - Increased oral mucus may lead to gagging and cyanosis
  - May have tachycardia
  - Bowel sounds present; may pass meconium and void for the first time
- Monitor temperature frequently; prevent heat loss by drying newborn immediately, protecting from drafts

Essential Newborn Assessment

A systematic assessment of the full-term newborn reveals findings in appearance, reflexes, and responses to the environment that are normal, a variation on normal, or abnormal (Figure 10.5). These findings also vary depending on the gestational age of the newborn. Assessment should include the following:

- Vital signs: Temperature is labile, prone to hypothermia due to large body surface area, not a reliable indicator of infection, and 36.5 to 37°C; blood pressure is 60/40 to 90/60 mm Hg; respiratory rate is 30 to 60; listen for heart rate at apex for 1 full minute (120–170 bpm when awake, 80–90 bpm when sleeping).
- Weight and length: Average weight is 3 500 g; average length is 50 cm.
- Skin: Skin is is erythematous (red) for a few hours after birth and then fades to its normal colour; body fat is present; acrocyanosis (bluish discoloration of extremities) is a normal finding for the first 7 to 10 days after birth due to poor peripheral circulation; waxy vernix is present in creases; lanugo (fine downy hair) is present; erythema toxicum or newborn rash and milia on the nose are common and resolve spontaneously. Birthmarks may be permanent, such as port wine stain, or they may resolve, as in strawberry hemangioma.
- Head: The head appears large compared with the flexed body. Measure the head circumference at the widest diameter of the occiput and over the eyebrows; average is 33 to 35 cm. Moulding resolves in the first week, anterior fontanelle is soft and pulsating and may be tense with crying. Assess for symmetrical facial features. Outer edge of eye should be in line with the top of the ear; eyes are slate blue and tearless and can focus 45 cm; ear cartilage springs back when folded. Palate in mouth is intact; Epstein's pearls (small white gum cysts) that look like teeth may be visible, but they disappear spontaneously.
- Chest: The chest moves in unison with the abdomen when breathing; it typically has a 32-cm circumference over nipple line. Engorged breasts are common due to maternal estrogen effect.
- Back and extremities: The back is smooth and straight; no dermal sinus or defect appears at base of the spine. The extremities are symmetrical and flexible; full-term nails extend beyond fingertips; skin creases are on soles of feet.
- Abdomen: The abdomen is cylindrical and protrudes, and bowel sounds are audible after 30 minutes of birth. The umbilical cord has two arteries and one vein, and it dries and falls off within 7 days. A patent anus passes meconium within 24 hours and voids within 24 hours. Reddish-brick dust spots in urine are harmless urate crystals.
- Genitals: In females, the labia majora covers the minora, and pseudomenstruation is common due to the effects of maternal hormones. In males, assess that both testes are in the scrotum and full-term scrotum has rugae; inspect penis for central position of the urethra.
- Reflexes in the full-term newborn include Moro (startle), rooting (turns head toward stroked cheek), grasp/palmar (grasps fingers around object), tonic neck (head turned to one side, same side arm and leg extend, opposite arm and leg flex), stepping (held upright, legs move as if stepping), and positive Babinski (when the sole of the foot is stroked upward, the toes extend outward).
- Behaviour states: These include crying, quiet, and alert (ideal time to interact, assess, feed), deep sleep (tunes out environment, very still, regular respiratory rate), and active alert (irregular breathing, easily startled, eyes wide, may cry, turns from eye contact).

Nursing Care, Parent Teaching, and Follow-Up Considerations

- Safety: Teach the parents to never leave the newborn unattended in a bath, on a change table, or with a family pet. Also, Canadian law requires that all newborns be transported in an approved car seat. The safest position is rear facing with the car seat in the back seat of the vehicle.
- *Candida albicans*: A pinpoint bright red diaper rash that does not resolve within 24 hours may be caused by *C. albicans* and should be assessed for antifungal skin treatment. Oral thrush (coated or red tongue and throat) will also require treatment.
- Sudden infant death syndrome (SIDS): Newborns should sleep on their backs, in their own crib, on a firm mattress with no pillows or thick blankets in the crib.
- Ongoing assessment: Following stabilization in the transitional stage, ongoing assessment at each shift and as needed includes monitoring of vital signs and skin colour and integrity; nutrition and elimination patterns; behavioural responses; and interactions with the mother and family.
- Vitamin K injection/eye prophylaxis: If not part of labour and birth procedures, administer vitamin K 1.0 mg IM within 6 hours of birth to prevent hemorrhagic disease of the newborn (into the middle one-third of the side of the thigh muscle—the vastus lateralis—using a 25-gauge needle) and eye prophylaxis (erythromycin [E-Mycin] ointment onto the lower lid of the eye).
- Hygiene: A sponge or tub bath daily or twice per week using mild soap is recommended. Prevent excess heat loss and assess water temperature (24°C) using a thermometer or dorsal part of the hand, not the fingers; do not use baby powder as particles may be aspirated. Bathing prior to feeding will avoid the risk of regurgitation and promote alertness for better feeding success.
- Client teaching on newborn conditions: Provide phone numbers and resources and teach parents to seek help if

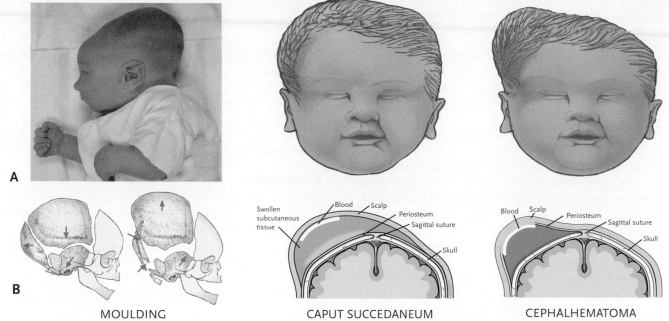

MOULDING
A. Significant moulding, soon after birth.
B. Schematic of bones of skull when moulding is present.

CAPUT SUCCEDANEUM
Caput succedaneum (left) and
cephalhematoma (right) are common birth injuries.

CEPHALHEMATOMA

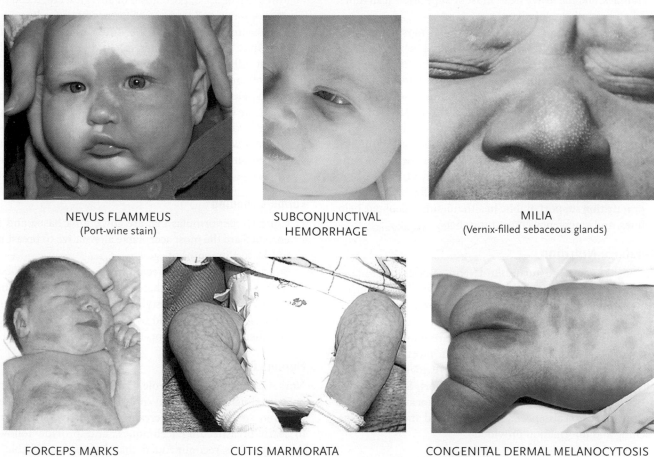

NEVUS FLAMMEUS
(Port-wine stain)

**SUBCONJUNCTIVAL
HEMORRHAGE**

MILIA
(Vernix-filled sebaceous glands)

FORCEPS MARKS

CUTIS MARMORATA
(Mottling)

CONGENITAL DERMAL MELANOCYTOSIS
Congenital dermal melanocytosis are common
in dark-skinned children. These bluish skin
discolorations should not be confused with bruises.

Fig. 10.5 Common variations in the newborn. (From **[top left]** Lowdermilk, D. L., Perry, S.E., Cashion, K., et al. [2020]. *Maternity & women's health care* [12th ed., p. 475, Figure 23-14]. Elsevier. **A,** Courtesy Kim Molloy, Knoxville, IA, United States; **[top right]** Bowden, V., Dickey, S., & Greenberg, C. [1998]. *Children and their families: The continuum of care.* Philadelphia: Saunders; **[middle left]** Zitelli, B. J., & Davis, H. W. [2002]. *Atlas of pediatric physical diagnosis* [4th ed.]. Mosby; **[middle centre]** Beischer, N. A., Mackey, E. V., & Colditz, P. B. [1997]. *Obstetrics and the newborn* [3rd ed.]. Baillière Tindall; **[middle right]** Beischer, N. A., Mackey, E. V., & Colditz, P. B. [1997]. *Obstetrics and the newborn* [3rd ed., p. 599]. Baillière Tindall; **[bottom left]** Leifer, G. [2007]. *Maternity nursing: An introductory text* [10th ed., p. 169, Table 10-1]. Saunders; **[bottom centre]** Keenan-Lindsay, L. [2020]. *Leifer's introduction to maternity and pediatric nursing in Canada* [1st ed., p. 280, Table 11.3]. Elsevier; **[bottom right]** Lowdermilk, D. L., Perry, S. E., Cashion, K., et al. [2020]. *Maternity and woman's health care* [12th ed., p. 471, Fig. 23.8]. Elsevier.)

the newborn is having difficulty breathing, not successfully feeding, not voiding six to eight wet diapers per day, crying inconsolably, lethargic, or jaundiced or appears unwell.

- Infection avoidance: Everyone having contact with the newborn should first wash their hands and avoid contact if they are infectious as the newborn immune system is immature.
- Diaper rash: Diaper rash may be treated with exposure to air (avoid cold stress), petroleum jelly or zinc oxide barrier products, and frequent diaper changes with each feeding.
- Umbilical cord care: The cord normally dries within 24 hours and falls off within 7 days. Teach the parent to dry around the cord carefully and report any signs of bleeding, foul odour, or discharge.
- Holding and positioning: Newborns require interaction and nurturing, ideally during quiet alert states. They are consoled by being contained in a moderately flexed body posture with a receiving blanket and with skin-to-skin contact covered with a blanket. Newborn necks have weak muscles, and the heavy head must be supported at all times when holding the infant.
- Male circumcision: Male circumcision is most often practised to comply with religious or cultural beliefs. Routine circumcision is not recommended (CPS, 2015). If circumcision is performed, teach the parents to observe for first voiding and complications including bleeding (apply direct pressure and seek medical help) and infection. Pain medication should be used during the procedure.
- Follow-up appointment and information on additional support: Upon discharge, ensure that the client and family have a follow-up appointment usually at week 1 or 2 and then monthly. Provide information for breastfeeding or nutrition support, public health nursing, telephone help lines, and emergency contact numbers.

Newborn Nutrition

Newborns require adequate fluids and calories to promote hydration and growth. Breastfeeding is widely recognized and recommended as the ideal feeding method to meet the newborn's nutritional requirements. There are few contraindications to breastfeeding, and there are numerous health advantages. Nurses support the client in meeting the newborn's nutritional needs by providing evidence-informed information, teaching, and practical support. Some parents, for a variety of reasons, will instead use formula feedings, and their decision also needs to be respected and appropriate teaching and information provided.

Requirements

- A healthy full-term newborn requires about 100 to 120 kcal/kg/day. Expected rates of growth include a weight gain of 15 g/kg/day or an average of 1 kg per month for the first 3 months of life. Growth charts are used to monitor acceptable growth patterns.
- Newborns go through growth spurts at 2 weeks, 4 to 6 weeks, 3 months, and 6 months, and demands to be fed will increase accordingly.

- Fluoride supplementation is not recommended in the first 6 months of life.
- Breastfed infants need vitamin D supplementation of 400 IU/day, available in infant drops. In areas of Canada north of 55° latitude (such as Edmonton) or for dark-skinned infants, 800 IU/day is needed between October and April, when sunlight levels are low (CPS, 2022).

Breastfeeding

Exclusive breastfeeding is recommended for the first 6 months of life and can be continued for 2 years and beyond (CPS, 2013; RNAO, 2018b).

- Contraindications include clients who are HIV positive, have undergone long-term chemotherapy, or have galactosemia, untreated infectious tuberculosis, or herpes simplex lesions on or near the nipple (Keenan-Lindsay, 2020).
- Breastfeeding is ideally suited to newborn metabolic needs and digestion and is associated with decreased infections, lower risk of SIDS, prevention of allergies, enhanced brain development, and lower costs for newborn feeding.
- Colostrum is available at the time of birth. It is rich in proteins, vitamins, minerals, and immunoglobulins. Breast milk is produced by day 3 or 4 postpartum under the influence of the hormone prolactin. Oxytocin hormone causes the letdown reflex that releases the milk when the baby begins to feed. The amount of milk produced is dependent on the breast being stimulated and emptied with frequent feedings. Clients are encouraged to feed on demand. Newborns may initially feed 8 to 12 times in 24 hours.

Formula Feeding

- Commercial formulas that are cow's milk based and iron enriched are the most acceptable alternative to breast milk until 9 to 12 months of age.
- Soy-based formulas are recommended only if dairy-based milk is not used for health, religious, or cultural reasons, as in the case of a vegan lifestyle or infants with galactosemia.
- Water for formula should be boiled to remove pathogens and then cooled for infants (Keenan-Lindsay et al., 2022).

Nursing Considerations

Nurses have an important role in promoting and supporting breastfeeding as the optimal choice for infant nutrition; educate and support parents, create a supportive environment to learn breastfeeding techniques, and provide follow-up resources. It is recommended that nurses use reliable and valid tools to ensure a consistent and systematic approach to assessments for the breastfeeding process. Examples of tools to use are Latch Breastfeeding Assessment tool and the Breastfeeding Self-Efficacy Scale–Short Form (BSES-SF). These tools can help to identify further support and assistance required to support initiation, exclusivity, and continuation of breastfeeding (RNAO, 2018b).

- Breast milk can be expressed and stored in glass bottles (or bisphenol A–free hard plastic containers) or plastic bags made for breast milk storage. Commercial bottle liners are not recommended for storage (Keenan-Lindsay et al., 2022). Breast milk can be stored at room temperature for 4 hours or 6 to 8 hours in very clean conditions. Examples of clean conditions include properly washed hands and properly cleaned pump parts and containers (Keenan-Lindsay, 2020).

- Breast milk may be stored in the back of the fridge (4°C where the temperature is the coolest) for up to 96 hours (4 days) or in the freezer (−4°C) for 6 to 12 months. It is important not to microwave breast milk because it destroys the antimicrobial agents and vitamin C.
- The newborn will feed best if correctly attached to or "latched on" to the breast. The client should be comfortable and supported. Signs a baby is feeding well include a wide-open mouth encircling the breast; movement of the baby's jaw, not just lips; the baby swallowing at regular intervals; the baby being content after feeding; the mother not being in pain; and the baby wetting six to eight diapers in a 24-hour period. Most newborns, properly latched, will empty the breast within 30 minutes. The client should break the seal by placing a clean finger between the breast and the baby's mouth. Upright burping will help release any swallowed air. Small amounts of regurgitation are normal.
- Nutrient-rich solid foods can be introduced at 6 months of age in addition to breast milk or formula feedings, including iron-fortified cereals, meat, or other protein sources. To prevent newborn botulism, no honey or honey products should be given in the first year of life. Herbal teas are not recommended. The CPS recommends offering non-choking forms of foods containing common allergens (e.g., peanuts, egg) at around 6 months of age, but not before 4 months, as this can be effective in preventing food allergy in some high-risk infants (CPS, 2019).
- Criteria for postpartum discharge should include demonstration of a clear understanding of feeding needs and techniques, written instructions, community resources and referrals, and at least two successful infant feedings independently performed by the client. Professional follow-up within 48 hours of discharge is recommended to assess infant hydration, feeding, and the presence of jaundice (CPS, 2018).

Hospital-Based Care for Child-Bearing Clients With Confirmed or Suspected COVID-19 and Their Newborn

Research data continue to show that COVID-19 is not commonly transmitted to newborns during pregnancy and when newborns do have COVID at birth, most are asymptomatic or experience mild to moderate disease (CPS, 2020).

The CPS (2020) recommends that child-bearing clients suspected or confirmed to have COVID-19 should not be separated from their newborns. There is some evidence to suggest newborns can get infected with SARS-CoV-2 postnatally. Therefore, rooming in should occur after proper health teaching of the risks and benefits, leaving the decision making with families and health care providers.

Preventing infection should focus on proper hygiene to limit the transmission:

- Child-bearing clients, should practise careful hand hygiene.
- Don a surgical/procedure mask within 2 metres of the newborn.
- Practise hand hygiene before skin-to-skin contact, breastfeeding, and routine newborn care.
- The main concern of a child-bearing client who is not vaccinated is transmitting the virus from themselves to the infant through respiratory droplets during breastfeeding. The child-bearing client should wear a mask and perform hand hygiene before placing the newborn to the breast. An added precaution for when a child-bearing client coughs or sneezes when the chest is exposed should be to cleanse the breast region with soap and water before feeding. Child-bearing clients may also choose to pump their breast milk, ensuring they do proper hand hygiene and the equipment is all clean (CPS, 2020).

Newborn Complications
Maturity and Size

Preterm or post-term newborns may be SGA (10th percentile), LGA (90th percentile), or average for gestational age (AGA; 50th percentile), depending on their percentile score against weight and age categories on a growth assessment chart. SGA newborns score below the 10th percentile, meaning that 10% of other newborns weigh less than them and 90% weigh more. LGA babies should be investigated as infants of mothers with diabetes. SGA newborns may be associated with conditions that impaired uteroplacental circulation during the pregnancy.

Preterm Newborn

Pathophysiology

- A preterm baby is one born after 20 weeks' and before the end of 37 weeks' gestation, regardless of weight. Assessment tools to determine age include the Dubowitz and Ballard scoring systems.
- The cause is often unknown. Preterm birth is the leading cause of morbidity and mortality; for maternal risk factors, see the section "Preterm Labour and Birth."
- Preterm complications are numerous depending on age and include an inability to establish and maintain independent respirations (respiratory distress syndrome [RDS]), heart murmurs, cold stress, electrolyte and calcium imbalances, increased risk of infection, poor skin integrity, hypoglycemia, risk of neurological impairment and bleeding, anemia, poor digestive ability and malnourishment, and retinopathy of prematurity.

Clinical manifestations. Physical characteristics are dependent on gestational age but may include extended body position, fine downy hair on the head, soft pliable ear without cartilage, lack of body fat, tissuelike or gelatinous skin with visible veins, lack of rugae on the scrotum, labia minor and clitoris visible on females, no sole creases, fine downy lanugo hair widely distributed, and vernix covering the body.

Nursing considerations

- Observe for signs of respiratory distress, including grunting, chest indrawing, nasal flaring, oxygen saturation of less than 85%, tachypnea, or apnea.
- Maintain a neutral thermal environment; monitor temperature, preventing cold stress using a hat and booties; and maintain skin integrity.
- Establish early frequent feedings to counter hypoglycemia. If the respiratory rate is greater than 60, nasogastric feedings will be required. Carefully monitor intake and output and weight gains or losses.
- Support parents in understanding the needs of the preterm infant, especially if intensive care is required; allay feelings of guilt, and anticipate grieving and the need for open discussion. Some hospitals have support groups for the parents of infants in NICUs.
- The birth of a preterm infant or high-risk infant affects the entire family. Nurses need to consider reactions and responses of not just the parents but also grandparents and siblings when providing family-centred care for the infant and family. Grandparents may worry about the well-being of their grandchild or have feelings of sadness and grief as they watch their own child struggling with the difficulties and challenges of a preterm infant. Siblings may be confused if the infant is not brought home but must remain in hospital. Nurses can support grandparents' and siblings' visits while the infant is in the hospital and help prepare the parents for possible reactions from siblings once the newborn is discharged home and requires a lot of parental attention (Lowdermilk et al., 2020).

Post-Term Newborn

Pathophysiology

- A post-term newborn is one born after 42 weeks' gestation, a condition associated with primiparas, history of postmaturity, and congenital anomalies, including anencephaly (lack of brain development).
- Morbidity and mortality risks are associated with increasingly poor uteroplacental circulation and hypoxia and include meconium aspiration, pneumothorax, hypoglycemia, hypothermia, asphyxia, and birth trauma.

Clinical manifestations. Physical characteristics include a long thin body with wasted appearance, little body fat, long nails, dry and cracked skin, meconium staining, and no vernix or lanugo.

Nursing considerations

- Monitor for uteroplacental insufficiency with regular NST beginning at pregnancy term.
- Be prepared for complications at the time of birth and the need for respiratory support.
- Closely monitor respiratory rate and effort, observe for complications, prevent cold stress, monitor for hypoglycemia and establish frequent regular feedings, and provide information for follow-up care in the community and referral to a pediatrician if needed.

Birth Trauma

Most instances of birth trauma are temporary and self-resolve over time. Trauma may result from medical interventions, including forceps, or be related to pelvic or fetal dystocia factors. Examples include the following:

- Cephalohematoma: It is a well-defined, soft, localized swelling, an accumulation of blood between the skull and periosteum that does *not* cross the cranial suture lines. It emerges on day 2 or 3 following birth and then slowly disappears over weeks or months. There is a risk of jaundice secondary to the blood loss and reabsorption.
- Caput succedaneum: It is a poorly defined, localized soft tissue edema caused by cervical pressure on the fetal head, present at birth, crosses the suture lines, and disappears within hours or days.
- Forceps injury: Facial bruising may be apparent over the cheeks from forceps application. Compression may cause one-sided facial nerve palsy, with one side of the newborn's face appearing asymmetrical, especially when crying. The bruising resolves within a few days. The facial paralysis is rarely permanent and usually resolves within a few hours or days.
- Brachial plexus injury: It is the most common nerve injury and is caused by traction on the nerves in the neck and head during birth. The affected arm is extended and limp, with absent reflexes. Recovery is within weeks with immobilization and physiotherapy. Some infants require surgical intervention. LGA infants with shoulder dystocia and breech infants are especially at risk.
- Fractured clavicle: Redness, swelling, or crepitus is noted over the collar bone, and the infant may be irritable and crying. The fracture is confirmed by X-ray and immobilized.
- Bruises and edema: The infant may have bruising and edema on the other parts of the body due to birth trauma, particularly in difficult deliveries, which disappears in a few days. These bruises can be mistaken for congenital dermal melanocytosis. Congenital dermal melanocytosis results in bluish-black areas of pigmented skin that can occur in babies of Mediterranean, Latin American, Asian, or African descent. They disappear eventually in months or years.

Hemolytic Disease

ABO and Rh blood incompatibilities in the fetus and newborn are caused by maternal immune reactions against blood group factors on the fetal RBCs. While fetal and maternal blood supplies are separate, minute amounts of fetal blood cross into maternal circulation with placental breaks and at the time of birth.

Pathophysiology

- ABO incompatibility affects about 20% of pregnancies of group A or B infants with group O mothers. Group O clients have natural anti-A or anti-B antibodies, or both, which initiate a hemolytic response against the fetal RBCs.
- Rh incompatibility affects about 2% of pregnancies. The child-bearing client is Rh-negative, while the fetus is Rh-positive. During the first pregnancy, the hemolytic

response is initiated when the child-bearing client's blood is sensitized and antibodies are produced. The first pregnancy may be unaffected, but unless treated, each subsequent pregnancy will result in a stronger immune hemolytic response with resulting destruction of fetal RBCs and stimulation of the fetal liver and spleen to produce more RBCs.

- Immunization and antibody formation can also occur with a spontaneous or induced abortion, amniocentesis, or ectopic pregnancy.

Clinical manifestations

- ABO incompatibility: Pathological or nonphysiological jaundice occurs in the first 24 hours, with mild anemia but rarely with an enlarged liver or spleen.
- Rh incompatibility: In affected pregnancies, jaundice occurs in the first 24 hours, with moderate to severe anemia, hepatosplenomegaly, cardiac or pulmonary failure, ascites, edema, or even stillbirth in severe cases.

Diagnostics and therapeutics

- ABO incompatibility: Diagnosis is via direct and indirect Coombs test (detecting maternal antibodies), bilirubin, and CBC. It usually resolves without complications using phototherapy.

- Rh incompatibility: Blood tests are the same as for ABO. Diagnosis may also require testing amniotic fluid for bilirubin levels or performing cordocentesis for fetal blood analysis.
  - Provide Rh-immune prophylaxis (Rhogam) for all at-risk clients to prevent and suppress the maternal antibody response.
- Exchange blood transfusion: The newborn's blood is replaced with type O blood, which will not react to the maternal antibodies. The newborn will revert to their natural blood type over time without a subsequent hemolytic reaction.

Nursing considerations

- Monitor antibody, bilirubin, and CBC levels in the child-bearing client and newborn.
- Provide information and teaching to the Rh-negative child-bearing client about the importance of receiving prophylaxis in all high-risk situations. It is given at 28 weeks' gestation, within 72 hours postpartum, or following the at-risk episodes noted earlier.
- Provide antenatal fetal monitoring for Rh incompatibility, including ultrasonography and amniocentesis.
- Assess the newborn for early-onset jaundice and implement appropriate treatment.

PRACTICE QUESTIONS

Case 1

Ms. Viraj gave birth to her first child 18 hours ago in an uncomplicated vaginal birth. She is preparing to be discharged home later today with her newborn son and her common-law partner. The baby has successfully breastfed several times since birth. The nurse is performing a postpartum assessment and preparing the family for discharge.

Questions 1 to 6 refer to this case.

1. The nurse notes that the lochia is a moderate amount of rubra on the perineal pad. She palpates Ms. Viraj's uterus and assesses that it is firm, 2 cm above the height of the umbilicus, and located toward the left side of the abdomen. What is the most likely cause for this assessment finding?
   1. Postpartum hemorrhage
   2. A uterine infection
   3. A full bladder
   4. Normal uterine involution

2. Ms. Viraj is concerned that she will not know if the baby is getting enough breast milk. Which of the following provides the best information for Ms. Viraj to assess if the baby is receiving enough nourishment?
   1. The baby is feeding every 3 to 4 hours.
   2. The baby has four to five wet diapers every day.
   3. The baby has frequent audible swallows while feeding.
   4. The baby is gaining 10 g per day.

3. The nurse explains to Ms. Viraj that while breast milk provides the ideal nutrition, she will need to give the baby supplemental drops. What nutrients, not found in adequate amounts in breast milk, will need to be supplemented?

   1. Vitamin D
   2. Iron
   3. Vitamin A
   4. Essential fatty acids

4. Ms. Viraj's partner tells the nurse that he can't understand why she keeps talking about what happened during the labour and birth, telling the story over and over again. Which of the following is the best response by the nurse to Ms. Viraj's partner?
   1. "You seem tired. Perhaps you should try to get some extra rest."
   2. "I can provide referral information for counselling services."
   3. "It's an essential part of the bonding experience for her."
   4. "Reliving the experience helps her with the reality of the experience and is a normal part of adjusting to parenthood."

5. The baby's physical assessment reveals a poorly defined, soft mass across the top of the head. The nurse explains to the parents that this is a temporary condition that will resolve over the next few days. What is this assessment finding called?
   1. Moulding
   2. Caput succedaneum
   3. Cephalohematoma
   4. Congenital dermal melanocytosis

6. Ms. Viraj and her partner have been discussing whether they are going to have their son circumcised. Ms. Viraj tells the nurse that she has heard it is healthier for the baby. The nurse's best response would include which of the following information?

1. Circumcision should be performed only for religious reasons.
2. The nurse's personal beliefs regarding the need for circumcision should be shared.
3. Circumcision is not recommended as a routine practice.
4. There is clear evidence that circumcision is beneficial and should be performed in infancy.

Case 2

Ms. Smitherman, age 42, gravida 1, para 0, is admitted to the labour unit at 33 weeks' gestation after she experienced painless vaginal bleeding that soaked through several sanitary pads. An ultrasonogram is ordered. Preparations are made for a possible early birth. Six hours later, Ms. Smitherman goes into premature labour and her vaginal bleeding worsens.

Questions 7 to 10 refer to this case.

7. What is the primary purpose for the ultrasonogram in this situation?
   1. To assess fetal well-being
   2. To detect fetal abnormalities
   3. To determine the location of the placenta
   4. To calculate fetal growth and gestational age
8. What is the most likely cause of Ms. Smitherman's painless vaginal bleeding in the third trimester?
   1. Placenta previa
   2. Placental abruption
   3. Spontaneous abortion (miscarriage)
   4. Hemolytic Rh incompatibility
9. The nurse prepares Ms. Smitherman for a Caesarean birth. Ms. Smitherman is anxious about this unplanned Caesarean surgery. She wants to know whether this will be the only way she can deliver future children. The nurse indicates that
   1. Her future deliveries will be by Caesarean birth.
   2. She should have a vaginal birth with the next pregnancy.
   3. Caesarean births are easier to recover from than vaginal births.
   4. She will need to discuss the possibility of a future vaginal delivery with the obstetrician.
10. In the operating room, a neonatal team of physician, nurse, and respiratory therapist attends to the premature infant when it is born. What is the most important assessment by the team after delivery?
    1. Respirations
    2. Apical heart rate
    3. Colour
    4. Identification of any congenital defects

Case 3

Mr. and Ms. Cane's full-term newborn son is 3 days old. Ms. Cane is recovering from a difficult birth. The baby has forceps bruising on his face and a cephalohematoma on the right side of his head. The morning assessment of the baby reveals that the sclera of the eyes, oral mucous membranes, and skin are yellowed. Blood work shows an elevated bilirubin. Phototherapy is prescribed for the baby.

Questions 11 and 12 refer to this case.

11. Mr. Cane asks the nurse whether the baby has a liver disease that caused the jaundice. In explaining physiological jaundice to the parents, which explanation would best describe this condition?
    1. It occurs after 24 hours in many babies who are in good health and will resolve in a few days.
    2. Physiological jaundice was caused by the bruising and cephalohematoma.
    3. Physiological jaundice occurs on the first day of life, and more tests will be needed.
    4. A blood exchange transfusion will be required to prevent brain damage.
12. What side effect of phototherapy should the nurse teach the parents to expect?
    1. Fluid requirements for the baby decrease by 10% while undergoing phototherapy treatment.
    2. The baby may experience constipation with fewer, firmer stools.
    3. The baby may be more awake, irritable, and difficult to settle.
    4. The baby's eyes will be covered for protection, but most of the skin will be exposed and may darken temporarily.

Independent Questions

Questions 13 to 25 do not refer to a particular case.

13. A client is 39 weeks' gestation with their first pregnancy. The client calls the obstetrician's office and tells the nurse they are having regular contractions 7 minutes apart, but their membranes have not ruptured. What advice would the nurse provide?
    1. Wait until their membranes have ruptured before going to the hospital.
    2. Have their partner drive them to the hospital.
    3. Walk around the house to see if the contractions become less regular.
    4. Come to the hospital when the contractions are 4 minutes apart.
14. By what physiological mechanism do newborns stay warm?
    1. Shivering
    2. Metabolizing brown fat stores
    3. Decreasing oxygen consumption
    4. Keeping an extended body posture
15. Which of the following is an indicator used in assessing gestational age?
    1. Weight
    2. Head circumference
    3. Ear cartilage
    4. Body length
16. During the transitional changes at birth when the newborn breathes independently, what causes the foramen ovale to close?
    1. Oxygen levels increase.
    2. The umbilical cord is clamped.
    3. Pressure in the left atria of the heart becomes greater than that in the right atria of the heart.

4. Pulmonary blood vessels constrict, and pulmonary blood pressure increases.

17. How frequently should prenatal appointments be scheduled for a client with an uncomplicated pregnancy?
    1. Every 3 weeks until the sixth month, then every 2 weeks until birth
    2. Every 4 weeks until the seventh month, after which appointments will become more frequent
    3. Monthly until the eigth month
    4. Every 2 to 3 weeks for the entire pregnancy

18. Rh-immune prophylaxis treatment with Rh immune globulin (Rhogam) should be administered in certain situations to prevent maternal antibody formation. In which one of the following situations would Rh immune globulin (Rhogam) be administered to the client who is Rh negative?
    1. Following the birth of an Rh-negative newborn
    2. Following a spontaneous or induced abortion
    3. Following all births, regardless of blood type and Rh factor
    4. Following an ABO-incompatible birth

19. Which instruction should be included in the discharge teaching plan to assist the postpartum client in recognizing early signs of complications?
    1. Palpate the fundus daily to ensure that it is soft.
    2. Notify the primary health care provider of any increase in the amount of lochia or a return to bright red bleeding.
    3. Report any decrease in the amount of brownish red lochia.
    4. The passage of clots as large as an orange can be expected.

20. A nurse is aware that a full-term infant is born with which of the following reflexes? **Select all that apply.**
    1. Moro
    2. Babinski
    3. Rooting
    4. Stepping
    5. Pincer grasping
    6. Tonic neck

21. Which of the following is a risk factor for the infant of a child-bearing client with gestational diabetes?
    1. Hypoglycemia
    2. Small for gestational age (SGA)
    3. Hyperglycemia
    4. Insulin resistance

22. A nurse is aware that which of the following are risk factors for a postpartum hemorrhage (PPH)? **Select all that apply.**
    1. Polyhydramnios
    2. Tachycardia
    3. Trauma
    4. Uterine atony
    5. Thromboembolism

23. The nurse is providing discharge teaching to a breastfeeding client who has been diagnosed with mastitis. Which of the following will the nurse recommend? **Select all that apply.**
    1. Limit fluid intake to 1 litre per day.
    2. Ensure frequent breastfeeding or pumping from the affected breast.
    3. Take warm showers prior to feeding.
    4. Wear a supportive bra.
    5. Use ice packs prior to breastfeeding.
    6. Take the prescribed antibiotic until symptoms improve.

24. The nurse educates prenatal clients about the threat of TORCH infections. Which infections are included in this classification? **Select all that apply.**
    1. Toxoplasmosis
    2. Toxemia
    3. Cytomegalovirus
    4. Rubella
    5. Herpes simplex

25. What are the functions of amniotic fluid? **Select all that apply.**
    1. Maintaining an even temperature
    2. Impeding excessive fetal movement
    3. Lubricating fetal skin
    4. Acting as a reservoir for nutrients
    5. Acting as a cushion for the fetus

REFERENCES

Astle, B., & Duggleby, W. (2024). *Potter and Perry's Canadian fundamentals of nursing* (7th ed.). Elsevier.

Battams, N. (2018). *A snapshot of family diversity in Canada.* The Vanier Institute of the Family. https://vanierinstitute.ca/a-snapshot-of-family-diversity-in-canada-february-2018/

Battams, N. (2021). *New Statistics Canada data show COVID is impacting fertility in Canada.* The Vanier Institute of the Family. https://vanierinstitute.ca/new-statistics-canada-data-show-covid-is-impacting-fertility-in-canada/

Beischer, N. A., Mackey, E. V., & Colditz, P. B. (1997). *Obstetrics and the newborn* (3rd ed.). Baillière Tindall.

Blackburn, S. (2017). *Maternal, fetal & neonatal physiology: A clinical perspective* (5th ed.). Saunders.

Bowden, V., Dickey, S., & Greenberg, C. (1998). *Children and their families: The continuum of care.* Saunders.

Burman, D. (2019). *Surrogacy and IVF in Canada: What you need to know.* City News on CityTV. https://toronto.citynews.ca/2019/01/09/surrogacy-and-ivf-in-canada-what-you-need-to-know/

Canadian Institute of Health Research. (2020). *Detailed documentation of the tiers of obstetric and neonatal service in Canadian hospitals: Report of the CIHR team on improved prenatal health care regionalization.* https://med-fom-phsr-obgyn.sites.olt.ubc.ca/files/2021/03/TOSDetailedJune2020.pdf

Canadian Midwifery Regulators Council. (2022). *About Canadian Midwifery Regulators Council.* http://cmrc-ccosf.ca/about-cmrc

Canadian Paediatric Society (CPS). (2013). *Practice point: Nutrition for healthy term infants: Birth to six months; an overview.* [Reaffirmed 2022] http://www.cps.ca/en/documents/position/nutrition-healthy-term-infants-overview

Canadian Paediatric Society (CPS). (2015). *Position statement: Newborn male circumcision.* [Reaffirmed 2022] http://www.cps.ca/en/documents/position/circumcision

Canadian Paediatric Society (CPS). (2018, updated 2021). *Position statement: Facilitating discharge from hospital of the healthy term infant.* https://cps.ca/documents/position/facilitating-discharge-from-hospital-of-the-healthy-term-infant

Canadian Paediatric Society (CPS). (2019, updated 2020). *Practice point: Timing of introduction of allergenic solids for infants at high risk.* https://cps.ca/en/documents/position/allergenic-solids

Canadian Paediatric Society (CPS). (2020, updated 2021). *Practice point: Breastfeeding and COVID-19.* https://cps.ca/documents/position/breastfeeding-when-mothers-have-suspected-or-proven-covid-19

Canadian Paediatric Society (CPS). (2022). *Position statement: Preventing symptomatic vitamin D deficiency and rickets among Indigenous infants and children in Canada.* https://cps.ca/en/documents/position/vitamin-d-deficiency-and-rickets-among-indigenous-infants-and-children

Centers for Disease Control and Prevention (CDC). (2022). *COVID-19 vaccines while pregnant or breastfeeding.* https://www.cdc.gov/coronavirus/2019-ncov/vaccines/recommendations/pregnancy.html

Dames, S., Luctkar-Flude, M., & Tyerman, J. (2021). *Edelman and Kudzma's Canadian health promotion throughout the life span* (1st ed.). Elsevier Inc.

Fostik, A., & Galbraith, N. (2021). *Statistics of Canada: StatCan COVID-19: What can fertility intentions tell us about the impact of the pandemic.* https://www150.statcan.gc.ca/n1/pub/45-28-0001/2021001/article/00041-eng.htm

Government of Canada. (2014). *Prenatal nutrition guidelines for health professionals: Gestational weight gain.* https://www.canada.ca/en/health-canada/services/canada-food-guide/resources/prenatal-nutrition/eating-well-being-active-towards-healthy-weight-gain-pregnancy-2010.html

Government of Canada. (2019). *Ultrasound.* https://www.canada.ca/en/health-canada/services/health-risks-safety/radiation/medical/ultrasound.html

Government of Canada. (2020). *Vitamin D and calcium: Updated dietary reference intakes.* https://www.canada.ca/en/health-canada/services/food-nutrition/healthy-eating/vitamins-minerals/vitamin-calcium-updated-dietary-reference-intakes-nutrition.html

Government of Canada. (2021a). *Family-centred maternity and newborn care: National guidelines.* https://www.canada.ca/en/public-health/services/publications/healthy-living/maternity-newborn-care-guidelines-chapter-1.html#a1

Government of Canada. (2021b). *Canada's food guide: Healthy eating when pregnant and breastfeeding.* https://food-guide.canada.ca/en/tips-for-healthy-eating/pregnant-breastfeeding/

Government of Canada. (2021c). *Canada prenatal nutrition program (CPNP).* https://www.canada.ca/en/public-health/services/health-promotion/childhood-adolescence/programs-initiatives/canada-prenatal-nutrition-program-cpnp.html

Government of Canada. (2021d). *Human papillomavirus vaccine: Canadian immunization guide.* https://www.canada.ca/en/public-health/services/publications/healthy-living/canadian-immunization-guide-part-4-active-vaccines/page-9-human-papillomavirus-vaccine.html#p4c8a5_d

Government of Canada. (2021e). *Canadian immunization guide part 4: Active vaccines: Varicella (chicken pox) vaccine.* https://www.canada.ca/en/public-health/services/publications/healthy-living/canadian-immunization-guide-part-4-active-vaccines/page-24-varicella-chickenpox-vaccine.html#p4c23a5c

Government of Canada. (2022). *Canada's food guide.* https://food-guide.canada.ca/en/

Information and Privacy Commissioner of Ontario. (2015). *Frequently asked personal questions: Personal Health Information Protection Act.* https://www.ipc.on.ca/wp-content/uploads/2015/11/phipa-faq.pdf

Keenan-Lindsay, L. (2020). *Leifer's introduction to maternity and pediatric nursing in Canada* (1st ed.). Elsevier.

Keenan-Lindsay, L., Sams, C. A., & O'Connor, C. (2022). *Perry's maternal child nursing care in Canada* (3rd ed.). Elsevier.

Leifer, G. (2018). *Introduction to maternity and pediatric nursing* (8th ed.). Elsevier Canada.

Lowdermilk, D. L., Perry, S. E., Cashion, K., et al. (2020). *Maternity & women's health care* (12th ed.). Elsevier.

National Aboriginal Council of Midwives (NACM). (2020). *Missions and values.* https://indigenousmidwifery.ca/mission-vision-values/

Ontario Ministry of Health and Long Term Care. (2018). *Health protection and promotion act: Regulation 557 communicable diseases–general.* https://www.health.gov.on.ca/en/common/legislation/opth_neo/default.aspx#facts.

Pfizer. (2021). *Product monograph including patient information: Depo-Provera (medroxyprogesterone acetate injectable suspension, USP).* https://www.pfizer.ca/sites/default/files/202201/Depo-Provera_PM_E_252963_17Dec2021.pdf

Registered Nurses Association of Ontario (RNAO). (2018a). *Best practice guideline: Assessment and interventions for perinatal depression* (2nd ed.). https://rnao.ca/sites/rnao-ca/files/bpg/Perinatal_Depression_FINAL_web_0.pdf

Registered Nurses Association of Ontario. (2018b). *Best practice guideline: Breastfeeding-promoting and supporting the initiation, exclusivity, and continuation of breastfeeding for newborns, infants, and young children* (3rd ed.). https://rnao.ca/sites/rnao-ca/files/bpg/breast_feeding_BPG_WEB_updated_Oct_2_1.pdf

Society of Obstetricians and Gynaecologists of Canada (SOGC). (2021). *SOGC statement on COVID-19 vaccination in pregnancy.* https://sogc.org/common/Uploaded%20files/Covid%20Information/SOGC_Statement_COVID-19_Vaccination_in_Pregnancy.pdf

Society of Obstetricians and Gynaecologists of Canada (SOGC) (2022a). *Before you conceive. Assisted reproduction.* https://www.pregnancyinfo.ca/before-you-conceive/human-reproduction/assisted-reproduction/

Society of Obstetricians and Gynaecologists of Canada (SOGC). (2022b). *Medications and drugs during pregnancy.* https://www.pregnancyinfo.ca/your-pregnancy/healthy-pregnancy/medications-and-drugs-during-pregnancy/

Society of Obstetricians and Gynaecologists of Canada (SOGC). (2022c). *Your pregnancy: Cancer during pregnancy.* https://www.pregnancyinfo.ca/your-pregnancy/special-consideration/cancer-during-pregnancy/

Statistics Canada. (2018). *First Nations people, Metis and Inuit in Canada: Diverse and growing populations.* https://www150.statcan.gc.ca/n1/pub/89-659-x/89-659-x2018001-eng.htm

Statistics Canada. (2019). *Families matters: Being common law, married, separated, or divorced in Canada.* https://www150.statcan.gc.ca/n1/daily-quotidien/190501/dq190501b-eng.htm

Statistics Canada. (2021a). *Live births, by age of mother.* https://www150.statcan.gc.ca/t1/tbl1/en/tv.action?pid=1310041601

Statistic Canada. (2021b). *A statistical portrait of Canada's diverse LGBTQ2+ communities.* https://www150.statcan.gc.ca/n1/daily-quotidien/210615/dq210615a-eng.htm

Statistics Canada. (2021c). *Projections of the Indigenous populations and households in Canada 2016 to 2041.* https://www150.statcan.gc.ca/n1/daily-quotidien/211006/dq211006a-eng.htm

Trojano, G., Raffaello Damiani, G. R., Olivieri, C., et al. (2019). VBAC: Antenatal predictors of success. *Acta Bio-Medica: Atenei Parmensis, 90*(3), 300309. https://www.ncbi.nlm.nih.gov/pmc/articles/PMC7233729/

Vanier Institute. (2022). *Definition of family.* https://vanierinstitute.ca/definition-of-family/

Zitelli, B. J., & Davis, H. W. (2002). *Atlas of pediatric physical diagnosis* (4th ed.). Mosby.

BIBLIOGRAPHY

Association of Ontario Midwives. (2022). *What is a midwife?.* https://www.ontariomidwives.ca/what-midwife

Canadian Nurses Association. (2008). *Joint statement on breastfeeding.* https://hl-prod-ca-oc-download.s3-ca-central-1.amazonaws.com/CNA/2f975e7e-4a40-45ca-863c-5ebf0a138d5e/UploadedImages/documents/JPS94_Breastfeeding_March_2008_e.pdf

College of Midwives of Ontario. (2022). *Midwives.* https://www.cmo.on.ca/

College of Nurses of Ontario. (2019). *Professional conduct: Professional misconduct* (publication No.42007).

Davidson, M., London, M., & Ladewig, P. (2019). *Old's maternal-newborn nursing and women's health across the lifespan* (11th ed.). Pearson Education.

Government of Canada. (2016). *Smoking cessation during pregnancy and relapse after childbirth in Canada.* https://www.canada.ca/en/public-health/services/publications/healthy-living/smoking-cessation-during-pregnancy-relapse-after-childbirth-canada.html

Government of Canada. (2017). *Human papillomavirus (HPV) prevention and HOV vaccines: Questions and answers.* https://www.canada.ca/en/public-health/services/infectious-diseases/sexual-health-sexually-transmitted-infections/hpv-prevention-vaccines-questions-answers.html

Government of Canada. (2020). *Perinatal health indicators.* https://health-infobase.canada.ca/phi/

Government of Canada. (2021). *Chapter 4: Care during labour and birth. Pain management: Non-pharmacological, pharmacological and epidural options.* https://www.canada.ca/en/public-health/services/publications/healthy-living/maternity-newborn-care-guidelines-chapter-4.html#a7

Jarvis, C., Browne, A. J., MacDonald-Jenkins, et al. (2024). *Physical examination and health assessment* (4th ed.). Saunders.

Office of AIDS Research National Institute of Health. (2022). *About the office of AIDS research.* https://www.oar.nih.gov/about

Perinatal HIV Guidelines Working Group. (2018). *Recommendations for use of antiretroviral drugs in pregnant HIV-infected women for maternal health and interventions to reduce perinatal HIV transmission in the United States. Maternal HIV testing and identification of perinatal HIV exposure.* https://clinicalinfo.hiv.gov/en/guidelines/perinatal/appendix-c-antiretroviral-counseling-guide-for-health-care-providers?

Society of Obstetricians and Gynaecologists of Canada. (2014). Practice guidelines: Diagnosis, evaluation, and management of hypertensive disorders of pregnancy. executive summary. *Journal of Obstetrics and Gynaecology Canada, 36*(5), 416–438. https://www.jogc.com/article/S1701-2163(15)30588-0/fulltext

Society of Obstetricians and Gynaecologists of Canada. (2022). *All of us against HPV. Take action to protect yourself and others. What is HPV.* http://hpvinfo.ca

Statistics Canada. (2019). *Census in brief: Diverse family characteristics of Aboriginal children aged 0 to 4.* http://www12.statcan.gc.ca/census-recensement/2016/as-sa/98-200-x/2016020/98-200-x2016020-eng.cfm.

Statistics Canada. (2020). *Births, 2019.* https://www150.statcan.gc.ca/n1/daily-quotidien/200929/dq200929e-eng.htm

WEBSITES

- **Government of Canada—Healthy Pregnancy for First Nations and Inuit** (https://www.sac-isc.gc.ca/eng/1581523249046/1581523302054): This Government of Canada site provides information specifically for First Nations and Inuit people on a variety of topics, including becoming a mother, eating well, and being active. It also includes links to additional resources.

- **Public Health Agency of Canada, Your Guide to a Healthy Pregnancy** (https://www.canada.ca/en/health-canada/services/healthy-living/healthy-pregnancy.html): This site has extensive information on healthy living during pregnancy.

- **Society of Obstetricians and Gynaecologists of Canada** (http://www.sogc.org): This site includes information on women's health, including pregnancy. The site includes many resources for health professionals.

Pediatric Nursing

This chapter on pediatric nursing encompasses the care of children of all ages, from newborns to adolescents, focusing on injury prevention and the promotion of optimal health in a variety of health conditions. An awareness of growth and development patterns in children, as well as the unique physical changes that occur at each stage of development, is essential to the delivery of quality pediatric nursing care.

Pediatric care is provided within the context of the family. Effective care is respectful of social and cultural differences and beliefs and involves the development of trusting and collaborative relationships between family members and the nurse.

FAMILY INFLUENCES ON CHILD HEALTH

Family is defined in many ways by scholars and individuals according to the individuals own frame of reference, values, and disciplines. There is no universal definition of family, a family is what an individual considers it to be. Biology emphasizes the family fulfilling the biologic function of perpetuation of the species. Psychology describes the interpersonal aspects of the family and its responsibility for personal development. Economics depicts the family as a productive unit that provides material for needs. Sociology views the family as a social unit that interacts in a larger society, creating the context within cultural values and identity is formed. Others define family in terms of the relationships of the persons who make up the family unit (Hockenberry et al., 2022). Refer to Chapter 10 for the Vanier's Institute definition of family, which is purposely broad and promotes respect and support for all types of families.

It is important to keep in mind that numerous social, cultural, religious, and economic factors influence the family as well as the health and well-being of the child. A family-centred care model is recognized to promote child health and well-being.

In pediatric nursing, a thorough family assessment is essential and should include the collection of data concerning both family structure and family function.

Family Structure

"The family structure, or family composition, consists of individuals, each with a socially recognized status and position, who interact with one another on a regular, recurring basis in socially sanctioned ways" (Hockenberry et al., 2022, p. 17). With the transition from the nuclear family to nontraditional family structures, the pediatric nurse is challenged to understand the influences each family structure has on the health and well-being of a given child. When members are added or lost through events such as marriage, divorce, abandonment, birth, death and incarceration, the family structure is changed, and roles must be redefined or redistributed. In a lifetime, it is not unusual for children to belong to many different family groups (Hockenberry et al., 2022).

Common Types of Family Structures

Nuclear family. A nuclear family (referred to as a *census family* by Statistics Canada, 2022a) has one of the following characteristics (each consists of persons living in the same dwelling):

- A married couple without children
- A married couple with one or more unmarried children
- A father with one or more unmarried children
- A mother with one or more unmarried children
- Couples living in consensual unions, who should be regarded as married couples
- Grandchildren living with their grandparent(s) but no parents (Statistics Canada, 2022a)

Nursing considerations for a dual-income nuclear family include developing strategies for the family to meet the conflicting demands of careers and child-rearing while promoting optimal health.

Blended family. A blended family has at least one step-parent, stepsibling, or half-sibling. In 2016, 10% of Canadian children aged 0 to 14 years were living with one biological or adoptive parent and one step-parent (Statistics Canada, 2019a).

Nursing considerations include providing resources for families on parenting styles and strategies to reduce conflicts that can arise between the stepchild and the step-parent.

Extended or multigenerational family. Multigenerational families consist of grandparents, children, and grandchildren living in the same household. In an extended family, household expenses and child-rearing responsibilities are shared with a couple and a grandparent. This type of family structure is common for recently immigrated families as well as working-class families. The unique functioning styles and family strengths are significant resources that make the family unit even stronger. For some groups, such as Indigenous peoples, the family network is an important resource for encouraging health and healing (Keenan-Lindsay et al., 2022).

Nursing considerations include ensuring that resources are in place for aging family members (e.g., an older grandparent) participating in child-rearing, who may have financial difficulties and increasing health conditions.

Lone-parent family. A lone-parent family is a household led by one parent by choice or following death, divorce, or separation. In 2016, 19.2% of Canadian children under the age of 15 years were being raised in a lone-parent family. In all, 81.3% of lone-parent families were led by the mother, and 18.7% were led by the father (Statistics Canada, 2019a).

Nursing considerations include focusing on resources for social, emotional, and financial support.

Same-sex parent families. Same-sex families consist of people of the same sex who live together with or without children. The children may be offspring from a previous heterosexual marriage, adopted children, or therapeutic insemination. The parents may be married or common-law. Same-sex couples in Canada represent 0.9% of all couples in 2016. There were slightly fewer female (48.1%) same-sex couples than male (51.9%) same-sex couples. In 2016, approximately 1.8 same-sex couples (12%) had children living with them, compared with about half (51.4%) of couples of opposite sex (Statistics Canada, 2019b). Transgender couples also form families and become parents, either through adoption, the use of fertility drugs, or transmen discontinuing the hormones they are taking so they can become pregnant themselves (Keenan-Lindsay et al., 2022).

Family Function

"*Family function* refers to the interactions of family members, especially the quality of those relationships and interactions" (Hockenberry et al., 2022, p. 19). Assessment of family strengths and unique functioning styles is important for a pediatric nurse, as these factors can promote a stronger family unit and will influence how a family copes with illness in their child.

Parenting

Parents assume a leadership role in the family to guide children to learn acceptable behaviours. Ideally, parents instill beliefs, morals, and cultural values in their children in an effort to develop socially responsible and contributing members of society. The parenting style, along with the child's personality traits, will influence a child's developmental outcomes.

Parenting Styles

There are three main parenting styles. Families will generally display one style but may assume a different style in certain situations.

Authoritarian parents
- Rules and standards of conduct are set by the parent and followed rigidly.
- Children do not participate in family decision making.
- Children develop with poor communication and negotiation skills.
- Children are generally shy and self-conscious.

Authoritative parents
- Firm controls and limits are set by the parent.
- Children participate in open discussions on family issues and decisions.
- Children develop a sense of high self-esteem and self-reliance.

Permissive parents
- Parents exercise little or no control over their children.
- Children are permitted to regulate their own activity as much as possible.
- Children often control the parents and are disobedient, rebellious, and aggressive.

Parenting in Special Circumstances

Even in ideal circumstances, parents encounter many challenges when raising their children. When the family unit deviates from the norm, parents and children can face challenges that can potentially lead to family disruption.

Adoption. Adoption is not merely a simple matter of the legal transfer of parental rights from one party to another but includes the social and emotional health of the adopted child, the birth parents, and the adoptive families. Nurses can support families by helping to identify sources of adoptive agencies, by assisting families in preparing other siblings for the arrival of the adoptive child, and by helping to integrate the adoptive child into the family system.

Divorce. Research has shown that divorce has a tremendous impact on children (Keenan-Lindsay et al., 2022). Potential effects on children are as follows (Hockenberry et al., 2022):
- Children may experience more emotional and behavioural conditions.
- Factors that influence the impact include the age and sex of the child, the outcome of the divorce, the quality of the parent–child relationship, and parental care following the divorce.
- Children may feel guilt, or feel they are being punished for misbehaving or abandonment. Their need for reassurance and love is paramount at this time.
- Children may feel more loyal to one parent and may become the "message carrier" between the divorced parents.

There are two types of custody arrangements: divided or joint custody. Joint custody falls under two types: Joint physical custody involves parents sharing the responsibilities legally regarding their physical care and control of their children. The other type of joint custody is joint legal custody where the children live with one parent but both parents participate in the child-rearing and are both legal guardians. Divided custody separates the custody of the siblings amongst both parents.

Child- and family-centered care. It is common practice in most pediatric centres to approach care using a child- and family-centred care philosophy. Families and health care providers work together to plan, provide, and evaluate care.

According to SickKids (2022), child- and family-centred care involves a holistic approach to health care that prioritizes the needs and preferences of the child or client and recognizes the central role of the family in the child's life. Family may include all those identified by the child and family as close to and engaged in the care and support of the child (e.g., parents, siblings, grandparents, friends and other social supports). The approach is based on several key principles:

Respect: Recognizing and embracing the unique strengths, vulnerabilities, and values of both children and their families. Health care providers deliver care that is personalized and compassionate, acknowledging the individuality and specific needs of each child and family they serve.

Communication: Effective communication is essential in child- and family-centred care. Health care providers actively engage with children and their families, listening to their concerns and preferences. Information is shared in a clear, understandable manner and families' questions and input are valued and validated throughout the care process.

Partnership: Children and families are considered active partners in the care process. Health care providers work collaboratively with them, respecting their preferences and involving them in decision making. Authentic engagement and participation of children and families are in all aspects of care.

The outcomes of implementing child- and family-centred care can be categorized into four main areas:

Promoting optimal health: Efforts are made to enhance the overall quality of life for children and their families. This includes addressing aspects such as growth and development, symptom control, and successful treatments of both acute and chronic illnesses. The well-being of the entire family is considered, including factors like sibling adaption, caregiver sleep, and family coping. By tailoring to the unique needs and preferences of each child and family, health care providers can work toward achieving the best possible health outcomes.

Ensuring client safety: Child- and family-centred care places a strong emphasis on minimizing harm and optimizing outcomes. Health care providers take all necessary precautions to ensure the safety of children and their families during the care process. This includes maintaining the highest quality of care possible to promote client safety.

Achieving health equity: The goal is to provide care that is just and fair for all children and families. This involves recognizing and addressing disparities in access to high-quality services. Health care providers strive to provide equitable access to care, regardless of child's background, socioeconomic status, or other potential barriers to health care.

Maximizing client experience: Children and families feel personally supported, respected, and valued throughout the health care process. They ideally perceive excellence in care delivery, which can have a significant impact on their emotional well-being and overall satisfaction with the health care process.

GROWTH AND DEVELOPMENT

It is essential to understand the stages of growth and development when caring for children. As children progress through infancy to adolescence, their nutritional, cultural, and social situations will impact their development. Pediatric nurses integrate their knowledge of growth and development in each encounter with a child, and care is delivered in an age-appropriate manner.

Key Terms Related to Growth and Development

- *Growth* refers to increases in physical parameters, for example, height, weight, and vital signs.
- *Development* refers to increases in capability or function, including motor, psychosocial, and cognitive functions.
- *Cephalocaudal* means developmental progression from head to toe. For example, a child gains control of the head and neck before the trunk and limbs.
- *Proximodistal* means developmental progress that proceeds from the centre of the body outward to the extremities. For example, a child gains control of the hands before the fingers.

Major Theories of Development

Many theorists have organized their observations of childhood development into stages based on these approximate age groups:

- Infancy: Birth to 1 year
- Toddler: 1 to 3 years
- Preschool: 3 to 6 years
- School-age: 6 to 12 years
- Adolescence: 12 to 18 years

A few of the major theories of childhood development follow.

Freud's Theory of Psychosexual Development

Freud's theory divides psychic energy into three components of personality: the id, ego, and superego. The id, the unconscious mind, is the inborn component driven by instincts. The ego, the conscious mind serves the reality principle. The superego, the conscience, functions as the moral arbitrator and represents the ideal (Keenan-Lindsay et al., 2022).

Freud's theory suggests that sexual energy is centred in specific parts of the body at certain ages. During childhood, certain areas of the body assume a prominent psychological significance as the source of new pleasures and new conflicts gradually shift from one part of the body to another at certain stages of development (Keenan-Lindsay et al., 2022).

Erickson's Theory of Psychosocial Development

Erickson's theory suggests that individuals progress through life experiencing developmental crises at certain stages in life. Critical developmental needs must be met at each stage in order to move on to future stages and prevent future maladaptive social relationships (Hockenberry et al., 2022).

Piaget's Theory of Cognitive Development

Piaget's theory suggests that children are greatly influenced by age, experience, and maturational ability. Children learn from new experiences by integrating these experiences into their learning base. The child will then manage new experiences through accommodation (Keenan-Lindsay et al., 2022). The three theories are summarized in Table 11.1.

Kohlberg's Theory of Moral Development

Kohlberg's theory explains the development of moral decision making and judgement. Older children and adolescents start to develop a value system that is autonomous from that of their parents and other authority figures. Attention is given to the conscience of the individual within the society. While rules still play an important role, varying them to meet the needs of a culture is examined (Keenan-Lindsay, 2020).

Kohlberg's theory of moral development is summarized in Table 11.2.

Spiritual Development (Fowler)

Spiritual beliefs are closely related to the moral and ethical portion of the child's self-concept and, as such, must be considered as part of the child's basic needs assessment. Children need to have meaning, purpose, and hope in their lives. Also,

TABLE 11.1 Developmental Theories of Freud, Erickson, and Piaget

Age Group	Freud	Erickson	Piaget
Infancy (birth to 1 year)	*Oral stage*: Understanding the world by exploring the mouth	*Trust versus mistrust*: Getting needs met. Tolerating frustration in small doses. Recognizing caregiver are distinct from others and self.	*Sensorimotor* (birth to 2 years): At birth responses are limited to reflexes; begins to relate to outside events; concerned with sensations and actions that affect self directly.
Toddler (1–3 years)	*Anal stage*: Learning to give and take	*Autonomy versus shame and doubt-* Trying out powers of speech. Beginning acceptance of reality versus pleasure principle.	*Sensorimotor* (ends at 2 years) *Preoperational* (2–7 years)-child is still egocentric; thinks everyone sees world as self does.
Preschool (3–6 years)	*Phallic stage*: Becoming aware of self as a sexual being	*Initiative versus guilt*: Questioning. Exploring own body and environment. Differentiation of sexes.	*Perceptual* (4–7 years): Capable of some reasoning but can concentrate on only one aspect of a situation at a time.
School age (6–12 years)	*Latency stage*: Focusing on peer relations: learning to live in groups and to achieve knowledge	*Industry versus inferiority*: Learning to win recognition by producing things. Exploring, collecting. Learning to relate to own sex.	*Concrete operations* (7–11 years): Reasoning is logical but limited to own experience; understands cause and effect.
Adolescence (12–18 years)	*Genital stage*	*Identity versus diffusion (confusion)*: Moving toward own identity; sexual identity emerges. Selecting vocation. Beginning separation from family. Integrating personality (i.e., altruism).	*Formal operational* (11–16 years): Acquires ability to develop abstract concepts for self; oriented to problem-solving.

From Keenan-Lindsay, L. (2020). *Leifer's introduction to maternity and pediatric nursing in Canada* (1st ed., p. 333). Elsevier.

TABLE 11.2 Kohlberg's Theory of Moral Development

Preconventional (4–7 years)	Decisions are based on the desire to please others and to avoid punishment.
Conventional (7–11 years)	A conscience or internal set of standards is based on beliefs and teaching of others, such as parents. Rules are important and to be followed to please others and "be good."
Postconventional (12 years and older)	The individual has internalized ethical standards on which to base decisions and uses awareness of the common good and ethical principles rather than relying on the standards of others. Social responsibility is recognized. The value in each of two offering moral approaches can be considered and a decision made.

From Hockenberry, M., Rodgers, C., Wilson, D., (2022). *Wong's essentials of pediatric nursing* (11th ed. p. 46). Elsevier.

the need for confession and forgiveness is present, even in very young children. Extending beyond religion (an organized set of beliefs and practices), spirituality affects the whole person, including the mind, body, and spirit.

Fowler (1981) identified six stages in the development of faith, four of which are closely associated with and parallel cognitive and psychosocial development in childhood.

Stage 0: Undifferentiated: This stage encompasses the period of infancy, in which there is no concept of right or wrong, no beliefs, and no convictions to guide behaviour. The beginning of faith is established with the development of basic trust through the relationship with the primary caregiver.

Stage 1: Intuitive-projective: Toddlers imitate the religious gestures and behaviours of others without comprehending any meaning or significance to the activities. In preschool years, children assimilate some of the values and beliefs of their parents. Parental attitudes toward moral codes and religious beliefs convey to children what they consider to be good and bad. Children still imitate behaviour at this age and follow parental beliefs as part of their daily lives rather than through an understanding of the basic concepts underlying those beliefs.

Stage 2: Mythical-literal: During the school-age years, spiritual development parallels cognitive development and is closely related to children's experiences and social interaction. Many children have a strong interest in religion. They may accept the existence of a deity, and petitions to an omnipotent being are important and expected to be answered; good behaviour is rewarded, and bad behaviour is punished. Their developing conscience bothers them when they disobey. They have reverence for thoughts and matters and are able to articulate their faith. They may question the validity of their faith.

Stage 3: Synthetic-convention: As children approach adolescence, they become increasingly aware of spiritual disappointments. They realize that prayers are not always answered (at least on their own terms) and may begin to abandon or modify some religious practices. They begin to reason, to question some of the established parental religious standards, and to drop or modify some religious practices.

Stage 4: Individuating-reflective: Adolescents are more skeptical. They compare the religious standards of their parents with those of others and attempt to determine which standards to adopt and incorporate into their own set of values. They begin to compare religious standards with the scientific viewpoint. They are uncertain about many religious ideas but will not achieve profound insights until late adolescence or early adulthood.

INFANCY: BIRTH TO 1 YEAR OF AGE

Biological Changes

Infancy is the most rapid period of growth, with increases in length, weight, and head and chest circumference and changes in fontanelles. Growth should be charted on standardized growth charts for boys and girls to observe for comparable gains in length, weight, and head circumference.

Length

- Increases in length occur in spurts rather than through slow and steady growth.
- Elongation of the trunk dominates, with height increasing by 2.5 cm per month during the first 6 months and then by 1.25 cm per month during the second 6 months.
- Length should increase by 50% by the end of the first year.

Weight

- Weight increases 680 g per month for the first 5 months, at which point, the birth weight is doubled.
- Weight increases at half this rate for the next 6 months, with an average of 340 g per month; by 12 months, the birth weight should have tripled.
- Breastfed infants tend to weigh slightly less than formula-fed infants during the second 6 months of life.

Head and Chest Circumference

- Head growth is rapid and is a major indicator of brain development.
- Head circumference increases on average 1.5 cm per month for the first 6 months, then 0.5 cm per month for the next 6 months.
- By the end of the first year, head size has increased, on average, 33%.
- Chest circumference is normally 2 cm less than head circumference.

Fontanelles

- The anterior (diamond-shaped) fontanelle typically measures 5 cm at birth and closes at between 12 and 18 months.
- The posterior (triangular-shaped) fontanelle typically measures 1 cm and closes at 1 to 2 months.

Vital Signs

Temperature. Body temperature measurements differ in children based on the method used.

- The rectal route gives the closest temperature to the core temperature.

- Rectal temperatures may lag behind a core temperature during rapid temperature changes.
- Rectal thermometers should not be used in newborns under 1 month due to the risk of anal perforation.
- The axillary route is recommended unless a core temperature is necessary.
- For safety reasons, use of an oral thermometer is not recommended for children under 4 years old.
- For accuracy reasons, use of a tympanic thermometer is not recommended for children under 2 years old (Hockenberry et al., 2022).

For further information on temperature-taking, refer to Chapter 7, page 92.

Heart rate
- Heart rate decreases as age increases.
- The apical impulse (heard through a stethoscope held to the chest at the apex of the heart) is most reliable.
- It is important to count the apical rate for 1 full minute, as young children may have irregularities in rhythm.

Respirations
- The rate decreases as age increases.
- It is important to count for 1 full minute due to irregular movements.
- Abdominal movements should be monitored since respirations are primarily diaphragmatic.

Blood pressure
- A healthy newborn infant's blood pressure is not routinely checked but if required it is measured with an electronic instrument (Keenan-Lindsay, 2020).
- The most important factor in accurate assessment is use of an appropriately sized cuff that covers three quarters of the upper arm.

See Table 11.3 for normal-range vital signs for newborns and infants.

Gross and Fine Motor Development

Gross motor development includes maturation in posture, head balance, sitting, creeping, standing, and walking. Fine motor development includes the use of hands and fingers to grasp objects. See Table 11.4 for a summary of growth and development during infancy.

Nutrition

Both the rate and the pattern of growth can be modified by nutrition.

- Breast milk is the most desirable, complete diet for infants during the first 12 months.
- Breastfed infants will feed on demand.
- Breastfed infants require a daily supplement of 10 mcg (400 IU) of vitamin D from birth until the equivalent amount is obtained from other dietary sources or until they reach 1 year of age. If the infant lives north of the 55th parallel (which is about the level of Edmonton), this level should increase to 20 mcg (800 IU) per day, year round (Canadian Paediatric Society [CPS], (2022a). Formula-fed infants receive vitamin D in formula but still require supplements of an additional 10 mcg (400 IU) if they live north of the 55th parallel. The

Canadian Paediatric Society (CPS) also recommends that pregnant and lactating persons consult their obstetrical health care provider about taking up to 2 000 IU of vitamin D daily to ensure adequate amounts (CPS, 2022b).

- An acceptable alternative to breastfeeding is a commercial iron-fortified formula.
- Formula-fed infants will take about 5 to 8 feedings every 24 hours.

TABLE 11.3 Comparison of Pediatric Differences in Vital Signs

	Temperature (°C)	Pulse (Bpm)	Respirations (number per minute)	Blood Pressure (mm Hg)
Newborn	37.5	100–180	35	65–80/40–50
1–12 months	37.5–37.7	80–150	30–40	95–100/60–70
1–3 years	37.7–37.2	70–110	20–30	90–105/55–70
3–6 years	37.2–37.0	65–110	20–25	95–110/60–75
6–12 years	36.7	60–95	14–22	100–120/60–75
12–18 years	36.6–36.8	55–85	12–18	110–135/65–85

bpm, Beats per minute.
Vital signs for pulse, respirations, and blood pressure from Keenan-Lindsay, L., Sams, C.A., & O'Connor, C. (2022). *Perry's maternal child care in Canada* (3rd ed., p. 1530). Elsevier. Temperature parameters from Hockenberry, M., Rodgers, C., & Wilson, D. (2022). *Wong's essentials of pediatric nursing* (11th ed., inside back cover). Elsevier.

TABLE 11.4 Growth and Development During Infancy

Age	Physical	Gross Motor Development	Fine Motor Development	Vocalization
1 month	Weight gain of 150–210 g (5–7 oz) weekly for the first 6 months Height gain of 2.5 cm (1 inch) monthly for the first 6 months Head circumference increases by 1.5 cm (0.5 inch) monthly for the first 6 months. Primitive reflexes present and strong Doll's eye reflex and dance reflex fading Obligatory nose breathing (most infants)	Can turn head side to side when prone Marked head lag when pulled from lying to sitting position	Hands predominantly closed Grasp reflex is strong Hand clenches on contact with rattle	Cries to express displeasure Small throat sounds Comfort sounds during feeding
2 months	Posterior fontanelle closed Crawling reflex disappears	Less head lag when pulled to a sitting position Can maintain head in same plane as rest of the body when held in ventral suspension When prone, can lift head almost 45 degrees off table When moved to a sitting position, head is held up but bends forward	Hands often open Grasp reflex fading	Vocalizes, distinct from crying Crying becomes differentiated Coos Vocalizes to familiar voices
3 months	Primitive reflexes fading	Able to hold head more erect when sitting but still bobs forward Has only slight head lag when pulled to a sitting position Able to raise head and shoulders from prone position to a 45- to 90-degree angle from the table Bears weight on forearms When held in a standing position, able to bear slight fraction of weight on legs Regards on hands	Holds rattle but will not reach for it Grasp reflex gone Pulls at blankets, clothes and own hands	Squeals aloud to show pleasure Coos, babbles, chuckles Vocalizes when smiling "Talks" a great deal when spoken too Less crying during periods of wakefulness

Continued

TABLE 11.4   Growth and Development During Infancy—cont'd

Age	Physical	Gross Motor Development	Fine Motor Development	Vocalization
4 months	Drooling begins Moro, tonic neck, and rooting reflexes have disappeared	Has almost no head lag when pulled to a sitting position Balances head well in sitting position Able to sit erect if propped up Able to raise head and chest off surface to angle of 90 degrees Rolls from back to side	Inspects and plays with hands; pulls blanket or clothing over face in play Tries to reach for objects but overshoots Cannot carry objects to mouth Grasps object with both hands Plays with rattle placed in hand and shakes it but cannot pick it up if dropped	Laughs aloud Makes consonant sounds n, k, g, p, b Vocalization changes according to mood
5 months	Beginning signs of tooth eruption Birth weight has doubled	No head lag when pulled to sitting position When sitting able to hold head erect and steady Able to sit for longer periods of time with back supported Can turn from abdomen to back When supine puts feet to mouth	Able to grasp objects voluntarily Takes objects directly to mouth Plays with toes Holds on cube while regarding a second one Uses palmer grasp, bidextrous approach	Squeals Makes cooing vowel sounds with interspersed consonants (e.g., "ah-goo")
6 months	Growth rate may decrease Weight gain of 90–150 g (3–5 oz) weekly for the next 6 months Height gain of 1.25 cm (0.5 inch) monthly for the next 6 months Teething may begin with two lower central incisors Chewing and biting occur	When supine, puts feet in mouth When prone, can lift chest and upper abdomen off surface, and bear weight on hands Rolls from back to abdomen Sits in highchair with back straight When held in a standing position, bears almost all of weight Hand regard absent	Grasps and manipulates small objects Drops one cube when given another Holds bottle Grasps feet and pulls to mouth	Begins to imitate sound Babbling resembles one-syllable utterances—"m," "mu," "da," "di," "hi" Vocalizes to toys and mirror images Enjoys hearing own sounds
7 months	Eruptions of upper central incisors	Bears full weight on feet Bounces when held in standing position Sits erect momentarily, sits leaning forward on both hands	Transfers objects from one hand to the other Holds two cubes more than momentarily Bangs cubes on table Rakes a small object	Produces vowel sounds and chained syllables (e.g., "baba," "dada," "kaka") Vocalizes four distinct vowel sounds "Talks" when others are talking
8 months	Begins to show regular bladder and bowel patterns Parachute reflex disappears	Sits steadily unsupported Readily bears weight on legs when supported and stands holding on to furniture Adjusts posture to reach an object	Has beginning pincer grasp Reaches for and pulls toys Rings bell purposely Releases objects at will Retains two cubes while regarding third cube Secures object by pulling on a string	Listens selectively for familiar words Makes consonant sounds t, w, d Utterances signal emphasis and emotion Combine syllables, such as "dada," but does not ascribe meaning to them

Continued

TABLE 11.4 Growth and Development During Infancy—cont'd

Age	Physical	Gross Motor Development	Fine Motor Development	Vocalization
9 months	Eruption of upper lateral incisor may begin	Creeps on hands and knees Pulls self to standing position by holding onto furniture Sits steady on the floor for prolonged time (10 minutes) Recovers balance when leaning forward but cannot do so when leaning sideways	Uses thumb and index finger in crude pincer grasp Shows preference for use of dominant hand Grasps third object Compares two cubes by bringing them together	Responds to simple commands Comprehends "no-no"
10 months	Labyrinth righting reflex is strongest (when in prone or supine position, infant is able to raise head)	Cruises by holding onto furniture Can change from prone to supine position Recovers balance easily while sitting When standing lifts one foot to take a step	Release of object from crude pincer grasp begins Grasps bell by handle	Says "dada" or "mama" with meaning Comprehends "bye bye" May say one word (e.g., "hi," "bye," "no")
11 months	Eruption of lower lateral incisors may begin	When sitting, will pivot to reach objects behind Cruises or walks while holding onto furniture or with both hands held	Examines objects more closely Has neat pincer grasp Drops object deliberately to be picked up Able to manipulate an object to remove it from tight-fitting enclosure	Imitates definite speech sounds
12 months	Birth weight has tripled Birth length increased by 50% Head and chest circumference equal (head circumference 46 cm (18 inches) Has six to eight deciduous teeth Anterior fontanel almost closed Landau reflex fading Babinski reflex disappears	Walks with one handheld and cruises well Can sit down from standing position without any help	Can turn pages in a book, many at a time Attempts to build two-block tower but fails Releases cube in a cup	Recognizes objects by name Imitates animal sounds Understands simple verbal commands (e.g., "give it to me") Says three to five words besides dada or mama Comprehends the meaning of several words (comprehension always precedes verbalization)

Adapted from Hockenberry, M., Rodgers, C., & Wilson, D. (2022). *Wong's essentials of pediatric nursing* (11th ed., p. 286a, Table 9.1). Elsevier.

- All drinking water and water used for formula must be boiled for 2 minutes and cooled to no less than 70°C and then the powder is added.
- Infant fluid requirements average 125 to 150 mL/kg/day from birth to 6 months of age and 120 to 135 mL/kg/day from 6 to 12 months.
- Use of a cup at 6 to 9 months will help reduce nursing bottle caries when diluted apple juice is introduced.
- Solids can be introduced at 6 months, starting first with rice cereal, which is easy to digest, contains iron, and rarely causes an allergic reaction.
- Other cereals, fruits, vegetables, and finally meats should be introduced one at a time and usually at intervals of 4 to 7 days apart to test for possible food allergies (Hockenberry et al., 2022).
- Finger foods such as toast, teething crackers, soft fruits, and cooked vegetables should be introduced at 6 to 7 months. Parents should be advised to monitor for choking.
- Chopped table food or commercially prepared junior food can be introduced around 9 to 12 months.
- Weaning from the breast or bottle to a cup may occur after 6 months and should be based on the readiness of the mother and infant.

Sleep

- Sleep patterns vary greatly among infants.

- Newborns have six sleep-wake states. As age increases, the sleep-wake states change, with increasing time spent in awake alert states and decreasing amounts in sleep time (Hockenberry et al., 2022).
- By 3 to 4 months, most infants will sleep 15 hours a day, of which 9 to 11 hours will be overnight.
- By 12 months, morning and afternoon naps are common.
- Breastfed infants will usually sleep for shorter periods than bottle-fed infants.

Dental

- Fluoride is an essential mineral to promote healthy teeth.
- Most Canadian municipalities add fluoride to drinking water
- Primary teeth erupt around 6 months of age, beginning first with the upper central incisors.
- Parents should begin a routine of good dental hygiene before teeth are present by using a soft-bristled toothbrush or a damp cloth with water rather than toothpaste. Swallowing too much toothpaste containing fluoride can lead to fluorosis (Hockenberry et al., 2022).
- To prevent dental caries, parents should avoid breast- and bottle-feeding while the infant sleeps and avoid fruit juices in a bottle, particularly before 6 months of age.
- Foods with concentrated sugar should be used in limited quantity.
- The practice of coating a pacifier with honey should be discouraged; this can cause infant botulism.
- The use of hard-candy pacifiers should be discouraged, not only due to the sugar content, but also as parts of the candy can break off and be aspirated.

Immunizations

Publicly funded immunization programs may vary by province or territory (Government of Canada, 2023a).

See Table 11.5A–B for the recommended Canadian routine immunization schedule.

Nursing Considerations

When administering immunizations, do the following:
- Ensure proper storage of the vaccine.
- Rotate sites and administer the injections as painlessly as possible.
- Consider use of topical anaesthetics such as EMLA cream to prevent a painful injection
- Give acetaminophen (Tylenol) at least 6 hours after a vaccination for fever or pain (Government of Canada, 2020b).
- If the infant or young child is breastfed, breastfeeding during the vaccine injection (for children 2 years of age or younger) is recommended for pain management.
- If the infant or young child is not breastfeeding during the vaccination, a combination of other strategies for pain management include skin to skin contact during the vaccine (1 month or less), holding during the vaccine or rocking the child after the vaccine, and administration of a sweet-tasting (sucrose) solution prior to vaccine injection for children age 2 years and younger (Government of Canada, 2020b).
- For children 3 to 12 years of age, pain management could include having the child sit up during the injection, topical anaesthetics as stated previously, presence of the parent/caregiver during vaccine injection, and education of the individual about pain management for vaccine injection on the day of the immunization (Government of Canada, 2020b).
- Monitor for signs of allergic reaction.
- Ensure adequate penetration of the muscle when administering intramuscularly.
- Provide adequate information to parents on the risks and benefits of immunizations. See Chapter 6, page 83, for more information on vaccinations and risk communication.
- Maintain accurate documentation in an immunization record for parents to keep.

Safety

- The most common cause of death amongst infants ages 6 to 12 months are from injuries (Hockenberry et al., 2022).
- Some of the leading causes of injury include suffocation, choking, strangulation, drowning, falls, poisonings, burns, and motor vehicle accidents.
- As the infant develops fine and gross motor skills and begins to explore the environment, the risk of injury should be addressed with parents with appropriate injury prevention teaching. See Table 11.6 for a list of preventable hazards for infants.
- The Government of Canada toy safety website provides consumer information on potentially hazardous products, particularly toys that present choking hazards and toxic compositions. This site also includes product recalls, for example, toys that are manufactured with unacceptable levels of lead paint. See the end of this chapter for this and other websites focused on child safety.

Play

- In infancy, play is mostly used for physical development and for gaining awareness of the environment.
- Play is basically solitary and will become more interactive during the first year.
- Toys should be simple to match the child's attention span.
- Toy safety is of primary concern, to prevent aspiration and injury.

See Table 11.7 for a list of suggested toys for infants.

Reactions to Illness and Hospitalization

The impact of hospitalization on an infant under 3 months is minimized if it is for a short time and there is a nurturing person who can meet the child's physical needs. At 4 to 8 months, the infant starts to recognize the parents as separate from itself and develops a fear of strangers, which can lead to separation anxiety if the child is hospitalized.

Nursing Considerations During Hospitalization

- Be present with the parents within sight of the infant to build a sense of safety in the child.
- Encourage parents to participate in the child's care as much as possible.
- Follow home routines as much as possible.
- Give the infant a sense of security by holding the child and moving gently, cuddling, talking, and responding to the child's reactions.
- Ensure that sensorimotor stimulation is provided.
- Provide physical care, comfort, and safety.
- Keep the infant warm and dry and plan treatments and tests around the home feeding schedule to prevent hunger and discomfort.
- Encourage breastfeeding or the use of the same type of formula used at home.
- Make sure crib rails are up and provide safe crib toys and an area to play in.
- Encourage cognitive stimulation through various stimulating toys, such as rattles, mobiles, and music boxes with different textures.
- Encourage vocal stimulation and language development by talking to the infant and making sounds.
- Develop and maintain a relationship with the parents and encourage parent participation throughout the hospitalization whenever possible.
- Encourage the parents to voice their concerns and address them as much as possible.
- Try to keep the same core nurses with the child as much as possible.

TODDLER: 1 TO 3 YEARS OF AGE

Biological Changes

Growth slows considerably during childhood compared to the first year. The toddler will experience steplike growth with spurts and lags versus the more linear growth of infancy.

Toddlers have a "pot-belly" abdomen as a result of underdeveloped abdominal muscles. Legs will remain slightly bowed in appearance due to the weight of a comparatively large trunk.

Height

- The rate of increase in height slows, with an average increase of 7.5 cm per year.
- Increase occurs mainly in elongation of the legs rather than the trunk.
- Adult height is about twice the height of the child at age 2.

Weight

- Average weight gain is 1.8 to 2.7 kg per year.
- Birth weight is quadrupled by age 2.5.

Head and Chest Circumference

Chest circumference surpasses head and abdominal circumferences, giving the toddler a taller, leaner appearance.

Vital Signs

See Table 11.3 for normal-range vital signs for toddlers.

Temperature
- Recommended routes include axillary, tympanic, temporal artery and rectal (if a core temperature is required).
- Use of an oral thermometer is not recommended in children under 4 years old.

Heart rate. A satisfactory radial pulse can be obtained in children over 2.

Gross and Fine Motor Development

- The major gross motor development of the toddler is locomotion.
- Fine motor development is demonstrated by increasingly skilful manual dexterity.

See Table 11.8 for a summary of growth and development during the toddler years.

Nutrition

- As growth slows, so will the toddler's requirements for calories, protein, and fluids.
- By 12 months, most children will eat the same food prepared for the rest of the family.
- Parents should be encouraged to follow *Canada's Food Guide* for children 2 years of age and older (Government of Canada, 2022a). (For more on *Eating Well with Canada's Food Guide*, see Chapter 6, page 74.)
- Toddlers will fully transition from the bottle to a cup by age 18 months, with some spilling.
- Proper control of a spoon is seen after 18 months of age.
- Emphasis should be placed on the introduction of a variety of foods and in developing healthy eating habits.
- Food should be presented in an appealing manner and served in small sizes; toddlers enjoy finger foods.
- By 18 months, most toddlers will display a phenomenon called *physiological anorexia*, evidenced by a decrease in nutritional needs and appetite.
- Toddlers become picky eaters and may eat voraciously one day and almost nothing the next; however, most toddlers will continue to consume enough nutrients for growth.
- Toddlers may experience "food fads" or "jags," eating one particular type of food for several days in a row and then suddenly refusing to eat it again.
- Toddlers need to feel a sense of control over food choices.

Sleep

- Total sleep decreases slightly during the second year, with an average of 12 hours per day.
- Most toddlers will require one nap per day and most often will give up napping by age 3.
- Toddlers will commonly experience difficulty going to bed and falling asleep as a result of separation anxiety.
- Parents should establish bedtime rituals with a consistent bedtime and the use of a transitional object such as a stuffed animal or a blanket for comfort and security.

TABLE 11.5A   Provincial and Territorial Routine and Catch-up Vaccination Schedule for Infants and Children in Canada

VACCINES							
Abbreviations	**Descriptions**	**BC**	**AB**	**SK**	**MB**	**ON**	**QC[(2)]**
DTaP-IPV-Hib	Diphtheria, Tetanus, acellular Pertussis, Inactivated Polio Virus, Haemophilus Influenzae type B vaccine	Age: 18 months	Age: 18 months	Age: 2, 4, 6, 18 months	Age: 2, 4, 6, 18 months	Age: 2, 4, 6, 18 months	Age: 12 months
DTaP-HB-IPV-Hib	Diphtheria, Tetanus, acellular Pertussis, Hepatitis B, Inactivated Polio Virus, Haemophilus Influenzae type B vaccine	Age: 2, 4, 6 months	Age: 2, 4, 6 months	N/A	N/A	N/A	Age: 2, 4 months
Tdap-IPV	Tetanus, Diphtheria (reduced toxoid), acellular pertussis (reduced toxoid), Inactivated Polio Virus vaccine	Age: 4–6 years	Age: 4 years	Age: 4–6 years	Age: 4–6 years	Age: 4–6 years	Age: 4–6 years
Tdap	Tetanus, Diphtheria (reduced toxoid), acellular pertussis (reduced toxoid) vaccine	Grade: 9	Grade: 9	Grade: 8	Grade: 8–9	Age: 14–16 years	N/A
Td	Tetanus, Diphtheria (reduced toxoid)	N/A	N/A	N/A	N/A	N/A	3rd year of high school
BCG	Bacille Calmette-Guerin (BCG) Vaccine	N/A	N/A	N/A	N/A	N/A	N/A
HAHB	Hepatitis A Vaccine, Hepatitis B vaccine	N/A	N/A	N/A	N/A	N/A	18 months
HB	Hepatitis B vaccine	HB is provided in a 3-dose combination vaccine (DTaP-HB-IPV-Hib) in infancy	Catch-up (3-dose) Grade: 6	(2-dose) Grade: 6	(2-dose) Grade: 6	(2-dose) Grade: 7	HB is provided in a 2-dose combination vaccine (DTaP-HB-IPV-Hib) in infancy 1 dose of HAHB at 18 months

PROVINCES AND TERRITORIES

NB	NS	PE	NL	YT	NT	NU
Age: 2, 4, 6, 18 months	Age: 2, 4, 6, 18 months	Age: 18 months	Age: 2, 4, 6, 18 months	Age: 18 months	Age: 2, 4, 6, 18 months	Age: 2, 4, 6, 18 months
N/A	N/A	Age: 2, 4, 6 months	N/A	Age: 2, 4, 6 months	N/A	N/A
Age: 4 years	Age: 4–6 years	Age: 4–5 years	Age: 4–6 years[3]	Age: 4–6 years	Age: 4–6 years[3]	Age: 4–6 years
Grade: 7	Grade: 7	Grade: 9	Grade: 9	Grade: 9	Grade: 7	Grade: 6
N/A	N/A	N/A	N/A	N/A	N/A	N/A
N/A	N/A	N/A	N/A	N/A	Age: 1 month	Age: 1 month
N/A	N/A	N/A	N/A	N/A	N/A	N/A
Age: At birth, 2, 6 months	(2-dose) Grade: 7	HB is provided in a 3-dose combination vaccine (DTaP-HB-IPV-Hib) in infancy	(2-dose) Grade: 6	HB is provided in a 3-dose combination vaccine (DTaP-HB-IPV-Hib) in infancy	Age: At birth, 1, 6 months	Age: At birth, 1, 9 months

Continued

TABLE 11.5A **Provincial and Territorial Routine and Catch-up Vaccination Schedule for Infants and Children in Canada—cont'd**

VACCINES							
Abbreviations	Descriptions	BC	AB	SK	MB	ON	QC[(2)]
MMR	Measles, Mumps, Rubella vaccine	Age: 12 months	N/A	N/A	N/A	Age: 12 months	N/A
Var	Varicella vaccine	Age: 12 months	N/A	N/A	N/A	Age: 15 months	Catch-up Age: 4–6 years
MMR-V	Measles, Mumps, Rubella, Varicella vaccine	2nd dose Age: 4–6 years	Age: 12, 18 months	Age: 12, 18 months	Age: 12 months, 4–6 years	2nd dose Age: 4–6 years	Age: 12, 18 months
Men-C-C	Meningococcal conjugate (Strain C) vaccine	Age: 2, 12 months	Age: 4, 12 months	Age: 12 months	Age: 12 months	Age: 12 months	Age: 18 months
Men-C-ACYW-135	Meningococcal conjugate (Strains A, C, Y, W135) vaccine	Grade: 9	Grade: 9	Grade: 6	Grade: 6	Grade: 7	N/A
Pneu-P-23	Pneumococcal polysaccharide (23-valent) vaccine	N/A	N/A	N/A	N/A	N/A	N/A
Pneu-C-13	Pneumococcal conjugate (13-valent) vaccine	Age: 2, 4, 12 months	Age: 2, 4, 12 months	Age: 2, 4, 12 months	Age: 2, 4, 12 months	Age: 2, 4, 12 months	Age: 12 months
Pneu-C-10	Pneumococcal conjugate (10-valent) vaccine	N/A	N/A	N/A	N/A	N/A	Age: 2, 4 months
Rota	Rotavirus vaccine	Age: 2, 4 months	Age: 2, 4, 6 months	Age: 2, 4 months	Age: 2, 4 months	Age: 2, 4 months	Age: 2, 4 months
HPV	Human Papillomavirus vaccine	(2-dose) Grade: 6	(2-dose) Grade: 6	(2-dose) Grade: 6	(2-dose) Grade: 6	(2-dose) Grade: 7	(2-dose) 1st dose in 4th year of primary school and 2nd dose in 3rd year of high school

CHAPTER 11 Pediatric Nursing 331

PROVINCES AND TERRITORIES

NB	NS	PE	NL	YT	NT	NU
N/A	N/A	N/A	N/A	Age: 12 months	N/A	N/A
N/A	N/A	N/A	N/A	Age: 12 months	N/A	Catch-up Grade: 6
Age: 12, 18 months	Age: 12, 18 months	Age: 12, 18 months	Age: 12, 18 months	2nd Dose Age: 4–6 years	Age: 12, 18 months	Age: 12, 18 months
Age: 12 months	Age: 12 months	Age: 12 months	Age: 12 months	Age: 2, 12 months	Age: 2, 12 months	Age: 12 months
Grade: 9	Grade: 7	Grade: 9	Grade: 4	Grade: 9	Grade: 12[1]	Grade: 9
N/A	N/A	N/A	N/A	N/A	N/A	Age: 2–3 years
Age: 2, 4, 12 months	Age: 2, 4, 12 months	Age: 2, 4, 12 months	Age: 2, 4, 12 months	Age: 2, 4, 12 months	Age: 2, 4, 6, 18 months	Age: 2, 4, 6, 15 months
N/A	N/A	N/A	N/A	N/A	N/A	N/A
Age: 2, 4, 6 months	Age: 2, 4, 6 months	Age: 2, 4, 6 months	Age: 2, 4 months	Age: 2, 4, 6 months	Age: 2, 4, 6 months	Age: 2, 4, 6 months
(2-dose) Grade: 7	(2-dose) Grade: 7	(2-dose) Grade: 6	(2-dose) Grade: 6	(2-dose) Grade: 6	(9–14 years: 2-dose 15 years+: 3-dose) Grade: 4–6	(2-dose) Grade: 6

[1]If attending postsecondary school out of territory.
[2]A catch-up program in the third year of high school evaluates student's vaccination history. Students will be provided any missed vaccination to protect against the following diseases: diphtheria, pertussis, tetanus, polio, measles, mumps, rubella, varicella, meningococcal serogroup C infections, hepatitis A and B, and human papilloma virus. In addition, children in the fourth year of primary school will be vaccinated against hepatitis A.
[3]DTaP-IPV-Hib may be substituted for DTaP-IPV in times of shortage for those who are 4–6 years of age.
N/A, Vaccine is not publicly funded in the province/territory.
Catch-up, A specific catch-up program is currently underway. A catch-up program is defined as a time-limited measure to implement a new vaccine program to a certain age cohort (e.g., an additional dose of vaccine is recommended, and a targeted program is put in place).

TABLE 11.5B   Recommended Immunizations Schedule, Children (less than 7 years of age), NOT Previously Immunized as Infants

Vaccine	First Visit	TIME AFTER FIRST VISIT						6–12 Months After Last Dose
		4 Weeks	8 Weeks	3 Months	4 Months	6 Months		
DTaP-IPV-Hib Or DTap--IPV	A		A		A			A B
Pneu-C-13	C		C					
Men-C-C	D							
MMR	E	E						
VAR OR	F			F				
MMRV	G			O				
HB	H	H				H		
Inf	I	I						

A. Diphtheria toxoid-tetanus toxoid-acellular pertussis-inactivated polio-*Haemophilus influenzae* type b (DTaP-IPV-Hib) or diphtheria toxoid-tetanus toxoid-acellular pertussis-inactivated polio (DTaP-IPV): 4 doses of DTaP-IPV containing vaccine. The number of doses of Hib-containing vaccine required varies by age at first dose. If first visit at 12–14 months of age: 1 dose of Hib-containing vaccine at first visit and booster dose at least 2 months after the previous dose. If first visit at 15 months–less than 60 months of age: 1 dose of Hib-containing vaccine. If first at 60 months of age or older, Hib-containing vaccine is not required.

B. Diphtheria toxoid-tetanus toxoid-acellular pertussis-inactivated polio (DTaP-IPV) or tetanus toxoid-reduced diphtheria toxoid-reduced acellular pertussis-inactivated polio (Tdap-IPV): if the fourth dose of DTaP-IPV vaccine was given before the fourth birthday, a booster dose of DTaP-IPV or Tdap-IPV vaccine should be provided at 4–6 years of age.

C. Pneumococcal conjugate 13-valent: 12–23 months of age, 2 doses, at least 8 weeks apart; 24–59 months of age: 1 dose.

D. Meningococcal conjugate monovalent: 12–59 months of age, 1 dose; 5–11 years of age, consider 1 dose.

E. Measles-mumps-rubella: 2 doses, at least 4 weeks apart; second dose after 18 months of age but should be given no later than around school entry.

F. Varicella: 2 doses, at least 3 months apart; second dose after 18 months of age but should be given no later than around school entry. A minimum interval of 4 weeks between doses may be used if rapid, complete protection is required.

G. Measles-mumps-rubella-varicella: 2 doses, at least 3 months apart; second dose after 18 months of age but should be given no later than around school entry. A minimum interval of 4 weeks between doses may be used if rapid, complete protection is required.

H. Hepatitis B: 3 doses—months 0, 1, and 6 (first dose = month 0) with at least 4 weeks between the first and second dose, 2 months between the second and third dose, and 4 months between the first and third dose.

I. Influenza: 2 doses, at least 4 weeks apart.

TABLE 11.6   Preventable Hazards for Infants

Hazard	Nursing Considerations When Educating Caregivers
Falls	Keep car seat or baby carrier on the floor rather than on a table or counter. Always use safety straps in strollers and highchairs. Avoid using the highchair until the child can sit well with support. Always raise crib rails. Never leave a child alone on a change table. Keep all supplies at hand. Be aware that wheeled baby walkers, which have been banned in Canada since 2004, should not be used as they can cause serious injuries to children, including falls, head injuries, and burns. Use a baby gate at the top of stairs; the baby gate must be fastened to the wall with screws, not suction.
Burns	Check the temperature of bath water and foods and liquids. Keep hot items out of reach. Place guards in front of fireplaces or heating devices. Avoid hanging tablecloths as children may pull down hot items. Avoid overexposure to the sun and use sunscreen if the infant is over 6 months of age. Do not leave child in a parked car Check surface heat of the car restraint before placing the child in the seat (Hockenberry et al., 2022).

TABLE 11.6   Preventable Hazards for Infants—cont'd

Hazard	Nursing Considerations When Educating Caregivers
Motor Vehicle Accidents	Motor vehicle crashes are the leading cause of preventable injury and death to children between one and nine years. In 2019, more than 91 000 children aged 12 and younger were injured and 608 children died in motor vehicle accidents (Centers for Disease Control and Prevention, 2021). The Transport Canada website provides information on child car seat requirements for Canada. The site includes installation instructions, airbag safety tips, and recall alerts. For children up to 10 kg, use rear-facing car seats. For children over 10 kg, use forward-facing seats until they outgrow the seats to at least 18 kg and are 2 years of age. Some forward-facing seats are made for children who weigh up to 30 kg. For children who have outgrown forward-facing seats, use booster seats until the child is able to use the seat belt safely (each province has a minimum age, weight, and height requirement). Use from when a child is a minimum of 18 kg to 145 cm tall and is at least 4 years old. (Parachute, 2021a). For children 36 kg or 145 cm tall and 8 years of age, use seat belts. The safest location for children 12 years or younger is in the back seat, away from airbags (Government of Canada, 2019).
Drowning	Backyard pools are the most common place for drownings for children under the age of 5 years old. The child was not supervised or the person supervising was distracted in 92% of the cases (Parachute, 2021b). Children can drown in as little as 5 cm (2 in) of water in just seconds. Never leave an infant alone in a bath, even for a few seconds. Avoid the use of a baby bath seat as it is not a safety device. Keep one hand on the child at all times in the tub. Keep bathroom door shut. Constant supervision is needed when children are near any source of water, such as buckets, toilets, and drainage areas (Hockenberry et al., 2022).
Poisoning	Do not store toxic substances in food containers. Keep medications locked up. Do not administer medications as candy. Keep the phone number of a poison control centre readily available.
Suffocation and Strangulation	Position infants to sleep on their backs. Do not place pillows, bumper pads, thick comforters, or stuffed toys in a crib. Do not use plastic in a crib. Keep all plastic bags out of children's reach. Avoid latex balloons. In Canada, cribs made before 1986 are dangerous and should not be used as the part supporting the mattress can fall, entrapping an infant. Crib bars should be no more than 6 cm (2.4 in.) apart to prevent the infant's head from getting caught in the bars. Keep the infant's crib away from windows as children have died when their heads got caught in the cords of blinds. Do not use pacifiers with cords attached. Make sure the infant does not have a bib, necklace or anything tied around their neck. Do not use baby gates made before 1990 as children have died when their heads were trapped in the gates (these are usually gates with large diamond- or V-shaped openings).
Choking	Hold infant for feeding and do not prop a bottle. Use pacifiers with one-piece contraction and a loop handle. Keep small objects such a buttons, beads, and small toys away from the infant. Avoid the use of baby powder. Use caution with toys and ensure that no small parts can come off and choke the infant.

Obtained information from Centers for Disease Control and Prevention. (2021). *Child passenger safety. get the facts.* https://www.cdc.gov/transportationsafety/child_passenger_safety/cps-factsheet.html; Government of Canada (2019). *Stage 4: seat belts.* https://tc.canada.ca/en/road-transportation/child-car-seat-safety/installing-child-car-seat-booster-seat/stage-4-seat-belts; Hockenberry, M., Rodgers, C., & Wilson, D. (2022). *Wong's essentials of pediatric nursing* (11th ed.). Elsevier; Parachute (2021b). *Car seats. Choosing the right car seat.* https://parachute.ca/en/injury-topic/car-seats/choosing-the-right-car-seat/; Parachute (2022). *Poisoning.* https://www.parachutecanada.org/en/injury-topic/poisoning/

TABLE 11.7 Suggested Toys for Infants

Age	Visual Stimulation	Auditory Stimulation	Tactile Stimulation	Kinetic Stimulation
Birth to 1 year	Nursery mobiles Unbreakable mirrors Contrasting coloured sheets	Music boxes Music mobiles Crib dangle bells Small-handled clear rattle	Stuffed animals Soft clothes* Soft or furry quilt* Soft mobiles**	Rocking crib or cradle Weighted or suction toy Infant swing
6–12 months	Coloured blocks Nested boxes or cups Books with rhymes and bright pictures Strings of big beads Simple take-apart toys Large ball Cup and spoon Large puzzles Jack-in-the-box	Squeaky toys and animals Rattles of different sizes, shapes, tones, and bright colours Recordings with light, rhythmic music	Soft, different-texture animals and dolls Sponge toys Floating toys Squeeze toys Teething toys Books with textures, such as fur and zippers	Activity box for cribs Push–pull toys Wind-up swing

*Toys must be removed from the crib when the infant is sleeping to avoid suffocation.
**Remove all toys strung across a playpen or crib (such as a mobile) as soon as the body starts to push up on their hands or knees or if the infant is 5 months old (whichever comes first).
Adapted from Hockenberry, M. J., Rodgers, C. & Wilson, D. (2022). *Wong's essential of pediatric nursing.* (11th ed. p. 286a, Table 9.1), Elsevier; Keenan-Lindsay, L. (2020). *Leifer's introduction to maternity and pediatric nursing in Canada* (1st ed. p. 356–360, Table 14.1), Elsevier; Parachute (2021d). *Home safety: Play time.* https://www.parachutecanada.org/en/injury-topic/home-safety/play-time/

TABLE 11.8 Toddler Growth and Development

Age	Physical	Gross Motor Development	Fine Motor Development	Language
12–15 months	Steady growth in height and weight Head circumference, 48 cm (19 inches) Weight, 11 kg (24 pounds) Height, 78.7 cm (31 inches)	Walks alone without help Creeps up stairs Kneels without support Assumes standing position without support	Can grasp a very small object Can drop a small object into a narrow opening Repeatedly throws objects and retrieves them Scribbles spontaneously with a crayon Cannot insert a particular shaped object into a matching hole Drinks from cup Uses spoon but will rotate it	Says 4–6 words Asks for objects by pointing Shakes head to denote "no" Understands simple commands Uses common gestures, such as putting cup to mouth when empty
18 months	Physiological anorexia from decreased growth needs Anterior fontanelles closed Physiologically able to control sphincters	Tries to run but falls easily Walks up stairs with one hand held Pulls and pushes toys Jumps in place on both feet Can throw a ball over head without losing balance	Can build a tower of 3–4 blocks Can insert a particular shaped object into the matching hole Turns 2 or 3 pages in a book at a time Manages spoon without rotation	Says 10 words or more Forms word combinations Points while naming the object
24 months	Chest circumference exceeds head circumference May be ready to start toilet learning to begin daytime control of control of bladder and bowel Primary dentition of 16 teeth	Walks up and down stairs on own with two feet on each step Runs fairly well, with wide stance Picks up an object without falling Kicks ball forward without overbalancing	Can build a tower of 6–7 blocks Imitates a circular and a vertical line with a crayon Turns door knobs and unscrews lids Turns pages in a book one at a time	Has a vocabulary of about 300 words Uses pronouns *I*, *me*, and *you* Refers to self by name Talks continuously Verbalizes the need for toileting, food, or drink
2 1/2 years	Quadruples birth weight May have bladder and bowel control during the day Primary dentition is complete at 20 teeth	Can jump using both feet Stands on one foot for a second or two Can take a few steps on tiptoe	Can build a tower of 8 or more blocks Holds a crayon with fingers rather than in fist	Gives first and last name Refers to self by appropriate pronoun Uses plurals Names one colour

Adapted from Hockenberry, M. J., Rodgers, C. & Wilson, D. (2022). *Wong's essentials of pediatric nursing* (11th ed., p. 347, Table 11.1). Elsevier Inc.

Dental

- The Canadian Dental Association encourages the assessment of infants by a dentist within 6 months of the eruption of the first tooth or by 1 year of age (Canadian Dental Association, 2022b).
- All 20 baby (or primary) teeth should erupt by age 2 to 3 years.
- Dental hygiene includes brushing with a soft-bristled toothbrush and flossing.
- As with infants, toothpaste should be avoided. Children under age 3 should have their teeth brushed by an adult (Canadian Dental Association, 2022a).
- Foods high in sugar should be limited.

Immunizations

See Table 11.5A–B for the recommended Canadian routine immunization schedule.

Safety

- Unintentional injuries are one of the major causes of death and morbidity for children aged 1 to 4 years (Hockenberry et al., 2022).
- Leading causes of injury include suffocation, choking, strangulation, drowning, falls, poisonings, burns, and motor vehicle accidents.
- As the infant develops fine and gross motor skills and begins to explore the environment, injury prevention should be addressed with parents.
See Table 11.9 for a list of preventable hazards for toddlers.

Play

- Toddlers engage in parallel play by playing alongside, but not with, other children.
- Toddlers will play freely and spontaneously without following rules.
- This is an active stage of development that involves intense exploration of the environment.
- Due to their short attention spans, toddlers will change activities often.
- Appropriate toys will help develop locomotion (push–pull toys), imagination, language, and gross and fine motor skills. See Box 11.1 for a list of appropriate toddler toys.

TABLE 11.9	Preventable Hazards for Toddlers
Hazard	**Nursing Considerations/Parent Education**
Falls	Due to a developing sense of balance, toddlers will quite often fall while climbing, jumping, or running.
	Parents should continue to keep crib rails up, monitor the toddler around stairs. Place gates at the top and bottom of stairs, and secure windows and screens with window guards.
	Apply nonskid decals in bathtub or shower.
	Remove unsecured or scattered rugs
	Never leave unattended in shopping cart or vehicle.
	Supervise playgrounds, select play areas with soft ground cover and safe equipment.
Burns	Keep hot items well back from the edge of a countertop as with increased height, the toddler can easily reach for items on top of counters.
	Turn pot handles in on stoves.
	Avoid hanging tablecloths as children may pull down hot items.
	Teach the toddler what "hot" means.
	Check bath water and do not allow the toddler to play with the faucets.
	Avoid overexposure to the sun and use sunscreen.
	Place guardrails in front of radiators, fireplaces, and other heating elements.
	Cover electrical outlets with protective plastic covers.
	Keep electrical wires hidden or out of reach.
Motor Vehicle Accidents	Rear-facing child seats are required for children up to 10 kg (22 lb), then front-facing seats are necessary until seats are outgrown.
	Supervise the toddler at all times during outdoor play and teach the safety rules around roads and parked cars.
	Head injuries are the number one cause of serious injury and death among children riding wheeled vehicles, including bicycles, in-line skates, scooters, etc. (Parachute, 2021c)
	Fit the toddler properly with a bike helmet that meets safety standards of the Canadian Safety Association (CSA). Supervise tricycle riding.
Drowning	Never leave a toddler alone in a bath, even for a few seconds.
	Supervise the toddler around all sources of water at all times, including buckets.
	Keep bathroom doors closed and toilet seats down.
	Have a fence with a locked gate around swimming pools.

TABLE 11.9	Preventable Hazards for Toddlers—cont'd
Hazard	**Nursing Considerations/Parent Education**
Poisoning	Poisonings by household chemical products, such as bleaches, laundry detergents (including single packets), paint thinners, ammonia, and abrasive cleaners, are among the top causes of injuries and deaths in children under the age of 5. Poisoning is the third leading cause of unintentional injury hospitalizations for children aged 0–14 years (Parachute, 2022).
	A small amount of a chemical product can be harmful to a child, and bad tastes and odours do not keep children away from chemical products. Place toxic substances on a high shelf or in a locked cabinet. Avoid storing in containers that are also used to store drinks and food.
	Keep other harmful products, such as cosmetics, drugs, vitamins, and first-aid treatment products, out of the sight and reach of children.
	Hang plants or place on a high surface out of reach of children and not on the floor.
	Keep cannabis, including edibles, locked up and out of reach of children and in child resistant packaging or containers.
Suffocation	Remove drawstrings from clothing.
	Dispose of old appliances properly by removing doors.
	Select safe toy boxes without heavy hinged lids.
	Keep window covering cords out of the toddler's reach.
Choking	Avoid giving toddlers foods that are choking hazards, such as whole hot dogs, large chunks of meat, fruit with pits, fish with bones, dried beans, chewing gum, nuts, popcorn, grapes, round candies, and marshmallows.
	Choose large, sturdy toys without small parts that can be removed and without sharp edges.
	Keep automatic garage door transmitters out of the toddler's reach.

Adapted from Hockenberry, M. J., Rodgers, C. & Wilson, D. (2022). *Wong's essentials of pediatric nursing* (11th ed., p. 347, Table 11.1). Elsevier Inc.

BOX 11.1   **Appropriate Toys for the Toddler**
• Dolls
• Play telephones, furniture, and dishes
• Puzzles with few, large pieces
• Pedal toys such as a riding truck or tricycle
• Push–pull toys
• Clay, sand box, crayons, finger paints
• Large blocks and pounding toys

Toilet Learning

One of the major tasks for the toddler to learn to use the toilet. See Box 11.2 for a summary of the factors involved in determining readiness for toilet learning.

Reactions to Illness and Hospitalization

The toddler age group has a poorly defined body image and body boundaries. Painful and invasive procedures can cause extreme anxiety. Toddlers react to pain in a similar way to infants but also can recall previous painful experiences. Most toddlers have separation anxiety and look at hospitalization as being abandoned.

Toddlers respond to stressful situations by using regression as a coping mechanism. They can have a feeling of loss of control when they are physically restricted, if there is a disruption of routines and rituals, or when there is a fear of injury, pain, or dependency. Separation anxiety occurs in children from 6 months to 2.5 years old (Hockenberry et al., 2022). The following are the three stages of separation anxiety:

BOX 11.2   **Assessing Toilet Learning Readiness**
Physical Readiness
• Voluntary control of anal and urethral sphincters, usually by 22–30 months of age
• Ability to stay dry for 2 hours, decreased number of wet diapers, waking dry from naps
• Regular bowel movements
• Gross motor skills of sitting, walking, and squatting
• Fine motor skills to remove clothing
Mental Readiness
• Recognition of urge to defecate and urinate
• Verbal or nonverbal communication skills to indicate when child is wet or has the urge to defecate or urinate
• Cognitive skills to imitate appropriate behaviour and follow directions
Psychological Readiness
• Expressing willingness to please parent
• Ability to sit on toilet for 5–8 minutes without fussing or getting off
• Curiosity about adults' or older siblings' toilet habits
• Impatience when in soiled or wet diapers, desire to be changed immediately
Parental Readiness
• Recognition of child's level of readiness
• Willingness to invest the time required for toilet learning
• Absence of family stress, such as a divorce, moving, new sibling, or imminent vacation

From Hockenberry, M. J., Rodgers, C. & Wilson, D. (2022). *Wong's essentials of pediatric nursing* (11th ed.) Elsevier.

- Protest: This is the usual reaction to hospitalization. The child cries for the parents, verbally or physically attacks others, tries to find parents, clings to them, and is inconsolable.
- Despair: The child shows disinterest in surroundings and play, passive reactions, depression, loss of appetite.
- Detachment or denial: The child appears to adapt to surroundings, but the adaptation is superficial, and the child remains detached. This adaptation usually happens after a long period of separation.

Nursing Considerations for Separation Anxiety

- Encourage the toddler to protest.
- Encourage parents to stay if possible.
- Encourage the use of transitional or parent objects associated with the parents that can be left with the child.
- Request that parents leave the room only when the child is awake and truthfully tell the child their return time.
- Try to keep to home routines, such as bedtime rituals, and use the words that the child is familiar with, such as "bye bye," to promote security.
- Provide activities and a play area to enhance muscle development.
- Encourage self-care with assistance in feeding, toileting, dressing, and hygiene.
- Encourage sensorimotor learning by imitation.
- Promote language skills by reinforcing mastered vocabulary and using activities that require language.
- Provide simple explanations to prepare for treatments.
- Enhance the toddler's sense of autonomy by offering choices.
- Use parents' photographs and encourage parental visiting.

PRESCHOOL: 3 TO 6 YEARS OF AGE

The preschooler has a slow and uniform rate of growth. Preschool children tend to be slight, sturdy, and nimble and have improved posture.

The major milestone for a preschooler is to prepare to enter school. Achievements that prepare them for school include gaining control of bodily systems, experiencing brief and prolonged periods of separation, ability to interact cooperatively with other children and adults, use of language, increased attention span, and memory preparation (Hockenberry et al., 2022).

Biological Changes

The rate of physical growth slows down and stabilizes:

- Increases in height remain steady at an increase of about 6.5 to 9 cm per year.
- Increases in weight continue to be steady as well at a rate of 2 to 3 kg per year.
- A typical 4-year-old will be 103 cm tall and will weigh an average of 16.5 kg.
- Boys and girls will have a similar body shape and size and may at times be distinguishable only by dress and hairstyle.

- Muscles and bones continue to mature as the preschooler gains strength by walking, running, and jumping.
- A balance of good nutrition, exercise, and rest is essential for growth and development.
- Blood pressure should be measured annually in children over 3 years of age.

Gross and Fine Motor Development

Gross motor skills improve and become more refined:

- An average preschooler can hop, skip, and run, which can lead to the introduction of a sport such as soccer, skating, or swimming.
- Encouraging physical activity in children of this age will help create a pattern that may benefit them for the rest of their lives.
  Fine motor skill advancement is most evident in improvements in the preschooler's ability to draw:
- The preschooler will begin to hold a pencil or crayon with the fingers rather than the fist.
- Drawings demonstrate advancements in perception of shape as well as developing fine motor skills.
  See Table 11.10 for a summary of growth and development in the preschooler years.

Nutrition

As they do in the toddler, the nutritional and fluid requirements in the preschooler continue to decrease slightly, with the exception of protein requirements, which will increase.

- Parents should be encouraged to follow *Canada's Food Guide: Healthy Eating for Parents and Children* to determine the correct amount and portions of each food group for young children (Government of Canada, 2022a).
- Preschool children will change their eating patterns daily, and parents may find that the quantity consumed varies day to day.
- Parents should be concerned with the quality versus the quantity of food as children have the ability to self-regulate their caloric needs and intake. What they do not eat at one meal they will make up at the next.
- An average preschool child will consume slightly more food than a toddler, or about half an adult portion.
- Food habits such as fad foods and strong food preferences will continue in the preschool years.
- At age 4, the child may become more rebellious and refuse to try new foods.
- By age 5, the child will become more open to trying new foods and will enjoy being included in food preparation with a family member.
- Parents should introduce table manners but should be cautioned not to be too strict. The preschooler may find it difficult to sit still for long periods of time.

Sleep

The preschooler will sleep an average of about 12 hours a night and very rarely naps during the day. It is common to see most sleep disturbances during the preschool years.

TABLE 11.10	Growth and Development During Preschool Years			
Age	**Physical**	**Gross Motor**	**Fine Motor**	**Language**
3 years	May have night-time control of bowel and bladder	Rides tricycle, jumps off bottom step, goes up stairs using alternate feet but may still come down the stairs using both feet may dance, stands on one foot for a few seconds	Builds tower of 9 to 10 cubes, builds bridge of 3 cubes, copies a circle, imitates a cross, names what has been drawn, cannot draw stick figure but may make a circle with facial features	Says 900 words, uses three- to four-word sentences, talks incessantly, asks many questions
4 years	Length at birth is doubled	Skips, jumps, goes downstairs using alternate feet, catches a ball reliably, throws a ball overhead	Uses scissors successfully to cut out picture following outline, laces shoes but may not be able to tie a bow, copies a square, traces a cross and diamond, adds three parts to stick figure	Says 1 500 words, uses four- to five-word sentences, tells exaggerated stories, sings simple songs; questioning is at its peak, names one or more colours, comprehends analogies, such as "If fire is hot, ice is __"
5 years	Permanent teeth may begin to erupt Handedness is determined (90% are right-handed)	Skips and hops on alternate feet, throws and catches a ball well, balances on alternate feet well with eyes closed, walks backward with heel to toe, good balance with skating	Ties shoelaces; uses scissors, simple tools, and pencil well; copies a diamond and a triangle; prints a few numbers, letters, or words such as first name, adds seven to nine parts to a stick figure	Says 2 100 words, uses six- to eight-word sentences, names four or more colours, knows days of the week and the months, names coins (dime, nickel, quarter), Can follow three commands in succession, describes a picture or drawing with much comment and enumeration

Adapted from Hockenberry, M. J., Rodgers, C. & Wilson, D. (2022). *Wong's essentials of pediatric nursing* (11th ed., p. 371, Table 12.1). Elsevier Inc.

- Mastery of autonomy, separation, and object permanence can lead to sleep disturbances (Hockenberry et al., 2022).
- Nightmares can occur and are typically defined as a scary dream followed by full waking. They typically occur in the second half of the night, when dreams are more intense. Once fully awake, the child will be aware of the parent's presence and can be comforted and reassured.
- Sleep terrors can also occur and are typically defined as a partial arousal from a deep sleep. They typically occur 1 to 4 hours after falling asleep. The child will not be aware of the parent's presence and hence is not easily consoled. The child should simply be observed during the sleep terror until it subsides, and the child returns to a calm state. They should be guided back to bed if needed.
- Establishing good bedtime routines is essential to promote good sleep patterns.
- Behaviour that delays bedtime and is determined to be attention-seeking should be ignored by the parent.
- Preschoolers can be very active during the day and slowing down before bedtime can lead to less resistance in going to bed.

Dental

The focus for preschoolers is on dental hygiene and prevention of decay:

- They should be encouraged to brush their own teeth, but they will require adult supervision of how well they manipulate the toothbrush.

- Professional care and routine follow-ups are encouraged every 6 months (Canadian Dental Association, 2022b).
- Dental injuries are not uncommon at this age and should be examined by a professional.

Immunization

See Table 11.5A–B for the recommended Canadian routine immunization schedule.

Safety

Preschoolers are less accident-prone than toddlers; however, injuries among children in this age group are common. The most common causes of injury in the home to children less than 5 years of age are falls from heights, burns, and scalds, and poisonings (Hockenberry et al., 2022).

- To reduce the risk of injury caused by falls from heights in this age group, ensure that there is a mechanism to prevent the child from falling downstairs or from opening windows more than 15 cm (Hockenberry et al., 2022).
- To reduce the risk of injury caused by burns and scalds, ensure that the maximum temperature of tap water is less than 49°C or less; cords do not dangle from the kettle or other appliances in the kitchen; there is a stove guard to prevent a child from grabbing pots; and matches and lighters are well out of reach.
- To reduce the risk of injury by fire, ensure that the home has functioning smoke detectors and fire extinguishers (Hockenberry et al., 2022).

- To reduce the risk of injury caused by poisonings, ensure that all choking hazards in the home are out of reach of the child; all bathroom supplies, cleaning supplies, and medications are out of reach; all bathroom bottles and medications have child-resistant lids (especially grandparents' and visitors'); and a functioning carbon monoxide detector is in the home (Hockenberry et al., 2022).

Play

Preschoolers engage in associative play. This age group enjoys group play in similar activities but without rigid organization or rules.
- Activities should promote physical growth and motor skills and include running, jumping, and climbing.
- Toys that help develop muscles and coordination include tricycles, wagons, gym and sports equipment, sandboxes, and wading pools.
- Activities to help promote muscle strength and coordination include swimming, skating, and skiing.
- Large blocks, puzzles, crayons, paints, and simple crafts can help develop fine motor skills.

Reactions to Illness and Hospitalization

Preschoolers still have poor differentiation between themselves and their environment. They still have a limited understanding of language and can see only one part of an object or situation at a time.

Preschoolers believe that unrelated events cause illness. They also have magical thinking that cause them to perceive illness as a punishment. There is also a fear of mutilation.

Reactions to hospitalization at this stage are primarily regression and a lack of co-operation as coping mechanisms for separation. Preschoolers can experience a loss of control because they feel a loss of their own power. Fear of injury and pain leads to a fear of mutilation and invasive treatments. They lack knowledge about the body. This creates, for example, a fear of castration from enemas or rectal thermometers or a fear that the insides of their body may leak out during the insertion of an intravenous (IV) line. They perceive hospitalization as a punishment and separation from parents as a lack of love.

Nursing Considerations for Separation Anxiety
- Use puppets and dolls to demonstrate treatments with an appropriate level of vocabulary.
- Use adhesive bandages to "stop the insides from coming out."
- Stay with the preschooler during treatments.
- Give rewards such as stars or stickers.
- Use hospital therapeutic play kits to work through anxieties.
- Help prevent a sense of guilt by reassuring the preschooler that they are not responsible for the illness.
- Provide motor stimulation and praise achievements.
- Promote autonomy by encouraging choices and self-care, such as a choice of clothing.
- Promote language skills by telling stories and teaching new words.

- Encourage parental involvement, rooming in with the child and visiting as well as contact with siblings and peers to decrease separation anxiety. A family centered care philosophy recognizes the family is an essential part of the child's care and illness experience.

SCHOOL AGE: 6 TO 12 YEARS OF AGE

At this age, the child has a slow and uniform rate of growth. This is a generally healthy age group with fewer visits to the pediatrician and fewer immunizations.
- It is important to focus on establishing good health habits, proper nutrition, and physical activity.
- There may be an increased risk of obesity at this stage.

Biological Changes

This is generally a period of gradual growth and development with a growth spurt at prepuberty.
- Height changes are slow and steady, adding 5 cm per year to gain about 30 to 60 cm.
- Weight will almost double, with increases of 2 to 3 kg per year.
- Boys and girls vary little during this phase, although girls will begin to surpass boys in both height and weight toward the end of the stage.
- At prepubescence (2 years preceding adolescence), the difference in girls and boys in biological terms can be as much as 2 years, with girls starting prepubescence first.
- In girls, prepubescence is a period of rapid growth, with puberty beginning at approximately age 10. This may cause anxiety in girls who develop earlier or later than their peers.
- In boys, prepubescence is a period of steady growth, with puberty beginning at approximately age 12.
- Changes in height and weight will differ greatly among children; therefore, some may appear older physically than their behavioural, emotional, or mental development would indicate.
- Heart rate and respirations tend to decrease, whereas blood pressure will increase in this stage.

Gross and Fine Motor Development

Generally, school-aged children are steadier on their feet and more graceful than those at the previous stage. Bodies will take on a slenderer look, and certain activities, such as biking and climbing, will be easier.

Muscle mass will increase, but it is important not to overwork muscles to the point of fatigue. See Table 11.11 for a summary of growth and development in the school-age years.

Nutrition

The focus for this age group is independence and forming good habits for the years to come. Children become more independent in their food choices at home and school, have strong likes and dislikes for foods, are exposed to choices of foods and are very influenced by friends and the media.

TABLE 11.11	**Growth and Development During the School-Age Years**			
Age	**Physical**	**Gross Motor**	**Fine Motor**	**Language**
6 years	Continues to grow slowly, loses first tooth, vision reaches maturity	A very active age with constant activity Demonstrates gradual increase in dexterity	Likes to draw, print, and colour	Develops concept of numbers, knows morning from the afternoon, defines objects in terms of use (e.g., fork, chair), knows left from right hand
7 years	Begins to grow at least 5 cm per year Jaw begins to expand to accommodate permanent teeth	More cautious approach to new performances Repeats performances to master them	Can copy a diamond	Notices certain items missing from a picture, repeats three numbers backward, develops concept of time More mechanical in reading, often does not stop at the end of a sentence, skips words such as it, the, and he.
8–9 years	Continues to grow at least 5 cm per year	Dresses self completely More limber, bones grow faster than ligaments Always on the go and hard to quiet down, movement fluid, often graceful and poised	Produces simple paintings and drawings	Gives similarities and differences Can count backward from 20 Describes common objects in detail, not just by use, repeats in order the days of the week and months, knows the date
10–12 years	Slow growth in height and rapid weight gain, possibly leading to obesity Posture more similar to that of an adult	Reaches adult levels	Continues to refine	Writes brief stories Writes occasional short letters to friends Reads for practical information or own enjoyment

Adapted from Hockenberry, M. J., Rodgers, C. & Wilson, D. (2022). *Wong's essentials of pediatric nursing* (11th ed., p. 406, Table 14.1). Elsevier Inc.

- Good choices and habits will lead to good nutrition and healthy weight gain, whereas poor choices and habits will lead to excessive weight gain and poor nutrition.
- Caloric needs tend to decrease.
- There are fewer stomach upsets, blood sugar levels balance out and are better maintained, and there is an increase in stomach capacity, meaning that food is retained for longer periods of time.

Sleep

It is very important for school-aged children to have enough energy for school and other activities.

- They begin to take charge of bedtime routines; however, they will need reminders to go to bed.
- They no longer take naps and will sleep through the night with typically 8 to 12 hours of sleep.

Dental

Many changes to the mouth at this stage require regular visits to the dentist.

- Most children lose their first tooth by age 6 (usually the front).
- Eventually, they will lose all 20 deciduous teeth, and permanent teeth will begin to erupt.

- Permanent teeth appear large in proportion to the rest of the face, a stage that is sometimes known as the "ugly duckling" phase.
- The jawline elongates, and the new teeth move into their new positions.
- Regular flossing, brushing, and dental visits will promote good oral hygiene.
- Sweets and sugary snacks should be limited.

Immunization

See Table 11.5A–B for the recommended Canadian routine immunization schedule.

Safety

School-aged children tend to have frequent minor injuries, such as falls from bikes. Injuries from skateboards, roller skates or in-line skates and scooters, skin rashes from environmental exposures, and bruises from ball sports.

- Due to the increasing need for independence, this age group tends to engage in activities without an adult. Therefore, it is important to teach about safety, risks, and consequences.
- Parents should ensure that children use protective gear, such as bike helmets (which are mandatory in most provinces).

- Parents should ensure that children use a booster seat until the vehicle seat belts fit correctly (Parachute, 2021b).
- Safety strategies should be put into place for "latch-key" children. Some employers, schools or communities have developed after school programs for children, so they do not have to be alone at home. Other programs include self-help skills for children, telephone hotlines to provide check-ins, and reassurance programs for children. Nurses need to be aware of these services provided and encourage parents to teach self-help skills to their children (Hockenberry et al., 2022).
- Street proofing and learning how to avoid abduction help children achieve independence and autonomy safely.
- Parents may participate in community programs in which fingerprints and other identification systems are organized in case the child is missing.
- After-school programs keep children occupied during times when parents are unavailable to supervise.
- Emergency numbers and contact people need to be readily available to the child.

Play

Learning good physical activity habits will influence future involvement in an activity or sport. A proper amount of physical activity will help with weight control, encourage good socialization, help develop gross and fine motor skills, and give the child a sense of accomplishment.

- Play involves increased physical skill, intellect, and fantasy.
- Groups and cliques foster a sense of belonging to a team or club, which leads to a sense of importance.
- Games now have well-established rules, and knowing the rules means belonging (conformity and ritual will guide play).
- Children have increased interest in complex games and electronic games.
- Children have increased interest in reading.
- Quiet and solitary play is valued at this stage as school-aged children enjoy collecting objects and toys, which they tend to keep in disorganized piles.

Mental Health

This is an age at which one's self-concept and self-esteem are developed (Hockenberry et al., 2022).

- Self-concept is the mental idea one has of oneself.
- Self-esteem reflects a positive self-concept.
- The family has a great influence on the child's development of self-esteem and self-concept.
- Children at this age are beginning to form a concept of sexuality and need to have good information and openness to discuss ideas, questions, misconceptions, and fears.
- They are beginning to develop ways to problem-solve situations and develop solutions, for example, around doing homework, making choices, or setting limits.
- This is the concrete stage of cognitive development; therefore, when teaching, provide opportunities to touch, feel, and become engaged in learning.

- Poor relationships with peers or a lack of group identification can contribute to bullying. Cyberbullying involves an electronic source to harm or bother another individual and can be more harmful because the attack instantly can reach a wider audience range while allowing the bully to remain anonymous. Children targeted by bullies often have a lower self-esteem, anxiety, depression, withdrawal, and reduced assertiveness that make them an easy target for bullying. Long-term consequences for victims include increased risks for low self-esteem, depression, anxiety, loneliness, feelings of insecurity, and poor academic performance (Hockenberry et al., 2022).
- Three types of temperament categories in this stage are as follows (Child Care State Capacity Building Center, 2018)
  - Easy: adapts readily to new situations
  - Slow to warm up: is uncomfortable with new situations and takes time to adapt
  - Active: is easily distracted and needs to be prepared for a situation and have varied routines (sleeping, eating etc.)

Reactions to Illness and Hospitalization

The school-aged child can be stressed by immobilization, fear of mutilation and death, and modesty. This child can also be stressed by necessary dependency, which gives a sense of loss of control. It may still be difficult for these children to be able to express themselves verbally, and they may be self-conscious with their care. However, they are curious about their body and are eager to learn about it.

Children at this stage think of illness as being caused by external forces. School-agers are aware of the implications of the different illnesses. They react to separation by exhibiting loneliness, boredom, isolation, and depression. They may show aggression, irritability, and inability to relate to siblings and peers.

Nursing Considerations for Illness and Hospitalization

- Encourage verbalization and reassure the child that it is acceptable to cry.
- Promote autonomy, self-care, and choices with participation in care.
- Celebrate successes when the child succeeds at tasks in order to enhance feelings of accomplishment.
- Encourage peer interaction and use group teaching.
- Provide diversions that help with the development of fine motor skills, such as computer skills, as well as with stress control.
- Increase understanding of bodily functions and the illness and prepare for procedures using pictures to teach the child about the body.
- Work through emotions and stress through various expressive means such as art, music, and drama therapy.

ADOLESCENCE: 12 TO 18 YEARS OF AGE

Adolescence is the second most rapid growth period. It is defined as the transition period between childhood and adulthood and is a time of development in which one makes educational and occupational choices for the future. It is common for adolescents to take chances and engage in risk-taking behaviour, which may lead to health concerns and injury.

Biological Changes

The period of development referred to as *puberty* involves complex biological, cognitive, psychological, and social changes—more so than any other time in life.

- Puberty involves a predictable series of hormonal and physical changes in both sexual maturation and physical growth.
- Puberty is triggered by a series of hormonal changes in the body controlled by the anterior pituitary gland in response to stimulus from the hypothalamus (Hockenberry et al., 2022).

The Tanner stages of development, which comprise five stages, depict the typical sequence of changes in external secondary sexual characteristics in females and males (Hockenberry et al., 2022). The Tanner stages are used to describe changes in females and males in the text that follows.

Changes in the Female

The primary sexual change in females is the buildup of enough estrogen to force the release of an egg, or ovum, from the ovaries every 28 days.

Female breast development
- Stage 1 is the prepubertal stage.
- Stage 2 is characterized by the development of breast buds.
- Stage 3 is characterized by the further enlargement of the breasts and areolae, with no separation of contours.
- Stage 4 is characterized by projection of areolae and papillae to form secondary mounds.
- Stage 5 is characterized by adult configuration.

Pubic hair development (male and female)
- Stage 1 is the prepubertal stage.
- Stage 2 is characterized by sparse, long, straight, downy hair.
- Stage 3 is characterized by darker, coarser, curly hair that is sparse over the entire pubis.
- Stage 4 is characterized by dark, curly, and abundant hair in the pubic area only.
- Stage 5 is characterized by an adult pattern.

Changes in the Male

The primary male sexual characteristic is the development of viable sperm.

- Follicle-stimulating hormone (FSH) and luteinizing hormone (LH) act on testicular cells to stimulate the production of testosterone and viable sperm.
- The production of viable sperms tends to follow the male's first ejaculation.

Male genitalia development
- Stage 1 is the prepubertal stage.
- Stage 2 is chaterized by enlargement of the scrotum and testes and rugation and reddening of the scrotum.

- Stage 3 is characterized by lengthening of the penis and further enlargement of the scrotum and testes.
- Stage 4 is characterized by an increase in the length and width of the penis, development of the glans, and darkening of the scrotum.
- Stage 5 is characterized by an adult configuration.

Gross and Fine Motor Development

In the adolescent, gross motor development reaches adult levels. Fine motor development continues to be refined.

Nutrition

Puberty marks the beginning of accelerated physical growth, which can result in as much as double the adolescent nutritional requirements for iron, protein, zinc, and calcium.

Many factors influence an adolescent's nutrition, including growing independence, the need for peer acceptability, concerns over physical appearance, and an active lifestyle.

- It is common for the adolescent to choose snacks of "empty calories," those devoid of any appropriate vitamins and minerals.
- Skipping breakfast or eating a breakfast that is nutritionally poor in quality is frequently a problem.
- Adolescents are at increased risk for obesity, as well as for eating disorders such as anorexia and bulimia.

Sleep

Adolescents commonly feel fatigued. Factors contributing to fatigue include rapid growth, overexertion, a tendency to stay up late, insufficient sleep, and poor nutrition. In an effort to catch up on missed sleep, many adolescents like to sleep in.

Dental

Continued dental hygiene must be encouraged, including proper brushing, flossing, and regular dental visits.
- Orthodontics are common and may lead to teasing and embarrassment.
- Good snack choices and reduce exposure to empty calories should be encouraged.

Immunization

See Table 11.5A–B for the recommended Canadian routine immunization schedule.

Safety

Adolescents rarely consider the risk or consequence of their actions and often feel invulnerable.
- The use of safety devices decreases in this age group, resulting in increased injury, such as the failure to use helmets or seat belts.
- Health teaching should focus on managing peer pressure to engage in risky activities.

Reactions to Illness and Hospitalization

For adolescents, hospitalization can have a significant impact, causing stresses due to issues around body image, separation from peers, and reduced independence due to necessary restrictions. In children up to 14 years, illness may still be viewed as a punishment.

Reactions to illnesses include the adolescent coping mechanisms of denial and displacement. A sense of a loss of control occurs because of dependency and loss of identity, causing the adolescent to react with rejection, uncooperativeness, self-assertion, anger, frustration, or possibly withdrawal, even from peers. Adolescents also fear mutilation and sexual changes, fears demonstrated by a lot of questioning, rejecting others, questioning adequacy of care, psychosomatic complaints, and sexual reactions. Separation, particularly from the peer group, may result in further withdrawal, loneliness, and boredom.

Nursing Considerations for Illness and Hospitalization

- Relate to adolescents at their level and be authentic.
- Allow them to wear their own clothes, keep their belongings, and decorate their rooms.
- Understand that staying connected through social media is important for family and peer interaction.
- Respect their privacy.
- Set limits.
- Teach about puberty-related issues such as personal hygiene, breast self-examination, testicular self-examination, sexuality and safer sexual practices, contraception, human immunodeficiency virus (HIV), and other relevant topics.
- Provide clear explanations based on science.
- Encourage as much mobility and exercise as possible.
- Encourage the adolescent to participate and be an active decision maker in their own health care.
- Promote independence.
- Explore body image and self-esteem.
- Encourage family participation and support.
- Encourage the teen to keep up with schoolwork and in contact with teachers and encourage career goals.

THERAPEUTIC RELATIONSHIP

A therapeutic relationship with the child and the family is the foundation of pediatric nursing. See Chapter 4, page 21, for more information on this topic. The hallmarks of effective communication are as follows:

- Establish trust.
- Respect and maintain confidentiality.
- Be truthful.
- Convey respect.
- Implement appropriate communication strategies.

Inherent in every group of nursing considerations in this chapter is the importance of the nursing role in developing therapeutic relationships, encouraging clients and families to participate in their care and verbalize their concerns, being a client and family advocate, teaching disease prevention and health promotion, providing support and counselling, and making ethical decisions. The impact of hospitalization according to the age and stage of development is outlined in the previous sections. These principles should be referred to in relation to each of the following health challenges.

PAIN MANAGEMENT

Pain management is an important aspect of pediatric nursing care. Nurses perform pain assessments and provide nonpharmacological and pharmacological pain-relieving interventions that bring relief and comfort to children and their families. Children's perception of pain and the meaning of pain varies from child to child. Unaddressed pain will only increase a child's fear and anxiety which will heighten their awareness of the pain. It can lead to potential long term physiologic, behavioural, or psychosocial effects. Both nonpharmacological approaches and pain medications are essential to providing adequate pain control for children (Hockenberry et al., 2022). Culture, community, and family also impacts a child's experience with pain management. Some of the challenges documented among non–English-speaking clients include the following:

- Making inadequate pain assessments
- Clients and families being reluctant to report pain or even take pain medication
- Being worried that increased pain means the disease is progressing
- Lack of commitment to taking the prescribed medication ordered
- Being worried about the adverse effects of and tolerance to the pain analgesia (Keenan-Lindsay et al., 2022)

Indigenous children's pain may not be accurately reported using Westernized pain assessment tools. It is important to create culturally safe spaces for the child, family, and the community in order to have a better understanding of their pain and coping mechanisms. Methods like Talking Circles and painting workshops have been shown to provide a safe space for them to share their feelings and understandings related to both emotional and physical pain (Keenan-Lindsay et al., 2022).

Physiological Measures of Pediatric Pain

Physiological reactions to pain, particularly in the nonverbal younger age groups and children with communication and cognitive impairments, can help nurses assess the child's level of pain.

Developmental Characteristics of Children's Responses to Pain

The response to pain depends on the child's developmental stage. Characteristics of pain response based on development are summarized in Box 11.3.

Pain Tools

Nurses can use a variety of pain tools to help assess children's level of pain. These tools are adapted to the different developmental stages and include behavioural, physiological, or self-report measurements.

Pain scale for preterm infants. Keenan-Lindsay (2020) examined various pain assessment tools for infants:

CRIES: This pain assessment tool involves a 10-point scale (with each component scored from 0 to 2) that includes facial expression, cry, movement of the arms and legs, ability to

BOX 11.3 Developmental Characteristics of Children's Responses to Pain

Young Infant
- Generalized body response of rigidity or thrashing, possibly with local reflex withdrawal of stimulated area
- Loud crying
- Facial expression of pain (brows lowered and drawn together, eyes tightly closed, and mouth open and square-shaped)
- No association demonstrated between approaching stimulus and subsequent pain

Older Infant
- Localized body response with deliberate withdrawal of stimulated area
- Loud crying
- Facial expression of pain or anger
- Physical resistance, especially pushing the stimulus away after it is applied

Young Child
- Loud crying, screaming
- Verbal expressions such as "Ow," "Ouch," "It hurts"
- Thrashing of arms and legs
- Attempts to push stimulus away before it is applied
- Lack of co-operation, need for physical restraint

- Requests termination of procedure
- Clings to parent, nurse, or other significant person
- Requests emotional support, such as hugs or other forms of physical comfort
- May become restless and irritable with continuing pain
- Behaviours occur in anticipation of actual painful procedure

School-Aged Child
- May exhibit all behaviours of young child, especially during actual painful procedure, but fewer in anticipatory period
- Stalling behaviour, such as "Wait a minute" or "I'm not ready"
- Muscular rigidity, such as clenched fists, white knuckles, gritted teeth, contracted limbs, body stiffness, closed eyes, wrinkled forehead

Adolescent
- Less vocal protest
- Less motor activity
- More verbal expressions, such as "It hurts" or "You're hurting me"
- Increased muscle tension and body control

From Hockenberry, M. J., Rodgers, C., & Wilson, D. (2022). *Wong's essentials of pediatric nursing* (11th ed., p. 114, Box 5–1). Elsevier Inc.

TABLE 11.12 Premature Infant Pain Profile (PIPP)

Ages of Use	Reliability and Validity	Variables	Scoring Range
28–40 weeks' gestational age	Internal consistency using Cronbach alpha = 0.75–0.59; standardized item alpha for six items = 0.71 Construct validity using handling versus painful situations: statistically significant differences (paired t = 12.24, two-tailed p <.0001, and Mann-Whitney U = 765.5, p <.0001) and using real versus sham heelstick procedures with infants aged 28–30 weeks' gestational age (t = 2.4, two-tailed p <.02, and Mann-Whitney U = 132, p <.016) and with full-term males undergoing circumcision with topical anaesthetic versus placebo (t = 2.6, two-tailed p <.02, or nonparametric equivalent Mann-Whitney U test, U = 145.7, two-tailed p <.02)	Gestational age (0–3) Eye squeeze (0–3) Behavioural state (0–3) Nasolabial furrow (0–3) Heart rate (0–3) Oxygen saturation (0–3) Brow bulge (0–3)	0 = no pain; 21 = worst pain

From Stevens, B., Johnston, C., Petryshen, P., et al. (1996). Premature Infant Pain Profile: Development and Initial validation. *The Clinical Journal of Pain, 12*(1), 13–22. Reprinted with permission.

console, and oxygen saturation in its scoring. Letters of the acronym are C = cry, R = requires oxygen, I = increased vital signs, E = expression on face, S = sleeplessness.

FLACC: This pain tool measures the pain of infants. The parameters include face, legs, activity, cry, and, if able, to console. Each parameter is scored from 0 to 2, with a higher cumulative score indicating increased distress.

PIPP: This is a unique pain scale developed for preterm infants (Premature Infant Pain Profile). There is a higher pain score for infants with a lower gestational age. Sleeping infants also receive additional points for reduced reactions. See Table 11.12 for a summary of the PIPP scale. This rates eye squeeze, nasal labial furrow, heart rate, oxygen saturation, and the brow furrow on a 0 to 3 scale, with 21 indicating the worst level of pain.

NIPPS: The Neonatal Infant Pain Scale rates facial expression, arm movement, cry, leg movement, respiration, and arousal on a 0 to 2 scale, with a score of 7 indicating the worst level of pain (Keenan-Lindsay, 2020).

Pain scale for 1- to 5-year-olds. CHEOPS, or Children's Hospital of Eastern Ontario Pain Scale, was developed for 1- to 7-year-olds by McGrath et al. (1985) in collaboration with recovery room nurses. Six categories of behaviours are identified: cry, facial, verbal, torso, touch, and legs. See Table 11.13 for a summary of this scale.

Pain scale for 3- to 12-year-olds. The Wong-Baker FACES® Pain Rating Scale is a self-reporting tool for children 3 to 12 years old. See Figure 11.1 for the FACES tool.

Pain assessment in the child with communication and cognitive difficulties. Children with communication and

TABLE 11.13 Children's Hospital of Eastern Ontario Pain Scale (CHEOPS)

Ages of Use	Reliability and Validity	Variables	Scoring Range
1–5 years	Interrater reliability = 90–99.5% Internal correlation = significant correlations between pairs of items Concurrent validity between CHEOPS and visual analogue scale (VAS) = .91; between individual and total scores of CHEOPS and VAS = 0.50–0.86 Construct validity with preanalgesia and postanalgesia scores = 9.9–6.3	Cry (1–3) Facial (0–2) Child verbal (0–2) Torso (1–2) Touch (1–2) Legs (1–2)	4 = no pain; 13 = worst pain

From McGrath, P. J., Johnson, G., Goodman, J. T., et al. (1985). The CHEOPS: A behavioural scale for rating post-operative pain in children. In H. L. Fields, R. Dubner, & F. Cervero (Eds.), *Advances in pain research and therapy* (p. 207). Raven Press. Reprinted with permission.

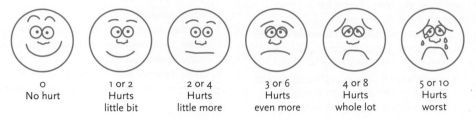

0	1 or 2	2 or 4	3 or 6	4 or 8	5 or 10
No hurt	Hurts little bit	Hurts little more	Hurts even more	Hurts whole lot	Hurts worst

Fig. 11.1 Wong-Baker FACES Pain Rating Scale. (Wong-Baker FACES Foundation (2020). Wong-Baker FACES® Pain Rating Scale. From WongBaker FACES.org.

cognitive difficulties present a significant challenge to nurses in accurately assessing their pain level. These children may not react in the usual way to pain. Parents are very important in helping nurses interpret the child's pain reactions. The most reported behaviours in this type of child are as follows (Keenan-Lindsay et al., 2022):

- Moaning, crying, or being irritable
- Inconsistent patterns of play and sleep
- Changes in facial expression
- Changes in behaviours of cooperation, activity, and eating
- Behavioural changes in engagement with family, friends, and others

Nonpharmacological Strategies for Pain Management

Many nonpharmacological strategies can be used to help children cope with pain. A number of these strategies are listed in Box 11.4.

Pharmacological Strategies for Pain Management

The following are routes used to deliver pain analgesics:

- Oral, sublingual, buccal, or transmucosal
- IV
- Subcutaneous, continuous
- Patient-controlled analgesia (PCA), family-controlled analgesia, or nurse-activated analgesia
- Intramuscular (this route is discouraged)
- Intranasal
- Intradermal
- Topical or transdermal

Groups of Drugs

Many types of medications can be used in pediatric pain control. See Chapter 8 for more specific information on those listed here. For the pediatric population, the types of drugs that can be used are as follows (Hockenberry et al., 2022):

- Nonsteroidal anti-inflammatory drugs (NSAIDs) approved for children
  - Indomethacin, ibuprofen, naproxen, diclofenac
- Acetaminophen
- Opioids formulated for children
  - Morphine, fentanyl, codeine, hydromorphone, hydrocodone, and acetaminophen, levorphanol, methadone, oxycodone
- Antidepressants
  - Amitriptyline, nortriptyline
- Anticonvulsants
  - Gabapentin, carbamazepine
- Anxiolytics
  - Lorazepam
- Corticosteroids
  - Dexamethasone
- Others
  - Clonidine, mexiletine

SKIN AND HAIR CARE

Pediculosis Capitis

Pediculosis capitis, or head lice, is an infestation in the hair and is a common condition that can be difficult to eliminate.

BOX 11.4 Nonpharmacological Strategies for Pain Management

General Strategies
- Use nonpharmacological interventions to supplement, not replace, pharmacological interventions and use for mild pain and pain that is reasonably well controlled with analgesics.
- Form a trusting relationship with the child and the family.
- Express concern regarding their reports of pain and intervene appropriately.
- Take an active role in seeking effective pain management strategies.
- Prepare the child before potentially painful procedures but avoid "planting" the idea of pain. Use "non-pain" descriptors when possible, such as "It feels like heat" rather than "It is a burning pain." This avoids suggesting pain and gives the child control in describing reactions. Avoid evaluative statements or descriptions such as "It will hurt a lot."
- Stay with the child during a painful procedure.
  - Allow parents to stay with the child if so desired by both child and parent and encourage the parent to talk softly to the child and to remain near the child's head.
  - Involve the parent in learning specific nonpharmacological strategies and in assisting the child with their use.
  - Educate the child about the pain, especially when explanation may lessen anxiety, and ensure that the child understands they are not responsible for the pain.
  - For long-term pain control, offer the child a doll, which represents "the client," and allow child to do everything to the doll that is done to them; emphasize pain control through the doll by stating, "Dolly feels better after the medicine."
  - Teach procedures to child and family for later use.

Specific Strategies
Distraction
- Employ play, music, computer games, singing, and rhythmic breathing.
- Have the child use deep breathing and blowing it out.
- Encourage the child to concentrate on yelling or saying "ouch."
- Have the child look through a kaleidoscope and concentrate on designs.

- Use humour by watching cartoons, telling jokes or funny stories, or acting silly with the child.
- Help the child read, play games, or visit with friends.

Relaxation
- Hold infant in a comfortable position and rock or sway back and forth.
- Repeat one or two reassuring words softly.
- Use relaxation techniques, such as going limp as a rag doll while exhaling or asking the child to yawn.
- Help child assume a comfortable position (e.g., pillow under neck and knees).
- Allow child to keep eyes open, since children may respond better if eyes are open rather than closed during relaxation

Guided Imagery
- During a painful episode, have the child identify and describe some pleasurable or imaginary experiences, including as many senses as possible.
- Write down or record a script.
- Combine the script with relaxation and rhythmic breathing.

Positive Self-Talk
- Teach the child positive statements to say when in pain.

Thought Stopping
- Identify positive facts about the painful event.
- Identify reassuring information.
- Condense positive and reassuring facts into a set of brief statements and have the child memorize them and repeat whenever they think about or are experiencing a painful event.

Behavioural Contracting
- May be used with children as young as 4 or 5, with stars, tokens, or stickers as rewards.
- Identify rewards or consequences that are reinforcing and goals that can be evaluated.
- Reinforce identified rewards or consequences.
- Use a formal written contract, dated and signed by all persons involved in any of the agreements.

Adapted from Hockenberry, M., Rodgers, C. & Wilson, D. (2022). *Wong's essentials of pediatric nursing* (11th ed., p. 121). Elsevier.

It can also spread to other family members. It occurs in all socioeconomic groups. Outbreaks can occur, particularly in elementary schools and day care facilities.

Pathophysiology

Head lice live only on humans and are transmitted by direct hair-to-hair contact or by sharing brushes, combs, towels, and so on. They can move quickly but do not jump. The female louse will lay her eggs along the hair shaft. The eggs, which stick to the hair and look like teardrops, hatch in 8 to 10 days.

Clinical Manifestations

The child will complain of severe itching of the scalp, and the scalp has the appearance of dandruff. Secondary infections can develop because of scratching lesions.

Therapeutics and Nursing Considerations

The CPS recommends a topical insecticide shampoo treatment, which contains pyrethrins or permethrin (Cummings et al., 2021). These pediculicides affect the lice but do not affect the nits (eggs); therefore, the treatment must be repeated to kill the hatched lice. Lindane shampoo may be used as a secondary treatment, but only with caution and not with children under 2 because of potential toxicity and resistance There are two noninsecticidal products that contains isopropyl myristate and cyclomethicone for use in children who are over 4 years old. Dimeticone solution is a noninsecticidal treatment that is used for children who are over 2 years old.

Dermatitis

Dermatitis is a skin inflammation that develops in response to various stimuli. The types of dermatitis that are the most common in children and adolescents are contact, diaper, seborrheic, and atopic, or eczema. A child's skin is sensitive, and it is important to keep the skin clean, moisturized, and protected from skin breakdown to prevent infections.

Contact Dermatitis

Contact dermatitis is an inflammatory reaction of the skin to an allergen or irritating substance. It commonly affects infants of 9 to 12 months.

Pathophysiology and Clinical Manifestations

The clinical manifestations are erythema, edema, pruritis, vesicles, or bullae that rupture, ooze, and crust over. Contact dermatitis is usually present only in the contact area, where fissures, dryness, scaling, and necrosis can also appear. Sometimes there is a rash that is distal to the originating area after about 1 week that can last about 3 to 4 weeks without treatment.

Irritants can cause an inflammatory response, and allergens can be absorbed into the skin, creating an initial sensitization. The allergen is carried to the T lymphocytes to create an immune memory. It takes repeated exposures to the allergen to create an allergic inflammatory reaction. The exception is poison ivy or poison oak, which requires only one or two exposures to elicit the immune reaction.

Therapeutics and Nursing Considerations

The treatment is to remove the irritant or allergen and wash the skin, decrease itching, and promote healing. The child may need patch testing for the allergen. Antihistamines, calamine lotion, wet dressings, or colloidal oatmeal–based bath products will help decrease the itching. Burow's solution soaks (aluminum acetate) will encourage drying. Topical corticosteroids after dressing soaks followed by an emollient will increase the absorption and decrease the itching. Mild to moderate severe cases may require a stronger topical corticosteroid over 2-week time frame and a systemic corticosteroid may be required for severe cases (Keenan-Lindsay et al., 2022).

Diaper Dermatitis

Diaper dermatitis is caused by a skin reaction to urine, feces, moisture, or friction that causes abrasion.

Pathophysiology and Clinical Manifestations

The skin reacts to the irritants and becomes increasingly permeable to the irritants and microbes. Irritants such as urine and stool can lead to a rash and subsequent skin breakdown. Common diaper rash, or diaper dermatitis, occurs frequently and affects approximately one-third of infants. Breastfed babies have a lower pH, which helps decrease the occurrence of dermatitis (Hockenberry et al., 2022).

The clinical manifestations are as follows:
- Red glazed plaques appear in the diaper area.
- In most cases, the rash is not in the skin folds of the groin area but affects the rest of the diaper region.

- If the rash becomes severe, it is characterized by a raised, red, and confluent rash, and pustules may also occur.
- *Candida albicans* infection can occur as a primary or secondary infection and is indicated by red, scaly plaques with sharp margins. Small papules and pustules can be present, including in the groin area.

Diagnostics

A skin scraping for microscopic testing with potassium hydroxide can be used to diagnose *Candida* (Kalyoussef et al., 2020).

Therapeutics and Nursing Considerations

A barrier cream with zinc oxide paste can treat a mild dermatitis. Moderate or severe dermatitis can by treated with a mild hydrocortisone cream (0.25–1%) with each diaper change for 5 to 7 days. For candidiasis, an antifungal cream such as clotrimazole can be added. Sometimes an oral antifungal medication may be used to decrease the candidiasis in the bowels (Horii, 2022).

It is important to teach the family how to prevent dermatitis. The following interventions can help (Keenan-Lindsay et al., 2022):
- Using superabsorbent disposable diapers, change the child every 2 hours during the day and once at night.
- Expose healthy or slightly irritated skin to air, not heat, to dry completely.
- Cleanse skin with mild soap and use diaper barrier creams frequently.
- Do not use tight diapers or waterproof pants.
- Avoid overwashing the skin. Wipe gently stool from the skin using mild soap and water.

Seborrheic Dermatitis

Seborrheic dermatitis is an inflammatory skin condition that recurs.

Pathophysiology and Clinical Manifestations

This form of dermatitis is probably caused by an overgrowth of *Pityrosporum* yeast, which is generally found near sebaceous glands in the scalp (cradle cap), forehead, postauricular and periorbital regions, eyelids, inguinal area, skin neck folds, or nasolabial folds. It often occurs in infants and adolescent age groups. It presents with the following manifestations (Hockenberry et al., 2022):
- A waxy, scaly rash with yellow-red patches
- Skin flakes (dandruff)

Therapeutics and Nursing Considerations

The treatment is as follows:
- In young babies, daily shampooing with a baby shampoo
- In the adolescent age group, antidandruff shampoo on the scalp with selenium sulphide or salicylic acid and baby shampoo on the eyes and eyebrows
- It often occurs on the scalp in the infant age group because parents may be reluctant to shampoo over the soft fontanelle. In this case, the scalp needs to be soaked with mild

soap or commercial baby shampoo, and then the scales are gently combed out and the area is shampooed. An antiseborrheic shampoo may be used that consist of ingredients containing salicylic acid and sulpher. The shampoo is applied and remains on the scalp until the crusts soften. Then the scalp is completed rinsed, and a fine tooth comb removes the loosened crusts from the infants' strands of hair after shampooing (Hockenberry et al., 2022). Nurses can provide support and education on proper cleansing of the scalp though a demonstration.

Eczema or Atopic Dermatitis

Eczema is a chronic, superficial inflammatory condition that is very itchy.

Pathophysiology and Clinical Manifestations

Eczema is due to a genetic predisposition and external triggers that cause T cells to activate and produce an excess amount of immunoglobulin E (IgE). A child with eczema tends to have allergies and has an increased risk of developing asthma. Frequent triggers are dust mites, animal dander, pollens, food allergies, soaps, chemicals, hormonal changes, and emotional stress. Flare-ups tend to be related to high or low temperatures, perspiration, scratching, and irritant fabrics, such as wool. Severe atopic dermatitis in the infant age group tends to be related to food allergies (Graham & Eigenmann, 2020).

The symptoms are as follows:
- Pruritis
- Erythematous patches with vesicles, exudate, and crusts
- Chronic symptoms, which include pruritis, dryness, scaling, and lichenification (thickening of the skin)

It occurs most often in dry or cold weather and usually on the face, upper arms, back, upper thighs, and back of the hands and feet. Skin folds are frequently affected.

Diagnostics

Eczema is diagnosed by family history and through the presence of a generalized rash without any known exposure to an allergen. Culture of the skin may be done if there is a secondary infection. A food elimination test can be done to see if food allergies are a factor. Most often, cow's milk, wheat, eggs, soy, citrus, and peanuts are the food allergens (Grace, 2020).

Therapeutics and Nursing Considerations

- Wet dressings or colloidal oatmeal cleansing will help decrease the itching; lubricate with emollients while the skin is still moist to enhance moisture trapping.
- If there is oozing, Burow's solution soaks (aluminum acetate) will encourage drying.
- Topical corticosteroids after dressing soaks followed by an emollient will increase the absorption and decrease the itching.
- In the case of a severe flare-up, oral corticosteroids may be required to decrease the inflammation and start the healing.

- Immunomodulators that inhibit T-lymphocyte action are a second line of topical medication that is more often used on the face.

Burns

Burns can range from a minor scald to a major, life-threatening deep tissue injury. In children under 5 years, burns comprised 60% of the scald injury cases reported in emergency departments (Parachute, 2021a). Thermal burns are the most frequent injuries, from scalding, flames, or contact with a heated object such as a hot cooking pot. Some of these burns are caused by child abuse. Because of the sensitivity of children's skin, it burns more quickly than that of.

Special age groups are at greater risk for certain types of burns, and they are as follows (Hockenberry et al., 2022):
- Infants: They are mostly injured by thermal burns as a result of scalding and house fires.
- Toddlers: They are mostly injured by thermal burns as a result of pulling hot liquids and grease onto themselves.
- Preschoolers: They are mostly injured by thermal burns as a result of scalding or hot objects such as irons or ovens.
- School-agers and adolescents: They are mostly injured by thermal burns (from matches, lighters, or fireworks). Other risks are electrical burns (due to climbing high-voltage towers and contact with electrical wires) and chemical burns (from combustion experiments).

Children are at more risk from fluid balance shifts and electrolyte imbalances that result with a burn because their bodies have a greater surface area. Refer to Chapter 9, pages 254-255, for burn treatment and nursing considerations for the nurse. Burns can be devastating to a child, causing pain, scarring, decreased range of motion (ROM), and damage to self-image and self-esteem.

FLUID AND ELECTROLYTE IMBALANCES

The percentage of body water varies with the age of the child:
- In the infant age group, total body water constitutes 80% of body weight.
- At age 3, total body water constitutes about 65% of body weight.
- At age 15, total body water constitutes about 60% of body weight.

The daily maintenance fluid requirements by body weight are shown in Table 11.14.

Fluid and electrolyte imbalances occur more often and more quickly in infants and young children. They are more at risk for these imbalances because of the following:
- A greater body surface area permits a higher proportion of water to be lost through the skin.
- A higher metabolic rate increases the water turnover, and the body fluid needs to be replaced.
- The immature kidney function and buffer system in young children make it harder for them to regulate homeostasis.
- There is a higher proportion of fluid in the extracellular spaces.

- There are higher insensible water losses through the skin and respiratory system.
- Young children lack the ability to control body temperature by sweating or shivering.

Dehydration

Dehydration is an excessive loss of water from the body tissues. It occurs in infants and children whenever total fluid intake is less than fluid output. It is caused by conditions that result in an increase in water loss from the kidneys and gastrointestinal (GI) system and insensible water loss from the skin and respiratory tract. Possible causes include the following:

- Excessive vomiting and diarrhea
- Insufficient oral fluid intake
- Prolonged high fever
- Diabetic ketoacidosis (DKA)
- Extensive burns

Pathophysiology

A child can become dehydrated and can lose both fluid and electrolytes, depending on the cause of the loss. Dehydration is categorized as isotonic, hypotonic, or hypertonic. For further information on fluid and electrolytes, see Chapter 9, page 171.

The degrees of dehydration can be estimated as a percentage of body weight lost. As with diarrhea, dehydration can be classified by severity as follows (Hockenberry et al., 2022):

- Mild dehydration: less than 3% in older children or less than 5% in infants
- Moderate dehydration: 5 to 10% in infants and 3 to 6% in older children
- Severe dehydration: more than 10% in infants and more than 6% in older children

Clinical Manifestations

Clinical manifestations of dehydration are summarized in Table 11.15.

Diagnostics

The following diagnostic tests are used to assess the level of dehydration:

- Abnormal values of serum electrolyte (sodium [Na^+], potassium [K^+], chloride [Cl^-])
- Decreased serum pH value if there is acidosis
- Increased hematocrit
- Increased blood urea nitrogen (BUN) level
- Urine is concentrated with a high specific gravity (>1.030) and high osmolarity
- Decreased urine sodium concentration

Therapeutics and Nursing Considerations

Nursing consideration goals are to correct fluid and electrolyte imbalances and to treat the underlying cause.

TABLE 11.14	Daily Maintenance Fluid Requirements
Body Weight	**Amount of Fluid Per Day**
1–10 kg	100 mL/kg
11–20 kg	1 000 mL plus 50 mL/kg for each kg >10 kg
>20 kg	1 500 mL plus 20 mL/kg for each kg >20 kg

From Hockenberry, M. J., Rodgers, C. & Wilson, D. (2022). *Wong's essentials of pediatric nursing* (11th ed., p. 680, Table 22.1). Elsevier Inc.

TABLE 11.15	Clinical Manifestations of Dehydration		
Manifestation	**Isotonic (loss of water and salt)**	**Hypotonic (loss of salt in excess of water)**	**Hypertonic (loss of water in excess of salt)**
Skin			
Colour	Grey/ashen gray appearance on black skin, more yellowish-brown colour in brown skin	Grey/ashen gray appearance on black skin, more yellowish-brown colour in brown skin	Grey/ashen gray appearance in black skin, more yellowish-brown colour inn brown skin
Temperature	Cold	Cold	Cold or hot
Turgor	Poor	Very poor	Fair
Feel	Dry	Clammy	Thickened, doughy
Mucous membranes	Dry	Slightly moist	Parched
Tearing and salivation	Absent	Absent	Absent
Eyeball	Sunken	Sunken	Sunken
Fontanelle	Sunken	Sunken	Sunken
Body temperature	Subnormal or elevated	Subnormal or elevated	Subnormal or elevated
Pulse	Rapid	Very rapid	Moderately rapid
Respirations	Rapid	Rapid	Rapid
Behaviour	Irritable to lethargic	Lethargic or comatose; convulsions	Marked lethargy with extreme hyperirritability on stimulation

From Hockenberry, M. J., Rodgers, C., & Wilson, D. (2015). *Wong's essentials of pediatric nursing* (11th ed., p. 685, Table 22.4, and p. 88, Table 4.6). Elsevier.

- Assess the child's health history, health assessment findings, and laboratory tests to help find the cause of the dehydration.
- Weigh the child to get an accurate initial weight and monitor weight changes indicating fluid balance increases and decreases.
- Administer oral rehydration solution (ORS) or other oral fluids in small quantities—about 30 to 60 mL (1–2 oz) every hour—and do not give a full diet to the child until the child's hydration has improved, the reason for the dehydration has been corrected, and the fluid balance is normal.
- If the child cannot drink enough fluid to rehydrate or has significant dehydration, start an IV line, and administer an appropriate replacement solution, as prescribed. Since dehydration (volume depletion) is a severe life-threatening complication, the first priority is the restoration of circulation by rapid expansion of extracellular fluid volume to treat or prevent shock. The solution selected is based on what is known regarding the probable type and cause of dehydration. The ordered solution is usually an isotonic solution of 0.9% sodium chloride or lactated Ringer's solution. These two solutions are close to the body's serum osmolarity of 285 to 300 mmol/kg. (Keenan-Lindsay et al., 2022). Sodium bicarbonate and K+ may be additives to balance the pH and electrolytes if needed.
- Observe the IV site frequently for signs of infiltration.
- Do not add K+ to the IV solution until the child voids.
- Assess the child's level of hydration by watching the fluid balance and watching for signs of dehydration.
- Observe and record accurate intake and output and urine specific gravity values.
- Prevent infection by using aseptic technique to insert the IV line and keeping the skin clean at the site.
- Maintain good handwashing and isolation techniques, if required, to prevent spreading infection.
- Slowly increase the child's diet until a full diet is tolerated and chart the response.
- Provide family teaching and support for the following:
  - Oral fluid rehydration and diet increases
  - Care of a child with an IV line
  - Cause and signs and symptoms of dehydration
  - Education regarding handwashing and other hygiene techniques
  - Follow-up medical appointments as necessary after discharge

Fever

Fever or hyperpyrexia occurs when there is an increase in the hypothalamic set point, the body's thermostat-like mechanism, and when the body's heat loss mechanism cannot dissipate excess heat production, leading to an abnormally elevated body temperature.

- Hyperthermia occurs when the body's set point is normal, but other internal or external conditions exceed the ability of the body to eliminate excess heat. These conditions could include heat stroke, Aspirin toxicity, and hyperthyroidism (Keenan-Lindsay et al., 2022).
- Frequent causes of pyrexia in pediatrics include otitis media, respiratory tract infections, general viruses, and enteric viral infections.
- More serious causes of fever include urinary tract infections (UTIs), bacteremia, meningitis, pneumonia, osteomyelitis, cancer, immunological disorders, septic arthritis, poisoning or drug overdose, and dehydration.

Pathophysiology

Fever most commonly results from interference with the hypothalamic set point as a result of allergy, infection, endotoxins, or tumour and leads to increased heat production and decreased heat loss. Clinical assessment of associated symptoms will help the nurse decide how serious the fever is. For example, infants, with their larger body surface, are at higher risk for fluid imbalances due to a fever.

Clinical Manifestations

- Temperature of 38.9 to 40.6°C by axilla (refer to Table 11.3 for normal-range pediatric vital signs)
- Reddened skin colour (for light skin) with diaphoresis and chills. More difficult to assess skin colour in darker skin tones. Therefore, palpations for warmth are a more accurate sign. (Hockenberry et al., 2022).
- Sluggishness or restlessness

Diagnostics

Laboratory tests and results will vary depending on the etiology of the fever.

Nursing Considerations

- Check the temperature as indicated. It is important for the nurse to remember that the degree of fever does not necessarily indicate the severity of the illness.
- Be aware that fever can be a serious concern, and the child needs immediate medical assessment in the following circumstances (Hockenberry et al., 2022):
  - Infant is under 3 months of age
  - Fever is over 40.5°C
  - Child is appearing or acting very ill
- Administer antipyretics as prescribed if the child has pyrexia.
- As prescribed, administer acetaminophen instead of Aspirin because of the association with Reye's syndrome. Acetaminophen is given as an antipyretic and to alleviate discomfort and can be given every 4 hours but not more often than five times per 24 hours.
- Administer NSAIDs or ibuprofen, if prescribed. Ibuprofen also is approved for reducing fever in children as young as 6 months.
- Know that loosening clothing, decreasing room temperature, applying a cool washcloth to the forehead, and increasing the amount of circulating air are effective measures if provided about 1 hour after an antipyretic drug, but only if the child is not shivering. Shivering increases the metabolic rate and can increase the core temperature.

- Teach parents how to take the child's temperature accurately and control fever.

Febrile Seizures

A febrile seizure is a seizure that is associated with an illness that has caused a fever. It is the most common seizure in children.

Febrile seizure affects approximately 2 to 5% of children. It usually occurs between 6 months and 5 years; with the peak incidence between 12 and 18 months (Hockenberry et al., 2022).

- Most children have only one seizure, but some will have recurrences, particularly if febrile seizure runs in families.
- The etiology is unknown, but it is usually associated with common childhood illnesses such as upper respiratory tract infections and UTIs.

Pathophysiology

Febrile seizure usually is a tonic–clonic seizure, associated with an acute febrile illness.

- Febrile seizure usually results when the child hits a peak temperature threshold over 38.8°C, which seems to be more important than the rapidity of the temperature increase (Potter et al., 2019).
- It is considered benign if the electroencephalogram (EEG) is normal and other neurological and physical abnormalities are not found.

Clinical Manifestations

Seizure activity generally ceases by the time the child is brought in for medical attention. Most seizures are tonic–clonic and last less than 1 minute.

Diagnostics

Diagnostic tests to check for other underlying problems that contributed to the seizure include lumbar puncture to rule out meningitis and an EEG to rule out a seizure disorder. Computed tomography (CT) and magnetic resonance imaging (MRI) are other tests that may be performed.

Therapeutics and Nursing Considerations

- Observe for signs and symptoms of illness.
- Provide a safe environment in case of a seizure, have suction and oxygen ready, and roll the child on their side to maintain a patent airway.
- Prepare the client and family for procedures and provide emotional support.
- Use temperature-reducing interventions, as noted earlier.
- Educate parents on how to lower a fever and how to protect the child during a seizure.
- Administer anticonvulsant therapy as prescribed if the child is still seizing when they arrive at hospital.

Diarrhea

Diarrhea is defined as frequent, abnormally watery stools. Diarrhea can be mild, moderate, or severe. There is also acute or chronic diarrhea, which can be inflammatory or noninflammatory. Diarrhea is a very common childhood illness that can be life-threatening if the child becomes dehydrated and has an electrolyte imbalance with hypovolemia. The children who are most at risk are young, attend day care centres, and have poor sanitation at home.

Pathophysiology

- Acute diarrhea is caused by a rotavirus, which is the most common nonbacterial gastroenteritis. Bacterial causes include *Escherichia coli*, *Salmonella*, *Campylobacter*, and *Shigella*. *Clostridium difficile* may occur after antibiotic treatment.
- Chronic diarrhea is commonly related to malabsorption syndromes, immune deficiencies, allergies, and inflammatory bowel disease.

In cases of infectious diarrhea, the pathogens produce enterotoxins that attack the intestinal walls and cause an increase in fluid and electrolyte secretions.

Clinical Manifestations

The severity of the diarrhea needs to be determined:

- Mild diarrhea is a slight increase in frequency with a liquid consistency.
- Moderate diarrhea is several loose or watery stools, possibly accompanied by nausea, vomiting, or irritability, which resolves in 1 to 2 days.
- Severe diarrhea is frequent or continuous stools with moderate to severe fluid and electrolyte imbalances, cramping, and irritability. The child may appear lethargic, with inappropriate responses, and may become comatose (Keenan-Lindsay et al., 2022).

Diagnostics

A stool specimen can be sent for culture and sensitivity to confirm the presence of an infectious or parasitic agent. A stool pH of less than 6 and the presence of reducing substances suggest carbohydrate malabsorption or a lactase deficiency. In stools with a fatty or oily appearance, a 3-day stool collection can determine fat malabsorption.

- Stool positive for occult blood can be an indicator of irritation or inflammation.
- It is important to also test for serum complete blood count (CBC), electrolytes, creatinine, and BUN.

Therapeutics

The fluid and electrolyte imbalances need to be corrected and the cause of the diarrhea treated. Premixed ORS is the initial treatment for mild or moderate dehydration. If there is significant dehydration and electrolyte imbalance, IV treatment is started. Reintroduction of a normal diet is done gradually as tolerated by the dehydrated child (Hockenberry et al., 2022). A child who is not dehydrated should be fed a normal diet.

Nursing Considerations

- Obtain an accurate history in order to identify the causative factor, such as travelling or eating contaminated foods.

- Assess the type of diarrhea.
- Assess for signs of dehydration, which are outlined in Table 11.15.
- Give ORS frequently to the child with dehydration, and increase the volume as tolerated.
- Check for specific gravity of urine and daily weights and maintain strict intake and output to monitor fluid balance.
- Administer prescribed parenteral fluid and antimicrobials if needed.
- Cleanse the skin area around the perineum and apply protective cream such as zinc oxide to prevent skin breakdown and reduce the potential for infection.
- Provide education to help the family assess the child's diarrhea and level of hydration and to know when to seek medical attention.
- Teach parents oral rehydration treatment with commercial products such as Pedialyte, Rehydralyte, Gastrolyte, Enfalyte, or Cera. It is important to instruct the family not to give the child water, fruit juices, carbonated beverages, gelatin, or any caffeine-containing products when rehydrating the child.
- Restart the child's normal nutrition, in particular breastfeeding and solids, unless the child has developed a lactose intolerance from the diarrhea. A lactose-free formula or half-strength lactose-containing product can be used briefly if there is intolerance until the bowel returns to normal.
- Teach proper handling of stools and hand hygiene to prevent the spread of infection.

Sepsis

Sepsis is a generalized bacterial infection with a systemic inflammatory response. Infants within the first year of life, particularly if they are low birth weight, have a high risk of developing sepsis. All neonatal infections are potentially opportunistic, and any bacteria are capable of causing sepsis. Group B *Streptococcus* is the most common bacteria, and *E. coli* and *Streptococcus viridans* are also common causes of sepsis (Hockenberry et al., 2022). The neonatal inflammatory and immune defence mechanisms are immature, which allows rapid invasion, spread, and multiplication of infecting microorganisms. The young infant is unable to localize infections.

Clinical Manifestations

The initial signs and symptoms may be subtle and may include temperature instability (the child may be hypo- or hyperthermic), tachycardia, poor peripheral perfusion with pallor, cyanosis or mottling, and respiratory distress. The manifestations may also include poor sucking and feeding, weak cry, lethargy, irritability, decreased pain response, hypotension, jaundice, dehydration, GI disturbances, seizures, hypotonia, tremors, full fontanelle, and cardiac arrest.

Late-onset sepsis (up to age 4 months) usually appears with meningitis.

Diagnostics

- Blood culture, urine culture, and lumbar puncture for cerebrospinal fluid (CSF) analysis are done to try to determine the focal site of the infection.
- CBC with an elevated white blood cell (WBC) count with increased immature neutrophils indicates infection, and C-reactive protein (CRP) levels may or may not be elevated.
- A chest X-ray is done when the infant has respiratory symptoms.

Therapeutics

The infant is treated immediately with antimicrobials after the cultures have been collected. Ampicillin and gentamicin are usually prescribed and are based on drug sensitivities to the common organisms cultured from the infant with sepsis. If the cultures are negative and the infant is asymptomatic after 48 to 72 hours, then the medication therapy can be discontinued (Hockenberry et al., 2022).

Nursing Considerations

Nursing management is focused on the following goals and is similar to that given to a high-risk newborn:

- Assess the newborn for signs and symptoms of onset infection and sepsis, particularly in infants having invasive procedures done that can elevate the risk of infection.
- Provide a neutral thermal environment due to the infant's immature abilities to regulate temperature.
- As prescribed, administer antibiotic therapy for 7 to 10 days if culture results are positive and discontinue therapy if culture results are negative (usually in 2 days).
- Monitor hydration and intake and output.
- Monitor the infant for signs of a worsening condition or shock (Hockenberry et al., 2022).

Meningitis

Meningitis is an inflammation of the meninges caused by a bacterial or viral infection. Neonates and infants are at increased risk of developing bacterial meningitis, and it can be fatal if not treated immediately. Viral meningitis is less virulent. The outcome of the meningitis depends on the organism, as well as the child's age and response to treatment.

- Most cases occur between 1 month and 5 years, with infants under 12 months being the most susceptible to bacterial meningitis. The risk of mortality is higher in adolescents and young adults.
- Meningitis in Canada has decreased significantly with the introduction of universal immunization programs delivering conjugate vaccines for *Haemophilus influenzae* type b (Hib), *Neisseria meningitidis*, and *Streptococcus pneumoniae*. Pneumococcal meningitis has also decreased significantly in all age groups following the introduction of the vaccine PCV7 (Centers for Disease Control and Prevention [CDC], 2022a).
- Viral meningitis or aseptic meningitis is caused mainly by enteroviruses and less commonly by arboviruses, herpes

simplex, cytomegalovirus, and varicella zoster. It is a self-limiting disease that lasts 7 to 10 days.

- In bacterial meningitis, the bacteria from a focal infection site, such as otitis media, enter the meninges through the bloodstream and spread through the CSF. The infection can also be introduced as the result of an invasive procedure or through a surgical or trauma site. The bacteria toxin creates a meningeal inflammatory response and causes a release of purulent exudates that spreads the infection rapidly. The brain surface becomes covered in exudate and is edematous. The ventricles can then become obstructed by pus, fibrin, or adhesions, blocking the CSF flow and potentially producing increased intracranial pressure (ICP). Serious damage to the brain cells, some of which can be permanent, is caused by necrosis (Hockenberry et al., 2022).

Clinical Manifestations

The manifestations vary depending on the child's age, the type of bacterial infection, and the onset of the infection. Newborns have nonspecific symptoms that are different from those of older children. Symptoms in this age group may include poor sucking ability, vomiting, or diarrhea. Newborns with meningitis tend to have poor muscle tone with little movement and a weak cry. The fontanelle may be bulging, but this is a late sign. The newborn may be irritable, lethargic, jaundiced, and drowsy and have seizures, apnea or irregular respirations, cyanosis, fever (varies with level of maturity), and weight loss. If the infant is not treated, there is deterioration leading to cardiovascular collapse, seizures, and apnea (Hockenberry et al., 2022).

Infants who are between 3 months and 2 years of age show signs of fever, poor feeding, vomiting, and a bulging or tense fontanelle and often have a high-pitched cry. Nuchal rigidity (resistance to neck flexion) and Brudzinski's and Kernig's signs are not usually present in children under 12 to 28 months of age. Older children may initially have respiratory or GI conditions and then develop nuchal rigidity (stiff neck), headache, and tripod posturing. Kernig's sign is present with meningitis when the supine or sitting child's knee is flexed, and there is pain and resistance upon extension of the knee. Brudzinski's sign is present with meningitis when the supine child's head is flexed, and the hips and knees flex involuntarily. A petechial rash may also appear.

Diagnostics

- A lumbar puncture is done in order to diagnose meningitis. CSF may be cloudy, with an elevated WBC count, elevated protein level, and decreased glucose level. The CSF is cultured, and a Gram stain is done to determine the causative agent. A CT scan may be done before this test if increased ICP is present to prevent brain herniation.
- CBC reveals increased WBC count.
- Blood culture may pinpoint the causative agent as well.

Therapeutics

The prognosis of meningitis depends on treating the infection before clinically severe disease ensues. Therefore, the timely administration of empirical antimicrobial therapy, specifically third-generation cephalosporin, is crucial (Hockenberry et al., 2022).

Nursing Considerations

Perform careful assessments to monitor the child for changes in illness and signs of complications.

- Monitor temperature, vital signs, and level of consciousness frequently, particularly for shock or respiratory distress.
- Accurately monitor intake and output and fluid and electrolyte balance; children with decreased levels of consciousness should receive nothing by mouth; others are allowed fluids and diet as tolerated.
- Assess neurological signs and level of consciousness, including signs of increased ICP. Measure head circumference to monitor for the development of subdural effusions and obstructive hydrocephalus.
- Administer antibiotics as prescribed (the type depends on the organism) and maintain IV line.
- Provide fever-reducing measures.
- Monitor for signs of a secondary infection.
- Know that steroids may be prescribed to relieve cerebral edema.
- Set up respiratory isolation for 24 to 48 hours after antibiotic administration begins.
- Be aware that the child will be sensitive to sound and bright lights; keep the room as quiet as possible to decrease environmental stimuli. Help the family limit the number and frequency of visitors until the child is improving.
- Assess the level of pain and give prescribed acetaminophen (Tylenol) with codeine as needed.
- Position the child in a side-lying position without a pillow with the head of the bed slightly raised to increase comfort from neck stiffness (Hockenberry et al., 2022).

PSYCHOSOCIAL AND MENTAL HEALTH CHALLENGES

Child Maltreatment

Child maltreatment refers to the harm, or risk of harm, that a child or youth may experience while in the care of a person whom they trust or depend on, including a parent, sibling, other relative, teacher, caregiver, or guardian. Harm may occur through the direct actions by the person (acts of commission) or through the person's neglect to provide a component of care necessary for healthy child growth and development (acts of omission).

The five types of child maltreatment are as follows:
- Physical abuse (assault): The application of unreasonable force by an adult or youth to any part of a child's body
- Sexual abuse: Abuse involving a child, by an adult or youth, in an act of sexual gratification, or exposure of a child to sexual contact, activity, or behaviour
- Neglect: Failure by a partner or caregiver to provide the physical or psychological necessities of life to a child

- Emotional harm: Adult behaviour that harms a child psychologically, emotionally, or spiritually
- Exposure to family violence: Circumstances that allow a child to be aware of violence occurring between a caregiver and their partner or between other family members

Child maltreatment is a very serious situation that has long-term implications for the child and the family. A full 32% of adults in Canada have reported having experienced some form of maltreatment as a child.

The COVID-19 pandemic safety measures have had a negative impact on some aspects of children's and adolescents' health. Physical abuse tripled during the early months of the pandemic for school age children (Mann, 2021). In 2020 to 2021, Statistics Canada reported a drop in admissions to shelter facilities but an increase in crisis calls for support outside their facilities (Statistics Canada, 2022d).

The resulting intergenerational trauma, ongoing socioeconomic inequalities, systemic barriers, and racism continue to place Indigenous women and children at an increased risk of victimization. Approximately 21% of women residents and 22% of accompanying children in shelters for victims of abuse were identified as First Nations, Metis, and Inuit (Statistics Canada, 2022d).

Based on 2016 police-reported data, of the children and youth who were victims of violence, 30% were victims of family violence—that is, acts perpetrated by parents, siblings, extended family members, or spouses (Government of Canada, 2018).

Three types of factors put a child at increased risk of being abused: parental factors, child factors, and environmental factors.

Parental factors
- Severe punishment as children
- Poor impulse control
- Free expression of violence
- Social isolation
- Poor social–emotional support system
- Low self-esteem
- Lack of knowledge of appropriate parenting skills
- Substance abuse

Child factors
- Temperament: doesn't "fit" as well into the family
- Illness, disability, or developmental delay
- Illegitimacy
- Hyperactivity
- Resemblance to someone the parent does not like
- Failure to bond
- Difficult pregnancy, delivery, or prematurity
- Other siblings who are not attached

Environmental factors. These factors apply to all socioeconomic groups.
- Chronic stress, such as divorce, poverty, unemployment, poor housing,
- alcoholism, drug addiction
- Frequent relocation
- Substitute caregivers who can be abusive (Hockenberry et al., 2022)

Clinical Manifestations

Physical abuse. Physical indicators include the following:
- Skin injuries, such as bruising, with different stages of healing in unusual locations and often shaped like the object that was used
- Burns, such as cigarette burns
- Fractures, such as spiral fracture
- Head injuries, particularly in a young child
- Abusive head trauma (AHT) without signs of external injuries caused by violent shaking, especially in infants and young children (Hockenberry et al., 2022)
- Subdural or retinal hemorrhages in the absence of external signs
- Traumatic eye injuries such as conjunctival hemorrhages
- Mouth injuries
- Poisonings
- Drowning
- Repeated accidents

Behavioural indicators:
- The child may be wary of adults and fearful of parents as well as afraid of going home.
- The child suffers pain without crying.
- The child has superficial relationships or is overly friendly.
- The child reports injury by parents.
- The child exhibits attention-seeking behaviour (Hockenberry et al., 2022).

Nursing Considerations

Nurses often identify potential or actual abuse situations. Any suspected child maltreatment must be immediately reported to the appropriate authorities, such as a hospital child abuse team or a children's aid society. The following interventions are critical to ensuring a child's safety, as well as helping the child and the child's family cope with the situation:
- Carefully perform a physical examination and history-taking for signs of abuse. This is essential.
- Know that accurate documentation is very important to preserve the facts.
- Encourage the child to verbalize concerns without any undue questioning.
- Encourage positive self-concept in the child.
- Use play to help the child work out stress.
- Collaborate with the interdisciplinary team and refer the family to social services.
- If the child has been apprehended, help the child cope with the loss of the family and ease their transition into foster care.

Emotional abuse. Emotional abuse is a deliberate attempt to destroy a child's self-esteem or confidence.

Indicators include the following:
- Failure to thrive, developmental delays
- Feeding issues
- Sleep issues
- Enuresis
- Habit disorders such as rocking, biting, or hair-pulling
- Withdrawn
- Unusual fearfulness

- Behavioural extremes, either withdrawal or aggression
- Age-inappropriate behaviours
- Attempted suicide (Hockenberry et al., 2022)

Neglect. The definition of the term *neglect* is to deprive a child of necessities.

Physical indicators include the following:
- Failure to thrive, malnutrition, constant hunger
- Poor hygiene and inappropriate clothing
- Bald patches on an infant's head
- Lack of adequate supervision, abandonment
- Poor health

Behavioural indicators include the following:
- Dull, inattentive infant
- Begging or stealing food
- School attendance issues
- Use of drugs and alcohol
- Delinquency
- Child reports having no caretaker (Hockenberry et al., 2022)

Sexual abuse. Sexual abuse includes incest, molestation, exhibitionism, child pornography, child prostitution, and pedophilia (Hockenberry et al., 2022).

The following are characteristics of the abuser and the child:
- Anyone can be an abuser, but usually it is a male whom the child knows.
- Child sexual abuse involves all socioeconomic groups.
- The abuser may be a prominent community member or someone who works with children, such as a teacher or coach.
- Pornography or prostitution can involve the parents or strangers.
- Stepfathers may put a child more at risk.
- The child is often a runaway.
- The child is often afraid to expose the abuser because of a fear of retaliation or that they will not be believed.
- Boys are less likely to report abuse (Hockenberry et al., 2022).

Physical indicators of sexual abuse include the following:
- In many children, no obvious signs
- Difficulty walking or sitting
- Torn, stained, bloody underwear
- Gross evidence of trauma (genital, oral, anal), pain, itching, sexually transmitted infections, discharge
- Pregnancy
- Weight loss, eating disorder
- Vague somatic complaints

Behavioural indicators include the following:
- Under age 5: Regression, feeding or toileting disruptions, temper tantrums, requests for frequent underwear changes, seductive behaviour
- Ages 5 to 10: School problems, night terrors, sleep problems, anxieties, withdrawal, refusal of physical activity, and inappropriate behaviours
- Adolescents: School problems, running away, delinquency, promiscuity, drug, and alcohol abuse, eating disorders, depression, and other significant psychological problems, such as suicide attempts (Hockenberry et l., 2022)

Munchausen syndrome by proxy. This syndrome occurs when a parent, usually the mother, induces the symptoms of an illness, such as poisoning, in a child. It is very hard to verify.

Indicators include the following:
- The history does not match the clinical findings.
- Unexplained, prolonged, or extremely rare illness that does not respond to treatment and occurs only when the parent is present. Common symptoms include seizures, nausea and vomiting, diarrhea, and altered mental status.
- The parent shows unusual interest in the health care team members and pays special attention to the child. In most cases the perpetrator is the biological mother with some degree of health care knowledge and training. Health care providers can easily become misled and unknowingly enable the perpetrator.
- The resolution of symptoms after separation from the perpetrator confirms the diagnosis (Hockenberry et al., 2022).
- The child and family need to be referred to the child abuse team. There can be significant physical effects that can potentially cause serious physical illness and death. As well, significant emotional trauma can be caused to the child.

Suicide

Suicide is taking action to intentionally end one's life. Suicide is the second most common cause of death among Canadian adolescents (Government of Canada, 2020a). The First Nations and Inuit populations and 2SLGBTQI+ youth are at a significantly higher risk (Government of Canada, 2021). The risk factors for suicide in this age group are as follows:
- Previous suicide attempts
- A friend who has tried to or has committed suicide
- School issues and grade changes
- Substance abuse
- Problems with a love relationship
- Depression, loneliness, hopelessness, and isolation
- Bullying (cyberbullying)
- Chronic family issues
- Chronic condition
- Change in behaviour or weight
- Family history of suicide
- Abuse: physical, emotional, sexual
- Low self-esteem
- Giving away possessions
- Impulsivity (physical aggression, risk-taking behaviours)
- Access to guns and ammunition
- Minority sexual practice (CPS, 2021b)

Clinical Manifestations
- Depression usually precedes suicide. Symptoms of depression may be obvious or subtle.
- Danger signs include lethargy, feeling unwell, insomnia or early-morning awakening, poor appetite or overeating, excessive crying, giving away important possessions, a preoccupation with death or death themes, and statement of intent.

Nursing Considerations

- Provide education for groups such as teachers, families, and youth about risk factors.
- Provide youth counselling, stress management, and problem-solving techniques.
- Assess if the child has a suicide plan.
- Arrange for counselling, crisis intervention, and hospitalization if necessary and refer the youth and family to a professional therapist.
- Provide counselling after a suicidal death for the adolescent's family and friends to help them understand and work through their bereavement.

Attention Deficit/Hyperactivity Disorder
Pathophysiology

Attention-deficit/hyperactivity disorder (ADHD) is a neurodevelopmental condition whose exact cause is unknown. Genetics is believed to be a factor associated with ADHD. Children born into families where there is a history of ADHD are more likely to be diagnosed with ADHD than children having no family history of ADHD. There is no conclusive evidence to link environmental factors as a cause of ADHD (Centre for Addiction and Mental Health (CAMH), 2022). It is a persistent pattern of inattention, and/or hyperactivity/impulsivity that interferes with functioning or development (American Psychiatric Association [APA], 2022). ADHD is very common; it is estimated that ADHD affects 7.2% of children worldwide (APA, 2022).

Clinical Manifestations

There are two presentations of ADHD. A child may be diagnosed with ADHD if, for the past 6 months, they have displayed six or more symptoms of either hyperactivity or impulsivity behaviours or inattention behaviours to a degree that is inconsistent with developmental level and that negatively impacts social and academic or occupational activities. For older adolescents (age 17 and older), at least five symptoms are required (APA, 2022).

Hyperactivity/Impulsivity presentation includes the following:

- Often fidgets with or taps hands or feet or squirms in seat
- Often leaves seat in situations when remaining seated is expected
- Often runs about or climbs in situations where it is inappropriate
- Often unable to play or engage in leisure activities quietly
- Is often "on the go," acting as if driven by a motor
- Often talks excessively
- Often blurts out an answer before a question has been completed
- Often has difficulty waiting their turn
- Often interrupts or intrudes on others (APA, 2022)

Inattention presentation includes the following:

- Often fails to give close attention to details or makes careless mistakes in schoolwork, at work, or during other activities
- Often has difficulty sustaining attention in tasks or play activities

- Often does not seem to listen when spoken to directly
- Often does not seem to follow through on instructions and fails to finish schoolwork, chores, duties in the workplace
- Often has difficulty organizing tasks and activities
- Often avoids, dislikes, or is reluctant to engage in tasks that require sustained mental health effort
- Often losses things necessary for tasks or activities
- Is often easily distracted by extraneous stimuli
- Is often forgetful in daily activities (APA, 2022)

A combined presentation is if both inattention and hyperactivity criteria are met for the past 6 months.

Children with ADHD may have delays in language, motor, or social development. Emotional dysregulation or emotional impulsivity commonly occur in children with ADHD (APA, 2022). Children with ADHD are at a greater risk for conduct disorders, oppositional defiant disorders, depression, and anxiety disorders (Hockenberry et al., 2022).

Therapeutics

Medication is an important component of the treatment ADHD. Medication is very effective for treating the symptoms, which improves behaviour in the classroom and in social situations. In turn, this improves children's relationships with their peers, teachers, and parents.

Behavioural treatment can help the child become responsible for their own behaviour and provide support in the process. It is important to address all areas of the child's life. This means making the child's whole environment supportive, including at home and in school.

A combination of both medication and behavioural treatment is recommended, as well as close follow-up and feedback from school personnel (Hockenberry et al., 2022).

Nursing Considerations

The nurse is an active member of the health care team in managing a child with ADHD and acts as a link between other health care providers and educators. In this role, they should do the following:

- Encourage parents to express their concerns and express their emotions.
- Participate in child and family teaching, arrange referrals to support groups, and discuss school settings and classroom placement for special assistance.
- Provide information on the medication and treatment plan.

Environment manipulation education is needed to help the family and the child. The use of organizational charts, decreasing distractions, and modelling positive behaviours in a consistent approach may help (Hockenberry et al., 2022).

Autism Spectrum Disorders

Autism spectrum disorder (ASD) is a complex developmental brain disorder. Researchers are investigating a number of theories, including a combination of genetic, medical, immune dysregulation or neuroinflammation, oxidative stress, and environmental influences (Hockenberry et al., 2022). Autism appears to have its roots in very early brain development. The etiology is still uncertain. However, the most obvious signs and symptoms of autism tend to emerge between 2 and 3 years of age. It is considered to be a lifespan disorder. An estimated 1 in 66 children and youth ages 5 to 17 years old are identified with ASD (Autism Speaks Canada, 2022b).

Clinical Manifestations

ASD is characterized by social-interaction difficulties, communication challenges, and a tendency to engage in repetitive behaviours. However, symptoms and their severity vary widely across these three core areas. Taken together, they may result in relatively mild challenges for someone on the high functioning end of the autism spectrum. For others, symptoms may be more severe, as when repetitive behaviours and lack of spoken language interfere with everyday life.

Some children with autism have an identifiable genetic condition that affects brain development. These genetic disorders include fragile X syndrome, Angelman syndrome, tuberous sclerosis, and chromosome 15 duplication syndrome and other single-gene and chromosomal disorders.

It is estimated that a range of physical and mental-health conditions co-occur with autism. Common issues include GI conditions, epilepsy, feeding issues, disrupted sleep, ADHD, obsessive compressive disorder (OCD), schizophrenia disorder, Down syndrome, bipolar disorder, and anxiety disorders (Autism Speaks Canada, 2022a).

Diagnostics

Diagnosis is based on the presenting deficits as well as the severity. The diagnose is based on two behaviour domains:
1. When the child exhibits persistent deficits in social communication and social interaction across multiple contexts:
   - Deficits in social-emotional reciprocity
   - Deficits in nonverbal communicative behaviours used for social interaction
   - Deficits in developing, maintaining, and understanding relationship
2. When the child demonstrates a marked restricted scope of interests and activities:
   - May demonstrate abnormal play activities
   - May exhibit preoccupation with certain objects and routines
   - May demonstrate restricted body movements
   - May have a very narrow range of interests

Severity is based on social communication impairments and restricted repetitive patterns of behaviour (APA, 2022).

ASD is about four times more frequently seen in boys than in girls. Many children with autism measure low on IQ tests. Motor skill development may be good, but the use of their motor skills is inappropriate. Many children with autism become functioning adults, whereas others are totally dependent for care (Bard et al., 2022).

Therapeutics

Early diagnosis, referral, and concentrated intervention are critical for the child to progress and increase the level of social development. Some children can improve when language and communication skills can be acquired. Intervention can include intensive behaviour modification treatments and medication. Early intensive behavioural intervention involves the entire family working closely with a team of professionals.

Nursing Considerations

Children with autism do not adapt easily to new situations and require directed activities, minimal stimulation, established routines, and close supervision. It is important to encourage the family to stay with the child when hospitalization is required because of the difficulties surrounding new people and situations. Effective communication should be at the child's developmental level. The objective in treatment is to promote positive reinforcement, increase social awareness of others, teach verbal communication skills, and decrease unacceptable behaviour. Providing a structured routine for the child to follow is the key to management (Hockenberry et al., 2022).

Complementary and alternative medicine has developed as a treatment for ASD, including horseback riding, massage therapy, implementation of elimination diets (casein-free diet, gluten-free diets), vitamin and omega-3 supplementation, and high-fat, low carbohydrate ketogenic diet. Further research is required to validate these various therapeutic approaches (Hockenberry et al., 2022).

The child and the family require highly specialized care and treatment. Programs are designed to meet the individual child's unique needs (Bard et al., 2022). They need to be referred to community treatment centres and support networks. Families need support and education on how to manage the child at home. The treatments can be very expensive and can be a significant drain on the family's finances.

Anorexia Nervosa and Bulimia Nervosa

Anorexia nervosa is a potentially life-threatening eating disorder that affects mainly females. The peak incidence is at 12 to 13 years; there is another peak again at 17 to 18 years. Bulimia nervosa also occurs mainly in females and with a teenage onset. See Chapter 12, pages 465-468.

Sudden Infant Death Syndrome

Sudden infant death (SIDS) (which is a component of sudden unexpected infant death [SUID]) is the sudden death of any infant younger than 1 year of age for whom a postmortem examination fails to determine the cause of death. The death usually occurs during sleep. From 2016 to 2020, Canada observed a 50% decrease in the rate of SIDS (Statistics Canada, 2022c). The drop in rates may be due to how infants' deaths are classified, but likely it is mainly due to the changes in recommendations for safe sleeping positions and safe sleep space for young infants.

The risk factors for infants are as follows:
- Sleeping position other than on the back
- Sleeping alone in a room
- Bed sharing with parents who are cigarette smokers
- Bed sharing with an adult who is extremely fatigued or impaired by drugs or alcohol

- Use of soft bedding, a pillow, and covers that can cover the head
- Sleeping with stuffed animals or toys
- Sleeping with an infant on a sofa, which is of particular high risk
- Bed sharing with someone other than parents or usual caregiver (Statistics Canada, 2021)

Infants who are at higher risk for SIDS include the following groups:

- Infants requiring cardiopulmonary resuscitation or vigorous stimulation with a combination of apnea, colour change, marked change in muscle tone to limpness, and choking or gagging
- Preterm infants with apnea spells when discharged home
- Siblings of two or more infants with occurrences
- Infants with certain types of diseases or conditions, particularly with central nervous system (CNS) disturbances and respiratory disorders such as bronchopulmonary dysplasia (Hockenberry et al., 2022)

The peak age for SIDS ranges from 2 to 3 months, with most cases occurring before 6 months. SIDS affects male infants more than females and usually occurs in winter.

Pathophysiology

The cause of SIDS is unknown, but the most accepted theory is an abnormality of the brainstem, the area that regulates the neurological system of cardiopulmonary control, which can cause sleep apnea, dysrhythmic breathing and impaired arousal to increased carbon dioxide and decreased oxygen. However, sleep apnea does not cause SIDS. There may be a genetic predisposition. Maternal smoking may be an important factor in SIDS. Prone sleeping is also a major factor, one that can impair arousal, cause oropharyngeal obstruction, and carbon dioxide rebreathing and affect thermal balance. Soft bedding may prevent infants from turning their heads to the side, creating the same dangers as prone sleeping (Hockenberry et al., 2022).

Clinical Manifestations

There are no characteristic findings before death. Usually, parents discover that the infant has died in the crib. The infant is often found with blankets over the head, face down, with frothy, blood-tinged secretions in the nose and mouth. The diaper usually has both urine and stool in it. The child's appearance causes acute distress to the family (Hockenberry et al., 2022).

Diagnostics

No laboratory tests are diagnostic of SIDS.

Nursing Considerations

- To decrease the risk of SIDS, teach families to place their infant on their backs to sleep and decrease exposure to smoking before and after the birth (Statistics Canada, 2021).
- Nurses need to educate parents and caregivers during postpartum discharge planning, newborn discharge planning, follow-up home visits, and well-baby clinic visits about the modifiable risk factors for SIDS.

- Encourage the family to verbalize concerns and validate feelings.
- Assess the family's grieving patterns and ability to cope.
- Refer the family for counselling if needed. Bereavement counsellors and support groups are often very helpful.
- Provide a supportive environment and time for the family to say goodbye to the child.
- Offer a memory package with a lock of hair, foot and hand prints, and other important mementos.

EAR DYSFUNCTION

Acute Otitis Media

Acute otitis media (OM) is inflammation of the middle ear, with the signs and symptoms of acute infection, fever, and ear pain. It is the most common reason that antibiotics are prescribed. It is usually caused by *H. influenzae*, *Moraxella catarrhalis*, or *S. pneumoniae*. The viral cause is usually respiratory syncytial virus (RSV) and influenza. It is one of the most prevalent illnesses of early childhood. Potential risk factors for OM are children attending day care and children who have siblings or parents with a chronic history of OM (Hockenberry et al., 2022).

Pathophysiology

Children more predisposed to OM are as follows:

- Children who have short, horizontally positioned eustachian tubes, which allow secretions to easily migrate into the middle ear
- Children with immaturely developed cartilage that lines the eustachian tube opening; this makes the tubes more likely to open up, allowing secretions to migrate into the middle ear
- Children who have immature immune systems, which increases the risk of infection
- Children with enlarged lymph tissue, which can block the eustachian tube openings
- Children who are in environments with smokers; passive smoking increases inflammation and decreases secretion drainage

Breastfed infants have a lower incidence because of their semiupright feeding position and immunity acquired from the mother, whereas bottle-fed infants who are fed in the supine position have a higher incidence of infection due to the possibility that formula may reflux into the eustachian tubes.

Treatment of OM with antibiotics remains controversial because of the risk of bacteria such as *S. pneumoniae* developing antibiotic resistance. Although controversial, antibiotic therapy is the main treatment, with amoxicillin being most frequently used, unless the child has been on antibiotics in the last month. Other antibiotics include amoxicillin–clavulanates (Clavulin), azithromycin (Zithromax), and cephalosporins (Cefazolin). It is generally agreed that waiting up to 72 hours for the infection to clear in healthy children is acceptable, but for children under 2 years, caution is needed because of the risk of sepsis (Hockenberry et al., 2022).

Possible complications include hearing loss, scarring of the tympanic membrane, tympanic perforation, chronic suppurative otitis media, mastoiditis, meningitis, and cholesteatoma, in which the epithelial lining forms scales and can destroy bone and middle ear structures.

Myringotomy tubes are tiny drainage tubes that may be inserted into the tympanic membrane to drain excess secretions in the middle ear and equalize pressure.

Follow-up is important to ensure that the antibiotic therapy has cleared the infection and that there are no complications, such as hearing loss.

Clinical Manifestations

Health history and physical assessment data may reveal the following:
- Irritability, pulling at the affected ear, and complaints of ear pain
- Fever
- Decrease in appetite
- Nasal congestion, rhinorrhea, cough, and vomiting and diarrhea, showing a concurrent infection
- Otoscopic findings, including erythematous tympanic membrane; bulging tympanic membrane, membrane with no visible landmarks, including no light reflex; or diminished tympanic membrane mobility and discoloured effusion
- Purulent discharge

Diagnostics

Culture and sensitivity tests may identify organisms in ear discharge. An audiology referral for hearing tests can be done if hearing impairment is suspected.

Nursing Considerations

- Reduce fever by administering antipyretics as prescribed and dressing the child lightly.
- Relieve pain with prescribed analgesics by offering soft foods to reduce chewing and through the application of local heat or warm compresses to the affected ear. Note that heat may aggravate the pain in some children. Ice packs on the affected ear may relieve pain by reducing edema.
- Facilitate drainage by having the child lie on the affected ear.
- Prevent skin breakdown by keeping the external ear clean and dry and by using a moisture barrier.
- Assess for hearing loss and recommend referral for audiological testing if indicated.
- Administer prescribed antibiotics; prophylactic antibiotic treatment may be prescribed for children with recurrent infections.

RESPIRATORY DYSFUNCTION

Upper Respiratory Infection

Upper respiratory tract infections include nasopharyngitis, pharyngitis, and tonsillitis.

Nasopharyngitis and Pharyngitis

Also called the *common cold*, nasopharyngitis is a viral infection of the nose and throat. It is usually caused by viruses such as rhinoviruses, RSV, adenoviruses, influenza, and parainfluenza viruses. Pharyngitis is an inflammation of the pharynx. Nasopharyngitis is the most common illness in infancy and childhood.

Pathophysiology

The disease course of upper respiratory tract infections is usually self-limiting and lasts from about 10 to 14 days with a peak on day 2 to 3 of the illness. If the infection is caused by group A beta-hemolytic *Streptococcus*, there is the potential for complications such as acute glomerulonephritis or rheumatic fever (Hockenberry et al., 2022). Young children are more susceptible to catching these infections because of their immature immune systems.

Clinical Manifestations

The symptoms often include fever, irritability, restlessness, decreased appetite and fluid intake, and decreased activity. Rhinorrhea and nasal congestion can occur because of inflammation and can lead to skin irritation from wiping away secretions.

Therapeutics

- Antipyretics and other fever-reducing measures are given.
- The CPS (2021a) recommends saline drops to help clear nasal congestion. Over-the-counter decongestants and cough medicines may not be very effective and are not recommended for children under 6 years unless recommended by a physician or nurse practitioner.

Nursing Considerations

Teaching family members to care for their children at home is important; considerations are as follows:
- Elevate the head of the bed to help the secretions drain.
- Provide suction with a nasal bulb to clear congestion and use vaporization.
- Ensure fluid intake, which is necessary to prevent dehydration.
- Be aware that preventing infection is difficult but necessary. When possible, keep children away from other infected people and encourage children and family members to wash their hands frequently. Teach everyone in the family about covering the mouth and nose with tissues or elbow when coughing or sneezing. They need to wash hands thoroughly or use hand sanitizer and avoid touching their eyes, noses, and mouths (Hockenberry et al., 2022).

Tonsillitis

Tonsillitis is inflammation of the tonsils and often occurs with pharyngitis. In young children, the tonsils commonly are enlarged and become smaller as the child ages. The infection can be caused by bacteria or viruses.

Clinical Manifestations

The symptoms are caused by inflammation and include the following:

- The child may have difficulty eating and swallowing because of swelling and pain. If the tonsils are very large, there can be breathing issues due to airway obstruction.
- The child's breath can have an odour, and they may have decreased ability to smell and taste.
- Frequent sore throats and ear infections can occur.
- There may be a muffled and nasal tone of speech if the adenoids are enlarged.
- Throat cultures may show streptococcal organisms; if so, the child needs to be treated with an antibiotic.
- Nonbacterial tonsillitis is mild and self-limiting. It is characterized by a gradual onset, low-grade fever, mild headache, sore throat, hoarseness, and a cough.
- Bacterial tonsillitis is marked by the rapid onset of high fever, headache, generalized muscle aches, and vomiting.

Nursing Considerations

- Tonsillectomy is not recommended unless there are recurrent, frequent streptococcal infections, a history of peritonsillar abscess, and/or sleep-disordered breathing (Hockenberry et al., 2022).
- Treatment is focused on symptom relief: Antibiotics are used if it is a bacterial infection, along with analgesics–antipyretics such as acetaminophen (Tylenol) or an opioid combination (Tylenol with codeine), salt-water throat gargles for older children, lozenges or hard candy, fluids or soft foods, and rest.

  If surgery is required:
- Preoperatively: Prepare the child and family for hospitalization and surgery as with any procedure, with the teaching adapted to the child's developmental level. Explain that the child will have a sore throat after surgery but will be able to talk and swallow normally.
- Postoperatively: Observe for unusual bleeding; monitor vital signs; assess child's colour; be alert for restlessness, which can indicate hemorrhaging; help prevent bleeding by discouraging the child from coughing, clearing the throat, and blowing the nose; until the child is fully alert after the anaesthetic, position them on the side or the abdomen to facilitate drainage from the throat.

  Clear fluids that are not red in colour, which could disguise bleeding, and that are cool or iced should be given first; milk products should not be used because they tend to coat the throat and cause throat-clearing; analgesics should be given on a regular basis (Hockenberry et al., 2022).

  Postoperative teaching:
- Avoid gargling and vigorous tooth-brushing.
- Avoid persons with infections.
- Provide a soft diet that does not include acidic, spicy, or other irritating foods.
- Avoid coughing and clearing the throat and do not use straws.

- Monitor for bleeding, especially immediately postoperatively and 5 to 10 days postoperatively, when tissue sloughing occurs. The most obvious sign of bleeding is the child's continuous swallowing of the trickling of blood. When the child is sleeping, note the frequency of swallowing. Return to hospital immediately if bleeding occurs (Hockenberry et al., 2022).
- Limit activity to decrease the risk of bleeding, including when the child returns to school.

Pneumonia

Pneumonia's main feature is an acute inflammation of the bronchioles, alveolar ducts and sacs, and alveoli that impairs gas exchange.

Pneumonia is classified according to the etiological agent and the location and extent of pulmonary involvement:

- Lobar pneumonia involves a large segment of one or more lobes; when both lungs are affected, it is called *bilateral pneumonia.*
- Bronchopneumonia begins in the terminal bronchioles, which become clogged with mucopurulent exudates, and then consolidates in patches in the nearby lobules.
- Interstitial pneumonia is an inflammation confined to the alveolar walls and peribronchial and interlobular tissues (Hockenberry et al., 2022).

Pathophysiology

Pneumonia most commonly results from infection from viruses, bacteria, mycoplasma, or fungi.

- In children less than 5 years old, viral pneumonia is the most common type, including RSV, adenovirus, rhinovirus, influenza, parainfluenza, and enterovirus.
- Bacterial pneumonia in the newborn is commonly caused by group B *Streptococcus* and *Chlamydia trachomatis.*
- In children over 5, bacterial pneumonia is most common and is most often caused by *Staphylococcus aureus* and *S. pneumoniae.*
- In school-aged children, *Mycoplasma pneumoniae* is a common cause of pneumonia.
- *H. influenza* type b and *S. pneumoniae* decreased as causative agents as a result of current immunizations against these agents (Hockenberry et al., 2022).
- Pneumonia typically begins with a mild upper respiratory tract infection. As the disorder progresses, lung inflammation occurs.
- Bacterial pneumonia flows through the bloodstream to the lungs, usually causing inflammation and edema with cellular debris and mucus, in turn leading to airway obstruction and consolidation within one lung.
- Viral pneumonia agents enter the lung through the upper respiratory system into the alveoli near the bronchi and spread to nearby lung tissue in a patch pattern. Infants' small airways make them vulnerable to atelectasis and edema.
- Aspiration pneumonia can be caused by a child aspirating formula or vomitus or experiencing gastric reflux and can

cause chemical injury and an inflammatory response that leads to pneumonia as a secondary infection.

Clinical Manifestations

Manifestations vary, depending on the causative agent. Common signs and symptoms in viral pneumonia include the following:

- Variations ranging from mild fever, slight cough, and malaise to high fever, severe cough, and prostration
- Nonproductive or productive cough with whitish sputum
- Wheezing or fine rales

Common signs and symptoms in bacterial pneumonia include the following:

- High fever
- Unproductive to productive cough with whitish sputum, tachypnea, wheezing, rales, dullness on percussion, chest pain, retractions, nasal flaring, pallor, or cyanosis (depending on severity)
- Irritability, restlessness, lethargy
- Nausea, vomiting, anorexia, diarrhea, and abdominal pain (Hockenberry et al., 2022)

Diagnostics

- Chest X-ray studies may show diffuse or patchy infiltrates, consolidation, disseminated infiltration, or patchy clouding, depending on the type of pneumonia.
- Blood tests may reveal an elevated WBC count.
- A causative agent may be grown in blood culture or Gram stain and culture of sputum.

Nursing Considerations

Administer medication as prescribed.

- Viral pneumonia: Treatment is usually supportive, with fever and pain control, although antibiotic therapy may be recommended to reduce the risk of a secondary bacterial infection.
- Bacterial pneumonia: Antibiotic therapy is indicated; oral amoxicillin (Amoxil) or a second-generation cephalosporin such as cefuroxime (Kefurox) should be given if the child is not completely immunized for *H. influenzae*. Erythromycin (Novo-Rythro) is given to older children and adolescents until *M. pneumoniae* has been diagnosed.

If the child is hospitalized:

- Be aware that humidified oxygen, chest physiotherapy, and deep breathing, as well as incentive spirometry may be helpful.
- Assess for respiratory distress by monitoring respiratory status and vital signs.
- Change the child's position frequently and elevate the head of the bed.
- Monitor fluid balance and encourage oral fluid intake to ensure hydration.
- Promote rest by maintaining bed rest and organizing nursing care to minimize disturbances.
- Provide client and family teaching.
- Discuss home care and follow-up measures.

Atypical Pneumonia

Some children have an atypical type of pneumonia that is caused by *M. pneumoniae*. It occurs commonly in the school-aged child who is living in crowded conditions.

A serious new form of atypical pneumonia appeared in Asia in 2003, called *severe acute respiratory syndrome* (SARS). SARS is caused by a previously unrecognized coronavirus called *SARS-CoV*. Although rare in Canada, persons who are in contact with clients with SARS, or who have travelled in areas where SARS is present, are at risk of being infected. Strict isolation with a fitted respiratory mask is required. The clinical manifestations include the following:

- Fever higher than 38°C
- Headache
- Cough, shortness of breath, difficulty breathing
- A dry, nonproductive cough after 2 to 7 days
- In the young child, milder symptoms and a runny nose and cough
- In the adolescent group, malaise, myalgia, chills, and rigour (Denison, 2005)

Some individuals may require ventilation. Treatment is mostly supportive, with no clear improvement from using steroids, antibiotics, or antivirals (Hockenberry et al., 2022).

Coronavirus (SARS-CoV-2)

COVID-19 is caused by infection with the severe acute respiratory syndrome coronavirus (SARS-CoV-2) virus strain (Keenan-Lindsay et al., 2022). Information provided below is currently what is recommended. Information may change based on ongoing studies and data related to safety and how well vaccines work over time and against new variants.

Clinical Manifestations

- Symptoms include fever or chills, shortness of breath or dyspnea, cough, fatigue, headache, muscle or body aches, sore throat, new loss of smell or taste, congestion or runny nose, nausea or vomiting and diarrhea. Children tend to have abdominal symptoms and skin changes or rashes (Keenan-Lindsay et al., 2022).

Nursing Considerations

- The Government of Canada recommends all children 6 months to 17 years get vaccinated against COVID-19. Two vaccine doses are recommended at least 8 weeks apart. The booster doses or an additional dose may be offered to youth 12 to 17 years of age. The booster dose should be given 6 months from the last dose of primary series (Government of Canada, 2022c).
- Provide health teaching that even if a child had COVID-19, they should still get vaccinated. Getting vaccinated is the best way to slow the spread of COVID-19 and to prevent infection by future COVID-19 variants.
- Prevention of COVID-19 includes proper wearing of a well-fitted mask, physical distancing (2 metres), vaccination, and frequent handwashing.
- It is important for children to stay home when sick and get tested as needed.

Parvovirus B19 (Erythema Infectiosum)

Parvovirus is a human infection that infects mainly children. It usually causes fifth disease or "slapped cheek illness," so named because of the facial characteristics of a mild rash on the cheeks of the affected child (Keenan-Lindsay et al., 2022).

Pathophysiology

- The person will develop the fifth disease usually within 14 days after getting infected with the parvovirus B19.
- It spreads through respiratory secretions when the infected person coughs or sneezes.
- It is most contagious when the person has a fever or cold and before the rash, joint pain, and swelling occur. Once the rash develops the person is less likely to be contagious.
- The disease usually has a low risk of having adverse effects on the pregnant client, fetus, or baby. Occasionally, a baby will develop severe anemia caused by it. Fetal hydrops and death from anemia and heart failure occur with early exposure (Keenan-Lindsay et al., 2022)

Diagnosis

- Diagnosis is based on assessment of the rash on the person's face.
- A blood test can determine if a person is susceptible or possibly immune to parvovirus B19 infection or if recently infected by the virus (CDC, 2019).
- Pregnant clients diagnosed with the infection will have serial ultrasonography to assess for fetal hydrops or anemia. Cordocentresis is done to determine need for intrauterine transfusion if hydrops is present. Aggressive cardiovascular and respiratory support is required for newborns with hydrops (Keenan-Lindsay et al., 2022).
- Pregnant health care workers should not care for clients who may be highly contagious.
- Occupational exposure should be minimized in pregnant clients without immunity (Keenan-Lindsay et al., 2022).

Clinical Manifestations

- Symptoms are usually mild and may include fever, runny nose, headache, and rash.
- The red rash is usually on the face, but some people develop a second rash a few days later on the chest, arms, legs, back and buttocks. The rash may be itchy, especially on the soles of the feet. The rash varies in intensity but usually goes away within 10 days. At times the rash will have periods of flare-ups and remissions for several weeks.
- The person can also develop pain and swelling in joints, which is more common in females.
- Some adults with fifth disease may only have painful joints in their hands, feet, or knees and no other symptoms. Joint pain usually lasts 1 to 3 weeks but can last for months or longer. It goes away without any long-term complications.
- Complications are chronic anemia. There is an increased risk for serious complications if the person has a weakened immune system from leukemia, cancer, organ transplant, or HIV infection (CDC, 2019).

Nursing Considerations

- There is no vaccine or medical treatment to prevent parvovirus B19 infection.
- Fifth disease is usually mild in children and adults who are healthy; otherwise, clients usually recover completely.
- Health teaching on preventive measures includes handwashing, avoiding contact with people who are sick, avoiding touching one's mouth, nose, or eyes, proper coughing etiquette, and staying home if ill.
- Follow strict infection control practices to prevent the spread of transmission.
- Any pregnant persons who have been exposed to parvovirus should seek medical attention as soon as possible. A pregnant person who is infected with the parvovirus can pass the virus to their fetus (CDC, 2019).

Asthma

Asthma is a chronic inflammatory respiratory disease that causes difficulty breathing following exposure to certain triggers. A trigger is anything that causes inflammation in the airways and is specific to the individual. Inflammatory triggers include dust mites, animals, cockroaches, moulds, pollens, viral infections, and certain air pollutants. Symptom triggers, which do not cause inflammation but instead provoke "twitchy" airways, include smoke, exercise, cold air, strong smells such as perfumes, food additives such as sulphites, air pollutants, moulds and mildew, dust, and intense emotions. Because it is a chronic condition, asthma must be monitored and controlled over a lifetime. Asthma is the third leading cause of pediatric admissions to hospitals in Canada (Hockenberry et al., 2022).

Pathophysiology

In response to triggers, the following changes occur in the airways:

- Bronchoconstriction, which is tightening and narrowing of the circular muscles in the airway
- Edema of the airways as an inflammatory response
- Mucus production, which is also part of the inflammatory response to triggers

The result is a narrowing of the airways primarily on expiration, causing restricted airflow and subsequent respiratory distress.

Clinical Manifestations

Children typically present with signs of asthma between the ages of 3 and 8. In younger children, an attack usually follows a respiratory infection. Symptoms typically occur at night or in the early morning. Asthma can vary in symptoms from mild or moderate to severe and can vary from person to person. The clinical manifestations are as follows:

- Wheezing on expiration is a classic sign.
- Suprasternal and substernal retractions
- Shortness of breath, dyspnea, increased respiratory rate
- Tightness in the chest
- Coughing that may be dry, nonproductive, or productive and that commonly occurs at night

- Diaphoresis, worried look, anxiety, pale skin
- Hunched shoulders, tripod position, refusal to lie down
- In more severe attacks, difficulty speaking, behavioural signs of hypoxia
- "Silent chest," an ominous sign of impending respiratory arrest

Diagnosis is typically determined on the basis of clinical manifestations, history, and physical examination. Generally, chronic cough in the absence of infection or diffuse wheezing during expiration is sufficient for a diagnosis.

Diagnostics

Peak flow measurements and spirometry test lung volumes and expiratory capacities are used. Pulmonary function tests are more comprehensive tests to determine airway parameters.

Therapeutics

- Controller medicines (usually inhaled steroids) stabilize the airways and decrease the inflammatory response. They are maintenance therapy and are of no use during an acute attack.
- Reliever medicines (usually inhaled bronchodilators) open the airways during attacks and are used prior to steroid inhalations to provide maximum airway dilation.
- Allergy desensitization has proven to be of little value.

Nursing Considerations

- Be aware that asthma can best be managed if an asthma plan is in effect. This plan is best formulated with the input of the health care team and family. The focus is on avoidance of triggers, appropriate and timely medication therapy, proper use of inhalers, avoidance of upper respiratory infections, symptom monitoring, involvement of the child and the family, and maintenance of a normal lifestyle.
- Ensure the proper use of inhalers as this is a frequent cause of poorly managed asthma. Use appropriate devices, such as a spacer, to improve medication delivery. Allow several minutes between bronchodilator inhalations.
- Know that the child may benefit from using the bronchodilator prior to exercise or in cold weather.
- Advise the child to rinse the mouth following steroid inhalation.
- Teach parents when to bring the child to hospital for emergency care.
  In hospital:
- Observe the chest, including size, shape, symmetry, and movement.
- Perform lung auscultation to assess for adventitious breath sounds.
- Take vital signs.
- Administer inhaled bronchodilator via a mask with compressed air or oxygen. Monitor the response to the inhalation.
- Maintain the child on clear and increased fluids.
- Know that extreme shortness of breath or the absence of breath sounds accompanied by a sudden rise in respiratory rate is an ominous sign indicating respiratory failure and imminent asphyxia.
- Provide support and reassurance: An asthma attack is very frightening for both the child and the parent.

Respiratory Syncytial Virus (RSV) and Bronchiolitis

RSV is the most common respiratory pathogen for bronchiolitis and pneumonia among infants and children under 2 years of age. RSV is the most frequent cause of hospitalization in children younger than 2 years of age. RSV is less frequent in breastfed children and more frequent in children who live in crowded conditions (Hockenberry et al., 2022). In many cases, RSV will cause symptoms similar to a cold; however, serious infection in the lungs can occur in premature infants, babies with chronic lung disease or congenital heart disease, or those infants who are immunocompromised. The infection rate rises in the late fall, peaks midwinter, and decreases in frequency in the spring in countries with temperate climates, such as Canada. This highly contagious pathogen is typically spread from hand to eye, nose, or other mucous membranes. The virus will live on surfaces such as clothing, toys, countertops, and facial tissues for hours.

Pathophysiology

RSV affects the epithelial cells of the respiratory tract, causing obstruction due to accumulated debris from infected cells, mucus, and exudate. This leads to small airway obstruction, air trapping, poor gas exchange, increased work of breathing, and a characteristic expiratory wheeze.

Clinical Manifestations

The signs and symptoms of RSV vary, depending on the age and condition of the child and the severity of the infection. Peak incidence of RSV bronchiolitis is 2 to 5 months. The infection progresses as follows:
- Early: Runny nose, sneezing, pharyngitis, coughing, wheezing, and crackles; there may be intermittent fever, or possible drainage from the eye or ear
- As illness progresses: Increased coughing and wheezing, shortness of breath, tachypnea and accessory muscle use, fever, and cyanosis
- In severe illness: tachypnea at more than 70 breaths per minute, listlessness, poor air exchange, significantly decreased breath sounds, and apneic spells, which may rapidly progress to respiratory failure
- Symptoms will appear 3 to 5 days after exposure and will last approximately 12 days.

Diagnostics

Positive diagnosis of RSV is based on the initial upper respiratory infection symptoms, the time of year (late fall to early spring), history of exposure, and an RSV antigen detection performed on a nasopharyngeal swab (Hockenberry et al., 2022).

Therapeutics

RSV infections are treated symptomatically with high humidity, adequate fluids, and caloric intake and rest.

Most children can be managed at home. Hospitalization is required for those with advanced symptoms of the illness or an underlying respiratory or cardiac disease. RSV immune globulin, or, less frequently, RSV monoclonal antibody, may be administered prophylactically for high-risk infants. Bronchodilators and steroids can be used but are controversial in terms of effectiveness (Hockenberry et al., 2022).

Nursing Considerations

- Monitor for respiratory distress, noting respiratory rate and rhythm, breath sounds, and adventitious sounds, especially wheezing.
- Assess skin colour and hydration status.
- Take appropriate isolation precautions.
- Administer prescribed medications.
- Ensure high humidity with oxygen as prescribed; increase fluids to maintain adequate hydration, offering small amounts frequently to prevent aspiration.
- Know that the child may need IV fluids if tachypnea creates a potential for aspiration.
- Maintain proper positioning to promote increased air exchange, usually high Fowler's.
- Provide support for parents.
  Treatment with ribavirin:
- Note that use of this medication is controversial as it may cause toxic effects in health care workers who inhale the aerosol, and the effectiveness in children has not been proven.
- Ribavarin (Virazole) may be used for high-risk children, such as premature or very young infants, and infants at increased risk for progressing from mild to severe disease.

Laryngotracheobronchitis

Laryngotracheobronchitis (LTB), or croup, is an inflammation and narrowing of the laryngeal and tracheal areas. The cause is usually viral, and the common infectious agents are RSV, influenza viruses, parainfluenza viruses, adenoviruses, and measles virus. As a result of effective immunization campaigns, the number of *H. influenzae* LTB infections has decreased. LTB also may be of bacterial origin (as in diphtheria or pertussis).

LTB affects boys more than girls, usually between the ages of 6 months and 3 years, and peaks in the winter months (Hockenberry et al., 2022).

Pathophysiology

LTB usually follows an upper respiratory infection, which may spread to the larynx, trachea, and sometimes the bronchi. The elastic larynx of a young child can go into spasm and can cause a significant airway obstruction. Severe airway edema can cause airway obstruction and seriously affect air exchange.

Clinical Manifestations

In spasmodic croup with rapid onset, the child wakes at night with a barklike or seal-like cough.

- Acute LTB: gradual onset from upper respiratory tract infection, progressing to signs of respiratory distress with pallor or cyanosis
- Hoarseness, inspiratory stridor, indrawing, and possibly severe respiratory distress
- Possibly low-grade fever
- Restlessness and irritability
- Wheezing, crackles, and localized areas of diminished breath sounds

Therapeutics

Treatment is commonly humidity with cool mist via a face mask or blow by mist even though it has not been shown to decrease subglottal edema.

- Racemic epinephrine, which causes vasoconstriction and decreases subglottal edema, is administered by nebulizer for children who are not improving.
- Steroids may be effective when administered orally or intramuscularly if oral steroid cannot be tolerated.

Nursing Considerations

- Assess for airway obstruction by evaluating respiratory status by colour, respiratory effort, evidence of fatigue, and vital signs.
- Know that in severe cases of LTB, intubation to manage the airway may be necessary.
- Administer oxygen and increase humidity to decrease hypoxia if oxygen saturation is below 92%.
- Administer IV or oral fluids as prescribed to ensure good fluid balance.
- Reduce the child's anxiety by maintaining a quiet environment and promoting rest and relaxation.
- Provide parental support and teaching.
- Teach home management with cool, moist air: For example, to decrease subglottal edema, measures include having the child breathe in the cool night air, taking the child to a cool basement, or having the child breathe in air from an open freezer.

Epiglottitis

Epiglottitis is an acute and severe inflammation of the epiglottis that causes a supraglottic airway obstruction. It is mainly caused by parainfluenza A and B, adenovirus, and RSV. *H. influenzae* immunizations have decreased the occurrence of that type of infection. Now it usually affects older children and is caused by viruses.

Pathophysiology

Swelling and inflammation of the soft tissue of the epiglottis cause life-threatening obstruction of the airway. Progressive obstruction results in hypoxia, hypercapnia, and acidosis, closely followed by decreased muscle tone, altered level of consciousness, and, if obstruction becomes complete, sudden death. Endotracheal intubation or tracheostomy usually is considered. IV antibiotics are initiated, and steroids may be used for edema.

Clinical Manifestations

- Sudden onset of fever, sore throat, dyspnea, and lethargy
- Restlessness and anxiety due to respiratory obstruction
- Hyperextension of the neck, drooling, severe sore throat with refusal to drink
- Stridor, hoarseness
- Rapid, thready pulse
- Adoption of a characteristic "tripod" position by the child: sitting upright, leaning forward with chin thrust out, mouth open, and tongue protruding
- Late signs of hypoxia: listlessness, cyanosis, bradycardia, decreased respiratory rate with decreased aeration
- A red and inflamed throat with a large, red, edematous epiglottis (Hockenberry et al., 2022)

Diagnostics

- Lateral neck X-ray shows epiglottal enlargement.
- Elevated WBC count and increased bands and neutrophils may be seen on the differential count.
- Causative bacteria may be identified by blood cultures (Hockenberry et al., 2022).

Nursing Considerations

If epiglottitis is suspected, throat examination should be by a specially trained person. Ensure that intubation and tracheostomy equipment is nearby, as the throat examination may cause laryngospasm and precipitate a complete airway obstruction. Provide care as for other respiratory conditions.

Cystic Fibrosis

Cystic fibrosis (CF) is a chronic autosomal recessive hereditary disorder that affects the pancreas, respiratory system, GI tract, salivary glands, and reproductive tract. Approximately 1 in every 3 600 Canadian children is born with CF (Keenan-Lindsay et al., 2022).

The gene responsible for CF was identified in 1989 on chromosome 7. Advancements in treatments with gene and protein therapy, in addition to aggressive chest physiotherapy, inhalation therapy with antibiotics, and nutritional support, have improved the prognosis. In Canada, people with CF live until they are about 50 years old, which is 20 years longer than they did in 1990 (Cystic Fibrosis Canada, 2020).

Pathophysiology

The underlying defect is in the *CFTR* gene, causing impaired chloride movement and abnormally viscous and thick mucus that obstructs bronchioles and ducts in the pancreas and other exocrine glands, creating multisystem problems. The child with CF has an increase in sodium and chloride in the saliva and sweat.

In the lungs, ciliary movement is slower, and the thickened secretions accumulate, creating obstruction, air trapping, and infection. Respiratory infections recur and cause bronchiectasis and fibrotic scarring. The pancreas becomes obstructed and significantly decreases production of the digestive enzymes, leading to major malabsorption of proteins and fats. The small intestine can become obstructed.

Clinical Manifestations

Manifestations vary with severity and time of emergence; they may appear at birth or take years to develop. The skin of children with CF often tastes salty because of the high salt content of their sweat.

Respiratory signs and symptoms:

- Wheezing, dyspnea, cough, cyanosis
- Respiratory infections that are usually caused by staphylococci, *Pseudomonas aeruginosa,* and, eventually, as the disease progresses, *Burkholderia cepacia*; the child can develop resistance to antibiotics
- Chronic sinusitis, bronchitis, bronchopneumonia, or ear, nose, and throat problems

As CF progresses, atelectasis and generalized obstructive emphysema result from mucus blockage in the small airways, producing a barrel-shaped chest and finger clubbing.

GI signs:

- Meconium ileus at birth; rectal prolapse (common); loose, bulky, frothy, fatty stools; large appetite; weight loss; marked tissue wasting; failure to thrive; distended abdomen; thin extremities; evidence of vitamin A, D, E, and K deficiencies

Reproductive signs:

- Females: Decreased fertility, apparently from increased viscosity of cervical mucus, which blocks the entry of sperm
- Males: Sterility in 95%, which may be caused by blockage of the vas deferens with abnormal secretions or failure of the vas deferens tubes to develop

Cardiovascular signs:

- Cor pulmonale, right-sided heart enlargement, and heart failure resulting from obstruction of pulmonary blood flow (Hockenberry et al., 2022)

Diagnostics

- Elevated chloride levels on the sweat test (iontophoresis with pilocarpine); chloride level is >60 mmol/L
- Absence of pancreatic enzyme activity
- Steatorrhea detected in stool analysis
- Generalized obstructive emphysema on chest X-ray
- Fetal diagnosis in utero (Hockenberry et al., 2022)

Therapeutics

The child with CF receives aggressive treatments for respiratory infections from oral, inhaled, and IV antibiotics. Aminoglycosides, such as tobramycin and gentamicin, and cephalosporins are often used. Sputum cultures are required because clients with CF become colonized with *P. aeruginosa* and then the more antibiotic-resistant strain of *B. cepacia*, and antibiotics must match the sensitivity of the organisms. Clients with CF who are colonized with *B. cepacia* have a poorer prognosis. Inhaled bronchodilators, which may include inhaled tobramycin, are used before daily chest physiotherapy sessions with postural drainage. Huff breathing techniques, positive expiratory pressure, use of a spirometer flutter valve, and high-frequency chest wall oscillation all help clear mucus and prevent infection. DNAse can also be given by nebulizer to help thin respiratory secretions. Exercise also helps clear the mucus.

Replacement pancreatic enzymes in the form of one to five capsules are given with meals to help improve digestion of food. Fat-soluble vitamins are needed because of the difficulty of digesting fat. Esophageal reflux is common and is treated as usual.

Breast milk or hydrolysate formula can be given. Lactulose may prevent early distal intestinal obstructions and prevent recurrence; abdominal obstructions are treated with propylene glycol electrolyte solution (Golytely). Constipation, which can contribute to obstruction, is treated as usual. A high-calorie, high-protein, and high-fat diet is important to prevent malnutrition (Hockenberry et al., 2022).

Nursing Considerations

- Perform pulmonary mucus clearance to help increase sputum clearance, such as chest physiotherapy, postural drainage, inhalation treatments with bronchodilators, and breathing exercises.
- Monitor respiratory status.
- Encourage good nutrition with meals high in fat and protein. Increasing salt intake is important when the child experiences increased salt losses through the skin, as when they are in a hot environment or have a fever.
- Assess nutritional status by doing calorie counts, monitoring intake and output, and recording daily weights.
- Administer medications as prescribed, pancreatic enzymes with food, fat-soluble vitamins (A, D, E, and K), bronchodilators, and antibiotics when prescribed for infections.
- Promote growth and development by providing activities that enhance developmental stages.
- Monitor for signs of infection; prevent infection by promoting good health and hygiene practices, as well as by avoiding exposure to people with infections.
- Encourage adequate rest by organizing nursing activities around rest periods.
- Help the child maintain a positive self-concept by active listening, encouraging verbalization, and identifying strengths and coping strategies.
- Foster communication and allow the family and child to express their feelings about the chronic nature of the disorder and its long-term implications, the potential need for a lung transplant, and death and dying.
- Provide client and family teaching regarding pulmonary care, dietary instructions, medication dosage, administration and adverse effects, infection prevention, and the need for routine follow-up (Hockenberry et al., 2022).

GASTRO-INTESTINAL SYSTEM DISORDERS

The GI system has numerous important functions. The major purposes are to break down and digest foods so that the nutrients may be absorbed through the digestive tract and waste products may be eliminated.

During fetal development, the GI system begins to form during the fourth week of the embryonic stage, starting with the mouth and anal tube. The GI tract becomes more mature in the last few weeks of development. If there is any interruption in normal fetal growth, then malformations can occur anywhere along the GI tract. Congenital anomalies of the GI tract can be present at birth or shortly after birth.

Obesity
Pathophysiology
Increasingly, obesity is becoming a health concern in Canada and around the world. As childhood obesity rates rise, so do unusual childhood complications such as type 2 diabetes. There is widespread concern that children with obesity will have significant health issues as adults as a direct result of their condition. Childhood obesity is a predictor of adult obesity; therefore, prevention is the best intervention.

There are many reasons for increasing obesity rates, including the following:
- Parental overweight
- Overweight at birth
- Physical inactivity
- Irregular snacking
- Poor food choices
- Lack of availability of a variety of nutritious foods (Hassink & Fairbrother, 2020).
  Complications of obesity include the following:
- Decreased levels of growth hormone prolactin in girls and testosterone in boys
- Increased rates of amenorrhea and dysfunctional uterine bleeding in girls
- Dyslipidemia and hypertension
- Choledocholithiasis
- Slipped capital femoral epiphyses, Legg–Calvé–Perthes disease
- Obstructive sleep apnea and Pickwickian syndrome (increased daytime sleepiness and hypoventilation)
- Increased respiratory illness in toddlers under 2 years of age
- Psychosocial disturbances, such as low self-esteem, abnormal body image, difficulty developing peer relationships, social withdrawal, and isolation
- Adult obesity

Diagnostics

Tests include random blood glucose, thyroid-stimulating hormone (TSH) and thyroxine (T_4) levels (if short in stature), and urinalysis for glucose and lipid profile. In addition, in adolescent girls with amenorrhea or dysfunctional uterine bleeding, pelvic ultrasonography should be performed to rule out polycystic ovaries.

Therapeutics and Nursing Considerations

Goals of the treatment are family centred and are designed to modify behaviour so that more energy is used by the child for growth, activity, and metabolic processes than is consumed. Nurses play an important role in planning, teaching, and monitoring the child's progress.

Considerations include the following:
- Decreased caloric intake and making healthier choices using *Canada's Food Guide* (Government of Canada, 2022a)

- Increased exercise over time
- Decreased time spent doing sedentary activities, such as watching television and playing video games
- Behavioural therapy
- Group involvement diet workshops, weight reduction programs
- Family involvement-nutritional education and counseling, family mealtimes, helpful attitudes
- A holistic treatment plan that treats the whole person physically, emotionally, and socially

Follow-up visits are necessary to monitor height and weight (Keenan-Lindsay, 2022).

Cleft Lip and Palate Conditions

The most common craniofacial malformation is cleft lip (CL), with or without a cleft palate (CP). These two malformations are the most common birth anomalies in Canada. There is a higher incidence in certain ethnic groups, including the Indigenous population (Keenan-Lindsay et al., 2022). CL with or without CP occurs more commonly in males, and CP alone occurs more in females. There is an increased occurrence in relatives and in monozygotic twins.

Pathophysiology

CL occurs in the upper lip when the tissue does not completely close during the sixth week of fetal development. CL can occur unilaterally or bilaterally, with varying degrees of depth. CP occurs when the embryonic palate plates do not completely close at about the seventh and twelfth weeks of gestation. CL and CP conditions can occur separately, or both malformations may be present in a newborn.

See Figure 11.2 for variations in clefts of the lip and palate at birth.

Clinical Manifestations

The defects are present at birth. Other investigations need to be done to rule out other midline birth malformations.

Diagnostics

CL is more apparent than CP. CP may not be identified right away without a thorough examination of the mouth. CP is detected through a visual examination of the oral cavity or when the examiner places a gloved finger directly on the palate (Hockenberry et al., 2022).

Prenatal diagnosis with a fetal ultrasound is not reliable until the soft tissues of the fetal face can be visualized at 13 to 14 weeks. Approximately 20 to 30% of infants with CL and CL/P are prenatally diagnosed through ultrasonography. (Hockenberry et al., 2022).

Therapeutics

The treatment for CP and CL is surgical intervention.
- Early surgical correction of CL within 2 and 3 month permits a more normal sucking pattern and increases parental bonding. It also promotes a more normal speech pattern.

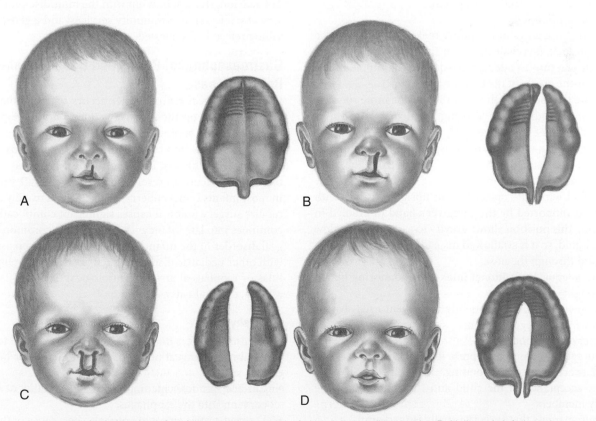

Fig. 11.2 Variations in clefts of lip and palate at birth. **A,** Notch in vermillion border. **B,** Unilateral cleft lip and cleft palate. **C,** Bilateral cleft lip and cleft palate. **D,** Cleft palate. (From Keenan-Lindsay, L., Sams, C.A., & O'Connor, C. [2022]. *Perry's maternal child nursing care in Canada* [3rd ed., p. 1209, Figure 46.6]. Elsevier.)

- For larger clefts, surgery for scar revision may be needed in the future.
- An extensive treatment plan developed by a multidisciplinary palate team is required for CP.
- The timing of surgical repair of the palate is controversial; it can be done in the neonate but is usually done before 12 months, before the incompletely fused palate can cause a speech impediment. A posterior pharyngeal flap is performed, and a bone graft may be done later to build up the palate density.
- The child with CP will have corrections performed in stages and usually requires speech therapy as well as orthodontics and prosthodontics to correct misaligned, missing, or malformed teeth.
- An obturator is a temporary appliance that blocks the defect in the palate until surgery is done, but it is controversial and may not be used.
- Ineffective eustachian tube function creates impaired drainage of the middle ear, with the result that recurrent bouts of OM can occur. Bilateral myringotomies may be required.
- There is the potential for damage to the child's self-image, particularly related to a speech impairment.
- Delayed development has also been observed.

Nursing Considerations

Nursing care involves facilitating feeding, providing emotional support, preoperative and postoperative care, and assisting parents through the health care system.

Feeding implications

- Know that openings in the palate make it difficult for the infant to suck. It is challenging for the child with CP to get enough pressure to adequately squeeze the nipple in the bottle or the areola of the breast.
- Be aware that babies with CL or CP may be more successful at breastfeeding than at using adaptive enlarged nipples, soft bottles, or syringes.
- During feeding, there is a risk of aspiration, so hold infants more upright and direct the milk away from the cleft, toward the side of the mouth.
- The infant with CP is placed in an upright position with the head supported by the caregiver's hand or cradled in the arm. This position allows gravity to assist with the flow of the liquid, so it is swallowed instead of resulting in a loss of liquid through the nose.
- Ensure adequate nutritional intake by monitoring height and weight gain.
- Feed slowly and burp frequently to prevent excessive air swallowing and regurgitation.

Psychosocial implications

- Encourage the family to express feelings and concerns to facilitate acceptance and bonding.
- Model acceptance of the child and the condition to the family members.
- Reassure parents that surgery usually is successful.
- Show the parents pictures of successful surgical repairs and refer them to a support group.

Postoperative care

- Assess airway clearance and vital signs to monitor for edema and respiratory distress.
- Place an infant with CL in a baby seat or on one side to avoid contact with the surgical site. Position a child with CP prone to facilitate drainage.
- Clean the suture line and apply prescribed antibacterial ointment for CL to prevent infection and help prevent scarring.
- Apply elbow immobilizers to prevent rubbing of the suture line. Remove immobilizers every 2 hours to provide ROM exercises and give skin care. The elbow immobilizers may be used for 7 to 10 days postoperatively.
- Feed the infant with adaptive devices such as droppers with a rubber tip, bulb syringes, Breck feeders, or soft bottle nipples, to help decrease pressure on the suture line.
- For older children, do not provide straws or sharp objects and try to keep them from rubbing the suture line with their tongue.
- Administer analgesics as prescribed to provide pain control.
- Check temperatures of warm liquids to prevent burns; the child with a new palate may lack nerve endings and sensation in the area.
- Provide mouth care to prevent the mucous membranes from drying out due to the child tending to mouth-breathe.

Family teaching requirements include care of the surgical wound; feeding strategies and positioning; prosthetic care if utilized; long-term follow-up with the multidisciplinary team services; referral to community services; and a genetic counseling referral, if requested.

Gastroesophageal Reflux and Gastroesophageal Reflux Disease

Gastroesophageal reflux (GER) occurs when stomach contents flow back up the esophagus due to an incompetent or relaxed cardiac sphincter. Gastroesophageal reflux disease (GERD) is reflux into the esophagus or oropharynx, causing symptoms. The highest incidence of GER occurs at 4 months of age, and it tends to resolve spontaneously by 1 year of age in most infants (Hockenberry et al., 2022). It usually does not require surgery unless it causes significant complications and continues into late infancy. This is the most common esophageal disorder in the infant age group. GER is often associated with other pediatric disorders, such as tracheoesophageal fistulas or esophageal atresia, neurological disorders, scoliosis, asthma, cerebral palsy, or CF.

Pathophysiology

The cause of GER is not known but may be related to immature lower esophageal neuromuscular function or hormonal control system.

- Cardiac sphincter incompetence allows reflux of stomach contents into the esophagus.
- Delayed gastric emptying may also be a cause of the reflux.
- Repeated episodes of reflux may harm the mucosal lining of the esophagus.

- Small amounts of reflux are considered normal in all age groups.
- Long-term GER can cause esophageal strictures from a scarred esophagus and recurrent respiratory problems due to aspiration.
- Usually, infants improve by 12 to 28 months of age and respond to conservative treatment.

Clinical Manifestations

The most common sign in infants is passive regurgitation or vomiting; occasionally, hematemesis is seen. Other manifestations include the following:
- Weight loss and poor growth
- Excessive crying, irritability, stiffening and aching of the back
- Aspiration and frequent respiratory infections
- "Blue spells" or apnea
- Esophagitis and bleeding due to gastric acid irritating the esophageal lining
- Melena stools
- Heartburn and abdominal pain

Diagnostics

- A history of vomiting and a health assessment examination can confirm the presence of GER.
- Barium swallow and upper GI radiology demonstrate reflux.
- An esophageal pH probe can measure the level of acidity, the timing of acid clearance, and the reflux amount. It can determine the impact of feedings and positioning.
- Intraesophageal pH monitoring measures reflux gastric acid from the stomach.
- Scintigraphy can detect delayed gastric emptying (Hockenberry et al., 2022).

Therapeutics

Most infants are treated conservatively until the reflux disappears. Small, frequent feedings of thickened rice cereal using enlarged bottle nipples and frequent burping decrease the number and volume of emesis. Placing the infant in the prone position decreases reflux but is controversial due to an increased risk of SIDS in infants placed in this position (Hockenberry et al., 2022).
- Pharmaceutical treatments include H_2 antagonists to treat the esophagitis and proton pump inhibitors to suppress gastric acid; as well, prokinetics are often prescribed to promote esophageal peristalsis and increase gastric emptying, but they are of limited value. Antacids are not generally recommended for children due to the aluminum content of the formulations, possible neurotoxicity, and lack of research.
- Surgery is performed on children who have not responded to conservative measures or when there are contributing anatomical anomalies.
- The most common surgical procedure is called a *Nissen fundoplication*, which creates an antireflux valve by bringing a portion of the fundus of the stomach around the esophagus.

Children with delayed gastric emptying may have a pyloroplasty.
- Fundoplications can result in complications including small bowel obstruction, no relief from GER, wrap hernia, retching, gas-bloat syndrome, and dumping syndrome (Hockenberry et al., 2022).
- For children who require long-term tube feeding, an alternative to a plication is the insertion of a percutaneous gastrojejunostomy.

Nursing Considerations

- Manage acute and chronic pain.
- Assess hydration and the frequency, amount, and characteristics of the vomitus.
- Assess whether positioning, postfeed handling, or the type of activity affects the vomiting.
- Provide small, frequent feedings of thickened formula and burp often.
- When the child is awake and observed, be aware that although positioning the infant upright after meals has not necessarily proven to be effective, it is generally used as a method to help prevent postfeeding reflux. Minimize handling of infants postfeeds.
- The supine position continues to be recommended for infant sleeping. Parents should not place infants on their sides as an alternative to fully supine sleeping (Hockenberry et al., 2022).
- Assess for signs of aspiration pre- and postfeeding.
- Monitor with a cardiac or apnea monitor if appropriate.
- Administer prescribed medications.
- Know that fundoplication requires routine abdominal postoperative care, including surveillance for wound infections, return of bowel motility, gagging, distension from gas, or intolerance of some foods, such as spicy meals. See Chapter 7, pages 122-124.
- Provide client and family teaching related to medications, hydration, nutrition, and feeding techniques.
- Be aware that treatment may involve temporary gastric decompression by nasogastric (NG) tube and gradual clamping of the tube until the infant tolerates the feeds.

Hypertrophic Pyloric Stenosis

Hypertrophic pyloric stenosis (HPS) occurs when a narrowed circular pyloric sphincter obstructs the flow of gastric contents into the intestine. It requires a surgical pyloromyotomy to correct the constricted valve and the obstruction. HPS is shown in Figure 11.3.

Pathophysiology

The narrowed pyloric sphincter leads to increasing hypertrophy of the valve. The pyloric canal narrows, leading to blockage of the pyloric sphincter, obstruction, gastric distension, and forceful vomiting. The cause is unknown but may be related to local innervation problems and can be associated with other conditions, such as intestinal malrotation and

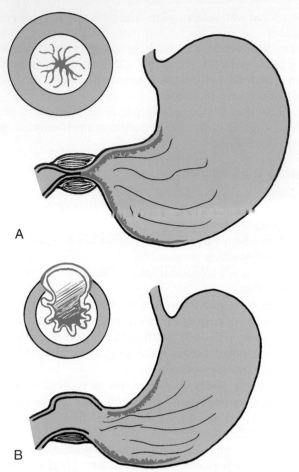

A

B

Fig. 11.3 Hypertrophic pyloric stenosis. **A,** Enlarged muscular tumour nearly obliterates pyloric canal. **B,** Longitudinal surgical division of muscle down to submucosa establishes adequate passageway. (From Hockenberry, M. J., Rodgers, C., & Wilson, D., [2022]. *Wong's essentials of pediatric nursing* [11th ed., p. 712, Figure 22.4]. Elsevier.)

esophageal and duodenal atresia. HPS occurs more commonly in first-borns, boys, and tends to run in families.

Clinical Manifestations

- Nonbilious vomiting usually begins at about 3 weeks of age, but the timing can vary.
- Vomiting increases in frequency and strength until it is projectile.
- Vomitus may be brown tinged from blood if gastritis develops.
- The infant is hungry and irritable.
- The condition progresses to dehydration, weight loss, and failure to thrive, with upper abdominal distension.
- Gastric peristalsis and the pylorus olive-shaped mass can be visible and palpable in the epigastrium to the right of the umbilicus.

Diagnostics

- HPS is often diagnosed by a history and physical exam. The olivelike mass is palpated when the stomach is empty, the infant is quiet, and the abdominal muscles are relaxed (Hockenberry et al., 2022).

- If diagnosis is incomplete from the history and physical exam, an ultrasonogram and upper GI series will show slowed gastric emptying with an abnormally stretched and thinned pylorus.
- The child has metabolic acidosis with increased serum pH and bicarbonate levels.
- There are decreased levels of serum chloride, sodium, and potassium due to vomiting.
- Dehydration leads to increased hemocrit, hemoglobin, and BUN levels.

Therapeutics

Rehydration and correction of electrolyte imbalance occur before surgery. A laparoscopic pyloromyotomy splits the pyloric muscle longitudinally. An NG tube may be inserted to decompress the stomach.

Nursing Considerations

- Maintain hydration and electrolyte balance by assessing for dehydration, monitoring intake and output and daily weights, evaluating urine specific gravity, and administering prescribed IV fluids of glucose and electrolytes (potassium is added to the IV fluid after voiding has occurred).
- Provide NG tube care if in situ. See Chapter 7, pages 118-119.
- Provide mouth care and a pacifier when a child is on a nothing by mouth (NPO) order.
- Start small amounts of clear fluids within 24 hours post-surgery; increase diet progressively, as tolerated, up to 48 hours postsurgery.
- Be aware that infants may be bottle- or breastfed for shorter-than-usual intervals.
- Feed slowly and burp frequently; place the child in a high Fowler's position on the right side after feeding.
- Administer analgesics as prescribed.
- Assess for wound infection as infants are more prone to wound-healing conditions.
- Encourage parent and family involvement in care; demonstrate feeding, positioning, and wound care.

Intussusception

Intussusception occurs when a portion of intestine invaginates, or folds into, an adjacent portion. This folding causes an obstruction that does not resolve and needs emergency medical intervention if the child is to survive.

Pathophysiology

Invagination usually begins close to or at the ileocecal valve. It can also occur in the ileum or the colon. Peristalsis pulls the invaginated section and causes edema and resulting obstruction that shuts off the flow of blood and lymph to the area. If intussusception is untreated for more than 24 hours, bowel strangulation can occur and cause ischemia, perforation, peritonitis, hemorrhage from venous engorgement, mucus buildup, and shock.

The cause of intussusception is usually not known but may be connected to viruses, intestinal polyps, lymphoma, CF, and

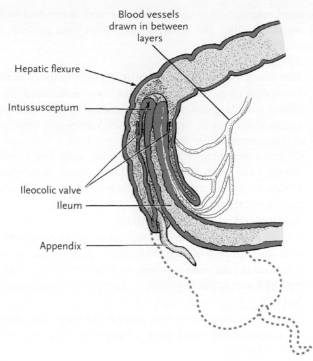

Blood vessels drawn in between layers

Hepatic flexure

Intussusceptum

Ileocolic valve

Ileum

Appendix

Fig. 11.4 Ileocecal valve (ileocolic) intussusception. (From Hockenberry, M. J., Rodgers, C., & Wilson, D. [2022] *Wong's essential of pediatric nursing* [11th ed., p. 713, Figure 22.5]. Elsevier.)

Meckel's diverticulum. It is one of the most common causes of bowel obstruction in children under 6 years, more common in males and in children under 2 years of age (Hockenberry et al., 2022).

Figure 11.4 shows the invagination of the bowel in a child with intussusception.

Clinical Manifestations

- Sudden, severe, spasmodic abdominal pain causes the child to cry and draw the legs up to the abdomen.
- As intussusception progresses, the child will vomit gastric contents and blood will appear in the stools.
- The classical presentation of a tender, distended abdomen, with a possibly palpable sausage-shaped abdominal mass and "currant jelly" stools, occurs in less than 30% of children.
- The child may present with a more chronic picture of diarrhea, anorexia, weight loss, occasional vomiting, and periodic pain. The older child may have only pain.
- If the obstruction is not relieved, symptoms are lethargy, "currant jelly" stool (containing blood and mucus), bile-stained or fecal emesis, and shocklike syndrome, which can progress to death (Hockenberry et al., 2022).

Diagnostics

- Frequently, subjective data lead to the diagnosis, which is confirmed with an ultrasound.
- A rectal examination produces mucus and blood and can detect a low intussusception.

Therapeutics

- Conservative treatment consists of radiologist-guided pneumoenema (air enema) with or without water-soluble contrast,

or an ultrasound-guided hydrostatic (saline) enema to decrease the defect. The advantage of an ultrasound-guided hydrostatic enema is that no ionizing radiation is required. Reoccurrence of intussusception is rare after having the conservative treatment. This procedure should not be attempted with prolonged intussusception, signs of shock, peritoneal irritation, or perforation (Hockenberry et al., 2022).

- IV fluids, NG decompression, and antibiotic therapy may be given before the hydrostatic enema.
- If the enema is unsuccessful in resolving the invagination, a surgical bowel resection is required.

Nursing Considerations

- Monitor vital signs, NG drainage, and signs of bowel bleeding.
- Postsurgery, monitor for return of bowel sounds, and then encourage clear fluid intake and increase diet as tolerated.
- Monitor for signs of infection; assess wound healing for redness, swelling, and drainage; and monitor temperature.
- Perform pain assessment and management.
- Provide parental support and discharge teaching for diet and wound care.

Appendicitis

Appendicitis is the most common condition that requires surgery in the pediatric population. The vermiform appendix becomes obstructed, leading to increased lumen pressure and bacterial infiltration with subsequent necrosis, perforation, and peritonitis.

Surgical removal of the appendix is required. Appendicitis occurs slightly more often in males and in older children, age 10 to 18 years. It is unusual in children under 5 years and is rare in infants less than a year. Perforation occurs more often in the younger child, possibly related to later detection.

Pathophysiology

The appendiceal lumen may become obstructed from a peritoneal skin fold, submucosal lymphoid tissue, fecaliths (hardened stool), foreign body, and parasites.

Clinical Manifestations

- The most common symptom is a spasmodic pain in the periumbilical area, which moves to the right lower quadrant near McBurney's point (located midway between the right anterior superior iliac crest and the umbilicus) with rebound tenderness.
- The pain causes difficulty with walking or when moving abdominal muscles over the inflamed area.
- Anorexia, nausea, and vomiting (common early sign but is less common in older children)
- Low-grade fever in the early stages; sharp rise with peritonitis
- Decreased or absent bowel sounds
- Constipation or small watery stools
- Irritability
- Complications can include perforation or peritonitis if appendicitis remains undiagnosed.

- Peritonitis leads to a sudden increase in fever, the release of and increase in pain, abdominal distension and guarding, tachycardia, rapid shallow breathing, and pallor, can be difficult to diagnose and can mimic other common conditions.

Diagnostics

- There is no definitive test; diagnosis is based mainly on history and physical examination.
- Blood tests mirror other common conditions.
- WBC count is elevated but is similar to counts for other types of infections.
- Urinalysis is done to rule out UTI.
- Ultrasonography and CT of the abdomen will visualize the appendix and show fluid around it.

Therapeutics

- Treatment for dehydration and electrolyte imbalance with IV therapy
- NG tube decompression if vomiting
- Preoperative antibiotics
- Appendectomy through an incision in the right lower quadrant removes the appendix.
- If perforated, abdominal lavage is done; the suture line may be left open for a drain, and a catheter may be inserted to instill antibiotics.
- Ampicillin, clindamycin (Dalacin C), metronidazole (Flagyl), or gentamicin (Garamycin) for 7 to 10 days if perforated, with an elective appendectomy at a later date

Nursing Considerations

- Preoperatively: Monitor hydration levels, administer prescribed IV fluid and electrolytes, assess the level of abdominal pain, perform light palpation only, and observe for signs of shock.
- Postoperatively: Maintain NPO, administer IV fluids and electrolytes, assess for abdominal distension and signs of peritonitis, listen for bowel sounds and observe for normal bowel movements, and provide pain management.
- If a drain has been left in to prevent infection, monitor drainage, assess for wound healing and signs of infection and fever, and apply saline-soaked wet dressings.

Constipation and Encopresis

Constipation is a common condition in pediatrics. Functional constipation occurs with disruption of the normal pattern of bowel movements, a change in regularity or consistency, or change in how easy it is to pass stool. This type of constipation has no underlying condition and occurs because of a brief illness, holding stool in due to a negative experience, or as a result of a diet lacking in fluid and fibre. Diet changes, enemas, and mild stool softeners usually solve the problem.

Pathophysiology and Clinical Manifestations

Constipation is diagnosed when a child has not passed a stool for more than 3 days, stool is hard and can be blood streaked, bowel movements may be painful, and stool is retained with or without soiling. All children have their own pattern of bowel movements.

Infants:
- Meconium should be passed within 24 to 36 hours of birth.
- Meconium plugs that have less fluid can be removed digitally or with irrigation and may be caused by lack of innervation in the bowel, hypothyroidism, meconium ileus, or obstruction resulting from CF.
- Other causes include low-fibre intake, mild cow's milk allergy, hard stools, infection of the perianal area, some antiseizure and diuretic medications, dehydration, CF, and anal or rectal anomalies.

Toddlers and school-aged children:
- Passing painful, hard stools may cause the child to withhold stool for fear of pain. This causes further dilation of the colon and decreases the urge to defecate. Subsequently, the child avoids passing stool, creating even more constipation.
- Encopresis can occur when stool is withheld and stool leaks around the stool plug, causing incontinence and embarrassment.
- When the child enters school, there is a change in toileting patterns, such as new daily schedules and a lack of privacy in the school toilets, and children can be teased if they are incontinent.
- Constipation can be caused by physical conditions such as disorders of the GI tract, neurological disorders, and decreased activity.

Diagnostics

The child needs to be assessed for any physical abnormalities or underlying psychological factors that are contributing to the constipation.

Therapeutics

- Mild constipation does not need treatment.
- Breastfed babies have fewer issues with constipation than formula-fed babies.
- Constipation usually improves when solids are introduced or fluids and fibre in the diet are increased.
- Stool softeners such as lactulose work well.
- Hard, impacted stool can be removed with suppositories, enema flushing, and occasionally propylene glycol electrolyte solution (Golytely) orally or by NG tube.
- Rectal stimulation is discouraged because it can be a negative experience and result in more constipation due to retention.
- Institute regular toileting routines for bowel relearning.

Nursing Considerations

Client and family teaching should cover diet changes to increase fibre, instituting a toileting routine, and the administration of medications, bowel irrigations, or other stool evacuation procedures.

Psychological factors need to be explored and a plan devised by the client and family.

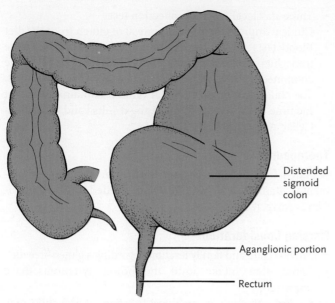

Distended
sigmoid
colon

Aganglionic portion

Rectum

Fig. 11.5 Hirschsprung's disease. (From Hockenberry, M. J., Rodgers, C., & Wilson, D. [2022]. *Wong's essentials of pediatric nursing* [11 ed., p. 698, Figure 22.2]. Elsevier.)

Hirschsprung's Disease

Hirschsprung's disease, or congenital aganglionic megacolon, is a lack of colon innervation that causes poor GI motility in the region of the colon or rectum and results in obstruction and dilatation. In rare cases, a child can be treated conservatively with stool softeners and enemas, but, generally, surgery is required to remove the aganglionic portion of the intestine. A temporary colostomy is created with a later pull-through procedure to close the colostomy.

Pathophysiology

Hirschsprung's disease is the absence of autonomic parasympathetic ganglia in one or many sections of the intestine. It may involve the entire intestine. As a result, intestinal contents collect in the abnormal part of the colon. The intestine then becomes distended because of the lack of GI motility and peristalsis.

Hirschsprung's disease is a congenital condition occurring in 1 in 5 000 births and about four times as often in males than in females. It is found in children with the genetic trait and less commonly in children with trisomy, Down syndrome, GI malformations, and craniofacial defects. There may be an accompanying tight anal sphincter, which interferes with the evacuation of stool. Figure 11.5 illustrates the dilated colon in Hirschsprung's disease.

Clinical Manifestations

Clinical manifestations vary, depending on the age of the child when diagnosed.

In neonates, symptoms are commonly as follows:
- Failure to pass meconium stools and abdominal distension in the first 48 hours
- Poor feeding and vomiting that is bile-stained
- Irritability

In infants, symptoms are commonly as follows:
- Poor weight gain
- Vomiting and bowel obstruction
- Abdominal distension, ribbonlike stools, constipation, and bouts of diarrhea

In older children, symptoms are commonly as follows:
- Chronic constipation, ribbonlike, foul-smelling bowel movements, abdominal distension, palpable fecal mass, observable peristalsis, malnourishment, and anemia and hypoproteinemia

A complication of Hirschsprung's disease is enterocolitis. The symptoms include explosive, watery stools, fever, and severe prostration. This complication can be life-threatening.

Diagnostics
- Rectal examinations show a lack of stool in the rectal area with stool overflow and a tight anal sphincter.
- Barium enema shows a dilated megacolon and a narrow distal portion in children over 2 months.
- Rectal biopsy demonstrates aganglionic cells.
- Anorectal manometry measures a lack of reflex relaxation.

Therapeutics

Most children affected with Hirschsprung's disease need to have surgical intervention. Very few can be managed with regular enemas and a low-fibre diet.

The surgery is usually very successful and is done in two stages. The bowel is resected, the aganglionic section is removed, and an ostomy is created. When the child has gained weight, a second-stage pull-through surgery eliminates the colostomy. If the bowel is not too distended, the ostomy may not be required. Some children who have a large part of the intestine involved may need a permanent ileostomy.

Following pull-through surgery, the child may have some incontinence or require bowel retraining or anal dilatation.

Nursing Considerations
- Neonate: Observe bowel movements and prepare parents for the surgery and colostomy.
- Child: Assess bowel history and patterns and observe for clinical manifestations of Hirschsprung's disease.
- If required, provide parental teaching regarding either pharmacy-prepared or correct homemade saline enemas.
- If the child is malnourished, the surgery may be delayed and managed with small, frequent, low-fibre, high-protein, and high-calorie meals; periodic enemas; and, if severely malnourished, total parenteral nutrition.
- Observe the bowel movement patterns and stool characteristics.
- Administer stool softeners and enemas as prescribed.
- Elevate the head of the bed to decrease discomfort, change the child's position frequently, and assess for respiratory distress due to abdominal distension.
- Preoperatively, prepare the child and the family for the surgery and resulting colostomy.
  - If enterocolitis develops, emergency care is required.

- Monitor the child's vital signs for signs of shock, check fluid balance and IV fluid and electrolyte therapy, administer blood derivatives if prescribed, and measure abdominal circumference and mark with a pen for accuracy.
- Assess for signs of bowel perforation, such as fever, increasing pain, irritability, dyspnea, and cyanosis.
- Postoperatively:
  - Perform NG tube decompression with suction and monitor fluid balance, including NG tube losses and stool from the ostomy.
  - Keep diapers below the suture line to prevent urine contamination.
  - Assess bowel sounds and bowel movements before oral fluids and solids are given.
  - Provide pain control.
  - Monitor wound healing and provide ostomy care.
  - Provide client and family teaching on ostomy care, signs of infection, wound care, monitoring bowel patterns and stool characteristics, signs of bleeding, and referral to home care for follow-up.

Celiac Disease

Celiac disease (CD) is a gluten-sensitive enteropathy in which the child has a permanent intolerance to grain gluten and associated proteins. Exposure to gluten causes villous atrophy in the small bowel. The most serious complication can be an increased risk of developing a lymphoma, particularly in the region of the small intestine. Management of diet with restricted intake of gluten will decrease the symptoms and the lymphoma risk. In Canada, CD occurs in approximately 1 in 100 people (Canadian Celiac Association, 2022).

Pathophysiology

CD is a genetic immune condition that causes an inability to digest the gliadin part of gluten found in wheat, barley, rye, and oats. As a result, the amino acid glutamine accumulates and is toxic to the intestinal mucosal cells. The resulting villous atrophy leads to malabsorption of nutrients due to decreased absorptive surface area.

Clinical Manifestations

- Symptoms usually appear at the age of 1 to 5 years, a few months after pasta and beans become part of the solid diet.
- Poor fat absorption causes steatorrhea and very foul-smelling stools.
- Poor absorption of nutrients can cause failure to thrive, weight loss, anemia, and muscle-wasting.
- Chronic diarrhea with abdominal distension, anorexia, vomiting, irritability, and abdominal pain is common.
- A lack of vitamin K due to malabsorption can cause epistaxis, bruising, or melena.
- Celiac crisis can occur episodically with acute, severe, watery diarrhea and vomiting.

Diagnostics

- Duodenal biopsy showing villous atrophy and hyperplasia of the crypts
- Three-day fecal fat stool collection test
- Clinical improvement with removal of gluten from the diet
- Blood tests show positive for immunoglobulin A tissue transglutaminase antibody (IgA-TTG) and need to be combined with serology tests to confirm the diagnosis. The child must be on a regular (gluten-containing) diet at the time of the testing to make the results valid (Canadian Celiac Association, 2022).

Therapeutics

A gluten-free diet is necessary for life. In addition, supplemental vitamins, iron, and folate are needed until malnutrition is corrected.

Nursing Considerations

- Provide child and family teaching regarding a gluten-free diet.
- Avoid fibre intake until the bowel symptoms have improved.
- Be aware that when the bowel is inflamed, the child may develop lactose intolerance.
- Provide a referral to a dietitian for nutritional counselling.
- Be aware that for a celiac crisis, an NG tube is inserted for decompression, and IV fluid and electrolyte imbalances are corrected.
- Teach the family that recognition of early symptoms of celiac crisis is important.

Hernias and Hydroceles

A hernia occurs when part of the bowel protrudes through an abnormal hole in the abdominal wall. In the pediatric population, it occurs most often at the umbilicus and in the inguinal canal. Hernias can occur in association with other congenital anomalies. Inguinal hernias occur most often in males than in girls and account for the majority of hernias. A hydrocele occurs when abdominal fluid is trapped in the scrotal sac.

Pathophysiology

In an umbilical hernia, the umbilical ring is not completely closed and results in parts of the omentum and intestine protruding through the opening. The opening closes spontaneously by 3 to 5 years. Surgical intervention is needed if the opening does not close or if the herniated bowel becomes incarcerated.

Inguinal hernias occur because the processus vaginalis does not close between the abdomen and the scrotum (or uterus in females), and a section of the intestine pushes downward. Incarceration results when the lower section becomes trapped in the hernia sac and the blood supply is reduced.

Emergency surgical intervention is required when a hernia is incarcerated. A hernia that is not incarcerated may still require elective surgical intervention.

There are two types of hydroceles. At birth, a noncommunicating hydrocele occurs when some peritoneal fluid is caught in the lower section of the processus vaginalis (the tunica vaginalis) with no communication with the peritoneal space. Normally, the fluid is reabsorbed and disappears in the first few months without any intervention.

A communicating hydrocele is often present with an inguinal hernia due to lack of closure of the opening in the processus vaginalis from the scrotum to the abdominal space. Surgical intervention is undertaken if the fluid is not absorbed by 1 year of age.

Clinical Manifestations

Hernias

- An umbilical hernia manifests as a soft protrusion around the umbilical region and usually can be reduced or decreased by pushing gently with a finger.
- An inguinal hernia is a painless, soft protrusion in the inguinal region that can be reduced and increases with crying, straining, coughing, or standing for long periods.
- An incarcerated hernia manifests with irritability, tenderness, anorexia, abdominal distension, and difficulty having a bowel movement. It can lead to a complete abdominal blockage, and a lack of blood flow can cause gangrene.

Hydroceles

- A noncommunicating hydrocele is a soft protrusion that does not increase with activity and is easily transilluminated.
- A communicating hydrocele is an inguinal protrusion that changes in size depending on the child's position and is not reducible.

Nursing Considerations

- Teach the family to avoid ineffective and potentially harmful home remedies such as taping a hernia.
- Teach early recognition of an incarceration.
- Inform the family that hernia repair is usually done as day surgery.

- Postsurgery family teaching: Change diapers as soon as they are damp, use an occlusive dressing to protect the incision and decrease the risk of irritation and infection, assess for signs of a wound infection, and administer analgesics as needed.
- Older children should avoid strenuous activity for about 3 weeks.

CARDIAC SYSTEM DISORDERS

Review of Circulation Changes at Birth

See Figure 11.6 for differences between prenatal and postnatal circulation.

Congenital Heart Defects

In Canada about 1 in 100 to 150 individuals are born with a congenital heart defect (CHD) (Canadian Institute of Child Health, 2022). In most cases, the cause of the CHD is unknown. Factors associated with the increased incidence of CHD include the following:

- Fetal and maternal infections in the first 3 months of gestation, especially rubella
- Chronic maternal illnesses, such as type 1 diabetes
- Exposure to toxins such as maternal use of alcohol or drugs with teratogenic effects
- Having a sibling or parent with CHD
- Chromosomal abnormality such as Down syndrome
CHDs are classified as *acyanotic* and *cyanotic*. These terms can be misleading because acyanotic cardiac conditions can also have cyanosis associated with the condition.

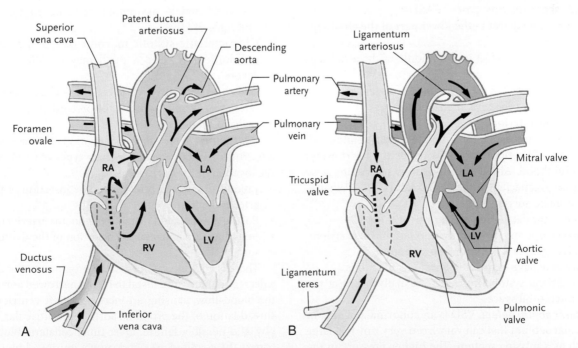

Fig. 11.6 Changes in circulation at birth. **A,** Prenatal circulation. **B,** Postnatal circulation. Arrows indicate direction of blood flow. Four pulmonary veins enter the LA; for simplicity, only two are shown here. *LA,* left atrium; *LV,* left ventricle; *RA,* right atrium; *RV,* right ventricle. (From Hockenberry, M. J., Rodgers, C., & Wilson, D. [2022]. *Wong's essentials of pediatric nursing* [11th ed., p. 737, Figure 23.2]. Elsevier.)

Acyanotic Cardiac Conditions

In acyanotic cardiac disorders, there is little or no reduction of blood flow to the lungs; therefore, deoxygenated venous blood does not enter the systemic arterial circulation. Defects that involve the left to right shunting of blood through an abnormal opening include patent ductus arteriosus (PDA), atrial septal defect (ASD), and ventricular septal defect (VSD). Malformations or lesions that obstruct or restrict ventricular outflow, such as aortic valvular stenosis, pulmonary stenosis, and coarctation of the aorta, are also acyanotic defects.

Pathophysiology and Clinical Manifestations

Patent ductus arteriosus defect. PDA occurs when the ductus arteriosus remains open, instead of closing, at about 3 to 4 days after birth. As a result, blood flows from the aorta through the PDA and back to the pulmonary artery and lungs. It usually affects premature infants but is seen in 5 to 10% of all cardiac anomalies and is more frequent in females.

Clinical manifestations

- Children with a small defect may be asymptomatic.
- A loud, machinelike murmur is common.
- The child may have frequent respiratory infections. The child may develop heart failure (HF) with tachypnea, failure to thrive, poor feeding, hepatosplenomegaly, and irritability.

Atrial septal defect. ASD occurs when atrial septal tissue does not fuse properly during fetal development, creating an abnormal opening. The pressure of blood within the heart is normally higher in the left atrium than in the right; therefore, blood shunts from the left to the right side of the heart through the abnormal opening. The right ventricle and pulmonary artery dilate because of the increased workload of more blood. There are three types of ASDs:

- Ostium primum: defect in the lower part of the atrial septum
- Ostium secundum: defect in the middle of the atrial septum
- Sinus venosus: defect in the upper part of the atrial septum near the superior vena cava and right atrium

Clinical manifestations

- Many infants are asymptomatic until early childhood; many small ASDs close on their own as the heart grows during childhood. About half of ostium secundum close on their own, especially if they are small (UCSF Pediatric Cardiothoracic Surgery, 2022).
- Symptoms vary depending on the size of the ASD.
- The usual symptoms are dyspnea and fatigue on exertion.
- Slow weight gain is also a common symptom.
- The child may have frequent respiratory infections.
- A characteristic systolic murmur is usually heard at the second intercostal space.

Ventricular septal defect. VSD is an abnormal opening in the ventricular septum that can vary from very tiny to a large defect, such as a missing septum. The higher pressure in the left ventricle causes the blood to flow through the abnormal opening to the right ventricle, leading to an increase in pulmonary vascular resistance and right heart enlargement.

Spontaneous closure of many VSDs (20 to 60%) occur especially in the infant's first year of life if they have small or moderate defects (Hockenberry et al., 2022).

Clinical manifestations. Manifestations vary, depending on the size of the VSD, the child's age, and the amount of resistance.

- The child is usually asymptomatic.
- The child fails to thrive.
- The child experiences excessive diaphoresis and fatigue.
- The child may have increased respiratory infections.
- The child may have signs and symptoms of HF.

Aortic valvular stenosis defect. A narrowing of the aortic valve causes an obstruction to the flow of blood from the left ventricle into the aorta. The long-term result is a left ventricular hypertrophy. Restricted and poor blood flow to the myocardium can develop because the oxygen need of the hypertrophied left ventricle is not met.

Clinical manifestations

- In infants with a severe defect, practitioners would expect to see decreased cardiac output, faint pulse, hypotension, tachycardia, and poor feeding.
- Older children may present with exercise intolerance, chest pain, and dizziness when standing for a long time.
- A characteristic systolic ejection murmur is heard at the second intercostal space.

Pulmonary stenosis. Pulmonary stenosis is a narrowing at the entrance of the pulmonary artery from the right ventricle. The obstruction to blood flow increases right ventricular pressure. Pulmonary atresia is the extreme form of pulmonary stenosis. Over time, right ventricular hypertrophy failure may result (Hockenberry et al., 2022).

Clinical manifestations

- The child may be asymptomatic or have a mild cyanosis and signs of HF.
- Characteristic systolic murmur may be heard over the pulmonic area, and a thrill may be felt if stenosis is severe.
- In a child with a severe defect, there is decreased exercise tolerance, dyspnea, pain in the precordial region, and generalized cyanosis.

Coarctation of the aorta. Coarctation of the aorta (COA) is a narrowing of the aorta. The three types of COA depend on the location of the narrowing:

- Preductal: Located proximal to the insertion of the ductus arteriosus
- Postductal: Located distal to the ductus arteriosus
- Juxtaductal: Located at the insertion of the ductus arteriosus

There is an increase in pressure proximal to the defect and a decrease in pressure distal to it. The narrowed aorta restricts the blood flow, causing an increase in left ventricular pressure, dilation of the proximal aorta, left ventricular hypertrophy, and possibly failure. Over time, collateral blood vessels bypass the coarcted area and supply improved blood flow to the lower part of the body.

Clinical manifestations

- The child may be asymptomatic.

- The child may have a marked difference in blood pressure and pulse quality between the upper and lower extremities. The upper extremity pulses are bounding with high blood pressure, and femoral pulses are weak or absent.
- The child may experience epistaxis, headaches, fainting, and lower leg muscle cramps.
- There is a risk of stroke, aneurysm, and ruptured aorta.
- A characteristic systolic murmur may be heard over the left anterior precordium and between the scapula posteriorly.

Diagnostics for Acyanotic Heart Defects

- Chest X-rays may show cardiac enlargement.
- Electrocardiograms (ECGs) may show an enlargement of the atria and ventricles, unclosed ductus arteriosus, size of shunts, and degrees of obstruction.
- Echocardiography can accurately detect specific cardiac conditions and may help the child avoid having to have a cardiac catheterization.
- Cardiac catheterization identifies defects and measures pressure variations.

Therapeutics

Patent ductus arteriosus defect

- This condition is managed either conservatively or surgically and has a risk of less than a 1% mortality rate (Hockenberry et al., 2022, p. 738).
- Medical management includes administration of prostaglandin–synthetase inhibitors, such as indomethacin, to stimulate closure of the open ductus.
- In clients with uncomplicated PDAs, nonsurgical management involves placing coils via cardiac catheterization to block the PDA.
- Surgical management involves ligating or dividing the PDA via a thoracotomy or clipping the PDA via video-assisted thoracoscopic surgery.
- Surgery is performed at 1 to 2 years old, or in infancy if HF is present.

Atrial septal defect

- This condition is managed either surgically or nonsurgically, with an operative mortality rate of less than 0.5% (Keenan-Lindsay et al., 2022, p. 1243).
- Nonsurgical treatment includes the placement via cardiac catheterization of a septal occluder for more centred and smaller defects.
- Surgical treatment includes the placement of a pericardial or Dacron patch, which requires a cardiopulmonary bypass and is usually done before school age.

Ventricular septal defect

- This condition is managed surgically or nonsurgically, with a mortality rate of less than 2% in uncomplicated VSDs (Hockenberry et al., 2022, p. 738).
- Nonsurgical treatment is using closure devices via cardiac catheterizations.
- Surgical treatment includes suturing small defects or placing a Dacron patch via cardiopulmonary bypass if the defect is larger.

- Palliative care, used only in children with complex cardiac anomalies, involves banding the pulmonary artery to decrease pulmonary blood flow.

Pulmonary stenosis

- This condition is managed surgically or nonsurgically and has a mortality rate of less than 1%, with a slightly higher rate in neonates (Keenan-Lindsay et al., 2022, p. 1246).
- The most common nonsurgical treatment is balloon angioplasty via cardiac catheterization. The balloon catheter is inserted into the narrowed valve, and the balloon is blown up and pulled back through the valve. The procedure dilates the pulmonary valve and improves blood flow.
- Surgical treatment consists of a pulmonary valvotomy, in which the valve is reconstructed via cardiopulmonary bypass.

Coarctation of the aorta

- This condition is managed surgically or nonsurgically, with a mortality rate of less than 5% in children with isolated coarctation (Keenan-Lindsay et al., 2022, p. 1245)
- Nonsurgical treatment, usually used in older children, is the balloon procedure to dilate the narrowed portion of the aorta.
- Surgical treatment is used in infants less than 6 months of age and in older children with a complex cardiac defect. The narrowed part of the aorta is removed, and the ends are reconnected. The alternative is to dilate the aorta using a prosthetic graft or a graft from a subclavian artery.

Nursing Considerations

Management of hypoxia

- Assess for signs of tachypnea, cyanosis, bradycardia, tachycardia, restlessness, cyanosis, grunting, nasal flaring, cough, and syncope:
  - Place the child in a knee–chest position.
  - Administer oxygen as prescribed.
  - Administer medication as prescribed.
  - Decrease the child's oxygen needs by organizing care around periods of rest, preventing crying, and providing quiet activities for the older child.

Cyanosis is apparent usually when the arterial oxygen saturation is between 80 and 85%. Cyanosis can display subjectively and varies depending on skin pigmentation, quality of light, colour of the room, and what clothing the child is wearing at the time. Children with severe anemia may not look cyanotic despite severe hypoxemia because the hemoglobin level may be too low to produce the characteristic blue colour (Keenan-Lindsay et al., 2022, p. 1255).

Management of nutrition

- Be aware that good nutrition, especially an iron-rich diet, is needed in these clients for normal growth patterns and electrolyte balance and to prevent anemia and infections.
- Provide a balanced diet rich in iron (to prevent anemia) and potassium and low in sodium.
- If the child is on potassium-losing diuretics, provide a high-potassium diet and administer potassium supplements when prescribed.

- Give small, frequent meals if the child tires easily.
- Know that the duration of breast- or bottle-feedings may need to be limited, or it may be necessary to feed the child more often for shorter periods to avoid fatigue.
- Evaluate weight gain daily.
  Assessing for signs of HF
- Observe for signs of bacterial endocarditis: fever, pallor, petechiae, anorexia, and fatigue.
- Antibiotics may be prescribed prior to dental work or before surgery or suturing repair.
- Observe for manifestations of thrombosis, including irritability, restlessness, seizure activity, coma, paralysis, edema, hematuria, oliguria, and anuria.
  Other nursing considerations:
- To decrease the risk of thrombosis, keep the child well hydrated.
- Institute infection control measures.
- Promote the child's self-esteem through self-care activities.
- Encourage activities within the child's exercise tolerance.
- Provide client and family education regarding hypoxic episodes, weight gain, exercise tolerance, avoiding infections, and medication management.
- Provide referrals to home care agencies, support groups, and follow-up care.

Cyanotic Cardiac Conditions

Cyanotic cardiac conditions are heart defects in which deoxygenated blood enters the systemic arterial circulation. Cyanotic heart defects include tetralogy of Fallot, transposition of the great vessels, truncus arteriosus, and hypoplastic left heart syndrome. In each of these defects, cyanosis is caused by the right-to-left shunting of blood through abnormal cardiac openings, resulting in a mixing of oxygenated and deoxygenated blood. Most cyanotic conditions require complex surgery.

Pathophysiology, Clinical Manifestations, and Therapeutics

Tetralogy of Fallot. Tetralogy of Fallot is the most common cyanotic heart defect, consisting of four major abnormalities: VSD, right ventricular hypertrophy, pulmonary stenosis, and aorta overriding VSD. The combination of these defects results in the aorta receiving blood from both the right and left ventricles.

Clinical manifestations and therapeutics. Manifestations vary, depending on the size of the VSD and the degree of pulmonary stenosis.

- Some infants are cyanotic at birth; others gradually develop cyanosis over the first year, with an increase in the degree of pulmonary stenosis.
- It is common for infants to have cyanotic spells, or "Tet spells," in which there is an acute cyanotic episode, especially during feeding or crying. These episodes can lead to a transient cerebral ischemia.
- After a cyanotic spell, there is a risk of emboli, seizures, and loss of consciousness.

- In older children, squatting is an adaptation that decreases the return of venous blood from the lower parts of the body, increases systemic vascular resistance, and increases pulmonary blood flow.
- The child fails to thrive.
- The child has clubbing of the fingers, exertional dyspnea, fainting, or slowness due to hypoxia.
- Characteristic pansystolic murmur is heard at the mid–lower left sternal border.
- The only treatment is surgery, either complete or palliative, if complete surgery cannot be done.
- A Blalock–Taussig shunt is inserted, which provides blood flow to the pulmonary arteries from the left or right subclavian artery via a tube graft. The shunt has the potential to distort the pulmonary artery.
- Complete repair is usually done during the first year, when there is an increasing level of cyanosis and Tet spells. A cardiopulmonary bypass and sternal entry are used. Improved techniques have reduced the surgical mortality rate to less than 3% (Hockenberry et al., 2022, p. 738).

Transposition of the great vessels. The pulmonary artery and aorta exit abnormally from the opposite ventricle. This abnormality leads to two separate circulatory patterns, in which the right heart manages systemic circulation and the left heart manages pulmonary circulation. To survive, the child must have an associated defect that allows oxygenated and deoxygenated blood to mix in the heart chambers. These infants are often referred to as "blue babies." There are many serious potential complications, including HF, endocarditis, brain abscess, and cerebrovascular accident resulting from hypoxia or thrombosis.

Clinical manifestations and therapeutics

- Varying degrees of cyanosis are seen, depending on the size of the associated defect.
- Cardiomegaly occurs within the first few weeks of birth.
- Severe cyanosis at birth
- In a child with associated defects, there is less cyanosis, but the child has HF symptoms.
- Failure to thrive
- No murmur is evident, or there is a murmur characteristic of an associated defect.
- This condition requires surgical intervention.
- Initial treatment is to provide mixing of oxygenated and deoxygenated blood.
- The administration of prostaglandin E keeps the ductus arteriosus open.
- A balloon atrial-septostomy may be performed to enlarge the ASD in order to increase the mixing of oxygenated and deoxygenated blood.
- Surgical intervention in the first few weeks of life involves performing an arterial switch, which re-establishes normal circulation, with the left ventricle acting as the systemic pump.
- The mortality rate varies, depending on the anatomy and the procedure; for neonates with intact ventricular septum, the operative mortality rate is 6% (Keenan-Lindsay et al., 2022, p. 1249).

- Long-term conditions include suprapulmonic stenosis and aortic dilation and regurgitation.

Truncus arteriosus. This is a defect of a single blood vessel instead of a separate pulmonary artery and aorta. Newborns with this abnormality may initially appear normal, but as pulmonary vascular resistance decreases after birth, severe pulmonary edema and HF usually develop. There are three types:

- Type I: A single pulmonary trunk arises near the base of the truncus and divides into the left and right pulmonary arteries.
- Type II: The left and right pulmonary arteries arise separately but in close proximity and at the same level from the back of the truncus.
- Type III: The pulmonary arteries arise independently from the sides of the truncus.

  Clinical manifestations and therapeutics
- Significant cyanosis, particularly when active
- Clinical manifestations of HF
- Left ventricular hypertrophy, dyspnea, significant exercise intolerance, and failure to thrive
- Characteristic loud systolic murmur best heard at lower left sternal border and radiating throughout the chest
- Treatment is performed in the first month of life.
- The condition requires a complex surgery that involves closing the VSD and forming conduits to establish continuity between the right ventricle and pulmonary artery.
- Postoperative complications include persistent HF, bleeding, pulmonary artery hypertension, dysrhythmias, and residual VSD.
- The mortality rate is higher than 10% (Keenan-Lindsay et al., 2022, p. 1250).
- Conduits do not grow with the child and may require one or more replacements.

  Hypoplastic left heart syndrome. Hypoplastic left heart syndrome involves a variety of abnormalities, including an underdeveloped or hypoplastic left ventricle, aortic valve, mitral valve, and ascending aorta. In order for the child to survive, the ductus arteriosus must remain open. When the ductus closes, low cardiac output leads to hypoxia and inevitable death.

  Clinical manifestations and therapeutics
- This condition is usually evident by 2 weeks of age.
- Mild cyanosis and HF become more severe with closure of the ductus.
- Signs and symptoms of HF
- Single S_2 heart sound
- Characteristic soft ejection murmur is present.
- Neonates require inotropes and stabilization with mechanical ventilation.
- Prostaglandin E is administered to maintain ductal patency and ensure adequate systemic blood flow.
- Complex two-stage surgical interventions are needed for the infant to survive.
- Prognosis for the first-stage operation varies from 5 to 10% (Keenan-Lindsay et al., 2022, p. 1250).
- If surgeries are unsuccessful, or if the defect is profound, heart transplantation may be the only option.

Heart Failure

HF results from an inability of the heart to produce enough cardiac output to meet the body's oxygen and metabolic needs. There is a decrease in myocardial contractibility, or the cardiac output is not sufficient to meet the needs of pathological conditions that require a higher cardiac output.

Pathophysiology

HF is caused by volume or pressure overload, decreased contractility, or a need for high cardiac output. There are two types of HF, right- and left-sided. Right ventricular failure occurs when the right ventricle is unable to pump effectively, causing pooling of systemic venous circulation and edema of the extremities. *Cor pulmonale* is the term for HF resulting from obstructive lung diseases such as CF or bronchopulmonary dysplasia. Left ventricular failure occurs because the left ventricle is unable to pump blood effectively into the systemic circulation. This leads to lung congestion, increased pulmonary pressure, and pulmonary edema.

Causes of HF. The primary cause in the first 3 years of age is CHD. Other causes include the following:

- Cardiomyopathies, arrhythmias, and hypertension
- Pulmonary embolism or chronic lung disease
- Severe hemorrhage or anemia
- Adverse effects of an anaesthetic or surgery, transfusions or infusions, or medications such as doxorubicin
- Increased body demands resulting from conditions such as fever or infection
- Severe physical or emotional stress
- Excessive sodium intake

Clinical Manifestations

It may be difficult to distinguish right- from left-sided ventricular failure because when one side of the heart is failing, it causes an impact on the other side.

The clinical manifestations are as follows:

- Weakness, fatigue
- Poor feeding, ascites, weight loss or weight gain from edema, and pleural effusions
- Irritability
- Pallor, cyanosis, and diaphoresis
- Dyspnea, tachypnea, orthopnea, wheezing, cough, weak cry, and grunting
- Tachycardia, cardiomegaly, and gallop rhythm
- Hepatomegaly and abdominal pain or distension
- Distended jugular, neck, and peripheral veins and edema

Diagnostics

- Chest radiology shows an enlarged heart and increased pulmonary vascular markings due to increased pulmonary blood flow.
- Blood values display dilution hyponatremia, hypochloremia, and hyperkalemia.
- Ventricular hypertrophy appears on an ECG.
- Echocardiology detects the cause of HF, such as a specific CHD.

Therapeutics

The aim of the therapeutic management program for a child with HF is to manage the HF and stabilize the condition until the underlying cause can be treated.

- Angiotensin-converting enzyme (ACE) inhibitors (such as Vasotec) reduce the afterload on the heart, making it easier for the heart to pump.
- Digoxin (Lanoxin) administered in an elixir or parenterally is the primary medication to improve myocardial contractility.
- Doses of digoxin must be exact and must be individually regulated for each client.

Nursing Considerations

- Monitor for signs of respiratory distress, suction as needed, administer oxygen as prescribed, keep the head of the bed elevated, and monitor arterial or capillary blood gas values.
- Monitor for signs of altered cardiac output, pulmonary edema, arrhythmias, including extreme tachycardia and bradycardia, and characteristic ECG and heart sound changes.
- Evaluate fluid balance by intake and output measurements, monitoring daily weights, assessing for edema and severe diaphoresis, and monitoring electrolyte and hematocrit levels, as well as maintaining fluid restrictions as prescribed.
- Prevent infections by using hand hygiene and keeping the child away from individuals with infections.
- Reduce cardiac demands by keeping the child warm, scheduling nursing interventions around rest periods, restricting infant feeding to less than 45 minutes at a time, and providing gavage feeding if the infant is fatigued or needs supplemental feeding.
- Help ensure adequate nutrition by feeding the child small, frequent, high-calorie, low-sodium meals as prescribed.
- Help decrease anxiety by providing developmentally appropriate explanations and encouraging parental involvement in the child's care as appropriate.
- Administer medications as prescribed: Digoxin is used to increase cardiac performance; diuretics such as furosemide, hydrochlorothiazide, and spironolactone to reduce venous and systemic congestion; and iron and folic acid supplements to improve nutritional status.
- Monitor for digitalis toxicity: Extreme bradycardia and increased serum levels are cardinal signs of toxicity; withhold digoxin if the child's heart rate falls below the normal range for their age.
- Provide referrals to follow-up community services as needed.
- Offer client and family teaching for signs and symptoms of HF, nutrition and fluid restrictions, and the dosage, administration, and adverse effects of prescribed medications.

HEMATOLOGICAL AND IMMUNOLOGICAL SYSTEM DISORDERS

Iron Deficiency Anemia

Iron deficiency anemia (IDA) is one of the most common nutritional disorders. IDA is most often caused by an insufficient quantity of iron in the diet, poor absorption of iron, or a significant loss of blood. Premature infants, children between the ages of 6 months and 3 years, and adolescents are most at risk. Infants fed cow's milk can develop intestinal irritation and lose blood through the stools.

Pathophysiology

- IDA is caused by an insufficient supply of iron that is required for normal red blood cell (RBC) formation.
- Lack of iron leads to smaller cells, a reduced RBC mass (microcytic), a decreased hemoglobin concentration, and decreased oxygen-carrying capacity of the blood.
- Over time, the depleted RBC mass leads to a decreased hemoglobin concentration and reduces blood capacity.

Clinical Manifestations

- The child may be asymptomatic.
- Pallor, irritability, fatigue
- Pica or eating nonfood items
- Tachycardia and systolic heart murmur
- Headaches and dizziness
- Muscle weakness and delayed growth
- Developmental delay may occur.
- Nail deformities

Diagnostics

Diagnostic blood tests include the following:

- CBC: RBC is normal or slightly decreased; hemoglobin and hematocrit are low; mean corpuscular volume (MCV) is decreased (microcytic); and mean corpuscular hemoglobin (MCH) is decreased (hypochromic).
- Erythrocyte protoporphyrin (EP) is greater than 0.75 mcml/L.
- Low serum iron capacity
- Elevated total iron binding capacity

Therapeutics

- The underlying etiology should be treated if it can be corrected.
- Adequate nutritional intake of iron is essential; boost iron intake via breast milk, iron-fortified formula, and cereal.
- Oral supplements of elemental iron should be provided to create iron stores. Ferrous iron is usually used because it is absorbed easily. Iron has adverse effects of nausea, GI irritation, anorexia, diarrhea, and constipation.
- Parenteral iron, administered intravenously or intramuscularly, is reserved only for children who do not respond to oral supplements and iron-rich diets as it is painful and expensive.
- Reticulocyte count is done after about 10 days to evaluate the effectiveness of the therapy.
- Blood transfusions are administered only to children with severe anemia.
- Supplemental oxygen is administered if the tissue hypoxia is severe.
- Some children have vitamin B_{12} deficiency and require intramuscular B_{12} injections.

Nursing Considerations

- Encourage sufficient intake of iron-rich foods, including iron-fortified formula and cereals, lean meat, fish, leafy dark green vegetables, beans, and whole-grain breads.
- Discourage milk as the predominant food source when the child is on solid food.
- Administer intramuscular injections of iron, using the Z-track method.
  Child and family teaching points regarding iron:
- Administer an oral iron supplement by giving it in two to three divided doses in a small amount of vitamin C–containing liquid (such as orange juice) before meals to enhance absorption and minimize adverse effects.
- Administer iron with a dropper to an infant or through a straw to an older child to minimize staining of the teeth.
- Brush the child's teeth after administration to minimize teeth staining.
- Be aware of the adverse effects of nausea and vomiting, diarrhea, or constipation, and dark green or black stools.
- Ensure safety precautions, as iron is very toxic.

Sickle Cell Anemia

Sickle cell anemia (SCA) is an inherited autosomal recessive disorder and a chronic, serious, hemolytic disorder found predominantly in people of African descent. With each pregnancy, there is a 25% chance of the child having sickle cell disease when both parents carry the trait. The sickle cell trait is not usually symptomatic unless there is an extreme or prolonged lower level of oxygen. SCA may lead to significant long-term complications. The major cause of death in children under age 5 with SCA is bacterial sepsis.

Pathophysiology

Low oxygen and pH in the blood trigger hemoglobin S (HgbS) to transform RBCs into a sickle (crescent) shape. Because of the sickle shape, the cells tend to clump, creating thrombosis, blockage of arteries, thickening of the blood, early breakdown of the cell, tissue anoxia, and necrosis. Acute and eventually chronic changes occur as the sickling progresses. Sickle cell crisis may be precipitated by infection, dehydration, fever, cold exposure, hypoxia, strenuous exercise, extreme fatigue, or extreme changes in altitude.

Clinical Manifestations

- Enlarged spleen because of clogging from sickled cells
- Enlarged liver, which causes pain due to poor blood flow
- Hematuria, inability to concentrate urine, enuresis, and occasionally nephritic syndrome, bone weakness, and dactylitis (symmetrical swelling of the hands and feet)
- Pain, often severe, especially during a vaso-occlusive crisis
  Complications include the following:
- Stroke
- Myocardial infarction (MI)
- Poor growth, delayed sexual maturation, decreased fertility, priapism
- Recurrent severe infections
- Splenic sequestration: A life-threatening condition in which the spleen collects a large amount of blood, causing a severe drop in blood volume and resultant shock. Symptoms include paleness, abdominal distension, pain and irritability, low blood pressure, and increased heart rate. Treatments are transfusions and splenectomy (Keenan-Lindsay et al., 2022, p. 1286).

See Figure 11.7 for the clinical features of sickle cell anemia from red cell obstruction and destruction.

Diagnostics

Blood tests:

- The Sickledex screening blood test can identify whether HgbS is present; however, hemoglobin electrophoresis is needed to differentiate between sickle cell trait and SCA.

Therapeutics

- Treatment varies depending on the specific complications for individual children.
- Standard immunizations for pneumococcal H. influenzae type b and meningococcal vaccine should be given.
- Prophylactic penicillin may be prescribed for the first 5 years to prevent life-threatening sepsis.
- Hydroxyurea decreases recurrent severe painful episodes. This may reduce long-term complications and prolong survival (Keenan-Lindsay et al., 2022, p. 1288). During vaso-occlusive crises:
  - Ensuring good hydration levels by administering IV and oral fluid to increase the blood fluid volume will help prevent sickling and, potentially, blood clots.
  - Electrolyte replacement is used to offset the acidosis caused by hypoxia, which can increase sickling.
  - Oxygen therapy is used to offset hypoxia.
  - Blood transfusions decrease the viscosity of the blood and treat anemia.
  - Morphine is administered for pain control, often via PCA, which may be used in children as young as 5 years.
  - Acetaminophen and codeine-containing compounds are administered for mild pain.

Nursing Considerations

- Monitor vital signs when the child is at rest and when active, particularly when there is reduced tissue perfusion.
- Assess for signs of HF.
- Monitor height, weight, and developmental status; growth can be delayed in children with SCA due to profound anemia.
- Carefully assess skin colour and mucous membranes, particularly in children with darker skin tones.
- Encourage bed rest or reduced activities as necessary to conserve energy and avoid overexertion to promote tissue oxygenation. Passive exercises promote circulation and ROM.
- Help the child develop coping strategies when under emotional stress and to increase oxygen perfusion.

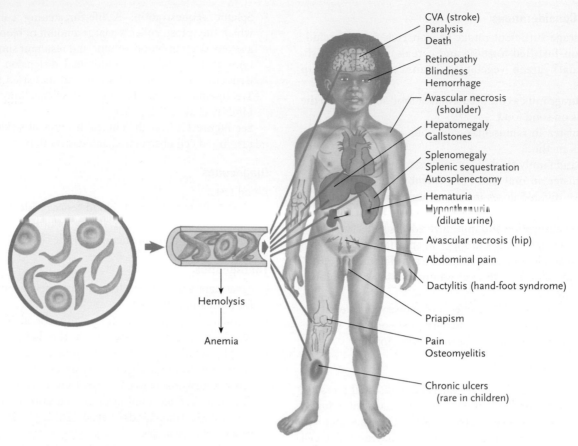

CVA (stroke)
Paralysis
Death

Retinopathy
Blindness
Hemorrhage

Avascular necrosis
(shoulder)

Hepatomegaly
Gallstones

Splenomegaly
Splenic sequestration
Autosplenectomy

Hematuria
Hyposthenuria
(dilute urine)

Avascular necrosis (hip)

Abdominal pain

Dactylitis (hand-foot syndrome)

Priapism

Pain
Osteomyelitis

Chronic ulcers
(rare in children)

Hemolysis

Anemia

Fig. 11.7 Clinical features of sickle cell anemia (SCA) from red blood cell (RBC) obstruction and destruction. *CVA,* Cerebrovascular accident. (From Hockenberry, M. J., Rodgers, C. & Wilson, D. [2022]. *Wong's essentials of pediatric nursing* [11th ed., p. 789, Figure 24.2]. Elsevier.)

- Perform pain assessment and management, with a PCA pump, if possible.
- Use pain control techniques such as heat to affected areas, relaxation, and meditation, as well as placing the child in the most comfortable position.
- Administer prescribed analgesics around the clock.
- Monitor for signs of dehydration and electrolyte imbalance and ensure adequate hydration by encouraging oral fluid intake or administering IV fluids; maintain strict intake and output and daily weight records.
- Provide a nutritionally balanced diet.
- Help the child avoid known sources of infection.
- Monitor for signs of infection and administer antibiotics as prescribed.
- Provide emotional support to the child and family, particularly in relation to issues around anger, self-esteem, positive body image, and the effects of chronic pain.
- Child and family teaching: Explain the disease process, genetic aspects, and early signs and symptoms of sickling crises and discuss home management measures for a mild crisis; how to avoid factors known to precipitate crises; the recognition of early signs of infection; the importance of regular health, dental, and eye examinations; and maintaining as normal a lifestyle as possible.
  - Provide referrals for possible genetic counselling.

Thalassemia

Thalassemia is the term used to describe genetic blood disorders characterized by insufficient synthesis of specific globulin chains of the hemoglobin molecule. The most common thalassemia is beta-thalassemia. The most serious form is thalassemia major (beta-thalassemia, or Cooley's anemia) and usually is seen in children of Mediterranean descent (particularly those of Italian and Greek heritage) or Asian descent.

Pathophysiology

- In thalassemia, a problem in the production of specific globin chains (beta) in hemoglobin ultimately results in the destruction of RBCs.
- The body tries to increase the production of RBCs to cope with the RBC destruction, but these cells are immature and break down quickly. The excess iron that is released when the RBCs disintegrate is stored in different organs, causing a condition called *hemosiderosis*.

Clinical Manifestations

- Thalassemia minor usually creates mild to moderate anemia that may be asymptomatic and often goes undetected.
- Thalassemia major produces clinical manifestations around the age of 6 months, when the protective effect of the fetal hemoglobin diminishes.

The following are signs of thalassemia (Hockenberry et al., 2022):

- Early signs include pallor, anemia, unexplained fever, poor feeding, poor weight gain, and an enlarged spleen or liver.
- Later signs include chronic hypoxia; headache; bone and precordium pain; decreased exercise tolerance; damage to the liver, spleen, heart, pancreas, and lymph glands from hemochromatosis, the excess storage of iron, which results in cellular damage in these organs; slight jaundice or a bronze skin colour; thick cranial bones with prominent cheeks and a flat nose; and growth delay and delayed sexual development.
- Long-term complications result from hemochromatosis, including splenomegaly, usually requiring splenectomy; skeletal complications, such as thickened cranial bones and an enlarged head; prominent facial bones, malocclusion of the teeth, and susceptibility to spontaneous fractures; cardiac complications, such as arrhythmias, pericarditis, HF, and fibrosis of cardiac muscle fibres; gallbladder disease; cirrhosis; jaundice and brown pigmentation due to iron deposits; growth delay; and endocrine complications, such as delayed sexual maturation and diabetes.

Diagnostics

- CBC shows abnormalities in hemoglobin and RBCs: decreased hemoglobin, hematocrit, and reticulocyte counts.
- Hemoglobin electrophoresis shows that HgbA and HgbF values are increased, confirming the type and severity of the hemoglobin variants.
- Increase in RBC precursors appears in bone marrow.
- Results show folic acid insufficiency.
- Prenatal screening is done through chorionic villus sampling or fetal blood cell analysis.

Therapeutics

- Supportive therapy with transfusions to maintain sufficient hemoglobin levels has the goal of preventing tissue hypoxia and promoting normal growth and development, more physical activity, decreased cardiomegaly and hepatosplenomegaly, and fewer bony changes and infections (Keenan-Lindsay et al., 2022, p. 1290).
- Three approved iron-chelating agents including deferoxamine, deferasirox, and deferiprone instead be used to minimize hemosiderosis (excess iron in tissues).
- Desferoxamine (Desferal), an iron chelator, is administered with transfusions.
- Home chelation therapy with desferoxamine is done 5 to 7 days a week via an IV infusion pump, usually during the night.
- Splenectomy may be necessary to decrease abdominal pressure from the enlarged spleen and increase the lifespan of RBCs.
- Amniocentesis sampling of fetal blood cells can diagnose thalassemia.
- Bone marrow transplantation (BMT) has been used with some success.

Nursing Considerations

- Administer blood transfusions and observe for complications of transfusions, which can lead to an overload of iron.
- Monitor for signs of iron toxicity related to blood transfusions: abdominal pain, vomiting, bloody diarrhea, decreased level of consciousness, shock, and metabolic acidosis.
- Administer chelation therapy and monitor vital signs, observing for hypotension or allergic reaction; visual acuity (ocular toxic) and hearing (ototoxic); intake and output; and colour of urine (may turn red).
- Provide information regarding splenectomy, if applicable.
- Administer folic acid as prescribed.
- Monitor for signs of infection and avoid sources of infection.
- Encourage the child to be careful with physical activities and to avoid situations of risk to prevent fractures.
- Promote adequate rest and good nutrition.
- Help minimize dietary iron ingestion as much as possible.
- Assess for signs and symptoms of hepatitis and iron surplus.
- Support and educate the child and family as to coping strategies and how to deal with a chronic illness and treatment protocols.
- Refer to family support groups as appropriate.
- Provide instructions for home chelation therapy (Keenan-Lindsay et al., 2022).

Hemophilia

Hemophilia is a group of hereditary bleeding disorders in which there is a deficiency in a blood clotting factor. The most common types of hemophilia are factor VIII deficiency (classic hemophilia, hemophilia A) and factor IX deficiency (Christmas disease, hemophilia B). From 80 to 85% of hemophiliacs have factor VIII deficiency. Hemophilia is mainly an X-linked recessive disorder transmitted by females or caused by a gene mutation. Hemophilia A affects less than 1 in 10 000 people or approximately 2 500 Canadians. Hemophilia B is even less common affecting around 1 in 50 000 people or approximately 600 Canadians (Canadian Hemophilia Society, 2018).

Pathophysiology

Hemophilia is classified as mild, moderate, or severe, depending on the degree of coagulation involved.

- In hemophilia A, there is a defect in the clotting function, although the factor VIII molecule is present.
- In hemophilia B, there is an impaired ability to form a fibrin clot caused by a defect or deficiency of factor IX (Hockenberry et al., 2022, p. 1290).

Clinical Manifestations

Hemophilia is initially suspected in the case of a newborn with excessive bleeding from the umbilical cord or after circumcision.

The manifestations of hemophilia include the following:

- Bruising easily and prolonged bleeding from wounds
- Nosebleeds
- Spontaneous hematuria
- Hemarthrosis (hemorrhages in the joints causing pain, swelling, and decreased ROM), which can be crippling

Complications of hemophilia include the following:

- Airway obstruction, which can occur due to bleeding into the neck, mouth, or thorax
- Bone changes, osteoporosis, and muscle atrophy from hemarthrosis
- Intracranial bleeding, which is a very serious potential complication that can lead to death
- GI hemorrhage, which can lead to intestinal obstruction
- Bleeding into the spinal cord, which can result in paralysis (Keenan-Lindsay et al., 2022, p. 1292)

Diagnostics

- The platelet count and bleeding time may be normal.
- Tests that evaluate clotting factor function, such as prothrombin time (PT), partial thromboplastin time (PTT), and whole blood clotting time, may be normal.
- Factor VII or IX level may be low.
- Prenatal diagnosis is done through amniocentesis and carrier identification.

Therapeutics

- Factor VIII concentrates acquired through genetic engineering or pooled plasma are used to replace the missing clotting factors. Home factor VIII treatments are taught to families and clients when children are old enough to perform self-administration.
- Corticosteroids are used to reduce joint inflammation and control hematuria.
- Anti-inflammatory drugs such as ibuprofen can be used for chronic synovitis but must be administered carefully because they inhibit platelets.
- Acetaminophen—with or without codeine—can be given for pain.
- Early intervention with home factor treatments is helping to prevent the severe joint damage from hemarthrosis that has occurred in the past. Exercise programs and physical therapy have also contributed to joint health.

Nursing Considerations

- Be vigilant for acute or chronic bleeding, particularly for signs of internal bleeding, such as hypovolemia and black, tarry stools, and signs of cranial hemorrhage, such as headache, slurred speech, vomiting, blurred vision, and decreased level of consciousness. This is very important.
- Assess for changes in neurological status: vision, hearing, and neurological development. This is very important.
- If there is bleeding into a joint from an injury, initiate factor treatment and the PRICE protocol (protection, rest, ice, compression, and elevation) immediately, followed by ROM exercises after the acute phase is over in order to prevent stressing and overstretching of the joint.

- Monitor for adverse effects of therapy.
- Implement a physical therapy program to help prevent joint dysfunction and injury.
- Encourage normal activities and noncontact sports.
- Support the child's self-esteem and positive self-image.
- Child and family teaching: Include home factor administration and information on support groups such as the Canadian Hemophilia Society.
  - Maintain good oral hygiene and avoid vigorous toothbrushing, which might cause gums to bleed. Recommend that clients clean their teeth by wetting a very soft toothbrush or using a sponge-tipped swab or water irrigation device.

Immune Thrombocytopenia (Idiopathic Thrombocytopenic Purpura)

Immune thrombocytopenia (ITP), formerly called *idiopathic thrombocytopenic purpura*, is an acquired hemorrhagic disorder in which the number of circulating platelets is reduced through the destruction of platelets (thrombocytopenia). There is excessive bruising or bleeding (mucosal bleeding, easy bleeding, petechiae) and the bone marrow, though normal, features an unusual number of large, young platelet cells. ITP occurs most frequently in children younger than 10 years of age with the highest incidence occurring between 1 and 6 years old. The etiology is unknown, but it is likely an autoimmune reaction and often occurs after an upper respiratory infection, measles, or chicken pox. The child usually recovers completely within 6 months. ITP can be either an acute illness, lasting 6 months or less (80%), or it can become a chronic illness that lasts longer than 6 months (20%) (Keenan-Lindsay et al., 2022, p. 1294).

Pathophysiology

The number of circulating platelets is reduced as a result of the action of an antiplatelet antibody that is produced in the spleen. This results in bleeding into the tissues. It is self-limiting.

Clinical Manifestations

- The child bruises easily, with petechiae, hematomas, and blood in the mucous membranes, stool, or urine.
- The child does not look sick.

Diagnostics

- Platelet count drops below 20×10^9/L.
- Blood tests that depend on platelet function, such as bleeding time, as well as clot retraction and tourniquet tests, are not normal.
- Several other tests may be performed to rule out disorders in which thrombocytopenia is a manifestation, such as leukemia and lupus.

Therapeutics

- Treatment is supportive, as ITP is usually self-limiting.
- Steroids can be prescribed for children at high risk for serious bleeding.
- Intravenous immunoglobulin (IVIG) may be used to increase platelet production.

- The anti-D antibody protects the platelets from destruction but can be used only if the child is not bleeding and meets specific criteria, such as having an Rh+ blood type.
- A splenectomy may be required if the child is unresponsive to treatment or if bleeding is severe (Hockenberry et al., 2022).

Nursing Considerations

- Observe for bleeding and new areas of petechiae and bruises.
- Focus on safety and injury prevention until the platelet count returns to normal.
- Avoid use of acetylsalicylic acid (Aspirin) or Aspirin-containing products, rectal temperatures, and intramuscular injections. Also, avoid antihistamines as they increase the risk of bleeding.
- Teach the importance of follow-up care to monitor the child's platelet level, usually every 1 to 2 weeks.

HIV and AIDS

HIV leads to a wide range of diseases and a variety of clinical courses. Acquired immune deficiency syndrome (AIDS) is the most serious condition of these diseases. Advances in treatments have been able to turn AIDS from a nonsurvivable disease into a chronic disease.

Pathophysiology

AIDS is caused by HIV, a retrovirus that infects a subset of T lymphocytes ($CD4^+$ T cells) and suppresses the immune system, reducing the number of $CD4^+$ T cells. Abnormal B-cell function can be detected early in pediatric HIV infection. The child with HIV cannot fight bacterial infections because helper T cells that control B-cell function have been reduced, decreasing cell-mediated and humoral immunity.

Modes of HIV transmission in children are as follows:

- Perinatally, mother-to-infant transmission occurs before or at birth and through breastfeeding. Most infected children are born to families in which one or both parents are infected. In Canada, the risk of infection for an infant whose child-bearing parent is HIV-positive is below 2%, if the pregnant person is treated during pregnancy and labour with the use of antiretroviral therapy medications (Keenan-Lindsay et al., 2022, p. 1303).
- Sexual contact from HIV-positive individuals can transmit HIV.
- Percutaneous exposure to contaminated needles can also transmit HIV.
- Transfusion of blood, blood components, or clotting factor concentrates is now a rare mode of transmission.

There is dissemination of the virus throughout the lymphoid organ. At the same time, the virus suppresses the function of the T lymphocytes, which no longer function effectively in the peripheral bloodstream. The suppression of the $CD4^+$ function creates an immune response that maintains the HIV plasma level. During the latency period, the virus does not increase in number, and in the adult population, this period can last at least 10 years.

The incubation period of a symptomatic HIV infection ranges from months to years. Over this time, the $CD4^+$ cells gradually continue to decrease in number, and, eventually, the child will develop opportunistic infections that can lead to death. In infants infected perinatally, the median age for onset of symptoms is 3 years, with the disease progressing more quickly because of the immaturity of the immune system.

Clinical Manifestations

The typical manifestations of HIV are as follows:

- Lymphadenopathy, hepatosplenomegaly, oral candidiasis, chronic or recurrent diarrhea, failure to thrive, developmental delay, and parotitis

The typical manifestations of AIDS are as follows:

- *Pneumocystis carinii* pneumonia (PCP), lymphocytic interstitial pneumonitis (LIP), recurrent bacterial infections, wasting syndrome, candidal esophagitis, HIV encephalopathy, cytomegalovirus disease, *Mycobacterium avium intracellulare* complex infection, pulmonary candidiasis, herpes simplex disease, and cryptosporidiosis (Keenan-Lindsay et al., 2022)
- Developmental disabilities: Many children with AIDS have developmental disabilities, including impaired motor skills, communication, use of language, memory loss, and behaviour changes (Keenan-Lindsay et al., 2022).

Diagnostics

- For children over 18 months, traditional enzyme-linked immunosorbent assay (ELISA) and Western blot assay tests are used.
- Accurate testing in infants is complicated due to the presence of maternal antibodies for up to 18 months; the result may be a false-positive ELISA. HIV cultures, detection of HIV–DNA sequences using the polymerase chain reaction (PCR) and identifying specific HIV antigens can be used for these infants. Most infants are diagnosed within 1 to 6 months of age.

Therapeutics

- There is currently no cure; management is primarily supportive, with treatment for opportunistic infections.
- Goals of therapy include slowing the growth of HIV, preventing and treating opportunistic infections, ensuring good nutritional support, and relieving symptoms.
- Medication regimens include combinations of the antiretroviral drugs that help prevent the production of new viral particles. New antiretroviral drugs are being developed, and the use of these in combination, as well as strict adherence to the medication regimen, prevents the development of drug resistance (Keenan-Lindsay et al., 2022, p. 1304).
- Trimethoprim-sulfamethoxazole (Septra) is prescribed as well as a prophylaxis medication of choice to prevent and treat PCP, the most opportunistic infection in this population, particularly in clients between 3 and 6 months of age.

- Children exposed to or infected with HIV should be immunized with pneumococcal, meningococcal conjugates, hepatitis A and B, and influenza vaccines as scheduled (Keenan-Lindsay et al., 2022, p. 1304).

Nursing Considerations

- Observe blood and excretion precautions (use gloves to change dressings; clean up spilled body fluids with a 1:10 bleach solution; keep garbage in a closed container; flush feces, urine, and other body fluids down the toilet; use proper containers for needles).
- Protect the child from infection, for example, by maintaining distance from people with infections, using hand hygiene, or through reverse isolation.
- Promote optimum nutrition.
- Administer antibiotics and other medications as prescribed.
- Assist the child in maintaining self-esteem, appropriate developmental tasks, and normalization of lifestyle.
- Assist with pain management.
- Provide health teaching concerning the disease and its transmission (particularly for sexually active adolescents); protection from infections; adherence to medication regimens, blood tests, and follow-up care; and referral to appropriate community agencies.
- Teach at-home body fluid precautions: Avoid mixing the ill child's secretions with those of the family; have separate linens, a separate toothbrush, a separate razor, and separate eating utensils.

Cancer

Childhood cancer is a rare occurrence in Canada, and most children diagnosed with cancer will survive. However, it is the leading cause of death from disease in children over 1 month of age. Males are more newly diagnosed with childhood cancer than females. Children less than 4 years old are twice as likely to be diagnosed with cancer than children between 5 and 14 years old. The incidence rate of childhood cancer is not increasing, the mortality rate is decreasing, and today the 5-year survival rate is on average 84%. Improved diagnostic methods and better treatment plans have improved this rate (Government of Canada, 2022b).

Cure criteria include cessation of therapy, continuous freedom from clinical and laboratory evidence of cancer, and minimal or no risk of relapse, as determined by previous experience with the disease. Time that must elapse is a period of 5 years since diagnosis (Hockenberry et al., 2022).

Pathophysiology

Categories of malignant cells include the following:
- Embryonal: Cells that arise from embryonic tissue, such as blastomas
- Lymphomas: Cells arising from the lymphatic system
- Leukemias: Cells that arise from blood-forming organs
- Sarcomas: Cells derived from connective and supportive tissue, such as bone
- Carcinomas: Those derived from epithelial cells

- Adenocarcinomas: Carcinoma of glandular tissue, such as breast tissue, prostate, lung

Properties of tumour cells include the following:
- The growth rate usually is rapid.
- Anaplasia is the loss of differentiation and organization of cells for a specific function.
- Invasion: Cancer cells invade adjacent tissue and replace normal cells.
- Metastasis: Cancer cells spread to distant sites (via the blood or lymphatic system, or by iatrogenic methods, such as biopsy) to form colonies of malignant growth.
- Competition: Cancer cells compete with normal cells for essential nutrients
- Expansion: Unrestricted growth of cancer cells compresses adjacent tissue and causes organ damage.
- Staging criteria and terminology are used.
- Criteria to describe and classify the extent of malignant neoplasms and their metastases depend on the specific tumour or treatment centre.
- Staging systems are used to guide therapy and evaluate progress (Hockenberry et al., 2022).

Clinical Manifestations

Specific clinical findings vary, depending on the particular body system involved.

The cardinal signs and symptoms of cancer in children are as follows:
- Prolonged unexplained fever, night sweats, illness
- Persistent, localized pain or limping
- Tendency to bruise easily
- Unusual mass or swelling
- Sudden changes in eye or vision
- Sudden, unexplained weight loss and anorexia
- Unexplained paleness and fatigue
- Frequent headaches, often with vomiting (Hockenberry et al., 2022).

Diagnostics

- CBC, such as increased production of immature cells, chemistry, and urinalysis
- Bone marrow aspiration or biopsy and other tissue biopsies for definitive diagnosis of cancer
- Lumbar puncture to analyze CSF for leukemic cells, as well as brain tumours and other cancers
- Imaging techniques (CT, ultrasonography, MRI, PET) to detect solid tumours and areas of metastases

Therapeutics

- Protocols may include the following therapies: surgery, chemotherapy or biotherapy, radiotherapy, immunotherapy, and hematopoietic stem cell transplant (HSCT).
- Supportive therapy, such as nutritional supplements, is needed when serious damage occurs to normal cells as the result of cancer treatment.
- Complications that may occur from therapy include oncological emergencies, such as acute tumour lysis syndrome,

hyperleukocytosis, superior vena cava syndrome, and infections (Hockenberry et al., 2022).

Nursing Considerations

- Childhood cancer has a significant impact on the family and profound psychosocial implications.
- The child and family need to adapt to living with the various phases of a life-threatening illness.
- The child's reaction largely depends on their age, the information they are given, and the physical impact of the disease on their energy level and coping skills.

Leukemia

Leukemia is the most common cancer found in children, affecting about one-third of all children with cancer. Leukemia may be diagnosed at any age but has a peak onset between 2 and 5 years. The etiology is unknown. Several genetic diseases have been associated with increased incidences of leukemia, including Down syndrome and Fanconi's hypoplastic anemia.

Leukemia is a proliferation of abnormal WBCs. There are different types of leukemia, based on the morphology of the cells and the course of the disease. Each type has a different prognosis and different characteristics.

Most leukemia in children is acute lymphoblastic leukemia (ALL), involving a proliferation of very immature WBCs, or blasts. Acute leukemia has a short history of symptoms and, without treatment, a rapidly declining course leading to death in 3 to 6 months. Acute myelogenous leukemia (AML) is less common (Canadian Cancer Society, 2022).

Pathophysiology

- Malignant leukemia cells arise from precursor cells in blood-forming elements.
- Cells accumulate and crowd out normal bone marrow elements, spill into peripheral blood, and eventually invade all body organs and tissues, depriving all body cells of nutrients necessary for survival.
- Replacement of normal hematopoietic elements by leukemic cells results in bone marrow suppression, marked by decreased production of RBCs, normal WBCs, and platelets.
- Bone marrow suppression results in anemia, decreased RBC production, the predisposition to infection due to neutropenia, and bleeding tendencies due to thrombocytopenia.
- Infiltration of reticuloendothelial organs (spleen, liver, and lymph glands) causes marked enlargement and, eventually, fibrosis.
- Leukemic infiltration of the central nervous system (CNS) results in increased ICP.
- Other possible sites of long-term infiltration include the kidneys, testes, prostate, ovaries, GI tract, and lungs (Hockenberry et al., 2022).

Clinical Manifestations

- Anemia from RBC suppression causes fatigue, tachycardia, and pallor.
- Bleeding from platelet suppression causes petechiae, purpura, hematuria, epistaxis, and melena stools.
- Immunosuppression from WBC suppression causes fever, infection, and poor wound healing.
- Reticuloendothelial involvement causes hepatosplenomegaly, bone pain, and lymphadenopathy.
- If CNS metastasis occurs, manifestations include headache, meningeal irritation, and signs of increased ICP.
- General symptoms include weight loss, anorexia, vomiting, and fever (Hockenberry et al., 2022).

Diagnostics

- CBC findings show a normal, decreased, or increased WBC count with immature cells (blasts), decreased RBCs, and decreased platelets.
- Diagnosis is confirmed with bone marrow aspiration showing extensive replacement of normal bone marrow elements by leukemic cells or biopsy.
- Lumbar puncture is performed to assess the migration of abnormal cells to the CNS.

Therapeutics

Therapy involves a combination of chemotherapy and possibly cranial irradiation therapy, provided at four levels:

1. Remission induction treatment is chemotherapy designed to eradicate the cancer cells.
2. Intensification or consolidation therapy involves the use of a combination of medications designed to eradicate any cancer cells that may remain after remission induction.
3. CNS prophylactic therapy prevents leukemic cells from invading the CNS and usually consists of intrathecal administration of chemotherapy.
   - Radiation to the brain, spinal cord, or testis is rarely done unless it is a high-risk client or there is existing infiltration of the CNS.
   - Prepubertal male clients may require androgen replacement therapy; sterility may also occur.
4. In the remission phase, maintenance chemotherapy is given to decrease the risk of recurrence.
   - If relapse occurs and leukemic cells appear in the bone marrow, reinduction therapy includes a combination of other medications not previously used. The prognosis worsens with each relapse.
   - HSCT, when successful, destroys leukemic cells and replenishes bone marrow with healthy cells. HSCT is usually done following a second relapse with ALL and is considered in the first phase for AML, which has a poorer prognosis (Keenan-Lindsay et al., 2022, p. 1298).
   - There are three categories of HSCTs:
     - *Allogenic* refers to tissue from a histocompatible donor, usually a sibling, but may also involve an unmatched donor. There is one in four chance that two siblings have two identical haplotypes and are perfectly matched. Umbilical cord blood stem cell transplantation is an established source of hematopoietic stem cells for use in children with cancer (Keenan-Lindsay et al., 2022, p. 1298).

* *Autologous* refers to tissue that is collected from the child's own tissue, frozen, and sometimes processed to remove undesired cells.

Nursing Considerations

Set realistic goals depending on the type of therapy prescribed:

* Prepare the child and family for diagnostic tests and treatments by assessing the child's level of understanding, addressing specific fears, providing information appropriate to the child's age and developmental level, and specifying what the child will see, smell, hear, and feel.
* Help prevent complications related to bone marrow suppression, such as infection, bleeding, and anemia.
* Promote optimal nutrition to maintain and rebuild healthy tissue.
* Promote adequate rest.
* Minimize the risk of infection secondary to diagnosis and chemotherapy: Avoid contact with others who have infections, monitor the child's temperature every 4 hours, practise handwashing, and avoid live plants and uncooked fruits and vegetables, which may contain pathogens.
* Prevent injury secondary to thrombocytopenia and chemotherapy.
* Minimize injections; when necessary, apply pressure to sites for 3 to 5 minutes to stop bleeding.
* Avoid rectal temperatures.
* Monitor hemoglobin and hematocrit.
* Monitor and report hemorrhagic bleeding.
* Minimize nausea and vomiting secondary to chemotherapy by administering an antiemetic 30 minutes before chemotherapy begins, continuing antiemetics as prescribed, and employing nonpharmacological measures such as visualization and music.
* Minimize discomfort from stomatitis secondary to chemotherapy by assessing the mouth frequently and providing mouth care every 2 hours using a soft toothbrush. Avoid potential irritants such as firm toothbrushes, commercial mouthwashes, and lemon–glycerine swabs, any of which can irritate the gums and mucous membranes; instead, offer cool, soothing, bland foods and liquids and administer anaesthetic mouthwashes.
* Minimize body image disturbances related to alopecia by reassuring the child that hair loss is temporary; educating them that the new hair may have different texture; using hats, soft cotton caps, scarves, and wigs; and avoiding the use of hair chemicals when hair grows back.
* Support the child and family by encouraging verbalization of concerns, fostering family support systems, and using appropriate resources.
  * Provide palliative care counselling as appropriate and use appropriate resources.
  * Encourage normal growth and development by fostering activities appropriate for the child's age and condition.
  * Provide child and family teaching.
  * Refer to appropriate home care and follow-up services (Keenan-Lindsay et al., 2022, p. 1301).

Wilms' Tumour (Nephroblastoma)

Wilms' tumour is a malignant neoplasm of the kidney, which is the most common intra-abdominal tumour in children. Wilms' tumour occurs most often in young children but may occur in adolescents. The median age at diagnosis is between 2 and 3 years, with 75% of cases under the age of 5. Siblings of children with Wilms' tumour have an increased risk of developing this cancer than do children in the general population (Keenan-Lindsay et al., 2022).

Pathophysiology

* The tumour originates in the renal parenchyma.
* It is well encapsulated in the early stages but may later extend into the lymph nodes and the renal vein or vena cava and metastasize to the lungs and other sites. Wilms' tumours are classified into five stages, from stage 1 (confined to one kidney) to stage 5 (involving both kidneys).
* Usually, the tumour is unilateral and occurs with other abnormalities, such as an absent iris or genitourinary conditions (Hockenberry et al., 2022).
* Children with stage 1 and 2 tumours (localized) have a 90% chance of cure with multimodal therapy (Keenan-Lindsay et al., 2022, p. 1327).

Clinical Manifestations

* There may be no symptoms.
* Characteristics may include a firm, nontender upper quadrant mass, fever, abdominal pain, hematuria, anemia (due to hemorrhage within the tumour), hypertension (due to secretion of excess renin from the tumour), anorexia, weight loss, and lethargy.
* If the tumour has metastasized to the lungs, shortness of breath, cough, dyspnea, and chest pain may be present.

Diagnostics

* Blood studies may show anemia secondary to bleeding from the tumour.
* Abdominal ultrasonography, CT, and MRI may disclose a mass or evidence of metastasis.

Therapeutics

* Nephrectomy, with removal of regional nodes and any resectable regional tumour, as well as the adjacent adrenal gland may be used.
* Chemotherapy may be used.
* Radiation may be used for high-risk Wilms' tumours, metastasis, residual postoperative disease, unfavorable histological characteristics, tumour rupture, or recurrence (Keenan-Lindsay et al., 2022, p. 1327).

Nursing Considerations

* Prepare the child for diagnostic tests and treatments.
* Help prevent rupture of an encapsulated tumour by avoiding abdominal palpation and by careful bathing and handling.

- Monitor bowel sounds and perform an assessment for signs and symptoms of intestinal obstruction resulting from abdominal surgery, vincristine-induced adynamic ileus, and radiation-induced edema.
- Help prevent infection by practising hand hygiene and limiting the child's exposure to persons with infections; observe for signs of infection.
- Monitor blood pressure.
- Help prevent postoperative pulmonary complications by providing frequent position changes and by encouraging coughing and deep-breathing exercises as well as ambulation.
- Therapeutic play can be beneficial in helping the child express their feelings and understand what they have experienced.
- Provide child and family teaching as for a child with leukemia.

Brain Tumours

Brain tumours include astrocytoma, medulloblastoma, brainstem glioma, and ependymoma. CNS tumours account for about 25% of all childhood cancers and are the most common solid tumors in children (Hockenberry et al., 2022).

Pathophysiology

- Tumours arise from anywhere in the cranium: glial cells (astrocytomas), nerve cells, neuroepithelium, cranial nerves, blood vessels, pineal gland, or hypophysis.
- About 60% are infratentorial, occurring primarily in the cerebellum or brainstem, and cause symptoms of increased ICP. The others are supratentorial and occur mainly within the midbrain structures (Hockenberry et al., 2022).

Clinical Manifestations

- Recurrent and progressive headache, especially on waking
- Loss of balance and coordination
- Increase in head circumference and tense fontanelles
- Behavioural changes such as irritability or lethargy
- Visual disturbances
- Severe morning vomiting and failure to thrive
- Cranial nerve neuropathy
- Signs of increased ICP
- Seizures

Diagnostics

- MRI is used to diagnose brain tumours and assess the growth of the tumour before and after treatment.
- CT permits direct visualization of the brain parenchyma, ventricles, and surrounding subarachnoid space.
- Angiography provides information about the tumour's blood supply.
- A definitive diagnosis is made by biopsy during surgery.

Nursing Considerations

- Assess for signs and symptoms when a diagnosis of brain tumour is suspected.

- Prepare the child and family for diagnostic tests and protocols.
- Prevent postoperative complications by monitoring vital signs, positioning, regulating fluids, and administering medication.
- Dressing needs to be observed for signs of drainage.
- Monitor for signs of increased ICP and seizures.
- For chemotherapy, follow the planning and interventions used for leukemia.
- Provide child and family teaching as for a child with leukemia.

ENDOCRINE SYSTEM DISORDERS

The endocrine system regulates energy production, growth, fluid and electrolyte balance, response to stress, and sexual reproduction. Most endocrine disorders are chronic in nature and require ongoing care related to health maintenance, education, development, and psychosocial needs.

Diagnostics

- Blood chemistry, including thyroid function tests and hormone, calcium, phosphorus, alkaline phosphatase, and electrolyte levels
- Urine studies, to evaluate sodium, calcium, phosphorus, and glucose levels and specific gravity
- Radiographic studies, to evaluate bone age and density and soft tissue calcification
- Genetic studies, to detect enzyme deficiencies, such as congenital adrenal hypoplasia (Hockenberry et al., 2022)

Nursing Considerations

There are important psychosocial implications for a child and family with an endocrine disorder:
- Young children may interpret treatments, such as hormonal injections, as punishment for wrongdoing.
- Injections may be a source of fear and may enhance a child's body mutilation anxieties.

Hypopituitarism

Hypopituitarism results from a diminished or deficient secretion of pituitary hormones, usually growth hormone (GH).

Pathophysiology

- Hypopituitarism may be caused by several conditions, including developmental disorders, lesions such as tumours, trauma, or certain hereditary or functional disorders, such as anorexia nervosa or dwarfism.
- The most frequent organic cause of undersecretion of GH is a tumour in the pituitary or hypothalamic region, especially a craniopharyngioma.
- Idiopathic hypopituitarism is usually related to GH deficiency.

Clinical Manifestations

- GH deficiency produces varied effects, depending on the degree of dysfunction, which include decreased linear growth, decreased muscle mass, thin hair, poor skin quality, delayed growth, excessive subcutaneous fat, hypoglycemia, and deficiencies of adrenocorticotropic hormone (ACTH), TSH, LH, and FSH, which produce effects related to the functions of these hormones.

- The chief presenting complaint is short stature.
- Children generally grow during the first year; then growth slows, remaining below the third percentile.
- Children with hypopituitarism appear younger than their chronological age.
- Premature aging is common later in life.
- Teeth may be malpositioned or crowded due to underdeveloped jaw.
- Sexual development is usually normal but delayed.
- Most children have normal intelligence.
- Emotional and academic problems are common.

Diagnostics

- Family history, including parental height, is an important predictor of the child's ultimate height.
- A history of the child's growth patterns and previous health status is required to rule out prenatal maternal disorders that affect growth, such as malnutrition, and to check for evidence of chronic illness in the child.
- Bone age is younger than chronological age.
- Definitive diagnosis is possible with a subnormal GH level.

Therapeutics

- Early diagnosis and treatment are crucial for children to achieve their genetic growth potential.
- The treatment of GH deficiency resulting from organic etiology is directed at correcting the underlying cause.
- Treatment for children with functional GH deficiency is replacement therapy. Other hormone deficiencies also require replacement therapy.

Nursing Considerations

- Monitor children for growth curves below the third percentile on growth charts.
- Prepare the child for diagnostic tests and procedures; explain that endocrine studies may require multiple blood draws.
- Monitor for early signs and symptoms of hypoglycemia, particularly during provocative tests for GH. If hypoglycemia occurs, increase the child's blood glucose level rapidly by giving orange juice.
- Administer GH replacement therapy at the same time of day.
- Assess for GH overdose, indicated by initial hypoglycemia followed by hyperglycemia.
- Promote the child's self-esteem and a positive self-image related to short stature.
- Provide realistic expectations for the child's growth and the effectiveness of GH replacement therapy and encourage the family to provide normal growth and development activities.

Diabetes Mellitus

Diabetes mellitus (DM) is a deficiency of pancreatic insulin that results in chronic high blood glucose levels and poor fat and carbohydrate metabolism. The differential diagnosis of DM has become more complex and now includes type 1 DM (T1DM), type 2 DM (T2DM), and monogenic and secondary forms of diabetes. DM is either a complete deficiency (T1DM) or a partial deficiency (T2DM) of the hormone. Type 2 diabetes in children has previously been rare, but the incidence is increasing due to the rise in childhood obesity.

T1DM is the most common endocrine disease of childhood. When pancreatic beta cells (which produce insulin) are destroyed, a lack of insulin is the result. T1DM has two forms. The first form of T1DM results from an autoimmune reaction, causing the destruction of pancreatic beta cells. This occurs when a child with a genetic predisposition is exposed to a trigger, most often a virus. The second form of T1DM is rarer and idiopathic, with no known etiology. In children with T2DM, obesity and genetic predisposition are factors. Children of Indigenous, African, Arab, Latin American, or Asian descent are at particular risk for this form of DM (Keenan-Lindsay et al., 2022). See Chapter 9, pages 211-219.

Secondary forms of DM can be due to an underlying medical condition such as CF or Cushing's syndrome. Other secondary forms are caused by treatments such as steroid and L-asparaginase. The latter form can resolve itself when the underlying conditions are treated or the medication treatments are finished. The early recognition and treatment of secondary diabetes can help improve the outcome and avoid longer term complications (Chwalba et al., 2020).

Pathophysiology

Insulin, produced by the beta cells of the pancreas, is needed to support carbohydrate, protein, and fat metabolism and to facilitate the entry of these substances into cells. The destruction of 90% or more of the pancreatic beta cells leads to a cascade of metabolic events, including hyperglycemia (increased glucagon, epinephrine, GH, and cortisol levels), lipolysis, fatty acid release, and ketone production.

- Excessive ketone production can cause diabetic ketoacidosis (DKA), a life-threatening condition characterized by marked hyperglycemia, metabolic acidosis, dehydration, and altered level of consciousness ranging from lethargy to coma.
- See the section in Chapter 9, pages 212-215, on T1DM.

Clinical Manifestations

The classic symptoms of T1DM are the three P's: polydipsia, polyuria, and polyphagia, along with fatigue. Other symptoms include weight loss, dry skin, and blurred vision. Some children present with an abrupt onset of DKA.

Diagnostics

- An 8-hour fasting blood glucose level >7.0 mmol/L or more

- A random blood glucose value of >11.1 mmol/L or more accompanied by classic signs of diabetes
- an oral glucose tolerance test (OGTT) finding of >11.1 mmol/L in the 2-hour sample
- Glycosuria
- In DKA, there is hyperglycemia, acidosis, glycosuria, and ketonuria.

Therapeutics

Treatment for T1DM in the child involves an interprofessional approach to manage the complexity of the disease and to foster self-care.

- Insulin therapy: The dose is calculated individually for each child based on carbohydrates to be consumed and blood glucose levels and is administered via subcutaneous injection or an insulin pump. Doses will be adjusted during stress, illness, exercise, growth, and puberty. Future therapies may include nasal administration of insulin and islet cell or pancreas transplantation.
- Glucose monitoring: Blood sugar must be monitored multiple times daily. There are many easy-to-use glucometers for home use.
- Glycosylated hemoglobin monitoring: Measuring glycosylated hemoglobin every 3 months is the best method for assessing glucose control.
- Nutrition: Food intake should be planned according to exercise, insulin injection times, and food preferences. Although concentrated sweets are not advised, there are no longer any absolute rules about foods that are not permitted.
- Exercise: Physical activity is encouraged; children will need to learn about food and insulin adjustments during exercise.

Nursing Considerations

- Nursing considerations are similar to those in the section "Diabetes Mellitus" in Chapter 9, pages 212-215.
- Know that children are able to learn at a young age about self-care: glucose testing, injection of insulin, and diet.
- Teach according to the developmental age of the child and include the child in health teaching.
- Teach the child and family about the signs and treatment of hypoglycemia.
- Know that children may have periods of fluctuating blood sugars with difficulty achieving stabilization. Glucose needs to be monitored frequently, along with increased follow-up with the diabetes team.
- Know that adolescents may rebel at the need for injections, glucose monitoring, and lifestyle changes. Parents and the health care team must be aware of the risk of nonadherence in these clients.

RENAL SYSTEM DYSFUNCTION

Kidney development is complete at the end of the first year. Glomerular filtration and absorption do not reach adult capabilities until between 1 and 2 years.

Kidney functions include maintaining body fluid volume, secreting erythropoietic stimulating factor (ESF), which stimulates the production of RBCs, and producing renin, which stimulates the production of angiotensin. Urine is formed in the nephron and then passes into the renal pelvis, through the ureter, into the bladder, and out of the body through the urethra.

Urinary Tract Infections

UTIs lead to inflammation, usually caused by bacterial infections, of the urethra (urethritis), bladder (cystitis), ureters (ureteritis), or kidneys (pyelonephritis). UTIs occur in 1% of boys and 1 to 3% of girls (Keenan-Lindsay et al., 2022). UTIs are more common in uncircumcised male infants younger than 3 months of age, and female infants younger than 12 months of age (Hockenberry et al., 2022).

Pathophysiology

- In uncomplicated UTI, inflammation usually is confined to the lower urinary tract.
- Recurrent cystitis may produce anatomical changes in the ureter that lead to vesicoureteral valve incompetence and resultant urine reflux, conditions that provide organisms with access to the upper urinary tract.
- Pyelonephritis usually results from an ascending infection from the lower urinary tract and can lead to acute and chronic inflammatory changes in the pelvis and medulla, with scarring and loss of renal tissue. Recurrent or chronic infection results in increased fibrotic tissue and kidney contraction.
- *E. coli* and other Gram-negative organisms account for most UTIs.
- In the neonate, the urinary tract may be infected via the bloodstream; in older children, bacteria ascend the urethra.
- There is an increased incidence of UTI in females due to the shorter urethra and proximity to the anus.
- The incidence of UTI in male infants is often due to congenital malformations of the urinary tract and should be investigated.
- Contributing factors include urinary stasis, urinary reflux, poor perineal hygiene, pregnancy, noncircumcision, indwelling catheters, tight clothes or diapers, bubble baths, antimicrobial agents that alter normal urinary tract flora, local inflammation, such as vaginitis, and sexual intercourse.

Clinical Manifestations

Manifestations vary, depending on age and the location of the infection. Approximately 40% of UTIs are asymptomatic.

- Infants: Fever, weight loss, failure to thrive, vomiting, and diarrhea
- Older children: Dysuria, frequency, urgency, incontinence, foul-smelling urine, abdominal pain, and possibly hematuria
- Pylenonephritis: Fever, chills, flank pain, and costovertebral abdominal tenderness

Diagnostics

- Urinalysis: Urine is tested for hematuria, proteinuria, and pyuria.
- Urine characteristically has a foul odour, cloudiness, and strands of mucus.
- Diagnosis is confirmed by bacteria in urine culture.

Therapeutics

- Antibiotics such as penicillins, sulphonamides (including trimethoprim-sulfamethoxazole [Septra]), cephalosporins and nitrofurantoin (Teva-Nitrofurantoin), are prescribed to treat a current disease or to provide prophylaxis, depending on the sensitivity identified through urine culture.
- All antibiotics can eventually cause resistant strains.

Nursing Considerations

- Evaluate urinary status by observing the appearance and odour of urine and by noting signs and symptoms such as frequency, burning, enuresis, urinary retention, or flank pain. Follow-up urine cultures may be required.
- Maintain sterile technique when performing urinary catheterization.
- Provide comfort measures: analgesics, antipyretics, and urinary anaesthetics.
- Encourage increased fluid intake to reduce fever and dilute urine.
- Employ and teach preventive measures, including good perineal hygiene, cleaning a girl from the urethra back toward the anus, avoiding irritants such as bubble bath and tight clothing, wearing cotton underwear instead of synthetics such as nylon, maintaining adequate fluid intake, voiding regularly and completely emptying the bladder with each urination, and maintaining acidic urine by drinking beverages such as cranberry juice and blueberry juice.
- Drinking cranberry juice or blueberry juice helps prevent bacteria from sticking to the bladder and urethra walls, in turn minimizing the incidences of UTIs. Research now shows that acidic urine is not the reason for UTIs but rather the sticking of bacteria. This nonsticking effect works to prevent UTIs.
- For the sexually active adolescent, teach the importance of voiding both before and after sexual intercourse.

Vesicoureteral Reflux

Vesicoureteral reflux (VUR) occurs when there is a backward flow of urine in the urinary tract when voiding. VUR does not cause UTI, but it does increase the risk that a lower UTI will develop into a pyelonephritis (Hockenberry et al., 2022).

Pathophysiology

- VUR usually occurs a result of an incompetent valvular mechanism at the ureterovesicular junction.
- VUR is graded according to the degree of reflux from the lower ureter to the kidney.
- VUR is a major cause of renal damage; refluxed urine ascending into the collecting tubules of nephrons initiates renal scarring from infective organisms.

- If the amount of refluxed urine is large, the child feels an urge to void shortly after having urinated.
- If the amount is small, it may remain in the bladder, causing urinary stasis and increasing the risk of infection.
  VUR causes:
- Primary reflux results from congenital abnormalities at the point of insertion of the ureters into the bladder.
- Secondary reflux results from infection and ureterovesicular junction incompetency; it may also result from neurogenic bladder or progressive dilation of ureters following surgical urinary diversion (Keenan-Lindsay et al., 2022, p. 1316).

Clinical Manifestations

- Dysuria
- Urinary frequency, urgency, and hesitancy
- Urine retention
- Cloudy, dark, or blood-tinged urine

Diagnostics

- Urinalysis may reveal RBCs or pyuria.
- Structural abnormalities may be detected by intravenous pyelogram (IVP), voiding cystourethrography, and cystoscopy.

Therapeutics

- Antibiotics and urinary antiseptics
- Possible antireflux surgery, involving the reimplantation of ureters

Nursing Considerations

- Administer or teach parents to administer prescribed medications, such as continuous low-dose antibiotics, usually given as nitrofurantoin (Teva-Nitrofurantoin) or trimethoprim-sulfamethoxazole (Septra).
- Encourage increased fluids to dilute urine and develop a regular (3-hour) voiding plan.
- Encourage a high-fibre diet to prevent constipation and to facilitate muscular relaxation, thereby helping to reduce residual urine.
- Some children with a lower grade reflux can have endoscopic correction instead of a surgical procedure.
- As appropriate, explain antireflux surgery, involving reimplantation of ureters.
- Provide preoperative and postoperative care after antireflux surgery:
  - Observe and protect urinary drainage tubes, in-dwelling catheters, suprapubic catheters, and ureteral stents.
  - Considerations are as in a child with UTI (Hockenberry et al., 2022).

Nephrotic Syndrome

Nephrotic syndrome can occur as a primary disease known as idiopathic nephrosis, childhood nephrosis or minimal-changed nephrotic syndrome (MCNS), a secondary disorder that is a clinical manifestation after or in association with glomerular damage that has a known or presumed cause; or a congenital form inherited as an autosomal recessive disorder (Hockenberry et al., 2022).

This disorder is characterized by massive proteinuria, hypoalbuminemia, dyslipidemia, altered immunity, and edema. MCNS is the most common type, and the prognosis is unusually good because it is self-limiting and usually responds to steroidal therapy (Hockenberry et al., 2022).

Pathophysiology

- Pathogenesis in MCNS is not understood, but a disturbance in the membrane of the glomeruli causes an increased permeability to protein.
- Proteins, especially albumin, leak through the glomerular membrane and are excreted in the urine.
- Once the albumin is excreted, colloidal osmotic pressure decreases, allowing fluid to escape from the intravascular spaces to the interstitial spaces, resulting in ascites in the abdomen.
- The plasma volume decrease stimulates the antidiuretic hormone (ADH) and aldosterone to reabsorb water and increase the intravascular volume.
- Secondary nephrotic syndrome usually occurs after glomerular damage of known or presumed cause (e.g., due to systemic lupus erythematosus, DM, or sickle cell disease).

Clinical Manifestations

- Manifestations may include periorbital, pedal, and pretibial edema initially, progressing to generalized edema (anasarca), weight increase, ascites, pleural effusion, decreased urine output, pallor, anorexia, fatigue, abdominal pain, and diarrhea.
- With significant edema, the child may appear pale and have respiratory distress.
- Blood pressure may be normal or slightly decreased.
- Children are more prone to infection from decreased immunity.

Diagnostics

- Urinalysis shows marked proteinuria, hyaline casts, few RBCs, and high urine specific gravity.
- The serum protein level is markedly decreased, especially the albumin level.
- A renal biopsy may be performed.

Therapeutics

- Diuretics such as loop diuretics, usually furosemide (Lasix) in combination with metolazone (Zaroxolyn), are sometimes effective, and restrictions are placed on high-sodium foods and salt to manage edema.
- Prednisone (Apo-Prednisone) is usually prescribed for 3 months to reduce proteinuria.
- Immunosuppressant therapy (usually cyclophosphamide [Procytox]) is recommended for the child who fails to respond to steroids. Immunosuppressants decrease the rate of relapse but can have long-term implications, particularly in terms of causing male sterility if used for more than 2 to 3 months.
- A broad-spectrum antimicrobial agent may be given if infection is present.

- Plasma expanders, such as salt-poor albumin, may be needed to manage severe edema (Hockenberry et al., 2022).

Nursing Considerations

- Assess for a decrease in blood volume by monitoring for increased edema and by measuring abdominal girth, weight, intake and output, blood pressure, and pulse rate. Test urine for protein and specific gravity.
- Monitor for signs of infection and take precautions to prevent infection (the child is susceptible to secondary infection because immunoglobulin is lost in the urine).
- Promote skin integrity by checking areas of edema for skin breakdown, ensuring frequent position changes, using scrotal supports for boys, and providing good skin care.
- Provide a high-protein, high-calorie diet without added salt. Fluids may be restricted if severe edema is present.
- Conserve the child's energy by encouraging bed rest and quiet activities.
- Perform urine testing for albumin.
- Provide parent and child teaching such as monitoring for relapses and signs of infection, medication administration, urine testing, and signs of skin breakdown.

Acute Glomerulonephritis

Acute glomerulonephritis (AGN) is an immune complex disease that may be a primary condition or can be symptomatic of a systemic disorder. It is likely caused by an immune injury secondary to *Streptococcus*, pneumococci, and viruses. Recovery occurs in most cases.

Acute poststreptococcal glomerulonephritis (APSGN) is the most common form. APSGN can occur at any age but is usually seen in school-aged children, peaking at 6 to 7 years. It is uncommon in children under the age of 2.

The majority of infections do not cause AGN. A latent period of 10 to 21 days occurs between the infection—usually of the throat or skin—and the onset of clinical symptoms.

Pathophysiology

It is speculated that the original infectious organism releases material into the circulation that is antigenic, and antibodies are formed in response. Antibodies interact with antigens that remain in the glomeruli, leading to immune complex formation and tissue injury, a decrease in filtration, and reduced excretion of sodium and water (Hockenberry et al., 2022).

Clinical Manifestations

Manifestations appear approximately 10 to 21 days after an infection, although some children do not appear to have been ill. These include mild to moderate or high blood pressure, pallor, irritability, fatigue, lethargy, periorbital and generalized edema, weight gain, oliguria, and hematuria (urine is brown—cola- or tea-coloured—and cloudy), costovertebral tenderness, and anorexia.

Diagnostics

- Urinalysis: Urine contains RBCs, epithelial cells, granular casts, WBCs, and protein.
- Serum chemistry: Results show elevated BUN and creatinine levels, elevated erythrocyte sedimentation rate (ESR), and elevated antistreptolysin O (ASO) titre and complement level (C3).
- Cultures of the pharynx are done on the child and family members, and if there is a positive culture of group A streptococci, all family members should be treated with an antistreptococcal agent.
- A renal biopsy is not usually performed unless an atypical nephritis is suspected.

Therapeutics

- Treatment usually includes medications to control hypertension, decrease fluid overload, and treat infection.
- Treatment for severe hypertension includes calcium channel blockers, beta blockers, or ACE inhibitors.
- Treatment for mild or moderate hypertension involves loop diuretics.
- Diuretics, usually furosemide (Lasix), are given for edema and fluid overload if no renal failure is present.
- The diet is usually no added salt; if edema is present or the client is hypertensive, there may be moderate sodium restrictions. During periods of oliguria, potassium is also restricted. Protein is restricted only if severe azotemia has developed due to prolonged oliguria.
- Antibiotics are used to treat an existing streptococcal infection.
- Rarely, dialysis may be required to manage severe AGN or heart failure.
- Caloric intake may be increased to balance protein breakdown.
- Diuresis indicates the beginning of recovery.

Nursing Considerations

- Assess fluid status by monitoring intake and output, recording daily weights, and monitoring for edema.
- Closely monitor blood pressure and respiratory rate to identify early signs of complications.
- Administer medications and observe for adverse and therapeutic effects.
- Maintain adequate caloric intake and nutrition with any dietary restrictions.
- Provide child and family teaching on the need for medical follow-up for urine testing and blood pressure monitoring, as well as on home care measures, including activity and diet instructions, infection prevention measures, and the signs and symptoms of potential complications.

Enuresis

Enuresis is repeated involuntary urination, usually at night, in a child who should have bladder control (usually by age 4 or 5). Enuresis is primary when the child has never achieved continence and secondary if the child starts bedwetting after continence is achieved. Boys are affected more than girls, and night-time bedwetting usually stops between the ages of 6 and 8 years. Nocturnal enuresis may have a familial component; 90% of children with enuresis have a first-degree relative with the condition (Hockenberry et al., 2022).

Pathophysiology

Enuresis is primarily a condition of delayed or incomplete neuromuscular maturation of the bladder. Most children with enuresis sleep long periods as infants and have a family history of enuresis. The condition is benign and self-limiting.

Therapeutics

- Bladder retention training, motivational therapy, or behaviour modification
- Drug therapy, such as imipramine, which has an anticholinergic effect on the bladder, or desmopressin (DDA VP) nasal spray, which decreases night-time output
- Urine-alarm mattresses, which sound an alarm when wet and can be very effective

Nursing Considerations

- Help the family accept the child's condition and avoid placing blame or adopting attitudes that may foster feelings of low self-esteem in the child.
- Discuss strategies to manage night-time incontinence, such as rubber sheets on beds. Suggest the use of incontinence "pull-ups," which do not look like diapers.

Hypospadias

Hypospadias occurs when the urethral opening is located below the glans penis or anywhere along the ventral surface (underside) of the penile shaft. The rate of occurrence is approximately 1 in 250 newborns. Testes are undescended in approximately 10% of boys with hypospadias, and inguinal hernias are a common associated finding.

Pathophysiology

- The urethral folds fail to fuse completely over the urethral groove.
- Ventral foreskin is lacking, and the distal segment looks like a hood.

Clinical Manifestations

- Abnormal placement of the meatus should be evident at birth.
- In mild cases, the meatus is just below the tip of the penis.
- In severe cases, the meatus is located on the perineum between the halves of the scrotum.
- Chordee (a ventral curve of the penis) results from the replacement of normal skin with fibrotic tissue and usually accompanies severe hypospadias.
- Severe hypospadias with undescended testes must be differentiated from ambiguous genitalia.

Therapeutics

Surgical repair improves the child's ability to stand when urinating and to urinate in a straight stream and improves the appearance of the penis, as well as preserving sexual adequacy. It is usually performed at 6 to 12 months of age to avoid issues with body image.

Nursing Considerations

- Inform the parents to avoid circumcision as the foreskin is usually used for surgical repair.
- Allow the parents to verbalize their feelings about the child's condition.
- Prepare the parents and child for the surgical procedures and the possibility of urinary diversion while the new meatus is being constructed.
- Prepare the parents for the expected cosmetic result and show them pictures of successful repairs.
- Monitor intake and output and urinary patterns, encourage fluids, maintain patency, and prevent and observe for infection if the child is catheterized postoperatively.

MUSCULO-SKELETAL AND NEUROMUSCULAR DYSFUNCTION

Bone growth occurs in diameter and length. Growth in bone length occurs at the epiphyseal plate, a vascular area of active cell division. These cells are highly sensitive to the impact of GH, estrogen, and testosterone. In adolescence, the epiphyseal plate turns to bone and growth stops.

In children, the epiphyseal plate represents an area of bone weakness that is prone to injury through fracture, crushing, or slippage. Injury to the epiphyseal plate can disturb bone growth. Because a child is still growing, some bony deformities due to injury can be remodelled or straightened over time. Conversely, this can also cause some deformities to worsen with growth.

Because a child's bones are more plastic than an adult's, more force is required to fracture a bone, and specific forces may produce different types of fractures. A child's bones generally heal much faster than those of an adult, often greatly reducing the time required for immobilization.

Pathophysiology

Physical activity is essential for the growth and development of bones and muscles. Conditions that may limit mobility include congenital defects, degenerative neurological disorders, integumentary disorders, musculo-skeletal trauma, imposed bed rest to assist healing and restoration, and mechanical restraint as part of therapy.

Clinical Manifestations

General signs and symptoms of musculo-skeletal disorders in children are as follows:
- Joint contracture and pain
- Muscular atrophy and weakness
- Fatigue

- Diminished reflexes
- Delayed healing
- Orthostatic hypotension
- Thrombus formation
- Shallow respirations
- Anorexia and constipation
- Renal calculi
- Urinary incontinence or signs of urinary infection
- Skin breakdown and pressure ulcers
- Sensory changes

Diagnostics

- Radiographs (the most common study to assess injury and healing)
- CT scan
- Bone scan
- Arthrography and arthroscopy
- Joint aspiration
- Electromyography (EMG)

Therapeutics

- Therapy is specific to the disorder.
- Immobilization may be required to stabilize disrupted muscle or protect bone integrity.

Nursing Considerations Related to Immobilization

- Know that treatment for musculo-skeletal conditions often require immobilization (casts, traction, or body frames), which can be frightening and painful.
- Know that play, social interaction, and self-care help the immobilized child gain self-esteem and independence and promote normal growth and development.
- Protect skin integrity by turning the child frequently and inspecting the skin for early signs of breakdown.
- Promote adequate hydration and nutrition by offering high-protein, high-calorie foods in small, frequent amounts.
- Promote bowel elimination by encouraging fluids and a high-fibre diet. Administer stool softeners as prescribed.
- Promote urinary elimination by encouraging fluids, monitoring intake and output, and assessing for bladder distension.
- Prevent respiratory complications by keeping the child well hydrated, changing the child's position frequently, and encouraging deep-breathing exercises.
- Protect the child from injury by moving and positioning the child carefully and by monitoring physical activities closely; postural hypotension and falling may result if the child resumes usual activities too quickly.
- Help prevent UTIs by keeping the child well hydrated, promoting frequent voiding, providing foods such as blueberry juice and cranberry juice, which prevents bacteria from sticking to the epithelium in the bladder area, and limiting high-calcium foods.
- Prevent contractures by maintaining proper body alignment and providing ROM exercises.

- Administer medications, which may include antibiotics to treat infection; diuretics to remove high levels of calcium; calcium-mobilizing drugs; anticoagulants to prevent clot formation; and stool softeners to prevent constipation. Be alert for the adverse effects of these medications.
- Be aware that preschoolers may view immobilization as punishment.
- Provide child and family teaching as appropriate, such as cast care, positioning, skin care, nutrition, and hydration to repair bone and muscle damage and prevent constipation and UTIs, as well as how to observe for thrombus and circulatory conditions and what medical follow-up is required.

Developmental Dysplasia of the Hip

Developmental dysplasia of the hip (DDH) is a spectrum of hip abnormalities that may arise in the fetus, infant, or child. Hip instability may involve subluxations and dislocations, which, if uncorrected, will lead to permanent disability. The etiology of DDH is unknown, but predisposing factors may be categorized as physiological (lax joints due to maternal hormones), genetic (family history), and mechanical (breech birth). DDH occurs most often in females and a positive family history increases a child's risk of having DDH (Hockenberry et al., 2022).

Pathophysiology

- Subluxation, the most common form of DDH, is defined as an incomplete dislocation, in which the femoral head remains in contact with the acetabulum, but a stretched capsule and ligament tears cause the head of the femur to be partially displaced.
- Dislocation describes the situation in which the femoral head loses contact with the acetabulum and is displaced posteriorly and superiorly over the fibro-cartilaginous rim.

Clinical Manifestations

- In the newborn: Ortolani's sign, Barlow's sign, asymmetrical gluteal folds, limited abduction of affected hip
- In older children: limp, Trendelenburg's sign

Diagnostics

- Radiographic examination is not reliable until between 3 and 6 months of age.
- Ultrasonography may be helpful in diagnosing dysplasia in the newborn.

Therapeutics

Newborn to 6 months. The infant is usually placed in a Pavlik harness, which centres the femoral head into the acetabulum in flexion and deepens the acetabulum by pressure.
- The harness is worn continuously until the hip joint is clinically and radiographically stable.
- By 3 to 6 months, the child usually is transferred to a protective abduction brace, which is worn for less than a year.

Six to 18 months. The child is placed in traction for gradual reduction, followed by cast immobilization until the joint is stable. If soft tissue blocks reduction, an open reduction is performed, followed by a spica cast for 4 to 6 months. Then an abduction splint is worn.

Older children. Correction is difficult because secondary changes create complications.
- Surgical reduction is required.
- Reduction and reconstruction are more challenging in children older than 6 years of age because of severe shortening and contracture of muscles and deformity of the femoral and acetabular structures (Hockenberry et al., 2022).

Nursing Considerations

- Provide care as indicated in the section "Nursing Considerations Related to Immobilization."
- Teach parents how to apply and maintain the reduction device.
- Be aware that children may be prone to putting toys, food, etc. inside the cast.
- Petal cast edges with waterproof tape, particularly in the diaper area.
- Place a disposable diaper beneath the entire perineal opening in the cast.
- Provide child and family teaching regarding holding techniques, moving, feeding, care of restrictive devices, and signs and symptoms of complications such as increased temperature, pain or blood on voiding, and difficulty breathing.

Cerebral Palsy

Cerebral palsy (CP) is a group of neurological disorders caused by injury or insult to the brain either before or during birth or in early infancy. CP has an early onset, and there is abnormal muscle tone and coordination. CP is the most common permanent disability in childhood. Risk factors include prematurity, asphyxia, ischemia, perinatal trauma, congenital and perinatal infections, and perinatal metabolic conditions, such as hyperbilirubinemia and hypoglycemia. Infection, trauma, and tumours can cause CP in early infancy. For most babies born with CP, the cause is unknown (Hockenberry et al., 2022). The estimated occurrence in Canada is 1.5 to more than 4 for every 1 000 births. CP can range from mildly hypertonic muscles to severe physical and neurological impairment (Hockenberry et al., 2022).

Pathophysiology

- Disabilities usually result from injury to the cerebellum, the basal ganglia, or the motor cortex.
- CP is nonprogressive but may become more apparent as the child grows older.
- It can be difficult to establish the precise location of neurological lesions because with a few exceptions, there is no typical pattern of pathology. In some children with CP, there is gross brain malformation, and in others, there is vascular occlusion, neuron loss, and laminar degeneration.

- Anoxia appears to be an important factor in neurological damage.
- CP is often secondary to a wide range of causative factors (Hockenberry et al., 2022).

Classification of CP

- Spastic: This type is the most common and may involve one or both sides. It involves upper motor neuron muscular weakness with intact reflex arc, increased stretch reflexes, increased muscle tone, and often weak muscles. Hallmarks include hypertonicity with poor control of posture, balance, and coordinated movement; impairment of fine and gross motor skills; and active attempts at motion increase abnormal postures and the overflow of movement to other parts of the body. In the infant up to 1 year, hypotonia is present; then spasticity begins to develop.
- Dyskinetic: This type is defined by abnormal involuntary movements that disappear in sleep and increase when the child is stressed; the major manifestation is athetosis (wormlike movement), in addition to dyskinetic movement of the mouth, drooling, dysarthria, and choreiform (jerky) movements.
- Ataxic: This type is characterized by a wide-based gait, rapid, repetitive movements performed poorly, and disintegration of movements of the upper extremities when the child reaches for objects.
- Mixed type: This type features a combination of spasticity and athetosis (Hockenberry et al., 2022).

Clinical Manifestations

- The most common clinical manifestation is universal delayed gross motor development.
- Additional typical manifestations include abnormal motor performance (early dominant hand preference, abnormal and asymmetrical crawl, poor sucking, feeding problems, and persistent tongue thrust), poor head control after 3 months, alterations of muscle tone (such as increased or decreased resistance to passive movements, the child feels stiff when they are being handled or dressed, difficulty in diapering, and opisthotonos), abnormal postures (such as scissoring the legs or persistent infantile posturing), and reflex abnormalities (persistent primitive reflexes, such as tonic neck or hyper-reflexia).
- Behavioural manifestations include extreme irritability, little interest in the environment, and sleeping for unusually long periods.
- Associated disabilities include intellectual delays, seizures, attention deficit disorder, and sensory impairment (Hockenberry et al., 2022).

Diagnostics

- Perinatal history
- Persistence of primitive reflexes
- Neurological examination
- Related diagnostic tests, such as MRI, to rule out other pathologies

- Assessment tools to evaluate muscle spasticity include Modified Ashworth scale, Functional Independence Measurement, elastography, and myotonometry.

Therapeutics

Although there is no cure, the child can be assisted to reach their optimum developmental potential.

- Therapeutic goals are as follows:
  - To establish locomotion, communication, and self-help
  - To gain optimal appearance and integration of motor functions
  - To correct associated deficiencies as effectively as possible
  - To provide educational opportunities based on the child's needs and abilities
  - Promote socialization experiences with affected and unaffected children
- Successful therapy relies on a multidisciplinary approach and collaboration among health care team members to manage various aspects of treatment.
- The child may require orthotic devices, such as braces, splints, or casting.
- The child may use assistive and adaptive devices, such as walkers, scooters, motorized wheelchairs, communication boards, and computers.
- Medications for spasticity, pain, seizures, and constipation may be required.
- Adaptive education and learning programs and educational support services should be investigated.
- Speech and language therapy may be employed.
- Physical and occupational therapy may be recommended.
- Some children may require surgery, such as tendon transfers, to correct deformities and decrease spasticity (Hockenberry et al., 2022).

Nursing Considerations

- Prevent injury by providing the child with a safe environment, appropriate toys, and protective gear (helmet, knee pads), if needed.
- Minimize physical deformity by ensuring the correct use of braces and other assistive devices and by providing ROM exercises.
- Promote mobility by encouraging the child to be involved with age- and condition-appropriate motor activities.
- Ensure good nutrition by providing a high-protein, high-calorie diet.
- Administer prescribed medications, which may include sedatives, muscle relaxants, anticonvulsants, and analgesics.
- Encourage self-care by urging the child to participate in activities of daily living (ADLs) that are appropriate for the child's age and condition; normalize as much as possible.
- Facilitate communication by talking to the child directly and slowly, using pictures to reinforce speech, and using communication devices.
- Encourage early speech therapy to prevent poor or maladaptive communication habits and to provide a means of articulate speech; technology, such as computer use, may help children with severe articulation impairments.

- Seek referrals as necessary for corrective lenses and hearing devices to decrease sensory deprivation related to vision and hearing deficits.
- Help promote a positive self-image in the child by praising their achievements and appearance, setting realistic goals, and encouraging their involvement with age- and condition-appropriate peer group activities.
- Refer the family to support organizations, such as the March of Dimes, or provincial or territorial cerebral palsy organizations.
- Discuss with the parents that achievement of new tasks will require patience and help from caregivers.
- Encourage the family to seek appropriate functional, adaptive, and vocational education for the child.
- Encourage family members to achieve balance in their lives between caring for the disabled child and pursuing other family and personal interests.
- Facilitate respite care as appropriate (Keenan-Lindsay et al., 2022).

Duchenne Muscular Dystrophy

Duchenne muscular dystrophy (DMD) is the most common and severe form of a group of disorders that cause progressive degeneration and weakness of skeletal muscles. Half of all cases are X-linked, and males are almost exclusively affected. Muscle weakness is progressive, and the disorder is eventually fatal, usually in adolescence, due to infection or cardiopulmonary failure. The incidence is 1 in 3 500 births (Hockenberry e al., 2022).

Pathophysiology

DMD occurs when a gene mutation occurs in the gene that encodes dystrophin. Dystrophin, a protein product in skeletal muscle, is absent in the muscles of children with DMD. This lack of dystrophin leads to a gradual degeneration of muscle fibres and is characterized by progressive weakness and muscle-wasting.

Clinical Manifestations

- Symptoms begin between the ages of 3 and 5, starting with weakness in the pelvic girdle.
- Key manifestations are delays in motor development; delayed walking and difficulties in running, riding a bicycle, and climbing stairs are among the first symptoms reported.
- Later, a waddling gait, lordosis, and difficulty sitting and standing up appear as muscles degenerate.
- Gowers' sign may appear: From a supine position, the child rolls over, kneels, and presses their hands against the ankles, shins, knees, and thighs in a "climbing" action to rise to a standing position.
- Profound muscular dystrophy appears in later stages, commonly with deformities and contracture in the large and small joints; by age 12, children with the disorder are usually unable to walk.
- Eventually, the diaphragm and accessory muscles are affected and cardiomegaly usually appears. Respiratory or cardiac failure is often the cause of death.

Diagnostics

- Blood test shows increased serum creatinine phosphokinase.
- Muscle biopsy discloses degeneration of muscle fibres and a lack of dystrophin through DNA analysis. The DNA can also be tested for genetic conditions by a serum sample.
- An ECG and pulmonary function tests may help diagnose compromise of heart and lungs.
- EMG results may show a decrease in amplitude and duration of motor unit potentials.

Therapeutics

Therapy is supportive to minimize deformity, prolong ambulation, and assist with ADLs.

Nursing Considerations

- Be aware that therapy is provided by an interprofessional team.
- Maintain optimal physical mobility by facilitating the maximum level of activity that the child can manage, including muscle strengthening and ROM exercises.
- Provide care as indicated in the section "Nursing Considerations Related to Immobilization."
- Monitor temperature when children with DMD receive an anaesthetic because they are at risk for malignant hyperthermia.
- Support the child and family in coping with this degenerative and fatal disorder.
- Refer the family to support agencies, such as Muscular Dystrophy Canada.
- Facilitate respite care for the family as required.
- Assist the family in obtaining genetic counselling.

Scoliosis

Idiopathic scoliosis is a lateral curvature of the spine. It may result from leg length discrepancy, hip or knee contractures, pain, neuromuscular disorders, or congenital malformations but usually is idiopathic. Scoliosis is often of unknown cause and usually is seen in females. Evidence points to a probable genetic autosomal dominant trait or to multifactorial causes. The most common spinal deformity, scoliosis is most noticeable during preadolescent growth spurt. (Hockenberry et al., 2022). The curvature can be minor, causing no disability, or severe.

Pathophysiology

- The deformity progresses during periods of growth, particularly during adolescent growth spurts, and stabilizes when vertebral growth is completed.
- As the spine grows and the lateral curve develops, the vertebrae rotate, causing rib asymmetry and thoracic hypokyphosis.
- The child attempts to maintain an erect posture, resulting in a compensatory curve.
- Vertebrae become wedge-shaped, and vertebral discs undergo degenerative changes.

- Muscles and ligaments either shorten and thicken or lengthen and atrophy, depending on the concavity or convexity of the curve.
- A hump may form as a result of the ribs rotating backward on the convex side of the curve.
- If the deformity is severe, the thoracic cavity becomes asymmetrical, leading to compromised respiratory function, decreased vital capacity, and potential pulmonary hypertension, cor pulmonale, and respiratory acidosis.

Clinical Manifestations

- If slight, scoliosis can be asymptomatic and can remain undetected until age 10.
- In more moderate to severe degrees of the condition, there may be a curve, asymmetry of the scapula and extremities, unequal distance between arms and waist, a pronounced hump, or twisting of the body.

Diagnostics

- Physical examination may detect scoliosis; when the child bends forward and dangles the arms, the curvature is apparent; or the child standing erect, observe from behind, noting asymmetry of shoulders, scapulae, waistline, and hips or distance that arms hang from the trunks.
- Radiographic examination reveals the degree and location of the curvature.

Therapeutics

- Early detection is important to prevent a more severe curvature.
- Exercise and bracing are used in milder idiopathic scoliosis to slow the progression of the curvature until growth is completed. Devices such as the Boston and Wilmington braces are plastic shells that mould to the body, and the thoracolumbosacral orthotic brace is a plastic mould that fits under the arms.
- In more severe cases, surgery may be attempted for spinal realignment and straightening by external or internal fixation and instrumentation combined with bony fusion of the realigned spine. Several surgical techniques are used in the surgery, and different instrument systems are available, such as the Harrington, Dwyer, Zielke, Luque, Cotrel-Dubousset, Isola, Texas Scottish Rite Hospital, and Miami–Moss systems.

Nursing Considerations

- Be aware that nurses are often the first to diagnose scoliosis during health assessments of adolescents (scoliosis is more common in females).
- Evaluate the child's acceptance of any prescribed brace and exercise to determine their compliance level and the need for further teaching.
- Emphasize the positive aspects of wearing the brace, including improved posture and symptom relief. Encourage the child to verbalize any concerns about wearing the brace in relation to body image, which is very important to adolescent females.

- Teach skin care to children wearing a brace: ensuring its proper fit, wearing a cotton shirt under the brace, and early treatment of skin breakdown.
- Provide the child and family with information about scoliosis and its treatment, including equipment.
- See Chapter 7, pages 123-124, for postoperative care.

Fracture

Fractures are breaks in the continuity of a bone when more stress is placed on the bone than it can resist. The bone is realigned or reduced by closed or open reduction followed by immobilization with a splint, traction, or a cast.

Pathophysiology

The fracture types that are most commonly seen in children are as follows:

- Plastic deformation: The bone bends to the breaking point and will not straighten without intervention. These are most commonly in the ulna and fibula.
- Buckle or torus : This fracture results from a compression of porous bone, with the bone telescoping on itself.
- Greenstick: The bone does not fracture completely through.
- Complete fracture: The bone divides into bone fragments that are subclassified as transverse, spiral, oblique, comminuted, or butterfly.
  Common sites include the following:
- The clavicle
- The humerus (in supracondylar fractures, which occur when a child falls backward onto the hands with the elbows straight, there is a high incidence of neurovascular compromise due to the closeness of the brachial artery and nerves to the fracture site)
- Radius, ulna, and femur (often associated with child abuse)
- Epiphyseal plates (with the potential for growth deformity)

  Precautions must be taken to prevent complications, such as cast syndrome, infections, and compartment syndrome. Fractures in children may be the result of falls, sports injuries, motor vehicle accidents, or child abuse.

Clinical Manifestations

Fracture manifestations vary, depending on the location, cause, and type of fracture. Usual symptoms are the six P's: pain, pulse, pallor, paraesthesia, pressure, and paralysis.

Other symptoms include deformity, swelling, bruising, muscle spasms, tenderness, pain, impaired sensation, loss of function, abnormal mobility, crepitus, shock, and refusal to walk or crawl (in small children).

Diagnostics

X-ray examination reveals the initial injury and subsequent healing progress. Ultrasonography, bone scan, and MRI might be required to further differentiate the injury.

Nursing Considerations

Emergency management includes the following:

- Assess the six P's.

- Determine the mechanism of injury.
- Immobilize the part, moving the injured parts as little as possible.
- Apply traction if circulatory compromise is present.
- Elevate the injured limb if possible.
- Apply cold to the injured area.
  Later treatment includes the following:
- Monitor the child for neurovascular status (circulation, sensation, and movement) and signs of compartment syndrome, edema and swelling, skin integrity, and signs of infection.
- Provide cast care, including cast petalling, keeping the cast dry, and checking for foul odour and soft spots. It is very important to check for tightness of the cast when edema is present as it can decrease circulation and cause nerve damage.
- Assist with pain management.
- Provide care as indicated in the section "Nursing Considerations Related to Immobilization."

Osteomyelitis

Osteomyelitis is an infection of the bone, most commonly caused by *S. aureus*. It may occur acutely as a result of a bloodborne organism or infection through a break in the skin or as a chronic condition that may lead to dead bone tissue and orthopedic disability. Typically, the joints and long bones of the leg are involved.

Pathophysiology

- In acute hematogenous osteomyelitis, organisms from sites such as infected tonsils and abscessed teeth travel through the bloodstream and infect the bone.
- In exogenous osteomyelitis, there is a direct inoculation of the organism through trauma close to the bone, for example, a fracture or puncture wound.
- Chronic osteomyelitis occurs when the infection is resistant to treatment, which may lead to dead bone or bone loss.

Clinical Manifestations

- Fever, pain, and tenderness manifests at the site of infection.
- There may or may not be signs of inflammation.

Diagnostics

- Cultures are ordered to identify the organism.
- Bone scans, CT scans, and MRIs are helpful in determining areas of infected bone.
- A bone biopsy may be done if necessary.

Therapeutics

- IV antibiotics are administered, usually for at least 4 weeks.
- Surgery may be required if there is a poor response to the antibiotics.

Nursing Considerations

- Assist with positioning and support of the painful limb.

- Know that weight-bearing activities should not be permitted until healing is established, to prevent stress fractures.
- Consider venous access devices for long-term IV antibiotic administration.
- Administer analgesics as required.
- Provide physical therapy and ROM exercises as indicated.
- Monitor for signs of improvement in the area of infection.

NEUROLOGICAL COGNITIVE DYSFUNCTION

Increased Intracranial Pressure

Increased ICP is excessive pressure from tissue or fluid volume within the rigid cranial vault that disrupts neurological function. While an infant's fontanelles are still open, the sutures can widen and expand slightly and compensate for some of the increased pressure.

Pathophysiology

- Normally, ICP remains relatively constant within a fluctuating range as a result of a system of compensatory mechanisms among the cranium's contents: the brain tissue, meninges, CSF, and blood.
- Any increase in the proportional volume of one component must be accompanied by an equivalent reduction in one or more of the others.
- After cranial sutures are fused, only two alterations can compensate for increasing intracranial volume: the displacement of CSF to the spinal subarachnoid space and increased CSF absorption.
- An increase in intracranial volume that exceeds the ability of these mechanisms to compensate produces clinical manifestations of increased ICP.
- Conditions that produce increased ICP include craniocerebral trauma, hydrocephalus, brain tumour, meningitis, encephalitis, and intracerebral hemorrhage.

Clinical Manifestations

Early signs and symptoms of increased ICP usually are subtle. Manifestations in infants include the following:
- A tense, bulging anterior fontanelle and separated cranial sutures
- Increased occipital frontal circumference
- "Setting sun" sign
- Macewen's sign ("cracked pot sound")
- Irritability and restlessness with a high-pitched cry
- Poor feeding
- Crying when picked up or disturbed
- Distended scalp veins
  Manifestations in older children include the following:
- Headache upon awakening that improves with emesis
- Anorexia, nausea, and vomiting, usually projectile
- Cognitive, personality, and behavioural changes, including irritability, restlessness, indifference, lethargy, decreased school performance, decreased physical activity and motor performance, drowsiness, increased sleeping, and inability to follow commands
- Diplopia, blurred vision

- Seizures

Late manifestations of extremely high ICP include the following:

- Confusion or decreased loss of consciousness (LOC), ranging from drowsiness to coma
- Decreased motor response to commands
- Decreased sensation to painful stimuli
- Decreased pupil size and reactivity
- Extension or flexion posturing
- Papilledema and strabismus
- Cheyne–Stokes respirations
- Bradycardia

Diagnostics

- ICP is measured by various devices, from a noninvasive transducer to the more commonly used invasive devices, such as a subarachnoid bolt, an epidural transducer, an intraventricular catheter transducer, and an anterior fontanelle pressure monitor.
- Normal pressure ranges are 0 to 15 mm Hg.

Nursing Considerations

- Assist in reducing intra-abdominal and intra-thoracic pressures, which contribute to ICP, by elevating the head of the bed by 15 to 30 degrees.
- Monitor for early changes in ICP by assessing vital signs (increased systolic blood pressure, wide pulse pressure, and bradycardia indicate increased ICP), LOC, respiratory status, motor activity, behaviour, and pupil size and reactivity.
- If appropriate, use a transducer to monitor ICP.
- Assist with treatments and supportive measures, such as hyperventilation, mechanical ventilation, and hypothermia.
- Prevent overhydration, which can lead to cerebral edema and can be fatal, and underhydration for adequate cerebral perfusion pressure; monitor intake and output, and impose fluid restrictions if prescribed.
- Avoid positions or activities that may increase the child's ICP, such as neck vein compression, flexion, or extension of the neck, turning the head from side to side, painful or stressful stimuli, and respiratory suctioning or percussion.
- Use a pressure mattress to avoid skin breakdown and use sand bags to keep the head midline.
- Avoid a noisy environment that can raise ICP and use touch to help decrease ICP.
- Promote normal bowel elimination to prevent an intra-abdominal pressure increase from straining.
- As appropriate, prepare the child for surgical intervention to relieve the increased ICP, such as a subdural tap, ventriculotomy, epidural evacuation, placement of ventricular shunt, decompressive craniectomy, or tumour resection.
- Administer medications as prescribed, including corticosteroids to decrease cerebral edema, osmotic diuretics such as mannitol or urea, sedatives for combative children, and antiseizure agents if seizuring.

- Control hyperthermia from fever with antipyretics and cooling devices to decrease oxygen needs.

Seizure Disorders

Seizures are interruptions in normal brain function resulting from excessive and disorderly abnormal electrical discharges in the brain, which can cause LOC, involuntary body movements, and changes in behaviours, sensation, and the autonomic system. Approximately 4 to 10% of children experience at least one seizure by adolescence (Hockenberry et al., 2022).

Pathophysiology

- Many conditions can cause seizures. They result from overly active and hypersensitive neurons in the brain that trigger excessive electrical discharges. Seizures are normally contained in a focal area, but if a specific trigger, such as hypoglycemia, is present, they can become generalized.
- The location of the hypersensitive cells and the pattern of discharges determine the clinical manifestations.
- There are three categories of seizures:
  - Generalized seizures involve both hemispheres of the brain, are bilateral and symmetrical, and do not have a local onset.
  - Partial, or focal, seizures involve a small area of the cerebral cortex and have a local onset; these seizures may be simple or complex.
  - Unknown-onset seizures, such as neonatal seizures, do not provide enough evidence to allow categorization, so they are put in this classification.
- Underlying possible causes include prenatal or perinatal hypoxia, infections, hemorrhages, allergies, syncope, congenital malformations, metabolic disturbances, lead poisoning, head injuries, drug abuse, alcohol misuse, or tumours.
- Most seizures are idiopathic.
- There is some evidence of a genetic etiological factor in which the seizure threshold is lower in affected individuals.

Clinical Manifestations

For generalized seizures:

- Generalized tonic–clonic seizures of unknown onset (formerly called *grand mal*): Tonic rigidity, extension of extremities, LOC, eyes roll up, fixed jaw and increased salivation, respiratory cessation, dilated pupils; clonic–rhythmic jerking of extremities, autonomic symptoms, possible incontinence
- Generalized absence seizures (myoclonic): Sudden brief contractions of muscle groups, similar in appearance to an exaggerated startle reflex
- Focal or generalized atonic seizures: Sudden, brief loss of muscle tone and postural control, and child falls
- Focal, generalized, unknown-onset epileptic spasms (formerly called *infantile spasm*): Brief flexion of the neck, trunk, or legs or, less frequently, extension

- Generalized absence seizures (formerly called *petit mal*): Brief periods of unconsciousness, may have tonic or atonic phase or automatisms (such as lip-smacking); often mistaken for daydreaming
  For partial seizures:
- Focal aware seizures (formerly called *simple partial*): Motor or sensory signs—consciousness is usually maintained; may include focal motor component (abnormal movement of leg); sensory component (tingling); autonomic (sweating) or psychic manifestations (déjà vu, anger)
- Focal impaired awareness seizures formerly known as *complex partial seizure*): Begin as a simple seizure but progress to unconsciousness, period of altered behaviour, amnesia of the event, complex sensory phenomena (aura)
- Status epilepticus involves recurrent, continuous, generalized seizure activity with the danger of cardiac arrest and brain damage.
- Some children experience an aura prior to the seizures, which is actually a partial seizure that reflects the area of abnormal activity. The aura occurs prior to the seizures and may take the form of odd smells, hallucinations, or a feeling of déjà vu.

Diagnostics

- EEG is done to document abnormal activity.
- Long-term video-EEG is performed to correlate observed seizures with brain electrical activity.
- Blood tests are done to screen for infections and metabolic imbalances.
- MRI may be performed to rule out a brain tumour.
- A lumbar puncture can rule out meningitis.
- A full physical examination and history are necessary.

Therapeutics

- Anticonvulsant medications may be prescribed to raise the threshold of neuronal excitability in predisposed persons. A few of the commonly used agents are phenobarbital, phenytoin, fosphenytoin, carbamazepine, valproic acid, clonazepam, and gabapentin, with the dosage adjusted as the child grows. Drug levels must be measured.
- Surgery may be indicated to remove the area of involvement if the seizures are caused by a cerebral lesion. For children with incapacitating refractory seizures that cannot be controlled by medication, surgery may be performed.
- A therapeutic diet, such as a ketogenic diet (high-fat, low-carbohydrate, low-protein diet, to induce ketosis), may be recommended in children with absence or other kinds of seizures; this diet is very difficult to maintain.
- Vagus nerve stimulation may be recommended as an additional treatment in clients 12 years of age and older with focal onset seizures. A subcutaneous signal stimulates the left vagal nerve at the onset of a seizure.

Nursing Considerations

- Obtain a thorough clinical history (birth trauma, medications, injuries, illnesses, family history, seizure descriptions).
- Maintain safety; provide a helmet, pad the bed's side rails, and have oxygen and suction equipment at the bedside.
- During a seizure, do not restrain the child, do not place anything in their mouth, remove harmful objects from the area, extend the neck to maintain the airway, position the child on one side to allow secretions to flow from the mouth, loosen clothing, and screen the child for privacy if possible.
- Document all seizure activity and encourage the family to keep a seizure journal, including the following:
  - The apparent trigger, if known or suspected
  - The child's behaviour before the seizure and whether or not there was an aura
  - The time the seizure began and ended
  - The clinical manifestations of the seizure
  - The child's postictal seizure behaviour and symptoms
- Help prevent seizures by preventing the child's exposure to known triggers, such as emotional stress or blinking lights.
- Use precautions with anticonvulsant medications and observe for adverse effects.
- Provide child and family teaching concerning the nature of the disorder and its possible triggers, seizure precaution measures, diagnostic tests and procedures, potential medication adverse effects, the importance of not discontinuing medication and of not switching to a different brand of the same medication, the need for periodic re-evaluation of medication effectiveness as well as follow-up and close monitoring of blood work, urinalysis, and vital signs; the importance of encouraging a normal lifestyle, activity limitations, the need to share information about the child's special needs with others, such as teachers and school nurses; adolescent needs, such as information about drugs and alcohol, peer pressure, dating, and getting a driver's licence.

Neural Tube Defects

Neural tube defects (NTDs) are a group of related defects of the CNS involving the cranium or spinal cord, which vary from mildly to severely disabling. NTDs include anencephaly, encephalocele, and spina bifida. Heredity and environmental factors have been implicated; NTDs have also been associated with the interaction of genetic predisposition and folic acid deficiency.

Pathophysiology

- During the third to fourth week of gestation, the embryonic neural plate closes to form the neural tube, which eventually forms the spinal cord and brain.
- The vertebral column develops, along with the spinal cord.
- Normally, the spinal cord and cauda equina are enclosed in a protective sheath of bone and meninges. If the sheath fails to close, leaving either a small opening or an opening the entire length of the spinal cord, this creates various degrees of defects.

Clinical Manifestations

Manifestations vary with the degree of the defect.

- The degree of neurological dysfunction is directly related to the anatomical location of the defect and thus to the nerves involved; sensory disturbances usually parallel motor dysfunction.

Diagnostics

- Diagnosis is made on the basis of a clinical examination; if the sac transilluminates, it usually is a meningocele.
- Other tests include ultrasonography, CT, MRI, and myelography.
- Prenatal detection involves ultrasonography and identifying elevated levels of alpha-fetoprotein in the amniotic fluid between 16 and 18 weeks.

Therapeutics

- No treatment is indicated for spina bifida occulta unless there is neurological damage; if a dermal sinus is present, it may need to be closed surgically.
- Meningocele requires closure as soon after birth as possible; the child should be monitored for postoperative complications that could include hydrocephalus, meningitis, and spinal cord disruption.
- Myelomeningocele requires management by a coordinated interdisciplinary team, including neurology, neurosurgery, pediatrics, urology, orthopedics, rehabilitation, and nursing.
- Skin grafting may be required, and shunting is performed for hydrocephalus.
- Antibiotics are initiated to prevent infection.
- The child will need correction of musculo-skeletal deformities and management of urological deficits and bowel control.

Nursing Considerations

For myelomeningocele:
- Before surgery, prevent infection by applying sterile, moist saline soaks to the sac or open lesion and keep them moist.
- Avoid placing a diaper or other covering directly over the lesion, to prevent infection from fecal contamination.
- Prevent trauma and tears to the sac by gently placing the infant prone in an isolette or warmer.
- Know that the infant may require clean intermittent catheterizations if neurogenic bladder is present.
- Help prevent hip subluxation by positioning the legs in abduction with a pad between the knees and the feet in a neutral position with a roll under the ankles.
- Monitor vital signs, measure head circumference, and monitor neurological status, including signs of ICP.
- After surgery, place the child in a prone position if a side-lying position, which is permitted by many neurosurgeons, aggravates the hips.
- Refer parents to the Spina Bifida and Hydrocephalus Association of Canada for resources.
- Provide family teaching for associated conditions in the growing child, such as neurogenic bladder and bowel, impaired mobility, skin breakdown, ICP, and possible neurological impairment related to hydrocephalus.

- Carefully assess the family's ability to care for the child and refer them for further assistance if needed.

Hydrocephalus

Hydrocephalus is a condition caused by a blockage to the flow of CSF, or an imbalance in the production and absorption of CSF in the ventricular system. When production exceeds absorption, CSF accumulates, usually under pressure, creating ventricular dilatation. Hydrocephalus is caused by congenital defects, such as myelomeningocele, or acquired conditions, such as intraventricular hemorrhage or CSF infection.

Pathophysiology

- CSF flows from the lateral ventricles through the foramen of Monro to the third ventricle, then through the aqueduct of Sylvius into the fourth ventricle through the foramen of Luschka, and the midline foramen of Magendie into the cisterna magna. From there, it flows to the cerebral and cerebellar subarachnoid spaces, where it is absorbed.
- Causes of hydrocephalus are varied but result in either impaired absorption of CSF within the arachnoid space or obstruction to the flow of CSF through the ventricular system

Therapeutics

- Surgery is the preferred intervention to remove the obstruction.
- A shunt provides primary drainage of the CSF to an extracranial compartment, usually the peritoneum.
- Ventriculoperitoneal shunts consist of a ventricular catheter, a flush pump, a unidirectional flow valve, and a distal catheter.
- Major complications of shunts are infections and malfunction; others include subdural hematoma caused by a too rapid reduction of CSF, peritonitis, abdominal abscess, perforation of organs, fistulas, hernias, and ileus.

Clinical Manifestations

- In infants: The child's head grows at an abnormal rate; signs and symptoms include a bulging fontanelle, a tense anterior fontanelle, often bulging and nonpulsatile; dilated scalp veins; Macewen's sign ("cracked pot sound"); frontal bossing; setting sun sign; sluggish and unequal pupils; irritability and lethargy with varying LOC; abnormal infantile reflexes; and possible cranial nerve damage.
- In children: Signs of ICP include headache on awakening with improvement following emesis; papilledema; strabismus; ataxia, irritability, lethargy, apathy, and confusion.

Diagnostics

- Ultrasonograms can diagnose hydrocephalus at 14 weeks' gestation.
- Cranial transillumination shows varying degrees of localized fluid accumulation.
- CT and MRI scans confirm fluid accumulation and enlarged ventricles.

Nursing Considerations

Preoperative considerations:

- Assess head circumference, fontanelles, cranial sutures, and LOC; also assess for signs of ICP: irritability, altered feeding habits, and high-pitched cry.
- Irritability, seizures, poor feeding, lethargy, and altered vital signs point to an advanced condition.
- Prepare the child and family for diagnostic procedures.
- Carefully support the head and neck when holding or repositioning the child.
- Provide skin care, particularly for the back of the head. Special pressure-sensitive mattresses and frequent position change help to prevent skin breakdown.
- Offer small, frequent feedings to decrease the risk of vomiting.
- Encourage parental participation in the child's care and promote bonding.

Postoperative considerations:

- Assess for signs of increased ICP.
- Measure head circumference daily; check the anterior fontanelle for size, tenseness, and fullness.
- Position the child on the side opposite the shunt to prevent pressure on the valve.
- Keep the child flat for the first 24 hours so as not to drain the CSF too quickly.
- Monitor dressings for bloody and clear drainage (the presence of glucose in drainage indicates CSF).
- Monitor the fluid balance.
- Promote natural bowel elimination in children with ventriculoperitoneal shunts, who may have constipation.
- Administer antibiotics as prescribed, IV or intraventricular.
- Monitor for infection, particularly CSF or peritonitis; watch for abdominal distension, which can mean peritonitis from the shunt insertion, or postoperative ileus because of shunt catheter placement.
- Administer osmotic diuretics as prescribed to reduce increased ICP.
- Provide child and family teaching concerning ICP, possible neurological impairment, skin care, and the need for frequent follow-up care.

Head Injury

A head injury is a pathological process that can involve the scalp, skull, or meninges. It can range from a mild injury to severe damage to the head.

Pathophysiology

- Pathophysiology and management are directly related to the force of the impact. Intracranial contents are damaged when the force is too great to be absorbed by the skull and the musculo-skeletal support of the head.
- Types of head traumas include skull fractures, contusions, diffuse injuries, and hematomas.
- Head injury is one of the most common causes of disability and death in children.
- Head injury is most frequently caused by motor vehicle accidents, bicycle or sport related injuries, abuse, falls, and birth trauma, with the etiology related to the child's age.

Clinical Manifestations

Skull fractures. The type, extent, and accompanying symptoms of skull fractures depend on the velocity, force, and mass of the object that struck the skull; the area of the skull involved; and the age of the child.

Skull fracture types include the following:

- Linear: This is the most common type of fracture. It resembles a thin line and is from a low-velocity blow. Most linear fractures are associated with an overlying scalp hematoma, particularly in infants younger than 2 years of age and in the parietal or temporal region (Hockenberry et al., 2022).
- Comminuted: This type has a "cracked eggshell" appearance and may also be categorized as depressed. It usually result from intense impact and may suggest maltreatment because it often results from repeated blows against an object (Keenan-Lindsay et al., 2022, p. 1349).
- Depressed: The skull is indented at the point of impact, which may cause compression on the brain, shifting of brain tissue, and intracranial damage; symptoms depend on the area damaged. This fracture may require surgery to lift the bone off the cerebrum. Bone fragments could also tear the dura and cause bleeding.
- Basilar: A linear fracture involving the basilar portion of the frontal, ethmoid, temporal, or occipital bones of the skull, often resulting in a dura tear. Classic signs are "raccoon eyes," "Battle's sign" (bruising behind the ear from bleeding into the mastoid sinus), and a possible blood or CSF leak into the ears, nasopharynx, or nose.
- Open fractures result in a communication between the skull and the scalp or the mucosa of the upper respiratory tract. There is increased risk of CNS infection with open fractures. When the open fracture involves the middle ear or paranasal sinuses it can lead to a leakage of CSF (rhinorrhea or otorrhea) (Hockenberry et al., 2022).
- Growing skull fracture is an unusual complication of head trauma. The fracture is accompanied by an underlying tear in the dura or brain injury that fails to heal properly. Most growing fractures occur before 30 months of age and occur in the parietal bone. Physical examination may reveal a swelling scalp and skull defect. Clinical neurological symptoms may be delayed for months to years after the initial skull fracture and include headache, seizures, hemiparesis, and learning and intellectual disabilities (Hockenberry et al., 2022).

Brain injury. Signs and symptoms depend on location and severity; post-traumatic syndromes (seizures, hydrocephalus, focal neurological deficits) and metabolic complications (diabetes insipidus, hyponatremia or hypernatremia, hyperglycemic hyperosmolar states) may occur; all of these may occur up to 2 years after the injury.

Hematomas. Epidural (between the skull and the dura) and subdural (between the dura and arachnoid layer) are the most common types.

- Epidural: life-threatening, with rapid onset, characterized by rapid deterioration, headache, seizures, coma, and brain herniation with compression of the brainstem

- Subdural: occurs within 48 hours of injury, characterized by headache, agitation, confusion, drowsiness, decrease in LOC, and increased ICP; chronic subdural hematomas may also occur

General manifestations of minor head trauma
- May or may not involve LOC
- Transient confusion
- Listlessness and irritability
- Pallor and vomiting

Signs of deterioration are as follows:
- Altered mental status
- Increasing agitation
- Significant changes in vital signs
- Reflexes hypo-responsive, hyper-responsive, or nonexistent

Diagnostics

Fractures may be visualized by X-ray; brain injuries and hematomas are viewed by CT or MRI.

Therapeutics

- Therapeutic interventions depend on symptoms, which must be closely observed and monitored.
- Surgical evacuation of hematomas may be needed and may be facilitated by burr holes for evacuation and relief of increased ICP; depressed skull fractures need to be elevated surgically.
- Scalp and dural lacerations may require sutures.

Nursing Considerations

- Promote prevention of injury, especially of falls.
- Promote safety practices, including the use of bike helmets, seat belts, and protective sports equipment; encourage safe driving.
- Perform neurological assessments of cerebral functioning (alertness, orientation, memory, speech), vital signs (check for increased blood pressure, decreased pulse), pupils, and motor and sensory function.
- Assess for cervical and other injuries.
- To help decrease cerebral edema, and if there is no cervical injury, raise the head of the bed to 30 degrees.
- Monitor for complications, which can develop rapidly; monitor vital signs and neurological status frequently; and check for increased ICP and for drainage (of CSF or blood) from the nose and ears.
- Be aware that seizures may occur for up to 2 years after injury.
- Be aware that the child may also require rehabilitation following an extensive brain injury.
- Provide child and family teaching:
  - Discuss complications and what to observe for in post-traumatic syndrome.
  - Refer family members to the Brain Injury Canada.

Intellectual Disability

Intellectual disability (ID), or cognitive impairment (formerly known as "mental retardation"), is part of a broad category of developmental disability. The condition is now defined by the American Association on Intellectual and Developmental Disabilities as "a disability characterized by significant limitations both in intellectual functioning and in adaptive behaviour as expressed in conceptual, social, and practical adaptive skills. This disability originates before the age of 18" (Hockenberry et al., 2022).

Pathophysiology

- Pathophysiology depends on cause.
- Early diagnosis and prompt treatment may be particularly important in cases involving an identifiable and possibly correctable cause, such as hypothyroidism phenylketonuria, malnutrition, or child abuse.
- A diagnosis of ID cannot be made on the basis of intellectual ability alone; there must be both adaptive (personal independence and social responsibility) and intellectual impairment.
- Causes include infection and intoxication, trauma, or physical agents, metabolic or nutritional abnormalities, gross postnatal brain disease, unknown prenatal conditions, chromosomal abnormalities, gestational disorders, psychiatric disorders with onset during the child's developmental period, such as autism, and environmental influences (Hockenberry et al., 2022).

Diagnostics

- Diagnosis usually is made after a period of suspicion, although it may be made at birth from recognition of a specific syndrome, such as Down syndrome.
- Diagnosis and classification are based on a variety of standardized IQ test scores.

Clinical Manifestations

Manifestations vary, depending on the classification or degree of disability.

Mild ID (50–75 IQ):
- Preschool: Often the child is not noted as having a disability but is slow to walk, talk, and feed themselves.
- School age: The child can acquire practical skills and learn to read and do arithmetic to a sixth-grade level; with special education, the child achieves a mental age of 8 to 12 years.
- Adult: Adults can usually achieve social and vocational skills, may need occasional guidance, and may handle marriage but have difficulty with parenting.

Moderate ID (35–55 IQ):
- Preschool: The child has noticeable delays, especially in speech.
- School age: The child can learn simple communication, health and safety habits, and simple manual skills; they have a mental age of 3 to 7 years.
- Adult: Adults can perform simple tasks under sheltered conditions and can travel alone to familiar places but usually need help with self-maintenance.

Severe ID (20–40 IQ):
- Preschool: The child exhibits marked motor delays and few communication skills; they may respond to training in elementary self-help, such as feeding.

- School age: The child usually walks with difficulty, has some understanding of and may respond to speech, can respond to habit training, and has the mental age of a toddler.
- Adult: Adults can conform to daily routines and repetitive activities but need constant direction and supervision in a protective environment.

  Profound ID (<20 IQ):
- Preschool: The child exhibits gross intellectual disability, has some capacity for function in sensorimotor areas, and needs total care.
- School age: The child displays obvious delays in all areas; shows a basic emotional response; may respond to skilful training in the use of the legs, hands, and jaws; needs close supervision; and has the mental age of a young infant.
- Adult: A profoundly delayed adult may walk but has primitive speech and needs complete custodial care; they usually benefit from regular physical activity.

Therapeutics

- The treatment goal is to promote optimal development.
- Preventive measures include regular prenatal care, support for high-risk infants, rubella immunization, genetic counselling, education, and injury reduction.

Nursing Considerations

- Support the family at the time of the initial diagnosis.
- Facilitate the child's self-care abilities through an early stimulation program, self-feeding, independent toileting, and independent grooming.
- Promote optimal development by encouraging self-care goals and emphasizing the universal needs of children, such as play, social interaction, and parental limit-setting.
- Assist the family in planning for the child's future needs.
- Refer parents to appropriate community agencies.
- Discuss the need for patience with the child's slow attainment of developmental milestones.
- Discuss stimulation and safety.
- Demonstrate communication strategies; accentuate non-verbal cues, such as facial expressions and body language, to help cue speech development.
- Explain the need for discipline that is simple, consistent, and appropriate to the child's development.
- Review an adolescent's need for simple, practical sexual information.
- Discuss the importance of positive self-esteem, built by accomplishing small successes, in motivating the child to accomplish other tasks.

Down Syndrome

Down syndrome is the most common chromosomal abnormality. This condition occurs in people of all economic levels and ethnicities. Approximately 1 in every 750 babies born in Canada has Down syndrome (Keenan-Lindsay et al., 2022).

Pathophysiology

- Approximately 95% of cases may be attributed to an extra chromosome on chromosome 21—hence the name *nonfamilial trisomy 21* (Keenan-Lindsay et al., 2022).
- Two out of three cases may be caused by translocation of chromosomes 15 and 21 or 22; this usually is hereditary and is not related to maternal age (Keenan-Lindsay et al., 2022).
- Children with Down syndrome are born to parents of all ages.
- There is a higher statistical risk for child-bearing clients over age 35, but most are born to child-bearing clients under this age, likely due to a higher fertility rate in younger clients and with prenatal screening for clients in older age groups as well as the option of abortion.
- The level of cognitive and physical impairment is related to the percentage of cells with the abnormal chromosome makeup.

Clinical Manifestations

- The most common findings include separated sagittal suture, oblique palpebral fissures, small nose, depressed nasal bridge, high-arched palate, skin excess and laxity, wide space between the big and second toes, plantar crease between the big and second toes, hyperextensible and lax joints, and muscle weakness.
- Other common findings include a small penis, short, broad hands (with a transverse [simian] palmar crease), protruding tongue, small ears, Brushfield spots, and dry skin.
- Associated impairments and features include the following:
  - Intelligence varies from severely disabled to low-normal but is generally within the mild to moderate range.
  - Social development may be 2 to 3 years beyond mental age; temperament range is similar to that of normal children.
  - Congenital heart disease can occur, especially septal defects, which are very common (Keenan-Lindsay et al., 2022).
  - Other defects include renal agenesis, duodenal atresia, Hirschsprung's disease, tracheoesophageal fistula, and skeletal deformities.
  - Sensory conditions include strabismus, nystagmus, myopia, hyperopia, cataracts and excessive tearing, and conductive hearing loss.
  - Other physical disorders may include altered immune function, respiratory infections, leukemia, thyroid dysfunction, and early aging.
  - Individuals have a shortened stature with a tendency for rapid weight gain.
  - Sexual development may be delayed, incomplete, or both.
  - Male genitalia and secondary characteristics are underdeveloped; males are infertile.
  - Female breast development is mild to moderate with menarche at an appropriate age; females may be fertile.

Diagnostics

Diagnosis is made by physical examination and chromosomal analysis.

Therapeutics

- Surgery may be used to correct some accompanying defects.
- Behaviour modification may be recommended for dealing with negative behaviours.
- Developmental, social, and educational supports will likely be required.

Nursing Considerations

- Implement nursing care as with ID.
- Support parental genetic counselling.
- Explain hypertonicity and joint hyperextensibility to parents.
- Know that feeding can take longer in the infant due to the large tongue and weak suck.
- For the older child, use a small, straight-handled spoon to push food to the side and back of the mouth.
- Monitor for common associated congenital anomalies, especially cardiac.

COMMUNICABLE DISEASES OF CHILDHOOD

Measles (Rubeola)

Rubeola, or "red measles," is a communicable disease that has been largely eradicated in Canada. Occasional outbreaks are primarily related to people who have been inadequately immunized.

Pathophysiology

- Rubeola, or measles, is a communicable virus that is usually transmitted by direct contact with droplets.
- Incubation time is 10 to 20 days, and infected individuals are contagious from 4 days before to 5 days after the rash appears.

Clinical Manifestations

- Stage 1: The prodromal stage includes fever and malaise; 24 hours later, acute rhinitis, cough, conjunctivitis with photophobia, and Kolick spots (white spots in the mouth) develop.
- Stage 2: Three to 4 days after the prodromal stage, a rash appears, causing red maculopapular lesions on the face and spreading down toward the trunk and extremities. The rash changes to a browner colour in 3 to 4 days; fine peeling of the skin begins in the more severely affected regions.
- Potential complications include otitis media, pneumonia, laryngotracheitis, and encephalitis.

Diagnostics

- Assessment of rash
- Antibody titres

Nursing Considerations

- Provide comfort measures, including antipyretics, skin care with oatmeal, cleansing the eyes if conjunctivitis develops, and sunglasses and dim lights for the photophobia.
- Promote childhood immunization. Rubeola is preventable with a vaccine.

Rubella

Rubella, or "German measles," is a communicable disease that, like rubeola, is now largely eradicated in Canada. However, outbreaks are of concern to the public as this disease may cause severe birth defects if contracted by pregnant women.

Pathophysiology

- The rubella virus is transmitted by direct and indirect contact.
- The incubation period is 14 to 21 days.
- The child is communicable for 7 days before to approximately 5 days after the rash appears.

Clinical Manifestations

- A reddish-pink maculopapular rash begins on the face and spreads downward to the trunk and extremities.
- The rash disappears first in the initial lesions.
- Symptoms also include a low-grade fever, malaise, and lymphadenopathy.
- Complications include possible damage to the fetus in a pregnant woman and, rarely, encephalitis, arthritis, or purpura.

Diagnostics

Diagnosis is generally based on observation of rash and antibody titres.

Nursing Considerations

- Provide comfort measures for the child.
- Advise the parents of the danger to pregnant women of exposure to a communicable child.
- Promote childhood immunization. Rubella is preventable with a vaccine.

Chicken Pox (Varicella)

Chicken pox is an uncomfortable, communicable disease of children and adults. It may leave scars and create a significant health risk for the immuno-compromised child.

Pathophysiology

- Varicella zoster is the communicable agent.
- Infection is transmitted by direct contact and via contaminated objects.
- The child is communicable for 1 to 2 days before the rash appears and remains infectious until all of the lesions are crusted over.

Diagnostics

Diagnosis is based on assessment of rash and antibody titres.

Clinical Manifestations

- The prodromal stage involves low-grade fever, malaise, and loss of appetite.
- Rash starts on the face with macules that turn to papules, then vesicles, then pustules, and finally crusts. The rash then spreads to the proximal extremities, with fewer lesions in distal areas.
- Lesions can also appear on the mucous membranes.
- The lesions cause severe itching.
- Other symptoms include fever, lymphadenopathy, and irritability from itching.
- Complications are secondary infections, such as encephalitis, pneumonia, and hemorrhagic varicella in immuno-compromised children.

Nursing Considerations

- Know that strict isolation until vesicles are dry is necessary to prevent spread.
- Provide comfort measures: a cool environment, cool oatmeal baths to soothe itchy and irritated skin and decrease the risk of secondary infection and scarring from scratching, loose clothing, antihistamines, and antipyretics.
- Know that zoster immune globulin (ZIG) and acyclovir are given to children who are immuno-compromised.
- Promote childhood immunization. Varicella is preventable with a vaccine.

Pertussis (Whooping Cough)

Pertussis is a potentially serious disease in the infant. Occasional outbreaks of pertussis occur in Canada despite adequate immunization.

Pathophysiology

- The infectious bacterium is *Bordetella pertussis*.
- The incubation period is 6 to 20 days, with an average of 7 days.
- Stage 1: The catarrhal stage, when the child has signs of an upper respiratory infection; 1 or 2 weeks later, the hacking cough increases in severity.
- Stage 2: The paroxysmal stage, which usually lasts 4 to 6 weeks. The child has the classic paroxysmal "whoop" cough, which usually occurs at night; the child is flushed or has a cyanotic face, bulging eyes, and a protruding tongue and coughs until they cough up a mucus plug, often vomiting afterward.
- Stage 3: The convalescent stage, in which the cough slowly decreases, vomiting stops, and strength returns.

- Complications include atelectasis, otitis media, seizures, hemorrhage, weight loss, and dehydration.
- In infants, apnea and respiratory arrest from a mucus plug can occur.

Diagnostics

Diagnosis is based on the characteristic cough and a throat swab for culture.

Nursing Considerations

- Maintain isolation.
- Use respiratory precautions.
- Provide a quiet environment, encourage fluids, and monitor for respiratory distress.
- Promote childhood immunization. Pertussis is preventable with a vaccine.

Mumps

Mumps is an infectious disease of the parotid glands. Occasional outbreaks occur in Canada despite adequate immunization.

Pathophysiology

- The infectious agent is paramyxovirus.
- Transmission is by direct contact or droplet.
- The incubation period is 14 to 21 days.
- The child is communicable immediately before the swelling occurs until immediately after.
- Symptoms of the prodromal stage are pyrexia, headache, and loss of appetite followed by earache, which worsens with chewing.
- The second acute stage occurs by the second day with parotid gland swelling, which is painful and peaks in 1 to 3 days.
- Complications include meningoencephalitis, orchitis, epididymitis, arthritis, myocarditis, meningitis, hepatitis, and, rarely, sterility in males.

Diagnostics

Mumps is generally diagnosed by the characteristic facial swelling produced.

Nursing Considerations

- Ensure isolation and bed rest with respiratory precautions.
- Administer analgesics and fluids and provide warmth and support for orchitis.
- Promote childhood immunization. Mumps is preventable with a vaccine.

PRACTICE QUESTIONS

Case 1

Simon is a 6-year-old boy who is brought by his parents to the emergency department of a local hospital. The triage nurse assesses that Simon has tachypnea, wheezing, and diminished air entry. The physician diagnoses asthma.

Questions 1 to 5 refer to this case.

1. In addition to wheezing and tachypnea, Simon manifests other clinical signs of an acute asthma attack. Which of the following are signs of respiratory distress seen in childhood asthma?

1. Tripod position with refusal to lie down
2. Harsh, barking cough on inspiration
3. Shallow breathing with periods of apnea
4. Continuous respiratory stridor

2. Simon's initial treatment is salbutamol (Ventolin) by inhalation. During the inhalation, Simon begins to shake. What should the nurse do?
   1. Stop the inhalation immediately.
   2. Reassure Simon that this is an adverse effect of the Ventolin.
   3. Provide Simon with a warm blanket.
   4. Reduce the flow of air or oxygen in the inhalation.

3. Which of the following is an appropriate and appealing diet for Simon while he is experiencing respiratory distress?
   1. Ice cream
   2. Macaroni and cheese
   3. Clear beef soup
   4. Ice pops (Popsicles)

4. Simon's parents ask the nurse how they can prevent further episodes of asthma. What would be the most appropriate response by the nurse?
   1. "We can discuss developing a plan to manage the asthma."
   2. "It is difficult to prevent asthma attacks in children Simon's age, so you need to know how to treat each attack."
   3. "You need to find out what particular triggers cause Simon's attacks."
   4. "Simon needs to take his asthma medications all the time, even when he is not wheezing."

5. The nurse assesses that Simon's environment has many potential allergens, for example, pet dander, dust, and second-hand smoke. Prior to discharge, the nurse reviews strategies for Simon's parents to modify the environment in order to reduce these allergens. Before discharge home, which of the following is the most important action that can be immediately implemented by the parents?
   1. Remove Simon's dog from the home.
   2. Stop smoking cigarettes in the car.
   3. Have a high-energy particulate air (HEPA) filter installed.
   4. Wet dust all floors and surfaces, particularly in Simon's bedroom.

Case 2

Leah is a healthy 9-month-old infant brought to the community health clinic by her parents. The nurse performs an assessment and health teaching.

Questions 6 to 10 refer to this case.

6. Leah's parents ask the nurse what to do when their daughter has a "cold" with a low-grade temperature. What would the nurse respond?
   1. Take Leah to the doctor if the symptoms continue for 2 days.
   2. Give her infant acetylsalicylic acid (Aspirin) as directed on the bottle.
   3. If she is uncomfortable, give her pediatric acetaminophen (Tylenol) or ibuprofen.
   4. Administer an over-the-counter cold remedy formulated for infants.

7. Leah's parents ask for advice on toys that are best for developing her motor abilities. Which of the following are most appropriate for motor development?
   1. Putting her in an infant walker with rollers
   2. Giving her several types of baby rattles
   3. Reading a book to her at bedtime every night
   4. Letting her play with kitchen utensils, such as bowls and spoons

8. The nurse discusses infant safety with Leah's parents. Which of the following safety precautions would the nurse advise?
   1. Do not give Leah finger foods until she is 18 months of age.
   2. Place pillows around Leah when she is in her crib.
   3. Dress Leah in clothes with Velcro fasteners.
   4. Check all toys for small movable parts.

9. As part of Leah's assessment, the nurse reaches out to Leah to take her vital signs. Leah begins to scream and cling to her father. What should the nurse do?
   1. Remove Leah gently from her father.
   2. Postpone the taking of vital signs for another visit.
   3. Talk softly at eye level with Leah.
   4. Hold her arms out and smile at Leah.

10. The nurse discusses developmental milestones with Leah's parents. She asks them about Leah's ability to vocalize and understand language. What vocalization milestone is appropriate for a 9-month-old infant?
    1. Responds to simple verbal commands and understands "no-no"
    2. Produces repetitive vowel sounds such as "baba" and "kaka"
    3. Begins to imitate sounds
    4. Says three to five words in addition to "mama" and "dada"

Case 3

Staff at a child care centre that provides care for children with health conditions ask a community nurse for a consultation about safe health practices.

Questions 11 to 15 refer to this case.

11. One of the children who attends the child care centre has a severe peanut allergy. What would the nurse recommend to best prevent potential sources of peanuts from coming in contact with the children?
    1. Do not allow parents to bring homemade food to share with the other children.
    2. Send home a letter to the parents informing them of a ban on foods containing peanuts.
    3. Identify all children at the child care centre who have a documented allergy to peanuts.
    4. Examine all food given to the children for sources of peanuts.

12. Many of the children develop communicable diseases, particularly upper respiratory infections and diarrhea during the fall and winter seasons. The nurse is asked about best practices for caregivers to reduce the incidence of infectious diseases with the children. Which of the following would the nurse recommend?

1. All workers should wash their hands with alcohol-based cleaner after changing diapers.
   2. Child care staff should wash their hands several times throughout the day.
   3. All equipment and toys should be washed with an antibacterial solution between uses by children.
   4. Any child who develops signs of a communicable disease during the day should be immediately separated from the other children.

13. Jayden is a 4-month-old infant with heart failure secondary to a congenital heart defect. The nurse discusses optimal feeding strategies for Jayden with the child care workers. Which of the following should the nurse advise?
    1. Feed Jayden on an every-2-hour schedule.
    2. Provide frequent rest breaks when feeding Jayden by bottle.
    3. Dilute formula feeds so that excess energy is not required for sucking.
    4. Gavage feed Jayden to conserve his energy.

14. The nurse has heard that there is a community outbreak of chicken pox. They are concerned about the children in the child care centre as many are immunocompromised. What immunization should the nurse ensure that each child has received?
    1. Varicella
    2. MMR
    3. Hib
    4. DTaP

15. Shobana, one of the children attending the child care centre, has been discovered to have head lice. What would the nurse recommend to the staff of the centre to control the spread of the head lice?
    1. Notify all families that Shobana has head lice and if their children have been playing with her, they should examine their children's hair.
    2. Send a letter to all parents about the outbreak with instructions for examining their child's hair and recommended treatment.
    3. Examine the hair of all children as they arrive at the child care centre and prohibit attendance if lice are found.
    4. Treat all of the children with the recommended pediculicide shampoo.

Independent Questions

Questions 16 to 25 do not refer to a particular case.

16. The nurse is preparing to admit a 3-year-old child with intussusception. What clinical manifestations should the nurse expect to observe? **Select all that apply.**
    1. Absent bowel sounds
    2. Passage of red, currant jelly-like stools
    3. Anorexia
    4. Tender, distended abdomen
    5. Hematemesis
    6. Sudden acute abdominal pain

17. What are the characteristics of diabetic ketoacidosis? **Select all that apply.**
    1. Pallor
    2. Acidosis
    3. Bradypnea
    4. Dehydration
    5. Hyperglycemia

18. What potential challenges will the nurse discuss with the parents of a newborn who has Down syndrome?
    1. Difficulty with feedings
    2. An increase in infections due to a decreased immune system
    3. An inability to respond to affection
    4. A gradual deterioration in developmental milestones

19. What clinical manifestations should the nurse recognize in an infant with increased intracranial pressure (ICP)? **Select all that apply.**
    1. High-pitched cry
    2. Poor feeding
    3. Setting-sun sign
    4. Sunken fontanel
    5. Distended scalp veins
    6. Decreased head circumference

20. A parent brings their 2-month-old infant to the health clinic, stating that the child has long episodes of crying with apparent abdominal pain and cannot be comforted. The infant is formula-fed. What would be an appropriate initial nursing intervention?
    1. Obtain a detailed history of the infant's diet, daily routine, and description of the crying episodes.
    2. Suggest a change to another formula as the symptoms are likely colic caused by an allergy to cow's milk.
    3. Discuss the advisability of initiating breastfeeding using techniques to re-establish the production of breast milk.
    4. Tell the parent that their infant is displaying classic manifestations of colic, and burping the infant more often along with comfort measures will correct the problem.

21. The nurse is caring for a 10-year-old child who has just returned to the surgical unit after a tonsillectomy for recurrent streptococcal infections. The nurse assesses the client. Based on the information provided, which initial action should the nurse take?

Vital Signs:	Nurse's Notes:	Physician Orders:
1045	1100	Ondansetron 4
Temperature: 36.8°C	Restless, vomiting	mg IV q6h for nausea
Pulse: 80 beats per minute	bright red blood.	Ibuprofen 200 mg po q6h for
Respirations: 18 breaths per minute	States throat is sore.	pain
Blood Pressure: 100/60		Clear fluids as tolerated

1. Position the client on their side.
2. Administer the ondansetron.
3. Notify the health care provider.
4. Administer the ibuprofen.

22. What clinical manifestations would be observed in a 2-year-old child with hypotonic dehydration? **Select all that apply.**
    1. Thick, doughy feel to the skin
    2. Slightly moist mucous membranes
    3. Absent tears
    4. Very rapid pulse
    5. Hyperirritability

23. A nurse works on a pediatric surgical unit with children experiencing postoperative pain. Which of the following is correct concerning pain in children?
    1. It is not possible to accurately assess pain in children.
    2. Use of narcotics in children is not recommended for pain control.
    3. Children are often undertreated for pain.
    4. Children always tell the truth about pain.

24. The nurse must administer a suspension of oral prednisone to a toddler. The prednisone solution is known to have a bitter taste. The child spat out the previous dose and is refusing to take the medicine. What is the most effective action to administer the prednisone?
    1. Have the parent assist the nurse in administering the prednisone.
    2. Ask the physician to change the liquid form to a suppository.
    3. Restrain the child and administer the prednisone via oral syringe.
    4. Mix the prednisone in applesauce.

25. A pediatric unit's philosophy is to provide family-centred care. Which of the following is an example of this approach to care?
    1. The family is included in the morning discussions with the health care team.
    2. The family receives lab values through the hospital website.
    3. Pediatric clients are given free access to the Internet to complete school work.
    4. Pediatric clients will need to follow a bedtime schedule based on their age.

REFERENCES

American Psychiatric Association (APA). (2022). *Diagnostic and statistical manual of mental health disorders* (5th ed.). American Psychiatric Publishing.

Autism Speaks Canada. (2022a). *Medical conditions associated with autism.* https://www.autismspeaks.org/medical-conditions-associated-autismAutism

Autism Speaks Canada. (2022b). *What is autism?* https://www.autismspeaks.ca/what-is-autism/

Bard, B., MacMullin, E., Williamson, J., et al. (2022). *Morrison-Valfre's foundations of mental health care in Canada.* Elsevier.

Canadian Cancer Society. (2022). *What is childhood leukemia?* http://www.cancer.ca/en/cancer-information/cancer-type/leukemia-childhood/childhood-leukemia/?region=on

Canadian Celiac Association. (2022). *Celiac disease: Overview.* https://www.celiac.ca/gluten-related-disorders/celiac-disease/

Canadian Dental Association. (2022a). *Cleaning teeth.* http://www.cda-adc.ca/en/oral_health/cfyt/dental_care_children/cleaning.asp

Canadian Dental Association. (2022b). *Your child's first visit.* http://www.cda-adc.ca/en/oral_health/cfyt/dental_care_children/first_visit.asp

Canadian Hemophilia Society. (2018). *Hemophilia A and B.* https://www.hemophilia.ca/hemophilia-a-and-b/

Canadian Institute of Child Health. (2022). *The health of Canada's children and youth: Congenital heart defects.* https://cichprofile.ca/module/8/section/7/page/congenital-heart-defects/

Canadian Paediatric Society (CPS). (2021a). *Caring for kids: Colds in children. what can I do if my child has a cold?* https://caringforkids.cps.ca/handouts/health-conditions-and-treatments/colds_in_children

Canadian Paediatric Society (CPS). (2021b). *Practice point: Suicidal ideation and behaviour.* https://cps.ca/documents/position/suicidal-ideation-and-behaviour

Canadian Paediatric Society (CPS). (2022a). *Caring for kids: Vitamin D. How much vitamin D should my baby receive?* https://caringforkids.cps.ca/handouts/pregnancy-and-babies/vitamin_d

Canadian Paediatric Society (CPS). (2022b). *Position statement: Preventing symptomatic vitamin deficiency and rickets among Indigenous infants and children in Canada.* https://cps.ca/en/documents/position/vitamin-d-deficiency-and-rickets-among-indigenous-infants-and-children

Centers for Disease Control and Prevention (CDC). (2019). *Parvovirus B19 and fifth disease.* https://www.cdc.gov/parvovirusb19/index.html.

Centers for Disease Control and Prevention (CDC). (2021). *Child passenger safety: Get the facts.* https://www.cdc.gov/transportationsafety/child_passenger_safety/cps-factsheet.html

Centers for Disease Control and Prevention (CDC). (2022). *Pneumococcal vaccination: What everyone should know. In depth.* https://www.cdc.gov/vaccines/vpd/pneumo/public/index.html

Centre for Addiction and Mental Health (CAMH). (2022). *Attention deficit hyperactivity disorder (ADHD). Overview.* https://www.camh.ca/en/health-info/mental-illness-and-addiction-index/attention-deficit-hyperactivity-disorder

Child Care State Capacity Building Center. (2018). *Planning for individual infants and toddlers in group care: Understanding and adapting to individual temperaments.* https://childcareta.acf.hhs.gov/sites/default/files/public/itrg_infants_and_toddlers_in_group_care_understanding_and_adapting_to_individual_temperaments.pdf

Chwalba, A., Dudek, A., & Otto-Buczkowska, E. (2020). Review article: Secondary diabetes. *Austin Journal of Nutrition and Metabolism, 7*(2), 1077. https://www.researchgate.net/publication/341463585_Secondary_diabetes

Cummings, C., Finlay, J. C., MacDonald, N. E., et al. (2021). *Practice point: Head lice infestations: A clinical update.* https://www.cps.ca/en/documents/position/head-lice

Cystic Fibrosis Canada. (2020). *Annual data report compiled by Canadian Cystic Fibrosis registry finds progress is being made, but there is still further to go.* https://www.cysticfibrosis.ca/news/annual-data-report-compiled-by-canadian-cystic-fibrosis-registry-finds-progress-is-being-made-but-there-is-still-further-to-go

Denison, M. R. (2005). Severe acute respiratory syndrome: Coronavirus pathogenesis, disease and vaccines: An update. *The Pediatric Infectious Disease Journal, 23*(Suppl. 11), S207–S214.

Fowler, J. (1981). *Stages of faith: The psychology of human development and the quest for meaning.* HarperCollins.

Government of Canada. (2018). *Family violence: How big is the problem in Canada?* https://www.canada.ca/en/public-health/services/health promotion/stop family violence/problem-canada.html

Government of Canada. (2019). *Stage 4: Seat belts.* https://tc.canada.ca/en/road-transportation/child-car-seat-safety/installing-child-car-seat-booster-seat/stage-4-seat-belts

Government of Canada. (2020a). *Suicide in Canada: Key statistics (infographic). Death and hospitalizations.* https://www.canada.ca/en/public-health/services/publications/healthy-living/suicide-canada-key-statistics-infographic.html

Government of Canada. (2020b). *Vaccine administration practices: Canadian immunization guide.* https://www.canada.ca/en/public-health/services/publications/healthy-living/canadian-immunization-guide-part-1-key-immunization-information/page-8-vaccine-administration-practices.html#p1c7a3d

Government of Canada. (2021). *Suicide in Canada. Higher risk populations.* https://www.canada.ca/en/public-health/services/suicide-prevention/suicide-canada.html

Government of Canada. (2022a). *Canada's food guide: Healthy eating for parents and children.* https://food-guide.canada.ca/en/tips-for-healthy-eating/parents-and-children/

Government of Canada. (2022b). *Childhood cancer counts in Canada.* https://www.canada.ca/en/public-health/services/publications/diseases-conditions/childhood-cancer-counts-canada.html

Government of Canada. (2022c). *Vaccines for children: COVID-19.* https://www.canada.ca/en/public-health/services/vaccination-children/covid-19.html

Government of Canada. (2023a). *Provincial and territorial immunization information.* https://www.canada.ca/en/public-health/services/provincial-territorial-immunization-information.html

Government of Canada. (2023b). *Recommended immunization schedule, children (less than 7 years of age), NOT previously immunized as infants.* https://www.canada.ca/en/public-health/services/publications/healthy-living/canadian-immunization-guide-part-1-key-immunization-information/page-13-recommended-immunization-schedules.html

Grace, V. (2020). *How eczema and food allergies are linked.* Very Well health. https://www.verywellhealth.com/foods-that-cause-eczema-1324065

Graham, F., & Eigenmann, P. A. (2020). Atopic dermatitis and its relation to food allergy. *Current Opinion in Allergy and Clinical Immunology, 20*(3), 305–310. https://doi.org/10.1097/ACI.0000000000000638

Hassink, S., & Fairbrother, G. (2020). Obesity and hunger threaten the foundations of child health. *Academic Pediatrics, 21*(3), 396–400. https://doi.org/10.1016/j.acap.2020.08.010

Hockenberry, M., Rodgers, C., & Wilson, D. (2022). *Wong's essentials of pediatric nursing* (11th ed.). Elsevier.

Horii, K. (2022). *Patient education: Diaper rash in infants and children (beyond the basics).* https://www.uptodate.com/contents/diaper-rash-in-infants-and-children-beyond-the-basics

Kalyoussef, S., Steele, R., Windle, M., et al. (2020). Pediatric candidiasis workup. laboratory studies. *Medscape.* https://emedicine.medscape.com/article/962300-workup

Keenan-Lindsay, L. (2020). *Leifer's introduction to maternity and pediatric nursing in Canada* (1st ed.). Elsevier.

Keenan-Lindsay, L., Sams, C., & O'Connor, C. (2022). *Perry's maternal child nursing care in Canada* (3rd ed.). Elsevier.

Mann, D. (2021). *Child abuse rose during COVID pandemic.* Health Day Us News. https://www.usnews.com/news/health-news/articles/2021-10-08/study-confirms-rise-in-child-abuse-during-covid-pandemic

McGrath, P. J., Johnson, G., Goodman, J. T., et al. (1985). CHEOPS: A behavioral scale for rating postoperative pain in children. In L. F. H, R. Dubner, & F. Cerveri (Eds.), *Advances in pain research and therapy* (pp. 395–402). Raven Press.

Parachute. (2021a). *Burns and scalds. Protect your child from scalds.* https://parachute.ca/en/injury-topic/burns-and-scalds/

Parachute. (2021b). *Car seats: Choosing the right car seat.* https://parachute.ca/en/injury-topic/car-seats/choosing-the-right-car-seat/

Parachute. (2021c). *Cycling. Protect your head: Wear a helmet.* https://parachute.ca/en/injury-topic/cyling/

Parachute. (2021d). *Drowning.* https://www.parachutecanada.org/en/injury-topic/drowning/

Parachute. (2021e). *Home safety. Play time.* https://www.parachutecanada.org/en/injury-topic/home-safety/play-time/.

Parachute. (2022). *Poisoning.* https://www.parachutecanada.org/en/injury-topic/poisoning/

Potter, P. A., Perry, A. G., Stockert, P., & Hall, A. (2019). *Canadian fundamentals of nursing* (6th ed.). Elsevier.

SickKids. (2022). *Our care philosophy: What is child and family-centred care?* https://www.sickkids.ca/en/patients-visitors/care-philosophy/

Statistics Canada. (2019a). *Census in brief: Portrait of children's family life in Canada in 2016.* https://www12.statcan.gc.ca/census-recensement/2016/as-sa/98-200-x/2016006/98-200-x2016006-eng.cfm

Statistics Canada. (2019b). *Census in brief: Same-sex couples in Canada in 2016.* https://www12.statcan.gc.ca/census-recensement/2016/as-sa/98-200-x/2016007/98-200-x2016007-eng.cfm

Statistics Canada. (2021). *Circumstances surrounding sudden and unexpected sleep-related infant deaths, 2015 to 2020.* https://www150.statcan.gc.ca/n1/daily-quotidien/211209/dq211209f-eng.htm

Statistics Canada. (2022a). *Census family.* https://www23.statcan.gc.ca/imdb/p3Var.pl?Function=UnitI&Id=1314048

Statistics Canada. (2022b). *A fifty-year look at divorces in Canada, 1970 to 2020.* https://www150.statcan.gc.ca/n1/daily-quotidien/220309/dq220309a-eng.htm

Statistics Canada. (2022c). *Leading cause of deaths, infants.* https://www150.statcan.gc.ca/t1/tbl1/en/tv.action?pid=1310039501

Statistics Canada. (2022d). *Many shelters for victims of abuse see increases in crisis calls and demand for external supports in the first year of the COVID-19 pandemic.* https://www150.statcan.gc.ca/n1/daily-quotidien/220412/dq220412b-eng.htm

Stevens, B., Johnston, C., Petryshen, P., et al. (1996). Premature infant pain profile: Development and initial validation. *The Clinical Journal of Pain, 12*(1), 13–22.

UCSF Pediatric Cardiothoracic Surgery. (2022). *Atrial septal defect (ASD): Types of holes in the heart.* https://pedctsurgery.ucsf.edu/conditions–procedures/atrial-septal-defect.aspx

BIBLIOGRAPHY

Astle, B., & Duggleby, W. (2024). *Potter and Perry's Canadian fundamental of nursing* (7th ed.). Elsevier.

Jarvis, C., Eckhardt, A., Browne, A., et al. (2024). *Physical examination & health assessment* (4th ed.). Elsevier.

Vanier Institute of the Family. (2022). *Definition of the family.* https://vanierinstitute.ca/definition-of-family/

WEBSITES

- **Canadian Paediatric Society** (http://www.cps.ca): This site was created by Canadian pediatricians to provide child health care information for physicians and other interdisciplinary health care providers.
- **Canadian Toys Regulations** (http://laws-lois.justice.gc.ca/eng/regulations/SOR-2011-17/FullText.html): This federal government site lists regulation requirements for toys sold in Canada.
- **Caring for Kids** (https://caringforkids.cps.ca/): Caring for Kids is a CPS site that provides child health and wellness information to families and children. It covers a variety of topics, such as pregnancy and babies, immunizations, care for sick children, and the use of natural products.
- **Clinical Practice Guidelines for Nurses in Primary Care: Pediatric and Adolescent Care** (https://www.canada.ca/en/health-canada/services/first-nations-inuit-health/health-care-services/nursing/clinical-practice-guidelines-nurses-primary-care/pediatric-adolescent-care.html): This federal government site includes pediatric clinical practice guidelines for nurses on different subjects, such as health assessment, prevention, fluid management, and child abuse.
- **Government of Canada: Toy Safety** (https://www.canada.ca/en/health-canada/services/toy-safety.html): This federal government site provides general toy safety tips and information on playing smart and playing safe.
- **Government of Canada: Transport Canada. Child car seat safety** (https://tc.canada.ca/en/road-transportation/child-car-seat-safety): This federal government site lists regulations and information on child car seats and booster seats.
- **Parachute** (https://www.parachutecanada.org/en/injury-topics/): This Canadian charitable organization is dedicated to preventing injuries and saving lives.

Mental Health Nursing

Mental health, like physical health, affects a person's well-being. Often the two go hand in hand due to the complex relationships among biological, genetic, psychological, and social or environmental factors. People with a mental illness often develop physical symptoms and vice versa. Mental illness does not discriminate among ages, cultures, or income or education levels. Each year, approximately 1 in 5 Canadians experiences a mental illness (Centre for Addiction and Mental Health [CAMH], 2022a).

Mental health and mental illness occur along a continuum, just as physical health and illness do. Consequently, just as we speak of health within illness, a person can have a mental illness but manage that illness in healthy ways. People may have varying qualities and experiences that could be designated as healthy or unhealthy, but only when the unhealthy outweighs the healthy will help be sought or required from a mental health professional. Nurses care for clients with mental health conditions in every type of setting and play an essential role in helping these clients and their families on the road to achieving their optimal level of health.

LEGAL, ETHICAL, AND INTERPERSONAL CONSIDERATIONS FOR MENTAL HEALTH NURSING

As professionals, nurses are bound by legal, moral, and ethical principles that govern their practice. Because laws, morals, and ethics are grounded in providing for the good of society, they offer guidelines that help nurses provide exemplary care for their clients. Sometimes, however, these guidelines are not completely clear, and often they can contradict one another. Ethical dilemmas occur when a practice decision must be made between two competing but imperfect and not completely desirable choices. Mental health practice challenges nurses to use their judgement to interpret the guidelines and make ethical decisions, often when the circumstances are ambiguous.

Canadian practical nurses uphold and promote a code of ethics. The Canadian Council for Practical Nurse Regulators (CCPNR, 2013) code of ethics states that a practical nurse's responsibilities are defined under the following five ethical principles:

1. Responsibility to the public
2. Responsibility to clients
3. Responsibility to the profession
4. Responsibility to colleagues
5. Responsibility to oneself

Registered and licensed practical nurses follow a code of ethics in conjunction with their provincial and jurisdiction standards and competencies, workplace policies, and the legal requirements that govern their practice and behaviour. The CCPNR code of ethics is discussed in more detail in Chapter 4. Refer to the CCPNR website, listed at the end of the chapter in the "Websites" section, for more information.

In Canada, health care is the responsibility of the provincial and territorial governments. Consequently, each province and territory has its own *Mental Health Act* outlining the regulations for voluntary and involuntary admission to hospital, consent for treatment, and the rights of (and safeguards for) clients with mental health disorders. Similarly, legislation defining guardianship and substitute decision makers varies across the country. Federal laws that impact clients with mental health disorders include the *Canadian Charter of Rights and Freedoms* and the *Criminal Code of Canada* (Bard et al. 2022; Halter et al., 2019).

Psychological, neurobiological, and genetic pathologies cause mental health disorders that result in disorganization and impairment of thinking, memory, mood, behaviour, or all of these. Consequently, people with a mental illness suffer significant distress and difficulties in everyday functioning.

Impairments of cognition and emotion can interfere with an individual's ability to make appropriate decisions in their own best interest, or they may cause the client to make decisions or exhibit behaviours that interfere with the rights of others. Thus, the client's condition may require nurses to make ethical and legal choices between competing values. For example, in the case of a client with a psychotic disorder, denying a client's right to autonomy may preserve their health or the rights and safety of others.

Mental illness does not discriminate; anyone can suffer from a mental illness. The characteristics of different population groups may pose particular legal and ethical issues for mental health nurses. Here, issues related to different cultures and people experiencing homelessness are discussed.

Cultural Differences

Mental health care in Canada is decidedly influenced by Western ideology and practices, yet we are a multicultural society, and people of different cultures may define normal and abnormal behaviour differently. Many people base their health care decisions on both scientific and cultural values. Traditional health practices explain disease culturally as an imbalance of energies. For example, Chinese cultures consider health to be a balance of positive and negative energy forces (yin and yang). An imbalance results in disease. African cultures view the mind and body are one and function in harmony with earth and the supernatural. Disease is caused by a state of disharmony (Bard et al., 2022). Indigenous health requires a balance among four components of the human: emotional, physical, spiritual, and mental. Poor health results from an imbalance or disharmony between the four components (Astle & Duggleby, 2024). Nurses need to understand and respect an individual client's traditional health beliefs and practices to promote effective mental health care in a culturally safe environment

Often health care providers require a translator to understand the client's history and health care needs. There is a difference between an interpreter and a translator. An *interpreter* is more likely to unconsciously try to make sense of (interpret) what the client is saying and therefore inserts their own understanding of the situation into the database. A *professional translator*, on the other hand, tries to avoid interpreting. Halter et al. (2019) strongly advises against the use of untrained interpreters such as family members, friends, and neighbours. These individuals might censor or omit certain content (e.g., profanity, psychotic thoughts, and sexual topics) due to fear or a desire to protect the client. They can also make subjective interpretations based on their own feelings, share confidential details with outsiders, or leave out traumatic topics because they hit too close to home for them (Halter et al., 2019).

To be culturally sensitive and competent, mental health nurses need to do the following:

- Critically examine their personal cultural beliefs, values, and any ethnocentric tendencies.
- Become familiar with a variety of different cultures and ethnic groups.
- Plan culturally congruent care after conducting a thorough cultural assessment (Bard et al., 2022).
- Assess how cultural groups define mental illness and what methods of healing are acceptable.
- Learn about cultural and religious rituals, protective symbols, and standards of modesty in various belief systems.
- Respect a person's dietary restrictions and customs.
- Exhibit sensitivity, openness, and flexibility in approach and interactions.
- Understand that cultural difference is not limited to a difference based on membership in an ethnic or racial group, but rather encompasses differences in experience, meaning, and what is significant to particular individuals and families (Bard et al., 2022).

Homelessness

The connections between mental illness and homelessness are many. The downsizing of mental hospitals over 50 years ago began a process of deinstitutionalization, when many people were discharged without appropriate community services and programs in place. Many who experience mental illness face multiple barriers (such as stigma and lack of social support) to achieving high levels of education or full employment. Reductions in social assistance eligibility, fewer opportunities for unskilled work, the lack of affordable housing, and a propensity for substance abuse are also factors leading to poverty and homelessness. Approximately 85% of people experiencing homelessness have concurrent conditions of addiction and a severe mental illness (Bard et al., 2022). Estimates of the proportion of people who are homeless with a mental illness vary widely across Canada, but in various cities they range from 23 to 67% (CAMH, 2022a).

The "not in my backyard" (NIMBY) syndrome is a common social attitude. Canadians want people experiencing homelessness off the streets but reject having services and housing for them located in their own neighbourhoods.

Factors to bear in mind about people experiencing homelessness with a mental illness:

- For some individuals, having a severe mental illness leads to being homeless; for others, the stress of being homeless leads to developing a mental illness.
- People experiencing homelessness with a mental illness are particularly vulnerable to being victimized in inner-city areas.
- Health care services for people experiencing homelessness with a mental illness involve assertive outreach programs that provide medical and psychiatric care, social assistance, meals, temporary shelters, and housing, vocational and life-skills training, and advocacy.
- Respecting the dignity and rights of the client according to the five ethical principles in the CCPNR code of ethics guides practical nursing practice with people experiencing homelessness with a mental illness.

Interpersonal Relationships With Clients With Mental Health Disorders

Establishing a therapeutic relationship with a client with a mental health disorder obligates the nurse to act in both ethical and legal ways. People with a mental illness are very vulnerable; their relationships with health care providers are often lengthy and very important to them. Conscientious nurses establish and maintain caring relationships but stay within their professional boundaries. Nurses must also be very aware of their relative power in those relationships and avoid abusing that power, while trying to balance a client's rights and safety with the societal rights of others.

Privacy and Confidentiality

- The CCPNR code of ethics states that personal, family, and community information must be protected and kept confidential. The only exceptions occur (a) when the practical nurse is legally required to disclose information and (b) when revealing information could prevent serious harm to the client or to others. In such cases, the practical nurse should try (where possible) to avoid actually identifying the client and to minimize any resulting stigma.
- If a client refuses to share information with family members, an ethical dilemma may arise, particularly if the family member is the person's primary caregiver outside the hospital.
- In most provinces, a family member must legally be notified when a client is admitted to or discharged from the hospital or scheduled to appear before a review board. The client nominates a family member or a near-relative (someone

who the client has identified as being equivalent to family) as the person who should be notified in these cases.

Clients' Rights

In Canada, unlike in the United States, there is no client's bill of rights. Clients with a mental illness, including those involuntarily admitted to hospital, are entitled to the same fundamental rights as all Canadians, under the *Canadian Charter of Rights and Freedoms*. All provincial and territorial *Mental Health Acts* must comply with the Charter (Bard et al., 2022).

Voluntary Admission to Hospital

- Most clients with a psychiatric illness in Canada are admitted voluntarily, by their own consent, under the same processes as other hospital clients.
- Voluntary clients may discharge themselves from the hospital when they wish.
- In most parts of Canada, for clients who are incapable of giving consent (such as a child or an incapable adult), consent may be provided by a parent, legal guardian, or substitute decision maker nominated by the client while well. In such cases, clients may not discharge themselves without the consenting person's agreement.

Involuntary Admission to Hospital

Admission to a psychiatric facility without the client's consent is often called *commitment* and usually happens in response to a crisis or need for emergency care. Although admission without consent contradicts the ethical value of promoting and respecting informed decision making, a client may be admitted when all three of the following conditions are met:

- The person refuses to be admitted or is incapable of making that decision.
- The person appears to have a mental health disorder.
- The illness is likely to cause harm or danger to the person or to others.

A physician completes a medical certificate that allows the person to be apprehended, transported to a mental health facility, and admitted for a specified period that varies across Canada from 1 to 3 days. Involuntary clients can only be admitted to hospitals that are defined by that province's *Mental Health Act* as mental health facilities.

If an individual meets these three criteria but refuses to see a doctor, the police may apprehend the person and take them to a hospital emergency department. There, a physician examines the person and completes the first certificate, if necessary.

To keep the client longer than the legally limited initial period, another physician or psychiatrist must complete a second certificate. In New Brunswick, however, the admission decision is made by a tribunal; in Quebec, by a judge; and in the Northwest Territories and Nunavut, by the Minister of Health. When the specified longer period of detention expires (between 2 and 4 weeks, depending on the jurisdiction), a renewal certificate must be completed or the client must be allowed to leave.

If a client who is involuntary admitted wishes to be discharged, they (or a substitute decision maker, if one is available) applies to a review panel. This board acts as a judge and can overrule the physician on the basis of evidence gathered. In the Northwest Territories, this review takes place in court. Review boards also meet at legally defined designated intervals for clients who are certified for long periods.

The Charter mandates that clients who are involuntarily admitted must be informed of their legal rights upon admission. Some provincial and territorial *Mental Health Acts* require this notification to be repeated each time a certificate is renewed. Clients must be informed of the following:

- Why they were admitted
- That they have the right to contact a lawyer
- That they can apply to a review board for a legal ruling on the involuntary admission (Bard et al., 2022).

There are many certificates (forms) under the *Mental Health Act*. These forms may vary depending on the province or territory. The following are a few regarding involuntary admissions to ensure the rights, assessments, and treatment of people experiencing mental health needs are being maintained.

Form 1: Application for Psychiatric Assessment (Admission Certificate)

- Provides detention to allow an assessment of a person's mental state
- This can occur when the medical physician reasonably believes the person is at risk of self-harm, harm to others, or unable to care for self without psychiatric treatment.
- Valid for up to 72 hours
- If a client leaves the facility without authorization the police can be notified to return the client.

Form 42: Notice to Person

- Notification to the client that they are now on a Form 1 and the reason why
- Completed by the medical doctor who is detaining the client at the psychiatric facility
- Must be given promptly to the client

Form 2: Order for Examination Under Section 16

- Filled out by a Justice of the Peace, based on the information presented by other members of the public (which can include but is not limited to a medical physician)
- Similar criteria as a Form 1: danger to self or others, inability to care for self secondary to a mental illness
- Valid for 7 days

Form 3: Certificate of Involuntary Admission

- Signed by a different medical physician than with Form 1; usually done by a psychiatrist
- This allows the client to have a second opinion assessment.
- Can last for up to 14 days

Form 4: Renewal Form of a Form 3

- Lasts longer and can be renewed
- Client now becomes an involuntary client

Form 30: Notice to Patient Regarding Right Advice

- Notification to the client that they are on a Form 3 and why
- Completed by medical physician who completed the Form 3 and given promptly to the client
- Client will get rights advice about the right to appeal

Informed Consent

For consent to be informed, a person must be provided with the following information to consider:
- Information about the condition
- Information about the proposed treatment
- The benefits to be expected from the treatment
- The risks and adverse effects of getting the treatment
- Any alternative treatments or courses of action
- The consequences to be expected from not receiving the treatment

Nurses value the right of people to make their own decisions about health care and services, without coercion, and to have sufficient information on which to base those choices.
- The CCPNR code of ethics stipulates that practical nurses must assist people to obtain complete current knowledge of their condition and also must respect a client's decision (or that of a legally approved substitute decision maker), even if it differs from the nurse's own beliefs and opinions. This includes respecting the right to refuse consent or withdraw consent at any time.
- Further, a nurse is responsible for providing care that goes against their personal values until a replacement care provider can be obtained.
- A person is considered incapable of providing consent if they cannot understand or appreciate the consequences of accepting or rejecting treatment.
- Involuntary admission does not necessarily mean that treatment can begin, although in some provinces or territories the physician or facility director can authorize treatment. In others, a tribunal must meet to approve treatment, and this may mean a delay lasting a few days.
- If the client has requested a review, no treatment can begin until the review panel upholds the involuntary admission, even if a substitute decision maker has signed the consent for treatment.

Treatment in the Least Restrictive Setting

Aggressive behaviour is common with some mental illnesses. It is also important to assess the client's history of aggression or violence. Most of our reactions to stimuli come from our previous experiences; therefore, identifying clients' triggers is essential. Initial and ongoing assessment of the client can reveal issues before they escalate to anger and aggression. Such assessment also leads directly to the appropriate nursing diagnosis and intervention (Halter et al., 2019). When a mental illness is well controlled, however, there is no greater risk of violence than there would be from the general population. Violence is most common when the illness is poorly controlled, as in the case of a client who has stopped taking their medications.

Restraints and Seclusion

When a client or someone else is likely to be harmed or property may be destroyed, seclusion or restraint may be necessary. The following restraint principles must be followed:
- The client is always entitled to the least restrictive alternative that ensures safety.
- Restraints should be released, and the client allowed out of seclusion, as soon as they have calmed down.
- Restraints require a physician's order.
- Clients in restraints or seclusion must be closely monitored at regular and frequent intervals, as often as every 5 to 15 minutes depending on the situation. Clients are assessed to ensure all physical needs are addressed, including safety, comfort, food, fluids, and elimination. Accurate and complete documentation is vital.
- Physical or chemical restraints (sedation) should not be used when a brief period of seclusion would suffice to calm the client and ease the situation.
- In most provinces and territories, the *Mental Health Act* provides legal protection for staff to give treatment or restrain individuals, if their health or safety is endangered or the safety of others would be compromised without that treatment or restraint (Bard et al., 2022).
- Restraints and seclusion should never be used as punishment or for staff convenience.
- Seclusion and restraints are contraindicated for people who are clearly suicidal and for those with delirium or dementia, for whom decreased stimulation is likely to increase agitation.

Managing Behavioural Crises

Behavioural crises can lead to client violence toward self or others and usually, but not always, escalate through fairly predictable stages. Staff in most mental health facilities practise crisis prevention and management techniques. Many general and psychiatric hospitals have special teams made up of nurses, psychiatric technicians, and other professionals who respond to psychiatric emergencies called codes. Each member of the team takes part in the team effort to defuse a crisis in its early stages. If preventive measures fail and imminent risk of harm to self or others persists, each member of the team participates in a rapid, organized plan to safely manage the situation. The nurse is most often this team's leader, not only organizing the plan but also timing the intervention and managing the concurrent use of prn medications (Halter et al., 2019).

Workplace violence toward nurses and other health care providers is an ongoing concern. Recommendations on how to deal with aggressive clients include creating a culture of safety, increasing the number of interventions, reporting incidents, and having skills on crisis intervention techniques (Halter et al., 2019). The following are ways nurses can keep themselves safe if anticipating aggressive behaviours:
- Nurses should stay at least an arm's length away (1.5 m) from the aggressive client and monitor the client for signs of losing control.
- Be aware of your physical environment. Know where the exits are and stand between the client and door for an unobstructive access to exit.

- Perform hourly rounds on the unit in pairs of two. Use a team approach.
- Have two nurses enter the room of a potential aggressive client or have one nurse enter the room and another nurse to stay by the door for immediate assistance if needed.
- If a client raises any verbal or nonverbal threat, stop solo intervention and retreat from the situation and, if needed, continue only as a team intervention.
- Nurses should not wear any lanyards or stethoscopes around their neck (Bard et al., 2022).
  De-escalation techniques are described in Box 12.1.

Duty to Report

People who are mentally ill are vulnerable to abuse. Nurses are legally and ethically obliged to report suspected or confirmed cases to the appropriate authorities in the following circumstances:

- Family abuse: Child abuse, elder abuse, and partner abuse are criminal acts and must be reported to the police and to the local child and family services office for suspected child abuse, neglect, injury, or abandonment.
- Abuse of clients: Staff who abuse clients should be reported to management, and criminal charges may be laid. Professional staff should be reported to their licensing bodies. Nurses have a duty to report any nursing colleague who abuses clients to the college or nursing association that registers/licenses nurses in their province or territory.
- Sexual abuse of a client is any sexual or romantic relationship with a client—even if it is perceived to be or is consensual, it is considered abusive. The staff who abuses the client sexually needs to be reported to management and criminal charges may be laid. Professional staff should be reported to their licensing bodies. Individuals or facilities may be fined if they do not make a report related to sexual abuse (College of Nurses [CNO], 2022).
- Unsafe nursing practices: Practical nurses are also obligated to report unsafe nursing practices to management and to the body that registers/licenses nurses in their province or territory.

BOX 12.1　De-escalation Techniques: Practice Principles

- Maintain the client's self-esteem and dignity.
- Maintain calmness (your own and the client's).
- Assess the client and the situation.
- Watch the client's body language (can indicate if client ready to hit or push).
- Identify stressors and stress indicators.
- Respond as early as possible.
- Use a calm, clear tone of voice.
- Invest time.
- Remain honest.
- Establish what the client considers to be their need.
- Be goal-oriented.
- Maintain a large personal space.
- Position yourself close to the door in case you have to escape quickly.
- Do not touch the client. Keep your hands free.
- Avoid verbal struggles.
- Give several options.
- Make the options clear.
- Utilize a nonaggressive posture.
- Use genuineness and empathy.
- Attempt to be confidently aware.
- Use verbal, nonverbal, and communication skills.
- Listen to the client. Restate what the client states in your own words.
- Be assertive (not aggressive).
- Assess for personal safety.
- Note location of call bells, alarms, and other security devices.
- If you are in the client's home, leave the house if you think you are in danger. Go to safe a place and call you supervisor. If cannot leave the house and feel threatened, call police 9-1-1.

Adapted from Halter, M. J., Pollard, C. L., & Jakubec, S. L. (2019). *Varcarolis's Canadian psychiatric mental health nursing: A clinical approach* (2nd Cdn. ed., Box 23-3, p. 519). Elsevier Canada.

The Nursing Process in Mental Health Nursing

Stuart (2013) describes the nursing process in mental health nursing:

The nursing process is an interactive, problem-solving process and a systematic and individualized way to achieve the outcomes of nursing care. When used with psychiatric clients, the nursing process can present unique challenges. Mental health problems may be vague and elusive, not tangible, or visible like many physiological illnesses. Many psychiatric clients may be unable to describe their problems. They may be withdrawn, highly anxious, or out of touch with reality. Their ability to participate in the problem-solving process also may be limited if they see themselves as powerless victims or if their illness impairs them from fully engaging in the treatment process. (p. 149)

The nursing process is a collaborative process that involves working with the client on developing client-centred, mutually agreed-upon goals and interventions.

SPECIFIC COMMUNICATION AND THERAPEUTIC APPROACHES WITH CLIENTS WITH MENTAL HEALTH DISORDERS

To fully understand mental health, mental illnesses, and therapeutic approaches in mental health nursing, the functions of the brain and central nervous system (CNS) are reviewed here.

Brain Structure and Function

The structure and function of the brain are illustrated in Figure 12.1.

Cerebrum

Two hemispheres are connected by the corpus callosum, where the pineal gland is located. The pineal gland regulates

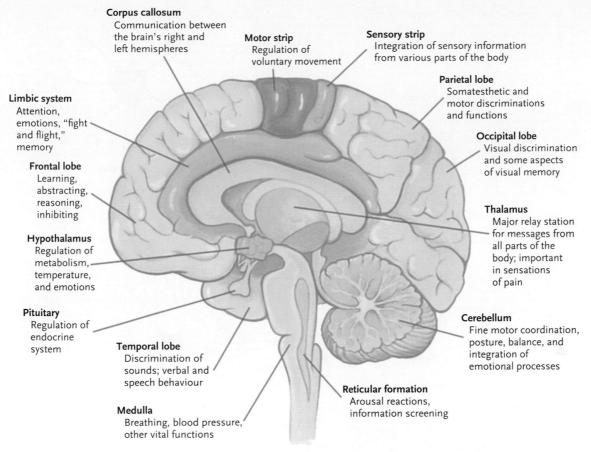

Corpus callosum
Communication between
the brain's right and
left hemispheres

Motor strip
Regulation of
voluntary movement

Sensory strip
Integration of sensory information
from various parts of the body

Parietal lobe
Somatesthetic and
motor discriminations
and functions

Occipital lobe
Visual discrimination
and some aspects
of visual memory

Limbic system
Attention,
emotions, "fight
and flight,"
memory

Frontal lobe
Learning,
abstracting,
reasoning,
inhibiting

Hypothalamus
Regulation of
metabolism,
temperature,
and emotions

Thalamus
Major relay station
for messages from
all parts of the
body; important
in sensations
of pain

Pituitary
Regulation of
endocrine
system

Temporal lobe
Discrimination of
sounds; verbal and
speech behaviour

Cerebellum
Fine motor coordination,
posture, balance, and
integration of
emotional processes

Reticular formation
Arousal reactions,
information screening

Medulla
Breathing, blood pressure,
other vital functions

Fig. 12.1 Structure and function of the brain. (From Stuart, G. W. [2013]. *Principles and practice of psychiatric nursing* [10th ed., p. 71, Figure 5-5]. Mosby.)

gonadal function and also produces melatonin, which influences the sleep cycle. Each hemisphere of the cerebrum contains the four lobes and other structures depicted in Figure 12.1. The following points describe the function of the structures within the hemispheres:

- Right hemisphere: Regulates creativity and intuition and controls the left side of the body
- Left hemisphere: Regulates logical, analytical thinking and controls the right side of the body
- Frontal lobes: Integrate and organize complex thinking for solving problems, producing speech, planning, and making decisions, regulating arousal, and focusing attention. Abnormalities in these lobes are found in schizophrenia, attention-deficit/hyperactivity disorder (ADHD), and dementia.
- Parietal lobes: Interpret taste and touch and help with spatial perceptions and balance
- Temporal lobes: Interpret hearing and smell and support memory, language comprehension, and the expression of emotions
- Occipital lobes: Help coordinate and interpret speech and vision

Cerebellum

The cerebellum coordinates movement and balance. Damage to the cerebellum is implicated in Parkinson's disease and dementia.

Brainstem

The brainstem structures control the following:
- Medulla oblongata: Controls cardiac and respiratory function
- Reticular activating system: Controls sleep and consciousness and relays motor neuron impulses
- Locus ceruleus: Is implicated in impulsive behaviour, related to stress and anxiety

Limbic System

The limbic system controls the following:
- Thalamus: Regulates mood, activity, and sensation
- Hypothalamus: Regulates temperature, appetite, hormones, and impulsive reactions, such as anger and excitement. The hypothalamus is involved in psychosomatic disorders and in stress response.
- Hippocampus and amygdala: Regulate emotions and memory Psychopathology of the limbic system includes dementia, mania, and other psychoses.

Ventricles

These spaces between the hemispheres and other structures are filled with cerebrospinal fluid (CSF), which cushions and nourishes brain structures. In many psychiatric disorders, enlarged ventricles imply the destruction and atrophy of surrounding brain structures.

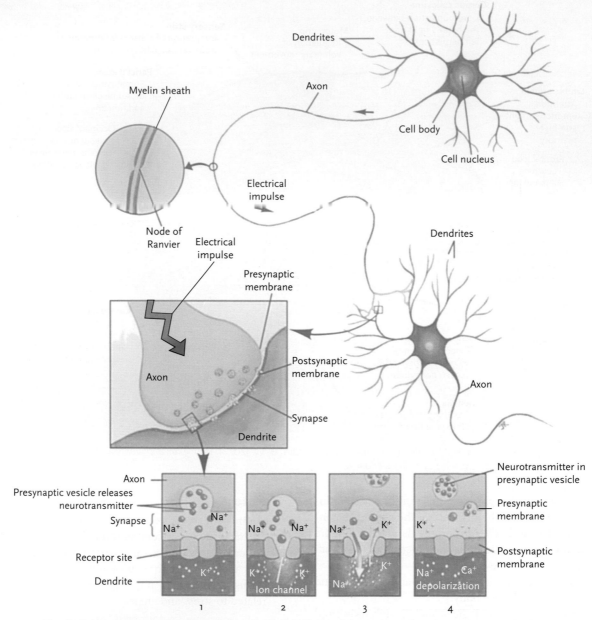

Fig. 12.2 Neurotransmission. (From Stuart, G. W. [2013]. *Principles and practice of psychiatric nursing* [10th ed., p. 75, Figure 5-7]. Mosby.)

Neural Structure and Function

Figure 12.2 illustrates the process of neurotransmission.

Neurotransmitters

Neurotransmission is the relaying of information in the synapse from neuron to neuron through electrical impulses and chemicals called neurotransmitters. Neurotransmitters and their function play an important role in many mental health conditions, as follows:

- Reuptake: After the message impulse is transmitted to the receptor cells, neurotransmitters return to the axon for storage or, alternatively, are inactivated and metabolized by enzymes, primarily monoamine oxidase (MAO).
- Psychiatric illnesses: They are characterized by abnormally high or low concentrations of certain neurotransmitters.

- Norepinephrine and epinephrine (noradrenaline and adrenalin): Found mainly in the brainstem, these chemicals control the stress response ("fight or flight") and influence the brain's reward system. Norepinephrine also helps regulate mood.
- Dopamine: It has mainly an excitatory effect on movement, emotions, motivation, and cognition. Dopamine is involved in movement disorders such as Parkinson's disease, as well as in schizophrenia and other psychotic illnesses.
- Serotonin: It has primarily an inhibitory effect. Serotonin is important in the regulation of sleep, appetite, and libido; therefore, serotonin-circuit dysfunction can result in sleep disturbances, decreased appetite, low sex drive, poor impulse control, and irritability (Halter et al., 2019). Serotonin also has been implicated in schizophrenia. It has a

modulating effect on dopamine. The first-generation atypical antipsychotic medications are combination serotonin/dopamine blocking agents, explaining their improved efficacy over the typical antipsychotics. Blocking serotonin in the limbic system increases frontal dopamine with a net effect of improving negative symptoms (Halter et al., 2019).

- Acetylcholine: It may be excitatory or inhibitory, affecting sleep–wake cycles, and signalling muscular activity. People with Alzheimer's disease have low levels of acetylcholine.
- Glutamate: It opens the calcium ion channel to allow electrical impulses through the synapse. Excessively high levels (such as those found in stroke, hypoglycemia, and ischemia and as a result of taking medications such as phencyclidine [PCP]) are toxic to brain cells.
- Gamma-aminobutyric acid (GABA): It is an inhibitory neurotransmitter that helps regulate other neurotransmitters. Benzodiazepines increase GABA to reduce anxiety and promote sleep.
- Endorphins and enkephalins: They are the brain's natural opiates. They have an inhibitory effect, reducing pain and stimulating pleasure by affecting the brain's reward system.
- Histamine: In addition to moderating allergic responses and reducing gastric and cardiac stimulation, histamine controls alertness. People with depression have low levels of histamine.

Diagnostics Tools and Therapeutics Used in Mental Health Nursing

Diagnosis

Criteria for diagnosing all psychiatric disorders and illnesses are defined in the *Diagnostic and Statistical Manual of Mental Disorders, 5th edition, Text revision* (DSM-5-TR; American Psychiatric Association [APA], 2022). It is the first published revision of the DSM-5. This dimensional diagnostic system correlates with treatment planning by using the DSM and International Classification of Disease (ICD) as the standards to how mental diseases are diagnosed and treated. Section II of the DSM-5-TR contains 22 different diagnostic criteria and codes. It identifies disorders based on criteria in clinical settings such as inpatient, outpatient, partial hospitalization, consultation–liaison, clinics, private practice, primary care, and community populations. The DSM-5-TR includes the addition of new disorders and psychiatric conditions, modifications and updated terminology, the refinement of diagnostic criteria, or specifier definitions for many disorders based on advances in literature and scientific research.

The DSM-5-TR organizes diagnoses for psychiatric disorders on a developmental hierarchy. Disorders seen in infancy, childhood, and adolescence appear in the first chapter, and neurodevelopmental disorders and disorders that occur later in life, such as neurocognitive disorders, appear later. The ICD sets the global health information standard for mortality and morbidity statistics. Clinicians and researchers use this classification system to define diseases, study disease patterns, monitor outcomes, and subsequently allocate resources based on the prevalence of disease.

The DSM-5-TR enables mental health care providers to communicate using a common diagnostic tool. It helps to implement effective interventions in order to improve clinical outcomes. It helps nurses in their assessment findings and in communicating clinical information to other health care providers, families, and clients. The DSM-5-TR classifies disorders, not people. In the DSM-5-TR, experts have integrated issues related to culture and mental illness into the discussion of each disorder. It is imperative to take the client's social and cultural influences into account during assessments and diagnoses. Frequently, when these illnesses are treated in culturally prescribed ways, the remedies are quite effective (Halter et al., 2019).

Psychological testing. Clinical psychologists administer many tests to measure intelligence and cognitive functioning, as well as aspects of personality, memory, impulse control, interpersonal behaviour, and self-concept. A common one is the Minnesota Multiphasic Personality Inventory (MMPI).

Electroencephalogram. Electroencephalograms (EEGs) are graphic tracings of the brain's electrical impulses, used to differentiate among neurological and psychiatric conditions and to evaluate various neurological symptoms, such as delirium, hallucinations, and altered states of consciousness.

Neuroimaging. Newer and more sophisticated technology for visualizing the brain includes the following:

- CT scans: Computed axial tomography uses X-rays, and sometimes a contrast agent such as iodine is used to produce sharply defined images of a "slice" through body tissues.
- MRI scans: Magnetic resonance imaging uses magnetic energy to discriminate among different tissue densities. This technique is contraindicated in pregnancy and for people with metal in their bodies, including pacemakers, metal plates, and bone replacements.
  - CT and MRI scans are used to detect structural abnormalities, such as tumours and hematomas.
- PET scans: Positron emission tomography aids investigation of brain function by measuring glucose consumption, that is, metabolic activity, in brain cells. Blood flow and synaptic activity can be distinguished. Common laboratory and diagnostic tests appear in Appendix D.

Pharmacotherapy

In general, medications used for psychiatric therapy regulate abnormal levels of specific neurotransmitters. Refer to Chapter 8 for medication action, adverse effects, and signs of overdose, with particular attention to the following classes of drugs:

- Antipsychotics: Typical and atypical
- Mood stabilizers: Lithium, antiepileptics
- Antidepressants: Tricyclic, selective serotonin/norepinephrine reuptake inhibitors (SNRIs), selective serotonin reuptake inhibitors (SSRIs), MAO inhibitors (MAOIs), atypical antidepressants
- Antianxiety medications: Also called *anxiolytics*

The major interactions of psychotropic drugs are reviewed in Table 12.1.

TABLE 12.1 Drug Interactions of Psychotropic Drugs

Drug Class	Interacting Drug(s)	Mechanism	Result
Anxiolytic Drugs			
Benzodiazepines	CNS (central nervous system) depressants (e.g., alcohol, opioids)	Additive effect	Enhanced CNS depression (e.g., sedation, confusion, ataxia)
	Oral contraceptives, azole antifungals, verapamil hydrochloride, diltiazem hydrochloride, opioids, valproic acid	Inadequate liver elimination of benzodiazepine	Enhanced benzodiazepine effects (e.g., CNS depression)
	Rifampin	Enhanced benzodiazepine clearance	Reduced therapeutic effects
	Theophylline	Antagonistic effects	Reduced sedative effects
	Phenytoin	Reduced clearance	Potential for digoxin toxicity and phenytoin toxicity
Miscellaneous			
Buspirone hydrochloride	CYP3A4 inhibitors, azole antifungals, verapamil hydrochloride, diltiazem hydrochloride	Reduced liver metabolism of buspirone hydrochloride	Enhanced buspirone hydrochloride effects
	Rifampin	Enhanced buspirone hydrochloride clearance	Reduced therapeutic effects
	MAOIs (monoamine oxidase inhibitors)	Unknown	Increased blood pressure
Selected Mood-Stabilizing and Antidepressant Drugs			
Mood Stabilizers			
Lithium salts	Thiazide diuretics, angiotensin-converting enzyme inhibitors, verapamil, diltiazem, NSAIDs (nonsteroidal anti-inflammatory drugs) caffeine (causes decreased lithium levels)	Decreased lithium excretion	Increased lithium toxicity
Antiepileptic Drugs			
Phenytoin	Amiodarone, benzodiazepine, azole antifungals, isoniated proton pump inhibitors, sulfonamide antibiotics, selective serotonin reuptake inhibitors (SSRIs)	Altered CYP450 enzyme metabolism	Reduced phenytoin clearance and increased effects
	Warfarin sodium	Displacement of warfarin from plasma protein binding sites	Increased free warfarin levels and bleeding risk
Carbamazepine	Azole antifungals, diltiazem, isoniazid macrolides, protease inhibitor antiretrovirals, SSRIs, valproic acid, verapamil	Altered CYP450 enzyme metabolism	Increased carbamazepine levels and toxicity
	Acetaminophen	Altered CYP450 enzyme metabolism	Increased hepatic metabolism of acetaminophen and toxicity risk and reduced efficacy
	Antipsychotics, antidepressants, benzodiazepines, cyclosporine, oral contraceptives	Altered CYP450 enzyme metabolism	Reduced efficacy, client response must be monitored
	MAOIs	Altered CYP450 metabolism	Increased MAOI toxicity risk
Valproic acid and divalproex sodium	Tricyclic antidepressants (TCAs)	Altered CYP450 enzyme metabolism	Increased TCA toxicity
Antidepressants			
First Generation			
Tricyclics (TCAs)	Carbamazepine, rifamycins	Enhanced TCA clearance	Reduced therapeutic effect

TABLE 12.1 Drug Interactions of Psychotropic Drugs—cont'd

Drug Class	Interacting Drug(s)	Mechanism	Result
	Carbamazepine	Reduced carbamazepine clearance	Potential for carbamazepine toxicity
	MAOIs	Enhanced serotonergic effects	Potential for serotonin syndrome
	Valproic acid	Reduced TCA clearance	Potential for TCA toxicity
	Anticholinergics	Additive anticholinergic effects	Potential for paralytic ileus
	Sympathomimetics	Enhanced sympathomimetic effects	Potential for cardiac dysrhythmias
Antidepressants *Second Generation* *Tetracyclics*			
Mirtazapine, maprotiline hydrochloride	Alcohol, CYP inhibitors	Additive effects	Increased toxicity
SSRIs (selective serotonin reuptake inhibitors)	MAOIs, linezolid, lithium, metoclopramide hydrochloride, buspirone hydrochloride, sympathomimetics, tramadol hydrochloride	Additive effects	Potential for serotonin syndrome
	Benzodiazepines	Reduced metabolism	Potential benzodiazepine toxicity
	Warfarin sodium, phenytoin	Protein binding displacement	Potential for warfarin sodium or phenytoin toxicity
	Propafenone hydrochloride	Increased propafenone levels	Potential for propafenone hydrochloride toxicity
SNRIs (Serotonin-Norepinephrine Reuptake Inhibitors)			
Duloxetine	SSRIs, triptans	Additive effects	Risk for serotonin syndrome
	NSAIDs, warfarin sodium	Additive effects	Risk for bleeding
	Alcohol	Additive liver toxicity	Increased risk of hepatotoxicity
Miscellaneous			
Trazodone, bupropion	Azole antifungals, phenothiazines, protease inhibitors	Inadequate hepatic metabolism	Increased effects
	Carbamazepine	Increased metabolism	Decreased therapeutic effects
	Alcohol, CNS depressants	Additive effects	Increased CNS depression
Selected Antipsychotics *Conventional and Atypical*	Alcohol, other CNS depressants	Additive drug effects	Enhanced CNS depression, dystonia with alcohol
	Antihypertensives	Enhanced antihypertensive effects	Potential for hypotension
Conventional Phenothiazines	Anticholinergics	Additive and antagonistic drug effects	Reduced phenothiazine efficacy, enhanced anticholinergic effects
	Beta blockers	Additive drug effects	Potential toxicity of either drug
	Opioids	Additive drug effects	Excessive sedation, hypotension
	Levodopa-carbidopa	Uncertain	Diminished antiparkinsonian effects
	Phenytoin	Uncertain	Can increase or reduce phenytoin levels
	Thiazide diuretics	Reduced diuretic clearance	Potential for hypotension
Atypicals	CYP3A4 inhibitors (e.g., ketoconazole)	Reduced antipsychotic clearance	Potential for antipsychotic toxicity
	Carbamazepine	Enhanced antipsychotic clearance	Reduced therapeutic effects

Adapted from Sealock, K., Seneviratne, C., Lilley, L., Rainforth, S., & Snyder, J. (2021). *Lilley's pharmacology for Canadian health care practice* (4th ed., p. 282, Table 17.3; p. 288, Table 17.6; p. 249, Table 15.5; p. 295, Table 17.11). Elsevier.

Common Psychiatric Treatments

Psychotherapy refers to various approaches to the psychological treatment of mental or emotional disorders, aimed at changing people's attitudes, feelings, and behaviour. These approaches are conducted by trained therapists.

"Talk therapy" approaches

- Psychoanalysis: Based on Freudian theory, this is a lengthy process of years of individual therapy aimed at uncovering repressed memories and other unconscious influences on thinking, behaviour, and relationships.
- Psychodynamic therapy: Also based on Freudian concepts but shorter in duration, this type of therapy can last weeks or months. The focus is on developing insight on particular issues thought to be causing the client's distress.
- Interpersonal therapy: This type of therapy is used to examine past relationship patterns to reveal ways of achieving more positive personal and interpersonal interactions.

Behaviour-oriented therapy.

Various techniques of behaviour modification focus on changing clients' behaviour patterns. Overall, positive behaviours are positively rewarded and negative behaviours are negatively rewarded. Examples include the following:

- Assertiveness training: Clients learn to express their wishes in a matter-of-fact way and to say no to unreasonable expectations without feeling guilty.
- Positive conditioning: Clients learn to associate desirable behaviours and the sources of any phobias with pleasurable outcomes and relaxation.
- Aversion therapy: Undesirable behaviours are associated with painful or negative stimuli.
- Desensitization: Clients are gradually exposed to situations that they fear.
- Thought stopping and thought switching: Clients practise controlling fears by stopping the negative thoughts (e.g., by using a verbal reminder) or switching to more positive ones.
- Token economy: Good behaviour is rewarded with tokens that clients can trade for privileges or desired objects.

Group therapy.

Small groups of people with similar conditions meet together, facilitated by a therapist, to discuss and work through their concerns. In community settings, many groups focus on self-help, with members helping one another along with the guidance and support of a professional facilitator.

Cognitive therapy and cognitive–behavioural therapy

- Cognitive therapy: It focuses on changing irrational beliefs, faulty reasoning, and negative self-statements that underlie behavioural conditions (Bard et al., 2022). Therapists help clients change their self-concept and coping skills by altering their thought patterns and behaviour.
- Cognitive–behavioural therapy (CBT): It uses techniques similar to those of behaviour modification, along with strategies for cognitive restructuring and reducing anxiety, coping skills, and problem-solving skills (relaxation training, biofeedback, role-playing). Clients have homework assignments for practising between sessions.

Communication Techniques

Therapeutic communication is the heart of mental health nursing. While nurses may focus on developing therapeutic verbal communication techniques, nonverbal communication is equally important. Nurses need to be aware of a client's nonverbal signals, just as clients are sure to be aware of the nurse's. Clients know when a nurse is being genuine, honest, and sincere. They can sense a nurse's respect and empathy (and they sense the opposite responses just as easily).

Managing therapeutic communication implies that nurses monitor all aspects of their own and their client's communication, such as movement, gestures, posture, facial expression, and body language. Be aware of vocal tone, pitch, and volume, as well as nervous habits, such as coughing or giggling. We also communicate a great deal about ourselves and our regard for clients through touch. Always remember that cultural patterns of communication may be different, especially with regard to boundaries of personal space and touching.

When it is necessary to confront a client about undesirable behaviour or attitudes, be assertive, but not aggressive or angry. Point out discrepancies in a matter-of-fact way between a client's self-interpretation of behaviour and how others may view those same actions. In Table 12.2, you will find a summary of therapeutic communication techniques. Refer to pages 21-22, for more ideas on how to develop therapeutic communication techniques and interviewing skills.

Assessing Mental Status

Evaluating the client's mental status is an important aspect of clinical assessment. Combining what the client can tell you with your own observations, the mental state assessment evaluates the client's current mental functioning, not their psychiatric history. Most organizations have a structured form to help the nurse recall the range of questions to ask and observations to make, to ensure that sufficient and appropriate information is collected. In general, assessing mental status includes describing the following characteristics:

- General description: Appearance, speech, motor activity, and interaction in the interview
- Emotional state, mood, and affect
- Experiences: Their perceptions of personal experiences
- Thinking: Thought content and thinking processes
- Sensorium (ability to sort information and cognition): Level of consciousness, memory, information and intelligence, level of concentration and calculation and evidence of judgement and insight.
- Further details on mental health assessment and neurological physical assessment appear in Chapter 5.

Milieu Therapy

Nurses help create a therapeutic community or milieu on the inpatient unit, in which clients become part of a community where they can learn new social skills, improve their coping mechanisms, and develop healthy interpersonal relationships. Establishing this type of environment to aid in social rehabilitation is more difficult in today's context of relatively brief

TABLE 12.2   Selected Therapeutic Communication Techniques

Technique	Definition	Example
Listening	An active process of receiving information, showing interest and acceptance	Maintain eye contact and convey positive nonverbal responses.
Broad openings	Asking questions that allow the client to select topics for discussion	"What are you thinking about?"
Restating	Repeating the client's main thought to have them validate what you heard and to emphasize important points	"You say that your mother left you when you were 5 years old."
Clarification	Asking the client to explain what they mean, to help the client examine issues in more detail	"I'm not sure that I fully understand. Could you tell me about that again?"
Reflection	Directing back the client's ideas, feelings, questions, and content to signify empathy and validate the nurse's understanding	"You're feeling anxious, and it's related to your conversation with your husband last night?"
Informing	Providing information for health teaching and self-care	"It's important for you to know how this medication works."
Focusing	Questions or statements that help the client expand on the topic, keeping the communication goal-directed	"I think we should talk more about your relationship with your father."
Sharing perceptions	Asking the client to verify your understanding of their thoughts or feelings, to clear up confusion	"You're smiling, but I sense that you are really very angry with me."
Identifying themes	Identifying issues or problems that the client repeatedly refers to in conversation, aimed at helping the client understand and explore important problems	"I've noticed that you have spoken often of being hurt or rejected by men with whom you have formed relationships. Do you think this is an underlying issue?"
Silence	Intentionally not initiating verbal communication, to allow time for thinking and reflection and to encourage the client to initiate communication	Sit with the client to nonverbally communicate support and interest.
Suggesting	Presenting alternative ideas for the client to consider in problem-solving, to increase possibilities and choices	"Have you thought about responding differently to your boss when he raises that issue with you? For example, you could ask him whether a specific problem has occurred."
Humour	Discharge of energy through comic enjoyment. Can promote insight by making conscious repressed material, resolving paradoxes, tempering aggression and revealing new options; is socially acceptable form of sublimation	"That gives a whole new meaning to the word nervous." Said with shared kidding between nurse and client.

Adapted from Bard, B., MacMullin, E., Williamson, J. & Morrison-Valfre, M. (2022). *Morrison-Valfre's foundations of mental health care in Canada* (p. 115, Box.10.6). Elsevier.

hospital stays; in outpatient settings, such as group homes, a therapeutic community is more easily established.

Family Therapy

Family nursing is important in mental health practice. Families are the context within which the client lives and may also require nursing care themselves. Often the family serves as caregiver and case manager for clients outside the hospital. Families need education about the client's illness and help with learning new patterns of interacting with the client. Different types of groups can help provide support to these families:

- Psychoeducational groups for families: They provide support to families coping with a member who has a severe mental illness. Families are taught about the signs and symptoms of the illness, medications, other options for therapy, sources of community help, and how to recognize signs of a relapse. In these groups, family members can share their experiences and successful strategies for managing the client at home.
- Self-help groups for families: They can be accessed through voluntary organizations, such as the Schizophrenia Society of Canada and the Canadian Mental Health Association

(CMHA). Such mutual aid groups empower families, reduce their isolation, and help them learn coping skills.

Community Mental Health Nursing

Because most people with a mental illness are treated outside the hospital, roles for community mental health nurses are expanding. Community treatment focuses clients on recovery, with a goal of helping clients learn to manage their illness and incorporate any limitations into a satisfying life. Social and functional-living skills (and, where possible, employment skills) enable clients to cope while living as independently as possible.

As members of interdisciplinary teams, nurses may work in a variety of models for community mental health services. Community outreach programs aim to assist clients where they live. Other services are provided in offices where clients must make and keep appointments. Many programs are a combination. Outreach programs may provide specific services for clients with mental illness and their families, or they may refer clients to other programs in the community. Examples of these services include the following:

- Assertive Community Treatment (ACT): A specific interdisciplinary team model for intensive community support.

Community programs and services may include client identification, mental health care and counselling, medical care, dental care, crisis response, social assistance, financial management, community education and advocacy, rehabilitation, housing, family support, and case management.

- Case management: Case managers develop caring and supportive therapeutic relationships with complex clients. They may be attached to an ACT team or a hospital outpatient service.
- Supported housing: This type of housing varies from apartments with a resident manager who has some mental health knowledge to group homes. Some group homes follow the club house model, where residents are members and collaborate with staff in running the house and its programs.
- Community Mental Health Centres (CMHCs): They provide outpatient clinics, mental health programs, and support services.
- Public health: In rural areas, the public health nurse may be the only source of community mental health outreach. In more urban areas, public health nurses are more likely to focus on prevention, such as stress management and parenting classes, school programming, or screening for depression. They make referrals to mental health programs and agencies.
- Addiction services: Street nurses may be the first point of contact for those with a mental illness and substance disorder.

MOOD DISORDERS: DEPRESSION AND BIPOLAR DISORDER

Mood disorders are also called *affective disorders*, "affect" meaning the expression of a person's mood. Emotional ups and downs are normal features of living; severe or prolonged changes in a person's mood may not be.

Abnormal mood ranges between two emotional extremes: depression and mania. Mania is an abnormally and persistently elevated mood state marked by hyperactivity, delusions, and lack of judgement. Depression is described in the next section.

Usually, hospitalized clients have either a severe depression or a bipolar illness, in which their mood swings between depression and mania.

Depression

Depression and anxiety are the most common psychiatric illnesses in Canada, with major depression affecting 5.4% of the Canadian population and anxiety disorders affecting 4.5% of the population (CMHA, 2021). All age groups can be clinically depressed, even children. Higher rates of depression and anxiety have been reported in Canadians during the COVID-19 pandemic due to struggling with many potential stressors such as social isolation, loneliness, job loss, the COVID-19 infection, and changes in relationships (Statistics Canada, 2021a).

Pathophysiology

Neurological, genetic, and psychosocial factors interact in complex ways to produce depression:

- Neurological factors: These include low levels of monoamines, such as serotonin and norepinephrine. Other neurotransmitters that are poorly regulated include dopamine, acetylcholine, GABA, and serotonin (5-HT). Serotonin also affects levels of growth hormone, cortisol, and prolactin, all of which are poorly regulated in people with depression.
- Brain: Brain scans can show decreased metabolic activity in the frontal and temporal lobes and increased blood flow to the amygdala.
- Genetic factors: People with a family history of depression have an increased incidence of depression. Genetic factors predispose people to develop depression when faced with environmental factors such as stressful life events.
- Endocrinology: Depression is commonly associated with Addison's disease, Cushing's syndrome, thyroid diseases, and abnormal estrogen levels. These hormonal imbalances disrupt the regulatory functions of the hypothalamus and pituitary glands. As well, the specifier for "with seasonal pattern" for major depression (previously called *seasonal affective disorder* [SAD]) may be linked to abnormalities in the hypothalamic control of circadian rhythms.
- Electrolytes: High levels of calcium, sodium bicarbonate, and either high or low levels of potassium are common with depression.
- Psychosocial factors: Factors such as multiple stressors or negative social interactions (criticism, anger, or bullying) are also risk factors for depression. By contrast, participation in physical activity and positive social support may offer some protection.

Clinical Manifestations

Depression is expressed as intense feelings of sadness, despair, and powerlessness, often as a consequence of loss. Depression can be brief and transient in the normal response to everyday disappointments or more prolonged, ranging from mild to moderate to severe chronic depression known as *depressive disorders*. Depressive disorders are severe enough to cause distress or impairment in the client's ability to function. These disorders include major depressive disorder, disruptive mood dysregulation disorder, persistent depressive disorder, premenstrual dysphoric disorder, substance/medication-induced depressive disorder, depressive disorder due to another medical condition, other specified depressive disorder, unspecified depressive disorder, and unspecified mood disorder. Moderate depression (dysthymic disorder) and severe depression (major depressive disorder) tend not to resolve without professional help.

People with depression share a number of common characteristics. They will tell you that they feel empty and extremely sad, with no hope for the future. Their pain is both emotional and physical, with diffuse aches and pains throughout their bodies. Previously enjoyable activities now provide no pleasure, and, not surprisingly, they can be irritable and socially withdrawn. However, there are differences in the duration, timing, and etiology of the various depressive disorders.

Normally, grief for a loved one is experienced as depression, with many of the same symptoms (with the exception of prolonged grief disorder as presented later on in this chapter).

Overwhelming sadness and hopelessness are manifested in sleep disturbances, changes in appetite and weight, and inability to concentrate or carry out usual activities. Unlike those experiencing chronic depression, grieving people (except those with prolonged grief disorder) recognize the reason for their feelings. Gradually, acceptance develops, the depressive symptoms resolve, and normal coping mechanisms resurface.

Depression is a common response with major loss, including the loss of health experienced with a chronic illness. Other risk factors include stressful life events, poor social support, substance disorder, and having a history of depression. Several specific depressive disorders are described next.

Major depressive disorder. Major depressive disorder (MDD; also called *major depression*) is persistent and devastating. The course of the disorder is variable. Some people with MDD can occur in a single episode, more frequently as recurrent relapses or as a chronic condition lasting longer than 2 years. It can be characterized by a continuous depressed mood lasting for a minimum of 2 weeks (Halter et al., 2019). In some, the symptoms are severe enough to cause psychosis (a psychotic break from reality) with delusions, hallucinations, and psychomotor impairment to the point of catatonia. (Bard et al., 2022). MDD is characterized by the following symptoms and must include one of the first two symptoms:

- Feelings of sadness and emptiness, hopelessness, with crying (in children this can be irritability)
- Loss of interest or pleasure in activities that were previously enjoyed (reported by the person or observed)
- Appetite changes accompanied by either weight loss or weight gain
- Sleep pattern changes (insomnia, or sleeping during the day)
- Lack of energy, extreme fatigue
- Feelings of worthlessness or inappropriate and excessive guilt
- Psychomotor agitation (restlessness) or impairment (slowed movement)
- Inability to concentrate or make decisions, difficulty thinking
- Recurrent thoughts of suicide or death (Bard et al., 2022)
- When a combination of these symptoms (including one of the first two symptoms) presents for a least 2 weeks and causes significant distress and impairment, it is called a *major depressive episode (MDE)*. The diagnostic criteria depend on the number of episodes (single versus recurrent), level of severity, presence of psychosis, and existence of remission (at least 2 months with no significant symptoms). Suicidal risk exists at all times during an MDE. The major risks factors are the history of attempts, threats of suicide, or both (Bard et al., 2022).

Disruptive mood dysregulation disorder. The main characteristics of disruptive mood dysregulation disorder are severe recurrent temper outbursts and aggression (physical, verbal, or both), temper outbursts occur three or more times a week and occur in a least two different settings (e.g., school, home, with peers), onset before the age of 10, persistently irritable or angry most of the day, nearly every day (even without outbursts) and is observable by others. This is a common diagnosis for inpatient children and adolescents in mental health units, and occurs more frequently in males (Bard et al., 2022).

Dysthymic disorder. Persistent depressive disorder (dysthymia) is a chronic low level of persistent depressive feelings for a least 2 years (for children and adolescents, the diagnosis may be made after 1 year). The somewhat milder symptoms are similar to major depression but not the same. If at any time the symptoms match those of major depressive disorder, then a separate diagnosis of major depressive disorder should be made in addition to the diagnosis of persistent depressive disorder along with the relevant specifier (e.g., with intermittent major depressive episodes, with current episode) (APA, 2022).

Individuals experiencing persistent depressive disorder feel depressed most of the time. When they are depressed, they also exhibit at least two of the following symptoms to meet the criteria: poor appetite or overeating, insomnia, or hypersomnia, low energy or fatigue, low self-esteem, poor concentration or difficulty making decisions and feelings of hopelessness. Social and occupational impairment are significant.

Postpartum depression. Some degree of depression affects more than half of all individuals who have given birth. Postpartum depression does not exist as a stand-alone diagnosis but is classified in the DSM-5-TR as a bipolar disorder or depression with a peripartum onset specification. A person suffering from postpartum depression has to meet the symptoms of a MDE. Postpartum depression is diagnosed when the depressive episode occurs before or after the birth of the person's child. "Fifty percent of postpartum major depression episodes actually begin prior to delivery. Thus, these episodes are referred to collectively as *peripartum episodes*" (APA, 2022, pp. 173 & 213). Although most individuals experience "baby blues" in the week or two after the birth, postpartum depression is more severe and lasts longer. Individuals with limited social support, previous episodes of depression, or perinatal complications are most at risk.

Postpartum depression greatly reduces a person's ability to care for their child, with negative consequences for both the childbearing person's health and that of their baby. In severe cases, the person can experience psychosis and may have thoughts of harming themself or their child. "Infanticide (a rare occurrence) is more often associated with postpartum psychotic episodes that are characterized by command hallucinations to kill the infant or delusions that the infant is possessed, but psychotic symptoms can occur in severe postpartum mood episodes without such specific delusions or hallucinations" (APA, 2022, p. 213).

Seasonal affective disorder. Seasonal affective disorder (SAD) is now classified in the DSM-5-TR as a specifier called "with seasonal pattern" for recurrent major depression disorders. In this disorder, changes in mood occur in response to a reduced exposure to daylight. In fall and winter, people with this disorder become clinically depressed. Depression generally resolves in the spring. Less commonly, there may be recurrent summer depressive episodes. The DSM-5-TR criteria for diagnosing depression with a seasonal pattern includes having these episodes for at least the last 2 years:

- "There has been a regular temporal relationship between the onset of major depressive episodes in major depressive disorder and a particular time of the year" (APA, 2022, p. 214).
- "Full remissions also occur at a characteristic time of the year (e.g., depression disappears in the spring)" (APA, 2022, p. 214).
- In the last 2 years, two major depressive episodes have occurred that demonstrate the temporal seasonal relationships defined above and no nonseasonal major depressive episodes have occurred during the same period" (APA, 2022, p. 214).
- "SAD (as described above) substantially outnumber the nonseasonal major depressive episodes that may have occurred over the individual's lifetime" (APA, 2022, p. 214).

Diagnostics

Along with a full history and physical examination to identify symptoms and comorbid illnesses, several rating scales are available to assess depression. Four of the most common rating scales are as follows:

- Beck Depression Inventory (BDI): A self-rating scale that clients complete
- Zung Self-Rating Depression Scale (ZSRD): Another self-report scale
- Hamilton Rating Scale for Depression (HAM-D): Completed by clinicians
- Geriatric Depression Scale (GDS): A self-reporting assessment scale for the older person

Therapeutics

Pharmacotherapy is the predominant mode of treatment for mood disorders. Remember that medications may take several weeks to be effective. See Chapter 8 page 138, for more details about antidepressants and mood stabilizing medications, including drug classifications, actions, and adverse effects. Chapter 8 also includes nursing implications for these drugs.

Medications for depression

- Tricyclic antidepressants (TCAs): Adverse effects are significant; therefore, these are used less frequently now.
- Selective serotonin reuptake inhibitors (SSRIs): They are considered first-line medications.
- Serotonin-norepinephrine reuptake inhibitors (SNRIs): They are often considered the next medication of choice after trying SSRIs.
- Norepinephrine-dopamine reuptake inhibitor (NDRI): A high dose may increase seizure risk.
- Monoamine oxidase inhibitors (MAOIs): They are usually reserved for clients with hard-to-treat MDD because of the medications' severe adverse effects.

Other newer antidepressants include serotonin modulators and stimulators (SMSs), serotonin antagonists and reuptake inhibitors (SARIs), tetracyclic antidepressants (TeCAs), mineral mood-stabilizing medications, anticonvulsant mood-stabilizing medications, and antipsychotic mood-stabilizing medications.

Nursing Considerations

Nursing assessment. Nurses working in all health care, occupational, and community settings should be attentive to signs of mood disorders. When a disorder is first suspected, the client may be asked to complete a self-assessment scale.

Assessment of depression. To assess for depression, the nurse determines whether the client has experienced the following:

- Previous history of depression or familial history
- Medical conditions that may increase risk of depression (hypothyroidism, Parkinson's)
- Recent life changes (divorce, unemployment, situational stressors)
- Misuse or overuse of alcohol, medications, or other drugs (marihuana, nicotine)
- Mental health conditions that may contribute to depression

The nurse also assesses whether the client is at risk of harming himself or herself or other people (see the section "Psychiatric Emergencies: Crisis, Suicide, Violence" in this chapter).

If the client has a history of depression, find out what worked then and what did not. Discuss with the client their level of knowledge about depression and whether supportive family or friends are available. Finally, assess whether the client needs referral to a primary care provider (physician or nurse practitioner).

The nurse–client relationship. The cornerstone of connecting with clients with mood disorders is spending time with the person to reinforce reality and provide support. Use a calm approach and moderate tone of voice—neither overly cheerful nor too serious—and active listening. Establishing rapport and communicating with people at either end of the mood spectrum present additional and different challenges, as follows:

- Be kind and compassionate: Just sitting with an isolated person is comforting and supportive.
- Use simple, direct language: Doing so can counteract slowed thinking processes.
- Be patient: Allow extra time for the person to follow directions and respond.
- Offer observations: Instead of questioning an individual who is not talkative, point out characteristics of the person and the immediate environment, for example, "Your blue dress matches your eyes" or "Your son brought you some fruit."
- Avoid common expressions that can discount a client's feelings, such as "Oh, things will be better soon; it just takes time."

Pharmacotherapy

Be aware of and monitor for adverse effects, adverse reactions, and interactions of major medications used for mood disorders. Clients with mood disorders may object to taking medications; be sure to supervise as they swallow oral medications.

Antidepressants. Nursing implications for antidepressant medication adverse effects are discussed in Table 12.3.

Preventing hypertensive crisis associated with MAOIs. MAOIs increase levels of serotonin, epinephrine, and norepinephrine in the brain. MAOIs can cause severe interactions with certain medications and foods, possibly leading to hypertensive crisis.

MAOIs and medications. Over-the-counter cold medications interact with MAOIs, producing a hypertensive crisis, a life-threatening condition manifested by tachycardia, sudden increase in blood pressure, severe headache and nosebleeds, stiff neck, nausea and vomiting, and cold, clammy skin. Clients can develop chest pains or a stroke and die. Emergency treatment for hypertensive crisis involves the following:

- Discontinue MAOI.
- Keep the client's head elevated.
- Reduce fever by external methods, such as fans, tepid baths, or ice packs.
- Administer a calcium channel blocker (such as nifedipine [Adalat]) sublingually, to promote vasodilation. Clients may be prescribed a 10 mg nifedipine capsule to carry in case of emergency.
- Administer 5 mg phentolamine (Rogitine) intravenously (Halter et al., 2019).

Other contraindicated drugs for people taking MAOIs include nasal and sinus decongestants, cold, allergy and hay fever remedies, inhalants for asthma, weight loss pills, narcotics, tricyclic antidepressants, antihypertensives, sedatives including alcohol, and legal or illegal stimulants such as amphetamines and cocaine.

Foods. In order to prevent a hypertensive crisis, the client also needs to avoid certain foods, particularly those with high levels of tyramine.

- Instruct the client *not to eat* any of the following foods: aged cheeses (cream cheese and cottage cheese are safe); red wine, sherry, cognac and liqueurs; beer, ale, over-ripe fruit; avocados, bananas, sauerkraut; pickled or smoked fish; dried fish, bologna, beef and chicken liver; fava and broad beans; canned figs, brewer's yeast; monosodium glutamate; meat tenderizers, salami, sausage and all fermented products.
- Instruct the client *to consume moderate amounts only* of white wine, beverages with caffeine, yogourt, soy sauce, raisins, chocolate, licorice, ginseng, and yeast.

Complementary and alternative medications. St. John's wort is an herbal product with proven effects against mild to moderate depression, SAD, and sleep disturbance. Melatonin supports circadian rhythm equilibrium, thus improving sleep. Many people explore natural remedies and self-medicate for the management of mood disorders. Clients using alternative or complementary medications should be encouraged to discuss this with their physician, nurse practitioner, or pharmacist as interactions can either reduce or increase the action of prescribed medications, potentially causing toxic effects.

Nursing Interventions

- Maintain client safety: Observe closely for self-harm or suicidal thoughts. Remove belongings that could be used for self-harm.
- Maintain nutrition: Give small, frequent meals, taking preferences into account.
- Maintain elimination: Add high-fibre foods and ensure adequate hydration to counteract constipation.
- Assist with personal hygiene: Encourage the client to gradually resume self-care.
- Encourage social interaction: Provide reassurance and positive reinforcement for gradually joining group activities.

Bipolar Disorder and Related Disorders

Bipolar disorders are less common than depressive disorders. There are different types of bipolar disorders. All of them involve changes in mood, energy, and activity levels. An older name for bipolar illness is *manic depression* (Halter et al., 2019).

Pathophysiology

A complex interplay of underlying biological factors can lead to the development of mania:

- Neurological factors: Neurotransmitter abnormalities, that is, high plasma levels of epinephrine and norepinephrine, can lead to mania.
- Brain: Brain scans show abnormalities in the white matter (fatty sheaths surrounding neurons), particularly in those areas of the brain responsible for emotions.
- Genetic factors: As with depression, higher rates of mania are found among first-degree relatives.
- Endocrinology: The biological clock is located in the hypothalamus. In mania, circadian rhythms are disrupted; sleep deprivation is common. Hypothyroidism is linked to bipolar illness.

Bipolar I Disorder

The main diagnostic feature of bipolar l disorder is a manic episode. The occurrence of at least one manic episode must be identified to diagnose bipolar l. A hypomanic or major depressive episode may occur before or after the manic episode (Bard et al., 2022).

Manic Episode

A manic episode is a distinct period of abnormally and persistent elevated, expansive, or irritable mood that causes a significant impairment in functions (or need for hospitalization to ensure safety) for at least 1 week. During the period, at least three of the following symptoms must be present:

- Being overly talkative (pressured speech)
- Inflated self-esteem or grandiosity
  - An increase in goal-related activity (either socially, at work, school, or sexually, or psychomotor agitation (purposeless, non–goal-directed activity)

TABLE 12.3 Nursing Considerations for Antidepressant Medication Adverse Effects

Adverse Effect	Nursing Care and Teaching Considerations
Anticholinergic Adverse Effects	
Blurred vision	Temporary; avoid hazardous tasks
Dry mouth	Encourage fluids, frequent rinses, sugar-free hard candy and gums; check for mouth sores
Constipation	Increase fluids, dietary fibre and roughage, exercise; monitor bowel habits; use stool softeners and laxatives only if necessary
Tachycardia	Temporary, usually not significant (except with coronary artery disease), but can be frightening; eliminate caffeine; beta blockers might help; provide supportive therapy
Urinary retention	Encourage fluids and frequent voiding; monitor voiding patterns; bethanechol; catheterize
Cognitive dysfunction	Temporary; avoid hazardous tasks; adjust lifestyle; provide supportive therapy
Cytochrome P-450 inhibition*	SSRIs inhibit the liver isoenzyme cytochrome P-450, which is instrumental in the metabolism of a variety of drugs (TCAs, trazodone, barbiturates, most benzodiazepines, carbamazepine, narcotics, neuroleptics, phenytoin, valproate, verapamil). This effect can be potentially life threatening because it increases serum concentrations as well as therapeutic and toxic effects of these drugs.
Dizziness or lightheadedness	Have client dangle the feet; provide adequate hydration, elastic stockings; protect from falls and ensure safety precautions, give at bedtime
ECG changes	Obtain complete cardiac history; obtain pretreatment ECG for clients over 40 and children; ST segment depression, T wave flattened or inverted, QRS prolongation; worsening of intraventricular conduction problems; do not use if recent myocardial infarction or bundle-branch block
Ejaculatory dysfunction	Dose after sexual intercourse, not immediately before
GI disturbances (nausea, diarrhea)	Take with meals or at HS; adjust diet if indicated, encourage good hygiene. Encourage fluids to 2500 mL/day, monitor intake and output
Hallucinations, delusions, activation of schizophrenic or manic psychosis	Change to another antidepressant class of drug; initiate antipsychotics or mood stabilizers if appropriate
Hypertensive crisis*	See the discussion of MAOIs in the section "Preventing Hypertensive Crisis Associated with MAOIs."
Hypotension	Obtain frequent BP; hydrate; provide elastic stockings; may need to change drug. For postural hypotension: obtain lying and standing BP, encourage gradual change of positions, protect from falls.
Insomnia	Dose as early in the day as possible; promote sleep hygiene; decrease evening activities; eliminate caffeine, relaxation techniques; sedative–hypnotic therapy
Memory dysfunction	Temporary; encourage concentration, make lists, provide social support, adjust lifestyle
Perspiration (excessive)	Suggest frequent changes of clothes, cotton or linen clothing, good hygiene; increase fluids
Priapism	Change dose, change drug
Psychomotor activation	Take drug in morning rather than HS; adjust lifestyle
Sedation/drowsiness	Administer drug at HS; avoid hazardous tasks, keep active during the day, institute safety precautions, instruct client to avoid operating machinery
Serotonin syndrome (SS)*	SS is a life-threatening emergency resulting from excess central nervous system 5-HT caused by combining 5-HT-enhancing drugs or administering SSRIs too close to the discontinuation of MAOIs. Symptoms are confusion, disorientation, mania, restlessness/agitation, myoclonus, hyper-reflexia, diaphoresis, shivering, tremor, diarrhea, nausea, ataxia, headache. Discontinue all serotoninergic medications immediately; anticonvulsants for seizures; serotonin antagonist drugs may help; clonazepam for myoclonus, lorazepam for restlessness or agitation, other symptomatic care as indicated; do not reintroduce serotonin drugs.
Sexual dysfunction	Dose after sexual intercourse; use lubricant if vaginal dryness is present; antidotes such as sildenafil, bupropion, or bethanechol
Tachycardia	See anticholinergic adverse effects
TCA withdrawal syndrome	Symptoms: malaise, muscle aches, chills, nausea, dizziness, coryza; when discontinuing drug, taper over several days or weeks
Tremors	Temporary; adjust lifestyle as indicated
Weight gain	Increase exercise; reduced-calorie diet if indicated; may need to change class of drug, monitor weight gain-weigh weekly

*Potentially life-threatening.

NOTE: Always educate the client and use the techniques in this table. Consider decreasing or dividing medication dose. Change medication only if necessary.

BP, Blood pressure; *ECG,* electrocardiogram; *GI,* gastro-intestinal; *HS,* at bedtime; *5-HT,* serotonin; *MAOIs,* monoamine oxidase inhibitors; *SSRIs,* selective serotonin reuptake inhibitors; *TCAs,* tricyclic antidepressants.

Adapted from Bard, B., MacMullin, E., Williamson, J., & Morrison-Valfre, M., (2022). *Morrison-Valfres foundations of mental health care in Canada.* (p. 257, Table 21.2). Elsevier.

- Rapid, often confusing speech patterns; "pressured speech" or "flights of ideas" or person feels their thoughts are racing
- Disturbed sleep patterns and seemingly needing very little sleep
- Over involvement in activities that have a high potential for painful consequences (e.g., engagement in money-making schemes or irresponsible spending, sexual indiscretions, or foolish business investments)
- Easily distracted by attention to unimportant or irrelevant external stimuli

Hypomanic Episode

Hypomanic episode characteristics do not cause marked impairment in functions, but an external observer can note a major change in functioning that is not characteristic of the individual. During this period the person may experience abnormally or persistent elevated, expansive or irritable mood, increased energy or activity, lasting at least 4 consecutive days and must be present the majority of days. Three or more of the following symptoms must be present:

- Inflated self-esteem or grandiosity
- Reduced need to sleep (e.g., feels rested after only 3 hours of sleep)
- More talkative than usual or pressure to keep talking
- Flight of ideas or clients subjective experience of racing thoughts
- Distractibility (attention drawn too easily to unimportant or irrelevant eternal stimuli)
- Major increase in goal-directed activity (social, sexual, or at work or school)
- Extreme overinvolvement in high-risk activities (e.g., engaged in unrestrained buying sprees, sexual indiscretions, or unrealistic business investments) that have a high potential for painful consequences (Bard et al., 2022)

Major Depressive Episode

A major depressive episode manifests when five or more of the following symptoms have been present during the same 2-week period and at least one of the symptoms is either depressed mood or significant decrease in interest or pleasure:

- Depressed mood most of the day, nearly every day, as reported by the person (sad, empty, hopeless) or through observations made by others (tearful) (in children and adolescents this can seem more like irritability)
- Significant decrease in interest or pleasure in most activities most of the day, nearly every day
- Weight loss when not dieting or weight gain (change of more of 5% of body weight in 1 month) or decrease in appetite most days
- Insomnia or hypersomnia most days
- Psychomotor agitation or impairment most days
- Fatigue or loss of energy most days
- Feelings of worthlessness or excessive or inappropriate guilt (may be delusional) nearly every day
- Decreased ability to think, concentrate, or make decisions nearly every day

- Recurrent thoughts of death, suicidal ideation without a specific plan, or a suicide attempt or a specific plan for committing suicide

Bipolar II Disorder

Bipolar ll disorder is a condition in which the person experiences at least one hypomanic episode and at least one major depressive episode. Individuals usually seek help during a major depressive episode but not during the hypomanic episode since it usually does not cause any significant impairment in functioning. Clients or even their families see no pathology in the hypomanic episode. Individuals with bipolar I disorder experience more hypomanic episodes than do individuals with bipolar II disorders. Individuals with bipolar II disorder experience more frequent and lengthier recurrent major depressive episodes than those occurring in bipolar I disorder.

"A common feature of bipolar II disorder is impulsivity, which contributes to suicide attempts and substance use disorders" (APA, 2022, p. 11).

Cyclothymic Disorder

Cyclothymic disorder has symptoms of hypomania alternating with symptoms of mild to moderate depression for at least 2 years in adults and one year in children and adolescents. The symptoms of hypomania and depression do not meet the criteria for a hypomanic and major depressive episode. The symptoms will still cause significant social and occupational impairment. Cyclothymic disorders usually begin in adolescence or early adult life. There is a 15 to 50% possibility that an individual with cyclothymic disorder will subsequently develop bipolar l or bipolar ll disorder (APA, 2022).

Diagnostics

Refer to the preceding symptoms in manic episode and major depressive episode.

Along with a full history and physical examination to identify symptoms and comorbid illnesses, several rating scales are available to assess depression (see the rating scales listed under "Diagnostics" in the section "Depression," page 428).

The symptoms of bipolar and related disorders usually happen in three phases: the acute phase (during an intense manic, hypomanic, or depressive episode), the continuation phase (when symptoms are controlled but the client's mental health status is still fragile), and the maintenance phase (when acute symptoms have subsided and the focus is on preventing relapse and limiting the severity and length of future episodes) (Halter et al., 2019, p. 284).

Medications for bipolar and related disorders

- Lithium carbonate
- Anticonvulsants, such as carbamazepine (Tegretol), valproic acid
- Anxiolytics
- Antipsychotics: Typical and atypical

See Chapter 8, page 138, for more details in the "Mood Stabilizers" section. Chapter 8 also includes drug classifications, actions, adverse effects, and nursing implications for these drugs.

Nursing Considerations

Nursing assessment of bipolar disorders. To assess for manic episodes, the nurse determines whether the client:

- Is a danger to themselves (exhaustion in severe mania can lead to death) or others (due to poor impulse control) and needs to be hospitalized
- Is spending money uncontrollably and engaging in overly risky behaviours
- Has comorbid medical conditions
- Misuses or overuses alcohol, medications, or other drugs (marihuana, nicotine)
- Requires information about bipolar disorder, medications, and support groups for the client or family

Communication during manic episodes

- Try to maintain a calm, nonstimulating atmosphere on the unit.
- Convey self-confidence when setting limits on the client's behaviour.
- Guard against being manipulated and ensure consistency with the rest of the team in your response to manipulative behaviour or acting out.
- Provide brief and concise explanations and statements since their comprehension is limited due to a short attention span.
- Hear and act on legitimate client complaints
- Firmly redirect the client's energy into more appropriate and constructive channels.

Pharmacotherapy

In the case of bipolar disorder, the medication dosage must be delicately balanced. Monitor clients' responses carefully; antidepressants can induce manic symptoms, and mood stabilizers may cause depression.

Lithium carbonate. Because achieving an adequate level of lithium in the body takes weeks or months, other mood stabilizers, antidepressants, or atypical antipsychotics may also be used for manic episodes until the therapeutic level of lithium is reached. Lithium toxicity is an abnormally high serum level of lithium. It can result from nonsteroidal anti-inflammatory drugs (NSAIDs), diuretics, vomiting, diarrhea, and other causes of fluid and electrolyte imbalance or from an overdose.

- Monitor clients for early signs of lithium toxicity: anorexia, nausea, diarrhea, drowsiness, muscle weakness, tremors, unsteadiness, and lack of coordination.
- If toxicity is suspected, monitor vital signs and level of consciousness. Push fluids.
- Be aware that more severe signs: fever, decreased urine, low blood pressure, electrocardiogram (ECG) changes, irregular heartbeat, seizures, and loss of consciousness—can cause death.
- To prevent lithium toxicity, encourage fluid intake of 2 to 3 L daily and replace any fluid loss from exercise, vomiting,

or diarrhea. Ensure a balanced diet with adequate salt intake. If a dose is forgotten or late, skip that dose and resume with the next scheduled dose.

Anticonvulsants

- Action: Medications such as carbamazepine, valproic acid, and lamotrigine stabilize mood by boosting the inhibitory effect of GABA on the stress response. Without inhibition due to GABA, high levels of epinephrine and norepinephrine heighten neural synapse activity. Anticonvulsant medications are often effective in treating mania, hypomania, and to a lesser degree, depressive symptoms.
  - Serious adverse effects: Carbamazepine can cause agranulocytosis. Divalproex (a valproic acid derivative) can cause thrombocytopenia. Overdoses can be lethal. It is important to monitor blood test results and observe the client for evidence of bruising and bleeding.

Nursing Interventions

- Maintain client's safety and that of other clients. Lock up sharp and hazardous possessions.
- Use seclusion, if necessary, when the client is argumentative and disruptive to other clients. Maintain close supervision and spend time with the client after they calm down, discussing their feelings and suggesting strategies to prevent future escalation of behaviour.
- Give emotional support and encourage rest periods.
- Set realistic limits on behaviour and reinforce socially appropriate conduct. For example, it may be necessary to impose controls on spending to prevent bankruptcy.
- Maintain nutrition and hydration: High energy levels require increased calories. Clients experiencing a manic episode need reminders to eat and drink. Provide high-calorie finger foods between mealtimes and, if the client is on lithium, salty snacks.
- Assist with personal hygiene; promote self-care.
- Suggest activities that suit the client's short attention span.

Electroconvulsive Therapy

Electroconvulsive therapy (ECT) involves passing electrical current through the brain, producing a tonic–clonic seizure lasting about 30–60 seconds. Researchers have been unable to pinpoint exactly how ECT works, but the current speculation is that it improves brain chemistry in a manner similar to that of mood-disorder drug treatments. Muscle relaxants confine most seizure activity to the brain, almost completely eliminating contractions elsewhere in the body (unlike the depictions of ECT in the media). ECT remains the treatment of choice for a major depression that does not respond to antidepressants and for an acutely suicidal depressed client. Similarly, ECT can be used for acute mania, if lithium or other mood stabilizers have proven ineffective, or if the mania has escalated to dangerous behaviour or exhaustion, which are life-threatening.

ECT has risks, especially for those with cardiovascular disease. Most memory loss is temporary, although permanent loss can occur. The electrodes are now commonly placed unilaterally rather than bilaterally, thus reducing the level of memory loss that clients experience.

Commonly, a series of three treatments weekly is given for 2–4 weeks. Reassurance, empathy, and teaching are necessary to allay a client's fears. Nursing care, before and after the procedure, is similar to that required by any client undergoing a general anaesthetic. Nursing considerations for clients receiving ECT therapy include the following:

- Before ECT, educate the client and family about the procedure and effects and encourage them to express any concerns. Allow nothing by mouth for several hours prior to the treatment. Remove valuables and dentures. Client should wear comfortable, loose-fitting clothing. Clients should urinate before the procedure.
- During the procedure, assist with monitoring vital signs and the electroencephalography.
- After ECT, monitor vital signs and maintain the client's airway until fully awake. Assist with ambulation and reorientation. Give analgesics and antiemetics as necessary. Reinforce teaching and ensure that family members understand the client's initial confusion or memory loss.

Transcranial Direct Current Stimulation

Transcranial direct current stimulation (tDCS) is a noninvasive, painless brain stimulation treatment that uses a mild electrical current to stimulate specific parts of the brain. Electrodes are placed on the client's scalp and a weak current is delivered for 20 to 30 minutes per session. Sessions occur several times a week over several months. No sedation or anaesthesia is required. Although still in the experimental stage, studies have shown encouraging results with improvement in depressive symptoms, memory and attention in both depression and bipolar disorders (Bard et al., 2022).

Repetitive Transcranial Magnetic Stimulation

Repetitive transcranial magnetic stimulation (rTMS) is a noninvasive procedure in which a changing magnetic field is introduced into the brain to influence the brain's activity. The field is generated by passing a large electrical current through a wire stimulation coil over a brief period. It is used frequently for mood disorders. When administered daily at the left prefrontal cortex, it has shown to be effective treatment for nonpsychotic depression. It may not be as effective as ECT for treatment resistant depression. Some clients may not be candidates for the treatment due to the strong magnetic fields involved. For example, clients with metal objects such as screws, plates, pacemakers, or other implants can prevent a client from receiving rTMS (Bard et al., 2022).

Therapies as Adjuncts to Medication

Therapies that are used as an adjunct to medications for treating clients with depression and bipolar disorders include the following:

- Individual psychotherapy: It is aimed at improved social functioning; therapy may focus on a client's interpersonal relationships, developmental delays, and role transitions.
- Group therapy: It provides peer support and education after clients are no longer acutely ill. Groups may be facilitated by professionals or peers. Peer-led groups are usually in community settings, often through voluntary agencies, such as the Mood Disorders Society of Canada and the CMHA.
- Family-focused therapy: It is aimed at education and at restoring adaptive and functional family relationships.
- Interpersonal and social rhythm therapy: It is aimed to regulate social routines and stabilize interpersonal relationships to improve depression and prevent relapse. Psychoeducation is an important feature of this therapy.
- CBT: It is aimed at guiding clients to examine the validity of their thinking and at modifying any distorted perceptions.
- Milieu therapy: The nurse may need to provide seclusion for highly manic bipolar clients.
- Phototherapy or light therapy for SAD: Regular exposure to broad-spectrum fluorescent lighting (which is of a higher intensity than normal indoor lighting) improves symptoms for most sufferers of SAD.

Teaching and Learning

For mood disorders, client and family teaching comes after ensuring the client's safety and addressing social needs. It is important to wait until the client is ready and able to learn.

Topics for the Family and Client Education

It is important for the nurse to educate the client and the family on the following topics:

- The illness, including the nature, causes, and symptoms of depression or bipolar disorder
- Medications, including the management of adverse effects and which adverse effects to report to the doctor
  - Emphasize the length of time required for medications to become fully effective, taking medications correctly and regularly, and diet restrictions for those on MAOIs.
  - For people on lithium, highlight having regular blood tests and reinforce the symptoms of lithium toxicity.
- Techniques for stress management, assertiveness (for depression), and anger management (for bipolar disorder)
- Available support services, including support groups, suicide hotline, and legal and financial assistance

ANXIETY DISORDERS, OBSESSIVE–COMPULSIVE DISORDER, AND POST-TRAUMATIC STRESS DISORDER

Anxiety and fear are normal stress responses to threatening situations. When anxiety is mild or moderate, people may have adaptive coping abilities to alleviate their concerns and overcome or avoid stressors. In contrast, with severe anxiety or panic, individuals experience considerable distress, the perceptive field narrows, and reactions are quite likely to be maladaptive and disorganized. In the DSM-5-TR, obsessive–compulsive disorder (OCD) and post-traumatic stress disorder (PTSD) have been moved from the "Anxiety Disorders" section to new sections to emphasize their differences from other anxiety disorders. Anxiety and fear are still a major part of these two mental illnesses.

Anxiety that is without a specific source or higher than expected for a given threat indicates an anxiety disorder. People with this disorder suffer excessive levels of anxiety, fear, or worry, causing them to avoid situations. The symptoms are persistent typically lasting 6 months or more (or shorter duration in children with separation anxiety disorder or selective mutism) according to the DSM-5-TR (APA, 2022). Many develop physical symptoms. In Canada, anxiety disorders are one the most common of all mental health conditions, especially among young people. Women have higher rates of mood and anxiety disorders (CAMH, 2022a). Many Canadians experienced higher rates of anxiety disorders from various stressors associated with the COVID-19 pandemic (Statistics Canada, 2021a).

Anxiety Disorders
Pathophysiology

The normal autonomic stress response is called "fight or flight" or the "general adaptation syndrome." It consists of three stages:

1. Alarm: The body prepares for defence or escape. The hypothalamus stimulates the adrenal glands to release adrenalin and norepinephrine for fuel and the liver to convert glycogen to glucose for cellular nutrition.
2. Resistance: The body adapts for survival, either by "fight or flight." The pupils dilate. Breathing and heartbeat accelerate, shunting highly oxygenated blood to the muscles. Once the person is out of danger, body responses relax.
3. Exhaustion: Unless resolved by adaptation during the resistance stage, emotional arousal continues until the body is depleted of stored energy, which will eventually cause death.

Anxiety disorders cause a prolonged and exaggerated stress response. Neurotransmitters of the limbic system (epinephrine, norepinephrine, dopamine, serotonin, and GABA) regulate anxiety. The biological mechanisms include the following:

- Excessive secretion of norepinephrine: It stimulates the cerebral cortex, the limbic system (especially the right temporal lobe), brainstem, and spinal cord, even without a source of fear.
- Low levels of GABA: GABA inhibits the excitatory neurotransmitters norepinephrine and dopamine, thus lessening emotional arousal and preventing disorganized responses.
- Abnormal serotonin functioning and glucose metabolism are also implicated.
- Genetics: Anxiety disorders cluster in families, indicating a genetic component.
- Neuroimaging shows anatomical brain changes contributing to (or resulting from) chronic stress. These include smaller frontal and temporal lobes and abnormalities of the amygdala (which regulates fear, memory, and emotion) and the hippocampus (the site of emotion and memory storage).

Clinical Manifestations

- All age groups are affected. In children, separation anxiety consists of an intense fear of losing their primary caregiver. Symptoms include refusing to attend school, fear of the dark and of going to sleep, stomach aches, headaches, nausea, and feeling faint. Other common anxiety disorders in children are social phobias and generalized anxiety syndrome.
- Older persons: There is a high prevalence of anxiety disorders in older persons, although the incidence is slightly less than in other age groups.

Examples of anxiety disorders

- Panic disorder: It is characterized by recurrent unexpected panic attacks. A panic attack is an abrupt surge of intense fear or apprehensive with palpitations, diaphoresis, shakiness, hyperventilating, nausea, chest pain, feelings of choking, distorted perceptions of reality, and fear of death (Halter et al., 2019).
- Agoraphobia: "Individuals with agoraphobia are fearful and anxious about two (or more) of the following situations: using public transportation; being in open spaces; being in enclosed places, standing in line or being in a crowd; or being outside of the home alone in other situations. The individual fears these situations because of thoughts that escape might be difficult or help may not be available in the event of developing panic-like symptoms or other incapacitating or embarrassing symptoms" (APA, 2022, p. 246).
- Generalized anxiety disorder: It is characterized by persistent and distorted apprehension and fear. The individual has excessive anxiety in many situations with the inability to concentrate, fatigue, irritability, tension, restlessness, and sleep disturbances (Halter et al., 2019).
- Social anxiety disorder (social phobia): It is characterized by marked anxiety or fear provoked by exposure to a social or performance situation (fear of being scrutinized or saying something foolish, performing on stage or public speaking, etc.). The individual goes to extremes to avoid the situation. Social anxiety is more than shyness (Halter et al., 2019).
- Substance-induced anxiety disorder: It involves symptoms of anxiety, panic attacks, obsessions, and compulsions that develop with the use of a substance or withdrawal of the substance. Diagnosis of this disorder involves a comprehensive review of the client's history and physical examination, and laboratory values indicating use of a psychoactive substance (e.g., cocaine, alcohol, heroin, hallucinogens) (Halter et al., 2019).

Defence Mechanisms Related to Anxiety Disorders

People use defence mechanisms to cope with anxiety. For the most part, defence mechanisms are employed unconsciously to preserve emotional stability and a sense of self. Sometimes, however, defence mechanisms are overused, or they promote reality distortion and self-deception, hindering the person's ability to cope realistically and practically. Nurses can help clients learn appropriate problem-solving and more effective coping strategies. Some common defence mechanisms include the following:

- Repression: Unconsciously blocking awareness of anxiety-provoking or painful perceptions
- Suppression: Similar to forgetting. It may be conscious or unconscious.
- Denial: Rejecting the reality of threatening situations, even with confirming evidence
- Projection: Attributing one's emotions, thoughts, and impulses to another person
- Introjection: Adopting the values and attitudes of others without questioning them
- Reaction formation: Stating the opposite of what one actually feels and thinks
- Displacement: Directing negative responses, such as anger, toward someone who is usually less threatening than the person who triggered the response
- Regression: Behaviour that characterizes an earlier developmental stage when the person may have felt more secure
- Withdrawal: Becoming passive and emotionally uninvolved

Diagnostics and Therapeutics

Diagnosis. Clients suffering from anxiety often present with the following concerns:

- They feel that they are doomed and likely to die.
- They have difficulties with problem solving and concentration.
- Their vital signs are indicative of the stress response: perspiring; increased blood pressure (BP), heart rate, and respirations; muscle tension; and dilated pupils.
- They exhibit somatic symptoms, for example, nausea, palpitations, frequent voiding or urgency, throat tightening, or a shaky voice.
- They complain of feeling tired and being short-tempered, disorganized, and unable to sleep.

While the above complaints clearly indicate anxiety, before concluding that it is a mental health condition, it is important to rule out whether the apprehension and worries stem from an underlying medical ailment. Medical illnesses causing anxiety may require urgent treatment. For example:

- Respiratory diseases such as chronic obstructive pulmonary disease (COPD), asthma, pulmonary edema, pulmonary embolism
- Cardiovascular diseases such as angina, heart failure, hypertension, hypotension, arrhythmias
- Endocrine diseases such as hyperthyroidism and hypoglycemia
- Neurological diseases such as delirium, Parkinson's disease, postconcussion syndrome
- Metabolic diseases such as hypercalcemia, hyperkalemia, hyponatremia

Treatment. First, treat any comorbid medical conditions. Then consider the following:

- CBT, including psychoeducation and cognitive restructuring

- Behavioural therapy, including relaxation, systematic desensitization, response prevention, flooding, and thought stopping.
- Psychotherapy, to help the client develop insight
- Animal therapy—using therapy animals to help the client feel more secure and to help decrease many of the physical responses to stress (Bard et al., 2022)
- Pharmacotherapy, including anxiolytics (especially benzodiazepines), buspirone which is an azapirones, antidepressants, beta blockers, Lyrica, an anticonvulsant medication, and antihistamines

The most common form of treatment is a combination of drug therapy and CBT.

Nursing Considerations

Nursing assessment. Begin with a full health history and physical assessment to ascertain whether there are concurrent medical conditions associated with the heightened anxiety. Ask about social activities and any worries, fears, or feelings of nervousness, tension, or insecurity. Does the person talk about a past traumatic experience?

- Several rating scales for anxiety are available, for example, the Hamilton Anxiety Rating Scale and the Patient Health Questionnaire (PHQ-9).
- Check vital signs (pulse, BP, respiratory rate, etc.), changes in appetite or weight, and other physiological symptoms, such as gastro-intestinal (GI) upsets, fatigue, diaphoresis, and insomnia.
- Assess the risk of self-harm or suicide (see the section "Psychiatric Emergencies: Crisis, Suicide, Violence").
- Inquire about cognitive capacity (ability to concentrate, disorientation, illogical thinking, narrowed perceptual field, etc.).
- Probe for any reasons for heightened anxiety.

The nurse–client relationship. Clients in any health care setting experience some level of anxiety. Reducing their anxiety to tolerable levels depends on a nurse's skill and patience in developing a trusting relationship. Be patient. There may not be much improvement for weeks or even months.

When communicating with clients with anxiety:

- Show respect by addressing your client using their preferred name.
- Use a calm, warmly accepting, and quiet approach.
- Encourage the client to talk about feelings and emotions.
- Convey compassion, empathy, and honesty.
- Speak slowly, wait patiently while your client responds, and then listen carefully.

Nursing Interventions

- Maintain a restful, nonstimulating environment or move the client to a quiet place and always stay with any person who is experiencing high levels of anxiety.
- Speak slowly in clear, simple language, repeating as necessary.
- Reinforce reality where there are distortions in the client's perception and understanding.
- Listen for themes in the client's communication.

- Monitor and encourage self-care activities for those clients with ritualistic and obsessive behaviours. Phobias and intense concentration on rituals can interfere with a client's personal hygiene and grooming, adequate nutrition and fluid intake, elimination, and sleep.
- Ensure client safety and protection from impulsive and destructive reactions based on fear.

Teaching and Learning

Teach relaxation techniques, either individually or in groups. Some examples of these techniques include the following:

- Deep muscle relaxation: Have the client lie down and tense and relax voluntary muscles, progressing from the toes upward and focusing attention on each area in turn.
- Controlled breathing or meditation or both
- Guided imagery of places and situations that the person has previously experienced as peaceful and restful
- Systematic desensitization of anxiety-causing situations, either through visualization, role-play, or repeated real exposure, while also engaging in controlled breathing or deep muscle relaxation techniques

Teach the client about anxiety and the client's specific diagnosis. Also provide information on the following:

- Support services: Provide resources on available community programs and services, such as support groups, crisis hotlines, and sources for individual psychotherapy.
- Medications: Teach clients and their families about medications and their adverse effects:
  - Clients should avoid working with dangerous equipment.
  - Clients should avoid both alcoholic and caffeinated beverages. Alcohol can enhance the effect of the medication, and caffeine can reduce it.
  - Clients should avoid pregnancy and breastfeeding when taking benzodiazepines.
  - Clients should be taught dietary restrictions for MAOIs.
  - Clients should be warned that stopping the medications abruptly may cause withdrawal symptoms, such as tremors, convulsions, confusion, insomnia, irritability, and nervousness.

Obsessive–Compulsive and Related Disorders
Clinical Manifestations

Obsessions refer to persistent, reoccurring thoughts, impulses, or images that cannot be let go from the mind. Examples include perfectionism, fear of losing control, fear of being responsible for the harm of others, concern with getting a disease, and fear of germs or contamination.

Compulsions are ritualistic behaviours or thoughts that people feel compelled to perform in an attempt to reduce their anxiety. The gain achieved by the ritual is only temporary, so the compulsive act must be repeated over and over again. Examples include washing and cleaning, repeatedly checking on things, or counting.

Obsessions and compulsions can occur independently from one another, but they often accompany one another (Halter et al., 2019). For an individual to be diagnosed with OCD, they must have obsessions or compulsions or both, that take up at least one hour per day or cause clinically significant distress or impairment in social, occupational, or other areas of important functioning (Bard et al., 2022).

Other Obsessive–Compulsive and Related Disorders

- Hoarding disorder: It is "characterized by persistent difficulty discarding or parting with possessions, regardless of their actual value, as a result of a strong perceived need to save the items and to distress associated with discarding them" (APA, 2022, p. 277). Hoarding disorder is not the same as collecting. Collectors look for certain items they may want to organize or display. Individuals with hoarding disorder randomly save items and store them all over the place. They excessively store, buy, or steal items not needed or have no area to store them in. Leading to clutter that accumulates dust, mold, and other health and safety concerns. The consequences of clutter can cause fire hazards, tripping hazards, and strained relationships with family members.
  - Hoarding disorder can also involve anxiety associated with parting with animals. Individuals can be deeply attached to their pets and find it difficult to let them go. Health issues may result from overcrowding living conditions with the animals, animal excrement, fleas and ticks, and animalborne illnesses.
- Trichotillomania (hair pulling) disorder: It is the impulse to pull out their hair resulting in hair loss. Individuals may pull out their hair when distressed as a way to decrease their anxiety. The hair pulling can lead to significant distress in social situations and functional impairment.
- Body dysmorphic disorder: It is "preoccupation with one or more perceived defects or flaws in physical appearance that are not observable or appear only slight to others, and by repetitive behaviours (mirror checking, excessive grooming, skin picking, reassurance seeking) or mental acts (of comparing one's appearance with that of other people) in response to the appearance concerns" (APA, 2022, p. 271).
- Excoriation (skin-picking) disorder: It is the urge to recurrently pick at one's own skin that can lead to skin lesions. The skin picking can cause severe distress or functional impairment.
- Substance/medication-induced obsessive–compulsive and related disorder: It "consist[s] of symptoms that must have developed during or soon after substance intoxication or withdrawal or after exposure to or withdrawal from a medication or toxin and the substance/medication must be capable of producing the symptoms" (APA, 2022, p. 289).

Treatment and Therapies for Obsessive–Compulsive Disorders

Medications, psychotherapy, or a combination of the two are used to treat obsessive–compulsive disorders. Refer to the "Treatment" section under "Anxiety Disorders" for treatments and therapies.

Nursing Interventions

Refer to the "Nursing Interventions" section under "Anxiety Disorders."

Trauma and Stressor-Related Disorder

Individuals' reactions to a psychological distress following exposure to a traumatic or stressful event may be very different for each person. Some people cope and move on, whereas others become anxious and fearful. "Trauma and stress related disorders include disorders in which exposure to a traumatic or stressful event is listed explicitly as a diagnostic criterion. These include reactive attachment disorder, disinhibited social engagement disorder, post-traumatic stress disorder (PTSD), acute stress disorder, adjustment disorders, and prolonged grief disorder" (APA, 2022, p. 295).

Post-Traumatic Stress Disorder

Clinical Manifestations

PTSD is triggered by a terrifying event or situation that a person has either experienced or witnessed. It involves exposure to trauma involving serious injury, threat of death or death, or sexual violence. Symptoms include flashbacks, nightmares, severe anxiety, or uncontrollable thoughts or feelings of being unsafe in the world as if experiencing the event in the present. Individuals may avoid triggers that remind them of the situation or event. They may experience symptoms of feeling very nervous all the time, irritability, and exaggerated startle. They may feel very numb or detached from others. They may have difficulty concentrating or sleeping. These symptoms can interfere with a person's normal daily tasks or create problems in social situations and relationships. Individuals with PTSD often have issues with developing trust (Halter et al., 2019).

Nursing Considerations

Nursing assessment. Assessment involves screening tools and PTSD checklists. Comprehensive assessments are done if they screen positive for PTSD. Detailed history is assessed regarding onset, frequency, course, severity, level of distress, and the degree of functional impairment. Further assessment is made for suicidal or violent ideation, family and social supports, insomnia, social withdrawal, functional impairment, current life stressors, medication, and past medical and psychiatric history. A mental status examination is also performed (Halter et al., 2019).

The nurse–client relationship

- The nurse should establish a therapeutic relationship through nonjudgemental acceptance and empathy.
- The nurse should interact with the client on regular intervals to display an opening, caring attitude that will allow the client the opportunity to talk. This will help develop a trusting relationship with the client.
- Using silence and listening communication techniques can encourage the client to express their feelings.
- One of the most helpful things a nurse can do is gently suggest to the client that they were not responsible for what happened (Halter et al., 2019).

Nursing interventions

- Initial education should include reassurance that reactions to trauma are common and that these reactions do not indicate personal failure or weakness.
- Strategies to improve coping, enhance self-care, and facilitate recognition of problems are essential.
- Relaxation techniques are helpful.
- The client should avoid caffeine and alcohol (Halter et al., 2019).

Treatments

- All clients should be informed of effective treatment options for PTSD and referred to an experienced licensed mental health practitioner.
- Treatments include group therapy, psychotherapy, imagery, animal therapy, and hypnosis.

Initial medication may include an SSRI such as fluoxetine (Prozac), paroxetine (Paxil), or sertraline (Zoloft), or an SNRI such as venlafaxine (Effexor) to decrease anxiety and decrease depressive symptoms (Halter et al., 2019).

ADJUSTMENT DISORDERS

Adjustment disorders are characterized as a recognizable response to a stressor that often occur during significant life transitions, such as starting school, entering adolescence, experiencing family breakup, facing job loss, dealing with financial problems, going through menopause, retiring, or encountering the death of a spouse. These stressors can give rise to emotional or behavioral symptoms that persist for a period of up to 3 months following the event. This disorder can affect individuals of all age groups. People who have underdeveloped social skills, inadequate coping mechanisms, or limited support from social networks may be especially susceptible. The resulting symptoms can significantly impact one's social, occupational, or overall functioning. Once the stressor or its consequences have subsided, it may take approximately 6 months for the symptoms to fully dissipate. It's important to note that this disorder carries a heightened risk of suicide (Bard et al., 2022).

Pathophysiology

No clearly defined biological causes or physiological changes are correlated with adjustment disorders, although when people exhibit depressive or anxiety-related behaviours, the expected pathophysiological changes for those conditions would be present. Theorists suggest that genetic factors may be implicated, at least for those persons with cognitive disorders or developmental challenges who respond poorly to stressful situations.

Clinical Manifestations

The behavioural and emotional symptoms of adjustment disorders can negatively affect functioning at work or school, and clients typically use a variety of defence mechanisms. Six subtypes of adjustment disorders are identified:

- Adjustment disorder with depressed mood: This is the most common adjustment disorder. Depressed mood, crying spells, and feelings of hopelessness are characteristic symptoms of a mood disorder; however, they are less severe than major depression.
- Adjustment disorder with anxiety: Some people who have an adjustment disorder also display nervousness, worry, and anxious feelings, and behaviour or separation anxiety is predominant.
- Adjustment disorder with mixed anxiety and depressed mood: Here, both anxiety and depression affect the person's ability to adapt to stressful events.
- Adjustment disorder with disturbance of conduct: Acting out inappropriately defines this type. Adolescents with a history of skipping school, fighting, vandalism, rebelling against all forms of authority, and getting into trouble with the law are often diagnosed with this disorder.
- Adjustment disorder with mixed disturbance of emotions and conduct: As the name implies, this is a mixture of the above types.
- Adjustment disorder unspecified: People with this disorder do not display the above symptoms but may withdraw socially or develop physical symptoms

Diagnostics and Therapeutics
Diagnosis
Diagnosing adjustment disorders requires a thorough personal history that shows a stressful event or social situation followed by the development of symptoms. These symptoms are more intense and last longer than usual, and all underlying physical or mental health disorders have been ruled out. Risk factors include social and environmental variables such as overprotective or abusive parents, frequent moves as a child, living in poverty, and being witness to wars and violence. Sometimes delayed or prolonged grief is classified as an adjustment disorder if the grief reaction does not meet the criteria for prolonged grief disorder.

Treatment
- Individual psychotherapy
- Family therapy
- Behavioural therapy
- Self-help groups
- Pharmacotherapy with antidepressants and anxiolytics

Nursing Considerations
Nursing Assessment
- Assess the level of anxiety or depression.
- Assess the client's support system, including family dynamics.
- Examine how the client perceives the condition or conditions.

The Nurse–Client Relationship
- Convey empathy and support.
- Avoid minimizing the client's struggle with empty reassurances, such as "You'll be fine" and "Everything will work out."

- Encourage the person to recognize that an issue exists and that it is important to talk together about their emotional reactions.
- Provide positive reinforcement for desirable behaviour. This helps increase self-esteem.

Nursing Interventions
- Have the client describe their life and lifestyle prior to the stressful event.
- Listen when the client expresses anger, fear, and other negative emotions.
- Encourage healthy self-care and lifestyle, such as eating well, adequate sleep, regular exercise, and enjoyable hobbies.
- Assist with problem-solving, providing alternatives for the client to consider.
- Assist the client to identify family members and friends who can provide support.
- Encourage family and friends to provide strong support.

Teaching and Learning
- Teach stress management techniques.
- Involve family and friends in teaching and learning opportunities.
  Explain to clients and families the following stages of grief:
- Numbness and shock: This stage is characterized by an inability to feel anything, sometimes alternating with extreme emotional outbursts.
- Yearning and searching: Expressions of anger, intense sorrow, and weeping as the reality of the loss sets in. There are often moments of imagining that the loved one will reappear.
- Despair and disorganization: This stage is characterized by emotions of hopelessness and acute loneliness, depression, and apathy.
- Reorganization and acceptance: Finally, there is gradual restoring of the self and a return to regular activities. Memories of the loved one become more comforting and less painful.
  Nursing responsibilities in assisting a person who is grieving include the following:
- Help the client identify their current stage of grief.
- Be accepting of expressions of anger. Accompany the client to a private and quiet area and stay with them.
- Try to engage the person in activities (keeping busy).
- Assess a client's spirituality and make a referral to a chaplain or minister if that is desired.
- Refer the person to a grief support group.

Prolonged Grief Disorder
The DSM-5-TR added a new diagnostic entity called *prolonged grief disorder*. Prolonged grief disorder is defined as "an intense yearning or longing for the deceased (often with intense sorrow and frequent crying) or preoccupation with thoughts and memories of the decreased, although in children and adolescents, this preoccupation may focus on the circumstances of the death" (APA, 2022, p. 323). These

grief reactions occur most of the day, nearly every day for at least a month. It can happen when someone close to the bereaved person has died within at least 12 months for adults (6 months for children and adolescents). At least three of following symptoms have occurred daily most of the day in the last month: identity disruption (e.g., feeling as though part of oneself has died), marked sense of disbelief about the death, avoidance of reminders that the person is dead, intense emotional pain related to the death, difficulty reintegrating into one's relationships and activities after the death, emotional numbness, feeling that life is meaningless as a result of the death, and intense loneliness as a result of the death (APA, 2022).

With the rising numbers of deaths caused by the COVID-19 virus and restrictions such as social distancing, reduced capacity at events, and hospital regulations, typical mourning processes and grief rituals were disrupted. Therefore, a greater chance of developing prolonged grief disorder has been reported from the reduced social connections and lack of psychological support systems (Szuhany et al., 2021).

SCHIZOPHRENIA SPECTRUM AND OTHER PSYCHOTIC DISORDERS

Schizophrenia spectrum and other psychotic disorders "are potentially devastating brain disorders that affect a person's thinking, language, emotions, social behaviour, and ability to perceive reality accurately" (Halter et al., 2019, p. 301).

Schizophrenia spectrum disorder is a disorder with a lifetime prevalence of 1%, both in Canada and worldwide (CMHA, 2022). The suicide rate for people with schizophrenia spectrum disorders is over 20 times higher than that for the general population (CAMH, 2022b). Thus, for a substantial proportion of clients, schizophrenia spectrum disorder is a terminal illness.

The DSM-5-TR includes a number of disorders in the category "Schizophrenia Spectrum and Other Psychotic Disorders," including schizophreniform disorder, schizoaffective disorder, delusional disorder, brief psychotic disorder, schizotypal (personality) disorder, schizophrenia substance/medication-induced psychotic disorder, psychotic disorder due to another medical condition, catatonia associated with another mental disorder, catatonia disorder due to another medical condition, unspecified catatonia, other specified schizophrenia spectrum and other psychotic disorder, and unspecified schizophrenia spectrum and other psychotic disorder. Although some people (and often the media) confuse dissociative identity disorder (DID) (previously referred to as *multiple personality disorder*) with schizophrenia, the two are distinctly different psychiatric illnesses, and DID is a much rarer condition.

Pathophysiology

Causation is complicated and involves many factors. Evidence is clear, however, that brain structure, balancing of neurochemical transmitters, and disrupted neural circuits underlie the development of schizophrenia. Although social and environmental factors may trigger the onset or exacerbation of schizophrenia symptoms, the psychosocial theories blaming dysfunctional families and parenting are both outdated and harmful. Some key factors include the following:

- Brain abnormalities: At the time of diagnosis, larger cerebral ventricles, atrophy of the cerebellum or frontal lobe, and a variety of other structural abnormalities can be seen; for example, the hippocampus may be smaller than normal. As the illness progresses, further degeneration is minimal. Abnormalities of the prefrontal cortex are associated with reductions in higher cognitive functions.
- Neurochemical transmitters: There is excessive dopamine activity. Serotonin, glutamate, and other neurotransmitters are also poorly regulated.
- Genetics: Decades of studies on twins provide ample evidence that inheritance is a factor. People with a parent or sibling with schizophrenia are at higher risk of developing schizophrenia. If both parents have schizophrenia, a child has almost a 40% risk of developing the disorder.
- Substances: Illegal drug use and substance misuse do not cause schizophrenia; however, when a person is genetically predisposed to schizophrenia, drugs and substances may initiate symptoms earlier and with more severity than would occur otherwise.

Clinical Manifestations

Schizophrenia affects males and females in equal numbers, although, on average, males are usually diagnosed in their late teens or early twenties, while women are often diagnosed during their mid-twenties. Males also tend to display more severe symptoms and more negative symptoms and be less responsive to pharmacological treatment, thus suffering a poorer outcome. Females, in contrast, are more likely to have a family history of schizophrenia but have less severe symptoms and cognitive impairment. Late onset, after the age of 40, occurs infrequently. Females and those with later onset tend to have better outcomes. Comorbid mental health conditions are common, especially depression and anxiety. As well, many people abuse substances, trying to relieve their symptoms through self-medication.

Schizophrenia is a lifelong illness for at least 95% of sufferers. Some people will have one severe episode for which they receive treatment but are then well stabilized on medications that they take for the remainder of their lives. A few are eventually able to function without antipsychotics. For many, however, the illness is marked by hospitalization during psychotic episodes interspersed with periods of community treatment. Over many years, the psychotic episodes may become further apart. A minority do not respond to antipsychotic medications and remain in psychiatric hospitals long term.

Diagnosis and Symptoms of Schizophrenia Spectrum Disorders and Psychotic Disorders

Many symptoms are visible to others and become a source of stigma against the disease, the people affected, and their families. Clients are often withdrawn and socially isolated, either to hide their illness or in an attempt to feel safe. Social isolation also is brought about by the ridicule and rejection that they experience, stemming from the stigma surrounding the illness and misunderstanding on the part of the public.

Positive symptoms. Positive symptoms are characterized by the exaggeration or distortion of normal functions. Sometimes positive symptoms are subdivided into psychotic and disorganized dimensions.

Psychotic symptoms

- Hallucinations: Distorted perceptions involving any of the five senses. Auditory hallucinations, in which the voices that clients hear are unusually threatening or disapproving, are particularly prevalent.
- Delusions: Unrealistic and unfounded beliefs. Common delusions are of grandeur, of being persecuted, or being controlled, or of having one's mind read.

Disorganized or catatonic behaviour

- When psychotic, the person's behaviour may be catatonic. Catatonia is defined as an increase or decrease in the rate and amount of movement. The most common form is a stuporous state in which the client may require complete physical nursing care, similar to that for a comatose client, sometimes with unpredictable outbursts of aggressive behaviour or strange posturing (Halter et al., 2019). Examples of catatonic behaviour include robot-like activity, complete immobility, or holding a position for long periods of time (waxy flexibility).
- Hostility and aggression may be present most often in response to paranoid and persecutory delusions. People who become violent while experiencing delusions are often trying to defend themselves.
- Cognitive disturbances are difficulties in processing information. Clients are often bombarded so rapidly with ideas that focusing on anything or sorting out what is relevant from what is not becomes impossible. Thoughts are illogical and disconnected. Terms used for cognitive disturbances include "thought disturbance," "loose associations," and "flight of ideas."
- Incoherent speech patterns reflect the disturbed thoughts and may be rapid, jumping from one topic to another. This is sometimes referred to as "word salad."

Negative symptoms

- Inappropriate affect: Emotions that are inconsistent with the occasion
- Flattened affect: Emotions or emotional responses that are diminished
- Alogia: A lack of speech or inadequate communication caused by an interruption in the thought processes
- Poor attention span: Inattentiveness and impaired concentration
- Anhedonia: An inability to experience pleasure from activities or social relationships
- Apathy: Physical inertia
- Avolition: An inability to persist with activities, including grooming and hygiene

A summary of the signs and symptoms of schizophrenia appears in Figure 12.3.

Phases of Schizophrenia

Schizophrenia usually progresses through predictable phases, although the presenting symptoms during a given phase and the length of the phase can vary widely. These phases tend to occur in sequence and appear in cycles throughout the course of the illness.

Prodromal (or prepsychotic) phase. The person has subtle symptoms where they are usually quiet, passive, obedient, and prefer to be alone. Hallucinations and delusions may be present, but behaviours are not completely disorganized yet. Family may report they feel the person is "is slipping away" in front of their eyes (Bard et al., 2022, p. 389).

Acute phase. Onset or exacerbation is characterized by florid, disruptive, symptoms such as delusions, hallucinations, marked distortion in thinking, apathy, withdrawal, and disorganized speech. The person exhibits disturbances in behaviours and feelings. Symptoms may progress to the point where the person requires hospitalization for acute care and treatment. Their functional ability may be severely impaired, and the person can be at risk of harming themselves and others (Bard et al., 2022).

Residual phase. The person's symptoms diminish and are less severe than in the acute phase. The person displays a lack of energy, no interest in goal-directed activities and has a negative outlook. Day hospitalization, or care in a residential crisis centre or supervised group home, may be required (Bard et al., 2022).

Remission phase. The symptoms are absent or diminished, and the person is nearing their baseline functioning. The person's level of functioning allows them to live in the community. The treatment goal is to maintain or improve functioning, improve quality of life, and facilitate personal recovery. There may be setbacks and struggles in the recovery phase; therefore, ongoing assessment and monitoring is required to accommodate any new issues or demands that arise (Bard et al., 2022).

Types of Disorders

Schizophreniform disorder. A person with schizophreniform disorder has the symptoms of schizophrenia but for less than 6 months, during which there are periods of functional, social and occupational activity.

Schizoaffective disorder. A person with schizoaffective disorder has schizophrenic symptoms and a concurrent major depressive or bipolar disorder, but no concurrent general medical disorder or substance abuse.

Delusional disorder. A person with delusional disorder experiences delusions for at least a month that contain either bizarre content (i.e., the person is not bizarre) or occur in real life, such as jealousy, persecution, delusions of grandeur, or having an infection or a somatic illness. The person can function socially and at work. There are specific types of delusions based on the predominant delusional theme: erotomanic, grandiose, jealous, persecutory, somatic, mixed, and unspecified types.

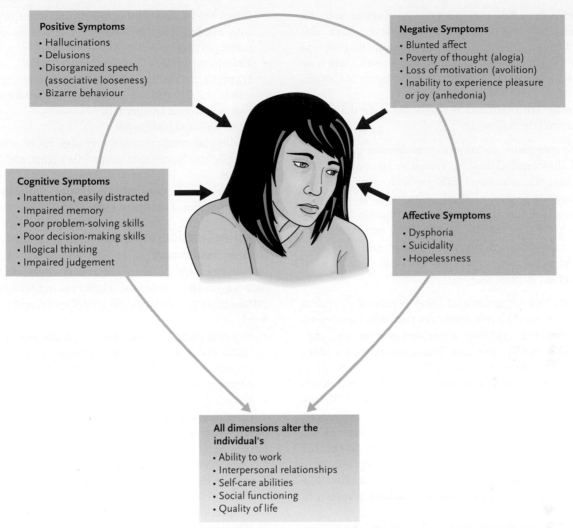

Positive Symptoms
- Hallucinations
- Delusions
- Disorganized speech (associative looseness)
- Bizarre behaviour

Negative Symptoms
- Blunted affect
- Poverty of thought (alogia)
- Loss of motivation (avolition)
- Inability to experience pleasure or joy (anhedonia)

Cognitive Symptoms
- Inattention, easily distracted
- Impaired memory
- Poor problem-solving skills
- Poor decision-making skills
- Illogical thinking
- Impaired judgement

Affective Symptoms
- Dysphoria
- Suicidality
- Hopelessness

All dimensions alter the individual's
- Ability to work
- Interpersonal relationships
- Self-care abilities
- Social functioning
- Quality of life

Fig. 12.3 The four main symptom group of schizophrenia. (From Pollard, C. L., & Jakubec, S. L. [2023]. *Varcarolis's Canadian psychiatric mental health nursing: A clinical approach* [3rd Cdn. ed., p. 277, Figure 15-1]. Elsevier.)

Brief psychotic disorder. Following a very stressful life event, a person suddenly experiences psychotic and disorganized symptoms. These symptoms last for 1 day to a month, after which the person returns to their usual functioning.

Substance- or medication-induced psychotic disorder. Psychosis may be caused by substances such as abuse of drugs, medications, alcohol, or toxins. The person may experience hallucinations or delusions (Bard et al., 2022).

Psychosis or catatonia associated with another medical condition or another mental disorder. According to Bard et al. (2022), "psychoses may also be caused by a medical condition (delirium, neurological or metabolic conditions, hepatic or renal diseases, and many others) as well as by mental illness such as post-traumatic stress disorder … or depression, particularly with coexisting victimization from sexual violence of bullying. … Medical conditions and substance abuse must always be ruled out before a diagnosis of schizophrenia or other psychotic disorder can be made."

Unspecified catatonia. The person has clinically severe distress or impairment in social, occupational or areas of functioning but not all, of the criteria for catatonia. There is also no known underlying medical or mental condition or insufficient information to make a more specific diagnosis (Bard et al., 2022).

Other specified schizophrenia spectrum and other psychotic disorder. The person has clinically significant distress in their life to due to the schizophrenia spectrum and other psychotic disorder symptoms, but these do not meet the full criteria of any of the above-listed conditions (Bard et al., 2022).

Unspecified schizophrenia spectrum and other psychotic disorder. The diagnosis is the same as above, but the clinician chooses not to communicate the reason why this condition does not meet any of the criteria for specific schizophrenia spectrum and other psychotic disorders (Bard et al., 2022).

Diagnostics and Therapeutics

Diagnosis

Diagnosing schizophrenia is complex for a number of reasons. Clients suffer from different combinations of symptoms, and none of the symptoms are completely confined to schizophrenia. In addition, the person in need of mental health help and treatment may be in such distress that they have a difficult time communicating. It often takes decades for people to be properly diagnosed with schizophrenia. As well, there is no single test for schizophrenia (Schizophrenia Society of Canada, 2022).

Commonly, schizophrenia is diagnosed once the person has experienced the following:

> at least one psychotic symptom such as delusions, hallucinations, disorganized thinking, speech, or behaviour. The person experiences extreme difficulty with or an inability to function in family, social, or occupational realms and frequently neglects basic needs such as nutrition or hygiene. Over a period of 6 months, there may be times when the psychotic symptoms are absent, and in their place, the person may experience apathy or depression.
> (Halter et al., 2019, p.302)

Schizophrenia spectrum and other psychotic disorders are complex mental health disorders that affect a person's language, thinking, emotion, social behaviours, and ability to perceive reality correctly. These disorders are identified by symptoms of psychosis. Psychosis is defined as a psychological break from reality. Associated behaviours include altered cognition and perception, great difficulty in functioning adequately, reduced level of awareness, and gross impairment in reality testing (Halter et al., 2019). Schizophrenia may be difficult to identify in the adolescent years since some of the early symptoms may be blamed on adolescent rebellion and immaturity. The DSM-5-TR diagnostic criteria for schizophrenia appear in Box 12.2.

Neuroimaging. CT, MRI, and PET scans may be used to narrow down the diagnosis.

Treatment

Antipsychotic medications. Antipsychotics are also called *neuroleptics* and *major tranquilizers.* There are two groups: the older typical antipsychotics and the newer atypicals (also called *novel antipsychotics*).

Typical antipsychotics
- Action: They block dopamine postsynaptic receptors in the hypothalamus, limbic system, brainstem, basal ganglia, and medulla.
- Effect: They provide some relief, primarily for the positive symptoms of schizophrenia.
  - Major adverse effects include neuromalignant syndrome and movement disorders (extrapyramidal symptoms [EPS]).
- Examples include chlorpromazine (Thorazine), thiothixene (Navane), trifluoperazine (Stelazine), loxapine (Loxapac), afluphenazine (Modecate), pimozide (Orap), perphenazine (Trilafon), flupenthixol (Fluanxol), zuclopenthixol (Clopixol), and haloperidol (Haldol).

Atypical antipsychotics
- Action: They block dopamine, serotonin, and other neurotransmitter receptors.

- Effect: They ease both the positive and negative symptoms, thus markedly enhancing quality of life for people with schizophrenia.
- Examples include clozapine (Clozaril), olanzapine (Zyprexa or Zydis), quetiapine (Seroquel), aripiprazole (Abilify), Ziprasidone (Zeldox), paliperidone (Invega), and risperidone (Risperdal).

  Other medical treatments
- Additional medications for symptoms of schizophrenia include antidepressants, antimania agents, and benzodiazepines.
- ECT is used for psychotic depression and for people who do not respond to antipsychotics.

Nursing Considerations
Nursing Assessment
Nursing assessment for psychosis is complex, but before focusing on the symptoms, try to rule out whether a medical condition or substance use is implicated, and think "safety first."
- Hallucinations: Assess especially if the person is hearing voices that order self-harm or harming others. If so, are the voices accepted as real, and is there intent to follow the commands?
- Delusions: Are there firm beliefs that are not reality based? Again, determine whether these could result in self-harm or harm to others and institute precautions if necessary.
- Co-occurring mental health disorders: These might include depression, suicidal thoughts, anxiety, substance abuse, or violent acts in the past.
- Medications: Has the individual been on any medications? If so, are they still being taken?
- Family: Is the family involved? In what way? Are they caring? Overprotective? Hostile? Suspicious? Does the family understand psychosis, the need for medication, and about support or respite services?

The Nurse–Client Relationship
Particular challenges in caring for someone who is psychotic involve communicating when a person is out of touch with reality. Mastering the following suggested communication skills will help the nurse establish a relationship of trust with these clients (Halter et al., 2019).

Communicating with a client experiencing delusions or hallucinations
- To overcome suspicion and gain trust, be present, straightforward, honest, and reliable.
- Ask directly about delusions and hallucinations. For example, "Are you hearing voices?" "What are you hearing?" "Tell me more about someone trying to hurt you."
- Observe for cues, such as the client's eyes searching around or staring at a particular empty space, and for events that appear to generate the delusions. Try to discuss these observations with the client.
- Do not argue with the voices and beliefs or react as though they are real. Instead, provide your own observations and

BOX 12.2 DSM-5-TR Diagnostic Criteria for Schizophrenia

A. Two or more of the following, each present for a significant portion of time during a 1-month period (or less if successfully treated). At least one of these must be (1), (2), or (3):
1. Delusions.
2. Hallucinations.
3. Disorganized speech (e.g., frequent derailment or incoherence).
4. Grossly disorganized or catatonic behaviour.
5. Negative symptoms (i.e., diminished emotional expression or avolition).

B. For a significant portion of the time since the onset of the disturbance, level of functioning in one or more major areas, such as work, interpersonal relations, or self-care, is markedly below the level achieved before the onset (or when the onset is in childhood or adolescence, there is failure to achieve expected level of interpersonal, academic, or occupational functioning).

C. Continuous signs of the disturbance persist for at least 6 months. This 6-month period must include at least 1 month of symptoms (or less if successfully treated) that meet Criterion A (i.e., active-phase symptoms) and may include periods of prodromal or residual symptoms. During these prodromal or residual periods, the signs of the disturbance may be manifested by only negative symptoms or by two or more symptoms listed in Criterion A present in an attenuated form (e.g., odd beliefs, unusual perceptual experiences).

D. Schizoaffective disorder and depressive or bipolar disorder with psychotic features have been ruled out because either (1) no major depressive or manic episodes have occurred concurrently with the active-phase symptoms, or (2) if mood episodes have occurred during active-phase symptoms, they have been present for a minority of the total duration of the active and residual periods of the illness.

E. The disturbance is not attributable to the physiological effects of a substance (e.g., a drug of abuse, a medication) or another medical condition.

F. If there is a history of autism spectrum disorder or a communication disorder of childhood onset, the additional diagnosis of schizophrenia is made only if prominent delusions or hallucinations, in addition to the other required symptoms of schizophrenia, are also present for at least 1 month (or less if successfully treated).

Specify if: The following course specifiers are only to be used after a 1-year duration of the disorder and if they are not in contradiction to the diagnostic course criteria.

First episode, currently in acute episode: First manifestation of the disorder meeting the defining diagnostic symptom and time criteria. An *acute episode* is a time period in which the symptom criteria are fulfilled.

First episode, currently in partial remission: *Partial remission* is a period of time during which an improvement after a previous episode is maintained and in which the defining criteria of the disorder are only partially fulfilled.

First episode, currently in full remission: *Full remission* is a period of time after a previous episode during which no disorder-specific symptoms are present.

Multiple episodes, currently in acute episode: Multiple episodes may be determined after a minimum of two episodes (i.e., after a first episode, a remission, and a minimum of one relapse).

Multiple episodes, currently in partial remission

Multiple episodes, currently in full remission

Continuous: Symptoms fulfilling the diagnostic symptom criteria of the disorder are remaining for the majority of the illness course with subthreshold symptom periods being very brief relative to the overall course.

Unspecified

Specify if: With catatonia

Specify current severity: Severity is rated by a quantitative assessment of the primary symptoms of psychosis, including delusions, hallucinations, disorganized speech, abnormal psychomotor behaviour, and negative symptoms. Each of these symptoms may be rated for its current severity (most severe in the last 7 days) on a 5-point scale ranging from 0 (not present) to 4 (present and severe).

From Bard, B., MacMullin, E., Williamson, J. & Morrison-Valfre, M. (2022). *Morrison-Valfre's foundations of mental health care in Canada* (p. 388). Elsevier. Based on American Psychiatric Association. (2022). *Diagnostic and statistical manual of mental disorders* (5th ed., Text Revision).

encourage the client to talk about feelings. For example, "I can't see what you do, but it seems to be upsetting you," or "It must be frightening to think that people are against you."

- Focus on reality-based, "here-and-now" activities such as conversations or simple projects. Tell the client, "The voice you hear is part of your illness; it cannot hurt you. Try to listen to me and the others you can see around you."
- If some aspect of the delusion or hallucination is real, validate that part, such as, "Yes, I heard Mr. Green talking on the phone, but he was discussing a movie he had seen. He didn't refer to you."
- Be alert to signs of anxiety in the client, which may indicate that hallucinations are increasing.
- Encourage the use of competing auditory stimuli such as listening to music through headphones.

- Address any underlying emotion, need, or theme that seems to be indicated by the hallucination, such as fear with menacing voices or guilt with accusing voices.
- Focus on the feelings or theme that underlie or flow from the delusions. For example, "You seem to wish you could be more powerful" or "It must feel frightening to think others want to hurt you" (Halter et al., 2019).

Interventions

Nursing interventions for schizophrenia vary depending on the stage of the client's illness. The focus for treatment and professional collaboration varies during each phase of schizophrenia. Interventions include crisis interventions, inpatient treatment teams, group therapies, cognitive enhancement therapy, CBT, social, vocational and self-care skills, medication maintenance education, psychoeducational interventions with families, community treatment agencies, and social support services.

Pharmacotherapy

Serious and sometimes permanent adverse effects occur with antipsychotic medications. In Table 12.4 nursing considerations for antipsychotic drug effects are described.

Drug interactions. Be aware of potential interactions with other medications. Note the following examples:

- Cimetidine (Tagamet), which is for acid indigestion, promotes liver detoxification of antipsychotics and thus decreases their effect.
- Other common antacids reduce absorption of oral antipsychotics. They should be taken 4 hours before or after the antipsychotic.
- Anticonvulsants lower the blood levels of antipsychotics, interfering with their efficacy.
- Epinephrine can produce severe hypotension if given with chlorpromazine.
- Lithium occasionally can produce neurological impairment when combined with antipsychotics. Clients should be monitored closely for neurological signs and symptoms.
- Some cardiac medications reduce the effectiveness of antipsychotics, increasing psychosis.

For more information on these medications, see Chapter 8.

Engaging With Families

Having a family member with schizophrenia is emotionally painful, exhausting, and frightening. Relatives, often the main caregivers when the client is not in hospital, should be consulted in treatment planning and decision making. Family caregivers generally know the client best.

When a client is first diagnosed, however, education for relatives is essential. A family educational plan for understanding psychoses appears in Table 12.5.

Community supports. Nurses should know what community resources and services are available and should assist families in accessing these services. The following two major community agencies provide comprehensive programs.

Schizophrenia Society of Canada. Provincial and local chapters are located across the country. Services and programs may include the following:

- Support groups and counselling services for family members; peer support for clients
- Monthly educational meetings and periodic conferences for family members
- Education programs for parents, siblings, and children of people with schizophrenia
- Public education programs for schools and other community agencies and service providers

CMHA. Services and programs may vary by location but may include the following:

- Educational programs for parents and families
- Community education programs

- Recreation and leisure opportunities for people with a mental health challenge
- Peer options for connecting people with a mental illness and reducing their isolation
- Supported housing
- Bereavement counselling

PERSONALITY DISORDERS

Personality "is an individual's characteristic pattern of relatively permanent thoughts, feelings, and behaviours that define their quality of experiences and relationships" (Pollard & Jakubec, 2023, p. 390). Each person develops unique personality traits from their biological constitution, psychosocial experiences, and environment. Personality traits become deeply engrained and stable, exerting control over a person's attitudes and behaviour.

When a person's character and behaviour deviate markedly from social and cultural expectations, causing functional impairment and distress, the person may have a personality disorder (PD). PDs vary from mild to severe, and people can function quite well when symptoms are mild or intermittent. In fact, most people occasionally display maladaptive characteristics identified with a PD, and some people are clearly eccentric. Health care providers need to take a person's cultural, ethical, and social background into account to prevent the risk of overdiagnosis of a personality disorder (Halter et al., 2019). Box 12.3 presents the DSM-5-TR categories for personality disorders.

The DSM-5-TR also include two other groups of personality disorders: "Personality change due to another medical condition and other specified personality disorder and unspecified personality disorder" (APA, 2022, p. 734).

The most common type of PD is obsessive–compulsive personality disorder (which is distinct from OCD). PDs typically become recognizable by adolescence or early adulthood, although some individuals may not seek clinical attention until much later. It is possible for a PD to become exacerbated after the loss of a significant supporting person or situation. The course of PD is relatively stable over time (Segal, 2021).

Pathophysiology

Some evidence exists for neurobiological abnormalities, but as for most psychiatric disorders, no clear-cut cause for PDs has been identified. A complex interaction of the following factors correlates with PD:

- Genetics: Some evidence exists for a genetic link for antisocial and criminal personality traits, as well as for schizotypal and paranoid PD.
- EEG evidence: Research evidence is mixed. Some studies show a relationship between PD and abnormal temporal and frontal lobe waves, but others do not.
- Neurotransmitters: Low dopamine and serotonin levels are found in aggressive and impulsive behaviours, as well as in suicidality.

TABLE 12.4 Adverse Effects of Conventional Antipsychotics and Related Nursing Interventions

CNS Adverse Effects	Nursing Care and Teaching Considerations
Extrapyramidal symptoms (EPS)	General treatment principles: • Tolerance usually develops by the third month. • Decrease dose of medication. • Add a medication to treat EPS, then taper after 3 months on the antipsychotic. • Use a medication with a lower EPS profile. • Give client education and support.
Acute dystonic reactions: oculogyric crisis, torticollis Onset: 1 to 5 days	Spasms of major muscle groups of neck, back, and eyes; occur suddenly; frightening; painful; parenteral medication works faster than PO; have respiratory support available; more common in children and young males and with high-potency drugs. Taper dose gradually when discontinuing antipsychotic drugs to avoid withdrawal dyskinesia. Administer antiparkinson agent (e.g., benztropine or trihexphenidyl)-give IM for rapid effect and because of swallowing difficulty. Also consider diphenhydramine hydrochloride (Benadryl) 25-50 mg IM or IV. Relief usually occurs in 5-15 minutes. Prevent further dystonia's with antiparkinson agent. Accompany person to a quiet area to provide support and comfort. Assist person to understand the event and avert distortion or mistrust of medication.
Akathisia: Onset 2 hours to 60 days	Cannot remain still; pacing, inner restlessness, leg aches are relieved by movement; rule out anxiety or agitation; medicate. Consult prescriber for possible medication change. Give antiparkinson medication. Tolerance to akathisia does not develop, but akathisia disappears when neuroleptic is discontinued. Propranolol (Inderal), lorazepam (Ativan), or diazepam (Valium) may be used. In severe cases, may be great distress and contribute to suicidality.
Pseudoparkinsonism: akinesia, cogwheel rigidity, fine tremor Onset: 5 hours to 30 days	More common in males and older persons; tolerance may not develop; medicate with DA antagonist amantadine (must have good renal function). Administer prn antiparkinson agent as above, if intolerable, consult prescriber for medication change. Provide towel or handkerchief to wipe excess salvia.
Tardive dyskinesia (TD) Onset: months to years	Can occur after use (usually long term) of conventional antipsychotics; stereotyped involuntary movements (tongue protrusion, lip smacking, chewing, blinking, grimacing, choreiform movements of limbs and trunk, foot tapping); if using typical antipsychotics, use preventive measures and assess often; consider changing to an atypical antipsychotic drug; there is no treatment at present for TD. Health care providers should encourage person to be screened for TD at least every 3 months. Onset may merit reconsideration of medications. Changes in appearance may contribute to stigmatizing response. Teach client actions to conceal involuntary movements (purposeful muscle contraction overrides involuntary tardive movements).
Neuroleptic Malignant Syndrome (NMS)* Onset- variable, progresses rapidly over 2–3 days	Potentially fatal: Fever, tachycardia, hypertension, sweating, muscle rigidity, tremor, incontinence, stupor, leukocytosis, elevated creatine phosphokinase (CPK), renal failure delirium, stupor, coma; more common with high-potency drugs and in dehydrated clients; discontinue all medications; supportive symptomatic care (hydration, renal dialysis, ventilation, and fever reduction as appropriate); bromocriptine can relieve muscle rigidity and reduce fever, arrhythmias should be treated, small doses of heparin may decrease possibility of pulmonary emboli., can treat with dantrolene or promocriptine; antipsychotic medications can be cautiously reintroduced eventually.
Seizures*	Potentially life-threatening: Seizures occur in approximately 1% of people taking these medications; clozapine has a 5% rate (in clients on 600 to 900 mg/day); may have to discontinue clozapine. Use seizure precautions. Document and report any seizure activity.
Adverse effects on other systems	
Agranulocytosis* Onset-during the first 12 weeks of therapy	This is an emergency: It develops abruptly with fever, malaise, ulcerative sore throat, agranulocytosis, and leukopenia. High incidence (1–2%) is associated with clozapine; must do weekly CBC/blood work for 6 months and then every 2 months and prescribe only 1 week of medication at a time; if test results are positive, discontinue medication immediately; may need reverse isolation and antibiotics. Teach person to observe for signs of infection.
Photosensitivity	Use sunscreen and sunglasses; cover body with clothing.
Anticholinergic effects	Symptoms: constipation, dry mouth, blurred vision, orthostatic hypotension, tachycardia, urinary retention, nasal congestion; see Table 11.3 for nursing care.
Weight gain	See Table 11.3 for nursing care.

*Potentially life-threatening.
CBC, Complete blood count; *CNS,* central nervous system; *DA,* dopamine; *PO,* oral tablet or capsule; *IM,* intramuscular; *IV,* intravenous.
Adapted from Halter, M.J., Jakubec, S. L., & Pollard, C. L. (2019). *Varcarolis's Canadian psychiatric mental health nursing, Canadian edition. A clinical approach* (2nd ed., p. 323, Table 15-8). Elsevier Canada.

TABLE 12.5 Family Education Plan: Understanding Psychosis

Content	Instructional Activities	Evaluation
Describe psychosis	Introduce participants and leaders State purpose of group Define terminology associated with psychosis	The participant will describe the characteristics of psychosis
Identify the causes of psychotic disorders	Present theories of psychotic disorders Use audiovisual aids to explain brain anatomy, brain biochemistry, and major neurotransmitters	The participant will discuss the relationship between brain anatomy, brain biochemistry, major neurotransmitters, and the development of psychosis
Define schizophrenia according to symptoms and diagnostic criteria	Lead a discussion of the diagnostic criteria for schizophrenia Show a film on schizophrenia	The participant will describe the symptoms and diagnostic criteria for schizophrenia
Describe the relationship between anxiety and psychotic disorders	Present types and stages of anxiety Discuss steps in reducing and resolving anxiety	The participant will identify and describe the stages of anxiety and ways to reduce or resolve it
Analyze the impact of living with hallucinations	Describe the characteristics of hallucinations Demonstrate ways to communicate with someone who is hallucinating	The participant will demonstrate effective ways to communicate with a person who has hallucinations
Analyze the impact of living with delusions	Describe types of delusions Demonstrate ways to communicate with someone who has delusions Discuss interventions for delusions	The participant will demonstrate effective ways to communicate with a person who has delusions
Discuss the use of psychotropic medications	Provide and explain handouts describing the characteristics of psychotropic medications that are prescribed for schizophrenia	The participant will identify and describe the characteristics of medications prescribed for self or family member
Describe the characteristics of relapse and the role of adherence to the therapeutic regimen	Help the participants describe their own experiences with relapse Discuss symptom management techniques and the importance of complying with the therapeutic regimen	The participant will describe behaviours that indicate an impending relapse and discuss the importance of symptom management and adherence to the therapeutic regimen
Analyze behaviours that promote wellness	Discuss the components of wellness Relate wellness to the elements of symptom management	The participant will analyze the effect of maintaining wellness on the occurrence of symptoms
Discuss ways to cope adaptively with psychosis	Lead a group discussion focused on coping behaviours and the daily problems in living with psychosis Propose ways to create a low-stress environment	The participant will describe ways to modify their lifestyle to create a low-stress environment

From Stuart, G. W. (2013). *Principles and practice of psychiatric nursing* (10th ed., p. 371, Table 20.8). Mosby.

- Autonomic nervous system (ANS): Dominance of parasympathetic over sympathetic impulses may amplify or jumble neural impulses, resulting in cognitive or affective conditions.
- Limbic system: Because of controlling emotions, the limbic system (amygdala, hippocampus) and its connections to the thalamus and hypothalamus are also implicated in PD.
- Psychosocial development: Strong attachments to supportive family, peer, and community networks may protect people from PD by enhancing coping skills and personal growth. Conversely, a history of abuse or neglect in childhood puts people at increased risk.

Clinical Manifestations

PDs usually arise in adolescence and early adulthood. Thus, if there is a biological predisposition, the social and developmental challenges of this life stage, related to gaining independence and separation from family, may trigger a PD.

PDs share features of other mental illnesses, but no single illness completely explains the long-standing maladaptive thinking and behavioural patterns of PD, some of which are as follows:

- Inappropriate emotions, with poor impulse and emotional control
- Disturbed self-concept and inappropriate perceptions of others and the environment
- Unhealthy or very limited personal relationships
- School or employment difficulties
- Often an associated depression or substance abuse, or both

PDs are classified into the three groups, or clusters, which are discussed next. Two additional groups exist as well. The first one is called *personality change due to another medical condition*. It is a persistent personality disturbance that is judged to be due to the direct physiological effects of a medical condition. The other group is called *other specified personality disorder and unspecified personality disorder*. It is a category provided for two situations:

BOX 12.3 DSM-5—TR Categorization of Personality Disorders

According to the American Psychiatric Association, there are 10 personality disorders. These 10 disorders are grouped into three clusters of similar behaviour patterns and personality traits. These clusters are:

Cluster A: (Eccentric) Individuals with these disorders share characteristics of eccentric behaviours, such as social isolation and detachment. They may also display perception distortions, unusual levels of suspiciousness, magical thinking, and cognitive impairment.
- Paranoid personality disorder
- Schizoid personality disorder
- Schizotypal personality disorder

Cluster B: (Erratic) People living with cluster B personality disorders show patterns of responding to life demands with dramatic, emotional, or erratic behaviour. Problems with impulse control, emotion processing and regulation, and interpersonal difficulties characterize this cluster of disorders. Insight into these issues is generally limited. To get their needs met, individuals with cluster B personality disorders may resort to behaviours that are considered desperate or entitled, including acting out, committing antisocial acts, or manipulating people and circumstances.
- Borderline personality disorder
- Narcissistic personality disorder
- Histrionic personality disorder
- Antisocial personality disorder

Cluster C: (Fearful) An individual with these types of personality disorders will demonstrate consistent patterns of anxious and fearful behaviours, rigid patterns of social shyness, hypersensitivity, need for orderliness, and relationship dependency.
- Avoidant personality disorder
- Dependent personality disorder
- Obsessive–compulsive personality disorder.

From Halter, M. J., Pollard, C. L., & Jakubec, S. L. (2019). *Varcarolis's Canadian psychiatric mental health nursing: A clinical approach* (2nd Cdn. ed., p.433). Elsevier. Based on American Psychiatric Association. (2022). *Diagnostic and statistical manual of mental disorders* (5th ed., Text Revision).

1. The individual's personality pattern meets the general criteria for a personal disorder, and traits of several personality disorders are present, but the criteria for any specific disorder is not met; or
2. The individual's personality pattern meets the general criteria for a personality disorder, but the individual is considered to have a personality disorder that is not included in the DSM-5 classification (e.g., passive-aggressive personality disorder)" (APA, 2022, pp. 733–734).

Cluster A: Eccentric

Odd and eccentric behaviour patterns are characteristic of three personality disorders, in which people tend toward social and emotional withdrawal. Descriptions of these three disorders follow.

Paranoid personality disorder. Symptoms include the following:

- Being suspicious and distrustful, misinterpreting others' motives as threatening, exploitive, or deceiving; often bears grudges
- Detachment and social isolation
- Overreaction to threats, even with no actual evidence of malice; has hostile outbursts often
- Fear of becoming close to others or confiding in anyone
- Hypervigilance and hyperactivity; is unable to relax
- Hypersensitivity and irritability; is often angry and jealous

Schizoid personality disorder. Symptoms include the following:
- Being a loner; is detached from social and family relationships
- Emotional detachment; prefers solitary activities, although the person may be lonely
- Avoidance of intimacy; is indifferent to the feelings or reactions of others
- Flattened affect, emotional coldness

Schizotypal personality disorder. Symptoms include the following:
- Acute discomfort in social relationships
- Eccentric and odd behaviour and appearance
- Strange beliefs or magical thinking (superstitions, clairvoyance, telepathy, distorted cognition, fantasies, and preoccupations) that is outside cultural norms
- Unusual patterns of speech (metaphorical, vague, very elaborate, and flowery), unusual perceptual experiences, including bodily illusions
- Having suspicious or paranoid ideation

Cluster B: Erratic

These four PDs are distinguished by behaviour that is overly emotional, dramatic, and erratic.

Borderline personality disorder. Symptoms include the following:
- Instability of mood, interpersonal relationships, and self-image
- Impulsive, reckless behaviour that is often self-damaging, such as substance abuse, spending binges, heightened sexuality, or binge eating
- Uncontrolled, inappropriate, or frequent anger episodes
- Fear of rejection and being alone; feels empty; frantically tries to avoid being abandoned
- Transient, stress-related paranoid ideation or severe dissociative symptoms
- Chronic feelings of emptiness
- Common threats of self-injury and suicide

Narcissistic personality disorder. Symptoms include the following:
- Feelings of superiority; is rude and arrogant
- Attention-seeking; requires constant admiration and special treatment
- Envy of those with high status; pursues friendships with them
- Lacking in empathy for others: It's all about me!
- Manipulative; is driven to succeed; takes advantage of others to achieve personal goals

Histrionic personality disorder. Symptoms include the following:

- Desire to be the centre of attention; craves excitement and instant gratification
- Consistent use of physical appearance to draw attention to self
- Speech that is excessively impressionistic and lacking in detail
- Rapid shifting and shallow expression of emotions—and exaggerated expression of emotions—overly sensitive to criticism; reacts with anger
- Provocative and sexually inappropriate behaviour
- Suggestibility (easily influenced by others)
- Belief that relationships are more intimate than they actually are

Antisocial personality disorder. Symptoms include the following:

- Persistent disregard for the rights of safety for self and others; shows contempt for other's feelings and rights
- Disregard for the law; has had frequent arrests
- Lack of remorse
- Impulsiveness and irresponsibility
- Irritability and aggressiveness; is involved in repeated fights or assaults
- Deceitful; chronically lies and misrepresents self but can appear very charming
- Evidence of conduct disorder with onset before 15 years old
- Being at least 18 years old

Older diagnostic terms for this disorder are *psychopathy* and *sociopathy*, or *dissocial personality disorder* referring to a lack of social conscience.

Cluster C: Fearful

The defining features of cluster C are anxious and fearful behaviour.

Obsessive–compulsive personality disorder (OCPD). Avoid confusing OCPD with OCD and related disorders. A person with OCD and related disorders exhibits considerable anxiety and distress. A person with OCPD desires perfection and order. The true obsessions and compulsions of a person with OCD are more intense and compelling.

Symptoms of OCPD include the following:

- Rigid desire for perfection and control, coupled with ruthless self-criticism
- Overattention to rules and regulations, schedules, and discipline
- Indecisiveness and inability to complete tasks; is afraid of making a mistake
- Inflexibility with ethics, thriftiness, and moral values, but not necessarily religious
- Diligent work habits and difficulty delegating work; is a "workaholic"

Avoidant personality disorder. Symptoms include the following:

- Low self-esteem; has feelings of inadequacy and of being a failure
- Being socially withdrawn; shows restraint within intimate relationships because of fear of being shamed or ridiculed
- Sensitivity to criticism and rejection

- Avoidance of personal risks, new activities, or relationships

Often individuals also suffer from general anxiety, depression and somatic disorder, or illness anxiety disorder

Dependent personality disorder. Symptoms include the following:

- Clinging behaviour; has pervasive need to be taken care of; fears separation
- Indecisiveness; requires excessive advice and reassurance; defers major responsibilities to others
- Craving approval and support; therefore, unable to disagree with others
- Low self-confidence; is unable to initiate activities
- Craving relationships; desperately seeks a new relationship when one has ended
- Feelings of worthlessness often motivate them to seek out relationships that are overprotective, dominating, or abusive

Diagnostics and Therapeutics
Diagnosis

Enduring but distressing behaviour patterns that deviate from cultural norms and that affect social and occupational functioning in a broad range of activities and social situations are identified. Diagnosis is challenging because of overlapping symptoms and the tendency for some people to have more than one PD. Therefore, it is good to keep in mind the criteria for a general personality disorder as a common denominator. Initially, one must rule out other mental or medical disorders and treatment or medication adverse effects.

Below is the characteristics of General Personality Disorder as outlined from the DSM-5-TR:

All criteria-**A, B, C, D, E and F** must be present.

A. An enduring pattern of behaviour that deviates markedly from the expectations of the person's culture. This pattern must be manifested in two (or more) of the following areas:
   1. Cognition: the way in which a person perceives self, others and events. This way of thinking is persistently different from the culture norms.
   2. Affect (emotional response to an event); the range of affect, liability, intensity, and appropriateness of emotional response is consistently outside of cultural norms.
   3. Poor interpersonal relationships (maladaptive behaviours, being hard to get along with)
   4. Poor impulse control; difficulty in controlling own urges to act

B. Persistent lack of flexibility across all life situations

C. The person's behaviour leads to significant impairment or distress in social, occupational, or other important areas of functioning.

D. The pattern is stable and of long duration and goes back to at least the adolescent years.

E. There is no other mental health illness that can explain that pattern of behaviour.

F. The enduring pattern of behaviour is not attributable to the physiological effects of a substance (e.g., a drug of abuse, a medication) or another medical condition (e.g., head injury) (Bard et al., 2022).

Treatment

Many PDs are difficult to treat because of the client's self-denial. Common treatments include intensive psychotherapy, behavioural, psychodynamic, family or group psychotherapy, along with psychopharmacology:

- Antipsychotics: For severe agitation or delusional thinking in paranoid, schizotypal, and borderline PD
- SSRIs, other antidepressants: For obsessive thoughts, anger, irritability, and unstable mood
- Anxiolytics: For cluster C disorders
- MAOIs: To decrease self-harm and impulsive acts
- Lithium carbonate, propranolol: For antisocial PD with violent episodes
- Dialectic behaviour therapy (DBT): Focuses on reducing the harmful behaviours by developing coping skills to improve affective (emotional) stability and emotional control
- Schema therapy: Combines several types of therapies into one integrated system or treatment. Its goal is to target "long lasting and self-defeating patterns that started early in life. Treatment is designed to help clients recognize and replace enduring negative thinking, feelings, and maladaptive behavioural patterns with healthy alternatives (Bard et al., 2022).

Nursing Considerations

Individuals with a PD have a significant and persistent impairment in their interpersonal relationships and other aspects of functioning. Therefore, the focus of care for clients with PD is to help clients identify and then become responsible for their own behaviours and to assist clients in developing satisfactory life goals (Bard et al., 2022).

The Nurse–Client Relationship

Nurses encounter PDs wherever they work, and establishing a therapeutic alliance challenges even very experienced nurses. These clients know just which "buttons to push." Pay special attention to professional boundaries and set realistic limits on the client's behaviour and your availability. Keep your communication clear and unambiguous, giving simple directions. Avoid power struggles or arguments, showing confidence in your abilities and decisions. Remember that for such enduring patterns of behaviour, improvement takes time.

Splitting behaviour, that is, setting staff members against one another, is common. Thus, professional teamwork is vital. Staff must support each other and be consistent with the client.

Nursing Interventions

Nursing care of people with PD involves providing them with structure and clear expectations for their behaviour. A contract may be helpful for encouraging specific behaviours. Communicate respect for the person. The behaviour is the problem, not the client—set mutually agreed-upon goals and stick to them. Help clients identify and voice their emotions. Some specific considerations for specific PDs follow.

Paranoid personality disorder

- Involve the client in planning care, thus helping the person feel in control.
- Teach clients to delay responding to others until they have validated their perceptions and assumptions. This helps them avoid acting on paranoid ideas.

Schizoid personality disorder

- Support the client's ability to function in the community (e.g., provide a referral to social services to arrange supportive housing).
- Be aware that these clients are likely to require case management, either a professional case manager or at least a family member who can arrange for services and assistance.

Schizotypal personality disorder

- Assist with development of self-care and social skills.
- Perform a detailed assessment to detect any other medical or psychological symptoms that may require intervention (suicidal thoughts).

Borderline personality disorder

- Ensure safety; negotiate a no self-harm contract with the client. The client agrees not to engage in injurious actions and to inform a nurse if they are losing control.
- Help the client identify moods, emotions, and situations that trigger self-harm activities and explore more effective coping strategies for those triggers.
- Provide structured daily activities that include health-promoting activities.

Narcissistic personality disorder

- Use a matter-of-fact approach as you try to gain the person's cooperation with treatment.
- Promote milieu therapy: Engage the individual in community activities (either the therapeutic community in the hospital or the larger community outside). Reinforce appropriate behaviour.

Histrionic personality disorder

- Provide social skills training, with factual feedback about their behaviour.
- Understand that seductive behaviour is a response to distress. Nursing interventions should display this understanding.

Antisocial personality disorder

- Teach effective problem-solving and anger management techniques.
- Confront the client when they overstep acceptable limits on behaviour.

Obsessive–compulsive personality disorder

- Engage in cognitive restructuring: Explore and encourage the client to accept outcomes that are "good enough" or "satisfactory."
- Assist the client with decision making and completing tasks.

Avoidant personality disorder

- Promote self-esteem by providing support and reassurance.
- Cognitive restructuring: Try positive self-talk, reframing situations, and decatastrophizing (e.g., ask, "What is the worst thing that could happen?" "How likely is that?").

Dependent personality disorder
- Encourage autonomy and self-reliance.
- Teach problem-solving and decision-making skills.

SUBSTANCE-RELATED AND ADDICTIVE DISORDERS

Substance-related disorders consist of two groups: substance-use disorders and substance induced disorders (intoxication, withdrawal, and substance-induced mental disorders).

Substance-related and addictive disorders refer to the consumption and excess consumption (by any route) of drugs and alcohol. Nurses often forget that the overuse of legally approved medications, both over-the-counter and prescription, also constitutes a substance disorder. Substance related disorders involve 10 classes of drugs that cause addiction: alcohol, cannabis, caffeine, hallucinogens, inhalants, opioids, sedative, stimulants, tobacco and other (or unknown) substances. In addition to the above substances, some types of behaviour may cause a strong addictive effective on individuals who are genetically predisposed to addiction. A few of these disorders that involve excessive behaviour include gambling addiction, shopping addiction, sex addiction, and internet gambling addiction (Bard et al., 2022).

Many Canadians use alcohol, some use illicit drugs, some use both, and many have developed a substance dependence to these substances. According to Statistic Canada, nearly 6 million Canadians aged 12 and over report heavy drinking at least once a month. One in five Canadians aged 15 years old or older met the criteria for alcohol abuse or dependence over a lifetime. It is reported that more Canadians may have long term and negative effects on their patterns and level of drinking since the COVID-19 pandemic. One in five who drink and are staying at home report drinking alcohol more often than before the start of the pandemic (Government of Canada, 2021a). Cannabis (marihuana) was legalized and regulated in 2018 and has remained the most used drug in Canada. In a 2019 report, cannabis use was more prevalent among young adults aged 20 to 24 years (45%) during 2018. It had increased from 2017 at (33%). There was no change among youth aged 15 to 19 years of age (19%) (Government of Canada, 2021b).

The comorbidity of mental illness and substance use disorder (also called a co-occurring disorder or *dual diagnosis*) is common. Some people use substances to ease their psychiatric symptoms; for others, substance use and dependency may promote the development or severity of a mental illness. For this reason, many health authorities combine mental health and addiction services into one department.

Pathophysiology and Clinical Manifestations

Addictive substances either depress or stimulate the CNS. Marihuana seems to do both. All interfere with neurotransmission and the limbic system, altering emotions and the brain's reward system.

Central Nervous System Depressants

Drugs that depress the CNS produce drowsiness and sedation. They include alcohol, opioids, sedatives, anxiolytics, and probably inhalants. Alcohol, accepted in many cultures, is also the most commonly used drug. People overuse these drugs because of the pleasant sensations of relaxation, euphoria, and reduced inhibition, commonly called being "high." Tolerance develops, such that higher and higher doses are required to produce the same effects, and eventually the person cannot function without the drug, experiencing cravings and physical dependence or addiction. Overdose can lead to respiratory or cardiovascular depression, coma, convulsions, and death.

Alcohol
- Alcohol, soluble in fat and water, is absorbed from the stomach and small intestine. It is quickly disbursed throughout the body and metabolized by the liver at the rate of one drink (one beer, 150 mL of wine, or 30 mL of hard liquor) per hour.
- Alcohol initially stimulates the release of naturally produced opioids (endorphins and enkephalins) and dopamine (the reward centres of the limbic system), producing feelings of pleasure. In higher concentrations, alcohol is toxic to nerve cells, producing poor emotional control, reduced muscle coordination, and then mental confusion and loss of consciousness. At very high concentrations, it produces coma, respiratory depression, and eventual death.
- Chronic alcoholism produces general body damage. Complications are dementia, hepatitis and cirrhosis, cardiomyopathy, gastritis, peptic ulcers, pancreatitis, and peripheral neuropathy.
- Withdrawal produces neural excitation, with tremors, agitation and anxiety, irritability, insomnia, and sometimes delirium tremens (DTs) with hallucinations, seizures, and delirium. This is a medical emergency and, without treatment, can cause death. Symptoms include high fever, hypertension, tachycardia, and seizures.

Opioids
- Opium derivatives are narcotics. Many are legally controlled, but heroin is illegal.
- Taken intravenously (IV) or nasally (snorting), they act on the reward centres of the brain, reducing neuron excitability, especially of the pain neurotransmitters, and producing analgesia and euphoria (a "rush"). Other effects include respiratory depression, constricted pupils, and constipation.

Sedative–hypnotics and anxiolytics
- These include the benzodiazepines and barbiturates, taken orally or intravenously.
- Tolerance, dependence, and withdrawal usually do not develop if taken for under a month.
- Withdrawal symptoms can be avoided by gradually tapering the dosage under medical supervision.

Inhalants
- These volatile substances are inhaled and include fuels, solvents, thinners, propellants, and nitrates.

- Inhalants produce a cheap "high" and are mostly used by youth. However, adverse effects from high doses or prolonged use are serious, damaging the brain, liver, kidneys, heart, and lungs.

Date rape drugs
- These are given to unsuspecting victims prior to rape.
- They include rohypnol (roofies), GHB (gamma-hydroxybutyrate), and ketamine (vitamin K).
- Effects are reduced inhibition and sedation, often enhanced by mixing with alcohol. Overdose depresses respirations or causes seizures, coma, and death.
- Rohypnol also produces amnesia.

Central Nervous System Stimulants

Stimulants produce alertness, excitation, and aggressiveness and reduce fatigue. Metabolism is increased, and appetite is suppressed. They include caffeine, nicotine, amphetamines, cocaine, and hallucinogens. The stronger drugs produce restlessness, overtalkativeness, anxiety, irritability, suspicion, paranoia, and hallucinations. Tolerance and dependence occur. Withdrawal symptoms, however, are less physiologically dangerous than those of alcohol or opiates. Withdrawal brings depressed mood, sleep disturbance, fatigue, and anhedonia (inability to experience pleasure).

Caffeine and nicotine
- Caffeine (coffee, cola soft drinks) can cause nervousness, anxiety, and difficulty sleeping.
- Nicotine (tobacco) is highly addictive. It became less socially acceptable with the recognition of the negative health effects, particularly for bystanders exposed to second-hand smoke. Effects include relaxation, excitement, and decreased appetite. Quitting smoking is very difficult, producing withdrawal (mood changes, anxiety, irritability, restlessness, and hunger).
- Vaping is the inhalation of a vapour created by a device like an e-cigarette. The device warms the liquid, so it is condensed into a gas to be inhaled. It usually contains nicotine. Vaping has become popular among young adults. Some of the health risks of vaping include bronchiectasis and emphysema. Vaping causes the same addiction and damage to the health as nicotine from regular smoking (Bard et al., 2022).

Amphetamines and cocaine
- The initial effect is stimulation, but CNS depression follows. Both drugs produce marked euphoria, but dangerous cardiovascular effects (tachycardia, arrhythmias, hypertension, vasoconstriction) that can cause heart failure, myocardial infarction, strokes, and renal complications can occur. First-time cocaine users have died. Continued use leads, however, to tolerance and some decrease in cardiovascular adverse effects.
- These drugs are absorbed directly into the bloodstream from direct injection into a vein and through mucous membranes (oral, nasal [snorted or smoked], or buccal membranes). Cocaine is the most addictive of all abused substances.

- Long-term sniffing causes ulcers in the nose and perforations of the septum; long-term smoking damages the throat, upper GI tract, and lungs.
- Crack cocaine is a purified, crystallized form. It is easily available with an immediate but very short effect (5–7 minutes) followed by profound depression, and there is a strong drive to relieve the depression with another "hit." The result is that crack is extremely addictive.

Hallucinogens
- These include lysergic acid diethylamide (LSD) MDMA (Ecstasy), peyote, and psilocybin.
- Effects are alterations in perception, including hallucinations with euphoria (a "trip") or frightening and depressing perceptions (a "bad trip"). People report awareness of themselves and surroundings but altered sensory perceptions of colours, time, arousal, body image, hearing, and so on.
- Sympathetic nervous system stimulation causes palpitations, increased BP, blurred vision, dilated pupils, and sweating. A bad trip may induce dizziness, anxiety, and panic.
- Flashbacks occur, perhaps more often if hallucinogens are combined with other substances.

PCP (Angel dust). Effects include hyperactivity, aggressiveness, impulsivity, unpredictable behaviour, feeling superhuman, and sometimes psychosis. Dangerous respiratory and cardiovascular adverse effects can lead to seizures, coma, and death.

Marihuana
- Also called *cannabis, hashish, tetrahydrocannabinol (THC), pot, weed, grass,* or *Mary Jane.*
- Spice is a synthetic form of cannabis known as K2 or Black Mamba.
- Marihuana has both CNS-stimulant and CNS-depressant effects through its influence on a variety of neurotransmitters and neurochemicals. Youth and young adults are more likely to experience harms from cannabis because their brains are still developing (until about age 25 years). The earlier a person consumes cannabis, the higher the risk for serious health conditions, including dependency and other mental health concerns (especially psychosis, schizophrenia and problematic substance use disorders) (Government of Canada, 2021c).
- Common effects are euphoria, relaxation, drowsiness, heightened or altered sensory perceptions, reduced coordination, dry mouth, tachycardia, red eyes, disorientation, and appetite stimulation.

Since Canada's legalization of cannabis there has been reported increased health and social issues, including greater rates of drug-impaired driving and motor vehicle accidents; child and some adult poisonings, primarily from edibles; increased criminal charges for public intoxication; increased rates of mental health issues such as anxiety and panic attacks, especially among adolescent users; and marihuana-associated cyclic vomiting syndrome (Public Safety Canada, 2022; Statistics Canada, 2021b).

Diagnostics and Therapeutics

Diagnosis

During a complete history and physical examination, special attention is paid to the manifestations noted earlier. The clinician may note needle tracks and bruising along arm and leg veins, signs of malnourishment, teary and reddened eyes, a runny nose, or frequent swallowing, indicating a postnasal drip. Laboratory tests may include toxicology urine screening, blood alcohol levels, or both, in addition to a full work-up for suspected complications. Denial is common with a person having a substance use disorder, making history-taking challenging.

Substance use disorder is classified as mild, moderate, or severe depending on how many of the diagnostic criteria a person meets. When at least two of the following 11 DSM-5-TR criteria exist for a 12-month period and cause significant impairment or distress, then a substance-use disorder diagnosis can be made (APA, 2022):

1. The substance is taken for longer than the intended period of time, and in larger amounts.
2. There is an effort to cut down the use of that substance but without success.
3. A significant amount of time is spent acquiring, using, or recovering from the substance.
4. There are cravings and urges to use the substance.
5. Use of the substance leads to the failure to fulfill basic functions and obligations (work, school, family obligations).
6. The individual continues to use the substance, even when it causes social or relationship problems.
7. Important social, family, occupational, or recreational activities are given up or significantly reduced because of substance use.
8. Recurrent use of the substance continues even when it places an individual in physical danger.
9. The use of the substance continues even when it causes or exacerbates physical and/or psychological challenges.
10. More of the substance is needed to achieve the same effect (tolerance).
11. Withdrawal symptoms are manifested when the substance is discontinued, and they can be eliminated when more of the substance is consumed (Bard et al., 2022).

Treatment

Treatment depends on the severity of the client's condition. First, treat an overdose and then address withdrawal symptoms. Only after stabilization can one begin to address addiction. Pharmacotherapy for treating chemical dependency varies according to the particular substance being abused. Some of the major pharmacological treatments follow.

Alcohol

- Benzodiazepines for alcohol withdrawal
- Naltrexone (ReVia) and Antabuse (disulfiram) to help maintain abstinence
- Thiamine to help prevent major brain damage complications (Wernicke-Korsakoff syndrome) for long-term alcoholics

Other central nervous system depressants

- Phenobarbital is given for withdrawal from sedative–hypnotics, benzodiazepines, and barbiturates.
- Methadone and clonidine are used to manage withdrawal from opiates. They reduce the severity of withdrawal symptoms by binding with opioid receptors.

Central nervous system stimulants

- Nicotine gum and nicotine patches replace smoking, with gradual tapering over time.
- Bupropion (Zyban, Wellbutrin) aids withdrawal from smoking by reducing cravings.
- Benzodiazepines and antipsychotics lessen psychotic reactions from hallucinogens and PCP.
- Naloxone hydrochloride (Narcan), an opioid antagonist, is used for narcotic overdose.
- Buprenorphine (Subutex), an opioid analgesic, is used for withdrawal from narcotics. It is less addicting than other narcotics.
- Currently, no specific medications are available for cocaine withdrawal or addiction, although antidepressants may ease mood changes due to abstinence; sedatives help with insomnia; anxiolytics reduce symptoms of anxiety and some anticonvulsant medications have been found to reduce some of the symptoms that occur during cocaine withdrawal and assist in the reduction of cravings. Antabuse is used to discourage cocaine use.

Treatment for chemical addiction is multifaceted and may include the following:

- Psychotherapy and counselling
- Education
- CBT
- Behaviour modification
- Motivational therapy
- Group therapy: Peer support groups in the community, for example, Alcoholics Anonymous (AA). Newer programs, often modelled on the AA 12-step program, have been developed for other addictions and may be accessed, depending on community availability (such as Cocaine Anonymous and Gamblers Anonymous).
- Indigenous healing lodge treatment approach is a 6-week residential program that takes a cultural perspective on treatment, including talking and healing circles. Talking circles are a form of group therapy where the person talks about issues causing pain. Other members of the circle give feedback and confront behaviours that are not helpful in the individual's recovery program. Some individuals may choose to smudge prior to joining the circle to find calmness from negative feelings by using medicines of sweet grass, sage, and cedar. Sweat lodges are also used by some individuals (Halter et al., 2019).

For dual diagnosis, successful treatment of the comorbid psychiatric diagnosis often reduces the individual's addictive behaviour.

Harm Reduction

Harm reduction is an evidence-informed approach to drug addiction, although it is not without political controversy. The first harm-reduction programs were methadone maintenance programs in the 1960s and 1970s. Recognizing the compulsion underlying dependence and that abstinence is difficult to achieve, the goal of these programs is to assist people who use substances in gaining better control of their health and enables them to take proactive and protective measures for themselves and their families. Harm reduction is one of the five pillars of the Canadian Drug and Substances Strategy (Bard et al., 2022). By providing such things as clean equipment and education about safe practices, they aim to achieve the following:

- Decrease overdoses, infections, hepatitis B and C, tuberculosis, other diseases such as HIV/AIDS, and deaths for injection drug users
- Reduce the violence and crime associated with the drug culture
- Reduce the use of impure street drugs that lack any quality control
- Provide access to community outreach, public health programs, education, detoxification programs, and other treatment
- Promote trust among drug users, their families, and health care providers

Some examples include needle-exchange programs, methadone replacement, supervised injection sites, heroin-assisted treatments, controlled drinking, managed alcohol programs, overdose prevention and education programs, and equipping automobiles with breathalyzer equipment that prevents ignition unless the driver "blows" below a specified alcohol level.

It is important to "create a substance-use care system that is built on harm reduction and continually moving people toward a path of recovery. The care provided must be integrated, because these approaches are stronger when used in combination rather than alone" (Johnson, 2017, p. 36).

Nursing Considerations

Nursing Assessment

Nurses should supplement their assessment of a client's physical and mental health with screening for substance use and dependence. Ask clients about their pattern of substance use and experiences of withdrawal. At the very least, determine the amount and frequency of alcohol or drugs used by clients. Some suggested questions include the following:

- "Are you interested in stopping the use of a substance?"
- "Do you have any physical complications from addiction?" Examples include AIDS, hepatitis, abscesses, tachycardia.
- "Do you know what community resources are available for safe detoxification, treatment, and client and family support? Do you know how to access them?"
- A common, easily remembered assessment tool for alcoholism that all nurses should know and use is the CAGE Questionnaire. If a client answers "yes" to two of the following four questions, it is an indication for further assessment of probable alcoholism:
  - Cut down: "Have you ever been told you should cut down on your drinking?"
  - Annoyed: "Has anyone annoyed you by criticizing your drinking?"

- Guilt: "Have you ever felt guilty or bad about your drinking?"
- Eye-opener: "Have you ever had a drink first thing in the morning to get over a hangover?"

The Nurse–Client Relationship

In order to develop an effective therapeutic relationship with a client who is a substance user, the nurse must examine their personal beliefs and overcome any prejudice toward the client. Otherwise, the nurse should refer the client to another staff member who can accept the client more openly and with whom the client will feel safe to communicate openly and honestly. Interacting with substance users requires patience, honesty, persistence, and acceptance of the potential for relapses. Principles underlying interacting with substance users include the following:

- Abstinence: Negotiate a contract with the client to abstain from substance use.
- Individualized treatment and goals: Negotiate a plan addressing the client's personal issues.
- Set appropriate limits: Include in your contract the conditions under which you will work together. Outline behaviour that is acceptable and unacceptable.
- Anticipate defensive reactions: Address the client by identifying or redirecting the behaviour and supporting appropriate responses.
- Patience: Acknowledge that recovery occurs in stages and that each stage takes time.
- Sharpen the focus: Focus on the benefits of giving up substance use that make abstinence worthwhile.

Nursing Interventions

When clients are ready for psychosocial interventions, that is, at the point at which overdose or withdrawal symptoms are stabilized, attention turns to overcoming addiction and maintaining abstinence.

Individual interventions. Use all opportunities with the client to engage in brief interventions, aimed at motivating change and supporting healthy behaviours. A helpful acronym for recalling the elements of these encounters is FRAMES:

- Feedback: Give personal feedback about client progress, including liver enzyme values.
- Responsibility: Emphasize that change is the client's responsibility, no one else's.
- Advice: Clearly provide supportive advice on the need to change. Avoid being judgemental.
- Menu: Allow clients to choose from a menu of addiction treatment options and programs.
- Empathy: Communicate warmth, respect, understanding, and support.
- Self-efficacy: Reinforce with the client that they have the ability to be successful (Stuart, 2013).

Group therapy. Encourage the client to attend group therapy, where available, but be available afterward to discuss and reinforce what clients learn about their addiction and themselves. Advantages of group therapy include mutual support and sharing of strategies for success. Interacting with other individuals who have maintained sobriety reduces isolation and encourages learning new social skills. Groups also offer opportunities for socializing that are not dependent on substance use.

Self-help groups. AA is the model for many other self-help groups that use the 12-step approach. Other groups are Narcotics Anonymous, Al-Anon for adult family members or friends of an alcoholic or chemically dependent person, and Alateen for teenage family members. (Some large urban centres also have Nar-Anon, a group specifically for families of those addicted to chemical substances.) Twelve-step programs require that members do the following:

- Admit to their powerlessness over the addictive substance and that they are unable to quit on their own, but require help from a power greater than themselves
- Accept responsibility for their own recovery
- Admit that no one and nothing else can be blamed for their addiction

In response to objections to the semireligious nature of AA, the organization has altered references to God to either "a power greater than ourselves" or "God, as we understand Him."

Teaching and Learning

In addition to information about the types of substances abused, education for families and clients may include concepts such as tolerance, dependence, intoxication, withdrawal, flashbacks, dual diagnosis, codependency, and the social and physical complications of substance abuse. Even more important may be education on managing recovery. Some examples for topics are healthy nutrition, techniques for relaxation, stress relief, and problem-solving, as well as the availability of community supports, including financial and legal assistance.

Relapse prevention. Avoid becoming discouraged when a client succumbs to temptation and relapses. Most clients will relapse, even when they are determined to succeed with abstinence. Nurses can help clients prevent relapses using the following strategies (Halter et al., 2019):

- Keep the program simple at first. Providing prompts and instructions for the client to review may help. Encouraging the use of the notebook to write important schedules, appointments, and quick review of information provided.
- Discuss difficult situations that the client has been able to handle relatively successfully.
- Discuss situations that the client has had little success in handling and rehearse some possible management strategies.
- Help the client recognize role models among their acquaintances.
- Help the client prepare for the possibility of a relapse through the following:
  - Identifying potential triggers to substance use
  - Learning skills to regain abstinence in the event of use
  - Adopting healthy coping, identity, and stress management skills to address triggers before they threaten sobriety

Engaging with Families

"Everyone in the family suffers, not just the client. Some problems that families experience include guilt, shame, resentment, insecurity, delinquency, financial troubles, isolation, fear, and violence" (Stuart, 2013, p. 466). Substance abuse can cause family breakup or become a self-sustaining pattern. Spouses and partners, if not already substance users, may become so, and many children learn patterns of addiction early. Many families, however, recognize the problems caused by substance abuse and seek education and help regardless of whether the substance user wants to overcome the addiction.

Codependency. Sometimes family dynamics evolve to enable the client with a substance use disorder to continue using. Family members try to preserve the peace, hoping that unconditional support will help the substance user become strong enough to quit. They may cover up dysfunctions to preserve the individual's or family's reputation and financial integrity. Two unintended consequences are as follows:

- Codependence: The family member's own needs for self-actualization and fulfillment are blocked in favour of catering to the needs and desires of the substance user.
- Enabling: Inadvertently, codependency reinforces substance use by protecting the addicted person from the consequences of their behaviour. Family members who assist a loved one to maintain an addiction need help to understand their own enabling behaviour patterns and to face the reality that the substance user, alone, must assume responsibility for quitting.

Self-help groups for partners and families. Nurses must be aware of self-help organizations so they can refer family members. Most communities have local chapters of Al-Anon and Alateen for families of alcoholics. Where self-help groups for drug addiction are located, such as Narcotics Anonymous and Cocaine Anonymous, associated programs for family members are also usually available.

SOMATIC SYMPTOM AND RELATED DISORDERS: CONVERSION DISORDER AND ILLNESS ANXIETY DISORDER

Most nurses agree that the connection between the mind and body is strong. Emotional stress often results in psychosomatic symptoms, producing or intensifying a physical illness. Conversely, having a disease or illness increases stress resulting in a wide variety of emotional responses. The expected conversion of mental states and experiences into physical symptoms is called *somatization*. People have a somatic symptom disorder if:

- Physical symptoms cannot be confirmed by laboratory tests or other medical evidence
- They have significant psychological issues or conflicts
- They are consciously unable to control the illness symptoms

Pathophysiology

Stressful psychophysiological responses were identified by Hans Selye as the *general adaptation syndrome* (GAS), or *stress response* (see the section "Anxiety Disorders"). The physiological results of stress can be confirmed by pathological changes; for example, chronic stress is implicated in heart disease. Without confirming pathology, however, the symptoms are presumed to be due to a mental health disorder. Nevertheless, health care providers must guard against this assumption until after a completed physical work-up, as true somatoform disorders are relatively rare.

Clinical Manifestations

- Somatic symptom disorder: This disorder is characterized by a combination of multiple symptoms such as pain, fatigue, and neurological, GI, and sexual complaints to the point of excessive concern, preoccupation, and fear. These clients suffer from pain that seems to be related to their psychological state and that cannot be relieved by analgesics.
- Conversion disorder (also called *functional neurological symptom disorder*): The client suddenly loses sensory or motor functions, resulting in paralysis or blindness. Often the client seems less concerned than one would expect (termed *la belle indifférence*). In such cases, the deficit actually brings relief by preventing the client from participating in an anxiety-provoking activity. Neurological testing is negative.
- Illness anxiety disorder (previously known as *hypochondriasis*): Clients become obsessed with the fear that they have a serious disease, often when they have misinterpreted minor symptoms.
- Factitious disorder: A person with *factitious disorder imposed on self* intentionally creates symptoms in order to gain attention. They may even inflict a self-injury. Perhaps the best-known factitious disorder is Munchausen syndrome, in which clients make up symptoms to gain hospital admission and emotional attention over and over again (Bard et al., 2022). When a person harms someone else or causes another person to be sick (so that they can be rewarded for caring for or saving the other person), the disorder is called *factitious disorder imposed on another* (previously known as *Munchausen's by proxy*). In the DSM-5-TR, this illness now appears in the category "Somatic Symptom and Related Disorders."
  - Malingering is a differential diagnosis classified under "Factitious Disorder" in the DSM-5-TR. It occurs when people fabricate physical symptoms for secondary gain. Either they want something (drugs, insurance payments), or they want to avoid something, such as going to work. The symptoms tend to dissipate after those hopes have been satisfied. This process of getting what they want is called *receiving a secondary gain*.

Diagnostics and Therapeutics
Diagnosis

Initially, a complete diagnostic workup is done to rule out medical conditions, reactions to substances, or other mental health disorders (such as an anxiety disorder) that may be suspected from the client's symptoms. An in-depth medical and social history may help rule out malingering. After a somatic symptom disorder has been diagnosed, healthcare providers must continue to observe for ongoing and new symptoms. There is a real danger of discounting legitimate medical conditions that the person may later develop and that require treatment.

Treatment

- Individual psychotherapy is aimed at helping the client gain insight into their stress and learn more adaptive coping strategies. The client can be encouraged to discuss feelings and conflicts rather than repress them.
- Periodic physical examination is an opportunity to provide verbal reassurance of the client's positive state of health.
- Cognitive therapy helps the client appraise stressful situations realistically and reduce attention on distorted body sensations and perceptions.

Nursing Considerations
Nursing Assessment

A thorough physical and psychological assessment is required. Because the client perceives the symptoms as real, carefully evaluate their daily living patterns. Some fabricated symptoms will interfere with basic needs, for example, nutrition, exercise, hygiene, rest, and so on. Evaluate how well clients are able to express their feelings. Estimate their level of stress and any opportunities for secondary gain through a full psychosocial assessment, including the following:

- Income
- Work
- Other daily activities
- Living arrangements
- Social support
- Self-care
- Stressful events

Addressing the client's health concerns at an early stage may prevent repeated consultations, multiple trails of medication, and medical examinations (Halter et al., 2019, p. 210).

The Nurse–Client Relationship

Caring for clients with somatoform ailments requires patience and understanding, to allow a trusting relationship to develop in which a client will be able to discuss their feelings and fears. Provide positive feedback when clients are able to express their feelings to others. Emphasize that you want to know your client as a person and not just about any physical symptoms. Acknowledge physical complaints, but do not allow the person to dwell on them. Instead, try to promote insight by encouraging the person to tell you what causes stress in their life. Then work together to problem-solve some ways of dealing with those stresses. Try to focus the conversation on positive aspects of the client's life and sources of satisfaction.

Nursing Interventions

- Give physical nursing care and explain all procedures fully, until physical illness has been ruled out by laboratory tests and other diagnostic investigation.

- Once a somatic symptom diagnosis has been confirmed, reduce opportunities for the client to achieve benefits from sick behaviour; for example, persuade the client to get out of bed and dress for the day, eat in the dining area, interact with others, perform self-care activities, and so on.
- Journal: Encourage the client to keep a diary, describing activities and interactions, occurrences that cause stress, and when symptoms appear. Help the client reflect on the relationship between stresses and symptoms. Explore other ways of achieving comfort and relieving symptoms rather than relying on medications and medical treatments.
- Encourage activities and exercise, both for promoting health and giving the client something to think about besides their complaints.
- Document any new physical complaints and report them to the medical staff for investigation.

Teaching and Learning

Client education focuses on learning about stress and about more adaptive coping strategies, including stress management techniques and establishing a healthy lifestyle. A client education plan (Halter et al., 2019) may cover the following:

- Define and describe stress, having the client share associated feelings and behaviours.
- Ask the client to describe and role-play stressful situations. Talk about the behaviours that you observe. What are some of the adaptive and maladaptive coping mechanisms observed?
- Provide alternative coping strategies. Teach stress reduction techniques such as relaxation, meditation, and mild physical exercise.
- Talk about events and experiences that are common stressors in everyday life. Try to have the client identify the elements in those experiences that heighten stress. Reinforce the client's strengths and problem-solving abilities. Help the client realize that needs can be met without resorting to somatic symptoms.
- Ask the client to choose one adaptive coping mechanism to practise for a day or a week and then review how it went at the end of the period and provide feedback.
- Teach assertive communication. Provide the client with a positive means of getting their needs met. This reduces the feelings of helplessness and need for manipulation.

Engaging With Families

Family education is essential. Once family members understand the reasons behind the client's symptoms, they can understand the importance of giving attention to the person when the client is not complaining of illness and reducing attention to their behaviour in the role of a sick person. Families and clients together can plan strategies for avoiding stress in the client's life and for reducing unavoidable stress. Family members may also need to learn the importance of expressing their feelings, as repressing emotions may be a long-standing family dynamic that the client has learned.

COGNITIVE DISORDERS: DELIRIUM AND DEMENTIAS, INCLUDING ALZHEIMER'S DISEASE

Cognition is the act or process of knowing. "It describes activities of the mind involved in thinking and the thought process. Cognition refers to intelligence, learning, judgement, reasoning, knowledge, understanding and memory—all of which are higher brain functions" (Bard et al., 2022, p.196). Cognitive ability is, for many people, synonymous with their sense of self. Two major classifications of cognitive impairment are dementia and delirium. Both of these conditions occur most often, although not exclusively in older persons. With Canada's aging population, cognitive disorders will constitute an increasing proportion of nursing practice.

The greatest known risk factor for dementia is increasing age, but not all older people will develop dementia. Most nurses recognize this to be an ageist attitude. In older persons, although physiological changes in the brain result in some cognitive decline, general intellectual capacity remains intact. Older persons retain their ability to learn, although processing new information and retrieving memories may take a little longer. Some older persons are more easily distracted. Thus, for older persons, cognitive functioning varies, just as it does for younger people. Only where significant cognitive deficits are noted should the nurse suspect a cognitive disorder.

Pathophysiology
Delirium

Although intellect is not markedly affected by age, the brain becomes less resistant to harm from factors such as electrolyte imbalance, medications, ischemia, hypoglycemia, and infections. The resulting cognitive impairment, called *delirium*, is also associated with many mental and physical illnesses, but, in general, the cognitive difficulties improve once the primary illness is resolved. Nurses on medical–surgical units frequently encounter delirium, especially following surgery or resulting from various other pathophysiological conditions that upset the biochemical balance of the CNS. In children and adolescents, the major causes are infection with a high fever, head trauma, drug toxicity, and brain tumours.

Dementias

In contrast, dementias involve progressive memory loss that is not reversible. Medications can slow the progression of the disease for a period of time but not reverse the symptoms. Alzheimer's disease is the most common form of dementia, followed by vascular dementia which occurs after a stroke. The third most common form of dementia is Lewy body dementia, which is type of progressive dementia that affects a decline in thinking, reasoning, and independent movements. Some of the physical symptoms of dementias affecting independent movement are loss of balance, rigid muscles and shuffling gait, and trouble initiating movements (Alzheimer's Society of Canada, 2022b).

In 2022, over 500 000 Canadians were living with Alzheimer's and other dementias (Alzheimer's Society of

Canada, 2022a). Alzheimer's disease accounts for 60 to 80% of all diagnoses of dementia (Alzheimer Society of Canada, 2022 c). There are many other conditions that can cause symptoms of dementia, including some that are reversible, such as thyroid conditions and vitamin deficiencies. While most changes in the brain that cause dementia are permanent and worsen over time, thinking and memory impairments caused by the following conditions may improve when the condition is treated or addressed: depression, medication adverse effects, excess alcohol, thyroid conditions, and vitamin deficiencies (Alzheimer's Association, 2022). The cerebral atrophy and deterioration of Alzheimer's disease are caused by the following:

- Amyloid plaques, which are microscopic deposits composed of degenerated neuron cells
- Neurofibrillary tangles of the hippocampus that affect memory and emotions
- Low acetylcholine levels resulting from insufficient levels of the enzyme necessary to produce acetylcholine, a major neurotransmitter
- A genetic defect involving at least four identified genes

Clinical Manifestations
Delirium

Symptoms of acute confusion and disorientation with bizarre behaviour patterns develop quickly, often at night. The person may be highly agitated or dazed, with hallucinations and aggressive behaviour (anger and lashing out). Speech may become incomprehensible. Over a 24-hour period, symptoms may fluctuate in intensity.

Dementias

Dementias are chronic and progressive. Onset is slow, with gradual deterioration of the cognitive and physical neurological systems. In the early stages, symptoms are often attributed to aging, stress, or mild depression. Symptoms may include forgetting, difficulty concentrating, limited problem-solving ability, apathy or irritability, and some language disturbance, such as searching for words. Over time, cognitive abilities decline and individuals become increasingly distressed, depressed, and debilitated, needing progressively more physical care, support, and supervision. The eventual outcome is death.

In Alzheimer's disease, the course of the illness, on average, is about 4 to 8 years. The progression (e.g., the rate of decline of cognitive functioning) of Alzheimer's disease varies from client to client and can range from 3 to 20 years (Sorrentino et al., 2022). Diagnosis usually is made between 40 and 65 years and, in general, the younger the person at diagnosis, the faster the deterioration. It is divided into four stages. The stages are outlined in Box 12.4.

Diagnostics and Therapeutics
Diagnosis

Diagnosing delirium usually involves diagnosing the underlying medical condition and identifying contributing factors, such as medications and substance abuse. There are many

different algorithms used to determine the presence or severity of delirium, such as the Confusion Assessment Method (CAM). It is a standardized tool that enables health care professionals to identify and recognize delirium quickly and accurately in a clinical setting.

It examines four key features of delirium:

BOX 12.4 Four Stages of Alzheimer's Disease

Early Stage: Mild
- Begins with the loss recent memory
- An inability to learn, process or retain information
- Language impairments
- Judgement and abstract thinking decline
- Experiences increased trouble with planning and organizing
- Forgets where they put things
- Begins to have difficulty performing activities of daily living (ADLs)
- Has difficulty coming up with the right word or name
- Difficulty in remembering names when introduced to new people
- Many individuals react to their loss of memory and control with irritability, agitation, or hostility
- Has difficulty performing tasks in social or work settings

Intermediate Stage: Moderate
- Obvious memory impairments; remote memory affected but not totally lost
- Gets confused about recent events or processing new information
- Aphasia: loss of language
- Apraxia: decreased ability to perform activities of daily living (ADLs)
- Visual agnosia (loss of recognition of previously known or familiar people or objects)
- Increasingly forgetful and may require assistance with toileting, bathing, dressing, and eating
- Feels moody or withdrawn, especially in socially or mentally challenging situations
- Agitation and physical aggression often occur
- Noticeable behavioural difficulties; compulsive repetitive behaviour like hand wringing or tissue shredding
- Increased tendency to wander and become lost
- Close supervision needed; still is ambulatory but at high risk for falls

Severe Stage: Severe
- Inability to do anything
- Incontinent, unable to walk, and entirely dependent on others for care
- Memory: recent and remote completely lost
- Inability to swallow: high risk for pneumonia, and malnutrition
- Many develop mutism (inability to speak) or communicate only in grunts

End Stage
- Slips into coma
- Death from pneumonia or other infection occurs

Adapted from Bard, B., MacMullin, E., Williamson, J. & Morrison-Valfre, M. (2022). *Morrison-Valfre's foundations of mental health care in Canada* (pp. 203–204). Elsevier.

1. Acute onset and fluctuating course
2. Inattention
3. Disorganized thinking
4. Altered level of consciousness

If features 1 and 2 and either 3 or 4 are present, then a diagnosis of delirium is suggested. A positive screening test result should lead to further investigation to identify and treat the underlying cause and provide supportive care (Registered Nurses Association of Ontario [RNAO], 2016).

Diagnosing dementia involves ruling out other illnesses and distinguishing among the various dementias. In addition to Alzheimer's disease, other dementia diagnoses include Lewy body dementia, Creutzfeldt-Jakob disease, Pick's disease, Huntington's disease, vascular dementia, and young-onset dementia. Dementia also occurs with advanced AIDS and Parkinson's disease.

Although delirium and dementias develop at different rates, symptoms overlap, and, not uncommonly, they are confounded. Postsurgical confusion is common in older persons, and too often, delirium goes unrecognized and the confusion is blamed on dementia. Untreated, the delirium can result in permanent damage. As well, depression (common in both delirium and dementia) is also very common for older persons. Thus, diagnosing cognitive disorders can be tricky. Table 12.6 provides a comparison of recognizing the three Ds: delirium, dementia, and depression.

Diagnostic tests. No single test provides a definitive diagnosis for delirium or dementia, but laboratory findings can help ascertain the cause of delirium, guide treatment decisions, and rule out other diagnoses. Neuropsychological testing may be used for either delirium or dementias to assess mental status.

The following laboratory results may be indicative of delirium:

- Serum electrolyte levels: Low calcium, low potassium, abnormal sodium
- High blood urea nitrogen (BUN), high creatinine, protein in the urine: To assess renal function and fluid levels
- Elevated prothrombin time, low hematocrit, abnormal blood gases: To assess for anoxia and poor circulation
- Urinary tract infections: Elevated leukocyte esterase, presence of nitrates in urine, increased white blood cells levels, positive urine culture and sensitivity samples
- Blood glucose, elevated aspartate transaminase (AST), and serum glutamic-oxaloacetic transaminase (SGOT): To assess metabolism

Physicians will order many laboratory tests when ruling out other medical conditions before settling on the diagnosis of dementia, including electrolytes, vitamin B_{12} level, thyroid function tests, EEG, ECG, HIV testing, and vision and hearing evaluation.

The diagnosis of dementia is usually confirmed through neuroimaging with CT scans, PET scans, an MRI, or some combination of these.

Treatment

Medical treatment of the underlying condition usually reverses delirium. All medication use in older persons should be carefully monitored for signs of overdose and adverse effects. This is vitally important to prevent both of the following:

- Drug interactions due to the high number of medications that many older persons routinely take (polypharmacy)
- Accumulation of toxic drug levels in the body due to less efficient and effective metabolism and excretion in older persons

Cholinesterase inhibitors. Donepezil (Aricept), rivastigmine (Exelon), and galantamine (Razadyne) are effective against some of the symptoms of Alzheimer's disease, slowing down the functional deterioration. By reducing the rate of acetylcholine metabolism, they may help preserve memory and learning and reduce anxiety. Other medications help ease behavioural symptoms, such as agitation (beta blockers, estrogen, anticonvulsants, SSRIs), anxiety (antidepressants, benzodiazepines), aggression (anticonvulsants), depression (antidepressants), and psychotic symptoms (SSRIs).

Nursing Considerations

Nursing Assessment

A number of assessment tools for evaluating a person's mental status are available. In many centres, nurses use the Mini-Mental State Examination. Refer to Chapter 5, page 37, for more information on mental status and neurological assessment.

Because of the acuity of most delirium and the temporary duration, assessment focuses primarily on the client's medical and mental condition. Monitor neurological status for fluctuating levels of consciousness. Ask the family about the client's normal cognitive status and whether there is a history of periods of confusion. Be alert for changes in medical signs and symptoms, monitoring vital signs, edema, intake and output, signs of jaundice, and pain level.

In contrast, much of the nurse's assessment for dementia is directed toward the client and family together. Determine the client's present cognitive functioning level, what medications are regularly taken, and the family's understanding of dementia. Discuss with family caregivers their concerns, coping abilities, safety issues in the home environment, and their knowledge of and access to community resources.

The Nurse–Client Relationship

Mental confusion is frightening to clients. Person-centred care is a philosophy of care built around the needs of the individual and contingent upon knowing the person through an interpersonal relationship (Fazio et al., 2018). Interaction, while challenging for the nurse, can be extremely frustrating for clients, who may search for words to communicate but often speak incomprehensibly. The nurse should approach clients calmly, speaking slowly and using simple language. Always introduce yourself at each contact and call the client by name, making certain that they can see your face. Ensure that clients who have hearing aids and glasses use them. Encourage them to tell you about themselves, their families, and their lives. Avoid arguing about their misperceptions

TABLE 12.6 Recognizing Delirium, Dementia, and Depression (3 D's)*

	Delirium	Dementia	Depression
Definition	Delirium is a medical emergency that is characterized by an acute and fluctuating onset of confusion, disturbances to attention, disorganized thinking, and/or decline in level of consciousness. Delirium cannot be accounted for by a pre-existing dementia; however, it can coexist with dementia.	Dementia is a gradual and progressive decline in mental processing ability that affects short-term memory, communication, language, judgement, reasoning, and abstract thinking. Dementia eventually affects long-term memory and the ability to perform familiar tasks. Sometimes there are changes in mood and behaviour.	*Depression* is a term used when a cluster of depressive symptoms (as can be identified using the SIG-E-CAPS mnemonic depression screening criteria) is present on most days, for most of the time, for at least 2 weeks, and when symptoms are of such intensity that they are out of the ordinary for that individual. Depression is a biologically based illness that affects a person's thoughts, feelings, behaviour, and even physical health.
Onset	Sudden, hours to days	Gradual deterioration over months to years	Recent, unexplained changes in mood that persist for at least 2 weeks
Course	Often reversible with treatment. Often fluctuates over 24-hour period and often worse at night	Slow, chronic progression, and irreversible	Usually reversible with treatment Often worse in the morning
Cognition	Fluctuations in alertness, thinking, perceptions, cognition, perceptions	Cognitive decline with memory impairments in memory, plus one or more of the following: aphasia, apraxia, agnosia and/or impaired executive functioning	Reduced memory, concentration, and thinking, low self-esteem
Sleep	Disturbed but with no set pattern	May be disturbed with an individual pattern occurring most nights	Disturbed Early morning awakening or hypersomnia
Mood	Fluctuations in emotions-outbursts, anger, crying, fearful	Depressed mood, especially in early dementia Prevalence of depression may increase in dementia; however, apathy is a more common symptom and may confused with depression.	Depressed mood Diminished interest or pleasure Changes in appetite (over- or undereating) Possible suicidal ideation/plan; hopelessness
Laboratory tests	Delirium workup includes the following tests: Hgb, WBC, Na, K, Ca, O_2 sats, blood gases, urea, creatinine, liver function tests, chest X-ray, urinalysis and culture, alcohol/drug/toxicology screen.	Dementia workup includes the following tests: CBC, TSH, blood glucose, electrolytes including Ca.	Depression workup includes the following tests: TSH, B12, folate, Ca, albumin, FBS, ferritin, ion, Hgb, K, ESR.
Next steps	Notify: Attending physician as soon as possible (consider delirium as a medical emergency; may require transfer to an emergency department)	Refer to: Attending physician Geriatric Mental Health Outreach Team Psychogeriatric Resource Consultant (PRC)	Refer to: Attending physician, and if suicidal risk, consider transfer to emergency department Geriatric Mental Health Outreach Team Psychogeriatric Resource Consultant (PRC)

*Individuals may have more than one D present at the same time, and symptoms may overlap.
B12, Vitamin B12; *Ca,* calcium; *CBC,* complete blood count; *ESR,* erythrocyte sedimentation rate; *FBS,* fasting blood sugar; *Hgb,* hemoglobin; *K,* potassium; *Na,* sodium; O_2 *sats,* oxygen saturation; *SIG-E-CAPS,* sleep, interest, guilt, energy, concentration, and appetite, psychomotor, and suicidal ideation; *TSH,* thyroid-simulating hormone; *WBC,* white blood cell count.
Adapted from Bard, B., MacMullin, E., Williamson, J., & Morrison-Valfre, M. (2022). *Morrison-Valfre's foundation of mental health care in Canada* (p. 198, Table 17.1). Elsevier.

and delusions; instead, reinforce what is real and gently try to change the subject. Distraction can help defuse anger and frustration, but always acknowledge the person's feelings. Above all, respect clients' humanity and never address them like children.

Nursing Interventions

Person-centred care is essential to good dementia care and is the underlying philosophy of the Alzheimer's Association dementia care practice recommendations (Fazio, et al., 2018).

Addressing fundamental areas in quality dementia care involves the following:

- Assessment
- Communication and understanding behaviour
- Social needs and activities
- Proper nutrition
- Reducing pain
- Falls
- Wandering
- Restraint-free care
- End-of-life care

Key components of person-centred dementia care include (a) holistic or person-centred care, (b) respect and value, (c) giving clients choice, (d) dignity, (e) self-determination, and (f) purposeful living. In all, it is clear that there is a shift in focus away from the traditional biomedical model in favour of embracing personal choice and autonomy (Fazio et al., 2018). Practice recommendations for a person-centred approach to caring for people with dementia and Alzheimer's disease appear in Box 12.5.

Restraints. Restraints are used to control a person's physical movement or behaviour and can be physical, environmental, or chemical (Astle & Duggleby, 2024). Restraints should be used as an absolute last resort. Restraints can cause emotional harm and serious physical injury. Confused persons react to restraints with agitation and anxiety, both of which provoke unsafe behaviour. The nurse must have a physician's order to use a physical or chemical restraint after consultation with the client's family (Sorrentino et al., 2022). Safety measures for using restraints are presented in Box 12.6.

Caring for clients with challenging behaviours. Clients with dementia often display behaviours that may make it difficult for the nurse to manage when providing care and can be disturbing for other clients around them. These challenging behaviours may develop from a reaction to a symptom from an infection, illness, or some form of physical discomfort (Sorrentino et al., 2022). The nurse's responsibility is to try and understand the reason for the challenging behaviour to help relieve the client's distress. Refer to Figure 12.4, the cycle of challenging behaviours.

Involving Families

For disoriented people, a familiar face can be soothing and help the individual to feel safe. If possible, a family member should stay while the client is in hospital to assist with the following:

- Reducing fear: Unfamiliar surroundings and strangers increase anxiety and agitation.
- Reducing disorientation: Even if the client is unable to recognize the family member, structuring the client's care in terms of personal preferences and routines is less disorienting. Informal caregivers often know a person's idiosyncrasies and can help with care planning. Request that the family bring in some familiar objects from home.
- Safety: Constant supervision helps maintain safety and avoids the use of restraints.

BOX 12.5 Dementia Care Practice Recommendations

1. **Know the person living with dementia.**
   The individual living with dementia is more than a diagnosis. It is important to know the unique and complete person, including their values, beliefs, interests, abilities, likes and dislikes—both past and present. This information should inform every interaction and experience.

2. **Recognize and accept the person's reality.**
   It is important to see the world from the perspective of the individual living with dementia. Doing so recognizes behaviour as a form of communication, thereby promoting effective and empathetic communication that validates feelings and connects with the individual in their reality.

3. **Identify and support ongoing opportunities for meaningful engagement.**
   Every experience and interaction can be seen as an opportunity for engagement. Engagement should be meaningful to, and purposeful for, the individual living with dementia. It should support interests and preferences, allow for choice and success, and recognize that even when the dementia is most severe, the person can experience joy, comfort, and meaning in life.

4. **Build and nurture authentic, caring relationships.**
   Persons living with dementia should be part of relationships that treat them with dignity and respect, and where their individuality is always supported. This type of caring relationship is about being present and concentrating on the interaction, rather than the task. It is about "doing with" rather than "doing for," as part of a supportive and mutually beneficial relationship.

5. **Create and maintain a supportive community for individuals, families, and staff.**
   A supportive community allows for comfort and creates opportunities for success. It is a community that values each person and respects individual differences, celebrates accomplishments, and occasions, and provides access to and opportunities for autonomy, engagement, and shared experiences.

6. **Evaluate care practices regularly and make appropriate changes.**
   Several tools are available to assess person-centred care practices for people living with dementia. It is important to regularly evaluate practices and models, share findings, and make changes to interactions, programs, and practices as needed.

From Fazio, S., Pace, D., Flinner, J., & Kallmyer, B. (2018). The fundamentals of person-centered care for individuals with dementia. *The Gerontologist, 58*(Suppl. 1), S10–S19.

Additional considerations:

- Be honest with family members about the diagnosis and future outcomes.
- Invite family caregivers to talk with you about their fears and emotions.
- If the client rejects family members, compassionately explain that it is not intentional.
- Assist families who may need help with financial and legal affairs and accessing community resources.

BOX 12.6 Safety Measures for Using Restraints

- Use the restraint specified in the care plan. The least restrictive device is used.
- Follow employer policies and procedures.
- Use only restraints that have manufacturer instructions and warning labels.
- Follow the manufacturer's instructions for snug fit and for specific use. Some restraints are safe for use with beds, chairs, and wheelchairs, whereas others are used only with certain equipment.
- Do not use sheets, towels, tape, rope, straps, bandages, or other items to restrain a client.
- Use only intact restraints. Check for tears, cuts, or frayed fabric or straps.
- Do not use restraints to position a client on the toilet.
- Do not use restraints to position a client on furniture that does not allow for the correct application. Follow the manufacturer's instructions.
- Position the client in good body alignment before applying the restraint.
- If mitt restraints are applied, you should be able to slide one or two fingers under the restraint. Check the client's circulation every 15 minutes. You should feel a pulse at a pulse site below the restraint. The client should have good circulation and movement. Remove the restraint if you cannot feel a pulse; the client's fingers are cold, pale, and blue; or the client complains of pain, numbness, and tingling in the restrained hand.
- Use a belt restraint with chairs and wheelchairs. Position the client in the chair so that hips are well back of the chair. Apply a belt restraint at a 45-degree angle over the hips. If a belt restraint is used, check the client at least every 15 minutes. The client should be able to breathe easily. Clients have slipped down in wheelchairs and choked or strangled themselves with a belt restraint.
- Bedrails are one type of environmental restraint. Use them only as indicated in the care plan. Check the care plan for instructions on when to lower or raise bed rails. According to the care plan, use bed rail covers or gap protectors, which prevent the client from getting trapped between the rails or the bed rail bars.
- Check the client at least every 15 minutes for safety and comfort.
- Remove the restraint and reposition the client every 2 hours. Meet the client's basic needs during this time, and whenever necessary, do the following:
  - Meet the client's elimination needs.
  - Give skin care.
  - Perform range-of-motion exercises or help the client ambulate. Follow the care plan.
  - Offer food and fluids.
  - Record what was done, the care given, your observations, and the time and details of what you reported. Follow your employer policy for reporting.
  - Keep the call bell within the client's reach.

Based on Sorrentino, S., Remmert, L., & Wilk, M. (2022). *Sorrentino's Canadian textbook for the support worker* (5th ed., p. 446). Elsevier.

- Know that families want to be helpful, but nurses must also remember that hospitalizing the client with dementia can provide respite for the primary caregiver. Encourage other family members to stay with the client to allow the primary caregiver frequent breaks and opportunities for rest.
- Help families identify and access community resources; for example, the Alzheimer Society of Canada and its local branches, the Caregiver Network, the CMHA, home care nursing services, home support services, respite care, Meals on Wheels, accessible transportation for disabled persons, and support groups for caregivers. Consult with the community health liaison nurse if your hospital has one.
- Express appreciation to family caregivers for their devotion and assistance.

SEXUAL DYSFUNCTION, PARAPHILIC DISORDERS, AND GENDER DYSPHORIA

Sexuality and identity are important sources of personality. Sexuality, sexual health, and reproduction contribute significantly to health and well-being throughout life. Nurses recognize that normal sexuality includes the curiosity and experimentation of children, as well as the need and desires for sexual relationships among older persons and people who have disabilities, either cognitive or physical.

Sexual orientation includes heterosexuality (people attracted to the opposite gender), homosexuality (gay or lesbian), bisexual attraction to both males and females, and asexual (people who do not experience any sexual attraction to anyone). In the not-too-distant past, cultural and moral standards limited acceptable sexual behaviour to heterosexual relations, preferably within marriage. Now, variations in sexual orientation and behaviour are considered to be mental health disorders only if a client defines them as such or wants to change, or if the client's sexual behaviour impinges on the rights of another.

In general, disorders of sexuality and identity can be divided into three categories:
- Sexual dysfunction
- Socially inappropriate or illegal methods of sexual expression
- Gender dysphoria

Pathophysiology

Sexual identity is largely determined genetically and manifested as male or female anatomy and physiology, although psychosocial factors (i.e., how people perceive of themselves and behave in a sexual role) also influence gender. Another biological influence on sexual expression is hormonal, as evidenced by puberty and the fact that for both men and women, libido is related to testosterone levels or high serum prolactin. In addition, high levels of androgens are found in people who exhibit inappropriate sexual arousal and hypersexual behaviour.

Sexual function, or the sexual response cycle, consists of four stages: desire, excitement, orgasm, and resolution. Disturbance at any stage can result in a sexual dysfunction, as can pain experienced with sexual intercourse.

A Preventing and Managing Resistive Responsive Behaviours When Attending to Activities of Daily Living (ADLs)

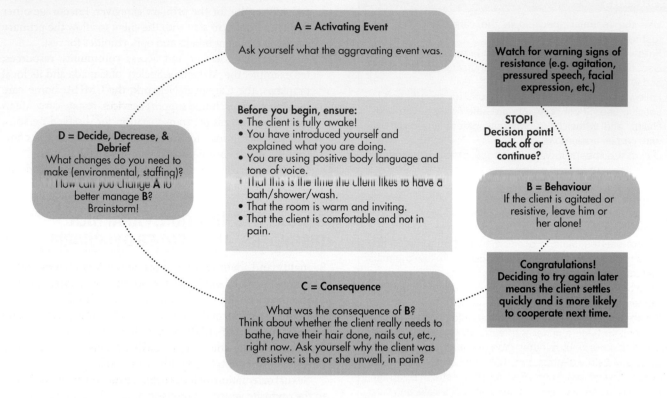

A = Activating Event

Ask yourself what the aggravating event was.

Watch for warning signs of resistance (e.g. agitation, pressured speech, facial expression, etc.)

STOP!
Decision point!
Back off or continue?

Before you begin, ensure:
- The client is fully awake!
- You have introduced yourself and explained what you are doing.
- You are using positive body language and tone of voice.
- That this is the time the client likes to have a bath/shower/wash.
- That the room is warm and inviting.
- That the client is comfortable and not in pain.

B = Behaviour
If the client is agitated or resistive, leave him or her alone!

D = Decide, Decrease, & Debrief
What changes do you need to make (environmental, staffing)? How can you change **A** to better manage **B**? Brainstorm!

Congratulations!
Deciding to try again later means the client settles quickly and is more likely to cooperate next time.

C = Consequence

What was the consequence of **B**? Think about whether the client really needs to bathe, have their hair done, nails cut, etc., right now. Ask yourself why the client was resistive: is he or she unwell, in pain?

B Preventing and Managing Aggressive Responsive Behaviours

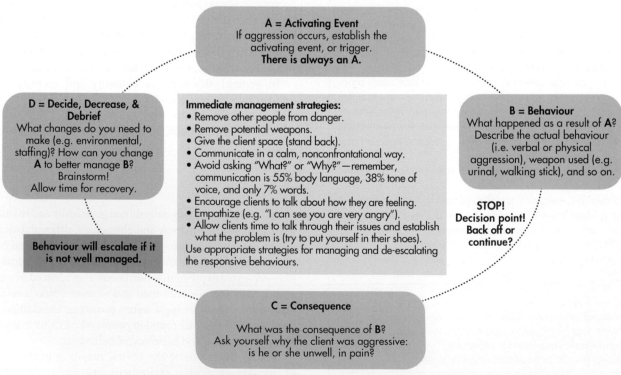

A = Activating Event
If aggression occurs, establish the activating event, or trigger.
There is always an A.

D = Decide, Decrease, & Debrief
What changes do you need to make (e.g. environmental, staffing)? How can you change **A** to better manage **B**? Brainstorm!
Allow time for recovery.

Immediate management strategies:
- Remove other people from danger.
- Remove potential weapons.
- Give the client space (stand back).
- Communicate in a calm, nonconfrontational way.
- Avoid asking "What?" or "Why?"—remember, communication is 55% body language, 38% tone of voice, and only 7% words.
- Encourage clients to talk about how they are feeling.
- Empathize (e.g. "I can see you are very angry").
- Allow clients time to talk through their issues and establish what the problem is (try to put yourself in their shoes).
Use appropriate strategies for managing and de-escalating the responsive behaviours.

B = Behaviour
What happened as a result of **A**? Describe the actual behaviour (i.e. verbal or physical aggression), weapon used (e.g. urinal, walking stick), and so on.

STOP!
Decision point!
Back off or continue?

Behaviour will escalate if it is not well managed.

C = Consequence

What was the consequence of **B**? Ask yourself why the client was aggressive: is he or she unwell, in pain?

Fig. 12.4 The cycle of challenging behaviours. **A,** Preventing and managing resistive responsive behaviours when attending to activities of daily living (ADLS). **B,** Preventing and managing aggressive responsive behaviours. (Source: Dementia Management Strategy 2009. Bendigo Health. Bendigo, Australia. Reprinted with permission of Bendigo Health).

Problems in relationships or unrealistic attitudes about sex may contribute to sexual dysfunction (Bard et al., 2022). Sexual functioning can also be affected by comorbid illness, physical injury, or the medications taken to contend with these.

- Depression, hypothyroidism, atherosclerosis, diabetes mellitus, and some urological infections and disorders, as well as neurological diseases such as epilepsy, multiple sclerosis, and Parkinson's disease, can negatively affect sexual functioning.
- Antihypertensives, antipsychotics, anxiolytics, anticonvulsants, antidepressants, and chronic alcohol or cocaine use may reduce levels of sexual desire and arousal.

Clinical Manifestations

Sexual Dysfunction

Sexual dysfunctions are a heterogeneous group of disorders that are typically characterized by a clinical disturbance in a person's ability to respond sexually or to experience sexual pleasure.

According to the DSM-5-TR, the following four subtypes of sexual dysfunction describes the onset of the difficulty:

- "*Lifelong* refers to a sexual problem that has been present from first sexual experiences.
- *Acquired* refers to sexual disorders that develop after a period of relatively normal sexual function.
- *Generalized* refers to sexual difficulties that are not limited to certain types of stimulation, situations, or partners.
- *Situational* refers to sexual difficulties that only occur with certain types of stimulation, situations, or partners" (APA, 2022, p. 477).

Frequently, a precise etiology of the sexual condition is unknown. It is important to first rule out conditions related to a nonsexual mental disorder, a substance effects or a medical condition, or whether the dysfunction is resulting from severe relationship distress, partner violence, or other stressors. For a diagnosis of a sexual dysfunction, the dysfunction must be present for more than 6 months and cause severe distress to the person (Bard et al., 2022).

A few of the various sexual dysfunctions are described next.

Female sexual interest or arousal disorders. These are characterized by emotional distress caused by absent or reduced interest in sexual fantasies, sexual activity, pleasure, and arousal. Some individuals experience these symptoms their whole lives, while others may gradually become less interested in sexual activities.

Erectile disorder. It is characterized by at least one of the three following symptoms:

- Marked difficulty in obtaining an erection during sexual activity
- Marked difficulty in maintaining an erection until the completion of sexual activity
- Marked decrease in erectile rigidity

It is considered a disorder if it happens on 75 to 100% of all sexual occasions, the symptoms have persisted for at least 6 months, and the symptoms cause significant distress in the individual. The sexual dysfunction is not better explained by a nonsexual mental disorder or as a consequence of severe relationship distress or other significant stressors and is not attributable to the effects of a substance or medication or another medical condition (APA, 2022).

Female orgasmic disorder. It is having difficulty experiencing orgasm or the inhibition of female orgasm. It is characterized by marked reduced intensity of the orgasmic sensation.

For the recognition of a clinically significant condition, it must persist for at least 6 months and must occur during the majority of sexual encounters (Halter et al., 2019).

Genito-pelvic pain or penetration disorder. The following two disorders have been combined to describe genito-pelvic pain or penetration disorder. It interferes with penile insertion during intercourse.

- Dyspareunia is recurrent or persistent pain during or after intercourse; it may occur in both females and males (Bard et al., 2022). This disorder may be caused by infection, irritation, vaginal dryness, or common skin disorders such as eczema.
- Vaginismus is the involuntary constriction of the vagina, preventing penetration and intercourse.

Individuals experiencing these problems become fearful that pain and spasms will occur during the next encounter. This fear enhances the condition further by increasing anxiety and muscle tension (Halter et al., 2019).

Paraphilic Disorders

Paraphilias are characterized by sexual arousal resulting from fantasies and behaviours. Often the fantasies involve nonhuman objects, painful or humiliating sexual activity, or sex without mutual consent. Generally, such fantasies and behaviours lead to arousal and orgasm, often assisted by masturbation. Paraphilias include exhibitionism, fetishism, frotteurism, pedophilia, sexual sadism, sexual masochism, voyeurism, transvestic disorder, other specified paraphilic disorders, and paraphilic disorders not otherwise specified. People engage in paraphilias secretly to avoid social sanctions, with the result that they are likely underdiagnosed. As with many mental health disorders, paraphilias may intensify when a person experiences stress.

Gender Dysphoria

Gender identity relates to a person's awareness of being male or female. Gender identity can be classified as cisgender or transgender. *Gender* refers to a person's identity and social classifications, often based on masculine or feminine qualities. *Transgender* refers to the broad spectrum of individuals whose gender identity and expression is different from their assigned sex at birth. *Cisgender* describes individuals whose gender expression is congruent with their birth assigned gender (also known as nontransgender) (APA, 2022). *Two-spirit* is used by some Indigenous individuals to describe their gender, sexual, or spiritual identity and refers to a person who embodies both a male and female spirit (Halter et al., 2019).

Gender dysphoria disorder occurs when biological sex and gender identity differ. From the outset, children with the disorder prefer opposite-gender playmates. With maturation, they become increasingly less comfortable with their assigned gender role. Individuals experiencing gender dysphoria disorder may face disapproval and rejection, which can lead to low self-esteem and impaired family and social interactions. As adults, wearing clothes of the opposite sex often helps decrease anxiety and depression and may or may not be accompanied by sexual excitement.

Often depressed and anxious from pressure to conform to their assigned sex role, people with a gender dysphoria may feel disgust toward their own bodies. Adolescents and adults may experience gender dysphoria, which is characterized by a person wishing to change their anatomical sexual characteristics to those of the opposite sex. The person often enters the mental health system requesting gender-affirming treatments. This is accomplished over a long period of psychological counselling, hormonal treatments, and major surgeries (Bard et al., 2022).

Diagnostics and Therapeutics

Diagnosis of sexual dysfunction, gender dysphoria, and paraphilic disorders requires a detailed general and sexual history and complete physical examination. The therapist probes for predisposing and developmental factors, as well as family and social history. A gender dysphoria disorder may be diagnosed when the discomforts interfere with activities of daily living (Bard et al., 2022).

Treatment

Treatment for sexual dysfunction, paraphilic disorders, and gender dysphoria includes the following:
- Individual or group psychotherapy
- Couples therapy
- Behaviour modification
- Pharmacotherapy with antianxiety medications or antidepressants, as necessary

More specific treatments differ depending on the classification of the disorder.

Sexual dysfunction
- Pharmacotherapy: Antidepressants, including SSRIs, have been successful against rapid ejaculation. Sildenafil (Viagra) and tadalafil (Cialis) are used for erectile dysfunction.
- Medications for female sexual disorders are less available, although studies with Viagra have shown some success when there is no history of sexual abuse.

Paraphilic disorder
- CBT may be used as treatment.
- Medications to lower testosterone levels, such as methoxyprogesterone, may be effective.

Gender dysphoria
- Hormone therapy for the development of opposite-sex secondary sexual characteristics may be used as treatment.
- Clients may undergo gender-affirming treatments after intensive psychotherapy and living as a member of the opposite sex for a significant period, usually at least 2 years. These are medical procedures (hormones or surgeries or both) that aim to align an individual's physical characteristics with their experienced gender (APA, 2022).

Nursing Considerations
Nursing Assessment
Prior to asking questions related to sexual history or sexuality, it is important for the nurse to develop a trusting, nonjudgemental, safe atmosphere. Clients with traumatic sexual histories or who may have faced previous discrimination and stigma may be reluctant to share information.

It is important to avoid making assumptions when talking about gender and sexuality with clients. Making heterosexist and gender assumptions could jeopardize the nurse–client relationship. When meeting a new client, ask which gender pronoun the client prefers you use. Inform the person that the information they provide is confidential and tell them about the limitations to confidentiality. Begin with a full health history, family history, and physical examination. A basic sexual health history includes the five P's: **P**artners, **P**ractices, **P**rotection from STIs, **P**ast history of STIs, and **P**revention of pregnancy (Bard et al., 2022). Include questions about sexual activity, number and gender of sexual partners, birth control, concern regarding HIV and other sexually transmitted infections (STIs), and whether there are any concerns about sexual functioning. Once you have established a relationship, you can ask more specific questions. The Public Health Agency of Canada offers suggestions on a variety of topics to include in a comprehensive assessment:
- Sexual knowledge, family attitudes, and sexual experience during childhood and adolescence
- Cultural and religious beliefs regarding sexuality
- The client's concerns and depth of understanding of their sexuality
- Concerns the client has about sexual or relationship violence or abuse
- Sexual patterns
- Self-esteem
- Anxiety and level of stress
- Social interaction
- Coping strategies
- Social and support networks (Government of Canada, 2021d)

The Nurse–Client Relationship
Culture, family background, societal values, and the media all contribute to the taboos surrounding sexual conduct and what is considered to be "normal." Assumptions and inferences about a client's sexual health may prove inaccurate and damaging to the nurse–client relationship. Nurses need to examine their own attitudes and values regarding sexual expression and sexual behaviour to minimize anxiety when discussing sexual matters. Awareness of one's personal attitudes, beliefs, and knowledge regarding sexuality is necessary before the nurse can set those issues aside to allow for an open and sensitive discussion, communicating warmth, acceptance, and positive regard. Because sexuality is one of the most private and personal aspects of our lives, few people will volunteer information, leaving it to the nurse to introduce the topic and guide the conversation.

Nursing Interventions

Sexual therapy is not within the scope of practice for a newly qualified nurse. For intensive therapy, the nurse should make a referral to a qualified sex therapist. The nurse's role includes assessment, education, and support to a client being treated for a sexual disorder. Some basic approaches that are helpful to clients with sexual conditions include the following:

- Active listening, allowing the client to explore sexual values and beliefs
- Helping the client set realistic goals
- Setting limits on the client's sexual behaviour, if included in the plan of care
- Relaxation techniques for stress and anxiety reduction
- Assisting with the behaviour modification plan by implementing the agreed-upon consequences for maladaptive behaviour

Teaching and Learning

If the client has a stable sexual relationship, include the partner in client education. Explore whether there are differences in their sexual beliefs and expectations as these can lead to conflict and misunderstanding. For example, the client's dissatisfaction with sexual desire and arousal may be less a matter of their personal lack of response than it is of not being able to match their partner's expectations.

Nursing Interventions Classification (NIC) interventions for sexual counselling appear in Box 12.7.

Responding to a Client's Sexual Advances

One very difficult aspect of caring for clients with paraphilic disorder is dealing with seductive advances and comments directed at the nurse. Sexually inappropriate behaviour toward nurses is not restricted to mental health settings but can be found in any health care environment. Inappropriate touching, asking for dates or personal contact information, and making explicit passes at the nurse cannot be tolerated, and the client must be so informed. The most professional response is to respond firmly and set clear limits.

FEEDING AND EATING DISORDERS: ANOREXIA NERVOSA AND BULIMIA NERVOSA

An eating disorder is an ongoing disturbance of eating or eating related behaviour that results in the altered consumption or absorption of food and that causes a significant impairment of a person's physical health or psychosocial functioning (APA, 2022). The continuum ranges from eating too little (anorexia nervosa), through disordered eating with binging and purging (bulimia nervosa), to chronic overeating causing obesity (binge eating disorder). Other disorders include pica, rumination disorder, and avoidant or restrictive food intake disorder. In our culture, however, obesity is not always considered a mental health condition, and most treatment consists of diet therapy only. Binge eating disorder often goes unrecognized. Anorexia and bulimia often overlap, with about half of people with anorexia displaying bulimic behaviours at times or developing bulimia later in their lives. Eating disorders are primarily identified in women (85–90%). However, the prevalence of bulimia in males may be underestimated because of their reluctance to seek treatment. Anorexia nervosa is not often seen before puberty and rarely appears after the age of 40 years. The average age of onset is about 17 years, but anorectic behaviours may be seen in children as young as 12 years old. Bulimia nervosa generally occurs later in adolescents (Bard et al., 2022).

Pathophysiology

Normal appetite regulation is a function of the hypothalamus, through several mechanisms that produce sensations of either hunger or satiety (feeling full). Hunger is experienced when the hypothalamus is stimulated by the following:

- Low blood glucose levels
- Contractions of an empty stomach (and possibly stimulation of the vagus nerve)
- High levels of neurotransmitters, such as serotonin
  Satiety is felt when the hypothalamus is suppressed. This occurs due to the following:
- High levels of fat and amino acids in the blood
- Slow emptying of the stomach and distension of the GI tract
- High cortisol levels (a physiological reaction to stress)

Clinical Manifestations

Eating disorders are closely related to body image and low self-esteem. Where thinness is admired and celebrated in all forms of the media, dissatisfaction with one's shape and size is widespread. Weight loss is big business, and some people engage in extreme measures to control their weight.

BOX 12.7 NIC Interventions for Sexual Counselling

Definition of *sexual counselling*: Use of an interactive helping process focusing on the need to make adjustments in sexual practice or to enhance coping with a sexual event or disorder.

Activities*:

- Establish a therapeutic relationship based on trust and respect.
- Provide privacy and ensure confidentiality.
- Discuss the effects of changes in sexuality on significant others.
- Discuss the knowledge level of the client about sexuality in general.
- Encourage the client to verbalize fears and ask questions.
- Provide reassurance and permission to experiment with alternative forms of sexual expression, as appropriate.
- Provide referral or consultation with other members of the health care team, as appropriate.

* Partial list.
From Halter, M. J., Pollard, C. L., & Jacubec, S. L. (2019). *Varcarolis's Canadian psychiatric mental health nursing: A clinical approach* (2nd Cdn. ed., p. 582). Elsevier. Data from Bulechek, G. M., Butcher, H. K., Dochterman, J. M., et al. (Eds.). (2013). *Nursing interventions classification (NIC)* (6th ed.). Elsevier.

Behaviours associated with eating disorders include the following:
- Binge eating: Consuming large amounts of food and excessive calories. The frequency of binging varies from occasionally to several times weekly or even many times each day.
- Dieting: Restricting food intake below what is necessary to maintain weight
- Fasting: Refusing to eat
- Purging: Inducing vomiting to lose weight or using over-the-counter laxatives or diuretics to stimulate fluid and waste excretion

Anorexia Nervosa and Bulimia

Individuals with anorexia nervosa refuse to maintain a normal body weight for their height and develop persistent behaviours that interfere with weight gain. Anorexia nervosa is a life-threatening condition. Symptoms include restriction of food intake, intense fear of gaining weight, and body image disturbance. The physiological effects of anorexia nervosa include constipation, cold intolerance, lanugo, lethargy, electrolyte imbalance, amenorrhea in females, and emaciation (Halter et al., 2019).

Bulimia nervosa is an eating disorder characterized by "recurrent episodes of binge eating and engage in inappropriate behaviours to avoid weight gain (e.g., self-induced vomiting), and are overly concerned with body shape and weight. However, unlike individuals with anorexia nervosa, binge eating/purging type, individuals with bulimia nervosa maintain body weight at or above a minimally normal level" (APA, 2022, p. 387). Clients who use recurrent vomiting to compensate for binge eating often experience changes to their teeth and oral mucosa, such as damage to tooth enamel and unexpected dental caries. Some clients may use laxatives or excessive exercise to avoid weight gain.

Complications of Eating Disorders

Without treatment, eating disorders cause medical complications in many body systems. Serious complications of starvation and dehydration include hypokalemia and hypoalbuminemia leading to hypotension, cardiac arrhythmias, and heart and renal failure, which are life-threatening. Frequent vomiting can cause stomach and esophageal ulcers, GI bleeding, tooth decay, and gum erosion. Amenorrhea is related to estrogen deficiencies that may result in calcium deficiency and osteoporosis. Deaths from eating disorders are tragic and much too frequent.

Diagnostics and Therapeutics
Predisposing Factors

There is no known specific cause for eating disorders. A number of risk factors have been identified such as biological factors (genetics, obesity), developmental factors (development of autonomy and control), and familial and social influences (lack of emotional support, child adversity, media influences). Criticism or teasing about one's weight from parents or peers can damage self-esteem, as can other family dysfunctions and a history of sexual or physical abuse.

Treatment

Unless there is a medical crisis, clients can be cared for as outpatients in community clinics, day treatment, or partial hospitalization. Selection of treatment setting is based on the severity of the illness as well as extent of comorbidities such as depression or life-threatening complications. Where possible, community care tends to be the best option, allowing clients to maintain autonomy while learning healthy self-control and a balanced lifestyle. Immediate medical intervention and possible hospitalization are required if the client presents with severe dehydration, cardiac damage, low blood glucose, and electrolyte imbalance, or if the client becomes psychotic, suicidal, or severely depressed. Sometimes people with an eating disorder may self-identify and ask to be admitted to the hospital.

Once in hospital, medical treatment to stabilize physiological health is the first priority, followed by behaviourally oriented interventions. Treatment may include the following:
- A healthy diet, possibly with liquid supplements
- Vitamin and mineral supplements
- Pharmacotherapy with anxiolytics (helpful for those with obsessive–compulsive features), tricyclics, and SSRIs (to decrease mood swings, depression, irritability, and food and fat obsessions). Sometimes appetite suppressants are used for bulimia, but only until new eating patterns have been established.
- Individual or group psychotherapy
- CBT
- Behaviour modification therapy
- Family therapy
- Stress management and self-monitoring

Nursing Considerations
Nursing Assessment
- The Eating Disorder Screen for Primary Care (ESP) is an eating disorder screening tool used to assess for a possible eating disorder. If the client identifies three or more abnormal responses, a more detailed assessment should be considered. The ESP asks the following questions:
  1. Are you satisfied with your eating pattern?
  2. Do you ever eat in secret?
  3. Does your weight affect the way you feel about yourself?
  4. Have any members of your family suffered with an eating disorder?
  5. Do you currently suffer with, or have you ever suffered in the past with an eating disorder? (Halter et al., 2019).
  The nursing assessment consists of a full health history, family history, and physical examination, placing emphasis on the following:
- Nutritional status and diet history, including food preferences, eating behaviours, and purging episodes
- Weight history, height, and weight measurement
- Signs of fluid and electrolyte imbalance
- Menstrual history, especially amenorrhea
- Frequency, type, and amount of exercise
- Mood and emotional state, for example, depression, anxiety, distress

- Evidence of obsession or compulsion, especially regarding food
- Evidence of disturbed body image, low self-esteem, self-criticism
- Risk of suicide
- Frequency, type, and amount of exercise
- History of dysfunctional family relationships
- Level of insight and motivation for treatment

The Nurse–Client Relationship

People with an eating disorder tend to be suspicious. The suspicion and mistrust are often a symptom of anxiety and fear. It is important for the nurse to develop a trusting, therapeutic relationship with the client. Focusing on identifying areas of strength not related to food or body image, assist in setting realistic goals, and avoid power struggles over food intake.

Nursing Interventions

The nurse encourages healthy eating by negotiating agreement on a target weight and a mutually determined recovery plan that includes the following:

- Adequate food intake
- Structured, time-limited meal times (e.g., three small meals a day)
- Food preferences
- Nutritious snacks between meals
  Monitor the client's eating and weight in an accepting and nonpunitive way.
- Stay with the client during meals and for an hour after to reduce opportunities for purging (in anorexia nervosa and bulimia nervosa) or stashing food (in bulimia nervosa and obesity).
- Ensure a pleasant and social atmosphere at mealtimes, discussing topics other than food.
- Encourage use of a food diary.
- Offer small amounts of food and drink frequently.
- Weigh the client daily in the morning, in the same clothing, after first voiding, and on the same scale. Be vigilant for attempts to artificially increase their weight, such as stuffing items into pockets or under clothes.
- Record intake and output.
- Assess for signs of dehydration, such as skin turgor, colour, and moistness of oral mucous membranes.
- Encourage rest times and appropriate exercise with supervision.

Teaching and Learning

Provide information about normal nutrition and balanced diet nutrients, such as teaching about normal growth and body development and that cutting out all fat is unhealthy. Discuss the nature of the illness (symptoms, causes, effects on the body) and the importance of expressing emotions and fears rather than holding them inside. What emotions and beliefs does the client associate with eating? Help people with anorexia set attainable goals. Setting unrealistic goals can result in feelings of failure and frustration. Regularly review the client's food journal and diet plan with them and explain how better nutrition will improve symptoms and prevent complications. Review the action, dose, and possible adverse effects of any mediation that the client is taking. Additional important components of teaching for clients with anorexia nervosa include the following:

- The physiologically damaging effects of dieting
- The identification and avoidance of triggers
- Techniques for self-monitoring
- Community resources
  Additional important components of teaching for clients with bulimia nervosa include the following:
- The effects on the body of the binging and purging cycle
- Adequate hydration
- Self-monitoring and the avoidance of cues
- Learning to set limits and appropriate boundaries
- Assertiveness (Bard et al., 2022)

Psychosocial Interventions

Behaviour modification

- Use a nurse–client contract to ensure that the client understands the illness and treatment involved and is committed to participating in making informed decisions to benefit their health.
  - Agreed-upon consequences for not adhering to the contract terms, such as loss of privileges, should be imposed consistently and in a matter-of-fact manner and voice tone.
  - Provide encouragement and positive reinforcement for adherence to the contract.
- Help the client identify any cues that stimulate harmful eating behaviour and explore ways of avoiding those situations or changing to a more adaptive response.

Body image perception

- Encourage the client to share their thoughts and feelings about body shape and weight.
- Avoid contradicting the client, but present alternative ideas and interpretations.
- Help the client reflect on and consider those alternative perceptions and explanations.
- Promote self-acceptance. Draw attention to positive physical characteristics.
- Encourage the client to use imagery and relaxation, which may reduce body-related anxiety.

Low self-esteem

- Explore the client's desire for perfection and encourage acceptance of what is good enough.
- Explore family and relationship history and the impacts on self-esteem and self-acceptance.
- Emphasize positive attributes and behaviours.

Interactions with families

- Include families in treatment team meetings and in planning care, in both the hospital and community phases of treatment.
- Be emotionally supportive but also candid about the client's state of health.
- Advise families to make their visits social occasions and to talk about topics other than eating.

- Encourage families to become informed about nutrition and about eating disorders.

In addition, there are self-help groups for treating eating disorders. Two mutual-help groups that focus on people with an eating disorder and offer face-to-face, online, and telephone meetings are as follows: Overeaters Anonymous (OA), which is based on the 12-step model, and Eating Disorders Anonymous (EDA), which is appropriate for anyone with an eating disorder.

PSYCHIATRIC EMERGENCIES: CRISIS, SUICIDE, VIOLENCE

In a highly stressful event or when confronted with a perceived threat for which the usual coping strategies are ineffective, people experience high levels of anxiety. This may escalate to a state of crisis. Crises may be developmental (such as adolescence, marriage, moving away from home to attend college) or situational (such as divorce or sudden unemployment). Extreme situational crises are sometimes called *adventitious*, indicating that the event is totally outside the person's control. Some examples include natural disasters, wars, or being the victim of a crime.

With no resolution of the crisis, behavioural reactions may continue to escalate. The most serious behavioural reactions include suicide and violence, neither of which are rare events. Although suicide deaths affect almost all ages, more than half of suicides involve people aged 45 years and older (CAMH, 2022a). Suicide is the second leading cause of death for young people between 15 and 34 years of age. The suicide death rate for men is three times as high as that for women. (Government of Canada, 2020).

Pathophysiology

For a description of the stress response, refer to the section "Anxiety Disorders."

- The limbic system is responsible for regulating emotions and aggression. The amygdala is involved in distinguishing between aversive and rewarding stimuli. Rage can be activated in animals by stimulating the amygdala.
- There is a correlation between low levels of serotonin and aggressive behaviour.
- Abnormalities in the temporal lobe may be related to aggressive responses.
- Some people are prone to aggressive behaviour after a traumatic brain injury.

Clinical Manifestations

Clients in crisis are overwhelmed by emotional pain and anxiety. After having attempted a number of solutions without success, they may reach the point of being "at their wit's end" and in a state of complete disorganization. Although people react to crises differently, common maladaptive behaviours include anger, apathy, somatic complaints, emotional outbursts, insomnia, fear, flashbacks, shock, hopelessness, helplessness, or substance use.

Diagnostics and Therapeutics
Diagnosis

Diagnosis is initially based on the client's behaviour and inability to control the source of extreme and intense anxiety. First, determine whether the person is suicidal or violent and initiate steps to ensure safety. Once safety is ensured, the nurse should try to identify the precipitating event or events. In psychiatric and community settings, the exacerbation of a mental illness often occurs when clients reject treatment. Apprehension under the *Mental Health Act* and certification for admission or treatment or both may be necessary (see the section "Legal, Ethical, and Interpersonal Considerations for Mental Health Nursing").

Nurses should know what services are locally available for crisis intervention and how to contact them. Some are as follows:

- "Crisis lines or Internet crisis services-telephone support by trained volunteers (for first aid or support) or professional (for assessment, triage, and referral).
- Mobile crisis outreach-outreach crisis response services often provided by collaborative teams, including police, mental health nurses and other first responders.
- Urgent or walk-in-crisis care-services where people can present their crisis needs to professionals for assessment, intervention, and referral.
- Psychiatric emergency care-services such as emergency mental health care in hospital triage; assessment; crisis counselling; emergency medical treatment, often for brief-stay admissions" (Halter et al., 2019, p. 486).

Treatment

Treatment varies depending on the root cause of the crisis. Treatment goals are to preserve the safety of the client and all those who could be exposed to danger, to prevent the client's anxiety from escalating, and to return the client to a precrisis state of being.

Psychopharmacology. Common medications for those prone to high levels of anxiety and impulsive behaviour include the following:

- Anxiolytics and sedative–hypnotics to manage agitation
- Antidepressants, especially SSRIs, to balance levels of serotonin
- Mood stabilizers to reduce aggressive behaviour
- Antipsychotics: The quick action of IM haloperidol combined with lorazepam (Ativan) is often used to calm people with escalating agitation. Atypical antipsychotics are given to reduce the incidence of violence in people at risk.

Nursing Considerations
Nursing Assessment

Assessment focuses on identifying the precipitating event, the client's interpretation of it, the client's coping resources, and the support systems available. Does the person in crisis require emergency psychiatric treatment or hospitalization? Whether you are a community nurse or in a hospital setting, your assessment will include several elements:

- Try to ascertain whether the person clearly understands the event that precipitated the crisis.
- What coping mechanisms may be helpful in this situation? Has the client used these coping strategies in the past?
- What or who are the client's current situational supports?
- Are there any cultural or religious beliefs or traditions that need to be taken into consideration?
- What is the appropriate level of intervention in this situation?
  - Primary intervention, such as education, changes in the environment, or new coping skills
  - Secondary, or crisis, intervention
  - Tertiary intervention, such as rehabilitation (Halter et al., 2019)

Suicide. The suicide rate is growing among the older population, and specifically among older men. In Canada, about 31 of every 100 000 older persons, especially those over 85 years, die by suicide. Most are white males, and most die through violent means (Sorrentino et al., 2022). The reasons for suicide include loneliness, loss of independence, deteriorating health, and wanting to avoid becoming a burden to families (Sorrentino et al., 2022).

Many social factors affect the incidence of suicide. Poverty and homelessness lead to depression and hopelessness. Suicide becomes an acceptable alternative when one is continually hungry, cold, ill, or living in fear. In Canada, suicide disproportionately impacts Indigenous peoples. The rate of suicide among First Nations is three times higher than among non-Indigenous Canadians, and nine times higher among Inuit (CMHA, 2021). To properly understand the elevated rate of suicide in Indigenous communities, the statistics must be considered alongside the historical trauma that has impacted Indigenous communities.

Veterans with combat experience and those with PTSD suffer higher suicide rates than does the general population.

It is important to be aware of social changes occurring in the world that impact the risk of suicide. Health care workers having an increased knowledge base that allows for offering early interventions is important to help decrease the attempts of self-harm by clients (Bard et al., 2022). Thoughts of suicide or suicide attempts should be suspected when clients appear alienated, disconnected, or in despair. In a kind but straightforward way, ask distressed clients if they are experiencing suicidal thoughts. If the answer is "Yes," ask whether the client has developed a plan. If so, evaluate whether the person has the ability and opportunity to carry it out.

Risk factors for suicide vary depending on the population group:

- Depressed adolescents with a family history of suicide and a personal history of legal trouble and substance abuse are at high risk.
- For older persons, high risk factors include a family member's death or having a serious or terminal illness.
- For depressed clients, times of greatest danger occur in the first few days following either admission to or discharge from the hospital. Clients are at high risk for suicide for the first few days following initiation of treatment with antidepressants or ECT. Psychomotor delay improves before mood improves. Thus, early in treatment, the client remains severely depressed but now has regained the motivation necessary to follow through with suicidal thoughts. Following discharge, some clients are more at risk of suicide when they return home to find that the things that initially caused their depression have not changed.
- People with schizophrenia disorder are at less risk for suicide when they are psychotic than when they begin to recover and may feel little hope for a satisfying life.
- Psychiatric clients who are at high risk for suicide are those who engage in self-directed harm, including self-mutilation to relieve tension, and those who stop taking their medications or otherwise do not adhere to treatment.
- People who misuse substances are at high risk, as are those who have been recently separated, divorced, or bereaved.
- Be especially wary of a severely disturbed client who suddenly becomes calm and rational. When people see suicide as the only escape from an intolerable existence, and when they have thought through a plan and have the means to carry it out, they may feel comforted by knowing their struggles are nearly over.

Violence. Nurses should be able to distinguish between assertive and aggressive behaviour.

Assertive behaviour: People who are assertive are direct, persuasive, and self-assured in their communications and interactions with other people. They convey respect for others.

Aggressive behaviour: People who are aggressive exert their own rights at the expense of the rights of others. They tend to express anger. They fight to get what they want and expect others to approach interactions in the same way. Aggressive behaviour can escalate to violence, and nurses should be aware that setting limits on clients' behaviour is sometimes an antecedent of aggressive behaviour by hospitalized clients. On the one hand, aggression is more common in psychiatric clients with active psychosis and in those with substance use disorders. On the other hand, people with schizophrenia disorder and mania are no more violent than ordinary citizens as long as they are well controlled on their medications. The best predictor of a person becoming violent is past violent behaviour.

The Nurse–Client Relationship

Connecting with violent and aggressive clients is challenging. Some nurses worry that their own behaviour could trigger a client's angry response. If a client is verbally abusive, the nurse's first response should be to leave the room. Of course, it is always best to prevent angry outbursts if at all possible. For clients with a history of violence or who are otherwise deemed to be at risk for violence, reward appropriate behaviour by giving time and attention to the person.

Identify client stressors and ways to avoid them and learn to recognize indicators that the client is becoming stressed. If so, the nurse draws on interpersonal skills for de-escalating the situation. Speak calmly and find out what the client needs or wants. If appropriate, help the client attain those wants. If not, then clearly state other more appropriate options from which the client might choose.

Be assertive and confident but also genuine and empathetic. Allow ample personal space between yourself and the client, continually assess for personal safety, and be certain that you have other nursing or security staff close by. Use medications for chemical restraint only when absolutely necessary and when less restrictive methods have been tried without success.

Nursing Interventions

Relieving acute stress involves helping the client process the traumatic event, emotionally and cognitively, and improve coping mechanisms. Ensuring the client's safety in a supportive environment always takes precedence. When a client feels safe, their anxiety should diminish, enabling the person to engage with the nurse, reflect on the experience, and explore alternative, more adaptive responses.

Suicide precautions. When suicide risk is high, toxic substances and sharp objects should be removed from the client's environment. No belts, neckties, or other articles of clothing that could be used for self-destruction should be worn, and the client should be monitored one-to-one at arm's length, 24 hours a day (never letting the client out of staff's sight). Communicate a caring presence and provide reassurance that you will help the client stay safe. Develop a safety plan in collaboration with the client. Safety plans include a description of how the client will keep their environment safe, how to recognize factors or events that that precipitated the suicidal thoughts, individual coping strategies, and identification of a nonmedical person (family, friend) who can help if coping strategies do not work; if that is not working, which clinicians to call; and if that also is not working, where to go for emergency help (Bard et al., 2022). Some clients will agree to a no self-harm contract, which is one way of helping clients begin to re-establish personal control. Encourage the client to express feelings and discuss ways for the client to manage those feelings and keep safe. If at all possible, provide for continuity of care, as establishing an emotional bond with someone could be a turning point toward suicide prevention.

Violence precautions. With violent clients, nurses must be hypervigilant of their own safety. A rule of thumb is to stay between the client and a door for escape. Call security to assist with violent episodes. Some behavioural strategies used with aggressive clients include the following:

- Setting limits: The nurse defines for the client acceptable behaviour patterns and the consequences of unacceptable behaviour. All staff must agree to monitor the behaviour and apply the agreed-upon consequences consistently.
- Behaviour contracts: The nurse and client negotiate and sign a contract outlining rewards for acceptable behaviour and the consequences of unacceptable behaviour.
- Time-outs: Socially unacceptable behaviour results in a time-out, removing the client from an overstimulating environment to a quiet area or the client's room. If the client

agrees to this and goes voluntarily when reminded by the nurse, it is not considered to be the same as seclusion.
- Token economy: The client can earn tokens or points that can be used to barter for privileges. The client loses tokens for unacceptable behaviour.

Teaching and Learning

Here are some ideas for teaching clients about anger and how it can be used appropriately.

- Focus on nonverbal expressions of anger, role-playing, and talking about angry feelings in the client's own words, allowing the client to demonstrate angry body language and facial expressions.
- Talk about situations where it is okay to feel angry and role-play those types of situations.
- Help the client identify real situations that cause anger. Role-play confronting the object or person that generates the anger. Give feedback on appropriate verbal and nonverbal responses.
- Give permission for the client to confront the real object of their anger. Provide a supportive presence if needed and debrief with the client afterward.

Families and Violence

Interpersonal violence and abuse in family contexts can affect all generations: children, intimate partners, and older persons. Each form of abuse is an instance of the abuser exerting control or power over the abused person (Halter et al., 2019).

- Forms of family abuse include physical abuse or neglect, forced sexual activity (including rape), psychological intimidation and threats, emotional maltreatment, and financial exploitation.
- Alcohol and drug abuse often underlie violence and neglect within families.
- Nurses are ethically and legally responsible for reporting evidence of all types of abuse involving vulnerable people and child abuse to the appropriate legal authorities.

Intimate-partner abuse

- "The cycle of violence" refers to the pattern of three phases of intimate-partner violence. In phase one, tension builds. In phase two, the actual incident of battering takes place. In phase three, the couple reconciles; this phase is also called "the honeymoon phase." The perpetrator vows that it will not happen again, with gifts and kindnesses to the victim as proof of love. Then the cycle begins again.
- Intimate-partner abuse is the most common form of family violence. Battered spouses tend to return and reconcile with their violent partner three times before they are able to leave permanently. Feminist theory suggests that patriarchy and sexual inequality make it difficult for women to maintain themselves independently, thus explaining the return to a dangerous home situation.
- Abusive partners are frequently pathologically jealous and prone to blame others for their own inadequacies.
- Victims suffer low self-esteem and feelings of helplessness and hopelessness and need help to make future plans. Nurses can teach victims of family violence strategies for

ensuring their safety. A safety plan for victims of domestic violence may include the following:

- Posting emergency numbers and teaching children to call 9-1-1
- Making a plan for at least two different places the client can go to be safe and storing extra clothes, cash, and copies of important documents there, even if the client hopes that the violence is over. Shelters and safe houses are available in many communities and are open 24 hours through hotline crisis information and shelter numbers.
- Providing a neighbour with a signal that will indicate they should call police
- If there is a restraining order, keeping it with the client at all times and giving a copy to a child's school or day care centre
- Connecting with a support group and with old friends

Child abuse

- Abusive parents often were abused as children. They have poor impulse control and ineffective coping and parenting skills.
- Sexual abuse may be suspected when children display the following dysfunctional behaviour patterns: excessive aggression, sexual activity that is inappropriate for their developmental stage, social withdrawal, poor performance at school, sleep disturbances, and low self-esteem.

See pages 353-355, for more details on pediatric abuse.

Elder abuse. Older persons are prone to abuse as their physical and mental health deteriorate, and they become dependent on their relatives. The types of elder abuse are as follows:

- Emotional abuse
- Financial exploitation
- Physical abuse
- Sexual abuse
- Neglect
- Violation of individual rights is another form of abuse involving failure to maintain clients' privacy or not allowing them to use the phone in private (Sorrentino et al., 2022).

Caregiver stress can lead to abuse in families that are dysfunctional in other ways or when caregivers are also at risk for mental health issues. Some of the types of abuse are harder to pinpoint but are prevalent and must be reported to the appropriate legal authorities.

Recognizing signs of family violence. Although the guidelines that follow refer specifically to clients who present in the emergency department, community nurses often will discover evidence of abuse during home visits or in ambulatory settings such as public health clinics. In any setting, signs of family stress could manifest as emotional and behavioural conditions, including increased aggression, inability to sleep, trouble in school, or being accident-prone. Pregnancy is a particularly vulnerable time for a childbearing client. Abuse may be suspected when people present to the emergency department with internal injuries, multiple contusions (especially facial or head and neck), burns (especially from cigarettes) and scalds, perforated eardrums, or miscarriage. There is often evidence of bruising at various stages of healing and a history of multiple emergency department or clinic visits with diffuse and varied complaints. Psychological trauma, anxiety, depression, and severe stress may be evident, and often the explanations fall short of matching the extent or seriousness of the injury. The type of abuse or neglect may be physical, sexual, emotional, or even financial (Sorrentino et al., 2022).

Interviewing victims of violence. Feelings of shame, fear, and worries of how to survive outside the family may make it difficult for victims of abuse to admit truthfully to the causes of their injuries. A health care provider who suspects abuse of a vulnerable client is obligated to report it and to validate the concerns to the greatest extent possible. Discuss issues of abuse with the client in a nonthreatening way in private; convey concern and understanding; reassure the client they are not at fault; and encourage the client to tell the story by using open-ended questions. It is not within the scope of the entry-level nurse to gather in-depth information on the possible abuse. If the suspected abuse involves an adult, the nurse should share information on supports and resources. The nurse must understand that they cannot disclose client information without the client's consent. If the suspicions of abuse involve a child, dependent adult, or person in care (hospital, facility, etc.), the nurse is responsible for documenting the observations factually and accurately and reporting the abuse to the appropriate agency either independently or in collaboration with another health care provider.

PRACTICE QUESTIONS

Case 1

Jason Beames, age 17 years, was brought to the emergency department by the police. His mother called the police after Jason violently attacked his father with no provocation. Jason is admitted to the psychiatric unit for investigation of his psychosis, with a provisional diagnosis of schizophrenia.

Questions 1 to 5 refer to this case.

1. What is the definition of *psychosis*?
    1. A psychological break from reality
    2. A group of mental health disorders characterized by various anxiety symptoms
    3. A disturbance of consciousness and change in cognition
    4. Another term for schizophrenia

2. The emergency department physician completes a certificate designating Jason an involuntary client because Jason would not consent to admission. Which of the following should the nurse tell Jason concerning his rights as an involuntary client?
    1. The physician is not legally permitted to admit Jason without his consent.
    2. Since Jason is only 17 years old, he does not have the same rights as an adult.
    3. Jason can apply to a review board for a legal ruling on his involuntary admission.

4. Jason has no legal rights since he has been certified as an involuntary psychiatric client.

3. Because of his violent behaviour, Jason is administered a chemical restraint. Which of the following statements is true with regard to using restraints in a psychiatric setting?
   1. Chemical restraints are preferable to other interventions for calming a psychotic client.
   2. Physical restraints are generally more effective than chemical restraints for psychotic episodes.
   3. Guidelines for the use of restraints apply to both chemical and physical restraints.
   4. A physician order for chemical restraints is generally not required in an emergency department setting.

4. Jason tells the nurse that the voices are yelling at him. What would be the most helpful response?
   1. "I don't hear the voices that you hear."
   2. "What are the voices yelling at you?"
   3. "You realize there are really no voices yelling at you."
   4. "Why do you think you are hearing voices?"

5. Jason's parents come to visit Jason. His mother asks the nurse if Jason has schizophrenia and will he have to be in the hospital for the rest of his life. What might the nurse respond to Jason's mother?
   1. "I can refer you to the local Canadian Schizophrenia Society. They will provide education for you about Jason's disease."
   2. "Because Jason is young, he will likely not have any further serious psychotic episodes."
   3. "I don't really know. We will have to wait to see how Jason responds to his medications."
   4. "Schizophrenia is a lifelong disorder, but antipsychotic medications allow most people to live and be treated outside the hospital."

Case 2

Marty Steele, age 42, has been diagnosed with borderline personality disorder. He is admitted to a psychiatric unit.
Questions 6 and 7 refer to this case.

6. Mr. Steele tells the nurse, Jeremy, that one of the other nurses, Sarah, is lazy and is not as good a nurse as Jeremy. What is this called?
   1. Narcissistic behaviour
   2. Schizoid behaviour
   3. Splitting behaviour
   4. Dependent behaviour

7. What is the priority assessment for the nurse to conduct with Mr. Steele?
   1. Potential for harm to himself or others
   2. Hallucinations
   3. History of child abuse
   4. Sexual orientation

Case 3

Tiffany Scolfield, age 15, comes to see the school nurse because she stopped menstruating several months ago. The nurse suspects an eating disorder.
Questions 8 to 12 refer to this case.

8. Which of the following statements about eating disorders is true?
   1. People can die from anorexia but not from bulimia.
   2. Men can suffer from bulimia but not from anorexia.
   3. Women who recover from anorexia often develop bulimia later.
   4. People with bulimia deny feelings of hunger.

9. The nurse assesses Tiffany for medical complications associated with her eating disorder. Which of the following physical assessments would it be most important to perform while Tiffany was in her office?
   1. Complete skin survey for breakdown
   2. Abdominal palpation for constipation
   3. Oral examination for dental caries
   4. Blood pressure monitoring for hypotension

10. Tiffany talks to the nurse about her feelings. The nurse uses clarification as a form of therapeutic communication. Which of the following responses is an example of clarification?
    1. "I'm not sure what you mean. Could you tell me about that again?"
    2. "Can you tell me more about what is bothering you?"
    3. "What do you think is causing you to feel this way?"
    4. "You've mentioned many things. Let's go back to how eating makes you feel."

11. The nurse arranges for Tiffany to come to the health office at regular intervals to monitor her weight. What would the nurse be aware of regarding the process of weighing Tiffany?
    1. Tiffany may drink excessive fluids to increase her recorded weight.
    2. Tiffany will probably refuse to be weighed.
    3. Tiffany should be weighed wearing her street clothes and shoes.
    4. Tiffany's parents must be informed about the monitoring of her weight.

12. Tiffany's weight decreases, and she is admitted to an eating disorders unit at a local pediatric hospital. What should be included in her care plan?
    1. Large meals at frequent intervals to improve her nutritional status
    2. Accurate input and output to monitor fluid status
    3. Leisurely meals to promote decreased stress while eating
    4. Segregation from other adolescents with eating disorders

Case 4

Nandini Balkan, age 48, is admitted to an inpatient psychiatric facility due to acute depression with suicidal ideation.
Questions 13 to 15 refer to this case.

13. With clients who have suicidal ideation, when is the person least likely to act on their suicidal impulses?
    1. On admission to a psychiatric facility
    2. On discharge from a psychiatric facility
    3. When symptoms of the depression are most severe
    4. As the symptoms, motivation, and energy begin to improve

14. The nurse finds Ms. Balkan curled in a fetal position, crying. Through her tears, she says to the nurse, "I really can't go on. I just want to end it all. Please, won't you help me die?" What is the most appropriate response by the nurse?
    1. "I am sorry you are feeling so badly today. Perhaps you will feel better tomorrow."
    2. "I see that you are terribly unhappy today. But you know I cannot help you to die."
    3. "You are feeling very badly today. Would you like to tell me about it?"
    4. "This feeling is just temporary. Why would you want to die?"

15. Ms. Balkan is prescribed fluoxetine hydrochloride (Prozac). The nurse would advise Ms. Balkan of which of the following about this medication?
    1. It may take up to 4 weeks to notice any improvement.
    2. There is increased risk of suicide after therapy is well established.
    3. Anxiety and nervousness will likely decrease in about 2 weeks.
    4. Herbal preparations are safe to take with his medication.

Independent Questions

Questions 16 to 25 do not refer to a particular case.

16. A client is receiving high doses of haloperidol (Haldol). What adverse effects would require the nurse to consult with the physician about stopping the drug?
    1. The client complains of feeling sleepy and tired.
    2. The client's skin and eye conjunctiva display a yellowish tinge.
    3. The client reports dizziness on standing.
    4. The client displays extrapyramidal symptoms.

17. Which nursing interventions will be implemented for a client who is actively suicidal? **Select all that apply.**
    1. Maintain arm's-length, one-on-one direct observations at all times.
    2. Check all items brought by visitors and remove risk items.
    3. Use finger foods, plastic utensils, and drinkware; count utensils upon collection.
    4. Remove the client's eyeglasses to prevent self-injury.
    5. Interact with the client every 15 minutes.

18. Which characteristic fits the usual profile of an individual diagnosed with gender dysphoria?
    1. Aggression
    2. Persistent low mood
    3. Promiscuous
    4. Attention seeking

19. Which assessment questions would be most appropriate for the nurse to ask a client with possible obsessive-compulsive disorder? **Select all that apply.**
    1. "Are there certain social situations that cause you to feel especially uncomfortable?"
    2. "Are you hearing voices?"
    3. "Have you been a victim of a crime or seen someone badly injured or killed?"
    4. "Is it difficult to keep certain thoughts out of your awareness?"
    5. "Do you do certain things over and over again?"

20. The plan of care for a client in the manic state of bipolar disorder should include which of the following interventions? **Select all that apply.**
    1. Touch the client to provide reassurance.
    2. Invite the client to lead a community meeting.
    3. Provide a structured environment for the client.
    4. Ensure that the client's nutritional needs are met.
    5. Design activities that require the client's concentration.

21. Which of the following is an important consideration when conducting a culturally sensitive mental health assessment?
    1. Nurses must treat clients according to the established beliefs of their specific culture.
    2. Some cultures are not accepting of mental illnesses among their population.
    3. Nurses must facilitate verbal expressions of feelings in cultures in which this is not a common practice.
    4. Regardless of culture, all people react to adverse stressors with similar behaviours.

22. The nurse is unsure if an older female adult is manifesting symptoms of delirium or dementia. What question might the nurse ask the client's family?
    1. "Do you think your mother has Alzheimer's disease?"
    2. "How long has your mother shown confused thinking?"
    3. "Does your mother have any family members with a history of dementia?"
    4. "Has your mother ever been violent?"

23. A nurse plans care for an individual diagnosed with antisocial personality disorder. Which characteristic behaviours will the nurse expect? **Select all that apply.**
    1. Reclusive behaviour
    2. Impulsivity
    3. Perfectionism
    4. Aggression
    5. Clinginess
    6. Anxiety

24. A client is an inpatient at a psychiatric facility. The nurse accompanies the client to a local restaurant for coffee during their hospitalization. Is this an appropriate behaviour for the nurse?
    1. It is appropriate if it is part of the care plan.
    2. It is appropriate if the friendship is mutual and non-sexual.
    3. It is not appropriate as the client has a mental health diagnosis.
    4. It is not appropriate as it is never ethical for a nurse to be in a social situation with a client.

25. A child was placed in a foster home after being removed from abusive parents. The child is apprehensive and overreacts to environmental stimuli. The foster parents ask the nurse how to help the child. Which interventions should the nurse suggest? **Select all that apply.**
    1. Use a calm manner and low voice.

2. Maintain simplicity in the environment.
3. Avoid repetition in what is said to the child.
4. Minimize opportunities for exercise and play.
5. Explain and reinforce reality to avoid distortions.

REFERENCES

Alzheimer Society of Canada. (2022a). *Dementia numbers in Canada*. https://alzheimer.ca/en/about-dementia/what-dementia/dementia-numbers-canada

Alzheimer Society of Canada. (2022b). *Other types of dementia*. https://alzheimer.ca/en/about-dementia/other-types-dementia

Alzheimer Society of Canada. (2022c). *What is Alzheimer's disease?*. https://alzheimer.ca/en/about-dementia/what-alzheimers-disease

Alzheimer's Association. (2022). *What is dementia? Causes*. https://www.alz.org/alzheimers-dementia/what-is-dementia

American Psychiatric Association. (2022). In *Diagnostic and statistical manual of mental disorders* (5th ed.). DSM-5-TR.

Astle, B., & Duggleby, W. (2024). *Potter and Perry's Canadian fundamentals in nursing* (7th ed.). Elsevier.

Bard, B., MacMullin, E., Williamson, J., et al. (2022). *Morrison-Valfre's foundations of mental health care in Canada*. Elsevier.

Bulechek, G. M., Butcher, H. K., & Dochterman, J. M., et al. (Eds.). (2013). *Nursing interventions classification (NIC)* (6th ed.) Elsevier.

Canadian Council for Practical Nurse Regulators (CCPNR). (2013). *Code of ethics for licensed practical nurses in Canada*. http://www.clpna.com/wp-content/uploads/2013/02/doc_CCPNR_CLPNA_Code_of_Ethics.pdf

Canadian Mental Health Association (CMHA). (2021). *Fast facts about mental health and mental illness: Who is affected*. https://cmha.ca/brochure/fast-facts-about-mental-illness/

Canadian Mental Health Association (CMHA). (2022). *Schizophrenia: Who does it affect*. British Columbia Division. https://cmha.bc.ca/documents/schizophrenia-3/

Centre for Addiction and Mental Health (CAMH). (2022a). *Mental illness and addiction. Facts and statistics*. https://www.camh.ca/en/driving-change/the-crisis-is-real/mental-health-statistics#:~:text=In%20any%20given%20year%2C%201,Canadians%20experiences%20a%20mental%20illness

Centre for Addiction and Mental Health (CAMH). (2022b). *Suicide rate for people with Schizophrenia spectrum disorders over 20 times higher than the general population*. https://www.camh.ca/en/camh-news-and-stories/suicide-rate-for-people-with-schizophrenia-spectrum-disorders

College of Nurses of Ontario (CNO). (2022). *Protect the public: Legal obligations*. https://www.cno.org/en/protect-public/employers-nurses/reporting-guide/legal-obligations/#sexualabuse

Fazio, S., Pace, D., Flinner, J., et al. (2018). The fundamentals of person-centered care for individuals with dementia. *The Gerontologist, 58*(S1), S10–S19. https://doi.org/10.1093/geront/gnx122

Fazio, S., Pace, D., Maslow, K., et al. (2018). Alzheimer's Association dementia care practice recommendations. *The Gerontologist, 58*(S1), S1–S9. https://doi.org/10.1093/geront/gnx182

Government of Canada. (2020). *Suicide in Canada: Key statistics (infographic)*. https://www.canada.ca/en/public-health/services/publications/healthy-living/suicide-canada-key-statistics-infographic.html

Government of Canada. (2021a). *Canadian alcohol and drug surveys: Summary of the results for 2019*. https://www.canada.ca/en/health-canada/services/canadian-alcohol-drugs-survey/2019-summary.html

Government of Canada. (2021b). *Cannabis in Canada, get the facts. Cannabis and your health*. https://www.canada.ca/en/services/health/campaigns/cannabis/health-effects.html

Government of Canada. (2021c). *Government of Canada supports national guidelines on high-risk drinking and alcohol use*. https://www.canada.ca/en/health-canada/news/2021/01/government-of-canada-supports-first-national-guideline-on-high-risk-drinking-and-alcohol-use-disorder.html

Government of Canada. (2021d). *Sexually transmitted and blood borne infections (STBBI) prevention guide*. https://www.canada.ca/en/public-health/services/infectious-diseases/sexual-health-sexually-transmitted-infections/canadian-guidelines/sexually-transmitted-infections/canadian-guidelines-sexually-transmitted-infections-17.html#a1

Halter, M. J., Pollard, C. L., & Jakubec, S. L. (2019). *Varcarolis's Canadian psychiatric mental health nursing: A clinical approach* (2nd ed.). Elsevier Canada.

Johnson, C. (2017). Harm reduction in the addiction continuum of care. *Canadian Nurse, 113*(3), 36.

Pollard, C. L., & Jakubec, S. L. (2023). *Varcarolis's Canadian psychiatric mental health nursing: A clinical approach* (3rd ed.). Elsevier.

Public Safety Canada. (2022). *Annual national data report to inform trends and patterns in drug-impaired driving 2021*. https://www.publicsafety.gc.ca/cnt/rsrcs/pblctns/2021-did-fad/index-en.aspx

Registered Nurses Association of Ontario. (2016). *Clinical best practice guidelines: Delirium, dementia, and depression in older adults: Assessment and care* (2nd ed.). https://rnao.ca/sites/rnao-ca/files/bpg/RNAO_Delirium_Dementia_Depression_Older_Adults_Assessment_and_Care.pdf

Schizophrenia Society of Canada. (2022). *Education: Diagnosing schizophrenia*. https://schizophrenia.ca/learn-more-about-schizophrenia/#learn2

Sealock, K., Seneviratne, C., Lilley, L., et al. (2021). *Lilley's pharmacology for Canadian health care practice* (4th ed.). Elsevier.

Segal, D. (2021). *Common personality disorders*. https://www.webmd.com/mental-health/features/common-personality-disorders#091e9c5e82253977-1-2

Sorrentino, S. A., Remmert, L. N., & Wilk, M. J. (2022). *Sorrentino's Canadian textbook for the support worker* (5th ed.). Elsevier.

Statistics Canada. (2021a). *Survey on COVID-19 and mental health, February to May 2021*. https://www150.statcan.gc.ca/n1/daily-quotidien/210927/dq210927a-eng.htm

Statistics Canada. (2021b). *Looking back from 2020, how cannabis use, and related behaviours has changed*. https://www150.statcan.gc.ca/n1/pub/82-003-x/2021004/article/00001-eng.htm

Stuart, G. W. (2013). *Principles and practice of psychiatric nursing* (10th ed.). Mosby.

Szuhany, K., Malgaroli, M., Miron, C., et al. (2021). Prolonged grief disorder: Course, diagnosis, assessment, and treatment. *Focus: The Journal of Lifelong Learning in Psychiatry, 19*(2), 161–172. https://focus.psychiatryonline.org/doi/10.1176/appi.focus.20200052

WEBSITES

- **Canadian Mental Health Association (CMHA)** (http://www.cmha.ca): This site provides information on many specific mental health conditions and explores ways in which to promote good mental health. CMHA has offices across Canada and national mental health programs.
- **Centre for Addiction and Mental Health (CAMH)** (provideshttps://www.camh.ca/): This site provides information on clinical care, research, education, policy development and health promotion to help transform the lives of people affected by mental illness and addiction. CAMH is fully affiliated with the University of Toronto and is a Pan American Health Organization/World Health Organization Collaborating Centre.
- **Code of Ethics for Licensed Practical Nurses in Canada (CCPNR)** (https://ccpnr.ca/about/): This document describes the code of ethics and ethical obligations of all licensed/registered practical nurses. The CCPNR is a federation of provincial and territorial members who are identified in legislation, and responsible for the safety of the public through the regulation of licensed/registered practical nurses.
- **eMentalHealth.ca** (http://www.ementalhealth.ca/site/ontario/index.php?m=1&ID=26): This Canadian mental health site provides a resource directory and event calendar with information relevant to both consumers and care providers. The site is an anonymous and confidential source of mental health information.
- **Mental Health Commission of Canada** (http://www.mentalhealthcommission.ca): This organization's goal is to integrate mental health services in Canada. The site follows the progress of the commission in terms of its projects and policies.
- **Mood Disorders Society of Canada** (https://mdsc.ca): This site describes different mood and anxiety disorders and their diagnosis and treatment. It is primarily designed for clients and their families and provides links to resources that may be useful for health care providers.
- **Public Health Agency of Canada: Mental Health** (https://www.canada.ca/en/public-health/services/health-promotion/mental-health.html): This site provides information on mental health issues encountered by Canadians. It also provides access to a range of materials on mental health promotion relevant to both consumers and service providers.

13

End-of-Life Care

End-of-life care refers to issues that relate to death and dying, the concluding phase of the normal lifespan. Nurses have always cared for dying clients. Nurses must understand and honour each client's and family's unique experiences near impending death, addressing the physical, emotional, and spiritual dimensions of their experiences through holistic end-of-life care that requires more than just physical tasks and basic knowledge. This compassionate care is guided by what is most important to the client and family at this time in their lives, helping them toward a peaceful death. Working with clients at the end of their life requires nurses to have knowledge of grief and bereavement services. With this in mind, this chapter provides a condensed summary of many end-of-life care topics to help students build on their knowledge and skills to promote quality of life and therapeutic relationships, as well as death with dignity, as an important aspect of nursing care.

The three main goals of end-of-life care are as follows:
- Providing comfort and supportive care during the dying process
- Improving the quality of the remaining life
- Helping ensure a dignified death

To provide appropriate and responsive nursing care, nurses must apply both critical thinking qualities and intellectual and professional standards. Critical thinking qualities and standards help nurses to apply information in a relevant and therapeutic way for the client's benefit. Guiding standards examples include those of the dying person's bill of rights (Box 13.1), the code of ethics for licensed practical nurses in Canada, and practice standards. These all provide evidence-informed guidelines for a thorough assessment and providing humane, compassionate nursing care (Astle & Duggleby, 2024).

BOX 13.1 A Dying Person's Bill of Rights

- I have the right to be in control.
- I have the right to be treated as a living human being until I die.
- I have the right to have a sense of purpose.
- I have the right to be cared for by those who can maintain a sense of hopefulness.
- I have the right to express my feelings and emotions about my approaching death in my own way.
- I have the right to have a respected spirituality.
- I have the right to participate in decisions about my care.
- I have the right to expect continuing medical and nursing attention even though "cure" goals have been changed to "comfort" goals.
- I have the right not to die alone.
- I have the right to be comfortable.
- I have the right to have my questions answered honestly.
- I have the right not to be deceived.
- I have the right to have help from and for my family in accepting my death.
- I have the right to die in peace and dignity.
- I have the right to laugh and to be angry and sad.
- I have the right to retain my individuality and not to be judged for my decisions that may contrary to beliefs of others.
- I have the right to be cared for by caring, sensitive, knowledgeable people who will try to understand my needs and will be able to gain some satisfaction in helping me face my death.

Adapted from Astle, B., & Duggleby, W. (2024). Potter and Perry's *Canadian fundamentals of nursing* (7th ed., p. 438, Box 26.1). Elsevier. Adapted from Barbus, A. J. (1975). The dying person's bill of rights. *American Journal of Nursing, 75*(99); and from Hospice RN. (2003). *Patient's bill of rights.*

END OF LIFE

Pathophysiology

Death occurs when all vital organs and systems cease to function. There will be irreversible cessation of circulatory and respiratory function. The body gradually slows down until all functions end. Generally, respirations cease first, with the heart stopping within a few minutes. Hearing and touch are the last senses to disappear. The vision may blur, the eyes may sink and glaze over, the blink reflex is absent, and the eyelids may remain half open. The skin of the hands, arms, feet, and legs becomes mottled and feels cold and clammy. There may be cyanosis on the nose, nail beds, and knees. A wax-like appearance of the skin suggests that death is imminent. Initially, there may be an increase in respiration, followed by Cheyne-Stokes respirations slowing down to terminal gaps of breathing (apneic spells) until respirations cease. Urinary output will gradually decrease. The client may be incontinent of urine or be unable to urinate. The digestive functions slow, with a possible accumulation of gas, resulting in abdominal distension and nausea. The client may experience a loss of sphincter control. A bowel movement may occur before imminent death, at the time of death, or not at all. The client will gradually lose the ability to move, and the jaw will sag as facial muscle tone is lost. Swallowing can become difficult, as can maintaining body alignment. The gag reflex will be lost. The heart rate may increase and then slow with a weakening pulse. The cardiac rhythm often is irregular.

Brain death occurs when the cerebral cortex stops functioning or is irreversibly destroyed. The cerebral cortex is

TABLE 13.1	Summary of Models of Grief and Bereavement	
Kübler-Ross (1969)	**Bowlby (1980)**	**Worden's Four Tasks of Mourning (1991)**
Denial	Numbness	Accepting the reality of loss
Anger/bargaining	Yearning and searching	Working through the pain of grief
Depression	Disorganization and support	Adjusting to an environment without the decreased
Acceptance	Reorganization	Emotionally relocating the deceased and moving on with life

Adapted from Sorrentino, S., Remmert, L., & Wilk, M. (2022). *Sorrentino's Canadian textbook for the support worker* (5th ed., p. 1122, Table 47.2). Elsevier.

responsible for voluntary movements and actions as well as cognitive functioning.

Psychosocial manifestations include the following:

- Altered decision making
- Anxiety about unfinished business
- Decreased socialization
- Fear of loneliness
- Fear of pain
- Fear of meaninglessness of one's life
- Helplessness
- Life review
- Peacefulness
- Restlessness
- Saying goodbyes
- Unusual communication
- Visionlike experiences
- Withdrawal (Tyerman & Cobbett, 2023).

Often the client and family feel overwhelmed, helpless, powerless, and tired. Clients at the end of life need time to ponder their thoughts, review their lives, and express their feelings. The client's needs and wishes must be respected.

Grief

Grief is the emotional and behavioural response to loss. Grief is an individual experience and can be manifested in many ways. The intensity of grief is driven by the individual's personality, the nature of the relationship with the dying person, concurrent life crises, coping resources, and the availability of support systems. Table 13.1 is a summary of models of grief and bereavement.

Grief is a complex process in which an individual attempts to make sense of the loss. Not everyone experiences all stages of grief, nor do they progress through the stages in a linear fashion. *Bereavement* is a term used to describe an individual's response to the loss of a significant person. Bereavement may begin prior to the actual death. The normal grief process may take months to years. Goals for the grief process include the following:

- Resolving emotions
- Reflecting on the dying person
- Expressing feelings of loss and sadness
- Valuing what has been shared

Unresolved grief, also termed *dysfunctional grief* or *complicated bereavement*, refers to unhealthy or ineffective grief reactions. The grieving person is unable to shift their attention from the loss to the realities of everyday life. They become so preoccupied with the loss that they are unable to function effectively. Complicated grief is a persistent yearning for the deceased person that often occurs without signs of depression. The symptoms may appear to be similar to those of normal grieving, but they are associated with impaired psychological functioning and disturbances with sleep, mood, and self-esteem. The grieving individual may idealize and search for the lost person or relive past experiences. Some may blame themselves for the death and wish to die so they can join the loved one. They may become intolerant of others and socially isolate (Bard et al., 2022). *Dysfunctional grief* refers to prolonged grief disorder. Adaptive grief is a healthy response, in which the person comes to accept the reality of death. See Chapter 12, page 438, for further information on prolonged grief disorder.

THE EXPERIENCE OF GRIEF FOR NURSES

Many nurses work with dying clients on a regular basis. Caring for clients and their families at the end of life is both challenging and rewarding. A connection may develop between the client, family, and nurse. The nurse needs to be aware of how grief will personally affect them. The nurse may feel sorrow, frustration, and guilt. It is important as a health care provider to recognize one's own attitudes, values, and feelings regarding death and dying in order to provide therapeutic interventions for the client and family. The nurse should share in the grief experience, but they need to remember the primary goal is to provide support for the remaining loved ones. Many health care facilities offer support groups or interdisciplinary team debriefings for nurses and other health care providers who work with dying clients in an effort to help them with their own grief experiences. Some interventions the nurse may try in order to help themselves through the grieving experience include learning to appreciate the experiences of dying and grieving clients, understanding the steps of the grieving process, and identifying ways to cope with losses. Nurses need to have a support system outside of the workplace and to find ways to renew their own energy through hobbies, exercise programs, and proper sleep (Bard et al., 2022).

CULTURALLY COMPETENT CARE

Canada is a multicultural society; therefore, health care providers need to be aware of the variables that may affect end-of-life care. These variables include attitudes and beliefs, as well as cultural, religious, and family influences, and often the client's beliefs and attitudes are based on their culture and religion. It may be common in some cultures and religions to experience and express emotions that are subdued and intensively private, whereas for others the experience may involve the community with a public expression of grief. Also, it is common is some cultures to shield or protect the dying client from information about their illness (Tyerman & Cobbett, 2023). However, health care providers must be vigilant not to assume that a person from a certain culture will always hold a particular set of cultural, religious, and spiritual beliefs and values. Nursing assessment must be completed on an individual basis to avoid stereotyping. Cultural assessments should be implemented and completed as a part of the holistic approach to care.

DEVELOPMENTAL STAGES AND REACTIONS TO END OF LIFE

Refer to the Chapter 11 in the Pediatric section (pages 343) regarding children's reactions to hospitalization based on their different developmental stages.

Infants and Toddlers

There is currently no consensus as to whether this age group grieves or mourns. Children in this age group will perceive that the family is very upset and sad even though they do not understand why. Instead of understanding death, this age group is more affected by any changes in lifestyle. Encourage the family members to stay with the dying child and provide physical comfort, such as cuddling and rocking. Establishing routines and rituals with familiar objects will give a sense of security.

Preschoolers

Children at this stage are familiar with the term *death*, but they see it as a going away or possibly as sleep. Preschoolers take statements literally; when family members tell a preschooler that they have put their dog to sleep, the child may fear sleeping. Death is equated with sleep, and separation and is reversible.

- In the magical thinking of preschoolers, the dead can be alive and do things such as breathing, eating, and sleeping.
- Preschoolers who have a seriously ill sibling may feel that their own actions have caused the death and that the anger and sadness of the family are being directed at them; as a result, they may view the illness as a punishment for their actions and thoughts.
- Separation from parents is the biggest fear for this group, and the preschooler may feel that the parents will go away and not come back.
- Encourage the family to minimize separations, use concrete language, and be alert for a sense of punishment and guilt.

School-Aged Children

For these children, death is only temporary and is personified by figures such as the "bogeyman" or the devil. The child may think that death can be avoided by being good. There are degrees of being dead; therefore, people are not really dead; life and death are transposable. By 9 to 10 years of age, there is a deeper understanding that death is universal and irreversible, and the child will defy death and joke about it.

When the school-aged child or a sibling has a terminal illness, the child fears the unknown and loss of control, which leads to a decreased sense of security and self-confidence. Clear explanations of what is going to happen will give the child a sense of control and maintain their self-esteem. The child at this stage can appear to be uncooperative or rude but is trying verbally to gain some sense of control and power.

- Encourage the child to express their feelings and provide physical activities to relieve stress.
- Provide as much choice and control as possible.
- Encourage parents to honestly answer questions about dying rather than avoiding the subject or fabricating an unrealistic answer.
- Encourage parents to share their moments of sorrow with their children
- Provide preparation for funeral and memorial services prior to death.

Adolescence

Adolescents normally respond with appropriate grief and react to death with an almost adult understanding. This age group is starting to look for the meaning in death and religious meaning, such as life after death.

- Adolescents are unable to prioritize their losses; therefore, the loss of a friend may be just as upsetting as the loss of a parent.
- A loss due to death can interfere with the search for identity, and physical changes in the body of a terminally ill adolescent can be more devastating than the actual illness.
- The ill adolescent is often isolated from their peer group; encourage contact and communication with friends because the child may be unable to communicate with their parents and get support. Peer support groups can be helpful.
- The nurse can facilitate communication between these groups and provide as much independence and control as possible.
- The nurse should their questions honestly, treating them as mature individuals and respecting their needs for privacy, solitude, and personal expressions of emotions

Adulthood

- Young adults may not relate to death unless forced to. Individuals in this age group typically expect to have a long life ahead of them and consequently do not think about death.
- People in middle adulthood report more fear of death than those in early and late adulthood. They may perhaps be caring for both children and older parents. They may feel anxiety about leaving them to care for themselves. They often have to deal with the death of parents.

Older Persons

- As people grow older, they begin to lose family and friends and must begin to face their own mortality.
- Nurses should not assume that older persons are comfortable with the idea of death.
- Coming to terms with death is often difficult and nurses play a key role in assisting the older client through the grieving process (Bard et al., 2022).

CLINICAL MANIFESTATIONS FOR CHILDREN

When evaluating a child's psychological state in relation to death and dying, assessment findings usually take into consideration the following:
- The developmental stage of the child
- Cultural and spiritual concerns
- Socioeconomic factors
- Support network and family connections
- Grief manifestations
- Unfinished business between parents and child
- Anticipatory grieving
- Dysfunctional grieving (Hockenberry et al., 2022)

Nursing Considerations for Children

The end of life is a very sensitive topic. The child and the family need guidance in understanding the process of death and dying and to maintain as healthy a grieving process as possible.

Nursing considerations for end of life are as follows:
- Encourage discussion of the child's past experiences with death and dying.
- Determine and develop strategies to help decrease anxiety.
- Determine comfort measures and objects and promote a sense of security.
- Encourage the use of the child's and family's rituals, routines, and customs.
- Provide a member of the clergy if the child and the family would like the referral.
- Encourage the child and the family to verbalize feelings and concerns.
- Refer the family to social services or community resources if the family needs financial assistance.
- Organize and help activate support systems.
- Refer the family to a grief counsellor if needed (Hockenberry et al., 2022).

ADVANCE DIRECTIVES

In Canada, it is recognized that mentally competent people have the right to make decisions regarding their health care, including the right to request or refuse life-sustaining treatment (Tyerman & Cobbett, 2023). Advance directives (or living will) give information about future health care and treatments and personal care. Health care includes all medical treatment: diagnostic, therapeutic, preventive and palliative. The advance directive specifies whether the client would like to die without heroic or extraordinary measures.

Advance directives are an important form of communication when the client is unable to communicate verbally.

"Most advance directives have a dual function:
1. They allow a person to appoint a representative (proxy) to make medical care treatment and personal care decisions.
2. They give written instructions about medical care and treatment and personal care" (Sorrentino et al., 2022, p. 1118).

The power of attorney for personal care will list the person(s) who may make health care decisions on the client's behalf should the client become unable to make informed decisions on their own (in which case a substitute decision maker [proxy] is chosen).

Clients do have the right to refuse life-sustaining measures. Advance care planning can help guide end-of-life care to ensure clients' wishes are honoured. If a do not resuscitate (DNR) order is in place, cardiopulmonary resuscitation (CPR) will not be attempted, but the DNR does not preclude the use of other forms of treatment. Another term that is being used to replace DNR or no code is *allow natural death* (AND). In this case, the client will still receive pain control and symptom management but no resuscitative treatment. Planning requires ongoing, open communication and documentation among the client, family, and health care providers. It can be initiated at any time along the client's health continuum. Clients can revise their advance directives at any time (Canadian Hospice Palliative Care Association [CHPCA], 2022a). Advance directives are still evolving in terms of their legal status, and there are some differences across the provinces and territories. Provincial and territorial legislation is not uniform across Canada, so each jurisdiction has its own guidelines related to substitute decision-making and instructional directives for treatment and care. Nurses need to know the legalities and regulations associated with advance directives as well as the nursing role responsibilities for their individual jurisdictions.

Ethical issues may arise regarding pain relief, in particular with clients who are terminally ill. According to the principle of nonmaleficence, the nurse is expected to prevent or reduce harm to the client and to provide adequate pain control to alleviate suffering in the terminally ill, even if a secondary effect of pain control is an earlier death. Medical assistance in dying (MAiD) is now legal in Canada for those who meet eligibility requirements.

One of the most important roles that nurses have is to work with and support clients and families as they make difficult end-of-life decisions. This is a complex issue that presents many legal and ethical dilemmas as well as nursing practice implications.

MEDICAL ASSISTANCE IN DYING (MAiD)

Nurses continue to play an important role in providing person-centred end-of-life care in palliative care and natural death, and MAiD nurses provide much of the care for clients who are at the end of their life.

The Canadian Nurses Association (CNA) (2022) developed a framework to help nurses understand changes in the federal law that now allows MAiD in Canada under certain circumstances and within defined regulatory standards. Bill C-14 came into effect in 2016 and amended the *Criminal Code* in relation to MAiD. Under Bill C-14, an individual who meets all the eligibility requirements may receive MAiD. See Box 13.2 for eligibility criteria for MAiD.

"The law developed safeguards for the clients and offers protection to health care providers who provide medical assistance in dying, along with people who assist in the process in accordance to the law" (CNA, 2017, p. 11). Section 241.1 of the act defines MAiD as follows:

(a) *the administering by a medical practitioner or nurse practitioner of a substance to a person, at their request, that causes their death; or*

(b) *the prescribing or providing by a medical practitioner or nurse practitioner of a substance to a person, at their request, so that they may self-administer the substance and in doing so cause their own death.* (CNA, 2017, p.11)

The law defines a client as having a grievous and irremediable medical condition only if:

- They have a serious and incurable illness, disease, or disability.
- They are in an advanced state of irreversible decline in capability. The loss of capability can be:
  1. either sudden or gradual
  2. ongoing or stabilized.
- The illness, disease, disability, or state of decline causes them enduring physical or psychological suffering that is intolerable to them and cannot be relieved under conditions that they consider acceptable (Government of Canada, 2022).

BOX 13.2   Who Is Eligible for Medical Assistance in Dying?

The criteria for determining eligibility apply whether natural death is reasonably foreseeable or not. In order to be eligible for medical assistance in dying, a person must meet **all** of the following criteria:

- The person must be eligible for health services funded by the federal government, or a province or territory.
- Generally, visitors to Canada are not eligible for medical assistance in dying.
- The person must be at least 18 years old and mentally competent. This means being capable of making health care decisions for themselves.
- The person has a grievous and irremediable medical condition.
- The person has made a voluntary request for medical assistance in dying that is not the result of outside pressure or influence.
- The person has given informed consent to receive medical assistance in dying after they were informed.

*Medical assistance in dying excludes cases where mental illness is the **only** underlying medical condition. This exclusion will remain in effect until March 17, 2023 when the government reviews this criteria with an expert panel.

The following outlines the various stages involved in MAiD:

Stage 1: Determine eligibility

Stage 2: Ensure safeguards are met

Stage 3: Obtain consent

Stage 4: Provide MAiD, either by a nurse practitioner (NP) or physician or self-administered by the client

NPs who may be providing MAiD (and RNs and RPNs or LPNs who may be supporting the process) must have a comprehensive understanding of these stages, including the risks, eligibility criteria, safeguards, and processes (College of Nurses of Ontario [CNO], 2021). The CNA framework outlines resources for all nurses involved in end-of-life care decision making and care around MAiD (CNA, 2017, p. 8). It is important for nurses to refer to the associated policies and guidelines in their jurisdiction and consult with their regulatory body and employer for specific instructions. Policies must be consistent with the law. Before assisting with MAiD, the nurse should confirm that the legal conditions for MAiD have been established.

Nurses can provide nursing care and skills such as the insertion of an intravenous (IV) line that will deliver the medication that will cause death of the client. Nurses require a doctor's order for the IV insertion. An NP or a physician is the only person who can administer any required medications for MAiD. They cannot delegate any of their roles to the nurse.

Nurses can assist in the education of clients regarding MAiD. When providing information to a client or family on MAiD, the nurse must ensure that they do not advise or persuade the client in any way to choose MAiD. The decision to take medication to end the client's life must be the client's own decision, with no encouragement or counselling from the nurse.

The nurse has the right to conscientiously object to participate in MAiD and transfer the care to another nurse who is agreeable to providing care for the client. A conscientious objector is to provide holistic nursing care to the client that is not connected to MAiD until a replacement nurse is found. At no time is the nurse to discuss their own personal beliefs or feelings regarding MAiD with the client.

Determining the eligibility of a client for MAiD is not the responsibility of a nurse. This falls under the scope of practice of the NP or physician along with obtaining informed consent. However, nurses do provide bereavement care to the family of the person receiving MAiD (CNA, 2017, pp. 17–18).

Caring for the palliative population requires palliative education to provide high-quality palliative care and adequate pain control. Nurses help decrease suffering and support a dignified and peaceful death. They make an important contribution to the health care team in the provision of palliative and end-of-life care. As well, they encompass the ethical principles of the Canadian Council for Practical Nurse Regulators (CCPNR) code of ethics so that they understand their role and responsibility when providing safe, competent, and ethical end-of-life care to clients undergoing MAiD.

PALLIATIVE CARE

Palliative care is supportive care or treatment that relieves or reduces the severity of symptoms rather than providing a cure. The CHPCA has defined palliative care as providing active, compassionate, and supportive care of the dying (CHPCA, 2022b). It is a philosophy of total care with the aim of relieving suffering, emphasizing dignity, and improving the quality of living and dying, from diagnosis to the end of life and bereavement.

Palliative care is intended to improve the quality of life of the client and their family as they manage a life-threatening illness, through identification and relief of suffering as well as through support (World Health Organization [WHO], 2020). Palliative care strives to remain sensitive to personal, cultural, and religious values, beliefs, and practices. The therapies provided during palliative care will change over the course of the illness according to the client's and family's concerns, treatment priorities, and goals of care. See Box 13.3 for further details on the goals of palliative care. Care is provided by a multidisciplinary team that consists of many care providers, such as nurses, physicians, social workers, chaplains, volunteers, pharmacists, physiotherapists, occupational therapists, and alternative therapists, such as massage therapists. Palliative care occurs in many settings, including hospitals, long-term care facilities, hospices, and clients' homes. Client and family needs are the focus of any interventions.

In Canada, the term *hospice palliative care* refers to the convergence of hospice and palliative care. Hospices exist to provide support and care for persons in the last phases of incurable diseases. This care is aimed at relief of suffering and improving the quality of life for these individuals. There are over 600 hospices in Canada, and they are organized under a variety of models. There are free-standing hospices, home hospice care, long-term care settings, and hospital-based palliative care units. Hospices are run by a medically supervised interdisciplinary team of professionals and volunteers, the hospice nurse being an integral part of this team. The nurse's role in hospice care is to meet the primary wishes of the dying client and to be amenable to the individual desires of each client. Nurses support a client's choice in maintaining comfort and dignity. When options are complicated by family needs, hospice professionals will try to work with the client's wishes (Astle & Duggleby, 2024). The hospice nurse plays a key role in educating the client and family on pain and symptom management. Grief support is incorporated into the plan of care for the family members and significant others during the illness and after the client's death.

The decision to begin hospice care is sometimes difficult due to a lack of information about hospice palliative care, difficulty in accessing palliative care services, the attitudes of health care providers who sometimes regard palliation as a personal failure, and the fact that clients and families may regard palliative care as "giving up." Coordination of palliative care focuses on the needs of the client and their family and significant others, as well as on education, counselling, advocacy, and support. The goals of palliative care focus on ensuring that the client is able to express and share their feelings with others and that comfort measures and physical maintenance care are provided during the last stages of life. Figure 13.1 shows how, over the course of an illness, the blend of therapies will vary, depending on the client's and family issues, their goals of care, and treatment priorities.

An *integrated palliative approach to care* or *community-integrated palliative* care involves meeting a person's and family's holistic needs at all stages of a life-limiting illness, not just at the end of life. This includes physical, psychosocial, and spiritual care along with the usual medical care. It is a shared model of care, one that shifts hospice palliative care from being a specialized service to a more generalized integrated service available to people with life-limiting conditions, regardless of where they live and receive care (Tyerman & Cobbett, 2023). It reinforces the client's autonomy and the right to be actively involved in their own care and strives to give the client and family greater sense of control. It helps to enhance their quality of life throughout the course of their illness or the process of aging. It provides key aspects of palliative care at appropriate times during the client's illness. As the client's illness progresses, it includes regular opportunities to review the person's goals and plan of care and referrals, if required, to expert palliative care services (Canadian Society of Palliative Care Physicians, 2022). In an effort to develop a national standard of palliative care, the CHPCA has produced "The Way Forward" as a national vision. Table 13.2 examines the success factors for an integrated palliative approach to care.

Education of the palliative client and family involves providing ongoing information about the disease, the dying process, the care needed and offered, coping strategies, and barriers to grief.

Nursing Considerations for Palliative Care

Nursing considerations for the dying client focus on comfort and improving the quality of life. Psychosocial care and physical care are interrelated for both the dying client and the family (Tyerman & Cobbett, 2023). Anxiety is a feeling of uneasiness caused by a source that is not easily identified. Anxiety in clients at the end of life is frequently related to fear. Anxiety and depression may be exhibited during the end-of-life period and can be caused by pain that is not well

---

BOX 13.3 Goals of Palliative Care

- Provide relief of symptoms, including pain.
- Regard dying as a normal process.
- Affirm life and neither hasten nor postpone death.
- Support holistic client care and enhance quality of life.
- Offer support to clients to live as actively as possible until death.
- Offer support to the family during the client's illness and in their own bereavement.

From Tyerman, J., & Cobbett, S. L. (2023). *Lewis's medical-surgical nursing in Canada: Assessment and management of clinical problems* (5th Cdn. ed., p. 202, Table 13-1). Elsevier. Reprinted from *Cancer*, WHO, WHO Definition of Palliative Care, Copyright 2018.

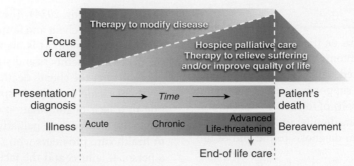

Fig. 13. 1 The role of hospice palliative care during illness. (From Lewis, S. M., Bucher, L., Heitkemper, M., Harding, M., Barry, M., Lok, J., Tyerman, J., Goldsworthy, S., Kwong, J., & Roberts, D. [2019]. *Medical-surgical nursing in Canada: Assessment and management of clinical problems* [4th Canadian. ed., p. 207, Figure 13.2]. Elsevier Canada. Source: Canadian Hospice Palliative Care Association. [2010]. *A model to guide hospice palliative care.* http://www.chpca.net/media/319547/norms-of-practice-eng-web.pdf).

TABLE 13. 2 **Success Factors for an Integrated Palliative Approach to Care**
Vision
• Commitment to person-centred care
• Focus on building capacity in the community
• Focus on changing organizational structure
• Senior management support
People
• Dedicated coordinators
• Interprofessional teams
• Strong role of and more support for family physicians
• Support for providers in long-term care facilities
• Key roles for nurses
• Relationships, partnerships, and networks
Delivery of Care
• Integration of primary, secondary, and tertiary care
• Cultural sensitivity
• Single access point and case management
• Round-the-clock community support and care
• Advance care planning
Supportive Tools
• Common frameworks, standards, and assessment tools
• Flexible approaches to education
• Shared records
• Research, evaluation, and quality improvement

From Tyerman, J., & Cobbett, S. L. (2023). *Lewis's medical-surgical nursing in Canada: Assessment and management of clinical problems* (5th Cdn. ed., p. 202, Table 13-02). Elsevier. Source: Canadian Hospice Palliative Care Association. (2013). *Innovative models of integrated hospice palliative care. The way forward initiative: An integrated approach to care.* http://www.hpcintegration.ca/media/40546/TWF-innovative-models-report-Eng-webfinal-2.pdf

controlled, psychosocial factors related to the disease process or impending death, altered physiological states, or the effects of medications. Encouragement, support, and education can help decrease some of the anxiety. Pharmacological and non-pharmacological measures may also be used.

Fear is a typical feeling for palliative clients. Fear of pain, loneliness and abandonment, and meaninglessness are common fears. Clients and families fear pain as they often associate death with pain. There is no physiological evidence that death is always painful. Psychologically, pain may occur based on anxieties. Terminally ill clients should receive enough analgesic so that they are comfortable. They should not be in physical pain, nor should they be deprived of the ability to interact with others.

There can be a real fear of loneliness and abandonment if the clients fear their loved ones cannot cope and will abandon them. Palliative clients appreciate loved ones comforting and supporting them at this stage. Holding hands, touching, and listening are greatly valued. Simply providing companionship allows the dying person a sense of security.

Fear of meaninglessness often leads palliative clients to review their lives, often examining their intentions and actions. Some clients may express regret, but many clients are able to recognize the value of their lives. Nurses should encourage clients and families to identify the positive qualities of the client's life. Nurses should also respect and accept practices and rituals associated with the client's life review without being judgemental.

Physical care centres around physiological and safety needs. Symptom management is key. The palliative client deserves the same care as people who are expected to recover from their illnesses. See Table 13.3 for the nursing management of physical care at the end of life.

Palliative Sedation

Strict guidelines are followed to intentionally produce sedation in order to relieve intractable symptoms in the last days of a client's life. MAiD should not be confused with palliative sedation. Palliative sedation is an infrequent and extraordinary intervention that requires interprofessional expertise. The goal of palliative sedation is to control unmanageable symptoms and suffering, not to shorten life or to hasten death. It is a nurse's ethical obligation to promote the relief of suffering, and it may include appropriate administration of medication (e.g., opioids) that have the potential to cause

TABLE 13.3   Nursing Management: Physical Care at the End of Life

Characteristic	Nursing Management
Pain • Pain may be a major symptom associated with terminal illness and is the most feared. • Pain can be acute or chronic. • Possible causes of bone pain: metastases, fractures, arthritis, and immobility • Physical and emotional irritations can aggravate pain.	• Assess pain thoroughly and regularly to determine the quality, intensity, location, and pattern, as well as the contributing and relieving factors. • Minimize possible irritants such as skin irritations from moisture, heat or cold, or pressure. • Administer medications around the clock in a timely manner and on a regular basis. • Provide complementary and alternative therapies, such as guided imagery, massage, acupressure, heat and cold, therapeutic touch, distraction, and relaxation techniques, as needed. • Evaluate the effectiveness of pain relief measures frequently to ensure that the client is on an adequate drug regimen. • Do not delay or deny pain relief measures to a terminally ill client.
Delirium • Delirium is characterized by confusion, disorientation, restlessness, clouding of consciousness, incoherence, fear, anxiety, excitement, and often hallucinations. • It may be misidentified as depression, psychosis, anger, or anxiety. • The use of opioids, corticosteroids, or both (as well as many other medications) in end-of-life care may cause delirium, or their withdrawal effects • The underlying disease process may contribute to delirium. • It is generally considered a reversible process.	• Perform a thorough assessment for reversible causes of delirium, including pain, constipation, and urinary retention. • Provide a room that is quiet, well lit, and familiar to reduce the effects of delirium. • Reorient the dying client to person, place, and time with each encounter. • Administer ordered benzodiazepines, sedatives, as needed. • Stay physically close to a frightened client. Reassure in a calm, soft voice with touch and slow stroking of the skin. • Provide family with emotional support and encouragement in their efforts to cope with the behaviours associated with delirium.
Anxiety or Restlessness • This may occur as death approaches and cerebral metabolism slows. • May occur with tachypnea, dyspnea or sweating.	• Assess for previous anxiety disorder. • Assess for spiritual distress or concerns related to death as causes for restlessness and agitation. • Do not restrain. • Use soothing music and slow, soft touch and calm, soft voice. • Limit the number of persons at the bedside. • Limit other stimuli and activity.
Dysphagia • This may occur because of extreme weakness and changes in level of consciousness. • Difficulty swallowing • Aspiration of liquids or solids, or both • Drooling/inability to swallow secretions	• Identify the least invasive alternative routes of administration for medications needed for symptom management. • If necessary, use alternative (rectal, buccal, transdermal) medication routes. • Modify diet as tolerated/desired (soft, pureed, chopped meats). • Suction orally as needed. • Hand feed small meals. • Elevate the client's head for meals and for at least 30 minutes after. • Discontinue nonessential medications. • Discuss risk of aspiration with the client/family.
Dehydration • Dehydration may occur during the last days of life, but hunger and thirst are rare. • As the end of life approaches, clients tend to take in less food and fluid.	• Assess the condition of mucous membranes frequently to prevent excessive dryness, which can lead to discomfort. • Maintain complete, regular oral care to provide for comfort and hydration of mucous membranes. • Encourage the consumption of ice chips and sips of fluids or use moist cloths to provide moisture to the mouth. • Use moist cloths and swabs for unconscious clients to avoid aspiration. • Apply lubricant to the lips and oral mucous membranes as needed • Do not force the client to eat or drink. • Reassure the family that cessation of food and fluid intake is a natural part of the process of dying.

Continued

TABLE 13.3 Nursing Management: Physical Care at the End of Life—cont'd

Characteristic	Nursing Management
Dyspnea • This is a subjective symptom, often accompanied by anxiety and the fear of suffocation. • An underlying disease process can exacerbate dyspnea. • Progressive difficulty with coughing and expectorating secretions	• Assess respiratory status regularly. • Elevate the head or position the client on one side to improve chest expansion. • Use a fan or air conditioner to facilitate the movement of cool air. Teach and encourage the use of pursed-lip breathing. • Administer supplemental oxygen as ordered. • Suction as necessary to remove accumulation of mucus from the airways. Suction cautiously when a client is in the terminal phase. • Administer expectorant as ordered.
Pooling of Secretions • Coughing and expelling secretions become difficult.	• Perform gentle oropharyngeal suctioning as needed to remove accumulated secretions. • Position the client on their side supported with pillows with head down, or in a semiprone position if there are excessive secretions. • Use anticholinergic medications (scopolamine or glycopyrrolate [Robinul]) as ordered.
Weakness and Fatigue • Expected at the end of life • Exacerbated by metabolic demands related to disease process	• Assess the client's tolerance for activities. • Time nursing interventions to conserve the client's energy. • Help the client to identify and complete valued or desired activities. • Provide support as needed to maintain client's positions in a bed or chair. • Provide frequent rest periods for the client.
Myoclonus • This is mild to severe jerking or twitching, which is sometimes associated with the use of large doses of opioids. • Clients may complain of involuntary twitching of the upper and lower extremities.	• Assess for the initial onset and duration of this effect and any discomfort or distress experienced by the client. • If myoclonus is distressing or becoming more severe, discuss possible drug therapy modifications with the health care provider. • Changes in opioid medication may alleviate or decrease myoclonus.
Skin Breakdown • Skin integrity is difficult to maintain at the end of life. • Immobility, urinary and bowel incontinence, dry skin, nutritional deficits, anemia, friction, and shearing forces lead to a high risk for skin breakdown. • Disease and other processes may impair skin integrity. • As death approaches, circulation to the extremities decreases, and they become cool, mottled, and cyanotic.	• Assess the skin for signs of breakdown. • Implement protocols to prevent skin breakdown by controlling drainage and odour and keeping the skin and any wound areas clean and dry. • Perform wound assessments as needed. • Follow appropriate nursing management protocol for dressing wounds. • Consider the use of special pressure-relieving air mattresses. • Follow appropriate nursing management protocol for a client who is immobile but consider realistic outcomes of skin integrity in relation to maintenance of comfort. • Follow appropriate nursing management to prevent skin irritations and breakdown from urinary and bowel incontinence. • Use blankets to provide warmth; never apply heat. • Prevent the effects of shearing forces.
Bowel Patterns • Constipation can be caused by immobility, the use of opioid medications, depression, a lack of fibre in the diet, and dehydration. • Diarrhea may occur as muscles relax or from a fecal impaction related to immobility, the use of opioids, or both.	• Assess bowel function. • Assess for and remove fecal impactions. • Encourage movement and physical activities as tolerated. • Encourage fibre in the diet if appropriate. • Encourage fluids if appropriate. • Use suppositories, laxatives, or enemas if ordered. • Assess client for confusion, agitation, restlessness, and pain, which may be a sign of constipation.

TABLE 13.3 Nursing Management: Physical Care at the End of Life—cont'd

Characteristic	Nursing Management
Urinary Incontinence • May result from disease progression or changes in the level of consciousness • Relaxation of perineal muscles soon before death	• Assess urinary function • Use absorbent pads for urinary incontinence • Follow appropriate nursing protocol for the consideration and use of in-dwelling or external catheters • Follow appropriate nursing management to prevent skin irritation and breakdown from urinary incontinence.

Anorexia, Nausea, and Vomiting
• They may be caused by complications of the disease process.
• Medications may contribute to nausea.
• Constipation, impaction, and bowel obstruction can cause anorexia, nausea, and vomiting.
	• Assess the client for complaints of nausea, vomiting, or both.
	• Assess possible contributing causes for nausea or vomiting.
	• Have family members provide the client's favourite foods.
	• Discuss modifications to the drug regimen with the health care provider.
	• Provide antiemetics before meals if ordered.
	• Offer and provide frequent meals with small portions of favourite foods.
	• Provide frequent mouth care, especially if the client has vomited.
	• Ensure uninterrupted mealtimes.
	  • If ordered, administer medications (e.g., megestrol, corticosteroids) to increase appetite.
	  • Teach family that appetite naturally decreases at the end of life.

Candidiasis • White, cottage cheese-like oral plaques • Fungal overgrowth in the mouth as a result of chemotherapy, immunosuppression, or both	• Administer oral antifungal nystatin if ordered. • Clean dentures and other dental appliances to prevent re-infection. • Provide oral hygiene and use a soft toothbrush.

Adapted from Tyerman, J., & Cobbett, S. L. (2023). *Lewis's medical-surgical nursing in Canada: Assessment and management of clinical problems* (5th Cdn. ed., p. 211, Table 13-11). Elsevier.

sedation. Careful titration of medication, which is based on the client's response, can improve the likelihood that the client will receive the correct proportion of medication and minimize the potential for harm. Refer to Chapter 7, page 21 for information on pain and comfort.

Using opioid medications for symptom management at the end of life is often misunderstood and feared by clients, families, and some health care providers. This fear can lead to the client not receiving adequate medication, which can lead to physical and emotional suffering from uncontrolled pain management. This is an opportunity for the nurse to educate the client and family about physical dependence on and tolerance of medications. A terminally ill client should not be concerned with physical dependence when the goal of treatment is comfort until death (Tyerman & Cobbett, 2023).

Therapeutic Communication

Therapeutic communication is an important nursing intervention that includes the essential components of empathy and active listening. Clients and their families should be allowed time to express their thoughts and feelings. Sometimes unusual communication by the client may take place at the end of life. The client's speech may be confused, disoriented, or garbled. The client may speak with family or friends who have predeceased them. At other times, the client may leave instructions for family members or speak of projects that have to be completed. Active careful listening allows identification of specific

patterns in the client's communication and decreases the risk for inappropriate labelling of behaviours.

The resolution of grief is the primary focus of interventions for anticipatory and dysfunctional grief. Specific interventions for both types of grief are similar and include providing an environment that allows the client to express their feelings. Clients should be free to express feelings of anger, fear, or guilt without others' judgement. Both the client and the family need to understand that the grief reaction is normal. The client's privacy should be respected. Honesty in answering questions and giving information is essential. Families and clients need encouragement to continue their usual activities as much as possible. Planning for the future or for the funeral may be needed based on the client's or family's coping abilities. Anger must be recognized as a normal response to dying. When a client or family member acts out in anger, the nurse must not react on a personal level. Nurses need to encourage realistic hope within the limits of the situation. A sense of power can be restored for the client by encouraging them to identify goals and make decisions pertaining to their own care.

Organ and Tissue Donation

Legally competent individuals who are 16 years of age and older may choose organ and tissue donation. Only clients who have sustained a nonrecoverable injury and are on life support may donate organs. However, all clients have the potential to donate tissue (e.g., eyes, bones, heart valves, and skin) after death (Tyerman & Cobbett, 2023). Nurses should be aware of ethical and legal issues and the client's wishes. Advance directives and organ donor information should be located in the client's medical record and identified on that record or in the nursing care plan. It is essential that nurses be familiar with provincial or territorial laws, as well as agency regulations (Tyerman & Cobbett, 2023).

Care of the Body

After the client is pronounced dead, the nurse prepares or delegates preparation of the body for immediate viewing by the family. Considerations when preparing the body include cultural customs, provincial and territorial laws, and agency policies and procedures. Box 13.4 summarizes the nurses' and physicians' responsibilities for care of the body after death. It is important to care for the client's body with dignity and sensitivity and in a manner consistent with the client's religious and cultural beliefs. The body undergoes many physical changes after death. Care must be provided as soon as possible to prevent tissue damage or disfigurement of body parts (Astle & Duggleby, 2024). Support of the family is important at the time of the client's death. After the death, it is acceptable to lower the head of the bed, to straighten the body, and attempt to gently close the eyes and mouth. Before the family views the body, it is beneficial for the nurse to explain to the family what they

---

BOX 13.4   Procedural Guidelines: Care of the Body After Death

Delegation Considerations

Care of the body after death can be delegated to unregulated care providers except in cases of organ and tissue donation. Check agency policy for which staff member is authorized to remove any invasive tubes or catheters.

Equipment

Bath towels, wash cloths, wash basins, scissors, shroud kit with name tags, bed linen, room deodorizer, documentation forms

Procedure

1. Physicians must complete the death certificate: causes of death, time when death was pronounced, therapy used, and actions taken. In some provinces, nurses may pronounce the death but may not complete the death certificate. (This may not be the policy in all agencies: follow your agency's policy).
2. Physicians may request an autopsy, especially for deaths under unusual circumstances.
3. Trained staff members offer survivors the option of donating organs or tissue of the deceased, personal, religious, and cultural needs should be included during this process.
4. Nurses work with sensitivity to preserve the client's and family's dignity.
   a. Check orders for any specimens or special orders needed by the physician.
   b. Make arrangements for staff, spiritual advisor, or others to stay with the family while the body is being prepared for viewing, find out whether other survivors have special requests for viewing (e.g., shaving, special gown, Bible in hand, rosary at bedside).
   c. Before shaving a client: Determine whether the family wishes the client unshaven if it is a custom to wear a beard. Determine whether client's religion or culture has a preference regarding facial hair.
   d. Remove all equipment, tubes, supplies, and dirty linen according to agency protocol. Exceptions to this process include organ donation (leave support systems in place), and unexpected sudden or unexpected deaths that necessitate coroner involvement or investigation (leave tubings and lines in situ but cut them near the body and clamp them).

   e. Cleanse the body thoroughly, apply clean sheets, and remove all trash from the room.
   f. Brush and comb the client's hair. Apply any personal hairpiece.
   g. Position according to protocol: The eyes should be closed by gently holding the client's eyelids closed for a few minutes; dentures should be in the client's mouth to maintain facial alignment.
   h. Cover the body with a clean sheet up to the chin with arms outside covers if possible.
   i. Lower the lighting and spray a deodorizer, if possible, to remove unpleasant odours.
   j. Give the family the option to view or not to view the dead body; clarify that either option is acceptable.
   k. If family members choose to view the dead body, go with them.
5. Encourage the family to say goodbye through touch and talk.
   m. Do not rush the goodbye process. Once the family is more comfortable, ask if they would like to be left alone. Remind them they call you if needed.
   n. Clarify which personal belongings should stay with the body and who will take personal items: documentation requires both a descriptor of the objects (e.g., rings, jewellery, electronics) and the name of each person who received them, with the time and date.
   o. Do not discard items found after the family is gone; call the family and tell them what was found and ask who might pick them up. Descriptions of the articles help the client's family make decisions accordingly.
   p. Apply name tags according to protocol, such as on the wrist, on the right big toe, or outside the shroud.
   q. Complete documentation in the nursing notes. Documents will vary, depending on the agency.
   r. Remain sensitive to other hospitalized clients or visitors when transporting the body, such as covering the body with a clean sheet, temporarily and gently closing doors to clients' rooms and watching to avoid visitors when moving the body to another part of the hospital or to the exit for the funeral home.
   s. Follow the protocol and policies to meet all legal requirements in caring for the body.

From Astle, B., & Duggleby, W. (2024). Potter and Perry's. *Canadian fundamentals of nursing* (7th ed., p. 450, Box 26.9). Elsevier.

may expect to see. Typically, a deceased person has a peaceful expression (as facial muscles have relaxed); however, the body feels cool to touch and appears greyish white. Within several hours, the body begins to stiffen as rigor mortis sets in. The body may have areas of pooled blood that appears bruised. The eyes and mouth may be partially open, but the mucous membranes will appear dry. This appearance may be difficult for some family members to observe (Astle & Duggleby, 2024).

PRACTICE QUESTIONS

Case 1

Mrs. Lin, aged 65, has end-stage breast cancer with metastases to her lungs and brain. Her family and the palliative care team are caring for her at home.

Questions 1 to 3 refer to this case.

1. Which of the following best describes palliative care for Mrs. Lin?
   1. Mrs. Lin will be kept comfortable and free from pain.
   2. Enteral feeds will be started to prevent starvation and malnutrition.
   3. Interventions will be focused only on the needs of Mrs. Lin.
   4. Services by the team terminate at the death of Mrs. Lin.

2. Mrs. Lin's daughter tells the nurse, "Mother doesn't really respond any more when I visit. I don't think she knows that I am here." Which of the following responses by the nurse is most appropriate?
   1. "You may need to cut back your visits for now to avoid overtiring your mother."
   2. "Withdrawal may sometimes be a normal response when preparing to leave life."
   3. "It will be important for you to stimulate your mother as she gets closer to dying."
   4. "Many clients don't really know what is going on around them at the end of life."

3. Mrs. Lin's family asks the nurse how they will know that Mrs. Lin's death is imminent. What would the nurse respond?
   1. "Her skin may become mottled."
   2. "Her respirations will be slow and deep."
   3. "Her pulse will increase."
   4. "Her temperature will decrease."

Case 2

Mrs. Dain, aged 60, has been admitted to the palliative care unit of the hospital with terminal lung cancer.

Questions 4 to 7 refer to this case.

4. Which of the following actions should the nurse include in the initial plan of care?
   1. Determine Mrs. Dain's wishes regarding end-of-life care.
   2. Emphasize the importance of addressing any family issues.
   3. Discuss the normal grief process with Mrs. Dain and family.
   4. Encourage Mrs. Dain to talk about any fears or unresolved issues.

5. Mr. Dain visits daily and cheerfully talks with Mrs. Dain about vacation plans for the next year. When the nurse asks about any concerns, Mr. Dain says, "I'm busy at work, but otherwise things are fine." Which of the following nursing diagnoses is appropriate?
   1. Ineffective denial related to threat of unpleasant reality
   2. Anxiety related to threat to current status
   3. Caregiver role strain related to inexperience with caregiving
   4. Hopelessness related to chronic stress

6. The nurse is discussing future treatments with Mrs. Dain. The nurse notes that she has not been eating and responds to the nurse's information by stating, "What does it matter?" What is the most appropriate nursing diagnosis for Mrs. Dain?
   1. Social isolation
   2. Hopelessness
   3. Denial
   4. Powerlessness

7. Mrs. Dain is very close to death and becomes restless. She keeps repeating, "I am not ready to die." Which of the following actions should the nurse take?
   1. Remind her that no one feels ready for death.
   2. Sit at the bedside and ask if there is anything she needs.
   3. Insist that family members remain at her bedside.
   4. Tell her that everything possible is being done to delay death.

Case 3

Krish Reddy, a 12-year-old boy is in the final phase of dying from leukemia.

Questions 8 to 12 refer to this case.

8. How might the quality of life for Krish and his family be enhanced by the nurse?
   1. Tell the family what is best.
   2. Leave the family alone to deal with their tragedy.
   3. Remain objective and uninvolved with family grieving.
   4. Advocate for and implement pain and symptom relief measures.

9. The nurse is providing support to Krish's family that is experiencing anticipatory grief related to their child's imminent death. What statement by the nurse is therapeutic?
   1. "Your other children need you to be strong."
   2. "You have been through a very tough time."
   3. "His suffering is over; you should be happy."
   4. "God never gives us more than we can handle."

10. When communicating with Krish, what should the nurse remember?
    1. Adolescent children tend to be concrete thinkers.

2. Games, art, and play provide a good means of expression.

3. When children can recite facts, they understand the implications of those facts.

4. If children's questions direct the conversation, the assessment will be incomplete.

11. Krish tells the nurse who is giving him opiates for pain that his grandfather is waiting for him. How should the nurse interpret this situation?

1. Krish is experiencing adverse effects of the opiates.

2. Krish is making an attempt to comfort his parents.

3. He is experiencing hallucinations resulting from brain anoxia.

4. He is demonstrating readiness and acceptance that death is near.

12. After Krish's death, several of his nurses tell their nursing supervisor that they want to attend the funeral. They say they felt especially close to both Krish and his family. The supervisor should recognize that attending the funeral serves what purpose?

1. It is improper because it increases burnout.

2. It is inappropriate because it is unprofessional.

3. It is proper because families expect this expression of concern.

4. It is appropriate because it can assist in the resolution of personal grief.

Independent questions

Questions 13 to 24 do not refer to a particular case.

13. Which of the following describes the engagement of nurses in in medical assistance in dying (MAiD)? **Select all that apply.**

1. Nurses have the right to share their views on MAiD with their clients.

2. Determining the eligibility of a client for MAiD is the responsibility of the nurse.

3. The law imposes a duty on nurses to participate in MAiD when the criteria set out in the legislation are met.

4. Organizations participating in MAiD should ensure that processes and policies are in place to support those health care professionals who do not want to participate.

5. Nurses provide bereavement care to the family of the person receiving MAiD.

14. Which of the following are therapeutic interventions for unresolved grief? **Select all that apply.**

1. Listening

2. Providing emotional support

3. Forcing the client to eat properly

4. Referring to appropriate resources

5. Encouraging return to work as soon as possible

15. What characterizes a school-aged child's concept of death? **Select all that apply.**

1. Have a mature understanding of death

2. Can respond to logical explanations of death

3. Personify death as the devil or the bogeyman

4. Have a deeper understanding of death in a concrete sense

5. Fear the mutilation and punishment associated with death

16. The newly graduated nurse is assigned to their first dying client. How can the nurse best prepare to care for this client?

1. Enrolling in a course dealing with death and dying

2. Controlling their own emotions about death

3. Drawing on the experience of the death of a loved one

4. Developing an understanding of their own feelings about death

17. What does the nurse recognize as physical signs of approaching death? **Select all that apply.**

1. Mottling of skin

2. Decreased sleeping

3. Cheyne-Stokes respirations

4. Loss of the sense of hearing

5. Decreased appetite and thirst

18. The nurse is caring for a client who has been diagnosed with metastatic cancer and plans a trip across the country "to settle some issues with my sisters and brothers." Which of the responses should the nurse recognize that the client is manifesting?

1. Restlessness

2. Yearning and protest

3. Anxiety about unfinished business

4. Fear of the meaninglessness of one's life

19. A client in the terminal stages of a disease experiences difficulty swallowing. Which of the following actions would the nurse take to provide comfort for this client? **Select all that apply.**

1. Give all medications subcutaneously.

2. Suction orally as needed.

3. Elevate the head of bed for meals and for 30 minutes after.

4. Do not force the client to eat or drink.

5. Change the diet to soft consistency.

20. Which of the following actions should the nurse perform before allowing the family of a deceased client to view the body?

1. Insert the client's dentures.

2. Lower the head of the bed.

3. Fold the arms and hands over the chest.

4. Leave all of the old dressings and tape in place.

21. Which is an appropriate nursing interventions when providing comfort and support for a client when death is imminent?

1. Limit interventions to palliative care.

2. Avoid playing music near the client.

3. Explain to the client the need for the constant measurement of vital signs.

4. Whisper to the client instead of using a normal voice.

22. Nurses respect the values of various cultures best by following which of the following practices?

1. Respectfully explaining to an Indigenous family that pipe ceremonies are not permitted because of fire risk
2. Ensuring that they are knowledgeable about the cultures of their clients
3. Ensuring their own values are understood by their clients so that there is no confusion about the care plan
4. Undertaking a comprehensive assessment of the client to understand their values and beliefs

23. Which is an appropriate nursing intervention for a client in the final stages of dying?
    1. Keep the client's room cool.
    2. Avoid catheterizing the client.
    3. Elevate the head of the bed as tolerated.
    4. Encourage the client to eat and drink more.

24. Which of the following statements is true when caring for a dying client who is experiencing severe pain?
    1. Addiction is not an issue when caring for the terminally ill.
    2. The client should be carefully assessed and monitored for signs and symptoms of addiction.
    3. Nonopioid analgesics are preferred for dying clients with a history of addiction.
    4. Addiction can be prevented with alternative pain management techniques.

REFERENCES

Astle, B., & Duggleby, W. (2024). *Potter and Perry's Canadian fundamentals of nursing* (7th ed.). Elsevier.

Bard, B., MacMullin, E., Williamson, J., et al. (2022). *Morrison-Valfre's foundations of mental health care in Canada*. Elsevier.

Canadian Hospice Palliative Care Association (CHPCA). (2022a). *Advance care planning*. https://www.chpca.ca/projects/advance-care-planning/

Canadian Hospice Palliative Care Association (CHPCA). (2022b). *Defining hospice palliative care*. https://www.chpca.ca/about-hpc/

Canadian Nurses Association (CNA). (2017). *National nursing framework: On medical assistance in dying in Canada*. https://www.virtualhospice.ca/Assets/cna-national-nursing-framework-on-MAiDEng_20170216155827.pdf

Canadian Nurses Association (CNA). (2022). *Medical assistance in dying*. https://www.cna-aiic.ca/en/policy-advocacy/advocacy-priorities/medical-assistance-in-dying#:~:text=Medical%20assistance%20in%20dying%20(MAiD,who%20have%20explicitly%20requested%20MAiD

Canadian Society of Palliative Care Physicians. (2022, March). *Key messages: Embedding a palliative approach to care in long term care facilities*. https://www.cspcp.ca/wp-content/uploads/2022/03/CSPCP-Key-Messages-LTC-March-2022-FINAL.pdf

College of Nurses of Ontario (CNO). (2021). *Guidance on nurses' role in medical assistance in dying*. https://www.cno.org/globalassets/docs/prac/41056-guidance-on-nurses-roles-in-MAiD.pdf

Government of Canada. (2022). *Medical assistance in dying: Eligibility*. https://www.canada.ca/en/health-canada/services/medical-assistance-dying.html

Hockenberry, M., Rodgers, C., & Wilson, D. (2022). *Wong's essentials of pediatric nursing* (11th ed.). Elsevier.

Lewis, S., Bucher, L., Heitkemper, M., et al. (2019). *Medical-surgical nursing in Canada: Assessment and management of clinical problems* (4th ed.). Elsevier Canada.

Sorrentino, S., Remmert, L., & Wilk, M. (2022). *Sorrentino's Canadian textbook for the support worker* (5th ed.). Elsevier.

Tyerman, J., & Cobbett, S. (2023). *Lewis's medical-surgical nursing in Canada: Assessment and management of clinical problems* (5th ed.). Elsevier Inc.

World Health Organization. (2020). *Palliative care: Key facts*. https://www.who.int/news-room/fact-sheets/detail/palliative-care

BIBLIOGRAPHY

Canadian Council for Practical Nurse Regulators. (2013). *Code of ethics for licensed practical nurses in Canada*. https://ccpnr.ca/wp-content/uploads/2021/03/IJLPN-CE-Final.pdf

Canadian Palliative Care Nursing Association. (2021). *About us. Our mission*. https://www.cpcna.ca/about-us

College of Nurses of Ontario. (2019). *Practice standard: Ethics* (Publication No. 41034). https://www.cno.org/globalassets/docs/prac/41034_ethics.pdf

Registered Nurses Association of Ontario. (2020). *Best practice guideline: A palliative approach to care in the last 12 months of life*.

WEBSITES

Canadian Hospice Palliative Care Association (https://www.chpca.ca/): This site offers information and advocates for quality end-of-life/hospice palliative care in Canada through public policy, education, knowledge translation, awareness campaigns and events, and collaboration. This site offers various resources, documents, and websites on research in hospice care, advance care planning, and caregiver education.

CPNRE Practice Exam: Book One

INTRODUCTION TO PRACTICE EXAMS

The following practice examinations are designed to be similar to those you will encounter in the Canadian Practical Nurse Registration Examination (CPNRE). The exam is organized into two books that contain 125 multiple-choice questions each, for a total of 250 questions. You may want to write the practice exam in a group with fellow students to help replicate an actual exam situation.

Instructions

Read each question carefully and then choose the answer that you think is the best of the four options presented. If you cannot decide on an answer to a question, proceed to the next one and return to this question later if you have time. Try to answer all the questions. Marks are not subtracted for wrong answers. If you are unsure of an answer, it will be to your advantage to guess. Allow yourself 3 hours for each book.

When you have completed both practice exam books, tally your scores and calculate your percentage for the total examination. See Chapter 2 for more details on test-taking skills.

PRACTICE QUESTIONS

Case 1

Nada Wasson delivered a healthy, 3 600-g baby boy, Sandu, a week ago. Mrs. Wasson attends the newborn infant clinic at her local hospital, where the nurse examines Sandu.

Questions 1 to 5 refer to this case.

1. The nurse takes Sandu's vital signs. Which of the following would be normal for a 1-week-old infant?
    1. Heart rate 100 bpm, respirations 26 breaths per minute, blood pressure 44 mm Hg systolic
    2. Heart rate 165 bpm, respirations 65 breaths per minute, blood pressure 94 mm Hg systolic
    3. Heart rate 140 bpm, respirations 40 breaths per minute, blood pressure 70 mm Hg systolic
    4. Heart rate 130 bpm, respirations 32 breaths per minute, blood pressure 100 mm Hg systolic
2. The nurse tests Sandu's Babinski reflex. What is the expected response by Sandu to the Babinski test?
    1. Dorsiflexion of the big toe
    2. Flexion and extension of the leg
    3. Flexion of the fingers
    4. Extension and adduction of extremities
3. The nurse obtains a weight of 3 450 g for Sandu. Mrs. Wasson is concerned about the weight loss, telling the nurse

that she is probably not producing enough milk. What would be the best response by the nurse?
    1. "This weight loss is normal in the first week. Continue breastfeeding at frequent intervals."
    2. "Although most newborns lose weight in the first week, you should probably supplement him with formula for the next few days."
    3. "This is not a significant weight loss, so don't be concerned."
    4. "To prevent further weight loss, you can increase your milk supply by drinking more liquids during the day."
4. Mrs. Wasson complains that her nipples are sore. What should the nurse suggest for care of the breasts?
    1. Air the nipples as much as possible.
    2. Use a lanolin-based cream after every feeding.
    3. Use plastic-lined breast pads.
    4. Begin nursing with the breast that is most painful.
5. Mrs. Wasson plans to express breast milk for use when she has a babysitter. She asks the nurse how she should instruct the babysitter to warm the bottle. What should be the nurse's response?
    1. Place the bottle in a pot of water and heat slowly on top of the stove.
    2. Place the bottle in a microwave oven and heat at a low temperature.
    3. Place the bottle in a bowl of lukewarm water.
    4. Warming is not necessary, as the bottle can be used directly from the refrigerator.

Case 2

Edgar is a 14-year-old boy who was diagnosed with type 1 diabetes at age 4 years. His blood sugar control has been poorly maintained for the past 2 months. It is suspected that the lack of control is related to an adolescent growth spurt and possible poor adherence to blood glucose monitoring, nutrition, and insulin administration. Edgar has been admitted to a short-stay unit in hospital for stabilization.

Questions 6 to 10 refer to this case.

6. When Edgar was diagnosed at age 4, he exhibited the cardinal symptoms of the three "polys." What are these manifestations?
    1. Polycythemia, polyuria, polymyositis
    2. Polydipsia, polyelectrolyte, polyneuropathy
    3. Polyopia, polyarthritis, polyphagia
    4. Polyphagia, polydipsia, polyuria

7. The nurse reviews insulin action, dosage, and administration with Edgar. What is the optimum insulin regimen for most children with diabetes?
   1. Twice-daily injections of rapid-acting and intermediate-acting insulins
   2. Multiple daily injections of rapid- and long-acting insulins
   3. Total dosage and percentage of regular- to intermediate-acting insulins determined individually
   4. Ratio and dose determined by weight in kilograms

8. Edgar admits to the nurse he has been experimenting with alcohol and binge drinking on the weekends. He states that his parents are "heavy drinkers" and are not aware of his behaviour. What is the most critical issue concerning Edgar's drinking of alcohol?
   1. Alcohol causes a rise in blood sugar, leading to a sustained period of hyperglycemia.
   2. Binge drinking can lead to inappropriate and dangerous behaviour.
   3. Alcohol causes a drop in blood sugar that could lead to severe hypoglycemia.
   4. Because Edgar's parents are "heavy drinkers," he is more likely to develop a dependency on alcohol.

9. Edgar injects seven units of regular (Humulin R) insulin at 1600 hours. When should the nurse caution him to be alert for a possible hypoglycemic episode?
   1. 1830 hours
   2. 2030 hours
   3. 2230 hours
   4. 2400 hours

10. The nurse assesses that Edgar has been non adherent to his diabetes management. What is the most appropriate nursing action to address Edgar's nonadherence?
    1. Ask Edgar's parents to supervise him more closely.
    2. Provide education to Edgar and his family about the potential dangers of poorly controlled diabetes.
    3. In private, explore Edgar's feelings about diabetes and the treatment regimen.
    4. Suggest to Edgar that he join an adolescent diabetes support group.

Case 3

A nurse works on an orthopedic surgery unit of a hospital. Many of the clients are older persons with increased risk for hospital-acquired infections.
   Questions 11 to 15 refer to this case.

11. A client's peripheral parenteral nutrition bag has run dry before the health care provider has ordered a new bag. The best action by the nurse is to hang which solution until the new bag arrives?
    1. 10% dextrose in water
    2. 20% dextrose in water
    3. 0.9% sodium chloride
    4. Lactated Ringer's solution

12. Mr. Carolis, age 81, has just had a total hip replacement. He has a history of poor nutrition. Postoperatively, he has an in-dwelling urinary catheter. Which of these factors puts Mr. Carolis most at risk for developing an infection?
    1. Age
    2. Poor nutrition
    3. Surgery
    4. In-dwelling urinary catheter

13. Mr. Carolis develops manifestations of an infection. Which of the following abnormal findings indicates that Mr. Carolis may have an infection?
    1. Leukocytosis
    2. Neutropenia
    3. Thrombocytosis
    4. Leukopenia

14. Mr. Carolis is ordered to have urine cultures and then is started on intravenous antibiotics. What action should the nurse take with regard to the specimen collection and antibiotic administration?
    1. Commence the antibiotics as soon as the medication is received from the pharmacy department.
    2. Ask the physician for the correct order for specimen collection and medication administration.
    3. Take the urine sample from the in-dwelling catheter, and then commence the medication.
    4. Administer the antibiotics, and then collect the urine sample from the urinary collection bag.

15. The nurse discovers that they have administered twice the ordered dose of a medication to Mr. Carolis. What is the most important initial action for the nurse to perform?
    1. Complete an incident report.
    2. Notify the ordering physician.
    3. Assess Mr. Carolis for adverse effects of the overdose.
    4. Report the error to the nurse administrator.

Case 4

Mr. Kassam has chronic renal failure, secondary to type 2 diabetes. He has been attending an outpatient renal clinic for several years, and recently his condition has deteriorated. The nurse sees Mr. Kassam in the clinic.
   Questions 16 to 21 refer to this case.

16. Which of the following laboratory blood test results would be of most concern to the nurse?
    1. Potassium: 7 mmol/L
    2. pH: 7.37
    3. Sodium: 142 mmol/L
    4. Blood urea nitrogen (BUN): 6.8 mmol/L

17. Mr. Kassam is on erythropoietin therapy. What is the rationale for this therapy?
    1. To treat the associated anemia
    2. To control hypertension
    3. To correct the acid–base balance
    4. To increase perfusion in the kidney

18. An important component of conservative treatment for chronic renal failure is diet therapy. Which of the following would be an appropriate lunch menu for Mr. Kassam?
    1. A 100-g cheese sandwich on whole wheat bread, a banana, and 200 mL of milk

2. Canned tomato soup, 250 mL, saltine crackers, and 400 mL of orange juice

3. Turkey, 60 g, on white bread with mayonnaise, an apple, and 250 mL of ginger ale

4. Grilled beefsteak, 300 g, a baked potato, cooked spinach, and chocolate milk

19. Following several months of dialysis, Mr. Kassam exclaims to the nurse, "I just can't do this anymore. I'd rather be dead!" What is the most therapeutic response by the nurse?

1. "You'd rather be dead?"

2. "This is very difficult treatment. Tell me about what is bothering you the most."

3. "Just hang on until we can get you a kidney transplant."

4. "Are you depressed?"

20. Mr. Kassam reveals to the nurse he has found an Internet site that provides kidney transplant surgery in another country for a significant amount of money. What is the nurse's professional responsibility in response to Mr. Kassam?

1. Tell Mr. Kassam it is illegal to buy or sell organs in Canada.

2. Tell Mr. Kassam he must wait until he can receive a kidney in Canada.

3. Ask Mr. Kassam for more details about the Internet site and details of the transplant service.

4. Inform Mr. Kassam that he should not waste his money.

21. Mr. Kassam's condition is deteriorating, and he decides to no longer take dialysis. He tells the nurse he just wants to die. He is considering medical assistance in dying (MAiD). Which of the following does *not* meet the criteria for MAiD?

1. The client is at least 18 years of age and capable of making decisions with respect to his or her health.

2. The client has a grievous and terminal medical condition.

3. The client has been encouraged by the physician and family members to request MAiD to end their suffering.

4. The client gave informed consent to receive MAiD after having been informed of the palliative care.

Case 5

Mrs. Dhillon, age 58, is suspected of having ovarian cancer. She has been referred by her family physician to an oncologist. The nurse consults with cancer clients in the physician's office.

Questions 22 to 26 refer to this case.

22. What are the early manifestations of ovarian cancer?

1. Vague or mild symptoms of abdominal pressure and digestive problems

2. Painful menstrual periods with increased bleeding

3. Sharp pain and swelling in the area of the affected ovary

4. Swollen inguinal lymph nodes

23. The oncologist plans a biopsy via laparoscopy. Mrs. Dhillon asks the nurse about this test. What should the nurse explain to Mrs. Dhillon?

1. "A laparoscopy is the insertion of a large needle through the abdomen into the ovary to collect cells for biopsy."

2. "A laparoscopy is an operation done through a surgical incision in the abdomen and can be used to take a biopsy of ovarian tissue or to remove any visible cancer."

3. "A laparoscopy is the insertion of a flexible tube through a small cut in the abdomen, through which small biopsy samples can be taken."

4. "A laparoscopy is the insertion of air into the fallopian tubes to enable ovarian cells to be withdrawn via the tubes."

24. The results of the biopsy determine that Mrs. Dhillon has stage 3, grade 2 ovarian cancer. The nurse explains that these results help determine which treatment will be most effective for her. Which of the following is the correct interpretation of stage 3, grade 2?

1. The cancer has spread to tissues in the pelvis but is slow growing.

2. The cancer has spread to organs of the abdomen and lymph nodes but is spreading at a moderate rate.

3. The cancer is confined to the ovaries but is highly likely to spread.

4. The cancer has spread outside the abdomen to distant parts of the body and is growing quickly.

25. The oncologist recommends surgery followed by chemotherapy to treat the cancer. Mrs. Dhillon telephones the nurse 2 days later, saying, "Surgery is too drastic, and the chemotherapy is poison that will destroy my body." She will, instead, try some special herbs she has heard about from a friend. What is the best response by the nurse to Mrs. Dhillon?

1. "These herbs have not likely been tested for safety or effectiveness, so it is not known whether they will harm you or be effective for your cancer."

2. "This is not recommended and will probably cause you to die sooner."

3. "At this stage, you are in denial, so call us back when you change your mind."

4. "You are right about the toxins in the chemotherapy, so it is a good idea to try the herbs first."

26. Mrs. Dhillon is experiencing difficulty deciding on a course of treatment for her cancer. She says to the nurse, "I am just so depressed. It doesn't matter what treatment I have; I'll die anyway." What is the most appropriate response by the nurse?

1. "Why do you feel this way?"

2. "Everyone diagnosed with cancer feels this way just after they receive their diagnosis."

3. "Everything will be fine as soon as you start your treatment."

4. "Let's talk about your prognosis and treatment options."

Case 6

A nurse works at a fitness centre. The nurse has been employed to perform health assessments, health counselling, and first aid as necessary.

Questions 27 to 32 refer to this case.

27. Reza Morhudi, age 32 years, has just run 10 km on a treadmill and asks the nurse to take his blood pressure (BP). The nurse obtains a reading of 146/90 mm Hg in Mr. Morhudi's right arm. What is the appropriate nursing action in response to this BP reading?
    1. Tell Mr. Morhudi to rest for 20 minutes and reassess the BP.
    2. Obtain a second BP reading in his left arm.
    3. Ask Mr. Morhudi if he has any history of hypertension.
    4. Tell Mr. Morhudi this is a normal reading for a man of his age and fitness level.

28. The nurse is called to see Valerya Dove, who is on the floor of the gym, crying and saying she has "twisted" her ankle. What interventions should the nurse perform while waiting for the health care provider to assess Ms. Dove's ankle?
    1. Heat, passive range of motion (ROM), analgesics
    2. Rest, ice, compression, elevation
    3. Cool compresses, partial weight-bearing, maintaining joint in flexion
    4. Immobilization of the joint, then sending Ms. Dove to the emergency department for an X-ray

29. Mr. Lackraj introduces himself to the nurse as a new client to the fitness centre. He is 54, obese, and flushed and appears short of breath. What should be the nurse's initial assessment question?
    1. "What has been your past pattern of exercise?"
    2. "What is your personal goal for an exercise plan?"
    3. "Have you consulted your physician about an exercise plan?"
    4. "Are you anticipating exercise will help you lose weight?"

30. A client has been taking haloperidol for 3 months for a psychotic disorder. Because the nurse is concerned about the development of extrapyramidal symptoms, the client will be monitored for which symptom?
    1. Cogwheel rigidity and blurred vision
    2. Drowsiness and dizziness
    3. Motor restlessness and muscle spasm
    4. Dry mouth and constipation

31. Chronic use of alcohol may result in which condition?
    1. Renal failure
    2. Stroke
    3. Korsakoff's psychosis
    4. Alzheimer's disease

32. The nurse has noticed that one of the adolescent clients, Bart Matthews, has developed acne and reduced body fat, with increased muscle size and strength. She suspects that he is using anabolic steroids to improve his sports performance. What would be the most appropriate approach for the nurse to initiate a discussion about the possible use of steroids?

1. "I've noticed that your muscle size has increased quite a bit and you have developed acne."
2. "Are you aware of the dangers of taking anabolic steroids?"
3. "Did you know that using anabolic steroids would disqualify you from sports competitions?"
4. "Are you taking any supplements to improve your performance?"

Case 7

Raize Manche is a 59-year-old woman who has been admitted to an inpatient psychiatric unit following a suicide attempt. She appears unkempt, lethargic, and tearful. She tells her primary nurse, "I'm no use to anyone. There's no point in me going on." Her diagnosis is dysthymia with suicidal ideation.

Questions 33 to 36 refer to this case.

33. During an interaction, Ms. Manche tells the nurse that no one cares about her, but she does love her grandchildren. What would be the most therapeutic response by the nurse?
    1. "Tell me more about your grandchildren."
    2. "I am sure that your family does care about you."
    3. "If you talk about your feelings, you will feel better and enjoy your grandchildren more."
    4. "Your grandchildren would be very upset if you harmed yourself."

34. Ms. Manche has not been eating during her depression and tells the nurse she "just isn't hungry." What would be an appropriate intervention by the nurse to encourage adequate nutrition?
    1. Have Ms. Manche's family bring in food from home.
    2. Consult with a dietitian about the most appropriate menu for Ms. Manche's anorexia.
    3. Offer Ms. Manche bland, high-protein foods.
    4. Ask Ms. Manche what foods and drinks she likes to eat.

35. After being on the unit for several days, Ms. Manche is asked to join a client discussion group. Ms. Manche states that she does not want to go because she has "nothing to say." How should the nurse respond to Ms. Manche?
    1. "You must go to the group, but you don't have to talk."
    2. "Perhaps you could participate by talking about your grandchildren."
    3. "You feel you have nothing to say?"
    4. "The group will be very therapeutic for you."

36. Ms. Manche's physician orders a selective serotonin reuptake inhibitor, sertraline (Zoloft). Ms. Manche tells the nurse she doesn't want to take any drugs because they "won't fix anything." How should the nurse respond?
    1. "No one likes to take drugs, but these might help you."
    2. "Zoloft helps correct the flaw in brain chemistry in depression and should relieve many of your symptoms."
    3. "You should speak with your psychiatrist about whether you can participate in psychotherapy without taking medications."
    4. "Zoloft is one of the newer antidepressants and does not have many side effects."

Case 8

A nurse works in a long-term care facility, Sunset Acres. The clients are primarily adults over 80 years of age, with physical and cognitive disabilities.

Questions 37 to 40 refer to this case.

37. The nurse finds Ms. Abetiu, a client with Alzheimer's disease and dementia, on the floor by her bed. The nurse examines Ms. Abetiu and finds no injuries. Throughout the day when she asks Ms. Abetiu if she has pain, Ms. Abetiu answers "No." The nurse documents the incident but takes no further action. The following day, the nurse notices Ms. Abetiu grimacing and occasionally crying out as if in pain. What is the most appropriate nursing action?
    1. Contact the facility health care provider.
    2. Call an ambulance to transport Ms. Abetiu to the hospital.
    3. Ask Ms. Abetiu if she is experiencing any pain.
    4. Contact Ms. Abetiu's family to report the incident and present manifestations.

38. Mrs. Ensoy is a newly admitted client with dementia. One morning, the nurse observes Mrs. Ensoy to be very agitated and aggressive. What action by the nurse may be of immediate help to manage Mrs. Ensoy's agitation?
    1. Sit and talk with Mrs. Ensoy to find out what is bothering her.
    2. Orient Mrs. Ensoy to the reality of her new environment.
    3. Hand Mrs. Ensoy a cloth and ask her to dust the furniture.
    4. Administer the ordered medication, risperidone (Risperdal).

39. Many of the clients at Sunset Acres have urinary incontinence. Evidence-informed practice suggests that which of the following is most effective in reducing urinary incontinence in people with dementia?
    1. Medication with cholinesterase inhibitors
    2. Reducing total fluid intake, especially in the evening
    3. Use of adult incontinence products, such as Attends or Depends
    4. Scheduled toileting and prompted voiding

40. The nurse is aware that her clients are at high risk for skin breakdown. Which of the following clients would be most at risk for a sacral pressure injury?
    1. Mr. Boston, age 92, who is fully ambulatory but has moderate dementia
    2. Mrs. Colorado, age 85, who is on bed rest and limited ambulation following total hip replacement
    3. Mrs. Carys, age 95, who has a fractured radius
    4. Mr. Cleveland, age 75, who has paraplegia and uses a wheelchair

Case 9

Anusha Satgun immigrated to Canada from Southeast Asia yesterday after a 12-hour flight. She felt unwell during the night, and her worried family took her to the local walk-in clinic the following day. The nurse sees Mrs. Satgun in the clinic.

Questions 41 to 44 refer to this case.

41. Mrs. Satgun does not have private insurance, nor is she eligible for care through the *Canada Health Act*. What is the necessary action by the nurse?
    1. They should refer to agency policies regarding provision of treatment to uninsured individuals.
    2. They should provide care based on professional humanitarian principles.
    3. They should advise Mrs. Satgun to arrange for health care insurance, after which care will be provided.
    4. They should refer Mrs. Satgun to the local community clinic that provides care for recent immigrants to Canada.

42. The nurse conducts an initial health screening with Mrs. Satgun. What would be the most important question to ask Mrs. Satgun?
    1. "What is your previous medical history?"
    2. "Have you had any coughs, colds, or fever in the past week?"
    3. "What medications are you presently taking?"
    4. "Have you consulted a physician in the past year?"

43. Mrs. Satgun is assessed by the nurse and then referred to a physician due to a possible immobility-induced deep vein thrombosis (DVT). What symptoms is Mrs. Satgun likely to have manifested?
    1. Severe, stretching-type pain in the inguinal area
    2. Pain, swelling, and erythema in the affected calf
    3. A dull ache and feeling of coolness in the affected thigh
    4. A line of erythema stretching from the popliteal area to the groin

44. What is the most serious complication of DVT?
    1. Gangrene in the affected limb
    2. Pulmonary embolism
    3. Varicose veins
    4. Cerebral thrombosis

Case 10

Matthew is a 5-month-old infant who was born with a large ventricular septal defect (VSD). He has a codiagnosis of failure to thrive related to the heart defect. He is admitted to hospital for evaluation and treatment of his symptoms.

Questions 45 to 49 refer to this case.

45. What is a VSD?
    1. An area of scar tissue in the left ventricle of the heart
    2. Failure of the aorta to develop, causing a stricture of blood flow in the ventricles
    3. Right ventricular hypertrophy
    4. An abnormal opening between the two ventricles of the heart

46. Nursing considerations during hospitalization of an infant include:
    1. Do not allow the parents to participate in the child's care if the infant has an IV and monitoring devices.
    2. Provide soft stuffed toys in the crib.
    3. Instruct parents that they need to keep the crib rails up only when they leave the room, otherwise the rails can be left down.

4. Encourage the parents to voice their concerns and address them as much as possible.

47. Matthew has a cardiac catheterization to help determine the extent of his VSD. During the procedure, cardiac output is determined. What is cardiac output?
1. The peak pressure in the left ventricle during systole
2. The amount of blood present in the left ventricle at the end of diastole
3. The amount of blood ejected from the heart in one contraction
4. The amount of blood ejected by the heart in 1 minute

48. Matthew returns to the unit after his cardiac catheterization. What assessment will be a priority for the nurse?
1. Level of consciousness
2. Pulses in both extremities
3. Pain
4. Temperature

49. Matthew's parents, Mai Kassaye and Jerome Dime, are both 15 years old. They are in a common-law relationship and live with Jerome's parents. Who may legally provide consent for Matthew's care?
1. Both Mai and Jerome
2. Jerome
3. Jerome's parents
4. Mai

Case 11

A nurse works in a hospice for people who are terminally ill with HIV/AIDS. One client is Georgia Wilcyska, who became HIV-positive many years ago as a result of intravenous heroin use. She was nonadherent to her antiretroviral therapy and is now receiving palliative care for late chronic infection and AIDS.

Questions 50 to 54 refer to this case.

50. Ms. Wilcyska talks to the nurse about the days when she was "turned on" to heroin by a male friend. What feeling would Ms. Wilcyska describe as a result of injecting heroin?
1. Increased alertness
2. Euphoria
3. Insomnia
4. Increased sexual drive

51. Prior to developing an addiction to heroin, Ms. Wilcyska was married with children and had a job. She states she "lost everything" because of her addiction. What is the most likely reason Ms. Wilcyska continued to take heroin in spite of the effects on her family life?
1. Neurophysical dependence
2. Uncomfortable withdrawal symptoms
3. Peer influence
4. Sociocultural factors

52. The nurse is aware that scientific evidence has shown that the practice of harm reduction reduces the financial and human costs of substance misuse. What might be included in harm-reduction strategies?
1. Education targeted to abstinence from chemical substances

2. "Tough on crime" law enforcement approach to drug dealers and users
3. Supervised injection of illicit drugs in designated environments
4. Segregated hostels for people addicted to harmful street drugs

53. Ms. Wilcyska has two children who were taken into care by child welfare authorities many years ago due to her heroin addiction, neglect, and physical abuse. Ms. Wilcyska tells the nurse she regrets she was not a better mother. How should the nurse respond?
1. "I'm sure your children know you tried your best."
2. "You must feel your life has been wasted."
3. "Would you like me to help you write a letter to them?"
4. "Do they have problems now due to the abuse and neglect?"

54. The nurse is trained in therapeutic touch, which she uses as therapy for Ms. Wilcyska. What is therapeutic touch?
1. Rebalancing of energy through the hands of the practitioner to the person
2. A group of therapeutic procedures that help the client redirect physiological responses
3. A type of therapeutic massage that increases blood flow and decreases tension
4. Directed attention to a single unchanging, repetitive stimulus to invoke relaxation

Case 12

Gabrielle French and her partner Jennifer Philips have conceived via in vitro fertilization. Ms. French has experienced an uneventful pregnancy and is now at 36 weeks' gestation. Ms. French and Ms. Philips plan to deliver their child at home with the assistance of a midwife and support from a doula.

Questions 55 to 60 refer to this case.

55. Ms. French's membranes spontaneously rupture at 36 weeks. After 12 hours, there are no contractions, and she becomes concerned. She contacts the midwife, who makes a home visit. Which classification of medication will the midwife most likely give her?
1. An antibiotic
2. An analgesic
3. An antipyretic
4. An oxytocic

56. Although Ms. French and Ms. Philips wish to stay at home, the midwife decides to admit Ms. French to the hospital as a precaution. Shortly afterward, Ms. French commences labour. On the antenatal unit, Ms. French has electronic fetal heart monitoring. The nurse performing the monitoring notes a pattern of early decelerations. What is this most likely caused by?
1. Head compression
2. Cord compression
3. Placental insufficiency
4. Uterine contractions

57. Gabrielle French is anxious, apprehensive, and upset that she will not be able to have a home delivery. Ms. Philips says to the nurse, "I don't seem to be able to help Gabrielle

as well as the nurses. Do you think I should leave?" What would be the best response by the nurse?

1. "As a woman, you should understand that Gabrielle needs you very much now."
2. "This is difficult for you. Let me help you to support her."
3. "Yes, you should leave if you are feeling unsure of the situation. Why don't you relax in the waiting room and come back when you are feeling better?"
4. "It's probably best for you to take a break because you will transmit your anxiety to Gabrielle."

58. As a precaution, an intravenous (IV) infusion is inserted in Ms. French's left arm. What is the most appropriate method of helping her to put on a hospital gown with the IV in situ?
    1. Disconnect the IV, quickly put on the gown, and reconnect the IV.
    2. Apply the gown through her right arm and drape the other sleeve over her right shoulder.
    3. Insert the IV bag through the sleeve from the inside of the gown.
    4. Apply the gown sleeves over both arms, keeping the tubing inside the gown.

59. Gabrielle French delivers a 36-week male infant with a 1-minute Apgar score of 3. Which of the following manifestations would be most likely to be observed in the baby?
    1. Muscle tone flaccid
    2. Heart rate 126 bpm
    3. Respirations 42 breaths per minute
    4. Blood pressure 60 mm Hg systolic

60. Ms. French is transferred to the postpartum unit 2 hours after the delivery. During the admission, Ms. Philips returns from visiting their newborn in the special care nursery. She reports that their infant's breathing sounded "grunty." The nurse explains that grunting respirations are a premature newborn's attempt to do which of the following?
    1. Remove fluid from the lungs
    2. Trap carbon dioxide in the lungs
    3. Decrease mucus obstruction
    4. Open the alveoli

Case 13

A nurse works in a palliative care hospice. One of the clients is Mr. Morrissey, who has terminal pancreatic cancer. Mr. Morrissey is weak and has been unable to move from his bed for several days. He has stopped eating and is not able to drink more than a few sips of water every few hours.

Questions 61 to 65 refer to this case.

61. What is the most important factor for the nurse to consider when developing end-of-life care for Mr. Morrissey?
    1. Cultural
    2. Spiritual
    3. Religious
    4. Individual uniqueness

62. Mr. Morrissey has not completed an advance directive. When he is no longer able to make decisions regarding his care, who should be the substitute decision maker (SDM)?
    1. Mr. Morrissey's former spouse
    2. Mr. Morrissey's eldest son
    3. Mr. Morrissey's adult children
    4. Mr. Morrissey's sister

63. Mr. Morrissey develops pain that is not adequately controlled by morphine. He moans and cries out. His family demands additional and more frequent doses of morphine. What is the most appropriate information for the nurse to communicate in this situation?
    1. "I understand your distress. Let's discuss this."
    2. "I will arrange a meeting with the pain team for us to find a solution."
    3. "I will speak with the physician to ask what to do."
    4. "I am not allowed, as a nurse, to administer increased doses of medication that will cause him to die more quickly."

64. Mr. Morrissey develops constipation. In consultation with the physician, what should be the nurse's initial intervention?
    1. Administer a cleansing enema.
    2. Remove fecal impactions.
    3. Administer a bulk-forming agent, such as Metamucil.
    4. Administer a stool-softening suppository.

65. In the last few days of his life, Mr. Morrissey becomes dehydrated. What should the nurse do?
    1. Apply lubricant to his lips and oral mucous membranes.
    2. Arrange for intravenous fluid replacement.
    3. Obtain an order for fluids via hypodermoclysis.
    4. Insert a nasogastric tube to administer fluids.

Case 14

In November, 5-month-old Sean is brought to the after-hours pediatric walk-in clinic by his parents. They do not have a vehicle, and the clinic was closer for the parents to seek out medical assistance than the children's hospital. He appears to be in respiratory distress, with dyspnea, chest retractions, and nasal flaring. He has a nonproductive, paroxysmal cough. His oxygen saturation is 94%. His parents report that he has had a "cold" with a runny nose for the past few days. The nurse performs a chest assessment and hears wheezing, crackles, and decreased breath sounds.

Questions 66 to 69 refer to this case.

66. Based on his signs and symptoms, the nurse should suspect that Sean has which of the following infectious viral conditions?
    1. Pharyngitis
    2. Croup
    3. Bronchiolitis
    4. Epiglottitis

67. The pediatrician indicates that Sean needs to go to the children's hospital. The nurse explains to the parents that Sean requires which of the following?

1. Antiviral agents
2. Humidified oxygen
3. Cough suppressants
4. Antibiotic agents

68. The nurse calls an ambulance to transport the infant to the hospital. Where is the most appropriate location for Sean and his parents to wait for the ambulance?
    1. In the waiting room to watch other children play
    2. In an office at the back of the clinic to maintain airborne precautions
    3. With adults in the waiting room
    4. In an examining room close by the nursing station to monitor Sean's respiratory status

69. Sean's parents are upset concerning Sean's illness and tell the nurse they would like to stay at the hospital with their son. What is the nurse's best response to this request?
    1. "It is best for Sean if you take a break, go home, and get some rest."
    2. "The children's hospital practises family-centred care, and parents are encouraged to stay."
    3. "It will help if you do stay at the hospital because there is a nursing shortage."
    4. "The pediatrician can write a prescription requesting that the children's hospital allow you to stay."

Independent Questions

Questions 70 to 125 do not refer to a particular case.

70. The nurse assists the physician to insert a peripherally inserted central catheter (PICC) line at the bedside of Mr. Blazevic. Immediately after the insertion, what should be the priority assessment?
    1. Hemorrhage at the insertion site
    2. Blood pressure monitoring
    3. Circulation distal to the insertion site
    4. Ability to withdraw blood from the catheter

71. The nurse teaches colostomy care to Mr. Singh following his colon resection surgery. Mr. Singh asks why he has to irrigate the colostomy. What should the nurse explain to him?
    1. Similar to colonic irrigations, irrigating a colostomy removes toxins from the gastro-intestinal tract.
    2. Irrigation helps regulate the evacuation of feces.
    3. Colostomy irrigations are necessary postsurgery to cleanse the surgical site.
    4. Routine irrigation prevents constipation.

72. Post-Caesarean birth, Ms. Urquhart has her urinary catheter removed. Six hours later, she has not voided. What should be the nurse's first action?
    1. Provide her with a bedpan and provide privacy.
    2. Assess her for abdominal distension.
    3. Recatheterize her for residual urine.
    4. Assist her to the bathroom and encourage her to void.

73. Mrs. Scales is experiencing a loss of peripheral vision. This is likely to be caused by which of the following eye conditions?
    1. Glaucoma

2. Cataracts
3. Macular degeneration
4. Detached retina

74. Ms. Kyrios buys a home pregnancy test kit 1 week after her first missed menstrual period. What hormone will the kit test for to determine if she is pregnant?
    1. Human chorionic gonadotropin (hCG)
    2. Estrogen
    3. Progesterone
    4. Follicle-stimulating hormone (FSH)

75. A client in the thoracic unit pulls out their right-side chest tube. What is the immediate action by the nurse?
    1. Place an occlusive dressing over the puncture site.
    2. Call for the on-site physician.
    3. Position the client on their right side.
    4. Place a saline dressing over the exit site.

76. Mr. Gupta has a tuberculin skin test at a physician's office. The nurse reading the test obtains a result of 7 mm induration. What should be the next action by the nurse?
    1. No action is required, as this is a normal finding.
    2. The nurse should refer Mr. Gupta to a health care provider for further investigation.
    3. The nurse should inform Mr. Gupta that he requires prophylactic medications that will be ordered by a physician.
    4. The nurse should repeat the test, as the result is inconclusive.

77. The nurse finds a client covered in blood after they have slashed their wrists in a suicide attempt. What should be the immediate action to manage the bleeding?
    1. Apply pressure to the laceration.
    2. Apply a tourniquet distal to the laceration.
    3. Determine whether the bleeding is arterial blood.
    4. Elevate the arm.

78. The nurse is about to administer vitamin K by intramuscular (IM) injection to newborn Jeremy. Which site should the nurse choose for the IM injection?
    1. Vastus lateralis
    2. Dorsogluteal
    3. Deltoid
    4. Rectus femoris

79. A nurse is concerned about the morbidity of tuberculosis in their city. Which of the following best defines the morbidity of tuberculosis?
    1. The rate of tuberculosis infection in a population
    2. The effect of tuberculosis on a defined group of individuals
    3. The death rate from tuberculosis
    4. The extent of communicability of tuberculosis within a community

80. Mr. Broadshaw has experienced an episode of renal calculi. The nurse teaches him dietary strategies to help prevent another attack. Which of the following should the nurse include in health teaching for this client?
    1. To increase his intake of clear fluids
    2. To decrease his intake of dairy products

3. To increase his intake of tea and hot chocolate

4. To increase his intake of high-sodium foods

81. Matthew, age 2 years, has chronic otitis media and has been on antibiotics eight times in the past year. What would the nurse be concerned about regarding the antibiotics?

1. He may develop antibiotic resistant microorganisms.

2. He may develop chronic diarrhea.

3. He will develop a hearing loss.

4. His immune system will become dependent on the antibiotics.

82. Mr. Shafikhani, age 25 years, has been recently diagnosed with epilepsy. The nurse speaks with him just after his health care provider tells him that he is no longer allowed to drive a motor vehicle. What is the most therapeutic statement to make to Mr. Shafikhani?

1. "Would you like a referral to the local Epilepsy Association?"

2. "How will not being able to drive affect your life?"

3. "I know this is difficult for you, but it is the safest option."

4. "Do you understand why you are not allowed to drive?"

83. Ms. Aubrey Gans, gravida 1, para 0, has a miscarriage at 10 weeks' gestation. Of the following, which is the most important question for the nurse to ask?

1. "Did you want this pregnancy?"

2. "Do you know if you are Rh-negative or Rh-positive?"

3. "Did you have difficulty becoming pregnant?"

4. "Did you take any medications while you were pregnant?"

84. The nurse is performing oropharyngeal suctioning on Mr. Abernethy. Which of the following would be a nursing consideration during the suctioning?

1. Encourage Mr. Abernethy to cough out secretions during suctioning.

2. Maintain sterile technique.

3. Measure the catheter from the mouth to the ear to the xiphoid process.

4. Moisten the catheter tip with a petroleum jelly lubricant.

85. An agency nurse is working their first shift in a long-term care facility where they are to administer evening medications to the residents. Residents do not wear identification armbands. It is not possible to identify residents from pictures in the medication record as the pictures are of poor quality. What is the initial action by the nurse to ensure safe administration of medications?

1. Ask residents their name and have them sign for the medication.

2. Refuse to administer the medications as it is not safe.

3. Contact the director of care for advice and directives.

4. Use a combination of the picture, clothing identification labels, and resident self-identification.

86. The nurse must instill mineral oil eardrops bilaterally to Mr. Lewis every 8 hours. The nurse directs him to lie in a side-lying position. What action should the nurse take to ensure successful instillation?

1. Instill the drops in the right ear, insert a cotton swab, reposition him, and then instill drops in the left ear.

2. Instill the drops in the right ear, and then 8 hours later, instill drops in the left ear.

3. Instill the drops in the right ear, have Mr. Lewis sit upright, and then instill drops in the left ear.

4. Instill the drops in the right ear, wait 10 minutes, and have him turn to the other side for the left eardrop instillation.

87. Ms. Samms has fatty liver disease, with resulting ascites. Which position would be best to assist her breathing?

1. Prone

2. Semi-Fowler's

3. Modified left lateral recumbent position

4. Supine

88. Harriet, a nurse, discovers her nursing colleague, Angie, smoking in the stairwell of the psychiatric facility where they work the night shift. Angie tells Harriet that she cannot last an entire shift without a cigarette, and it is too cold for her to go outside. What should Harriet do?

1. Remind Angie that smoking is against agency policies and that unless Angie stops this behaviour, she will have to report this to nursing management.

2. Understand that if Angie is on a scheduled break, Harriet has no responsibility to interfere with Angie's smoking.

3. Caution Angie about the dangers of smoking in an unapproved area and the potential dangers to the clients of second-hand smoke.

4. Discuss with Angie her addiction to cigarettes and provide support to establish a strategy that may assist her to quit smoking.

89. A nurse suspects one of their colleagues has falsified their credentials as a licenced practical nurse. What should the nurse do?

1. Talk with the colleague and ask to see their registration.

2. Report their suspicion, with rationale, to the nurse manager.

3. Report their suspicion to the provincial registration body.

4. Intervene to stop the colleague from performing nursing care.

90. Mrs. Verde experiences frequent urinary tract infections (UTIs). What should the nurse advise to decrease the incidence of these infections?

1. Drink orange juice daily.

2. Do not wear cotton underpants.

3. Empty the bladder before and after sexual intercourse.

4. Treat vaginal yeast disorders promptly.

91. Mrs. Brankston has had colon resection surgery due to Crohn's disease. Physician orders include "NPO until bowel sounds are heard." What is the rationale for this order?

1. There is a risk of emesis following gastro-intestinal surgery.
2. Bowel sounds are an indication that peristalsis has resumed.
3. Eating any food will disturb the operative site.
4. It is intended to prevent nausea associated with anaesthetic administration.

92. On the postpartum unit, it is the nurse's responsibility to weigh the newborn prior to discharge and compare this weight to the birth weight. The parents ask why the second weight is required. The nurse's best response is as follows:
    1. It is required to double check the birth weight for accuracy that will be used on the newborn's growth chart.
    2. Weight loss of greater than 10% requires closer monitoring.
    3. Weight gain of greater than 10% indicates the infant is being overfed.
    4. The amount of weight gain or loss will determine whether to supplement a breastfed baby's diet with formula.

93. Ms. MacLeod has received 760 mL of IV fluid and has had 140 mL of tea. She has voided 540 mL of urine and vomited 110 mL. What is Ms. MacLeod's fluid balance?
    1. +900 mL
    2. +250 mL
    3. −650 mL
    4. −110 mL

94. Which of the following is an example of the defence mechanism "displacement"?
    1. Ms. Colm repeatedly tells her nurse, Reena, how much she admires her, when in fact Ms. Colm does not like Reena.
    2. Ms. Henry yells at the nurse after the physician is rude to Ms. Henry.
    3. Mr. Patrick forgets to make an appointment with his physician when he feels a lump on his testicle.
    4. Mrs. Miyagi refuses to believe that her sister has a diagnosis of terminal lung cancer.

95. Mrs. Townsend is 20 weeks pregnant. She tells the nurse that she has twin girls at home but had a miscarriage prior to this pregnancy. What is her pregnancy classification?
    1. Gravida 4, para 2
    2. Gravida 3, para 3
    3. Gravida 3, para 2
    4. Gravida 2, para 1

96. What supplement is recommended for child-bearing persons to take during their reproductive years to help decrease the risk of neural tube defects in newborns?
    1. Iron
    2. Folate
    3. Vitamin A
    4. Calcium with Vitamin D

97. Mr. Brendan asks the occupational health nurse why he always looks pale when he is cold. What should the nurse explain to Mr. Brendan?

1. When you are cold, you have less melatonin.
2. In a cold environment, blood vessels in your skin constrict to save heat.
3. If your skin looks pink in warm weather, it is likely because you have mild sunburn.
4. In cold weather, surface capillaries dilate and make the skin appear whitish.

98. A child at the Tiny Tots child care centre has been diagnosed with impetigo. What advice should the nurse working at the day care centre provide to the centre's child-care workers?
    1. Place the child care centre under quarantine.
    2. Close the child care centre until complete cleaning has been performed.
    3. No special precautions are required.
    4. Suspend attendance for the infected child for 48 hours.

99. Which of the following behaviours would be considered to be a boundary violation of the nurse–client relationship in a mental health setting?
    1. Asking the client about their sexual history
    2. Sharing coffee and cookies with the client during a therapeutic session
    3. Nodding and smiling at the client
    4. Honouring a request by the client to keep a secret from the health care team

100. Brad Shaw tells the nurse he has been finding bright red blood on the toilet paper when he has a bowel movement. What should be the nurse's first response to Mr. Shaw?
    1. "Do you have abdominal bloating or cramping?"
    2. "We need to book you for a colonoscopy."
    3. "I will give you a test kit for fecal occult blood."
    4. "Are your stools hard, or are you constipated?"

101. A first-year nursing student about to enter their first clinical practice experience has artificial nails. The nursing professor tells the student that the policy states they must have the artificial nails removed. What is the most appropriate rationale for this policy?
    1. Artificial nails are too long and may injure the client.
    2. Artificial nails may accidentally be ripped off during client care, injuring the nurse.
    3. Artificial nails are not professional looking.
    4. Artificial nails may harbour microorganisms.

102. Troy, age 16, tells the school nurse that he frequently feels tired during the day and sometimes falls asleep during his classes. What would be the most appropriate initial question for the nurse to ask Troy?
    1. "Are you taking any medications that would make you drowsy?"
    2. "How often do you exercise?"
    3. "When was the last time you had a complete physical exam?"
    4. "How much sleep do you get at night?"

103. Ms. Alexandra has 20/40 vision on the Snellen eye chart. She will most likely need which of the following assistive devices or services?

1. Large-print books
2. Instruction in Braille
3. Referral to an ophthalmologist
4. Corrective lenses

104. Which of the following is the most widespread sexually transmitted infection (STI) in Canada?
    1. Gonorrhea
    2. HIV/AIDS
    3. Nongonococcal urethritis (NGU)
    4. Chlamydia

105. Mr. Schloss, a client with heart failure, is ambulating in the hall when he suddenly collapses. What is the priority assessment by the nurse?
    1. Check for injuries caused by the fall.
    2. Take an apical pulse to assess cardiac status.
    3. Assess for breathing.
    4. Observe for or establish a patent airway.

106. A physician has written the following order for pain relief for Mr. Madrigan: "meperidine (morphine), 10 mg, oral, q3–4h, prn." What is the appropriate practical nursing action?
    1. Administer the meperidine after completing the five rights.
    2. Perform a pain assessment on Mr. Madrigan.
    3. Calculate that this is an appropriate dose of meperidine for Mr. Madrigan.
    4. Contact the physician for clarification of the drug.

107. Jennie, age 18 months, is brought by her parents to the emergency department of her local community hospital. Jennie has bilateral otitis externa with enlarged tonsils and adenoids. She is mouth breathing and diaphoretic and appears febrile. What method should the nurse choose to take Jennie's temperature?
    1. Tympanic
    2. Axillary
    3. Oral
    4. Rectal

108. Mr. Rivers asks the nurse why he is being discharged home with community nursing care only 1 day after an uncomplicated appendectomy. What would be the nurse's best response?
    1. "You do not require acute care facilities."
    2. "Your condition is stable, so, with support, it is better to recover at home."
    3. "It is too expensive to have people stay in hospital to recover after surgery."
    4. "The trend in health care is to discharge clients as soon as possible."

109. The nurse tells Mr. Bartholomew, age 65, that his temperature is 36.6 degrees Celsius. He responds: "I only know Fahrenheit. Is 36.6 degrees Celsius the same as 98.6 degrees Fahrenheit? Is it normal?" What should the nurse tell Mr. Bartholomew?
    1. "Yes, it is the same as 98.6 degrees Fahrenheit."
    2. "It is about 98, almost the same as 98.6 degrees Fahrenheit, and is normal."

3. "No, it is 99.7 degrees Fahrenheit and is slightly elevated."
4. "It is quite a bit lower than 98.6 degrees Fahrenheit and shows you are cold."

110. Mr. Constant, a client in a psychiatric unit, tells the nurse: "The voices are saying bad things about me." What would be an appropriate response?
    1. "I do not hear the voices."
    2. "I understand you are frightened by the voices, and I will stay with you."
    3. "Why don't you sit with the other clients and watch TV?"
    4. "Don't listen to what the voices tell you."

111. Prior to the infusion of antibiotics for cellulitis, Mrs. Collins tells the nurse she is allergic to penicillin. What should be the nurse's first action?
    1. Place an allergy band on Mrs. Collins's wrist.
    2. Notify the prescriber of the allergy.
    3. Check that the ordered antibiotics do not contain penicillin.
    4. Ask Mrs. Collins what happens when she has penicillin.

112. Teklie, age 2 years, has had two episodes of watery diarrhea. What should the nurse recommend to Teklie's parents?
    1. Encourage constipating foods such as cheese.
    2. Administer an over-the-counter antidiarrhea medicine.
    3. Offer clear fluids, ice pops, and crackers.
    4. Continue with Teklie's normal diet.

113. Mrs. Bennett requires transfer from her wheelchair to the commode. She tells the nurse that usually two people perform this lift. The nurse has not previously cared for Mrs. Bennett but assesses that one person can perform the lift. What should the nurse do?
    1. Use a mechanical lift so she does not require two people.
    2. Ask Mrs. Bennett for more details about why two people are required for the lift.
    3. Find another co-worker to assist with the lift.
    4. Begin the lift to see how difficult it will be.

114. Mrs. Sheyer, age 87 years, is brought to the walk-in clinic by her family because she has had a fever for several days. The health care provider feels Mrs. Sheyer may be exhibiting early signs of delirium. What would be the most important step of data collection for the nurse to apply to help determine the possible cause of the delirium?
    1. Review Mrs. Sheyer's medication profile.
    2. Interview the family to determine cognitive function prior to admission.
    3. Assess Mrs. Sheyer's level of hydration.
    4. Take Mrs. Sheyer's temperature.

115. A nurse in a community mental health clinic is in the midst of a counselling session with Mr. Olan. Ms. Isabelle approaches the nurse and asks to speak with them. How should the nurse respond to this situation?

1. "What can I help you with, Ms. Isabelle?"
2. "Excuse me, Mr. Olan, I need to speak with Ms. Isabelle."
3. "Ms. Isabelle, I am with Mr. Olan until 10. I will see you directly afterward."
4. "Ms. Isabelle, you should not interrupt Mr. Olan and me."

116. A nurse is grocery shopping when she observes a young toddler experiencing a prolonged tonic–clonic seizure. What is the nurse's first responsibility in this situation?
    1. Call 9-1-1.
    2. Insert any safe object in the child's mouth to maintain an airway.
    3. Observe the seizure and protect the child from injury.
    4. Reassure the parents.

117. Ten-year-old Nicholas has just been diagnosed with a brain tumour. His parents tell the nurse Nicholas is not to be informed about the tumour. What is the nurse's most appropriate response to this request?
    1. "At Nicholas's age, he is not able to understand the diagnosis, so this is a wise decision."
    2. "Let's talk about the reasons why you don't think he should be told."
    3. "The policy of this hospital is that children have a right to age-appropriate information."
    4. "Children are very intuitive, and Nicholas probably already knows about the tumour."

118. The charge nurse on a busy surgical unit must assign care for Mr. Michener, age 27, who is 1 day postsurgery from an appendectomy. Mr. Michener's vital signs are stable, and the wound is approximated and shows no signs of infection. Mr. Michener is to be discharged the following day and requires health teaching. What category of health care worker is the most appropriate and cost-effective to be assigned to Mr. Michener?
    1. Registered nurse (RN)
    2. Registered practical nurse/licensed practical nurse (RPN/LPN)
    3. Expanded role nurse/nurse practitioner/clinical nurse specialist
    4. Unregulated care provider (UCP)

119. Mrs. Fraser, a pale-skinned woman of European descent, age 59 years, comes to the clinic. What is the most important observation by the nurse when performing a skin assessment on Mrs. Fraser?
    1. Areas of dry, flaky skin
    2. A reduction in skin elasticity
    3. A change in a mole or lesion
    4. Senile lentigines

120. The nurse obtains a thermometer reading of 39.6 degrees Celsius on Nick, age 4 years. His previous temperature 2 hours ago was 36.3 degrees Celsius, he does not feel hot, and he states that he feels well. What is the appropriate nursing action?

1. Take the temperature again in another hour.
2. Take a rectal temperature to obtain a core temperature.
3. Administer the ordered antipyretic.
4. Use a different thermometer to retake the temperature.

121. Mrs. Ginger has an amputation of her left leg. The afternoon following surgery, the nurse finds Mrs. Ginger lying in bed, in a fetal position, crying. What is the most appropriate documentation of this event?
    1. "Lying in a fetal position, crying"
    2. "Displaying manifestations of postsurgical depression"
    3. "Grieving observed due to loss of leg"
    4. "Client upset, manifesting sadness related to amputation"

122. Andre, age 6 years, is about to have an injected immunization. He is very tearful and apprehensive about how much the needle will hurt him. Which of the following would be the most effective method to reduce the pain of an injection for Andre?
    1. Using a topical anaesthetic cream
    2. Distracting Andre during the injection
    3. Having the parent hold Andre during the injection
    4. Providing postinjection analgesics, such as acetaminophen (Tylenol)

123. A nurse manager is concerned about the incidence of work-related accidents on the unit, causing many staff nurses to be on long-term disability. What is the first action the manager should take to address these problems?
    1. Compile a list of all data on staff accidents for the past 2 years.
    2. Tour the unit to observe hazardous workplace habits or environments.
    3. Interview all staff on long-term disability to find out how they were injured.
    4. Interview all staff for their opinions and observations about workplace hazards.

124. What part of the SBAR report does the following information fall under? Mrs. Rose's pain in the left lower leg is increasing for the past 1 hour. She has hypertension and type 2 diabetes. She is on metformin hydrochloride 500 mg bid. She is allergic to sulpha drugs.
    1. Situation
    2. Background
    3. Assessment
    4. Recommendation

125. A client who is on estrogen therapy should be counselled that smoking may cause what?
    1. An increased incidence of nausea
    2. An increased tendency to bleed during menstruation
    3. Increased level of triglycerides
    4. An increased risk for thrombosis

ANSWERS AND RATIONALES FOR BOOK ONE

The correct answer is set off in boldface.

1. **C: Foundations of Practice T: Knowledge**
   1. These values are all low. See choice 3.
   2. These values are too high. See choice 3.
   3. **Normal vital signs for a 1-week-old infant are heart rate 120 to 160 bpm, respirations 30 to 60 breaths per minute, and median blood pressure generally 65 to 80 mm Hg by Doppler (but can increase during crying or agitation).**
   4. Heart rate and respirations are within normal ranges, but blood pressure is too high.

2. **C: Foundations of Practice T: Knowledge**
   1. **The Babinski reflex is elicited by stroking the outer sole of the foot upward from the heel across the ball of the foot, causing dorsiflexion of the big toe and fanning of the toes.**
   2. This is the response from the dance, or step, reflex.
   3. This is the expected response from the grasp reflex.
   4. This is the part of the expected response from the Moro, or startle, reflex.

3. **C: Professional, Ethical, and Legal Practice T: Application**
   1. **This response best addresses Mrs. Wasson's concerns. A weight loss of up to 10% is expected 3 to 4 days after birth. Adequate breast milk supply is best facilitated by frequent feedings.**
   2. It is well established that the use of supplemental formula feedings before breastfeeding is to be avoided.
   3. This is true but does not answer Mrs. Wasson's concerns about milk production.
   4. Increased fluids have not been proven to increase milk supply.

4. **C: Foundations of Practice T: Application**
   1. **Airing the nipples as much as possible, and using heat, will help dry the nipples and decrease discomfort.**
   2. Creams and oils are to be avoided.
   3. Plastic-lined breast pads may trap moisture, increasing the risk of skin breakdown.
   4. Nursing should start with the least affected breast.

5. **C: Foundations of Practice T: Application**
   1. Breast milk or infant formula does not need to be heated.
   2. It is unsafe and unnecessary to warm milk in the microwave because the heat is not evenly distributed. The bottle may remain at a cooler temperature than the liquid, and the liquid may burn the baby.
   3. **Warming a bottle in lukewarm water is sufficient to bring it to room temperature.**
   4. Infants are used to body temperature milk from the breast and may not adjust to cold milk.

6. **C: Foundations of Practice T: Knowledge**
   1. Polycythemia (an increase in red blood cells) and polymyositis (an inflammation of many muscles) are not manifestations of diabetes.

   2. Polyelectrolyte (many charged electrolytes) and polyneuropathy (a disorder of the peripheral nerves) are not manifestations of diabetes.
   3. Polyopia (a defect in sight) and polyarthritis (an inflammation of more than one joint) are not manifestations of diabetes.
   4. **Polyphagia (excessive hunger and eating), polydipsia (excessive thirst), and polyuria (excessive urination) are cardinal manifestations of type 1 diabetes.**

7. **C: Foundations of Practice T: Application**
   1. This regimen involves insulin administration in the morning before breakfast and before the evening meal. It may not suit all people with diabetes, particularly during illness, stress, growth spurts, and so on.
   2. Some children require frequent dosing of insulin. Administration may be with multiple injections or the use a continuous subcutaneous infusion (pump). After individual assessment, this may be the optimum regimen.
   3. **The precise dose of insulin and optimum regimen cannot be predicted and need to be individualized for every child. Insulin requirements do not remain constant, changing with growth, activity, and pubertal status.**
   4. Although many pediatric medication dosages are calculated per kilogram, insulin dosages are not.

8. **C: Foundations of Practice T: Application**
   1. Alcohol causes a drop, not an increase, in blood sugar.
   2. This could be a serious problem, but more significant is an immediate and severe drop in blood glucose.
   3. **Alcohol causes hypoglycemia. The manifestations of slurred speech and antisocial combative behaviour are similar to those of being intoxicated; thus, Edgar may not receive appropriate life-saving treatment.**
   4. There is a family pattern to alcohol dependence, but this is not the most critical issue at this time.

9. **C: Foundations of Practice T: Application**
   1. **The peak action for regular insulin is 2 to 4 hours after administration; therefore, a hypoglycemic episode may occur between 1800 and 2000 hours.**
   2. This is past the time of peak action.
   3. The insulin would likely not be in the bloodstream at this time.
   4. There should be no effects from the insulin at this time.

10. **C: Collaborative Practice T: Application**
    1. This may need to occur but is not the best initial approach.
    2. Both Edgar and his parents may require more education, but an assessment of Edgar's needs and particular reasons for nonadherence must be explored first.
    3. **Prior to implementing interventions, the nurse must be aware of the reasons for Edgar's**

nonadherence. The nurse should discuss this with him in private, as he may speak more freely when his parents are not present.

4. This may be appropriate but does not address Edgar's individual needs with his present nonadherence.

11. C: Foundations of Practice T: Application

1. **If parenteral nutrition is discontinued abruptly, rebound hypoglycemia may occur. This complication can be prevented with an infusion of 5 to 10% glucose in situations in which parenteral nutrition must be discontinued immediately.**

2. For peripheral solutions, the proportion of dextrose must not be more than 12.5%

3. This solution would not prevent rebound hypoglycemia from occurring.

4. As in choice 3.

12. C: Foundations of Practice T: Critical Thinking

1. Age is a risk factor, as older persons generally have a decreased immune system; however, it is not as great a risk as a urinary catheter.

2. Poor nutrition may lead to poor immunity, but this is not as great a risk as a urinary catheter.

3. Surgery is a risk; however, the surgery should have taken place under strict sterile techniques.

4. **An in-dwelling urinary catheter, even though it is a closed system, places Mr. Carolis at risk for a urinary tract infection and should be discontinued at the earliest opportunity.**

13. C: Foundations of Practice T: Application

1. **Leukocytosis is an abnormal increase in white blood cells and is indicative of an infection.**

2. Neutropenia is an abnormal decrease in neutrophils. During an infection, there is an increase in neutrophils.

3. Thrombocytosis is an abnormal increase in platelets and may be indicative of malignancies or blood disorders.

4. Leukopenia is an abnormal decrease in white blood cells and may indicate bone marrow suppression.

14. C: Foundations of Practice T: Application

1. Antibiotics may interfere with accurate results from cultures.

2. It is not necessary to consult with the physician. This is nursing judgement.

3. **This is the correct sequence. Culture specimens can be inaccurate if taken after antibiotics are given.**

4. Sterile urine specimens must be taken from the catheter port, not the collection bag. The specimen must be taken before the antibiotics are administered.

15. C: Professional, Ethical, and Legal Practice T: Critical Thinking

1. Incident reports are specific agency documents. They are important for quality assurance purposes for the institution but are not the most important initial action for Mr. Carolis.

2. This must be done but is not the first action.

3. **The immediate action must be to address client safety. Administration of medication that is twice the ordered dose could have severe effects, particularly in an older client, and the nurse's first responsibility must be to assess Mr. Carolis.**

4. This must be done but is not the first action.

16. C: Foundations of Practice T: Knowledge

1. **Hyperkalemia, caused by decreased excretion by the kidney, is the most serious electrolyte disorder associated with kidney disease. A level of 7 mmol/L could result in a fatal arrhythmia.**

2. This is a normal value.

3. This is a normal value.

4. This is a normal value.

17. C: Foundations of Practice T: Knowledge

1. **Administration of erythropoietin intravenously or subcutaneously is effective in treating the anemia that results from the decrease in erythropoietin production occurring with kidney failure.**

2. An adverse effect of erythropoietin may be hypertension.

3. Erythropoietin will not affect the acid–base balance.

4. Erythropoietin will not increase perfusion in the kidney.

18. C: Foundations of Practice T: Critical Thinking

1. Cheese has high sodium and high protein. Banana and milk are high-potassium foods. Sodium, protein, and potassium are restricted in renal failure.

2. Canned soups are high in sodium, as are saltine crackers. Orange juice is high in potassium. Fluids are restricted: 400 mL is too much fluid at one meal.

3. **Nutrition therapy in renal failure is complex. It requires the expert determination by a nutritionist of menus that comply with guidelines of low sodium, protein, and phosphorus; restricted fluids; and unlimited carbohydrates and fats to ensure sufficient calories. Turkey, mayonnaise, bread, an apple, and ginger ale comply with these guidelines.**

4. The beefsteak provides too much protein, and the baked potato, cooked spinach, and chocolate milk are high in potassium.

19. C: Collaborative Practice T: Application

1. This reply does not necessarily allow Mr. Kassam to discuss his feelings.

2. **This open-ended response confirms Mr. Kassam's feelings and invites him to share them.**

3. This response closes the conversation and does nothing to help develop coping strategies. Kidney transplant may not yet have been discussed with him.

4. This is not a therapeutic response and does not allow for Mr. Kassam to discuss his feelings.

20. C: Professional, Ethical, and Legal Practice T: Critical Thinking

1. Although this is true, it is not pertinent, as the transplant surgery is being offered in another country.

2. It is neither the ethical nor the professional responsibility of the nurse to tell the client what he must do.

3. **This response provides the nurse with more information about a potentially dangerous, illegal, or unethical situation. It allows for a respectful discussion between the nurse and Mr. Kassam.**

4. As in choice 2.

21. C: Foundations of Practice T: Knowledge

1. This meets the criteria for MAiD.

2. This meets the criteria standard for MAiD.

3. **This is not a criterion for MAiD. Clients must voluntarily request MAiD with no external pressure.**

4. This meets the criteria for MAiD.

22. C: Foundations of Practice T: Knowledge

1. **Ovarian cancer in its early stages may not cause symptoms, or they may include mild pressure in the abdomen, pelvis, or back of the legs. There may be abdominal swelling or gastro-intestinal symptoms, such as indigestion, nausea, and bloating.**

2. This is not a manifestation of ovarian cancer but more likely of uterine cancer. At age 58, Mrs. Dhillon would likely be postmenopausal and thus not menstruating.

3. This is not a manifestation of ovarian cancer.

4. This is not a manifestation of early ovarian cancer.

23. C: Foundations of Practice T: Application

1. This is a needle biopsy.

2. This is a laparotomy.

3. **This is the correct definition of laparoscopy. It may be preferable to laparotomy as it is less invasive, is less painful, and only requires a local anaesthetic.**

4. This is not the definition of laparoscopy.

24. C: Foundations of Practice T: Application

1. This is grade 2, stage 1.

2. **This is the correct interpretation of grade 3, stage 2.**

3. This is grade 1, stage 3.

4. This is grade 4, stage 4.

25. C: Collaborative Practice T: Application

1. **This is factual information that will assist Mrs. Dhillon to make an informed decision about her treatment.**

2. The herbs are probably not recommended, but it is not a therapeutic response to tell Mrs. Dhillon that they will cause her to die sooner, especially as Mrs. Dhillon may not be aware of the possibility of a terminal diagnosis.

3. This is not a therapeutic response. It presumes she is in denial and presumes that she will change her mind. It does not provide information to assist her in making her decision.

4. This is an incorrect and potentially life-threatening response.

26. C: Collaborative Practice T: Application

1. Mrs. Dhillon has a type of cancer that has a very poor prognosis. It is evident why she is depressed.

2. This is patronizing and does not address Mrs. Dhillon as an individual. It ends the conversation.

3. This is probably not true and would not encourage further discussion.

4. **This is an open-ended response that invites further discussion with Mrs. Dhillon about her cancer and her feelings about the situation.**

27. C: Foundations of Practice T: Application

1. **Physical activity increases the cardiac output and thus increases the BP. Twenty to 30 minutes of rest following exercise is indicated before a resting BP can be considered reliable.**

2. This is not necessary. A BP in the left arm is likely to be the same as in the right arm.

3. This action would be indicated if, after resting, Mr. Morhudi's BP remained elevated.

4. A normal BP for Mr. Morhudi would be 120/80 mm Hg.

28. C: Foundations of Practice T: Application

1. Ice, not heat, is recommended for a muscle sprain. Heat may be applied after 24 hours. The ankle should be rested initially. Analgesics may be required once the RICE therapy has been initiated.

2. **This is RICE treatment. Movement should be limited, cold is applied to produce hypothermia, compression with an elastic bandage limits swelling, and the limb is elevated to impede edema formation.**

3. Ice is more effective than a cool compress. Ms. Dove will be encouraged to move the ankle joint once it is supported with a bandage. There is no rationale for maintaining the joint in flexion.

4. This is not necessary unless the nurse assesses there has been a possible fracture.

29. C: Professional, Ethical, and Legal Practice T: Application

1. This is an appropriate question but is not the most important initial data collection.

2. As in choice 1.

3. **Mr. Lackraj appears to have risk factors for cardiovascular disease. All clients should consult with their physician prior to initiating an exercise plan.**

4. As in choice 1.

30. C: Foundations of Practice T: Application

1. This is not an example of extrapyramidal symptoms.

2. As in choice 1.

3. **Extrapyramidal symptoms are involuntary motor symptoms similar to those associated with Parkinson's disease. This drug-induced state is known as *pseudoparkinsonism* and is characterized by symptoms such as akathisia (distressing motor restlessness) and acute dystonia (painful muscle spasms).**

4. As in choice 1.

31. C: Foundations of practice T: Application

1. This is not a condition that results from chronic alcohol use

2. As in choice 1.

3. Chronic use of alcohol may lead to a variety of serious neurological and mental disorders, such as Korsakoff's psychosis and Wernicke's encephalopathy, in addition to cirrhosis.

4. As in choice 1.

32. **C: Collaborative Practice T: Application**
1. **This initial answer is a statement of facts and does not accuse Mr. Matthews. It will likely lead to a discussion of the causes of his muscle bulk and acne.**
2. This accuses Mr. Matthews without any proof and will cause him to feel defensive.
3. As in choice 2.
4. This approach calls for a yes or no answer, is accusing, and is not likely to lead to a meaningful discussion.

33. **C: Collaborative Practice T: Application**
1. **The depressed client often has difficulty acknowledging any positive aspects of his or her life. By asking about the grandchildren that Ms. Manche loves, the nurse is reinforcing that she has worthwhile relationships.**
2. This ignores Ms. Manche's feelings and closes off the discussion.
3. This provides false reassurance and applies pressure on Ms. Manche to talk.
4. This answer is not therapeutic, as it may cause Ms. Manche to feel guilty.

34. **C: Collaborative Practice T: Application**
1. This may be appropriate but does not consider Ms. Manche's preferences. She did not eat at home when these foods were available.
2. There is no need to consult with a dietitian at this time. When Ms. Manche's food preferences have been established, a dietitian may be consulted.
3. This does not consider Ms. Manche's preferences.
4. **Ms. Manche is more likely to eat foods that she prefers.**

35. **C: Collaborative Practice T: Application**
1. While this reassures Ms. Manche that she does not have to talk, it does not lead to a therapeutic discussion.
2. This is a helpful response but may not lead to Ms. Manche exploring her feelings.
3. **This allows the nurse to further explore Ms. Manche's feelings of low self-worth and may lead to a discussion about the therapeutic effects of the group discussion.**
4. This response is autocratic, gives advice, and does not allow Ms. Manche to explore her feelings.

36. **C: Foundations of Practice T: Critical Thinking**
1. Ms. Manche has not said that she does not like to take drugs. This response makes the use of antidepressants appear to be of limited effectiveness.
2. **Antidepressant therapy benefits about 65 to 80% of people with depression. This response is factual and explains that depression is a chemical condition.**

3. The antidepressant is a first-line agent in the treatment of depression and should be combined with psychotherapy. This response negates the role of the nurse.
4. Ms. Manche has not asked about adverse effects; she has said she doubts the drugs will work.

37. **C: Foundations of Practice T: Critical Thinking**
1. **Ms. Abetiu is manifesting symptoms of pain and needs to be assessed by the health care provider for any possible injury that could have occurred due to the fall.**
2. The initial action is to contact the agency physician, if available, who should examine Ms. Abetiu. If there were no agency physician, the appropriate action would be to call for an ambulance for transport to a hospital.
3. People with dementia have difficulty communicating symptoms of health conditions or pain. While the nurse could ask Ms. Abetiu if she is experiencing pain, it is not likely that Ms. Abetiu would be able to provide accurate information, especially considering that she had previously denied pain. Health care staff must take the responsibility for assessment and diagnosis.
4. This will be necessary but is not the most appropriate action at this time.

38. **C: Foundations of Practice T: Application**
1. This is not likely to calm Mrs. Ensoy's agitation. In an agitated phase, logical discussions about feelings and cause and effect are not likely to be successful.
2. While reality orientation is helpful with clients who have dementia, in the agitated state, this would not be effective.
3. **Redirection is often helpful when dealing with difficult behaviour. Performing an activity such as dusting, which would be a familiar activity to Mrs. Ensoy, may calm her.**
4. Risperidone is helpful in managing disruptive behaviour; however, nonpharmacological therapies should be attempted initially.

39. **C: Foundations of Practice T: Application**
1. These drugs do not affect urination or continence.
2. This practice is dangerous with older persons. It is necessary to ensure that older persons have sufficient fluid intake.
3. Use of these products helps manage urinary incontinence but does not reduce incontinence.
4. **Evidence-informed practice has determined that behaviour modification, in the form of routine toileting and prompting the client to void, reduces urinary incontinence in people with dementia.**

40. **C: Foundations of Practice T: Application**
1. People who are ambulatory have a low risk for pressure injuries.
2. Mrs. Colorado is still able to change positions and ambulate.
3. A fractured radius will not lead to a pressure injury in the sacral area.

4. With paraplegia, there is decreased sensation and immobility, both of which are risk factors for pressure injuries.

41. **C: Professional, Ethical, and Practice T: Critical Thinking**
    1. **The most appropriate action is to refer to agency policies. There is likely to be an appropriate policy that will address ethical, financial, and legal implications of provision of treatment for nonresidents.**
    2. If Mrs. Satgun's condition were life-threatening, the humanitarian principle would be to provide emergency care.
    3. Mrs. Satgun may not be able financially to obtain the necessary medical insurance. Her condition could potentially deteriorate during the time it takes to obtain the insurance.
    4. This may ultimately be the solution; however, it is dependent on the policies of the agency.

42. **C: Foundations of Practice T: Critical Thinking**
    1. This is important but is not the most immediate concern.
    2. **This is the most important question, particularly as Mrs. Satgun has recently arrived in Canada from a foreign country. This question helps screen for recent communicable diseases, which may be a hazard to the rest of the clients, community, and staff in the clinic and may require specific isolation precautions.**
    3. This is important to develop a profile of Mrs. Satgun's health status but is not the most important question.
    4. This is important as it may reveal underlying conditions that are important for Mrs. Satgun's subsequent treatment; however, it is not as important as knowing her recent communicable disease status.

43. **C: Foundations of Practice T: Knowledge**
    1. DVT, particularly after a long air flight in a confined space, is most likely to occur in the calf.
    2. **In this type of DVT, the inflammatory response causes pain in the calf and swelling, and the area feels warm.**
    3. Mrs. Satgun may feel a dull pain but is likely to feel warmth rather than coolness, and it is not likely to be in the thigh.
    4. The swelling and erythema of DVT are generally not linear and are generally not in the popliteal–groin area.

44. **C: Foundations of Practice T: Knowledge**
    1. If untreated, the DVT could lead to necrosis and gangrene, but this is neither the most likely nor the most serious complication.
    2. **Pulmonary embolism is a life-threatening complication of DVT.**
    3. Varicose veins are not caused by DVT and are not as serious as pulmonary emboli.
    4. Cerebral thrombosis is serious and life-threatening; however, if the thrombus in the leg were to enter the venous circulation, it would first travel to the lungs.

45. **C: Foundations of Practice T: Knowledge**
    1. This is not the definition of VSD. It is not scar tissue.
    2. Coarctation of the aorta is failure of the aorta to develop, causing reduced systemic blood flow below the level of the defect.
    3. A large VSD may cause right ventricular hypertrophy but is not the actual defect.
    4. **This is the definition of a VSD.**

46. **C: Foundations of Practice T: Application**
    1. It is important to have parents actively participate in their child's care. Client- and family-centred care is a beneficial partnership that engages family as essential members of the health care team. It promotes health teaching and information sharing.
    2. Stuffed toys in an infant's crib are a suffocation risk.
    3. Crib rails need to be up when an infant is in the crib. They should never be left down when not attending to the infant. Infants can easily roll off beds. It is important to keep one hand on the infant at all times when giving care and the crib rails are down.
    4. **Parent collaboration helps parents feel in control, safe, and more comfortable caring for their child.**

47. **C: Foundations of Practice T: Knowledge**
    1. This is the definition of systolic left ventricular pressure.
    2. This is the end-diastolic volume.
    3. This is stroke volume.
    4. **This is the definition of cardiac output.**

48. **C: Foundations of Practice T: Critical Thinking**
    1. Matthew may need to be sedated for the procedure and may be sleepy, but this is not the priority assessment.
    2. **The catheter is inserted into either the femoral vein or the femoral artery. There is risk of vasospasm or thrombus formation, which could interfere with blood flow to the extremities. Thus, assessment of pulses is the priority assessment.**
    3. Matthew may be experiencing pain, but this is not the priority assessment.
    4. Matthew may be somewhat hypothermic if the temperature in the catheterization laboratory is reduced. It is not, however, the priority assessment.

49. **C: Professional, Ethical, and Legal Practice T: Application**
    1. **Both parents have equal rights and are considered emancipated minors because they have a child.**
    2. Jerome has no greater rights to provide consent than Mai. Both are emancipated minors.
    3. Jerome and Mai are emancipated minors and may provide consent for treatment for their son.
    4. Mai does not have greater rights than Jerome.

50. **C: Foundations of Practice T: Knowledge**
    1. Injection of heroin is more likely to cause detachment from the environment.
    2. **After injection of heroin, users feel a strong sense of euphoria.**

3. Following the euphoria, users are more likely to feel drowsiness than insomnia.

4. Heroin users often have a decreased libido.

51. **C: Foundations of Practice T: Critical Thinking**

1. **Current research shows that addictive drugs appear to increase the availability of dopamine in the pleasure area of the brain. Without the substance, the individual experiences depression, anxiety, irritability, and an intense craving for the drug. To feel "normal," the individual must take increasingly large doses of heroin.**

2. While the withdrawal symptoms (such as nausea, pain, vomiting, and so on) are unpleasant, the physical addiction is the primary difficulty.

3. Peer influence is a documented influencing factor associated with drug misuse but is not as direct a factor as the physical addiction.

4. Sociocultural factors affect the incidence of substance misuse however are not as direct a factor as physical addiction.

52. **C: Foundations of Practice T: Application**

1. Abstinence is not part of a harm-reduction strategy.

2. This is a societal view that seeks to punish those who use illicit drugs.

3. **This is a part of a continuum of strategies that aims to reduce the adverse health and social effects of problematic drug use.**

4. This is repressive.

53. **C: Collaborative Practice T: Application**

1. This is patronizing and is unlikely to help Ms. Wilcyska.

2. This confirms to Ms. Wilcyska that she was a poor mother, and it is not therapeutic.

3. **Reaching out to her estranged children may help Ms. Wilcyska. Writing letters to her children may bring the comfort of knowing that something of her may survive after her death.**

4. This further emphasizes to Ms. Wilcyska that she was a poor mother and is not therapeutic.

54. **C: Foundations of Practice T: Knowledge**

1. **With the hands of the practitioner either on the body or close to the body, energy flow is redirected and brings the person back into energy balance. It may be of value to reduce anxiety and pain.**

2. This is biofeedback.

3. Therapeutic touch is not a type of massage.

4. This is meditation.

55. **C: Foundations of Practice T: Knowledge**

1. **With ruptured membranes, there is a risk of ascending infection, particularly group B *Streptococcus*. If the infant is not delivered, the risk of infection increases relative to the time that has passed since the membranes ruptured; therefore, antibiotics are given to the mother.**

2. This is not indicated.

3. This is not indicated.

4. Labour will likely not be induced unless the infant is in distress.

56. **C: Foundations of Practice T: Knowledge**

1. **Head compression may cause early decelerations.**

2. Cord compression may cause variable decelerations.

3. Placental insufficiency will cause late decelerations.

4. Uterine contractions may cause fetal tachycardia.

57. **C: Collaborative Practice T: Application**

1. This statement is judgemental and patronizing.

2. **This acknowledges the fears of Ms. Philips. Both parents require additional support from the nurse at this time.**

3. Ms. French needs the support of her partner at this time. Generally, partners will not be asked to leave unless they are in the way during the emergency.

4. This does not help Ms. Philips fulfill her role in supporting Ms. French and may make Ms. Philips feel that she is failing her partner.

58. **C: Foundations of Practice T: Application**

1. This is not safe, as there is potential for introducing pathogens into the IV.

2. This would be uncomfortable for Ms. French.

3. **This ensures that the bag and tubing are safely put through the arm of the gown, with no unsafe breaks in the system or tension applied to the tubing.**

4. This would place the IV tubing inside the gown, where it is not in view, it may become kinked, and it may create tension on the insertion site.

59. **C: Foundations of Practice T: Knowledge**

1. **An Apgar score of 3 indicates severe distress. Of the listed manifestations, this is the only abnormal finding. It is given a score of 1 on the Apgar.**

2. This is normal. With an Apgar score of 3, the heart rate would likely be lower.

3. This is normal and would likely be associated with an Apgar score of 7 to 10.

4. Blood pressure is not a component of the Apgar score.

60. **C: Foundations of Practice T: Application**

1. There may be fluid in the lungs, but it is not removed by grunting.

2. The lungs require oxygen, not carbon dioxide.

3. There is no mucus obstruction in neonatal respiratory distress.

4. **With neonatal respiratory distress, the alveoli collapse due to insufficient surfactant. Grunting is an attempt by the body to open up the alveoli.**

61. **C: Professional, Ethical, and Legal Practice T: Critical Thinking**

1. Cultural, spiritual, and religious factors will influence end-of-life care; however, each person is a unique individual.

2. As in choice 1.

3. As in choice 1.

4. **Although a person's cultural, spiritual, and religious background must be included in end-of-life**

care, assumptions cannot be based on these factors. **All people are unique.**

62. **C: Professional, Ethical, and Legal Practice T: Application**
    1. If they are no longer legally married, the former spouse cannot be the SDM unless Mr. Morrissey has designated her as the SDM.
    2. There is no provision in the legislation that states that the eldest child, whether male or female, should be the SDM.
    3. **The adult children are the legal next of kin and will be the SDMs. The children should agree upon decisions, and in practice, the child who has been most involved with the parent may have more influence.**
    4. The sister is not the next of kin, unless she has been designated as the SDM.

63. **C: Collaborative Practice T: Application**
    1. This is a patronizing answer and does not find a solution to the pain-management problem.
    2. **This is an action-oriented response. It is the role of the palliative care team to appropriately manage pain and the ethics of increased morphine.**
    3. This implies that the nurse does not have a professional role in pain management.
    4. Depending on the specifics of the situation, this may or may not be true. However, it does not solve the problem of Mr. Morrissey's pain management.

64. **C: Collaborative Practice T: Application**
    1. This should not be the initial action as it may be unpleasant for Mr. Morrissey and may not be necessary.
    2. This may be necessary depending on a thorough assessment of the constipation. It would be a last resort for impacted feces that did not respond to a suppository.
    3. Bulk-forming agents require the person to ingest larger amounts of fluids, which Mr. Morrissey is not able to do. They also require time to achieve results.
    4. **This is the most appropriate and comfortable initial action. The suppository may soften the stool so that Mr. Morrissey will be able to pass it with limited effort.**

65. **C: Foundations of Practice T: Application**
    1. **Skin dryness can lead to discomfort. Lubricating the lips and mucous membranes is soothing.**
    2. This is likely not appropriate close to death, unless he has requested an IV.
    3. Injections of saline under the skin are not appropriate to maintain hydration, unless he or the family has requested it.
    4. This is not appropriate unless requested.

66. **C: Foundations of Practice: Application**
    1. Clients with pharyngitis usually present with sore throat ranging in severity from "scratchy" to severe pain that makes swallowing painful. The pharynx is red and edematous, with or without patchy exudates.

2. Symptoms of croup include a barky cough with low-grade fever. The voice may be harsh, but the client is able to speak and swallow.
3. **Bronchiolitis, most often caused by the respiratory syncytial virus (RSV), is common in infants during the fall and winter. It often begins with an upper respiratory infection. Symptoms include dyspnea, paroxysmal nonproductive cough, tachypnea with retractions and nasal flaring, and wheezing.**
4. Epiglottitis is most commonly found in children between the ages of 2 and 5 years. Signs and symptoms include sudden onset of high fever, difficulty breathing, severe sore throat, difficulty swallowing, drooling, and muffled voice, but no cough.

67. **C: Foundations of Practice T: Knowledge**
    1. Antivirals are not used with this condition.
    2. **Mist therapy is generally combined with oxygen to alleviate the dyspnea and hypoxia.**
    3. Cough suppressants are not recommended for children.
    4. Antibiotics are of no use with viral illnesses.

68. **C: Foundations of Practice T: Application**
    1. Respiratory syncytial virus (RSV) is very contagious, and Sean should not be with other infants.
    2. Sean does require isolation to prevent transmission to others, but also needs to be monitored by the nurse.
    3. Although adults are not as severely affected by RSV, being in the waiting room will not guarantee he will be isolated from children.
    4. **The nurse will need to monitor Sean's condition by having him close by and isolate him from the other children in the clinic.**

69. **C: Foundations of Practice T: Knowledge**
    1. This is not the philosophy of family-centred care. It is not the nurse's role to tell the parents it is best for them to leave their son.
    2. **This is the appropriate response and validates family-centred care and the role of his parents in Sean's care.**
    3. The nurse should not imply the hospital nursing staff would not be able to adequately look after Sean if they do not stay. This will not promote trust in the hospital's nursing care.
    4. The pediatrician does not need to write a prescription for the parents to stay at Sean's bedside.

70. **C: Foundations of Practice T: Critical Thinking**
    1. **This is the priority assessment. As with any invasive procedure, bleeding from an arterial access device carries considerable risk and could be life-threatening.**
    2. This is important but not a priority postprocedure. Blood pressure should be taken on the arm opposite the insertion site.
    3. This is an important observation postinsertion and will need to be assessed at all times while the device

is in situ. Immediately postprocedure, it is not the priority assessment.

4. This must be determined by the physician at the time of insertion and monitored thereafter by the nurse, but it is not the most critical assessment postprocedure.

71. **C: Foundations of Practice T: Application**
    1. This is not true, either for colonic irrigations or colostomy irrigations.
    2. **The primary purpose of irrigating a colostomy is to promote regular bowel movements.**
    3. It is not necessary to cleanse the anastomosis site.
    4. Constipation is not a common occurrence with a colostomy. Regular irrigation may help prevent constipation, but it does so by promoting regular bowel movements.

72. **C: Foundations of Practice T: Critical Thinking**
    1. The inability to void may be due to residual effects from an anaesthetic. As well, voiding into a bedpan is not easy for many clients, so this would not be the optimal strategy, unless Ms. Urquhart is unable to ambulate.
    2. **This should be the first action. If Ms. Urquhart has a full bladder, further and more immediate action will be required. If the bladder is not distended, the situation is less urgent.**
    3. This may happen but is not necessary until the bladder is assessed for distension.
    4. This should be done after Ms. Urquhart is assessed for bladder distension.

73. **C: Foundations of Practice T: Knowledge**
    1. **Glaucoma is manifested by loss of peripheral vision, producing "tunnel vision" and halos around lights.**
    2. With cataracts, vision loss is generally progressive blurring or haziness.
    3. With macular degeneration, close vision tasks become difficult.
    4. A detached retina may cause loss of vision in the affected area, blurring, or spots and flashes of light.

74. **C: Foundations of Practice T: Knowledge**
    1. **This hormone is produced by the chorionic villi of the developing embryo and is present in the blood and urine of a pregnant person.**
    2. Estrogen prepares the uterus for pregnancy. An elevation in estrogen occurs later in pregnancy and does not necessarily indicate pregnancy.
    3. Progesterone helps maintain the pregnancy and prepare the breasts for lactation but is not the hormone detected in pregnancy tests.
    4. Follicle-stimulating hormone (FSH) helps mature follicles but is not the hormone detected in pregnancy tests.

75. **C: Foundations of Practice T: Critical Thinking**
    1. **An occlusive dressing is needed to prevent air from entering the pleural space.**

2. The physician will need to be notified to reintroduce the tube; however, the initial action must be to occlude the puncture site.
3. This will not be as effective as the occlusive dressing.
4. This will not prevent air from entering the pleural space.

76. **C: Collaborative Practice T: Application**
    1. Five to 10 mm of induration may be significant. This is not normal.
    2. **This is the appropriate action as it is the health care provider's responsibility to further interpret the results and decide on further diagnostics.**
    3. This is not a definitively positive test. It is presumptive to tell Mr. Gupta that he requires prophylactic treatment.
    4. Although the protocol on repeating inconclusive tests varies among agencies, in this situation, it is not apparent that the nurse has the authority to repeat the test without consulting the health care provider.

77. **C: Foundations of Practice T: Critical Thinking**
    1. **This is the correct emergency action. Pressure to the site of bleeding will help control the bleeding.**
    2. This should not be done as it may compromise arterial blood flow.
    3. This is important, but the priority is to control the bleeding.
    4. Elevating the arm will help control the hemorrhage but is not as important as pressure at the site.

78. **C: Foundations of Practice T: Application**
    1. **The vastus lateralis is the best-developed muscle in infants and is the safest for IM injections.**
    2. This is not a well-developed muscle in the infant.
    3. As in choice 2.
    4. As in choice 2.

79. **C: Foundations of Practice T: Knowledge**
    1. **Morbidity refers to the incidence of disease within a defined population.**
    2. Morbidity does not refer to disease effects.
    3. This is the definition of mortality.
    4. This refers to the ability of an infectious disease to spread within a population.

80. **C: Foundations of Practice T: Application**
    1. **Calculi are more likely to form when the urine is concentrated. Increased fluids help dilute the urine.**
    2. Dairy products were routinely restricted in the past, however recent research suggests, high dietary calcium intake may actually lower the risk of the development of calculi.
    3. Tea and chocolate have high levels of oxalate and should be reduced in the diet.
    4. Dietary sodium should be restricted to reduce the risk of the development of calculi.

81. **C: Foundations of Practice T: Critical Thinking**
    1. **A concern about overuse of antibiotics is that they will lose their effectiveness and create drug-resistant strains.**

2. Some antibiotics cause diarrhea, but they will not cause chronic diarrhea.

3. Hearing loss may occur due to the chronic otitis media, but not due to the family of antibiotics used for otitis.

4. Antibiotics do not cause dependence.

82. **C: Collaborative Practice T: Application**

1. While a referral is a good option for Mr. Shafikhani, this does not address the immediate concern of not being able to drive.

2. **This open-ended question deals practically and emotionally with the issue of a young male no longer being able to drive.**

3. The nurse does not know Mr. Shafikhani's feelings. This sounds patronizing and does not invite therapeutic communication.

4. This is a closed question. The nurse may only get a yes or no answer. He may infer that the nurse thinks he is not intelligent enough to understand.

83. **C: Foundations of Practice T: Critical Thinking**

1. Emotional reactions to the pregnancy loss must be explored, but this question is inappropriate and insensitive.

2. **Aubrey's Rh status must be identified. If she is Rh-negative, she will require administration of RhoGAM within 72 hours of the miscarriage to prevent antibody formation in future pregnancies.**

3. This is an appropriate question but is not as important as determination of the mother's Rh status.

4. This may be an important question if Aubrey requires a D&C (dilation and curettage), but it is not important at this stage and may imply that Aubrey was at fault for the miscarriage.

84. **C: Foundations of Practice T: Application**

1. **Coughing moves secretions from the lower airway into the mouth and upper airway and may decrease the amount of suctioning required.**

2. Oral suctioning does not require sterile technique.

3. This is a measurement for a nasogastric tube.

4. Oil-based lubricants are not to be used as they are not water soluble and may be aspirated.

85. **C: Professional, Ethical, and Legal Practice T: Critical Thinking**

1. This is not a safe option, as some residents may answer to any name.

2. This is not a professional option.

3. **The director of care is responsible for policies and care in the agency and needs to be consulted regarding the safest option. This may involve the director administering the medications.**

4. This may be safer than the photos or self-reporting alone, but it does not necessarily guarantee the correct resident would receive the medication.

86. **C: Foundations of Practice T: Critical Thinking**

1. Cotton may be ordered post–eardrop instillation, but it will not prevent the mineral oil from flowing back out of the right ear during immediate instillation in the left ear.

2. This would be a medication error, as the drops must be instilled in both ears every 8 hours.

3. This will not prevent the drops from flowing back out of the right ear.

4. **This is the correct procedure. Mr. Lewis must remain in the side-lying position for at least 10 minutes in order for the drops to effectively be delivered to deeper ear structures.**

87. **C: Foundations of Practice T: Application**

1. This may compromise her breathing.

2. **The semi-Fowler's position reduces the pressure of the enlarged abdomen on the diaphragm.**

3. This will assist breathing somewhat but is not the most effective.

4. This may compromise breathing.

88. **C: Professional, Ethical, and Legal Practice T: Application**

1. **Angie's behaviour is unprofessional: smoking on health care premises is contrary to agency policies and most municipal bylaws. As well, Angie is placing the clients at risk from second-hand smoke. Harriet must report Angie's disregard of policies, the law, and client safety.**

2. Angie is on agency property; whether she is on a scheduled break is not pertinent.

3. It is likely that Angie is already aware of agency policies and the dangers of second-hand smoke. This does not address her unprofessional behaviour.

4. This discussion may be held at a different time. The professional responsibility for Harriet is to stop and report the behaviour.

89. **C: Professional, Ethical, and Legal Practice T: Critical Thinking**

1. This is potential fraud and needs to be reported.

2. **This is the appropriate chain of command. The nurse manager will investigate.**

3. This will be done by the nurse manager.

4. This could be done, but only if the nurse views unsafe practice.

90. **C: Foundations of Practice T: Application**

1. Cranberry juice, not orange juice, can help prevent UTIs.

2. Cotton, not synthetic, underpants are recommended.

3. **Sexual intercourse can "milk" bacteria from the vagina and perineum into the urethra. Emptying the bladder before and after intercourse may help flush out the introduced bacteria.**

4. Vaginal yeast disorders do not predispose clients to UTIs, unless related itching causes skin breakdown.

91. **C: Foundations of Practice T: Critical Thinking**

1. There may be a risk of vomiting, but this is not the primary rationale. The answer must provide a rationale for both the NPO and the detection of bowel sounds.

2. **Anaesthesia slows peristalsis. Hearing bowel sounds is an indication that peristalsis has returned. If Mrs. Brankston is fed when the bowel**

is not moving, the food would remain in the upper GI system, possibly leading to vomiting, obstruction, discomfort, and potential aspiration.

3. Unless there is peristalsis, it is not likely that any food will reach the operative site.

4. An adverse effect of anaesthesia is nausea; however, this is not a postoperative rationale for NPO until bowel sounds are heard.

92. **C: Foundations of Practice T: Critical Thinking**
    1. The weight of the infant 24 hours postdelivery will be less than the birth weight and should not be substituted.
    2. **Weight loss up to 10% is expected. More than 10% indicates feeding has not been well established. Possible delay in discharge may occur to assist the parents in feeding.**
    3. Weight gain within the first 24 hours is unusual. It is not the reason for taking a discharge weight.
    4. It is not recommended to use formula as a supplement. More frequent breastfeeding will accomplish the same outcome.

93. **C: Foundations of Practice T: Application**
    1. +900 mL: incorrect calculation
    2. **+250 mL: 760 mL + 140 mL = 900 mL; total intake 540 mL + 110 mL = 650 mL total output. For fluid balance, subtract output from intake: 900 mL − 650 mL = 250 mL positive balance**
    3. −650 mL: incorrect calculation
    4. −110 mL: incorrect calculation

94. **C: Foundations of Practice T: Knowledge**
    1. This is reaction formation.
    2. **This is the definition of displacement. Ms. Henry is displacing her anger at the physician toward the nurse.**
    3. This is repression.
    4. This is denial.

95. **C: Foundations of Practice T: Application**
    1. This would indicate four pregnancies, but Mrs. Townsend has been pregnant only three times.
    2. This would denote three pregnancies, which is correct, but also three living children. Mrs. Townsend has only two living children.
    3. **Gravida 3 is correct: the present pregnancy, the pregnancy that resulted in twin births, and the previous miscarriage. Para 2 is correct: Mrs. Townsend has two living twin children.**
    4. This would indicate two pregnancies and one living child.

96. **C: Foundations of Practice T: Knowledge**
    1. Iron is recommended to support and increase maternal red blood cell production.
    2. **Folate (folic acid) supplements decrease the risk for neural tube defects in the newborn. Folate is recommended before and during pregnancy to prevent some major birth defects that can happen in the first few weeks of pregnancy, often before a client finds out they are pregnant (400 mcg of folic acid is recommended daily). All child-bearing-aged clients should take folic acid.**
    3. This is not recommended. Vitamin A increases the risk for birth defects at intakes of 10 000 IU daily.
    4. Calcium and vitamin D are necessary for the development and maintenance of bone mass both prior to and during pregnancy. Adequate intake is required for fetal development.

97. **C: Foundations of Practice T: Application**
    1. This is not necessarily true. Melatonin is increased in response to sun exposure, not when someone feels hot or cold. Also, people vary in the amount of melatonin they have naturally.
    2. **This is a physiological response to cold. The constriction of the blood vessels to conserve heat means that there is not as much blood close to the skin surface, with the result that the skin appears a paler colour.**
    3. This may occur, but this is not what Mr. Brendan asked.
    4. This is the opposite of what occurs.

98. **C: Foundations of Practice T: Application**
    1. This is an extreme measure and not necessary.
    2. Although thorough cleaning is necessary at any child care centre, in this situation, it is not necessary for the centre to close. Transmission is most likely via contact with the infected child.
    3. This is not true. See choice 4.
    4. **Impetigo is an infection of the skin caused by *Streptococcus* or *Staphylococcus* bacteria and is transmissible to other children. The child with impetigo must be isolated from other children until 24 to 48 hours after treatment has started.**

99. **C: Professional, Ethical, and Legal Practice T: Application**
    1. This may be an important part of the client assessment, depending on the situation and client's condition.
    2. This may help put the client at ease.
    3. This is a therapeutic response.
    4. **This is crossing a boundary. It implies a special relationship between the client and the nurse. The nurse must inform the client that all relevant information must be shared with other members of the health care team.**

100. **C: Foundations of Practice T: Application**
    1. These are manifestations of irritable bowel disease, which does not cause rectal bleeding.
    2. This may be necessary once hemorrhoids or constipation is ruled out as a cause for the bleeding.
    3. This is not a necessary test, as Brad has said the blood is visible.
    4. **The most common cause of minor rectal bleeding is tearing of the rectal mucosa due to constipation and hard stool.**

101. **C: Professional, Ethical, and Legal Practice T: Critical Thinking**

1. Artificial nails may be trimmed to an appropriate length that would not scratch or injure a client.

2. This is possible, but not likely, and would not be the most appropriate reason for the policy.

3. Artificial nails, if kept well-trimmed and without polish, may be professional in appearance.

4. **Studies have shown that artificial nails, especially if not well maintained, may have crevices that enable microorganisms to flourish.**

102. **C: Foundations of Practice T: Critical Thinking**

1. This question could be asked as some prescription and nonprescription drugs cause drowsiness as an adverse effect. However, medications are not the most frequent cause of adolescent fatigue.

2. Lack of exercise may lead to fatigue during the day but is not the most common cause of adolescent fatigue.

3. This may be important information to obtain but should not be the initial question.

4. **The most common cause of daytime fatigue at all ages is inadequate sleep. Most teenagers do not know they need approximately 9 hours of sleep each night.**

103. **C: Foundations of Practice T: Application**

1. Large-print books are needed for people who have severe vision impairments.

2. Instruction in Braille is not necessary. Vision of 20/40 is mild vision loss.

3. While an ophthalmologist can prescribe corrective lenses, generally, for simple near-sightedness, referral is not required.

4. **A score of 20/40 indicates vision that will likely respond well to corrective lenses, either glasses or contact lenses.**

104. **C: Foundations of Practice T: Application**

1. This is a common STI in both sexes but is not the most prevalent.

2. This is not the most prevalent STI in Canada.

3. This is the most common STI in males but not in the general population.

4. **Chlamydia is the most widespread STI in Canada.**

105. **C: Foundations of Practice T: Critical Thinking**

1. Injuries occurring from the fall will need to be assessed, treated, and documented, but this is not the most important initial action.

2. Circulation is not the first priority.

3. Breathing is assessed after assessing for a patent airway.

4. **The priority of assessment is according to the ABCs: airway, breathing, and circulation. A clear airway is necessary for breathing and must be the initial assessment.**

106. **C: Professional, Ethical, and Legal Practice T: Critical Thinking**

1. Meperidine should not be administered, as there is confusion concerning the correct drug.

2. This should not be done until the correct drug is clarified.

3. This could be done once the drug is clarified.

4. **Meperidine is the generic name for Demerol, not morphine. The ordered dose is within the normal dosing range for morphine. The medication order must be clarified with the prescriber prior to any other action.**

107. **C: Foundations of Practice T: Critical Thinking**

1. Tympanic thermometers should not be used with clients who have ear infections or ear pain.

2. **An axillary temperature is not as accurate as tympanic, oral, or rectal temperature, but in this situation, it is the most appropriate approach. The thermometer should be kept under the axilla for 5 minutes.**

3. Oral thermometers should not be used with an 18-month-old child. In addition, a child who is mouth breathing may not be able to keep their mouth closed for the required time, and this may lead to an inaccurate reading.

4. Rectal temperatures should not generally be used with children due to the risk of rectal injury and the discomfort and distress related to the procedure.

108. **C: Collaborative Practice T: Application**

1. This does not answer Mr. Rivers question.

2. **This reassures Mr. Rivers that he is well enough to be discharged, he will have support by nurses in his home, and this is better for him.**

3. This may be true but will not be reassuring for Mr. Rivers.

4. This is true but does not answer Mr. Rivers question or reassure him.

109. **C: Foundations of Practice T: Application**

1. It is not exactly the same, and the nurse has not answered that it is a normal temperature.

2. **The conversion of 36.6 degrees Celsius to Fahrenheit is 97.9, or 98 degrees.**

$$\frac{36.6 \times 9}{5} + 32 = 97.9$$

This is **considered a normal temperature. Many clients who were not educated in the metric system prefer to use the Fahrenheit scale.**

3. This is an incorrect conversion and is not elevated.

4. It is lower, but not significantly, and is still considered to be a normal temperature.

110. **C: Collaborative Practice T: Application**

1. The voices are real to Mr. Constant, so this is not therapeutic.

2. **The voices are real and frightening to Mr. Constant. Acknowledging this, and staying with him, demonstrates concern and may reduce his fears.**

3. Mr. Constant will not be able to concentrate on the TV because of his fears.

4. Mr. Constant is not able to separate the voices from reality.

111. **C: Professional, Ethical, and Legal Practice T: Critical Thinking**

1. This will need to be done once the nurse assesses the type of allergic reaction.
2. As in choice 1.
3. This is important, but the nurse initially needs more information about the allergy.
4. **It is important to first obtain more information from Mrs. Collins about the allergy. Some clients have a sensitivity reaction; with others, it may be anaphylactic.**

112. **C: Foundations of Practice T: Application**
1. Milk-based foods are likely to irritate the gut and cause further diarrhea.
2. This is not appropriate for a child.
3. **With mild diarrhea, clear fluids will maintain hydration and will not irritate the gut. Crackers are also appropriate and will decrease Teklie's hunger.**
4. A normal diet may be resumed once the diarrhea has stopped.

113. **C: Professional, Ethical, and Legal Practice T: Critical Thinking**
1. This may help, but generally two people are required for a mechanical lift.
2. **The nurse needs more data, as what the client is telling her is different from the nurse's assessment.**
3. The nurse will probably have to obtain assistance, but it is best to find out first from Mrs. Bennett more information about the lift.
4. This could potentially be dangerous for both Mrs. Bennett and the nurse.

114. **C: Foundations of Practice T: Critical Thinking**
1. Medications can trigger delirium, but this is not the most important step in the data collection.
2. **All of these responses are important when assessing the cause of Mrs. Sheyer's delirium. By obtaining a baseline understanding of Mrs. Sheyer's cognitive function, it can be better determined how, or if, her behaviour has changed and what particular triggers may have been involved.**
3. Dehydration can cause delirium in an older person but is not the most important step in the data collection.
4. Fever or infection may trigger delirium, but this is not the most important step in the data collection.

115. **C: Collaborative Practice T: Application**
1. This allows Ms. Isabelle to continue with inappropriate behaviour and is not therapeutic toward Mr. Olan.
2. As in choice 1.
3. **This response is clear, provides exact information without appearing punitive toward Ms. Isabelle, and demonstrates respect for both clients.**
4. This response is punitive.

116. **C: Professional, Ethical, and Legal Practice T: Critical Thinking**
1. This is important; however, the nurse's expertise is needed with the toddler. It is more appropriate for the nurse to delegate another to call 9-1-1.

2. The nurse should observe for a patent airway, but this is not a safe option. It may cause damage to the mouth and teeth.
3. **The safest option with a child is to observe the seizure, make sure the child is not injuring themself, and ensure that they are maintaining a patent airway and not to actively intervene or attempt to restrain the child. These observations will be helpful when emergency medical personnel arrive at the scene.**
4. This is not the priority action. It may be appropriate once the seizure is over.

117. **C: Collaborative Practice T: Critical Thinking**
1. This is not true. At age 10 years, Nicholas would have an understanding of the diagnosis.
2. **This response opens up communication with the parents.**
3. This may be true but closes communication.
4. This may be true but may upset the parents and may not encourage communication.

118. **C: Professional, Ethical, and Legal Practice T: Critical Thinking**
1. This category of nurse is appropriate; however, the knowledge and skills of an RN would be more appropriately used for a more acutely ill, unstable client.
2. **The RPN or LPN is the most appropriate caregiver as the nurse provides care to clients such as Mr. Michener, whose conditions are stable and whose outcomes are predictable. The nurse has the competency to perform discharge health teaching, and assigning this task to them is more cost-effective than assigning it to an RN.**
3. While this category of nurse is certainly competent to provide care, their knowledge and skills would be more appropriately used for an acutely ill or complex client; therefore, this is not the most cost-effective option.
4. The UCP would be appropriate to provide some basic care for Mr. Michener but would not have the knowledge to provide discharge health teaching or wound assessment.

119. **C: Foundations of Practice T: Application**
1. This is a normal finding in the skin of a 59-year-old woman.
2. As in choice 1.
3. **This could be a possible finding of skin cancer and should be further investigated.**
4. These are more commonly known as "age spots" or "liver spots" and may be seen in adults starting in their late 40s or 50s.

120. **C: Foundations of Practice T: Critical Thinking**
1. There is no reason to wait an hour. The elevated temperature must be confirmed as soon as possible as temperatures in children can rise rapidly.
2. It is neither appropriate nor necessary to obtain a rectal temperature. The use of a rectal thermometer would be very upsetting and intrusive for a 4-year-old.

3. This action should not be taken until the temperature is confirmed. Other evidence suggests that Nick may not have a fever.

4. **As part of the assessment phase of the nursing process, the nurse validates data collected. Nick does not display manifestations of a fever; therefore, it is possible that the thermometer is malfunctioning or requires recalibration. The temperature should be confirmed using another thermometer.**

121. **C: Foundations of Practice T: Application**
    1. **This is factual documentation of observed behaviour.**
    2. This is an assumption and interpretation of behaviour. Documentation requires the inclusion only of observable facts.
    3. As in choice 2.
    4. As in choice 2.

122. **C: Foundations of Practice T: Critical Thinking**
    1. **Topical anaesthetic creams are effective in preventing pain from immunization and may help prevent future fear of needles.**
    2. Distraction techniques may help decrease stress and minimize pain, but they are not as effective as the anaesthetic cream.
    3. As in choice 2.
    4. Postinjection analgesics are often prescribed but are most useful with children who develop swelling and fever postimmunization. They do not prevent the pain of injections but treat it after the fact.

123. **C: Professional, Ethical, and Legal Practice T: Critical Thinking**
    1. **All responses could be correct. This is the first action, as the manager needs objective data: the number of accidents and types of accidents on the unit.**
    2. This is a good action but is not as important as the actual accident statistics.
    3. The manager should know this information. Not all accidents may cause staff to be on long-term disability.
    4. As in Choice 2.

124. **C: Foundations of Practice T: Knowledge**
    1. The situation describes what is going on with the client. It is a concise statement of the problem.
    2. **The information provided is the background report of a SBAR. This information is the clinical background. It describes the information and history that is relevant to the situation.**
    3. Assessment describes what one finds and considerations of options. It includes a physical assessment of the client along with the vital signs and lab reports.
    4. Recommendation is what action is needed to correct the problem or what one wants.

125. **C: Foundations of Practice T: Application**
    1. Smoking does not cause increased nausea in clients taking estrogen.
    2. An increased tendency to bleed during menstruation would not be caused by smoking when taking estrogen.
    3. Smoking would not cause an increased level of triglycerides in clients taking estrogen.
    4. **Smoking should be avoided during estrogen therapy because it adds to the risk for thrombosis formation.**

CPNRE Practice Exam: Book Two

PRACTICE QUESTIONS

Case 1

A nurse is employed by a hospital-based palliative care team that includes a physician, a pharmacist, and a social worker. The nurse is supporting the family of Mrs. Haliburton, who is terminally ill with stomach cancer and has chosen to die at home.

Questions 1 to 5 refer to this case.

1. The family asks the nurse how they will know Mrs. Haliburton's death is imminent. What should the nurse respond?
   1. "Her skin may become mottled."
   2. "Her respirations will become slow and deep."
   3. "Her pulse will increase."
   4. "Her temperature will decrease."

2. One morning when the nurse visits, the nurse finds the family sitting around Mrs. Haliburton's bed, crying. They tell the nurse that she stopped breathing 30 minutes ago. The nurse examines Mrs. Haliburton and finds no respirations, no heart rate, and no pupillary reaction, and her body is cooling. What should be the first action by the nurse?
   1. Confirm to the family that Mrs. Haliburton has died.
   2. Pronounce death and document it in the health record.
   3. Call the health care provider so that they can complete a death certificate.
   4. Notify the funeral home.

3. Mrs. Haliburton's health record had been kept in her home during her palliative care. What should the nurse do with Mrs. Haliburton's health record after her death?
   1. Leave it with the family.
   2. Put it in a sealed envelope for the health care provider.
   3. Take it to the agency that employs the palliative care team.
   4. Destroy the record, as it is no longer needed.

4. Several days later, the family calls the nurse to ask him what to do with Mrs. Haliburton's leftover morphine. What should the nurse say to them?
   1. "Take it to your pharmacy."
   2. "I will pick it up."
   3. "Dispose of it in the biohazard container I left."
   4. "Keep it just in case another family member requires morphine."

5. The nurse has been working in palliative care for several years and is surprised when they feel tremendous sadness at Mrs. Haliburton's death. What should the nurse initially do to cope with these emotions?
   1. Examine their patterns of dealing with grief.
   2. Arrange for time off or a vacation.
   3. Reflect on the need to change to another specialty in nursing.
   4. Make an appointment with a psychiatrist who specializes in palliative care.

CASE 2

Jean Cetaine, age 68, is golfing with his friends when he develops severe chest pain and shortness of breath. His friends call an ambulance, and he is transported to hospital, where he is diagnosed with unstable angina.

Questions 6 to 9 refer to this case.

6. Upon Mr. Cetaine's arrival in the emergency department, which of the following is a "first-line" medication he will likely receive?
   1. Nitroglycerin (Nitrolingual)
   2. Propranolol (Inderal)
   3. Tissue plasminogen activator (t-PA)
   4. Captopril (Capoten)

7. Which of the following tests will best evaluate the extent of Mr. Cetaine's coronary artery disease?
   1. Chest X-ray
   2. Cardiac ultrasonography
   3. Electrocardiography (ECG)
   4. Angiography

8. It is decided that Mr. Cetaine requires coronary artery bypass graft (CABG) surgery. What is the purpose of CABG surgery?
   1. To provide a new circuit for blood flow to get to the heart muscle
   2. To repair damage to the heart muscle
   3. To provide new vessels bringing blood to the right atrium
   4. To provide a route for blood to flow past obstructions in the ascending aorta

9. Nursing care within the first 3 days postsurgery for Mr. Cetaine would include which of the following?
   1. Complete bed rest
   2. Care for two surgical sites
   3. Administration of oxygen via nasal cannula at 3 L/min
   4. Prn analgesia

CASE 3

A nurse educator provides an orientation session about documentation to recently hired nurses.

Questions 10 to 13 refer to this case.

10. The nurse educator reviews the purpose of documentation. Of the following, which is the most important reason for client documentation?
    1. To facilitate communication concerning the client
    2. To demonstrate nursing accountability and professional practice
    3. To provide a source of data for evidence-informed practice
    4. To identify the type and amount of care clients require

11. The nurse educator presents a case scenario about a client who requests information from their health record. When care is provided through an agency, who owns and has access to the health record?
    1. The agency owns the health record, and the client has access only in exceptional circumstances.
    2. The client owns the health record and must provide consent to agency staff for its use for purposes related to care.
    3. The agency and the client co-own the health record, and both have equal access to the information.
    4. The agency owns the health record, but the client has legal access to the information according to agency policies.

12. The nurse educator cautions the nurses to only record care they personally provide. When is it acceptable to document care provided by another nurse?
    1. When the other nurse is not registered or licensed
    2. During an emergency when more than one nurse is involved
    3. When two or more nurses care for a client, only one nurse is required to document
    4. There are no exceptions to the practice of never documenting for another

13. The nurse educator presents another case scenario to the group. A postmastectomy client, Ms. Scharfe, has been crying, refuses to eat, and will not speak to her husband. The nurse educator asks the group to record this behaviour. What is the best documentation of this client situation?
    1. "Ms. Scharfe shows manifestations of depression."
    2. "Ms. Scharfe is upset due to her mastectomy."
    3. "Ms. Scharfe is crying, refuses food, will not talk to her husband."
    4. "Ms. Scharfe experienced an emotional postoperative day, with periods of weeping and anorexia due to pain and anaesthetic and was ignoring her husband."

CASE 4

Glen Martin has a history of alcohol dependence with a high daily intake of alcohol for 15 years. He has made several attempts to stop drinking, has attended Alcoholics Anonymous and private counselling, and has told his wife that he no longer drinks. She arrives home one day to find him confused, smelling of alcohol, and with hand tremors. She takes him to the local emergency department.

Questions 14 to 19 refer to this case.

14. The health care team tells Mrs. Martin that her husband is experiencing acute alcohol withdrawal and must be admitted to hospital. What is the most important reason alcohol-dependent people need to be monitored carefully while withdrawing from alcohol?
    1. Cardiac failure
    2. Acute organ failure
    3. Seizures
    4. Risk of suicide

15. Mrs. Martin says that she can't understand why her husband was drinking because he had promised her he had stopped. What should the nurse respond to Mrs. Martin?
    1. "Because of the effects of alcohol on the brain, he likely did not know what he was doing."
    2. "Why do you think he was lying to you?"
    3. "Your husband is trying to change a long-term habit, and lapses are sometimes to be expected."
    4. "He probably can't help himself."

16. After Mr. Martin's successful detoxification, the health care team notices that he has jaundice. Tests are ordered to confirm a diagnosis of cirrhosis of the liver. Which test should be ordered to confirm the level of jaundice?
    1. Alkaline phosphatase
    2. Serum bilirubin
    3. Alanine aminotransferase (ALT)
    4. Prothrombin time (PT)

17. Mrs. Martin asks the nurse why her husband is yellow. What would be the most appropriate answer by the nurse?
    1. "Your husband has jaundice."
    2. "There is inadequate hepatodetoxification of cellular metabolites resulting from scleroses related to alcohol."
    3. "The effects of alcohol on the liver have interfered with the ability to remove a yellow pigment that is released when red blood cells break down."
    4. "Pressure of the liver on the kidneys prevents them from filtering urine effectively, so it builds up in his system, causing the yellow colour."

18. The nurse teaches Mr. and Mrs. Martin about therapeutic nutrition related to cirrhosis. Which of the following breakfast menus should the nurse recommend?
    1. Toast, margarine, and banana
    2. Cheese omelette
    3. Bagel and peanut butter
    4. Ham, eggs, and hash brown potatoes

19. Mr. Martin is ready to be discharged home, with a referral to an outpatient alcohol rehabilitation program. He has refused alcohol aversion medications. Mrs. Martin is concerned that he will start drinking again. She states that she will consent to giving him disulfiram (Antabuse) but tells him that it is a vitamin. How should the nurse respond?
    1. "Can you arrange to be made his substitute decision maker so that you can consent to the Antabuse?"
    2. "Mr. Martin cannot be given Antabuse without his consent."

3. "That would be helpful, but I don't think you would be allowed to consent for him."

4. "Perhaps you can get the doctor to order it for you and then give it to your husband."

CASE 5

Mr. Ian Lewis is an 83-year-old man who has been referred to the respiratory clinic. He has chronic obstructive pulmonary disease (COPD) and asthma, with poor symptom control for the past few months. Mr. Lewis is frail but lives alone and independently.

Questions 20 to 23 refer to this case.

20. The nurse reviews Mr. Lewis's health history. The nurse asks him about his use of over-the-counter (OTC) medications. What medication would be of most concern to the nurse?
    1. Aspirin (ASA)
    2. Acetaminophen (Tylenol)
    3. Ibuprofen (Advil, Motrin)
    4. Loratadine (Claritin)

21. Mr. Lewis reports that he takes a combination inhaler that contains a long-acting beta$_2$-agonist as well as a steroid. What is the therapeutic action of these two medications?
    1. The medications act in combination to decrease airway inflammation.
    2. They work in combination to decrease airway bronchoconstriction.
    3. They provide bronchodilation and reduced airway inflammation.
    4. The two medications potentiate each other and provide longer-acting symptom control.

22. The nurse asks Mr. Lewis to demonstrate the use of his aerosol metered-dose inhaler (MDI) and observes that he has difficulty using the MDI effectively. What should the nurse recommend to Mr. Lewis?
    1. He should consult with the pharmacist about taking his medications in a form other than the inhaled route.
    2. There are oral forms of the medications that are just as effective and easier for him to take.
    3. A spacer used with the MDI is easier to use and will provide better delivery of medication to his airway.
    4. He will need to be re-educated in the use of inhaled medications.

23. Mr. Lewis tells the nurse he becomes quite frightened when he has a "bad attack" of asthma. He becomes very short of breath, wheezes, and feels as if he is drowning. What should the nurse teach him about the first thing he should do for a serious acute episode of shortness of breath?
    1. Take his combination inhaled drugs to relieve the bronchoconstriction.
    2. Call 9-1-1 to take him to the hospital for emergency respiratory therapy.
    3. Breathe cool, humidified air to liquefy secretions and open the airways.
    4. Use his "rescue inhaler" and wait for about 10 minutes to assess if it restores normal breathing.

CASE 6

A nurse provides primary nursing care to clients at a busy family practice clinic.

Questions 24 to 27 refer to this case.

24. Ryan Fraser is a new client to the clinic. He brings his health record from his previous health care provider and asks the nurse who will have access to his health record at this clinic. What should the nurse tell Mr. Fraser?
    1. "Only the health care provider has access to your record."
    2. "Any of the staff working in the clinic may see your record."
    3. "The health care provider, clerical staff, and I are able to view your health record."
    4. "You may keep your record if you are concerned about confidentiality."

25. Which of the following would be the correct procedure when taking the blood pressure of a hypertensive client who is monitored at the clinic once a week?
    1. Ensure that the client has not had caffeine within the last 5 hours.
    2. Allow the client to rest for 5 minutes prior to taking the blood pressure.
    3. Use manual rather than electronic blood pressure devices.
    4. Alternate arms for each visit.

26. Ms. Shannon has had disabling knee pain for several months and is booked to have magnetic resonance imaging (MRI) in several months. She does not want to wait this long and asks the nurse how she can get the test done earlier. What should the nurse respond?
    1. "Only clients with life-threatening illnesses can have immediate MRI scans."
    2. "You could call the MRI clinic to ask to be put on the cancellation list."
    3. "In Canada, there are not sufficient MRI machines, so you will have to wait until one is available."
    4. "It is not likely that your knee pain is serious, so be reassured that waiting will not contribute to a worsening of your condition."

27. A family visits the health clinic. The father tells the nurse, "I have read on several websites that there is scientific evidence vaccines are not effective, so I will not consent to immunizing my child." What would be the best response by the nurse?
    1. "Has your child, or any child you know, ever had a serious adverse effect after an immunization?"
    2. "Do you have any cultural religious, or personal beliefs regarding immunization?"
    3. "Which vaccines have you read about that are not effective?"
    4. "I agree there is much conflicting information. Can you tell me more about what you read?"

CASE 7

Tom Rutlege, 63 years old, has had surgery for a ruptured aortic aneurysm. The repair was successful, and after stabilization in the Critical Care Unit, he is transferred to a cardiovascular surgical unit.

Questions 28 to 32 refer to this case.

28. The nurse takes and records Mr. Rutlege's vital signs on admission to the unit: temperature 36.4°C; blood pressure 100/60 mm Hg; pulse 90 beats/minute; respirations 20 breaths/minute; oxygen saturation 96%. What should be the nurse's action in response to Mr. Rutlege's vital signs?
    1. Cover him with a warm blanket.
    2. Increase the oxygen, within medical directives.
    3. Continue to monitor the vital signs.
    4. Call the surgeon.

29. Which of the following would be of concern to the nurse when providing postoperative care to Mr. Rutlege?
    1. Urinary output of less than 30 mL per hour
    2. Absent bowel sounds
    3. Pain from the incision site
    4. Scant serosanguinous drainage from the incision

30. Mr. Rutlege has chest tubes attached to a Pleur-evac chest drainage system. The nurse is aware that care of this type of chest tube drainage system includes which of the following?
    1. Ensuring continuous bubbling in the water seal chamber
    2. Taping the connection between the chest tube and drainage system
    3. Adding sterile water to the suction control chamber every 8 hours
    4. Maintaining the system above waist level

31. Mr. Rutlege is ordered a type and cross-match prior to a blood transfusion. What is the purpose of the type and cross-match test?
    1. To determine whether Rh agglutinins are present
    2. To determine whether there is ABO incompatibility
    3. To determine the presence of A or O antigens
    4. To determine the compatibility of his blood with donor blood

32. Mr. Rutlege recovers from surgery and is to be discharged home. He will be caring for his incision himself. How should the nurse best evaluate his ability to perform incision care?
    1. Have him explain how to care for the incision.
    2. Have him demonstrate how to care for the incision.
    3. Ask him questions based on the instructional DVD he has viewed.
    4. Ask him if he has any questions about the care of his incision.

CASE 8

Four-year-old Sam has fallen out of a tree. His mother calls a neighbour, who is a nurse, for help. The nurse observes Sam lying on the ground, moaning and crying. He has several abrasions and a 1-cm cut on his forehead.

Questions 33 to 37 refer to this case.

33. The nurse assesses Sam for injuries. What is the priority assessment?
    1. Signs of head injury
    2. Evidence of limb fracture
    3. Sam's pulse
    4. Other injuries that may not be visible

34. The nurse needs to examine Sam's left leg. What would be the most appropriate initial action to determine whether there is a fracture?
    1. Ask Sam to stand on his left leg.
    2. Rotate the leg and ankle.
    3. Ask Sam to point to where his leg hurts.
    4. Apply pressure to the injured area to assess for bone integrity.

35. The nurse determines that Sam probably has a fracture close to or at the ankle. What is the most appropriate first aid to apply before transporting him to the hospital?
    1. Wrap the leg in a soft blanket.
    2. Immobilize the foot, ankle, and lower leg in a rolled magazine.
    3. Splint the left leg against the right leg.
    4. Apply ice to the fracture site.

36. At the hospital, Sam is seen by a nurse practitioner who orders tests to determine whether Sam has a fractured bone in his leg. What test will the nurse practitioner most likely order?
    1. X-ray
    2. Bone scan
    3. Bone densitometry
    4. Computed tomography (CT) scan

37. It is determined that Sam has a fracture, and his leg is encased in a plaster of Paris cast. Which of the following should be instructions to Sam's parents regarding cast care in the first 24 hours?
    1. Wrap the cast in a plastic bag to prevent it from getting wet or dirty.
    2. Expose the cast to air until dry.
    3. Lift and support the wet cast with the fingertips.
    4. Use a hair dryer to speed the drying process.

CASE 9

Roberta Wilmot, age 54 years, has osteoarthritis. Ms. Wilmot, who admits to being overweight, is a postal worker who walks a route to deliver mail. She is the single mother of an adult son with a disability and must work to maintain health benefits.

Questions 38 to 41 refer to this case.

38. Which of the following manifestations of osteoarthritis is Ms. Wilmot most likely to experience?
    1. Pain in her knees
    2. Sudden onset of pain in most joints
    3. Swelling and erythema in her feet
    4. Paraesthesia in her fingers

39. The nurse counselling Ms. Wilmot discusses lifestyle changes to help with the osteoarthritis. Which of the

following should the nurse most appropriately recommend to Ms. Wilmot?

1. Change of job
2. Weight loss
3. Assistance with her son
4. More exercise

40. Which of the following medications will be of greatest help to alleviate moderate to severe osteoarthritis pain?
1. Muscle relaxants
2. Nonsteroidal anti-inflammatory drugs (NSAIDs)
3. Antibiotics
4. Acetaminophen (Tylenol)

41. An interprofessional team works with Ms. Wilmot to manage her osteoarthritis. In addition to the nurse and physician, which of the following health care workers would be most important to include on the team?
1. Pharmacist
2. Naturopath
3. Social worker
4. Physiotherapist

CASE 10

Meredith Marshall is a 42-year-old woman who is 22 weeks pregnant with her fifth child. She attends the antenatal clinic for her prenatal care.

Questions 42 to 44 refer to this case.

42. What is the most important assessment for the nurse at this visit?
1. Mrs. Marshall's blood pressure
2. Presence of ketones in Mrs. Marshall's urine
3. Estimate of fetal growth
4. Weight gain or loss

43. It is determined that Mrs. Marshall has pre-eclampsia. What is the recommended treatment for mild pre-eclampsia?
1. Complete bed rest in hospital
2. Restricted activity at home
3. Sodium-restricted diet
4. Administration of magnesium sulphate

44. Which of the following questions related to pre-eclampsia should the nurse ask Mrs. Marshall?
1. "Do you have headaches or visual disturbances?"
2. "Are you constipated or bloated?"
3. "Have you experienced any vaginal bleeding or mucus discharge?"
4. "Have you felt any mild contractions or tightening in your abdomen?"

CASE 11

Ross is a 14-year-old adolescent in foster care. Ross was diagnosed as HIV-positive when he was an infant. He has been generally well, except for occasional acute infections that have required hospitalization. Ross is adherent to his antiretroviral therapy. He attends the HIV clinic every 2 months. The clinic nurse notes that Ross's CD4 counts have been dropping (below 500 cells) over the past few months.

Questions 45 to 49 refer to this case.

45. When Ross has his appointment at the clinic, which of the following initial actions, specific to his HIV status, should the nurse implement?
1. Performing hand hygiene
2. Gloving when she examines Ross
3. Placing him in a room separate from infectious clients
4. Asking him if he has been taking his medications

46. The nurse weighs Ross and notes that he has lost 2 kg since his last appointment. What would be an appropriate initial comment to Ross about his weight loss?
1. "What has your appetite been like in the past 2 months?"
2. "Have you had any episodes of diarrhea?"
3. "This may be a sign that your condition is getting worse."
4. "It's good to see you are not one of these obese children we've been reading about."

47. Which of the following is an appropriate topic for the nurse to discuss with Ross at this clinic visit?
1. Feelings and concerns about sexuality
2. Pain management
3. Education regarding transmission of HIV
4. Stress-management techniques

48. Which of the following is a principle of drug therapy for HIV infection?
1. Clients with chronic HIV do not require treatment if they are asymptomatic.
2. Treatment regimens should be individualized depending on CD4 counts.
3. It is preferable to begin treatment with single-drug therapy.
4. Pediatric treatment is limited due to fewer antiretrovirals that are safe for children.

49. The health care provider in the clinic discusses starting a new research medication with Ross. The nurse is not sure whether Ross is able to consent to the research drug because he is 14 and in foster care. What knowledge should the nurse have in this situation?
1. Ross is an emancipated minor and may provide his own consent for the research drug.
2. Foster parents are legally able to provide consent for minors.
3. Agency policies for consent guidelines regarding age and research drug protocols
4. An assessment of Ross's understanding of the proposed treatment

CASE 12

Mr. Ford has been seriously burned in an industrial fire. His condition is stabilized in hospital, but he is only able to manage small sips of fluid by mouth and is not able to maintain adequate nutrition. The health care provider orders total parenteral nutrition (TPN) of protein electrolyte, vitamin, trace elements, and fat emulsion via a peripherally inserted central catheter (PICC).

Questions 50 to 56 refer to this case.

50. The nurse practitioner inserts the single-lumen PICC line at Mr. Ford's bedside. What precautions are necessary for this procedure?
    1. A tourniquet placed around his upper arm
    2. Sterile conditions
    3. Intravenous infusion of midazolam (Versed) for light anaesthesia
    4. Mr. Ford positioned with his head to the side to facilitate subclavian access

51. What must be done by the nurse prior to the first infusion of the TPN solution?
    1. Ensure correct catheter placement is verified by chest X-ray.
    2. Educate Mr. Ford about the PICC line and TPN.
    3. Warm the solution for a minimum of 3 hours.
    4. Add ordered electrolytes and trace elements to the solution.

52. Mr. Ford is ordered an intravenous antibiotic. How should the nurse administer this medication?
    1. Add the antibiotic to the protein and electrolyte solution.
    2. Administer it in the fat emulsion solution.
    3. Administer it via Y-tubing to the PICC line.
    4. Commence an additional peripheral intravenous line in a separate vein.

53. The nurse is aware that they need to observe many safety measures related to Mr. Ford's PICC line and the TPN infusion. Which of the following is a nursing action related to client safety?
    1. Change all TPN tubing lines every 24 hours.
    2. Label the tubing and filter with the date and time they were changed.
    3. Change the dressing at the catheter insertion site once per shift.
    4. Send the tubing for culture once per week.

54. How should the nurse best evaluate Mr. Ford's tolerance of the TPN?
    1. Daily weights
    2. Positive balance for intake and output
    3. Improved healing of his burns
    4. Laboratory values

55. Several days later, Mr. Ford tells the nurse he still doesn't really understand the PICC line and where it is in his body. What would be the most appropriate response by the nurse?
    1. "Let me draw you some pictures of where the PICC line is in your body."
    2. "The PICC line is a flexible catheter that sits inside the large vein leading to your heart."
    3. "The manufacturer's monograph provides most of the information you need."
    4. "The nurse practitioner who inserted the line will explain it to you."

56. Mr. Ford's TPN solution is stopped one day because he is off the unit for tests. He is behind a total of 500 mL of solution. The solution is running at 200 mL per hour. What should the nurse do, in accordance with agency policies, in this situation?
    1. Do not make up the 500 mL.
    2. Increase the ordered flow to 220 mL until the 500 mL is made up.
    3. Take the solution off the infusion pump and increase the rate to 300 mL per hour.
    4. Offer Mr. Ford increased fluids by mouth.

CASE 13

Jennifer and Ronald Buxton are clients at a family practice clinic. Mr. and Mrs. Buxton have lived together in a "stormy" relationship for 10 years. A nurse at the clinic has often suspected intimate-partner violence and has spoken with Mrs. Buxton about it, but Mrs. Buxton has denied any abuse.

Questions 57 to 61 refer to this case.

57. One day, the nurse receives a phone call from Mrs. Buxton, who is hysterical and crying, saying, "Ronnie is beating me up." What should be the nurse's first response to Mrs. Buxton?
    1. "How long has he been abusing you?"
    2. "You need to come to the doctor's office right away."
    3. "How badly has he beaten you up?"
    4. "Are you in a safe place?"

58. Mr. Buxton is arrested by the police and subsequently convicted of assault. His sentencing requires him to have mandatory counselling. During the first session with the counsellor, who is a mental health nurse, what is the nurse's most important initial therapeutic goal?
    1. Establishing trust between himself and Mr. Buxton
    2. Determining the causative factors involved in the abuse of Mrs. Buxton
    3. Developing healthy and open patterns of communication
    4. Ensuring that Mr. Buxton understands that counselling is mandatory

59. Mr. Buxton tells the mental health nurse that he has absolutely no memory of hitting Mrs. Buxton. What defence mechanism is this an example of?
    1. Splitting
    2. Repression
    3. Introjection
    4. Compensation

60. Mr. Buxton eventually admits to abusing Mrs. Buxton. He tells the mental health nurse that it is all because she "nags" him. What would be a therapeutic response by the mental health nurse?
    1. "That is no excuse to hit Mrs. Buxton."
    2. "Does hitting Mrs. Buxton make her stop nagging?"
    3. "I'm not sure what you mean; please explain that to me again."
    4. "Why does Mrs. Buxton nag you?"

61. As the mental health nurse learns more about Mr. Buxton, he finds that Mr. Buxton has some typical characteristics of abusers. Which of the following is most characteristic of perpetrators of abuse?
    1. A history of alcohol abuse
    2. Low socioeconomic status
    3. Cultural factors
    4. A family history of abuse and authoritarianism

Case 14

Aubrey Hudson and her partner, Christof Peters, are a couple in their 30s who have experienced fertility problems. After taking clomiphene (Clomid) for several months, Ms. Hudson becomes pregnant. An ultrasonogram at 8 weeks' gestation confirms that Ms. Hudson is expecting twins. Ms. Hudson attends a health clinic routinely for prenatal care and counselling.

Questions 62 to 69 refer to this case.

62. Ms. Hudson is likely expecting fraternal twins. Which of the following is a characteristic of fraternal twins?
    1. A single ovum has divided into two embryos.
    2. They will be the same sex.
    3. They are more likely to occur in younger women.
    4. There are two placentas.

63. During her second trimester, Ms. Hudson asks the nurse what to do about constipation. What should be the first action the nurse recommends?
    1. Increase fluids, fresh fruits, and vegetables in her diet.
    2. Increase exercise.
    3. Use a natural laxative.
    4. Take a stool softener, such as docusate sodium (Colace).

64. Ms. Hudson will be monitored carefully during the pregnancy because of the previous fertility problems and multiple gestation. She will deliver in hospital rather than the birthing centre. Which of the following is a significant risk for individuals with a fraternal twin pregnancy?
    1. Preterm labour
    2. Twin to twin transfusion
    3. Conjoined twins
    4. Oligohydramnios

65. During the latter half of the second trimester, situations in the third trimester that require immediately notifying the health care provider are reviewed with the client. Which of the following would be a danger sign during a pregnancy?
    1. Dyspnea
    2. A weight gain of 0.5 to 0.75 kg in the third trimester
    3. Leg cramps
    4. Fewer than 10 fetal movements in 12 hours

66. Ms. Hudson has brown eyes, and her partner, Mr. Peters, has blue eyes. Ms. Hudson asks the nurse what colour the babies' eyes will be. What should be the nurse's response?
    1. Both babies will likely have blue eyes.
    2. Both babies will most likely, but not certainly, have brown eyes.
    3. One baby will have brown eyes, and the other will have blue eyes.
    4. Eye colour is genetically random, and it is not possible to predict.

67. As the pregnancy progresses, Ms. Hudson develops edema in her ankles. What should the nurse recommend to reduce the edema?
    1. Fluid restriction
    2. Keeping her legs uncrossed
    3. Elevating her legs
    4. Range-of-motion exercises

68. Ms. Hudson tells the nurse that although she is happy to have twins, she is disappointed because she will not be able to breastfeed two infants. What should the nurse respond?
    1. "You could breastfeed one and formula-feed the other."
    2. "Perhaps if you are able to get pregnant again, you could breastfeed the next baby."
    3. "It is very difficult to breastfeed twins, and most women are not successful."
    4. "With planning and extra nourishment, you may be able to breastfeed both infants."

69. At 36 weeks, Ms. Hudson delivers twins by Caesarean birth. Each twin has a separate health care team in the delivery room. What is the first assessment each nurse would perform with the infants?
    1. Heart rate
    2. Temperature
    3. Respirations
    4. Blood pressure

Case 15

A nursing teacher is assisting student nurses who are conducting a blood pressure clinic at a local shopping mall.

Questions 70 to 72 refer to this case.

70. The nursing teacher instructs a student nurse how to correctly perform blood pressure monitoring by auscultation. Which of the following should the teacher demonstrate as the proper technique?
    1. Have the client lie down with the arm extended.
    2. Use a cuff width that is 80% of the length of the client's upper arm.
    3. Quickly inflate the cuff to 10% above the client's expected blood pressure.
    4. Place the bell of the stethoscope over the brachial artery.

71. The nursing teacher instructs a student how to perform self–blood-pressure monitoring using an electronic device. What would be the most effective evaluation of the teaching?
    1. The student is able to correctly perform blood pressure monitoring on another student.
    2. The student is able to verbalize the correct procedure for blood pressure monitoring.
    3. The student is able to state normal blood pressure values.
    4. The student is able to demonstrate the technique on themselves.

72. One of the students takes Mr. Brown's blood pressure using the portable electronic blood pressure monitor and obtains a reading of 186/110 mm Hg. The student retakes the blood pressure but obtains the same result.

Mr. Brown tells the teacher and the student that although he takes antihypertensives, to his knowledge, his blood pressure has previously been within normal limits. What should be the nursing teacher's first action?

1. Retake the blood pressure with a manual device.
2. Ask Mr. Brown to lie down and relax and then take the blood pressure again.
3. Find out from Mr. Brown which antihypertensive medication he takes.
4. Replace the batteries in the electronic monitor.

Independent Questions

Questions 73 to 125 do not refer to a particular case.

73. Which of the following drugs may depress a client's immune system?
    1. Meperidine (Demerol)
    2. Cefazolin (Ancef)
    3. Prednisone (Apo-Prednisone)
    4. Salbutamol (Ventolin)

74. What is the primary reason why nurses should be involved in social justice issues?
    1. Socioeconomic and political issues have an impact on health.
    2. Social justice will improve the working conditions of nurses.
    3. Advocacy is part of the role of the nurse.
    4. Politicians will change laws based on nursing input.

75. Ms. Hope, mother of 5-month-old Isabelle, asks the nurse when Isabelle will be able to pull herself to a standing position. What should the nurse tell her?
    1. "It should be any time now."
    2. "Infants generally pull themselves up onto furniture at about 6 to 7 months."
    3. "Isabelle will probably stand holding onto a table by about 8 to 10 months."
    4. "I don't think you should expect Isabelle to stand until about 11 to 12 months."

76. When are antilipidemic medications such as atorvastatin (Lipitor) most appropriately ordered?
    1. In people over 65 years of age
    2. In people who do not exercise sufficiently
    3. In people for whom dietary measures have not lowered cholesterol
    4. In people who have elevated cholesterol for over 2 months

77. Health Canada recommends that all individuals who could become pregnant take a folic acid supplement. What is the reason for this recommendation?
    1. It helps prevent neural tube defects in the fetus, should the individual become pregnant.
    2. It maximizes the nutritional status of the individual prior to becoming pregnant.
    3. It prevents the occurrence of cleft lip and palate, which occurs early in pregnancy.
    4. It is necessary for the adequate formation of estrogen and progesterone.

78. A community nurse is concerned because many of their chronically ill clients do not have a primary care provider. What short-term solution should the nurse suggest to the clients?
    1. Advise them to go to the local community walk-in clinic as necessary.
    2. Provide them with a list of all the community health care providers for them to call.
    3. Advise them to call the provincial telephone health information line for advice.
    4. Provide the clients with comprehensive health care to the best of their ability.

79. Manifestations of sickle cell disease may include which of the following?
    1. Anemia
    2. Fever
    3. Vomiting
    4. Bradycardia

80. Ms. Blatchberg has leukopenia. Which of the following should the nurse include in client teaching?
    1. Her gums may bleed when she brushes her teeth.
    2. She should try to eat green leafy vegetables.
    3. She should ensure she receives the influenza vaccine.
    4. She should avoid people with communicable diseases.

81. Mr. Skinner has sustained a C6 spinal cord injury and has developed autonomic dysreflexia. Which of the following is the most common precipitating cause of autonomic dysreflexia?
    1. Distended bladder or rectum
    2. Nasal congestion
    3. High dietary fibre
    4. Low blood pressure

82. Ms. Benjamin, age 52 years, is scheduled for an elective hysterectomy. She has a prosthetic mitral valve and was advised by her health care provider to discontinue her daily dose of Aspirin (ASA) prior to surgery. What property of Aspirin forms the rationale for this action?
    1. Analgesic
    2. Antipyretic
    3. Anti-inflammatory
    4. Antiplatelet

83. A nurse reviews client data when arriving on shift. The nurse notes that one of their clients, Mr. Barry, routinely takes Advair, which is a combined inhaled steroid and bronchodilator. Which of the following would be a priority assessment for the nurse to perform on Mr. Barry?
    1. Cardiovascular
    2. Gastro-intestinal
    3. Neurological
    4. Respiratory

84. Which is the proper method of mixing IV solutions and medications?
    1. Shaking the bag or bottle vigorously
    2. Holding the bag or bottle and gently turning it end to end

3. Inverting the bag or bottle just once after injecting the medication

4. Allowing the IV solution to stand for 10 minutes to enhance even distribution of medication

85. Ms. Brette is voluntarily admitted, on a short-term basis, to a psychiatric unit for management of her anxiety disorder. She experiences a severe anxiety attack while she is in the client lounge. What should the nurse do?

1. Comfort Ms. Brette by holding and hugging her.

2. Move Ms. Brette closer to other clients.

3. Administer her ordered prn lorazepam (Ativan).

4. Take her to her room.

86. A nurse is on an airplane flight and is asked to come to the aid of a fellow passenger. The nurse assesses a man who is approximately in his 60s, diaphoretic, and complaining of severe pain in his chest. What should be the nurse's first action?

1. Tell airline staff the passenger may be having a heart attack.

2. Ask the man if he has any history of heart disease.

3. Take the man's vital signs with equipment provided by the airline.

4. Administer oxygen via passenger mask.

87. A nurse receives a telephone call from her neighbour Mrs. Dunlop, who tells the nurse that her husband is experiencing chest pain and is sweating. Which of the following should the nurse recommend?

1. Call 9-1-1.

2. Call 9-1-1 and give her husband an Aspirin (ASA) if available.

3. Call 9-1-1 and place her husband in a knee-chest position.

4. Call 9-1-1 and cover her husband with a blanket.

88. Dina Shpak, age 54, has chronic stable angina pectoris. Her health care provider orders nitroglycerin in the form of a spray (Nitrolingual sublingual spray). The nurse teaches Dina about the use of the spray. Which of the following should the nurse include in teaching?

1. The aerosol should be inhaled as she takes a deep breath.

2. If she experiences headache, she should immediately notify the physician.

3. She will experience pain relief in approximately 30 minutes.

4. The spray should be taken before exercise or stressful physical activity.

89. Mrs. Wiesenthal, a client on a chronic care rehabilitation unit, has a positive test for *Clostridium difficile* (*C. difficile*). What organism-specific manifestation is she most likely to experience?

1. Fever

2. Vomiting

3. Chills

4. Diarrhea

90. After many years of symptoms and diagnostic tests, Ms. Drummond has been diagnosed with fibromyalgia. Which of the following is characteristic of this condition?

1. It is primarily a psychiatric diagnosis.

2. There is no effective treatment.

3. There are neither manifestations nor diagnostics specific to the disease.

4. Pain and fatigue become progressively worse.

91. A nurse wishes to join an organization to protest social and economic inequality. Another nurse asks what this has to do with health. What is the nurse's best response?

1. "Economics is a social determinant of health."

2. "People at the lower end of the socioeconomic scale have proven poorer health than those at the upper end."

3. "Health care must be equal and available to all."

4. "Nurses have an obligation to be advocates for all levels of society."

92. Mr. Hardacre has just returned to the surgical unit following tracheotomy surgery. What is the priority nursing action?

1. Observing for hemorrhage

2. Maintaining a patent airway

3. Performing frequent suctioning

4. Taking vital signs

93. Mr. Scott is diagnosed with hepatitis A after returning from a tropical vacation. He asks the nurse how he got the virus. What should the nurse respond?

1. "Did you have any sexual encounters when you were on vacation?"

2. "Because of the air circulation in planes, it is likely you got the virus on the flight."

3. "Hepatitis A is endemic to tropical countries."

4. "You most likely ingested contaminated food or water."

94. A nurse has difficulty sleeping after working a 12-hour night shift and feels chronically sleep-deprived. Which of the following may be a recommendation to help the nurse obtain more sleep?

1. Eat a main meal consisting of high protein and low fat toward the end of the night shift.

2. Wear dark sunglasses before leaving work after her night shift.

3. Perform aerobic exercise for 30 minutes after working the night shift.

4. Advocate for a minimum of 12 hours off between rotating from night to day shift.

95. Mrs. Bedford, the mother of 4-month-old Garth, asks the nurse, "Which of my son's teeth are going to come in first?" What should the nurse respond?

1. "The upper two teeth, the frontal incisors."

2. "The bottom two teeth, the central incisors."

3. "The two 'eye teeth,' or canine teeth."

4. "His primary molars."

96. The nurse notes that Mr. Varcoe's nasogastric tube has not drained for several hours, and his abdomen appears distended. What should be the nurse's first action?

1. Irrigate the tube.

2. Instill saline in the tube.

3. Remove the tube.

4. Notify the health care provider.

97. Ms. Bacci is 10 weeks' gestation with her third pregnancy. She tells the nurse, "I make big babies. My other two were over 4.5 kg when they were born." What screening test, related to this statement, would be most appropriate for Ms. Bacci?
    1. Fasting blood glucose
    2. Amniocentesis
    3. Maternal nutrition analysis
    4. Pelvimetry

98. A 48-year-old female client has been started on estrogen hormone therapy after experiencing the symptoms of menopause. Which condition is a contraindication to the administration of estrogen for this client?
    1. Osteoporosis
    2. Uterine bleeding
    3. Thrombophlebitis
    4. Atrophic vaginitis

99. Which individual is at high risk for an altered response to anaesthesia?
    1. A 30-year-old male who has never had surgery before
    2. A 45-year-old female who stopped smoking 10 years ago
    3. A 20-year-old male who is to have a lymph node removed
    4. A 78-year-old female who is to have her gallbladder removed

100. A pregnant person has just received results indicating that they are HIV-positive. The person says to the nurse, "How am I going to tell my boyfriend that I have AIDS?" What is the most appropriate response by the nurse?
    1. "Is there a chance you got HIV from your boyfriend?"
    2. "You do not have AIDS; let's talk about being HIV-positive."
    3. "It is more important at this time to think about protecting your baby from HIV."
    4. "He will have to know you are HIV-positive; let's talk about how to tell him."

101. A nurse works in a multilingual environment. In many instances, the nurse cannot communicate with their clients and knows they are not providing optimal care. What is the nurse's best action for a long-term solution to this problem?
    1. Communicate to all clients to bring a family member to interpret.
    2. Advocate for the purchase of English translation dictionaries for the most common languages.
    3. As part of their reflective practice, enroll in classes to learn the most common languages.
    4. Speak with the agency representative regarding purchase of an on-site telephone or video-link interpreter service.

102. A nurse who works in a corrections facility has been called as a witness for an inquest into the death of an inmate. What is the purpose of a medical inquest?
    1. To determine criminal liability in an unexpected medical event
    2. To determine civil liability in a suspicious death
    3. To prosecute persons or agencies suspected of neglect with regard to their clients
    4. To make recommendations to improve the health care system in the future

103. Which of the following people, according to their body shape and body mass index (BMI), have the highest risk of cardiovascular disease (CVD) and type 2 diabetes?
    1. Mark: apple shape, BMI 24
    2. Consuelo: apple shape, BMI 31
    3. Pedro: pear shape, BMI 27
    4. Christa: pear shape, BMI 18

104. Aisha has anorexia nervosa. She has severely restricted fat in her diet. If Aisha were to eat 12 g of fat and a total of 1 100 kcal per day, what percentage of her daily intake would be from fat?
    1. 8%
    2. 10%
    3. 12%
    4. 15%

105. Mrs. Carnegy is hospitalized for pneumonia. She tells the nurse that she would like to continue to take peppermint, an herbal preparation, which she finds is effective for her irritable bowel syndrome (IBS). What should the nurse do?
    1. Consult with the health care team to see if they agree to include peppermint in the plan of care.
    2. Tell Mrs. Carnegy that herbal preparations cannot be administered while she is in hospital.
    3. Agree to provide Mrs. Carnegy with peppermint, as it is a recognized complementary therapy.
    4. Recommend that Mrs. Carnegy consult with her health care provider about other prescription medications that may be more effective than peppermint.

106. A nurse visits an older persons' residence in northern Saskatchewan. What would be an important safety precaution the nurse should suggest to the residents?
    1. Stay inside during icy winter days.
    2. Place area rugs on bare floors.
    3. Use a stove to warm food rather than microwave ovens.
    4. Take over-the-counter cough preparations at the first sign of a chest cold.

107. What is the most conclusive screening test for colorectal cancer?
    1. Fecal occult blood
    2. Sigmoidoscopy
    3. Colonoscopy
    4. Barium enema

108. A 2-year-old child in respiratory distress has the following health care provider order: "Give oxygen by face mask to keep the O_2 saturation above 95%." The nurse notes that the oxygen saturation has fallen to 80%. What should be the initial action by the nurse?
    1. Double-check the order with the health care provider.
    2. Administer additional oxygen.
    3. Arrange for arterial blood gases to confirm the O_2 saturation reading.
    4. Perform a chest assessment.

109. Mr. Patrick has had seasonal allergies for many years. Recently he has found his usual over-the-counter allergy medication is not working as effectively. He asks the nurse what he should do. What would the nurse initially suggest?
   1. Speak with his pharmacist.
   2. Make an appointment with the nurse practitioner.
   3. Arrange for allergy testing with a medical allergist.
   4. Discuss environmental controls with a respiratory therapist.

110. Mr. Price is admitted to hospital for investigation of abdominal pain. The nurse notes that one of Mr. Price's medications is clozapine (Clozaril), an antipsychotic. What action should the nurse take prior to administration of the Clozaril?
   1. Ask Mr. Price why he is taking an antipsychotic medication.
   2. Look in the medical record for information related to why he is on an antipsychotic drug.
   3. Perform an orientation to reality assessment on Mr. Price.
   4. Ensure that safety measures are in place prior to entering his room with the medication.

111. What is a frequent complaint of older persons who are beginning to experience age-related hearing loss?
   1. Ringing in the ears
   2. Other people mumbling when they talk
   3. Not being able to hear men's voices
   4. Not being able to hear themselves speaking

112. Mr. Braham has been on the rehabilitation unit for 2 days. He has been identified by the nurses as being a "demanding" client. He rings the call bell frequently for what are felt to be minor concerns and complains he is not receiving enough attention. When Mr. Braham calls for his nurse the fourth time within 1 hour, what is the best intervention by the nurse?
   1. Tell Mr. Braham that he is not allowed to ring the call bell more often than once an hour, unless it is an emergency.
   2. Sit with Mr. Braham and ask him to describe his feelings and concerns.
   3. Alternate care with the other nurse on duty so that he feels he is receiving more attention.
   4. Set limits by telling Mr. Braham his physical condition does not require the attention he is demanding and his behaviour is not appropriate.

113. Mr. Hill is a caregiver for his wife, Verna, who has dementia. He expresses frustration to the nurse because of difficulties communicating with Verna. What communication technique would be most effective for the nurse to suggest to Mr. Hill?
   1. Speak slowly and loudly.
   2. Use written rather than verbal communication.
   3. Speak in short, simple sentences.
   4. Repeat phrases several times.

114. Ms. Enright, a client newly admitted to a mental health facility, says to the nurse, "Do you have a boyfriend?" What is the most appropriate response by the nurse?
   1. "Let's talk about you. Are you dating anyone?"

   2. "I am not allowed to tell you about my personal life."
   3. "Yes, I do. We have been together for three wonderful years."
   4. "This interview is about you, not me."

115. Mr. Dovgan has just been admitted to the neurology unit. Mr. Dovgan is recovering from a brain injury and also has unstable bipolar disorder. When the nurse enters the room to assess Mr. Dovgan, he says to her, "Get out of here or I am going to kill you." What should be the primary action by the nurse?
   1. Document and report to the nurse in charge the facts of the verbal abuse and threat.
   2. Recognize that the behaviour is related to Mr. Dovgan's diagnosis and not take the abuse personally.
   3. Implement safety strategies to protect herself.
   4. Obtain support from nursing colleagues who are involved in Mr. Dovgan's care.

116. A nurse works at a suicide prevention telephone hotline. Which of the following callers would the nurse consider to be most at risk for suicide?
   1. Lindsay, age 16, who says she is going to buy razor blades to cut her wrists
   2. Ahmet, age 21, who tells the nurse he is going to use his gun to shoot himself
   3. Florence, a 40-year-old woman who expresses the desire to overdose on antidepressants but has agreed to go to the hospital
   4. Fred, an older person who is recently widowed and says he no longer wants to live

117. Mrs. Scales is a resident of a long-term care facility. She has advanced dementia, no spontaneous mobility, and severe contractures of her hands. The family asks how often splints are applied to her hands. What is the most appropriate response by the nurse to their question?
   1. The splints are ordered to be applied for 4 hours a day.
   2. The physiotherapist has recommended the splints be applied 4 hours a day.
   3. I have just assessed Mrs. Scales, and she has the splints on.
   4. The nurse's documentation shows the splints are applied 4 hours a day from 8 in the morning to noon.

118. The nurse is planning a teaching session about nutrition with a group of children. What must the nurse initially assess prior to the teaching session?
   1. What the children know about nutrition
   2. What the children normally eat
   3. What the developmental level of the children is
   4. What the learning outcomes should be from the session

119. Douglas, age 3, has recently been diagnosed with autism. What is a priority goal for Douglas's development?
   1. Provision of appropriate pharmacological treatment
   2. Intensive early intervention and education therapy
   3. Referral to a pediatric psychiatrist
   4. Safety assessment of the home

120. Antonia Chaley, age 6, experiences frequent epistaxis, particularly in cold, dry weather. What should the nurse advise Antonia and her parents for first aid treatment?
    1. Pinch both nostrils closed just below the nasal bone and hold for 10 to 15 minutes.
    2. Tilt the head back and hold the bridge of the nose.
    3. Blow the nose gently and repeatedly until the bleeding stops.
    4. Pack the nose with tissue or cotton balls.

121. Martina is a preceptor for a nursing student in their final clinical placement. The student has difficulty finishing their work before the end of the shift and has not been able to accurately assess client acuity. Martina has never been a preceptor before. What should be her initial action to address the situation with the student?
    1. Discuss with the student their learning goals, present performance, and past experience.
    2. Consult with the faculty advisor concerning the expected level of performance for students in the final clinical placement.
    3. Discuss the student's performance with the unit nurse educator.
    4. Refer to written material, provided by the nursing school, concerning student and preceptor expectations.

122. Ms. San explains to Ms. Ryerson, a nurse at a health clinic, that she has always taken ibuprofen (Advil) for aches, pains, and mild headaches but now finds that it bothers her stomach. Which of the following medications could be considered as an alternative?
    1. Naproxen (Aleve)
    2. Celecoxib (Celebrex)
    3. Acetaminophen (Tylenol)
    4. Acetylsalicylic Acid (Aspirin)

123. Liam Douglas is receiving intravenous (IV) fluids of 0.9% sodium chloride at 40 mL per hour. His nurse must hang a 2-L bag of IV fluid as no smaller bags are available. The nurse is not certain how long they can safely leave the bag hanging before changing it. What is the most appropriate action by the nurse?
    1. Change the bag of IV solution after 24 hours.
    2. Label the date and time of hanging the bag.
    3. Consult agency policies regarding IV solution "hang times."
    4. Change the bag when it is empty.

124. A moderately active female requires 18 kcal per 0.45 kg to maintain an ideal weight. How many kilocalories would a 56.7 kg woman require per day?
    1. 1 021 kcal
    2. 1 936 kcal
    3. 2 268 kcal
    4. 2 420 kcal

125. Following hip replacement surgery, Ms. Cakebread, age 92, develops pneumonia. She is receiving intravenous antibiotics and oxygen via a nasal cannula. Which of the following manifestations would be of most concern to her nurse?

1. Respiratory rate of 20 breaths per minute
2. Productive cough
3. Restlessness
4. Arterial pO_2 of 90 mm Hg

ANSWERS AND RATIONALES FOR BOOK TWO

The correct answer is set off in boldface.

1. **C: Foundations of Practice T: Application**
    1. **As death approaches, the skin becomes cool, clammy, and mottled due to diminished circulation.**
    2. Respirations are often rapid and shallow, progressing to Cheyne-Stokes respirations.
    3. The pulse becomes weak, but the rate does not increase.
    4. Although the skin feels cool to the touch, body temperature often increases prior to death.

2. **C: Professional, Ethical, and Legal Practice T: Critical Thinking**
    1. **The nurse will need to perform all the listed actions. Because the family is right there, the first action is to confirm for them that Mrs. Haliburton has passed away. It would be inappropriate to document or make calls before speaking with the family. The nurse can offer them time alone with the body while performing other duties.**
    2. The nurse must do this after speaking with the family.
    3. As in choice 2.
    4. As in choice 2.

3. **C: Professional, Ethical, and Legal Practice T: Critical Thinking**
    1. The health record does not belong to the family.
    2. The health care provider is part of the palliative care team. They do not own the health record.
    3. **The health care record belongs to the agency, in this case, the agency that employs the palliative care team. The nurse must take the record to the agency for legally specified storage.**
    4. This is not legal. Records must be maintained by the agency for a length of time as specified in legislation.

4. **C: Professional, Ethical, and Legal Practice T: Application**
    1. **The morphine is the legal property of the Haliburtons. They have no means to dispose of it safely. Pharmacies will safely dispose of unused medications.**
    2. The nurse should not be transporting narcotics. This is not a practical nursing responsibility.
    3. It is not optimum for a narcotic to be disposed of in a biohazard container.
    4. This is not safe advice. One person should not use medications prescribed for someone else.

5. **C: Professional, Ethical, and Legal Practice T: Application**
    1. **The nurse's initial action should be to reflect on their coping mechanisms for grief and whether these have been effective in the past. Once they have analyzed their reactions, they may choose one of the other options.**

2. This may be an option after self-reflection.

3. Reflection may determine a need to change to another specialty.

4. This is not likely to be necessary at this stage, only if the nurse experiences further emotional difficulties.

6. **C: Foundations of Practice T: Application**

1. **Nitrates are first-line therapy for treatment of acute anginal symptoms. They will dilate peripheral blood vessels and coronary arteries, increasing blood flow to the heart.**

2. Beta-adrenergic blockers reduce the heart rate and contractility and reduce afterload. They are not first-line drugs in emergency angina care.

3. This would be given only if the presence of thrombi were confirmed.

4. Angiotensin-converting enzyme inhibitors are useful with heart failure, tachycardia, myocardial infarction, and hypertension. They are not first-line drugs for unstable angina.

7. **C: Foundations of Practice T: Critical Thinking**

1. A chest X-ray will be taken to assess cardiac enlargement, cardiac calcification, and pulmonary congestion. It does not allow for visualization of the coronary arteries.

2. Cardiac ultrasonography is not of significant use with angina.

3. An ECG is obtained to determine abnormalities of electrical function in the heart. In Mr. Cetaine's case, it will likely be used to rule out myocardial infarction but does not confirm the extent of angina.

4. **Coronary angiography allows visualization of the coronary arteries and helps determine appropriate treatment.**

8. **C: Foundations of Practice T: Knowledge**

1. **The construction of new conduits beyond the coronary obstruction restores blood flow to the myocardium.**

2. CABG cannot repair damage to the myocardium but can help prevent further damage.

3. CABG provides new blood vessels to the myocardium, not the right atrium.

4. The obstruction is in the coronary artery, not the aorta.

9. **C: Foundations of Practice T: Application**

1. Complete bed rest is rarely indicated postsurgery as it is likely to increase postoperative complications. Mr. Cetaine likely would be permitted to gradually resume a limited degree of activity.

2. **CABG requires a graft from another site, most often the saphenous vein, internal mammary artery, or radial artery; thus, there would be a chest and a graft site.**

3. Oxygen will be ordered according to oxygen saturations. It may not necessarily be required.

4. Pain management is important, particularly if there is a thoracotomy. Narcotics are used; however, they are administered around the clock, not prn.

10. **C: Professional, Ethical, and Legal Practice T: Critical Thinking**

1. **The primary purpose of documentation is to communicate client information among care providers. Documentation is communication that reflects the client's health and well-being, the care provided, the effect of care, and the continuity of care. All health care providers need ongoing access to client information to provide safe and effective care and treatment.**

2. Documentation does demonstrate nursing accountability and gives credit to nurses for their professional practice. However, the primary purpose is to communicate information about the client.

3. Health records can be a valuable source of data for research and quality assurance purposes; however, this is not the primary purpose.

4. Data from nursing documentation can indicate the care and services provided to clients and the efficiency of the care. However, this is not the primary purpose of documentation.

11. **C: Professional, Ethical, and Legal Practice T: Application**

1. The agency does own the health record, but the client has the right of access to the information, not just in exceptional circumstances.

2. The client does not own the record. Consent for disclosure to agency staff for purposes related to care is implied upon admission.

3. Only the agency owns the record.

4. **When care is provided by an agency, the actual record belongs to that agency. With very few exceptions, clients have right of access to their own records. Agencies generally have policies about what to do if clients ask for their health records.**

12. **C: Professional, Ethical, and Legal Practice T: Application**

1. The term *nurse* is applied only to registered or licensed individuals. Although student nurses are not yet registered or licensed, and there may be others who have not yet received confirmation of registration/licence, those people must document the care they provide.

2. **This is the exception. The nurse who documents the care provided by another nurse in such situations would have been involved and have had personal knowledge of the situation. This most frequently occurs in emergency or "code" situations, in which one nurse may be designated as the recorder.**

3. This is not true. Both nurses are required to document the care they provided.

4. There is an exception, as noted in choice 2.

13. **C: Professional, Ethical, and Legal Practice T: Application**

1. This is a judgement and not fact.

2. As in choice 1.

3. **This is an accurate description of the facts concerning Ms. Scharfe's behaviour. Information should be recorded concisely and accurately and focus on facts rather than assumptions.**

4. This entry is too wordy and makes assumptions.

14. C: Foundations of Practice T: Critical Thinking

1. **Alcohol withdrawal delirium, or delirium tremens (DTs), may lead to death caused by hyperthermia, peripheral vascular collapse, and cardiac failure.**

2. This does not occur in alcohol withdrawal.

3. Seizures may occur but are not as serious as cardiac failure.

4. The client in alcohol withdrawal is unlikely to be able to commit suicide.

15. C: Foundations of Practice T: Application

1. This is not likely. He would be aware of his drinking.

2. This is not a therapeutic response.

3. **This is a factual response. It may help Mrs. Martin understand the disease and that support, although not acceptance, will be most helpful to her husband's recovery.**

4. Alcohol is a strong addiction; however, if Mr. Martin wishes to stop drinking, he has the ability to help himself.

16. C: Foundations of Practice T: Knowledge

1. This is a test for liver enzymes.

2. **Bilirubin metabolism abnormalities with cirrhosis are responsible for the deposit of yellow pigment in the skin (jaundice).**

3. As in choice 1.

4. Prothrombin time is a reflection of clotting factors.

17. C: Foundations of Practice T: Critical Thinking

1. This does not explain why Mr. Martin is yellow.

2. This is too complex an answer for Mrs. Martin.

3. **This is the correct physiological rationale for the jaundice and is at a level that Mrs. Martin can understand.**

4. This is not physiologically correct.

18. C: Foundations of Practice T: Application

1. **Cirrhosis interferes with the liver's ability to eliminate ammonia. Protein is converted to ammonia; therefore, Mr. Martin requires a low-protein diet. This breakfast is low in protein.**

2. This is a high-protein meal.

3. This is a high-protein meal.

4. This is a high-protein meal.

19. C: Foundations of Practice T: Application

1. There is no reason to assume that Mr. Martin is not cognitively able to make his own treatment decisions.

2. **This is a factual answer. Giving Mr. Martin Antabuse without his consent is unethical.**

3. This implies that an unethical practice is condoned and that the nurse is not sure of the legal and ethical implications.

4. This is an unprofessional and unethical response.

20. C: Foundations of Practice T: Application

1. **Aspirin can trigger asthma attacks in 20% of adults.**

2. There are no contraindications for the use of acetaminophen in clients with asthma.

3. There are no contraindications for the use of ibuprofen in clients with asthma.

4. Many people with asthma have seasonal allergies and use antihistamines such as loratadine for symptom control. These drugs are not contraindicated except during an acute attack.

21. C: Foundations of Practice T: Application

1. Beta$_2$-agonists do not decrease airway inflammation.

2. Inhaled steroids do not decrease bronchoconstriction.

3. **The long-acting beta2-agonist provides bronchodilation for up to 12 hours. The inhaled steroid decreases inflammation. Combining the two medications provides a convenient dosing regimen for the client.**

4. The medications do not potentiate each other, nor is it necessary to combine the drugs in one inhaler to provide longer-acting symptom control.

22. C: Foundations of Practice T: Application

1. Inhaled medications are the preferred therapy for asthma. Other forms are not as effective and may have increased adverse effects.

2. As in choice 1.

3. **Many people have difficulty using the MDI properly. A spacer is a tube that attaches to the MDI. Drugs are inhaled from the tube, resulting in better delivery of the medications into the airway.**

4. This is a possibility; however, the use of a spacer is easier for Mr. Lewis and is most likely to be successful.

23. C: Foundations of Practice T: Critical Thinking

1. The combination drugs need to be taken to stabilize and control chronic symptoms. They are not effective during an acute attack.

2. Mr. Lewis may need to do this if the rescue inhaler is not effective.

3. This is of value in croup but will not produce the bronchodilation necessary during an asthma attack.

4. **Short-acting bronchodilators (also known as "rescue" medications) provide temporary relief of bronchospasm and should help restore normal breathing within 10 to 15 minutes. Another puff may be taken if optimum breathing does not resume.**

24. C: Professional, Ethical, and Legal Practice T: Application

1. Any health care worker who provides care to Mr. Fraser has access to the record.

2. Only health care providers who are caring for Mr. Fraser have access to his record.

3. **These people are legally entitled to view the health record. While clerical staff may not be considered health care workers, they must view the chart in order to insert and maintain the information.**

4. This is unrealistic. The family practice clinic is responsible for initiating and maintaining relevant information and maintaining confidentiality. Mr. Fraser may have copies if he wishes.

25. C: Foundations of Practice T: Application
1. Caffeine can cause false elevations in blood pressure lasting up to 3 hours. There should be no effect after 5 hours.
2. **Relaxation facilitates a more accurate blood pressure reading.**
3. Electronic monitoring devices, if properly calibrated, are as reliable as manual devices. Care should be taken if interchanging the devices or if the electronic reading shows significant variance in comparison with previous readings.
4. The same arm should be used at each visit.

26. C: Foundations of Practice T: Application
1. While this is true, it does not answer Ms. Shannon's question.
2. **If Ms. Shannon asks the clinic to put her on the cancellation list, she may be able to take a spot that opens up, allowing her to have the scan earlier.**
3. This is true, but Ms. Shannon may be able to have the test earlier if she accesses the cancellation list.
4. This may not be true and does not advocate for Ms. Shannon to be involved with her plan of care.

27. C: Foundations of Practice T: Critical Thinking
1. This is important to know, but the nurse requires more information about what the father has read.
2. As in choice 1.
3. As in choice 2.
4. **This response validates the father's findings and invites him to discuss with the nurse what he has read.**

28. C: Foundations of Practice T: Application
1. Mr. Rutlege's temperature is within normal limits. A blanket may be used for comfort if he wishes but is not necessary.
2. The oxygen saturation is within normal limits. There is no reason to increase the oxygen.
3. **The vital signs are within normal limits for a post-operative client and should be monitored as per protocol.**
4. There is no reason to contact the physician.

29. C: Foundations of Practice T: Application
1. **An adult's urinary output should be a minimum of 30 mL per hour. Urinary output below this level may indicate inadequate perfusion of the kidneys, or urinary retention.**
2. This is normal following abdominal surgery.
3. This is a normal finding postsurgery.
4. This is a normal finding.

30. C: Foundations of Practice T: Application
1. There should not be any bubbling in the chamber. This indicates a leak.
2. **Taping connections prevents accidental disconnection.**
3. Sterile water is added only as necessary to replace evaporation.
4. The system should be maintained below waist level.

31. C: Foundations of Practice T: Knowledge
1. Type and cross-matching determines more than Rh information.
2. Type and cross-matching determines more than ABO information.
3. Type and cross-matching determines more than ABO information.
4. **Type and cross-matching provides a complete blood profile to determine the compatibility with donor blood.**

32. C: Foundations of Practice T: Critical Thinking
1. He may be able to explain the care but not able to actually perform care.
2. **This is the most appropriate method to evaluate his ability to care for the incision.**
3. This does not demonstrate competence.
4. This does not demonstrate competence. Most clients will not want to admit that they do not understand instructions and so may tell the nurse they do not have questions.

33. C: Foundations of Practice T: Critical Thinking
1. **With a fall from a height, there is the danger of head injury. In view of the fact that Sam is moaning, and therefore can breathe, and there is no evidence of critical hemorrhaging from the small cut, the most important assessment is for signs of head injury.**
2. This assessment would be made after assessing for head injury.
3. Because Sam is crying, this is evidence that he has an adequate, although likely elevated, pulse. The pulse should be taken, but it is not the priority.
4. These should be assessed after the level of consciousness.

34. C: Foundations of Practice T: Critical Thinking
1. This is not appropriate if there is a fracture as it may cause further injury.
2. The injured limb should be moved as little as possible.
3. **The initial practical nursing efforts are directed at calming the child. It is best not to touch children initially but to ask them to point to the painful area.**
4. Sam will be frightened and upset. Applying pressure to the area will cause unnecessary pain and make the remainder of the assessment difficult.

35. C: Foundations of Practice T: Critical Thinking
1. It is better to immobilize the limb and joint in a rigid rather than a soft splint.
2. **A rolled magazine may be used for a young child to form a rigid splint to keep the ankle in alignment and prevent further injury, especially to soft tissues.**
3. This can be done if no splint is available.
4. This can be done, but it is more important to immobilize the area of fracture.

36. **C: Foundations of Practice T: Knowledge**
    1. **In this situation, the diagnosis can be easily and most cost-effectively determined with an X-ray.**
    2. A bone scan is isotope imaging and is not required for what is believed to be a simple fracture.
    3. Bone densitometry is used to determine osteoporosis.
    4. A CT scan is not necessary for a fractured limb.

37. **C: Foundations of Practice T: Application**
    1. This will slow the drying process. The cast may be put in plastic after it is dry for purposes of bathing the child.
    2. **A plaster of Paris cast does not fully dry for up to 72 hours. Until then, it must be left exposed to the air to speed the drying process.**
    3. The cast should be handled with the palms of the hands rather than the fingers to prevent indentations.
    4. Dryers are not to be used because they may cause the cast to dry on the outside but remain wet on the inside, thus becoming mouldy.

38. **C: Foundations of Practice T: Knowledge**
    1. **Osteoarthritis is a joint disorder primarily affecting weight-bearing joints such as the knees.**
    2. The onset of osteoarthritis is more gradual.
    3. This occurs with osteomyelitis.
    4. Paraesthesia, or a "pins and needles" feeling, occurs more often in rheumatoid arthritis.

39. **C: Foundations of Practice T: Critical Thinking**
    1. Ms. Wilmot may not be able to change her job as she needs the health insurance benefits.
    2. **A modifiable factor in Ms. Wilmot's osteoarthritis is reducing the weight on her knees.**
    3. There is no evidence that Ms. Wilmot needs assistance in caring for her son.
    4. Ms. Wilmot obtains exercise by walking her postal route. She more likely may need rest during a period of acute inflammation.

40. **C: Foundations of Practice T: Application**
    1. These are used for muscle spasms, not osteoarthritis.
    2. **NSAIDs have been shown to provide greater relief than acetaminophen (Tylenol) in clients with severe pain from osteoarthritis.**
    3. Antibiotics are not useful in osteoarthritis.
    4. NSAIDs provide greater pain relief than does acetaminophen (Tylenol).

41. **C: Collaborative Practice T: Critical Thinking**
    1. Unless Ms. Wilmot experiences difficulties or lack of therapeutic effect with her medications, there is no need for a pharmacist.
    2. A naturopath would not necessarily be part of the team unless requested by Ms. Wilmot.
    3. There is no evidence that at present Ms. Wilmot requires the services of a social worker.
    4. **Physiotherapy is useful in planning appropriate exercise programs and recommending necessary assistive devices.**

42. **C: Foundations of Practice T: Critical Thinking**
    1. **Pregnancy-induced hypertension occurs after 20 weeks' gestation, more frequently in high-risk pregnancies. It can result in pre-eclampsia and eclampsia, which are dangerous to the pregnant individual and the fetus.**
    2. This is an indication of diabetes that is not controlled. The nurse would be testing for protein in the urine, a sign of pre-eclampsia.
    3. This is important but not as vital as the blood pressure determination.
    4. This may be important as an indication of fetal well-being but is not as important as the blood pressure.

43. **C: Foundations of Practice T: Knowledge**
    1. Hospitalization is not necessary. Bed rest has proven to be controversial and may have adverse physiological outcomes.
    2. **Most pregnant individuals with mild pre-eclampsia may be managed at home with restricted activity and mild exercise.**
    3. Because pregnant individuals with hypertension have lower plasma volume than do normotensive individuals sodium restriction is not necessary.
    4. Magnesium sulphate is used to prevent or control convulsions in individuals with eclampsia. It is not necessary in mild pre-eclampsia.

44. **C: Foundations of Practice T: Application**
    1. **These are signs of more severe pre-eclampsia.**
    2. Constipation is not related to pre-eclampsia.
    3. This may be a sign of early labour, not pre-eclampsia.
    4. These are signs of early labour, not pre-eclampsia.

45. **C: Foundations of Practice T: Critical Thinking**
    1. This is mandatory prior to all client care, not specific to clients with HIV.
    2. Gloves are not necessary unless the nurse is handling blood or body fluids.
    3. **Ross is at risk of infection and thus must have restricted contact with persons who have infections.**
    4. This may be an appropriate question later on during the appointment, particularly as adolescents are often nonadherent to taking medications. It is not important initially.

46. **C: Foundations of Practice T: Application**
    1. **Weight loss and a decrease in growth are potential complications in children with HIV/AIDS. Weight loss may also be part of normal adolescence. The initial question for data collection should be to determine the reason for the weight loss.**
    2. It may be that the weight loss is due to diarrhea, but this should not be the initial question.
    3. This is insensitive and may not be true.
    4. While a relatively high percentage of Canadian children are considered obese, this is not an appropriate comment to make with an HIV-positive client.

47. C: Foundations of Practice T: Application

1. **At Ross's age, he will have normal age-related concerns about sexuality. He needs to have anticipatory education about safe, healthy expressions of sexuality considering his HIV status.**
2. There is no indication that Ross is experiencing pain.
3. At age 14, if Ross has had HIV for his entire life, he is likely well aware of the modes of transmission.
4. This may be appropriate, but Ross has not indicated to the nurse that he is experiencing stress.

48. C: Foundations of Practice T: Application

1. Guidelines for the use of antiretroviral agents in HIV-infected adults and adolescents recommend that asymptomatic HIV-positive clients should be treated.
2. **Because rates of disease progression differ among individuals, treatment decisions should be individualized by the level of risk indicated by CD4 T-cell counts and plasma HIV RNA levels.**
3. The most effective means to suppress HIV replication is by combination antiretroviral therapy.
4. Many drugs are available for pediatric use.

49. C: Professional Practice T: Application

1. Ross is not an emancipated minor.
2. In many cases, foster parents are not legal guardians and may not provide consent.
3. **The nurse must know agency policies that will provide specific direction for investigational drugs and age of consent.**
4. The health care provider is recommending the treatment; thus, it is their responsibility to provide the necessary information.

50. C: Foundations of Practice T: Application

1. A tourniquet helps the nurse practitioner examine the antecubital fossa to select a suitable vein but is not necessary.
2. **Placement of a PICC line is performed under sterile conditions with preparation of the insertion site according to institution policy.**
3. There is no need for light anaesthesia. A topical anaesthetic cream is usually used at the insertion site.
4. A PICC line is not inserted in the subclavian vein.

51. C: Foundations of Practice T: Application

1. **An X-ray is necessary to confirm placement of the catheter in the superior vena cava prior to administration of the TPN.**
2. Education is appropriate before insertion of the PICC line, not after.
3. The solutions are to be refrigerated until 30 minutes before use. Leaving the solutions at room temperature for longer encourages microbial growth.
4. The solutions are prepared by the agency pharmacy, and nursing staff make no additions.

52. C: Foundations of Practice T: Application

1. Once established for TPN, a single-lumen catheter is not to be used for administration of blood or antibiotics or the drawing of blood samples.
2. As in choice 1.

3. As in choice 1. Use of Y-tubing will infuse the antibiotic into the PICC line.
4. **An additional intravenous line is required for the administration of antibiotics.**

53. C: Foundations of Practice T: Application

1. This creates an unnecessary break in the system. Canadian Infection Control Guidelines recommend that all intravascular delivery system components up to the hub should be changed at 72-hour intervals and lipid emulsions every 24 hours.
2. **This not only identifies the tubing but also is a reminder to other nursing staff when the tubing will need to be changed.**
3. Dressing changes are per institution protocol and usually not more often than once every other day.
4. This is not necessary. Only if there are signs of infection is the tubing cultured.

54. C: Foundations of Practice T: Critical Thinking

1. Weight gain or loss may be an indication of fluid shift, edema, or diuresis and does not evaluate tolerance of the TPN.
2. This evaluates his hydration status, not his tolerance of the TPN.
3. This will be a result of the improved nutrition but is not an ongoing accurate assessment of tolerance of the TPN.
4. **Blood glucose, electrolytes, urea nitrogen, complete blood count, and hepatic enzyme studies are performed at routine intervals. Assessment of these values will assist the nurse in evaluating Mr. Ford's tolerance of parenteral nutrition.**

55. C: Foundations of Practice T: Critical Thinking

1. **Visuals, such as drawings and pictures, will increase Mr. Ford's understanding.**
2. A picture, rather than a verbal description, would improve Mr. Ford's understanding.
3. Manufacturers' monographs are written at a technical level not suitable for most clients.
4. If the explanation were requested prior to insertion, the nurse practitioner would be responsible for the education in order to obtain informed consent. After insertion, the nurse has the knowledge to explain the PICC line.

56. C: Foundations of Practice T: Critical Thinking

1. If possible, the 500 mL should be made up to maintain normal blood values and nutrition.
2. **The flow of parenteral solutions can be increased by no more than 10%; thus, this is an appropriate option to make up the lost amount.**
3. TPN solutions should never be taken off an infusion pump and, due to their hypertonicity, may not run any faster than at 10% above the ordered rate.
4. Mr. Ford is not able to ingest sufficient fluids; therefore, this may not be possible.

57. C: Foundations of Practice T: Critical Thinking

1. This is not the most important information at this time.

2. Mrs. Buxton may not be able to come to the doctor's office. Other information needs to be determined first.

3. This is an important question, but the nurse first needs to determine whether Mrs. Buxton is safe.

4. **The initial priority is Mrs. Buxton's safety. The nurse needs to determine whether she is somewhere that Mr. Buxton can find her and continue the beating.**

58. **C: Foundations of Practice T: Critical Thinking**
    1. **Establishing trust is essential when counselling any client.**
    2. This may come out later on in the counselling but is not the most important initial goal.
    3. Communication is important, but it is an ongoing process and is likely to be facilitated by trust between the mental health nurse and Mr. Buxton.
    4. This puts the mental health nurse in an authoritative rather than a therapeutic relationship.

59. **C: Foundations of Practice T: Knowledge**
    1. Splitting is viewing people and situations as either all good or all bad.
    2. **Repression is the involuntary exclusion from awareness of a painful or conflictual thought, impulse, or memory. It is the primary ego defence. Mr. Buxton does not want to believe that he beats Mrs. Buxton.**
    3. Introjection is intense identification with another.
    4. Compensation is a process by which a person makes up for a perceived deficiency by strongly emphasizing a feature thought of as an asset.

60. **C: Foundations of Practice T: Application**
    1. This is a punitive response.
    2. This could be viewed as a sarcastic response.
    3. **This is the therapeutic communication technique called clarification. Attempting to put into words Mr. Buxton's unclear thoughts helps clarify his feelings, ideas, and perceptions.**
    4. This avoids the topic and is not therapeutic.

61. **C: Foundations of Practice T: Application**
    1. Some abusers blame their behaviour on alcohol, but this is a myth. Abuse is a learned behaviour, not the result of the loss of inhibitions.
    2. This may be a contributing factor, the hopelessness of poverty, but is not the most characteristic. Most people with a low socioeconomic status are not abusive.
    3. While there are cultures that may appear to ignore or condone family violence, there are no specific cultural factors that are most characteristic of abusers.
    4. **This is the most frequent finding in perpetrators of family violence. There is a history of violence, neglect, or emotional deprivation. The role model is abusive.**

62. **C: Foundations of Practice T: Knowledge**
    1. Identical twins begin with a single ovum that has been fertilized with one sperm and divides into two embryos.
    2. Identical twins are the same sex. Fraternal twins may be the same or different sexes.
    3. Older individuals are more likely to release two ova.

4. Fraternal twins are two ova that have been fertilized by two sperm. They develop as two fetuses and will have two placentas.

63. **C: Foundations of Practice T: Application**
    1. **Fluids and roughage in fruits and vegetables increase the fluids in stool, making them softer and more easily passed through the colon.**
    2. Exercise does help constipation; however, because of the twin pregnancy, the physician should clear this. It would not be the first approach.
    3. Laxatives, whether or not they are natural, should not be used without consulting the physician. They are not the first approach.
    4. The first approach would not be taking a stool softener, and a physician must order it.

64. **C: Foundations of Practice T: Application**
    1. **Individuals with a multiple gestation are at high risk for developing preterm labour.**
    2. This is a rare complication of twin pregnancy but occurs in monozygotic twins.
    3. This is a rare occurrence in monozygotic twins, when the division of the embryo occurs very late, causing incomplete cleavage.
    4. With twin pregnancy, there is more likely to be hydramnios, or an excess of amniotic fluid. Oligohydramnios is a decrease in amniotic fluid and may be associated with fetal kidney disorders.

65. **C: Foundations of Practice T: Application**
    1. Dyspnea is a common discomfort, particularly in the latter half of the third trimester and in multiple births. It is caused by pressure of the enlarged uterus on the diaphragm.
    2. This is normal weight gain.
    3. Leg cramps are a common discomfort of pregnancy, caused by a calcium to phosphorus imbalance.
    4. **A decrease in fetal movement is an ominous sign that indicates a loss of vitality in one or both infants. In a twin pregnancy, this is a greater risk, and it may be difficult for the client to determine whether one or both infants are not moving or are moving less.**

66. **C: Foundations of Practice T: Application**
    1. Blue eyes are a recessive genetic trait; therefore, it is not as likely for both infants to have blue eyes.
    2. **Brown eyes are a dominant trait; therefore, it is most likely that both infants will have brown eyes.**
    3. This is possible, but not as likely as both infants having brown eyes.
    4. Eye colour is not a random genetic trait. Brown eyes are dominant.

67. **C: Foundations of Practice T: Application**
    1. Fluids should not be restricted in pregnancy.
    2. Legs should be uncrossed as much as possible to help prevent varicosities, but this is not likely to be of benefit for ankle edema.
    3. **Elevating the legs will help venous return and decrease ankle edema.**

4. Range-of-motion exercises may be of limited benefit but are not as helpful as elevating the legs.

68. **C: Foundations of Practice T: Application**
    1. This is a possibility but is not necessary. Both infants can be breastfed.
    2. With Ms. Hudson's fertility problems, this may not happen, and they may not want more than two children. She is able to breastfeed twins.
    3. It is more difficult to breastfeed twins, but it is not true that most women are not successful.
    4. **While breastfeeding twins does require planning and adaptation, she may be able to successfully breastfeed twins, either simultaneously or one at a time.**

69. **C: Foundations of Practice T: Critical Thinking**
    1. This would be the second assessment.
    2. Because the infants are preterm, they have a greater risk for hypothermia. However, this is not the most important assessment just after birth.
    3. **Respirations are the most important initial assessment. Adequate respiratory effort is necessary for transition to extrauterine life.**
    4. Blood pressure is not a necessary assessment in the delivery room.

70. **C: Foundations of Practice T: Application**
    1. It is not necessary for the client to lie down. They may sit, with the arm extended at heart level.
    2. The cuff width should be at least 40% of the length of the client's upper arm.
    3. The cuff should be inflated to 30% above the expected systolic pressure.
    4. **The brachial artery is used for blood pressure determination. The teacher will demonstrate palpation of the brachial artery and place the bell of the stethoscope over the pulse point.**

71. **C: Professional, Ethical, and Legal Practice T: Critical Thinking**
    1. This is a valuable step in learning how to manage the equipment, but being able to perform blood pressure monitoring on themselves is more effective.
    2. Verbalizing the procedure is not as effective as actually being able to demonstrate the skill.
    3. This is important but is not an evaluation of the skill.
    4. **This is the most effective evaluation as the nursing teacher will be able to determine whether the student can manipulate the equipment on themselves.**

72. **C: Professional Ethical, and Legal Practice T: Critical Thinking**
    1. **The second step of the nursing process is to validate data. The best way to validate the high reading, and reassure Mr. Brown, is to take the blood pressure again using a manual device that is not dependent on correct calibration.**
    2. This would be the next step if the high blood pressure were confirmed by the manual method.
    3. This question should be asked but is not the first step.
    4. This is likely required, but it may be that the monitor requires recalibration. Also, this will not quickly reassure Mr. Brown.

73. **C: Foundations of Practice T: Knowledge**
    1. Meperidine, an analgesic, does not depress the immune system.
    2. Cefazolin, an antibiotic, will not depress the immune system.
    3. **Prednisone, a corticosteroid, has recognized immunosuppressive effects.**
    4. Salbutamol, a bronchodilator, does not have immunosuppressive effects.

74. **C: Foundations of Practice T: Critical Thinking**
    1. **Developing an awareness of social justice involves socioeconomic and political issues that can contribute to poor health in disadvantaged populations.**
    2. This may occur but is not the primary reason.
    3. This is true but does not answer the question of why nurses should be social justice advocates.
    4. The purpose of advocacy in social justice is to improve conditions for all people. It does not necessarily involve changes in law. Nurses may influence politicians, but it is not a given that laws will be changed based on nursing input.

75. **C: Foundations of Practice T: Application**
    1. This is too early for an infant to pull themselves to a standing position.
    2. This is too early for most infants to pull themselves to a standing position.
    3. **While there is considerable variation among infants with regard to milestones, this is the approximate age at which an infant can pull themselves to a standing position holding onto furniture.**
    4. If a child is not able to pull themselves to a standing position by 11 to 12 months, they should be further evaluated.

76. **C: Foundations of Practice T: Application**
    1. Lipid-lowering medications are ordered depending on lipid levels, not age.
    2. Exercise is only one factor influencing lipid levels.
    3. **Generally, diet therapy is attempted prior to medications.**
    4. Only chronically elevated cholesterol levels with failure of conservative lifestyle measures require medications.

77. **C: Foundations of Practice T: Application**
    1. **Folic acid is recommended to prevent neural tube defects during pregnancy. Individuals who could become pregnant should take it prior to becoming pregnant as it is necessary from the early stages, when the individual may not be aware they are pregnant.**
    2. This is not the role of folic acid.
    3. As in choice 2.
    4. As in choice 2.

78. **C: Professional, Ethical, and Legal Practice T: Critical Thinking**
    1. **The clinic will have health care providers who can manage chronic health problems.**
    2. This may take a long time and may not be successful.
    3. The nurse will have better information on availability of health care providers in the community.

4. The client may have needs beyond the scope of practice of the nurse.

79. **C: Foundations of Practice T: Knowledge**
    1. **Sickle cell disease, often termed *sickle cell anemia,* is a chronic inherited condition that results in abnormally shaped hemoglobin, resulting in anemia.**
    2. Fever is not a manifestation of sickle cell disease.
    3. Vomiting is not a manifestation of sickle cell disease.
    4. Children with sickle cell disease are more likely to be tachycardic, in response to red blood cell destruction and anemia.

80. **C: Foundations of Practice T: Application**
    1. Thrombocytopenia, not leukopenia, causes gums to bleed.
    2. There is no particular reason to eat these foods with leukopenia.
    3. Clients with leukopenia should not be immunized except on the judgement of their health care provider.
    4. **Leukopenia is reduced white blood cells (WBCs). With fewer WBCs, the immune system is depressed, causing the client to be at risk for communicable diseases.**

81. **C: Foundations of Practice T: Critical Thinking**
    1. **This is the most common cause of autonomic dysreflexia.**
    2. Nasal congestion is a symptom of autonomic dysreflexia.
    3. A high-fibre diet may decrease the risk of occurrence of autonomic dysreflexia by reducing risk of constipation.
    4. Low blood pressure does not cause autonomic dysreflexia.

82. **C: Foundations of Practice T: Application**
    1. There would be no rationale for discontinuing an analgesic prior to surgery.
    2. There would be no rationale for discontinuing an antipyretic prior to surgery. If she did have a fever, surgery would likely be cancelled.
    3. There is no rationale for discontinuing an anti-inflammatory drug prior to surgery.
    4. **People with prosthetic heart valves are at risk for thrombus formation. Aspirin decreases platelet aggregation, preventing formation of thrombi. However, during surgery, there is an increased risk of hemorrhage if the client is taking an antiplatelet medication; thus, the medication should be stopped prior to surgery.**

83. **C: Foundations of Practice T: Critical Thinking**
    1. Although the bronchodilator has cardiovascular adverse effects, the priority assessment is respiratory.
    2. These are respiratory drugs.
    3. As in choice 2.
    4. **Advair, which is a combination of fluticasone (an inhaled steroid) and salmeterol (an inhaled bronchodilator), is commonly used in clients with asthma. A respiratory assessment would be a priority to form a baseline and to assess the therapeutic effects of the drugs.**

84. **C: Foundations of Practice T: Comprehension**
    1. This is not the proper method and is unnecessary.
    2. **When adding medications to IV fluid containers, mix the medication and the IV solution by holding the bag or bottle and gently turning it end to end.**
    3. Inverting just once may not adequately mix the medication or IV solution.
    4. As in choice 1.

85. **C: Foundations of Practice T: Application**
    1. This is an invasion of Ms. Brette's personal space and not an appropriate therapeutic technique.
    2. This may prove to be too stimulating for Ms. Brette. She requires a calm, quiet environment.
    3. **Antianxiety medications are commonly used to bring the anxiety to a manageable level.**
    4. Ms. Brette may view this as punishment unless she initiates moving to her room.

86. **C: Foundations of Practice T: Critical Thinking**
    1. Airline staff will need to know this information so a decision can be made regarding landing at the closest airport or obtaining on-ground medical advice. It is not, however, the priority action.
    2. This is an important question, but it can be asked after oxygen is administered.
    3. As in choice 2.
    4. **If the man is experiencing a myocardial infarction, the heart muscle is being deprived of oxygen. The oxygen supply to the heart must be increased immediately to prevent heart damage.**

87. **C: Foundations of Practice T: Critical Thinking**
    1. Mr. Dunlop is displaying manifestations of myocardial infarction (MI); thus, 9-1-1 must be called. This is not the most complete answer.
    2. **This is the most complete answer. ASA is a fibrinolytic that may help break up thrombi that contribute to MIs. It is recognized to be part of appropriate first aid treatment if myocardial infarction is suspected.**
    3. There is no need to put Mr. Dunlop in a knee-chest position.
    4. A blanket may provide increased comfort for Mr. Dunlop, but administration of ASA is more important.

88. **C: Foundations of Practice T: Application**
    1. The spray is directed under the tongue, not inhaled.
    2. Headache is an expected adverse effect.
    3. Pain relief should be within 2 minutes. If there is no significant relief within 15 minutes, she should notify her physician.
    4. **Exercise creates cardiovascular demand. Administration of nitroglycerin prior to physical activity will increase blood flow to the heart, increasing tolerance for the activity.**

89. **C: Foundations of Practice T: Application**
    1. Fever is likely to be manifested, but it is not the classic symptom of *C. difficile* infection.
    2. Vomiting sometimes, but not always, accompanies a *C. difficile* infection.

3. Chills often accompany the fever but are not specific to *C. difficile*.

4. **Overgrowth of *C. difficile* in the colon causes diarrhea that is usually watery and voluminous.**

90. **C: Foundations of Practice T: Knowledge**
    1. Fibromyalgia is not a psychiatric disorder. Depression and anxiety may be involved, possibly due to living with chronic pain and fatigue.
    2. While fibromyalgia cannot be cured, there are treatments, including antidepressants, physiotherapy, rest, and analgesics.
    3. **A definitive diagnosis of fibromyalgia is difficult to establish as there are no specific diagnostic tests. Often the diagnosis is achieved by ruling out other conditions. Manifestations may be similar to many other conditions.**
    4. The pain and fatigue are not progressive.

91. **C: Professional, Ethical, and Legal Practice T: Critical Thinking**
    1. True, but this does not answer the question.
    2. **This explains why nurses support political advocacy for social determinants of health.**
    3. This is part of the *Canada Health Act* but does not answer the question.
    4. This is true but does not answer the question.

92. **C: Foundations of Practice T: Critical Thinking**
    1. This is an important nursing action but not the priority.
    2. **Maintaining a patent airway is the priority action based on the type of surgery and the ABC principles of care.**
    3. This is one action that will assist in maintaining the patent airway.
    4. As in choice 1.

93. **C: Foundations of Practice T: Application**
    1. Hepatitis A is not transmitted by blood or body fluids.
    2. Hepatitis A is not an airborne virus.
    3. This does not explain the mode of transmission. While there may be more cases of hepatitis A in tropical countries, it is not necessarily considered endemic.
    4. **Hepatitis A is transmitted by the fecal–oral route, most commonly in contaminated food and water. It may be more prevalent in countries where there is a warmer climate and poor sanitation practices.**

94. **C: Professional, Ethical, and Legal Practice T: Application**
    1. This meal should be eaten around 0100 of the night shift. Large meals eaten shortly before going to bed after a night shift do not facilitate sleepiness.
    2. **This may help prevent the circadian rhythm from being triggered by the morning light.**
    3. Because of its potentially stimulating effects, shift workers are advised to avoid strenuous activity just before bedtime.
    4. A 24-hour time period is recommended between shifts for those who rotate shifts.

95. **C: Foundations of Practice T: Application**
    1. These are generally the second set of teeth to erupt.
    2. **The lower central incisors are generally the first teeth to erupt, at about 6 to 8 months of age.**
    3. The canine teeth do not generally erupt until about 20 months.
    4. The first molar does not generally erupt until 14 to 18 months.

96. **C: Foundations of Practice T: Critical Thinking**
    1. **The tube must be assessed for patency. Irrigating can be done by instilling, and then withdrawing, saline.**
    2. Instillation may not determine patency and may add to the residuals in the stomach.
    3. The tube should not be removed as this may not be necessary and should not be done without a physician's order.
    4. The physician does not need to be notified until the patency of the tube has been determined.

97. **C: Foundations of Practice T: Application**
    1. **Pregnant persons with gestational diabetes often deliver large infants. It is important to determine the maternal baseline blood sugar level as early as possible.**
    2. Amniocentesis is not indicated for large infants unless there had been previous anomalies with the infants.
    3. Maternal diet can be related to the size of the infant at term but is not the most important test at this time.
    4. Pelvimetry will determine the size of the pelvis but does not predict whether Ms. Bacci will be able to deliver a large baby vaginally.

98. **C: Foundations of Practice T: Application**
    1. Osteoporosis is an indication for the use of estrogen
    2. Uterine bleeding is an indication for the use of estrogen
    3. **The most serious adverse effects of the estrogens are thromboembolic events; therefore, thrombophlebitis is a contraindication to the use of estrogens.**
    4. Atrophic vaginitis is an indication for the use of estrogen.

99. **C: Foundations of Practice T: Critical Thinking**
    1. Young adult clients are not at high risk for an altered response to anaesthesia.
    2. Middle-aged clients are not at high risk for an altered response to anaesthesia.
    3. As in choice 2.
    4. **The older client is more affected by anaesthesia because of the effects of aging on the hepatic, cardiac, respiratory, and renal systems.**

100. **C: Foundations of Practice T: Application**
    1. This avoids the question and puts the blame on the boyfriend.
    2. While this is true, the woman has expressed concern about telling her boyfriend, and this is the subject that needs to be discussed.
    3. As in choice 2.
    4. **This introduces the legal and ethical implications of telling the boyfriend and encourages**

communication about how to approach the discussion.

101. C: Foundations of Practice T: Critical Thinking

1. This may help in the short term, but it is best not to use family.
2. This may help, but there are too many languages and staff may not be able to effectively use a written dictionary.
3. The nurse may want to learn the most common languages, but it is not reasonable to be fluent in all.
4. **This is the best long-term option. Telephone and video link call centres with health care interpreters are available around the clock.**

102. C: Professional, Ethical, and Legal Practice T: Knowledge

1. Inquests are not held to determine criminal liability, although evidence provided may lead to formal charges.
2. Inquests are not held to determine civil liability.
3. Inquests are not held to prosecute persons or agencies.
4. **Inquests are held to provide recommendations that may be used to improve systems or practices in health care. They must answer how the person died and the manner of death.**

103. C: Foundations of Practice T: Application

1. A person with an apple body shape carries weight around the waist, which creates a higher risk of developing CVD and type 2 diabetes. However, Mark's BMI is within the normal range.
2. **An apple-shaped person carries weight around the waist, which creates a higher risk of developing CVD and type 2 diabetes. A BMI above 25 indicates that Consuelo is overweight.**
3. A pear shape indicates that the person carries weight around the hips and thighs and is not as unhealthy as someone who carries weight around the waist. The BMI indicates that Pedro is only slightly overweight.
4. Christa has a pear shape, but her BMI indicates that she is slightly underweight, which may not be a risk factor for CVD and type 2 diabetes.

104. C: Foundations of Practice T: Application

1. This is an incorrect calculation.
2. **The correct calculation is 12 grams × 9 kcal/gram = 108 kcal. 1 100 kcal divided by 108 kcal = 10.1, or 10%.**
3. This is an incorrect calculation.
4. This is an incorrect calculation.

105. C: Foundations of Practice T: Application

1. **Nurses should consult with the health care team before starting a complementary therapy. If the team agrees, the peppermint may be added to the plan of care.**
2. This is not true.
3. The nurse needs to consult with the health care team prior to providing Mrs. Carnegy with the peppermint.

4. Mrs. Carnegy has found the peppermint to be effective, so there may be no need to consult with the physician about an alternative medication.

106. C: Foundations of Practice T: Application

1. **Falls are the leading cause of injury in older persons. In icy winter conditions, there is a greater risk of falls with severe injuries.**
2. Area rugs may be a safety hazard. Bare floors decrease the likelihood of tripping, falling, and slipping due to rugs that may not be firmly attached to the floors.
3. An open element on a stove is more dangerous than a microwave, provided that the microwave is properly used.
4. Over-the-counter cough medications are not recommended for children or older persons. These clients should, more appropriately, drink fluids and take acetaminophen (Tylenol) for discomfort. The nurse or physician should assess them if their symptoms worsen.

107. C: Foundations of Practice T: Critical Thinking

1. A fecal occult blood test (FOBT) or a fecal immunochemical test (FIT) is recommended for people over the age of 50. However, they are not as conclusive as a colonoscopy.
2. A sigmoidoscopy looks only at the sigmoid colon.
3. **A colonoscopy is direct visualization of the entire colon from rectum to cecum. Because polyps and cancerous growths actually can be seen, colonoscopy is the recommended screening test.**
4. A barium enema is an X-ray of the lower bowel following the insertion of barium contrast medium. It can be used to see areas of obstruction; however, it is not as conclusive as the colonoscopy.

108. C: Foundations of Practice T: Critical Thinking

1. This is not necessary as the order is clear to provide oxygen. The nurse may want to further consult with the health care provider regarding the child's decreasing O_2 saturation.
2. **This is the first action as it is has been ordered by the health care provider, and the child is in need of supplemental oxygen.**
3. This may occur but is not the initial action.
4. This should occur and will be ongoing; however, the first action is to provide additional oxygen.

109. C: Professional, Ethical, and Legal Practice T: Critical Thinking

1. **The pharmacist has the specific scope of practice to best recommend effective over-the-counter antihistamines to Mr. Patrick.**
2. The nurse practitioner may be able to recommend effective therapies, but the pharmacist would be the most appropriate first choice.
3. This may be an alternative, but it would be better for Mr. Patrick to first consult with a pharmacist concerning effective medications.

4. A respiratory therapist might be an appropriate referral if Mr. Patrick were experiencing breathing difficulties.

110. **C: Professional, Ethical, and Legal Practice T: Application**

1. Although, in some situations, it is appropriate to discuss with the client their medication regimen, the professional nurse must display knowledge of the rationale for the medications being administered. Having to ask Mr. Price may create a lack of trust in the nurse's knowledge.

2. **This is the appropriate resource to determine the rationale for the antipsychotic. The nurse must have this knowledge prior to administration of the medication.**

3. This may be part of the psychiatric assessment but is not the first action.

4. Because Mr. Price is receiving an antipsychotic medication, this is not a reason to assume that he will be violent or that the nurse will need safety measures when performing care.

111. **C: Foundations of Practice T: Application**

1. This is not a manifestation of presbycusis.

2. **With age-related hearing loss, the ability to hear high-pitched consonants decreases, and sound becomes muffled. It seems to the person that others are not speaking clearly.**

3. The higher-pitched sounds of women's voices are lost initially.

4. People are able to hear their own speech.

112. **C: Foundations of Practice T: Application**

1. This is setting limits to behaviour, and in this case, it may make Mr. Braham more anxious. Demanding behaviour is often an attempt to decrease anxiety.

2. **All behaviour has meaning. The nurse needs to determine what is causing Mr. Braham's demanding behaviour. By sitting with him and asking open-ended questions, she may be able to determine the underlying problems.**

3. Maintaining continuity of care with one nurse is optimum to developing a trusting relationship between Mr. Braham and the nurse.

4. This is confrontational and will likely escalate the demanding behaviour. It is not a therapeutic response.

113. **C: Foundations of Practice T: Application**

1. The person with dementia is not necessarily deaf, and Mr. Hill does not have to speak loudly.

2. The person with dementia will not understand written communication any better than verbal communication.

3. **The person with dementia has lost some ability to interpret complex language. Short, simple sentences may enable the client with dementia to comprehend the spoken word.**

4. Repeating the communication will not aid in comprehension of what has been spoken.

114. **C: Professional, Ethical, and Legal Practice T: Application**

1. **A nurse may or may not decide to answer a question that may be a natural conversational question for a client. If the nurse chooses to respond, it should be a brief answer. The most appropriate response, however, is to refocus the conversation to the client. In this scenario, Ms. Enright may be using the question to open the topic of who she is dating.**

2. This response indicates that rules rather than professional judgement direct her practice.

3. This response provides too much personal information about the nurse. It may be considered a boundary crossing.

4. This response may sound harsh and punitive to the client. There are better words to redirect the client.

115. **C: Professional, Ethical, and Legal Practice T: Critical Thinking**

1. This is necessary, as most threats against health care workers are underreported. It is not, however, the primary action.

2. This is true; however, it is not the primary action or consideration.

3. **The nurse must first protect themselves from verbal abuse that may turn to physical abuse. Once safeguards are in place, the nurse may address documentation, support, communication with colleagues, and methods to provide care to Mr. Dovgan.**

4. This is important to obtain support and assistance in devising methods for caring for Mr. Dovgan. It is not, however, the primary action.

116. **C: Foundations of Practice T: Critical Thinking**

1. Lindsay is asking for help, but she does not actually have the razor blades, so the suicide risk is not imminent.

2. **Young men have a high risk of suicide, often by violent means. Ahmet has the gun and is able to act on his impulse immediately.**

3. Florence has agreed to treatment.

4. Older persons are at risk for suicide, but Fred may be feeling a grief reaction that will improve. He has not formed a plan.

117. **C: Foundations of Practice T: Critical Thinking**

1. This is the order, not what might be actually occurring.

2. This is the recommendation by the physiotherapist, but not what might be actually happening.

3. This is current but may not be what occurs all the time.

4. **Only this response specifically answers the family's question.**

118. **C: Foundations of Practice T: Critical Thinking**

1. This is an important assessment, but the developmental stage must first be determined.

2. As in choice 1.

3. Developmental level is essential in assessing children's ability and level of understanding. **It must be determined prior to a teaching plan.**

4. As in choice 1.

119. **C: Foundations of Practice T: Critical Thinking**
   1. Autism is not treated with medications, although some drugs appear to alleviate particular symptoms in individuals.
   2. **This is the cornerstone of treatment for autism and assists clients to achieve their potential.**
   3. Autism is not considered to be a psychiatric disease and cannot be helped with psychiatric treatment. In the past, it was viewed to be maladaptive parenting, which may have responded to psychiatric treatment.
   4. While a safety assessment is important, it does not help achieve developmental goals.

120. **C: Foundations of Practice T: Application**
   1. **This is the most effective method for stopping a nosebleed.**
   2. The head should not be tilted back as the blood may flow down the back of the throat. Holding the bridge of the nose is ineffective.
   3. This may increase the bleeding.
   4. This is a last resort, and cotton balls should not be used.

121. **C: Professional, Ethical, and Legal Practice T: Application**
   1. **The initial step in any type of conflict is to discuss the situation with the people involved. By discussing the student's performance with her, it provides an opportunity to clarify both appropriate roles and expectations.**
   2. This is a correct action but should occur after the discussion with the student.
   3. The nurse educator may be a valuable resource, but the initial action is for Martina to speak with the student.

4. Martina should have read this information prior to the beginning of the preceptorship.

122. **C: Foundations of Practice T: Application**
   1. Naproxen may cause stomach irritation.
   2. Celecoxib is used for pain related to arthritis.
   3. **Acetaminophen is generally considered to be a safe analgesic and is appropriate for mild aches, pyrexia, and headache.**
   4. Aspirin may cause stomach irritation.

123. **C: Professional, Ethical, and Legal Practice T: Application**
   1. This is not necessary.
   2. This is an expected nursing action but does not answer when the bag will need to be replaced.
   3. **There are no recommendations by the Centers for Disease Control and Prevention or the Public Health Agency of Canada for the "hang time" of IV fluids. It is the responsibility of each agency to develop policies, which the nurse will need to consult.**
   4. The bag will not be empty for several days. This may be contrary to agency policies.

124. **C: Foundations of Practice T: Application**
   1. This is an incorrect calculation.
   2. This is an incorrect calculation.
   3. **Correct calculation: 56.7 kg / 0.45 kg = 126 × 18 kcal = 2268 kcal.**
   4. This is an incorrect calculation.

125. **C: Foundations of Practice T: Critical Thinking**
   1. This is a slightly elevated respiratory rate and should be monitored.
   2. A productive cough is expected and aids the lungs in clearing mucus.
   3. **Restlessness is a cerebral manifestation of hypoxia.**
   4. This may be normal in an older person but should be monitored.

REx-PN Practice Exam: Book One

INTRODUCTION TO PRACTICE EXAMS

The following practice examinations are designed to be similar to those you will encounter in the Regulatory Exam–Practical Nurse (REx-PN). The exam is organized into two books that contain 250 questions each, for a total of 500 questions. You may want to write the practice exam in a group with fellow students to help replicate an actual exam situation.

1. A mother confides to the nurse that her live-in boyfriend pushed her 2-year-old child because he was crying too much. She begs the nurse not to tell anyone because her boyfriend has agreed to take anger management classes. What should the nurse do?
   1. Abide by the mother's wishes because this information was provided in confidence.
   2. Arrange for the earliest available counselling for the boyfriend.
   3. Advise the mother to take the child away from the boyfriend and find alternative housing right away.
   4. Report the incident to the child protection agency.

2. A hospitalized female client is unable to mobilize to the bathroom. What action should the nurse take to assist the client to void?
   1. Provide the client with adult incontinence briefs.
   2. Offer the client a female urinal or bedpan.
   3. Insert a urinary catheter.
   4. Request assistance from a colleague to carry the client to the washroom.

3. The nurse is admitting a client with suspected COVID-19 infection. The nurse applies an oxygen pulse oximeter to obtain an immediate diagnostic of the client's oxygen level. Where would the nurse apply this monitoring device?
   1. On the client's upper arm
   2. On top of the client's chest
   3. Over the client's mouth
   4. Around the client's finger

4. The nurse is preparing to administer alendronate to a client with osteoporosis. Which of the following actions will the nurse implement initially?
   1. Ensure the client has recently eaten.
   2. Ask about any leg cramps or hot flashes.
   3. Assist the client to sit up at the bedside.
   4. Administer the prescribed calcium carbonate.

5. The nurse is reviewing literature related to a potential problem that has been identified on the unit. The nurse realizes that nursing research is important in that it is designed to do which of the following? **Select all that apply.**
   1. Enhance the nurse's chance at promotion.
   2. Identify new knowledge.
   3. Improve professional practice.
   4. Enhance effective use of resources.
   5. Lead to decreases in budget expenditures.

6. A family who are Jewish wishes to have their newborn son circumcised. What is the nurse's best response to this request?
   1. "Circumcision is no longer recommended for male infants."
   2. "This is something you will have to ask the doctor about."
   3. "I will arrange for the circumcision to be scheduled."
   4. "I will find out which health care or religious practitioners perform circumcisions."

7. The nurse caring for an older client notices that they are not using the cane properly. Which of the following statements by the nurse would most likely elicit a positive response?
   1. "You're doing that all wrong. Let me show you how to do it."
   2. "I don't know who showed you how to use the cane like that, but you're not doing it right. Let me show you again."
   3. "You appear to be having trouble using your cane. Do you mind if I show you an easier way?"
   4. "If you use the cane that way you will fall. I'll show you the right way to do it."

8. The home health nurse who visits a client with a tactile impairment is concerned about injury related to the client's inability to feel harmful stimuli. The nurse determines that the client is able to care for themselves safely when they demonstrate which action?
   1. Places coloured stickers on faucet handles to indicate temperature and keeps a thermometer near the tub
   2. Asks the nurse to test the temperature of the water before entering the bath
   3. Replaces all lace-up shoes with Velcro closures
   4. Dispenses all medications onto a plate for easy access in the morning

9. The nurse instructs a client about performing an at-home fecal occult blood testing kit as a screening for colon cancer. Which of the following would the nurse include in the instructions? **Select all that apply.**
   1. Do not perform during a menstrual period.
   2. Do not eat red meat 2 days prior to the test.

3. Be sure to read instructions included in the kit.

4. Stop any antihypertensive medications 3 days prior to the text.

5. Defecate into the toilet as usual, scoop the stool out with the enclosed spoon.

6. Obtain a fecal smear with the enclosed applicator and apply to the hemoccult slide.

10. A 6-year-old child with severe anemia requires a unit of red blood cells (RBCs). The nurse explains to the child that the transfusion is necessary for which reason?

   1. Allows their parents to come visit them
   2. Fights the infection that they now have
   3. Increases their energy so they will not be so tired
   4. Helps their body stop bleeding

11. The nurse is providing discharge teaching for a client who will need dressing changes at home. Their caregiver does not feel comfortable performing the dressing changes. What action should the nurse take?

   1. Complete a referral for home care services.
   2. Ask the caregiver if there is anyone else who can help.
   3. Cancel the discharge.
   4. Discuss with the caregiver the reason they are not comfortable with the dressing changes.

12. What is the most important factor the nurse must perform prior to initiating an intermittent feed to a client via a nasogastric tube?

   1. Warm the formula.
   2. Ensure medications are infused prior to the feed.
   3. Assist client to sit at a 30-degree angle.
   4. Perform checks to ensure tube is in the correct position in the stomach.

13. A pregnant client asks the nurse about their due date. They say the first day of their last menstrual period was November 20. Using Naegele's Rule, what will the nurse calculate to be the client's expected date of delivery? Fill in the blank.

14. The nurse is caring for a client who is becoming increasingly short of breath. The nurse decides to call the health care provider. Which of the following should the nurse initially say when speaking with the health care provider?

   1. State the problem.
   2. Tell what is needed.
   3. State the client's allergies.
   4. Relate the client's background.

15. A client arrives at a medical walk-in clinic 7 days after abdominal surgery, saying that the incision site looks like it has come apart. The nurse assesses the client, and determines the bowel is protruding from the incision. What action should be taken by the nurse?

   1. Cover the wound with sterile gauze soaked in normal saline.
   2. Attempt to return the bowel back into the abdomen.
   3. Apply steristrip bandages to close the incision.
   4. Advise the client to remain standing, holding the abdomen.

16. A nurse works at a summer camp for children with developmental delays. A student nurse, who is a volunteer at the camp, asks the nurse for information about children with autism spectrum disorders. Which of the following would the nurse teach the student nurse? **Select all that apply.**

   1. Speak slowly and clearly while making eye contact with the child.
   2. If the child seems bored, redirect them with imaginative play.
   3. Maintain the child's routines as much as possible.
   4. Implement safety precautions for self-injurious behaviours.
   5. Observe the child's use of gestures to communicate.
   6. Assess specific ways the child communicates.

17. A nurse instructs a visually impaired hospitalized client on the most appropriate method to contact a nurse for assistance. How would the nurse facilitate this communication?

   1. Place a raised Braille sticker on the call button and instruct the client to press for assistance.
   2. Instruct the client to yell loudly to get the attention of the staff.
   3. Explain to the client that a staff person will stop by once an hour to see whether the client needs anything.
   4. Provide unit-based cell phone numbers assigned to each nurse.

18. A first-time parent is concerned that when they take their baby home, they will have difficulty breastfeeding. What should the nurse say to them?

   1. "Don't worry, all first-time parents feel like this."
   2. "There is a community breastfeeding clinic, I will get the information for you."
   3. "You should get help from your friends who have been successful at breastfeeding."
   4. "If your baby doesn't take to the breast, you can always give the baby formula."

19. The nurse is caring for a client in respiratory distress. The client has multiple monitoring systems that constantly beep and make noise. The client is becoming agitated over inability to sleep with all the noise. Which action by the nurse is most appropriate for this client?

   1. Giving the client a therapeutic back rub
   2. Turning off the alarms on the monitoring devices
   3. Administering an opioid medication to help the client sleep
   4. Providing the client with earplugs

20. A client has had a cystoscopy and biopsy of the bladder for possible bladder cancer. Which of the following are post-procedure nursing interventions? **Select all that apply.**

   1. Monitor for pink tinged urine.
   2. Assess urine characteristics.
   3. Monitor for potential allergic reactions to the dye.
   4. Expect bladder spasms and administer analgesics as ordered.
   5. Check client's perineum every 5 minutes for frank bleeding.
   6. Inform client that burning urination is expected.

21. A 16-year-old client informs the nurse that they are gender fluid. Which of the following statements will help the nurse establish a trusting relationship with the client?

   1. "Don't worry. It's just a phase you will grow out of."
   2. "Those are abnormal impulses. You should seek therapy."

3. "At your age, it is normal to be curious about both genders."

4. "Tell me what it means to you to be gender fluid."

22. The nurse is working at a first aid centre for a charity marathon run. The nurse screens each runner's vital signs prior to the beginning of the race. Evaluate the vital signs for a 40-year old experienced marathon runner.

Temperature	36.4°C
Pulse	50/min
Respirations	11/min
Blood Pressure	129/76

1. Normal findings
2. Bradycardia
3. Hypotension
4. Hypothermia

23. The nurse provides health education for an adult experiencing sleep deprivation. Which instruction has the highest priority?

1. "It's important to limit your driving to short periods. Sleep deprivation increases your risks for serious accidents."

2. "Sleep deprivation is usually self-limiting. See your health care provider if it lasts more than a year."

3. "Turn the radio on with a soft volume as you prepare for bed each evening. It will help you relax."

4. "Three glasses of wine each evening helps many clients who suffer from sleep deprivation."

24. The nurse works at a health unit in an Indigenous community. A 9-month-old infant who has been vomiting is brought to the health unit by the parents. The nurse determines the infant is dehydrated. What intervention would be taught to the parents?

1. Give the infant a carbonated beverage as often as possible.

2. Advise the parents to keep the infant NPO until the vomiting has stopped.

3. Provide oral rehydration therapy in the form of a pediatric electrolyte solution.

4. Place the infant in a cool environment with minimal clothing.

25. The nurse is preparing to insert a urinary catheter and is donning sterile gloves. Which of the following steps are included in this process? **Select all that apply.**

1. Lay glove package on clean flat surface above waistline.

2. Remove outer glove package by tearing the package open.

3. Glove the dominant hand first.

4. While putting on the first glove, touch only the outside surface of the glove.

5. With gloved dominant hand, slip fingers underneath second glove cuff.

6. After second glove is on, interlock hands.

26. The client's child asks to view the documentation in their parent's health record. What is the nurse's best response to this request?

1. "I'll be happy to get that for you."

2. "You will have to talk to the physician about that."

3. "You will need your parent's permission."

4. "You are not allowed to see it."

27. A 5-year-old client with respiratory syncytial virus (RSV) has a fever of 39.5°C. The child's parent asks the nurse for advice to help reduce their fever. The nurse will likely suggest which medication?

1. Acetylsalicylic acid (Aspirin)
2. Ketorolac
3. Indomethacin
4. Ibuprofen

28. A client asks the nurse what their body mass index (BMI) is. BMI is calculated by dividing weight by height squared. The client weighs 65 kg, and their height is 1.65 metres. Calculate the client's BMI. **Fill in the blank.**

Answer: BMI _____.

29. The nurse must remove interrupted sutures from a leg wound. What is the correct procedure for this skill?

1. Slip scissors under the suture, snip just below the knot.

2. Pinch the skin while lifting the knot with the forceps.

3. Snip both ends of the suture then pull through the skin.

4. Grasp knot of suture with forceps, pull up knot, cut the suture distal to the knot.

30. A client has experienced a stroke. Before initiating oral nourishment, the client must be evaluated for their swallowing ability to ensure they do not aspirate. What health care provider is most appropriate to assess swallowing?

1. Speech-language pathologist
2. Nurse
3. Physician
4. Physiotherapist

31. A health care provider orders 1 000 mL of normal saline (NS) to be infused intravenously (IV) at a rate of 50 mL/hr. The nurse determines that it will take how many hours for 1 litre to infuse. **Record your answer using a whole number. Fill in the blank.**

Answer: _____hour(s)

32. The nurse is caring for a client with *Clostridium difficile (C. difficile)* infection. Which of the following nursing actions is most efficient in preventing the spread of bacteria?

1. Monthly in-service education about contact precautions

2. Placing all contaminated items in biohazard bags

3. Mandatory cultures for all clients

4. Proper hand hygiene techniques

33. A 41-year-old primipara client attends the antenatal clinic at 38 weeks' gestation. The client reports decreased urine output, "spots" in their eyes, and headaches. What would be the first action by the nurse?

1. Take the client's blood pressure.

2. Report the findings to the on-site health care provider.

3. Arrange for immediate fetal monitoring.

4. Perform urine testing for protein by dipstick.

34. The nurse on the pediatric unit calculates the medication dose for an infant as prescribed and determines that the dose is twice what it should be. The pediatrician is contacted and says to administer the medication as ordered. What is the next action that the nurse should take? **Select all that apply.**

1. Notify the designated nursing authority.
2. Check the chain of command policy for such situations.
3. Give the medication as ordered.
4. Give the amount calculated to be correct.
5. Contact the pharmacy for clarification.

35. A client reports to the nurse he is experiencing insomnia and would like to try a sleep aid supplement. While cautioning that all complementary supplements should be discussed with their health care provider, which of the following would the nurse suggest?
   1. Echinacea
   2. Melatonin
   3. Ginko
   4. Peppermint oil

36. A client has used buffered acetylsalicylic acid (Aspirin) for several years as treatment for osteoarthritis. However, the client's symptoms are worsening. The health care provider prescribes a nonsteroidal anti-inflammatory drug (NSAID) and misoprostol. The client asks the nurse why two pills now have to be taken for the arthritis. Which is the nurse's best response to the client?
   1. "Misoprostol in combination with an NSAID will also reduce the symptoms of arthritis."
   2. "Misoprostol potentiates the action of the NSAID so that it will work better."
   3. "Misoprostol reduces the mucous secretions in the stomach, which reduces gastric irritation."
   4. "Misoprostol may help to prevent gastric ulcers that may occur when taking NSAIDs."

37. Identify the cardiac rhythm strip abnormality from this picture

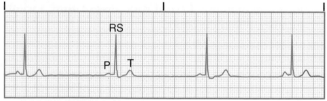

   1. Sinus bradycardia
   2. Premature ventricular contractions
   3. Ventricular tachycardia
   4. Atrial fibrillation

38. The nurse performs postoperative colostomy care. Which of the following are normal observations?
   1. The stoma is red and moist.
   2. Large amounts of formed stool are passed.
   3. The stoma drains moderate amounts of blood.
   4. There is no flatus in the pouch.

39. The nurse knows that which in-dwelling catheter procedure places the client at greatest risk for acquiring a urinary tract infection?
   1. Emptying the drainage bag every 8 hours or when half full
   2. Kinking the catheter tubing to obtain a urine specimen

3. Placing the drainage bag on the side rail of the client's bed
4. Failing to secure the catheter tubing to the client's thigh

40. A postmenopausal woman visits the sexual health clinic. She says she has multiple male sexual partners, and that although she realizes she no longer requires birth control, she would like information regarding "safer sex." Which of the following options would the nurse advise? **Select all that apply**.
   1. Take an oral antiviral to protect herself from HIV.
   2. Use a condom with all sexual partners.
   3. Restrict herself to only one sexual partner.
   4. Discuss with each partner their relative sexual history.
   5. Ensure twice annual testing for sexually transmitted diseases.
   6. Use a spermicidal barrier foam during intercourse.

41. A client with osteoporosis phones the family practice unit saying they have had a fall in their house, coming down hard on one foot. The foot is now swollen, painful, and the client cannot put weight on it at all. What advice should the nurse give to this client?
   1. Call an ambulance to take them to hospital.
   2. Arrange for transport to the hospital fracture clinic for an X-ray.
   3. Come to the family practice unit for the health care provider to assess the foot.
   4. Wrap the foot in an elastic bandage, call the family practice unit tomorrow if the foot is not better.

42. Which of the following is a requirement for a new nurse in delegating tasks to an unregulated care provider (UCP)?
   1. Obtaining the UCP's voluntary acceptance of the task
   2. Communicating the task in understandable terms
   3. Functioning with a laissez-faire style of leadership
   4. Always supervising the UCP

43. Which of the following are methods to reduce the risk of needle-stick injury? **Select all that apply.**
   1. Recap the needle after giving an injection.
   2. Use needleless systems when available.
   3. Use two hands to dispose of sharps into the disposal.
   4. Never force a needle into the sharps disposal.
   5. Clearly mark sharps disposal containers.

44. A client with an infection is being by monitored by the nurse for therapeutic results of antibiotic therapy. Which laboratory value indicates the effectiveness of this therapy?
   1. Increased red blood cell (RBC) count
   2. Increased white blood cell (WBC) count
   3. Decreased WBC count
   4. Decreased platelet count

45. The home care nurse visits a client to perform abdominal wound assessment and packing. Which of the following is a correct action for packing a wound?
   1. Moisten the packing material with povidone-iodine.
   2. Use woven gauze to pack the wound.

3. Tightly pack the wound and fix the wound closed with tape.
4. Lightly fill the wound with the moistened packing material.

46. The client is receiving 75 mL of Lactated Ringer's solution per hour. At what rate should the nurse set the drip rate if the intravenous tubing delivers 15 gtt/mL? **Record your answer using a whole number. Fill in the blank.**
Answer: ___gtt/min

47. When ambulating a client in the hall, the nurse notices that the client is beginning to fall. What should the nurse do?
1. Hold the client tightly to prevent the fall.
2. Gently lower the client to the floor.
3. Step back and let the client fall naturally.
4. Move the client against the wall and guide them to the floor.

48. Which referral will be most helpful for a person who was severely beaten by their intimate partner, has no relatives or friends in the community, is afraid to return home, and has limited financial resources?
1. A support group
2. A mental health centre
3. A shelter for victims of intimate partner violence
4. Vocational counselling

49. Which of the following are nursing interventions when caring for a postsurgical client with a closed drainage system (e.g., Hemovac, Jackson-Pratt, ConstaVac)? **Select all that apply.**
1. Empty the drainage device when it is half full.
2. Never disconnect the vacuum seal.
3. Place a safety pin in the drain just at the level of the skin.
4. Ensure that all drainage tubes are patent.
5. Report wound drainage on the client fluid balance record.
6. Determine if drain tube needs self-suction, wall suction, or no suction, according to health care provider's prescription.

50. When a drain is present at a surgical site, how should the nurse cleanse the area?
1. Use a circular stroke, start with the area immediately next to the drain.
2. Using sterile gauze, clean with up and down strokes perpendicular to the drain.
3. Cleanse from the further out from the drain to the area immediately next to the drain.
4. A drain site should not be cleansed unless there is a specific order from the health care provider.

51. The nurse counsels a 50-year-old client regarding immunization. The client expresses surprise that any "shots" are necessary at this age. What are the recommended immunizations for this client?
1. Tetanus toxoid every 10 years, recombinant Zoster Vaccine, annual influenza, COVID-19 according to schedule
2. Pneumococcal polysaccharide 23 valent, annual influenza, COVID-19 according to schedule

3. Tetanus toxoid every 10 years, rotavirus, biannual influenza, COVID-19 according to schedule
4. Measles-mumps-rubella, pneumococcal polysaccharide 23 valent, COVID-10 according to schedule

52. A nurse is assessing a client who is receiving a blood transfusion and documents the following findings. The nurse recognizes that the client is experiencing which transfusion complication?

Vital signs	Temperature: 36.9°C
	Pulse (beats per minute): 110
	Respiratory rate (breaths per minute): 28
	Blood pressure: 140/90 mmHg
	Oxygen saturation: 94%
Respiratory assessment	Crackles in both lung bases
	Dry cough
Nurse's notes	Restless in bed
Cardiovascular assessment	Distended neck veins

1. Anaphylactic shock
2. Septicemia
3. Fluid volume overload
4. Hemolytic reaction

53. A client is treated in hospital for an eating disorder, severe anorexia nervosa. A treatment plan is developed with the client prior to discharge. The nurse assesses the client 1 week after discharge to evaluate the effectiveness of the plan of care. What would be the most important evaluative factor?
1. The client states they are complying with the meal plan.
2. The client has not lost any weight post discharge
3. The client has participated in group therapy.
4. The client understands their personal triggers for refusing food.

54. A health care provider prescribes heparin 2 000 units/hr IV for a client diagnosed with a deep vein thrombosis. The medication label states: "Heparin 20 000 units of heparin in 500 mL D5W". How many mL will infuse per hour? **Record your answer using a whole number. Fill in the blank.**
Answer: _____ mL

55. The nurse is creating a plan of care for a client with glaucoma. Which nursing diagnosis addresses the visual impairment that places the client at greatest risk for injury?
1. Risk for falls
2. Body image disturbance
3. Social isolation
4. Fear

56. A nurse interviews a 17-year-old client who has been admitted to a drug rehabilitation program by court order. The client says, "I really don't belong here, but I guess I am messed up." What might be the most therapeutic response by the nurse?

1. "You will have to stay here because you are required to by law."
2. "How do you feel?"
3. "What is one thing about you that is messed up?"
4. "You can leave after you have completed treatment."

57. Which drug is commonly used to induce total cleansing of the bowel before diagnostic or surgical bowel procedures?
    1. Polyethylene glycol
    2. Lactulose
    3. Mmineral oil
    4. Milk of magnesia

58. Which of the following are grief behaviours in children ages 2 to 5 years. **Select all that apply.**
    1. See death as reversible
    2. Regressive behaviour may occur
    3. Aggressive behaviour may occur
    4. Concern about who will look after them
    5. Grief response only occurs with death of significant other
    6. May feel responsible for the occurrence

59. A nurse counsels a woman who would like to start oral contraceptive pills. The woman has been smoking for 21 years, and presently smokes 25 cigarettes a day. What is the risk for female smokers who use oral contraceptives?
    1. Myocardial infarction
    2. Bladder cancer
    3. Malignant melanoma
    4. Liver disorders

60. Which of the following clients should be the priority admission to the psychiatric unit?
    1. The client who feels anxious and sad after separation from a spouse of 10 years
    2. The client who self-inflicted a superficial cut on the forearm after a family argument
    3. The client experiencing a dry mouth and tremor related to taking haloperidol (Haldol)
    4. The client who is a new parent and hears voices saying, "Smother your baby."

61. When the nurse creates a plan of care for a client who is experiencing alterations in mobility, which of the following is true?
    1. The nurse cannot delegate interventions to unregulated care providers.
    2. The nurse is solely responsible for modifying activities of daily living (ADLs).
    3. The nurse consults other health care team members to help plan therapy.
    4. The nurse consults wound care specialists only when wounds are apparent.

62. The nurse obtains a tympanic temperature of 37.7°C on a newly admitted 42-year-old client. Which of the following is most correct when assessing this temperature?
    1. The client has a fever.
    2. This is a normal temperature.
    3. Within a range of 36°C to 38°C, no single temperature is normal for all people.
    4. There are sometimes incorrect readings based on improper positioning of the tympanic probe.

63. Which newborn reflex is demonstrated by this infant?

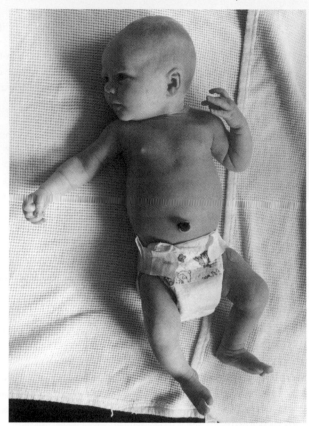

From Hockenberry, M. J., Wilson, D., & Rodgers, C. C. [2019]. *Wong's nursing care of infants and children* [11th ed.]. Mosby. Courtesy Paul Vincent Kuntz, Texas Children's Hospital.

1. Babinski
2. Rooting
3. Startle
4. Tonic neck

64. The nurse visits a 93-year-old client who lives independently at home. Upon entering the house, the nurse notices an odour of stale urine and feces. What should the nurse do?
    1. Ask the client if they wear adult incontinence underwear.
    2. Ask the client how they manage their personal hygiene.
    3. Suggest to the client they need to have a bath or shower.
    4. Do not say anything to the client as this will embarrass them.

65. A client has been prescribed an inhaled respiratory corticosteroid medication. What should the nurse tell this client about the proper method for taking this medication?
    1. Rinsing of the mouth after using the inhaler is recommended.
    2. The tubings and mouthpieces should be cleaned with only hot water.
    3. The medication is to be inhaled deeply, with the head tipped backward to maximize opening of the airway.
    4. After taking an inhaler medication, the client should remove the inhaler and hold their breath for at least 20 seconds.

66. During antibiotic therapy, the nurse should monitor the client closely for signs and symptoms of a hypersensitivity

reaction. What may be an indication of a hypersensitivity reaction? **Select all that apply.**
1. Wheezing
2. Diarrhea
3. Shortness of breath
4. Swelling of the face, tongue, or hands
5. Itching or rash

67. The nurse is teaching the family of a child with type 1 diabetes about insulin. What should the nurse include in the teaching session? **Select all that apply.**
1. Unopened vials are good for 60 days.
2. Insulin should not be left in a hot environment.
3. Insulin can be placed in the freezer if not used every day.
4. After it has been opened, insulin is good for up to 28 to 30 days.
5. Insulin vials that have been opened should be stored at room temperature or refrigerated.

68. A 70-year-old client is overweight, has a BP of 129/84, a blood sugar of 7 mmol/L, says he feels weak, unhappy, and spends most of his time lying on the sofa watching TV. What will the nurse counsel the client as a first step strategy for improving his mood and health?
1. Start a Mediterranean diet.
2. Purchase a blood glucose monitoring system.
3. Speak with the health care provider about medications for his high blood pressure.
4. Go for a daily walk in the outdoors.

69. An antihistamine diphenhydramine HCl (Benadryl) and an epinephrine auto injector (epi pen) are prescribed for an adolescent following a severe allergic response to a wasp sting. The adolescent is taught the use of both. The adolescent tells the nurse they will keep the Benadryl in their backpack and ensure their parents keep the epi pen safe at home. The nurse evaluates the adolescent's plan.
1. This is an effective plan as the Benadryl would always be close by and is effective until the epi pen is available.
2. This is an effective plan because the parents should be responsible for the epi pen.
3. This is not an effective plan as the epi pen is the most effective for anaphylaxis and needs to be readily available.
4. This is not an effective plan because the adolescent is not taking responsibility for managing a potential anaphylactic event.

70. A client arrives in the emergency department with a recent history of chest pain. Bloodwork demonstrates elevated troponin levels. The client is quite agitated. The nurse obtains vital signs as seen in the graph below. What is the priority action by the nurse at 2245?

Time	2200	2230	2245
Pulse	90 bpm	102 bpm	114 bpm
Respirations	18 breaths/min	26 breaths/min	34 breaths/min
Blood pressure	136/82 mmHg	110/72 mmHg	94 /68 mmHg

1. Apply a pulse oximeter.
2. Arrange for an ECG.
3. Contact the on-duty health care provider.
4. Reassure the client.

71. The nurse is caring for a client whose cultures were positive for *Clostridium difficile*. Which of the following nursing actions would be appropriate for this client?
1. Instructing assistive personnel to use soap and water rather than sanitizer to clean hands
2. Placing the client on droplet precautions
3. Wearing an N95 respirator when entering the client room
4. Teaching the client cough etiquette

72. A child is in palliative care at a hospice. Which of the following should be an aspect of care for the dying child and the family?
1. Organize care to minimize contact with the child in case it causes pain.
2. Ensure adequate oral intake to promote comfort.
3. Advise family that hearing may be the last sense to stop functioning.
4. Provide all care by the nurse as it is easier for the family.

73. The manager of a long-term care facility recognizes that the nursing staff are coping with tremendous stress due to the COVID-19 pandemic. They must wear full personal protective equipment (PPE), work with the fear of contracting COVID-19, provide care to many dying clients, cope with distressed families, and work many double and extra shifts because they are short staffed. What can the nurse manager do to most effectively help the staff with their immediate stress within the confines of the pandemic?
1. Hire additional staff.
2. Supply staff with gifts of appreciation.
3. Implement daily debriefing and strategy sessions.
4. Provide staff with extended vacation time and days off.

74. The nurse is performing a health assessment with an Indigenous client. What are health risks that affect the Canadian Indigenous population? **Select all that apply**
1. Tuberculosis
2. Diabetes
3. Alcohol and substance abuse
4. Cardiovascular disease
5. Arthritis
6. Bowel disorders

75. A client with cancer is scheduled for chemotherapy. The nurse discusses with the client the potential for mucositis. Which of the following would the nurse advise?
1. Use saline or prescribed oral rinses for mouth sores.
2. Use over-the-counter alcohol-based mouth washes.
3. Use acetylsalicylate acid (Aspirin)-based analgesics for painful lesions.
4. Use dental floss routinely.

76. The client requires temperatures measured every 2 hours. Which of the following cannot be delegated to an unregulated care provider (UCP)?
1. Selecting appropriate route and device
2. Obtaining temperature measurement at ordered frequency
3. Being aware of the usual values for the client

4. Assessing changes in body temperature

77. A client is prescribed one half of a unit of packed red blood cells (PRBCs) over 4 hours. The PRBCs half unit (125 mL) has been obtained from the blood bank. The administration set delivers 15 gtt/mL. At what rate should the IV infuse? **Record your answer using a whole number. Fill in the blank.**

    Answer: _____ gtt/min

78. A nurse who works in a magnetic resonance imaging (MRI) diagnostic area is aware that clients having an MRI may need which of the following?
    1. A lead apron to protect them from radiation
    2. An intravenous line (IV) to provide contrast dye
    3. Noise-cancelling headphones
    4. A warming blanket

79. The nurse is providing anticipatory guidance to parents of a 4-month-old infant on preventing an aspiration injury. What should the nurse include in the teaching? **Select all that apply.**
    1. Keep buttons and other small objects out of reach.
    2. Inspect toys for removable parts.
    3. Allow the infant to take a bottle to bed.
    4. Teething biscuits can be used for teething discomfort.
    5. The infant should not be fed hard candy, nuts, or foods with pits.

80. The single father of an 11-year-old girl tells the nurse he is worried because he has not spoken with his daughter about puberty. How should the nurse respond?
    1. "Do you have personal or religious reasons for not discussing puberty?"
    2. "You must feel uncomfortable speaking with her about it."
    3. "Do you have a trusted female friend or relative you could ask to speak with her?"
    4. "Don't worry, she will likely learn from her friends at school."

81. After 6 hours of total parenteral nutrition (TPN) infusion, the nurse checks the client's capillary blood glucose level and finds it to be 6.7 mmol/L. Which of the following actions should the nurse take?
    1. Obtain a venous blood glucose specimen.
    2. Slow the infusion rate of the TPN infusion.
    3. Recheck the capillary blood glucose in 4 hours.
    4. Notify the health care provider of the glucose level.

82. A nurse is caring for six clients on a postsurgical unit. The nurse hears a code blue being called on one of their assigned clients and runs to the client's room. When the nurse arrives, a code leader has been established. What is the first thing this nurse should do?
    1. Introduce themselves as the client's nurse, offering their specific knowledge and skills.
    2. Immediately join the code team and assist with the airway.
    3. Stand back, observe the situation and wait to be given a role by the code leader.
    4. Acknowledge that the situation is under control and go back to their other five clients.

83. After a natural disaster, an emergency worker referred a family for crisis intervention services. One family member refused to attend the services, stating, "No way, I'm not crazy." The best response the nurse can give is which of the following?
    1. "Many times, disasters can create mental health problems, so you really should participate with your family."
    2. "Crisis intervention is a short-term problem-solving type of help, and seeking this help does not mean that you have a mental illness."
    3. "You may not be crazy, but you need a trained psychiatrist to help you now"
    4. "Crisis intervention will help your family communicate better."

84. An order is written for phenytoin (Dilantin), 500 mg IM q3–4h prn for pain. The nurse recognizes that treatment of pain is not a standard therapeutic indication for this drug. The nurse believes that the prescriber meant to write for hydromorphone (Dilaudid). What should the nurse do?
    1. Give the client hydromorphone (Dilaudid), as it was meant to be written.
    2. Call the prescriber to clarify and justify the order.
    3. Administer the medication and monitor the client frequently.
    4. Refuse to give the medication and notify the nurse supervisor.

85. Which of the following circumstances represents examples of a nurse respecting a client's autonomy? **Select all that apply.**
    1. Posting pictures on social media with identifying information
    2. Documenting the client's refusal of treatment for an infected wound
    3. Stopping a treatment midway through a procedure because the client has requested it
    4. Discussing the client's refusal of a blood transfusion for religious reasons with the team
    5. Documenting the client's refusal to take a prescribed medication
    6. Counselling a client that in order to get better, they must follow the health care provider's orders for care

86. An infant who experienced neonatal apnea for several weeks, is being discharged from the nursery. The nurse instructs the parents about infant CPR. Which of the following would be included in the teaching plan?
    1. Obtain a pulse check on the carotid artery.
    2. Perform chest compressions using the palm of the hand, about 30 per minute.
    3. After the first 10 compressions, place mouth over baby's nose and give two breaths.
    4. Compression to ventilation ratio for one rescuer is 30:2.

87. Which intervention is correct when a nurse is administering a gastrostomy feeding by gravity to an adolescent client?
    1. Discard the residual and increase the volume of feeding by the amount of residual.

2. Flush the gastrostomy tube with 60 to 80 mL of water before the feeding.
3. Refill the syringe with formula after it has been completely emptied.
4. Position the client on the right side or in Fowler's position after the feeding.

88. Which of these nursing actions for the client with heart failure is appropriate for the nurse to delegate to experienced unregulated care providers (UCPs)?
    1. Assess for shortness of breath or fatigue after ambulation.
    2. Instruct the client about the need to alternate activity and rest.
    3. Obtain the client's blood pressure and pulse rate after ambulation.
    4. Determine whether the client is ready to increase the activity level.

89. The nurse is assessing a client prior to administration of the 0800 medications. Based on the information provided, which medication would the nurse hold and notify the health care provider?

Client history	Type 2 DM
	Hypertension
	Heart failure
Vital signs	Temperature: 37°C
	Pulse (beats per minute): 88
	Respirations (breaths per minute): 18
	Blood pressure: 150/90 mmHg
	O_2 sat: 97%
Lab values	Hb A1C: 5.8%
	Blood glucose 2.9 mmol/L
	K^+: 4 mmol/L

1. Potassium
2. Digoxin
3. Glyburide
4. Metoprolol

90. The nurse is caring for a client who has been receiving total parenteral nutrition (TPN) containing amino acids and dextrose for the past 24 hours. The nurse observes that about 50 mL remain in the TPN container. Which of the following actions by the nurse is most appropriate?
    1. Ask the health care provider to clarify the written TPN order.
    2. Add a new container of TPN using the current tubing and filter.
    3. Hang a new container of TPN and change the IV tubing and filter.
    4. Infuse the remaining 50 mL and then hang a new container of TPN.

91. The nurse is admitting to hospital an older client with a mobility impairment who has an acute illness. Which of the following interventions should the nurse perform first?

1. Orient the client to their room.
2. Administer the prescribed prn sedative medication.
3. Ask the health care provider to order a vest restraint.
4. Place the client in a "geri chair" near the nurse's station for observation.

92. A senior university student contacts the campus health clinic about a first-year student living on the same dormitory floor. The senior student reports that the first-year student is crying and is not adjusting to university life. The clinic nurse recognizes this as a combination of situational and maturational stress factors. What would be the best comment to the senior student?
    1. "I'd better call 9-1-1 because your friend is suicidal."
    2. "Give her this list and discuss with her university and community resources."
    3. "You must make an appointment for the student to obtain medications."
    4. "I'd recommend you help the student pack her bags to go home."

93. A client has received mild procedural sedation with propofol for a colonoscopy. Prior to the client being discharged home, which of the following would the nurse ensure? **Select all that apply.**
    1. Ability to walk independently without assistance
    2. Awareness to read and understand postprocedure instructions
    3. Successfully cough and deep breath
    4. Ability to void
    5. Successfully pass stool
    6. Presence of a friend or family member to transport the client home

94. The nurse must remove a client's nasogastric (NG) tube. The nurse understands that during removal the tube must be kinked while it is withdrawn from the client. What is the most important reason for kinking the tube?
    1. It will prevent aspiration of gastric contents.
    2. It will prevent leakage of fluid from the tube.
    3. It promotes client comfort.
    4. It reduces transmission of microorganisms.

95. The nurse is caring for a client in a hospice palliative care program who is experiencing continuous, increasing amounts of pain. Which of the following time schedules should the nurse implement for the administration of opioid pain medications?
    1. Around-the-clock routine administration of analgesics
    2. Prn doses of medication whenever the client requests
    3. Enough pain medication to keep the client sedated and unaware of stimuli
    4. Analgesic doses that provide pain control without decreasing respiratory rate

96. Which of the following strategies promote empowerment in the client receiving care? **Select all that apply.**
    1. Assess the client's level of understanding of their health issues.
    2. Provide discharge information on the day they are leaving the hospital.

3. Use medical terminology in describing the health information.

4. Accept the client's values and decisions, even if you disagree with them.

5. Encourage autonomy in the decision-making process.

97. The nurse has been caring for a client in the perioperative area for several hours. The surgical mask the nurse is wearing has become moist. Which of the following is the nurse's best next step?
1. Change the mask.
2. Air-dry the mask while on a break and reapply.
3. Ask for relief, step out of the surgical area, and apply a new mask.
4. Leave the mask in place if the nurse is comfortable.

98. A client who has just had a pacemaker implanted is very nervous that the pacemaker will stop working or that the battery will run out. What would the nurse say to reassure the client?
1. "You should keep a supply of lithium batteries on hand in case this happens."
2. "Your heart will keep beating even if the battery power runs out."
3. "Your pacemaker battery will last for 10 to 20 years."
4. "Your pacemaker is the latest model and is very reliable."

99. The case manager plans to discuss the treatment plan with a client's family. Select the case manager's first action.
1. Determine an appropriate location for the conference.
2. Support the discussion with examples of the client's behaviour.
3. Obtain the client's permission for the exchange of information.
4. Determine which family members should participate in the conference.

100. A client has been diagnosed with Alzheimer's disease (AD). Which of the following behaviours are characteristic of the moderate stage of AD? **Select all that apply.**
1. Forget events or own personal history
2. Become moody or withdrawn, especially in socially or mentally challenging situations
3. Experience some difficulty in word finding
4. Misplace articles such as keys
5. Unable to recall their own address or telephone number
6. Become confused about where they are or what day it is

101. A client is nauseous, anorexic, and weak postsurgery and chemotherapy for lung cancer, saying "I just don't feel like eating, it makes me feel sick." What diet would the nurse advise?
1. High-protein drinks
2. High-calorie drinks
3. High protein, high calorie drinks

4. Carbonated water

102. A client who is HIV-positive is taking antiretroviral medications. Which information is most important for the nurse to address when planning care for this client?
1. The client's blood glucose level is 10 mmol/L
2. The client complains of feeling "constantly tired."
3. The client is unable to state the adverse effects of the medications.
4. The client states, "Sometimes I miss a dose of zidovudine (AZT)."

103. A client on an 1 800 calorie per day diet. The following is the client calorie count up to dinner time.

Breakfast	325 calories
Midmorning snack	80 calories
Lunch	470 calories
Midafternoon snack	125 calories

How many calories should the client consume for the rest of the day, dinner, and evening snack? Fill in the blank.

104. When caring for a client with a temporary radioactive cervical implant, which action by the student nurse indicates that the unit nurse should intervene?
1. The student flushes the toilet once after emptying the client's bedpan.
2. The student stands by the client's bed for 30 minutes talking with the client.
3. The student places the client's bedding in the laundry container in the hallway.
4. The student gives the client an alcohol-containing mouthwash to use for oral care.

105. A trauma survivor is requesting sleep medication because of "bad dreams." Concerned about post-traumatic stress disorder (PTSD), the nurse would ask which of the following?
1. "Do you have trouble falling back to sleep after your dreams?"
2. "Are you concerned you will harm yourself?"
3. "Do you have a history of phobias?"
4. "Can you describe your bad dreams to me?"

106. An adolescent asks the nurse about the "safety of getting a tattoo." The nurse explains to the adolescent that it is important to find a qualified operator using proper sterile technique because an unsterilized needle or contaminated tattoo ink can cause which of the following? **Select all that apply.**
1. Hepatitis C virus
2. Hepatitis B virus
3. Hepatitis E virus
4. Human immunodeficiency virus (HIV)
5. *Mycobacterium chelonae* skin infections

107. A client who is about to have a bronchoscopy says to the nurse, "The doctor has told me what a bronchoscopy is, but I still don't really understand. What is a bronchoscope?" What would the nurse say to the client?
1. "It is a flexible tube that goes into your bronchi, your breathing tubes."

2. "It is a large stiff tube that goes down your throat and into your lungs."

3. "It is a soft tube that goes into your esophagus."

4. "It is a very small tube that goes through your nose and into your trachea."

108. A client is to receive medication through a nasogastric tube. What is the most important nursing action to ensure effective absorption?
    1. Thoroughly shake the medication before administering.
    2. After all medications are administered, flush tube with 15 to 30 mL of water.
    3. Position client in the supine position for 30 minutes.
    4. Clamp suction for 30 to 60 minutes after medication administration.

109. The nurse is discussing testicular cancer with a male client. Which of the following teaching points would the nurse discuss? **Select all that apply.**
    1. He should perform testicular examination after a warm shower.
    2. He should perform testicular self-examination every 6 months.
    3. The testicles should feel like a firm egg.
    4. Testicular cancer is more prevalent in men over 50 years.
    5. Testicular cancer is more prevalent with a history of undescended testicles.
    6. Notify his primary health care provider if there are any changes from one exam to the next.

110. A 2-year-old child who weighs 12 kg requires ibuprofen for fever of 39.0°C and discomfort associated with an ear infection. There is a countrywide shortage of pediatric ibuprofen, so none is available in any of the local pharmacies. What would the nurse advise the parent?
    1. Call the office of the health care provider to see if they have any pediatric Advil.
    2. Take the child to the hospital.
    3. Provide alternate comfort strategies, such as sponging with cool water.
    4. Crush one half of an adult 200 mg ibuprofen, mix with jam, and give to the child.

111. A nurse has been assisting a client to develop effective coping skills. Which of the following demonstrates effective coping behaviours by the client?
    1. Stating feeling better after talking with his family and friends
    2. Restricting consumption of alcohol to several drinks per day
    3. Discontinuing support group meetings
    4. Reducing time in bed to several naps per day

112. The primary health care provider writes these new orders for a resident in a nursing home: 2 G sodium restricted diet, restraint as needed. Limit fluids to 1 800 mL daily, Milk of Magnesia 30 mL PO once if no bowel movement for 3 days. Which order should the nurse question?
    1. The fluid restriction
    2. The order for restraint

3. The order for Milk of Magnesia
4. The sodium-restricted diet order

113. A client receiving chemotherapy and radiation for cancer completes daily blood work at the oncology outpatient lab. The nurse reviews the bloodwork as shown in the table below. Which of the laboratory values would the nurse report to the health care provider?

Hemoglobin	124 g/L
Hematocrit	41%
Platelet	162 X 10^9/L
White blood cell	3 600 X 10^9/L

1. Hemoglobin (Hg)
2. Hematocrit (Hct)
3. Platelets
4. White blood cell (WBC)

114. The nurse is caring for a client who has been taking antibiotics for several days and develops watery diarrhea. Which of the actions should the nurse take first?
    1. Notify the health care provider.
    2. Obtain a stool specimen for analysis.
    3. Provide education about handwashing.
    4. Place the client on contact precautions.

115. A client has returned to the unit after abdominal surgery. Which action would the nurse delegate to the unregulated care provider (UCP)?
    1. Initial vital sign monitoring
    2. Assessing the intravenous (IV) site
    3. Comfort measures
    4. Pain assessment

116. A 10-year old cares for siblings while the parents work because the family cannot afford a babysitter. A community health nurse performs a home visit and speaks with the child who says, "My father doesn't like me. He calls me stupid all the time." The mother says the father is easily frustrated and has trouble disciplining the children. The nurse should consider which resources as priorities to stabilize the home situation? **Select all that apply.**
    1. Parental sessions to teach child-rearing practices
    2. Anger management counselling for the father
    3. Continuing home visits to give support
    4. A safety plan for the wife and children
    5. Placing the children in foster care

117. A nurse prepares to administer a scheduled injection of haloperidol decanoate (Haldol) to an outpatient with schizophrenia. As the nurse swabs the site, the client shouts, "Stop! I don't want to take that medicine anymore. I hate the side effects." Select the nurse's best action.
    1. Assemble other staff to restrain if necessary and proceed with the injection.
    2. Stop the medication administration procedure and say to the client "Tell me more about the adverse effects you've been having."
    3. Proceed with the injection but explain to the client that there are medications that will help reduce the unpleasant adverse effects.

4. Say to the client, "Since I've already drawn the medication in the syringe, I'm required to give it, but let's talk to the doctor about delaying next month's dose."

118. A nurse is priority setting before a client's discharge from a residential substance abuse treatment program. Which of the following would be an appropriate priority for a client?
   1. Identifying community self-help groups before being discharged from the program
   2. Staying away from all triggers that cause substance abuse
   3. Stating a plan to never be tempted by illicit substances after discharge
   4. Identifying personal areas of weakness to grow stronger

119. Correct body alignment reduces strain on musculoskeletal structures and contributes to balance. Balance control is attained by which of the following? **Select all that apply.**
   1. Keeping the body's centre of gravity high
   2. Maintaining a wide base of support
   3. Keeping the body's centre of gravity low
   4. Maintaining correct body posture
   5. Maintaining immobility to prevent falls

120. A voluntarily hospitalized client tells the nurse, "Get me the forms for discharge. I want to leave now." Select the nurse's best response.
   1. "I will get the forms for you right now and bring them to your room."
   2. "Since you signed your consent for treatment, you may leave if you desire."
   3. "I will get them for you, but let's talk about your decision to leave treatment."
   4. "I cannot give you those forms without your health care provider's permission."

121. A 14-year-old client, who has received a hit while playing hockey, arrives in the emergency department. The client complains of feeling anxious, short of breath, and scared. On assessment, the nurse determines breath sounds are diminished on the left side compared to the right, and the oxygen saturation is 81%. Which of the following is the priority action by the nurse?
   1. Administer oxygen, as per unit protocol.
   2. Notify the health care provider.
   3. Determine the nature of the hit from the hockey game.
   4. Reassure the client.

122. Which statements about antiepileptic drug (AED) therapy are true? **Select all that apply.**
   1. AED therapy can be stopped when seizures are under control.
   2. AED therapy is usually lifelong.
   3. Consistent dosing is key to control of seizures.
   4. A dose may be skipped if the client is experiencing adverse effects.
   5. Abrupt withdrawal from AEDs may cause rebound seizure activity.

123. A child has just died following a long illness due to cancer. The nurse sits with the grieving family. What is a priority action for the nurse in supporting this family?
   1. Reassure them their child is in a better place.
   2. Counsel them that their grief will ease in about a year.
   3. Encourage the family to express their feelings and reminisce about their child.
   4. Recognize that because the child has been ill for a long time, the grief process will be easier for them.

124. A health care provider has prescribed depot injections every 3 weeks at the clinic for a client with a history of medication noncompliance. For this plan to be successful, which factor will be of critical importance?
   1. The attitude of significant others toward the client
   2. Understanding by the client of the need for depot injections
   3. The level of trust between the client and the nurse
   4. The availability of transportation to the clinic

125. The nurse is administering an oral antihistamine at bedtime to a child with atopic dermatitis (eczema). Which antihistamine should the nurse expect to be prescribed at bedtime?
   1. Cetirizine (Zyrtec)
   2. Loratidine (Claritin)
   3. Fexofenadine (Allegra)
   4. Diphenhydramine (Benadryl)

126. The nurse is providing care to a client who has been diagnosed with terminal cancer and has a poor prognosis. When the client's partner comes into the hospital cafeteria during a busy period, the nurse approaches him and openly expresses sympathy to the man for his partner's terminal illness. He bursts into tears and says that he did not know about the diagnosis. This nurse's action exemplifies which of the following violations? **Select all that apply.**
   1. Intentional tort
   2. Unintentional tort
   3. Invasion of privacy
   4. Negligence
   5. Battery

127. A client who has just given birth states their preference is to formula feed their newborn. What should the nurse planning discharge tell the client to help suppress lactation and promote comfort?
   1. Wear a well-fitting bra continuously for several days.
   2. Stand in a warm shower, letting the water spray over the breasts.
   3. Express small amounts of milk from the breasts several times a day.
   4. Massage the breasts when they ache.

128. An older person has serious vision problems and is no longer allowed to have a driver's licence. The client has been independent until this time. Which nursing diagnosis is most appropriate for this situation?
   1. Chronic confusion
   2. Ineffective coping

3. Risk for low self-esteem
4. Dysfunctional grieving

129. A client is transferred to a new unit within the hospital. The admitting nurse will perform the medication reconciliation. Which statement defines this process?
   1. Adjusting the time of medication administration for any medications scheduled at nonstandard times
   2. Ensuring the medications have been transferred with the client from the previous unit
   3. Comparing medications the client took on the previous unit with the current medication orders
   4. Assessing the client's adherence to all medications taken at home

130. The following blood gases were obtained on an 85-year-old client

pH	7.31
pO_2	94 mm Hg
pCO_2	37 mm Hg

Which value would concern the nurse?
   1. The pH
   2. The pO_2
   3. The pCO_2
   4. All values are within normal limits.

131. A confused client is restless and continues to try to remove their oxygen and urinary catheter. What are the priority nursing diagnosis and intervention to implement for this client?
   1. *Risk for injury:* Prevent harm to client; use restraints if alternative strategies fail.
   2. *Deficient knowledge:* Explain the purpose of oxygen therapy and the urinary catheter.
   3. *Disturbed body image:* Encourage client to express concerns about body.
   4. *Caregiver role strain:* Identify resources to assist with care.

132. Who is/are the expert in the understanding and management of client illness?
   1. The nurses
   2. The physicians
   3. The client
   4. The interprofessional team

133. A client returns to the recovery area after electroconvulsive therapy (ECT) for severe resistant depression. Which of the following would be most therapeutic to the client post procedure?
   1. Reassuring them that the ECT will likely have cured their depression
   2. Reporting to the client their vital signs are stable
   3. Assessing orientation with reminders that confusion is normal post-ECT
   4. Providing pain medication, as ordered

134. Which of the following is true concerning acquired immunodeficiency syndrome (AIDS)? **Select all that apply**
   1. It is caused by the human immunodeficiency virus.
   2. It is curable with newer forms of antiretroviral therapy.

3. It is considered to be a chronic illness.
4. The virus kills T cells, increasing susceptibility to infection and neoplasms.
5. It has a short incubation period.
6. It is more prevalent in high-risk groups, such as intravenous drug abusers.

135. The nurse is teaching a client self-injection of insulin. Which of the following is the most effective teaching-learning method?
   1. Provide written pamphlets for instruction.
   2. Show a video and allow the client to practise as needed on their own.
   3. Verbally explain the procedure and provide written handouts for reinforcement.
   4. Demonstrate the procedure, then allow the client to do several return demonstrations.

136. The nurse determines that the client may need a restraint and recognizes which one of the following?
   1. An order for a restraint may be implemented indefinitely until it is no longer required by the client.
   2. Restraints may be ordered on an as-needed basis.
   3. No order or consent is necessary for restraints in long-term care facilities.
   4. Restraints are to be periodically removed to have the client re-evaluated.

137. The nurse inspects a 10-day postamputation midthigh stump of a debilitated client with diabetes. The nurse observes black tissue at the wound site. The nurse evaluates the black tissue as a sign of which of the following?
   1. Dead or necrotic tissue
   2. Infected tissue
   3. Tissue staining from antiseptic solutions
   4. Normal healing

138. Which of the following statements are true concerning dementia? **Select all that apply.**
   1. Close to 100% of dementias are due to Alzheimer's disease.
   2. Lewy Bodies, frontotemporal, vascular, and traumatic brain injuries are types of dementia.
   3. It refers to a collection of symptoms rather than a specific disease.
   4. It manifests as a progressive deterioration in cognitive function.
   5. It presents as primarily an impairment in memory.
   6. When in the mild early stages, it does not interfere with the individual's functions.

139. A nurse is planning an education session for new nurses on an inpatient psychiatric setting. Which of the following would the nurse include as an example of a violation of client rights?
   1. Prohibiting a client from using the telephone
   2. In the client's presence, opening a package mailed to the client.
   3. Remaining within arm's length of a client with homicidal ideation
   4. Permitting a client with psychosis to refuse oral psychotropic medication

140. Equipment-related accidents are risks for clients in the health care agency. The nurse assesses for this risk when using which of the following?
    1. IV pumps
    2. A measuring device that measures urine
    3. Computer-based documentation
    4. A manual medication-dispensing device

141. Which of the following nursing actions demonstrates appropriate clinical decision making for groups of clients? **Select all that apply.**
    1. Identifying the nursing diagnosis of each client
    2. Prioritizing care based on urgency and complexity of problems
    3. Delaying family-centred care until the nurse has more time
    4. Combining activities to resolve more than one client problem at a time
    5. Delegating basic care activities to unregulated care providers

142. The home care nurse visits a client who is receiving peritoneal dialysis. The client has a fever of 39.0°C, there is abdominal tenderness, and the outflow is cloudy. Which of the following is an appropriate nursing intervention?
    1. Obtain a sample of the outflow for culture and sensitivity.
    2. Advise the client they will have to be admitted to hospital for antibiotic therapy.
    3. Discontinue the peritoneal dialysis.
    4. Reassure the client most dialysis infections are not serious.

143. The nurse is caring for a client in restraints. Which of the following must be documented by the nurse in the health record? **Select all that apply.**
    1. The client states that their gown is soiled and needs changing.
    2. Previous attempts to distract the client with television were unsuccessful.
    3. The client was placed in bilateral wrist restraints at 0815.
    4. Bilateral radial pulses present, 2+, hands warm to touch
    5. Released from restraints, active range-of-motion exercises complete

144. The pregnant client is assessed by the nurse on their first visit to the prenatal clinic at 8 weeks' gestation. Which of the following would be of concern to the nurse as potential maternal risk factors? **Select all that apply.**
    1. Nausea in the morning
    2. Breast tenderness
    3. Age of 16 years
    4. Hemoglobin of 90 g/L
    5. Frequent urination
    6. Genital warts

145. An infant with respiratory distress caused by bronchiolitis is placed in an oxygen mist tent. The infant cries constantly, worsening the respiratory distress, and the

parents are quite upset. What action should the nurse implement?
    1. Consult with the health care provider to provide sedation for the infant.
    2. Ask the parents to leave, as they are upsetting the infant.
    3. Encourage the parents to hold their infant, and provide oxygen via humidified face mask.
    4. Promote infant relaxation by darkening the room and decreasing environmental noise.

146. The nurse teaches a colleague that light therapy may be used with clients who have which of the following conditions?
    1. Ulcerative colitis
    2. Seasonal affective disorder
    3. Inflammatory diseases
    4. Stress and anxiety

147. Which of the following are clinical signs of fluid volume deficit. **Select all that apply.**
    1. Dry conjunctiva
    2. Blurred vision
    3. Weak pulse
    4. Excessive salivation
    5. Oliguria
    6. Increased urine specific gravity

148. The nurse determines that a confused older client is at high risk for falls. Which of the following interventions is most appropriate for the nurse to take?
    1. Place the client in restraints.
    2. Lock beds and wheelchairs when transferring.
    3. Place a bath mat outside the tub.
    4. Silence fall-alert alarm upon request of family.

149. A client is diagnosed with stage IV pancreatic cancer. The oncologist has suggested a palliative care referral for the client. The adult children of the client are very upset and tell the nurse they cannot consider palliative care, as that would show they were "giving up" and that it was "near the end." How should the nurse respond?
    1. "That is correct, it is probably too soon for palliative care."
    2. "It is a decision for your father to make, not the family."
    3. "Palliative care would relieve your father's symptoms and improve quality of life. It does not mean that death is imminent."
    4. "You must think of your father, that his pain will be better controlled by the palliative care team."

150. Which conditions are general contraindications to the use of oral laxatives? **Select all that apply.**
    1. High ammonia levels due to liver failure
    2. Abdominal pain of unknown origin
    3. Nausea and vomiting
    4. Pregnancy
    5. Acute surgical abdomen
    6. Familial risk for colon cancer

151. Which situation will require the nurse to obtain a telephone order?
    1. As the nurse and primary care provider leave a client's room, the primary care provider gives the nurse an order.

2. At 0100, a client's blood pressure drops from 120/80 to 90/50 and the incision dressing is saturated with blood.

3. At 0800, the client and primary care provider make rounds and the primary care provider tells the nurse a diet order.

4. A nurse reads an order correctly as written by the primary care provider in the client's medical record.

152. Which technique should the nurse use to facilitate the administration of a rectal suppository?

1. Having the client lie on the right side of the body, unless contraindicated

2. Having the client hold the breath during insertion of the medication

3. Lubricating the suppository with a small amount of petroleum-based lubricant

4. Encouraging the client to lie on the left side of the body for 15 to 20 minutes after insertion

153. The nurse educator is reviewing hand hygiene for a group of new nurses. What are the rationales for hand hygiene? **Select all that apply.**

1. Provides an uninterrupted chain of infection.

2. Decreases the incidence of health care-associated infection.

3. Protects the nurse from transmission of microbes.

4. Decreases the transmission of microbes to other clients.

5. Decreases the drying effects of soap.

154. A client expresses interest in alternative therapies and asks the nurse, "What is guided imagery?" Which of the following statements is the most accurate response?

1. "It is a technique where the person focuses on an image to relieve stress."

2. "It involves relaxation of every muscle in sequence."

3. "The person enters a hypnotic state to promote relaxation."

4. "It is provided by a practitioner who provides therapy through guided touch."

155. When using evidence-informed practice, the nurse is doing which of the following?

1. Integrating clinical knowledge into nursing practice

2. Applying knowledge from best research evidence, clinical experience, judgement, and the person's values and beliefs

3. Problem-solving approach informed by the best evidence from research

4. Applying evidence from randomized control trials and meta-analyses into practice

156. The nurse is conducting an in-home assessment at the request of a family for a person who has been diagnosed with dementia. Which of the following is the priority evaluation?

1. The person's current level of cognitive and daily functioning

2. Safety of the person's home environment

3. Review of medications, including herbs and complementary agents

4. Needs of the family for teaching and guidance

157. The nurse is caring for a client who has had a recent stroke and is paralyzed on their left side. The client has no respiratory or cardiac issues, but they cannot walk. They become extremely frustrated when they cannot button their shirt and cannot feed themselves because they were left-handed. The client has shown no signs of dysphagia, but they have been eating very little and have lost 0.9 kg (2 pounds). The client asks the nurse, "How can I go home like this? I'm not getting better. I can't ask my partner to take care of me like a baby." Of the following list of health care team members, which member would the nurse need to consult? **Select all that apply.**

1. Physiotherapy

2. Occupational therapy

3. Respiratory therapy

4. Cardiac rehabilitation

5. Psychology services

158. The nurse reviews postoperative instructions with the parent of a 3-year-old child who has had insertion of myringotomy tubes. Which of the following would be included in these instructions?

1. Show the parent the tube so that it will be recognized if it falls out.

2. Advise the parent the child may not blow their nose for 2 days after surgery.

3. Keep warm wet compresses over the ears.

4. Do not allow the child to swim for 2 weeks.

159. The nurse needs to reposition a 136.1 kg (300-pound) client. Which of the following strategies is most likely to prevent back injury?

1. Turn the client alone using the lift pad and applying pillows.

2. Put the bed in the Trendelenburg position and pull from the head of the bed.

3. Assess and obtain the number of people needed to help.

4. Bend at the waist and pull the lift pad, using the arms.

160. The nurse is preparing to initiate a continuous subcutaneous infusion (hypodermoclysis). Which condition(s) are contraindications in the use of hypodermoclysis? **Select all that apply.**

1. Mild dehydration

2. Marked edema

3. Renal failure

4. Fluid overload

5. Limited IV access

161. An adult child of a parent with dementia expresses frustration to the nurse concerning their parent's confusion because it causes a lot of stressful arguments between the parent and adult child. In order to decrease these stressful situations when the parent is confused, the nurse advises the adult child to do which of the following?

1. Orient the parent to person, place, and time.

2. Question the parent about the facts of what they are saying,

3. Affirm with the parent that what they are saying is confusing and untrue.

4. Try distraction, such as "Let's have a cup of tea."

162. A client with asthma is to begin medication therapy with a metered-dose inhaler. What important reminder should the nurse include during teaching sessions with the client?
    1. Repeat subsequent puffs, if ordered, after 5 minutes.
    2. Inhale slowly while pressing down to release the medication.
    3. Inhale quickly while pressing down to release the medication.
    4. Administer the inhaler while holding it 7.5 to 10 cm away from the mouth.

163. An experienced nurse says to a new graduate, "When you've practised as long as I have, you know exactly how to take care of sick people." What information should the new graduate consider when analyzing this comment? **Select all that apply.**
    1. New research findings should be integrated continuously into a nurse's practice to provide the most effective care.
    2. The experienced nurse may need to be reminded of the importance of professional Standards of Nursing Practice.
    3. Experience provides nurses with the essential tools and skills needed for effective professional practice.
    4. Experienced nurses have learned the best ways to care for clients through trial and error.
    5. An intuitive sense of clients' needs guides effective nurses.

164. A client diagnosed with delirium is experiencing perceptual alterations. Which environmental adjustment should the nurse make for this client?
    1. Provide a well-lit room without glare or shadows. Limit noise and stimulation.
    2. Maintain soft lighting day and night. Keep a radio on low volume continuously.
    3. Light the room brightly day and night. Awaken the client hourly to assess mental status.
    4. Keep the client by the nurse's desk while awake. Provide rest periods in a room with a television on.

165. A competent client becomes angry, insists on leaving against medical advice, and refuses to sign the waiver acknowledging that they have been advised that leaving is not recommended at this time. What should the nurse do?
    1. The nurse should call security to restrain the client.
    2. The nurse should let the client go but alert the police.
    3. The nurse should refuse to give the client their personal effects.
    4. The nurse should allow the client to leave.

166. A client with acute surgical pain who has never received opioids in the past is ordered opioids through a patient-controlled analgesia (PCA) pump. Which of the following nursing actions regarding opioid administration are appropriate at this time? **Select all that apply.**
    1. Assessing for signs that the client is becoming addicted to the opioid
    2. Monitoring for therapeutic and adverse effects of opioid administration
    3. Emphasizing that the risk of some opioid adverse effects increases over time
    4. Educating the client about how analgesics improve postoperative activity level
    5. Teaching about the need to decrease opioid doses by the second postoperative day

167. A nurse says, "I am the only one who truly understands this client. Other staff members are too critical." The nurse's statement indicates which of the following?
    1. Boundary blurring
    2. Sexual harassment
    3. Positive regard
    4. Advocacy

168. Several cases of measles have been reported in the community. Which of the following terms is used to describe a communicable disease that occurs among a cluster of individuals?
    1. Epidemic
    2. Outbreak
    3. Pandemic
    4. Mitigation

169. The nurse is caring for a hospitalized 12-year-old child who is on fall precautions secondary to seizures. What interventions should be included in the child's care plan? **Select all that apply.**
    1. Place a call light and desired items within reach.
    2. Keep the bed in the highest position with the two side rails up.
    3. Turn off the lights and television at night.
    4. Keep personal belongings and clutter contained in one area of the floor.
    5. Have the child wear an appropriate-size gown and nonskid footwear.

170. When asked about their Indigenous cultural affiliation, a client responds, "That's personal, why do you want to know?" Which of the following is the most appropriate nursing response?
    1. "You need not answer my question if you prefer not to share that information."
    2. "By knowing your cultural background I can best meet your specific needs."
    3. "All information that you provide will be kept in strict confidence."
    4. "I did not mean to offend you; we ask that question of all of our new admissions."

171. The nurse is caring for a client who has an order to change a dressing twice a day, at 0600 and 1800. At 1400, the nurse notices that the dressing is saturated. What is the nurse's next action?
    1. Wait and change the dressing at 1800 as ordered.
    2. Revise the plan of care and change the dressing now.
    3. Reassess the dressing and the wound in 1 hour.
    4. Discontinue the plan of care.

172. The nurse caring for a client with a stage 2 pressure injury and understands the need for a multidisciplinary approach. The nurse evaluates the need for

several consults. Who of the following should always be included in the consults? **Select all that apply.**

1. Registered dietitian
2. Enterostomal and wound care nurse
3. Physiotherapist
4. Case management personnel
5. Pharmacist

173. A client is taking a combination of antitubercular drugs for the treatment of tuberculosis (TB). What should the nurse say about this drug therapy to the client? **Select all that apply.**

1. "You are considered contagious for most of the illness and must take precautions to prevent spreading the disease."
2. "The medications may be stopped if you have severe adverse effects."
3. "Alcoholic beverages should be avoided while on this therapy."
4. "If you notice reddish-brown or reddish-orange urine, stop the drug and contact your doctor right away."
5. "If you experience a burning or tingling in your fingers or toes, report this to your health care provider immediately."

174. A nurse finds a client with moderate-stage dementia crying in the bathroom of the long-term care facility, holding a toothbrush in their hand. The client states they want to brush their teeth but says, "I don't know what to do." What should the nurse say?

1. "Here is the toothbrush. Pick up the toothpaste. Now, put the toothpaste on the brush and rub your teeth with the brush."
2. "Don't be upset, I will brush your teeth for you."
3. "You don't need your teeth brushed just now, you have already done that today."
4. "This is something you know how to do, see if you can remember."

175. A terminally ill client tells the nurse that they are afraid to speak up regarding their desire to end care for fear of upsetting their spouse and children. Which nursing code of ethics principle ensures that the nurse will promote the client's cause?

1. Responsibility
2. Advocacy
3. Confidentiality
4. Accountability

176. A nurse is providing a change-of-shift report. Which information is critical for the nurse to communicate? **Select all that apply.**

1. The client had a good day with no complaints.
2. The family is demanding and argumentative.
3. The client has a new pain medication, hydromorphone hydrochloride (Dilaudid).
4. The family is poor and had to go on social assistance.
5. The client reports the pain is relieved when positioned on their side.

177. The nurse has become aware that narcotics are missing in the client care area. Which ethical principle obligates the nurse to report the missing medications?

1. Advocacy
2. Responsibility
3. Confidentiality
4. Accountability

178. A nurse attends a sporting event in an arena. One of the spectators collapses, the nurse assesses there is no breathing and no pulse. The nurse is aware there is an automated external defibrillator (AED) in the building. What should be the priority action by the nurse?

1. Start CPR, tell an onlooker to obtain the AED.
2. Obtain the AED, follow the voice prompts.
3. Determine if the spectator has a history of cardiac problems.
4. Administer acetylsalicylic acid (aspirin) 81 mg under the tongue.

179. Which action by a nurse constitutes a breach of a client's right to privacy? **Select all that apply.**

1. Documenting the client's daily behaviour during hospitalization
2. Releasing information to the client's employer without consent
3. Discussing the client's history with other staff during care planning
4. Asking family to share information about a client's prehospitalization behaviour
5. Providing information to police

180. Choose the correct information about intimate partner violence. **Select all that apply**

1. Most clients will not spontaneously provide information about family violence.
2. Abuse is a life-threatening public health concern.
3. Clients must be reassured all information will be confidential.
4. Both partners should be present for the assessment interview.
5. Abuse tends to decrease during pregnancy.
6. Threatening is common and not likely to lead to physical abuse.

181. A client with a history of a transient ischemic attack (TIA) has been instructed to take one 81-mg tablet of acetylsalicylic acid (Aspirin) each day. When the nurse is administering the medications, the client says, "I don't need the Aspirin today. I don't have any aches or pains." Which of the following actions should the nurse take?

1. Document that the Aspirin was refused by the client.
2. Tell the client that the Aspirin will prevent aches.
3. Explain that the Aspirin is ordered to decrease stroke risk.
4. Call the health care provider to clarify the medication order.

182. A client who has recently completed routine baseline blood work at a local community lab is curious about the results. The client asks the nurse who works in the

lab how best to obtain the results. What would the nurse respond?

1. "Your health care provider will schedule a virtual appointment to review your results."
2. "Call your health care provider in two days to discuss the results."
3. "You may call or visit the lab next week to receive a report of your results."
4. "Here are the instructions to access our digital health portal that allows you to see your results."

183. In which situations would a nurse have the duty to intervene and report? **Select all that apply.**
    1. A nursing colleague has difficulty writing measurable outcomes
    2. A health care provider gives a telephone order for medication
    3. A team member who is in an alcohol-impaired state provides client care
    4. A team member violates relationship boundaries with a client
    5. A client refuses medication prescribed by a health care provider
    6. A nursing colleague shares client information with the news media without consent

184. The nurse needs to transfer the client from the bed to the chair. Which of the following safety measures should the nurse implement?
    1. Avoid using a transfer or gait belt around the client's waist before transfer.
    2. Do not allow the client to help in any way.
    3. Assess for the need of a mechanical lift and assistance by a colleague.
    4. Ensure that the client has socks on the feet for transfer.

185. The nurse is interviewing a 90-year-old client. What teaching strategies which are appropriate? Select all that apply.
    1. Sit facing the client.
    2. Speak loudly.
    3. Keep a low tone of voice.
    4. Focus on a single topic.
    5. Assume the client will have difficulty understanding.
    6. Ensure a family member joins the discussion.

186. What is the proper technique for administering ear drops to a 2-year-old child?
    1. Administering the drops without altering the ear canal direction
    2. Straightening the ear canal by pulling the lobe upward and back
    3. Straightening the ear canal by pulling the pinna down and back
    4. Straightening the ear canal by pulling the pinna upward and outward

187. Which of the following are signs of dehydration in a 5-year-old child? **Select all that apply**
    1. Decreased pulse
    2. Sunken fontanelle
    3. Irritable
    4. Dry mucous membranes
    5. Decreased urine output
    6. Capillary refill over 4 seconds

188. According to hospital policy the nurse must dress an IV site with a gauze dressing. The nurse has done a literature review and believes that evidence-informed practice dictates the use of a transparent dressing to prevent catheter dislodgement. What should the nurse do?
    1. Begin to use transparent dressing instead of gauze dressings.
    2. Bring findings to the policy and procedure committee.
    3. Use transparent dressings on half of their IV starts and gauze on the other.
    4. Continue following hospital policy without saying anything.

189. What is the best method to reduce the incidence of pressure injuries? **Select all that apply**
    1. Use of the Braden Risk Assessment Scale
    2. Use of the Norton Scale
    3. Turning the client every 6 hours
    4. Clinical judgement
    5. Critical thinking
    6. Targeted interventions

190. A nurse works in a retirement home. An 82-year-old resident comes to the nurse's office asking for information about sexuality and sexual intercourse. What would be the nurse's first response?
    1. "Do you have a new partner?"
    2. "I do not believe you have reason to be concerned about sexuality."
    3. "Let's talk about what you would like to know."
    4. "Are you worried about sexually transmitted diseases?"

191. The nurse has been closely observing a client who has been displaying escalating and aggressive behaviours. Which nursing interventions are most beneficial to the client at this time? **Select all that apply.**
    1. Initiate confinement measures.
    2. Acknowledge the client's behaviour.
    3. Assist the client to an area that is quiet.
    4. Maintain a safe distance from the client.
    5. Allow the client to take control of the situation.
    6. Contact agency security.

192. A recent immigrant who does not speak English or French is alert and requires hospitalization. What is the initial action that the nurse must take to obtain informed consent?
    1. Ask a family member to translate what the nurse is saying.
    2. Notify the health care provider that the client does not speak English or French.
    3. Request an official interpreter to explain the terms of consent.
    4. Use hand gestures and medical equipment while explaining in English.

193. A client tells the nurse, "I am bipolar." What is the best response by the nurse?
    1. "What are your symptoms?"
    2. "When were you diagnosed with bipolar disorder?"
    3. "How does being bipolar affect your life?"
    4. "Have you felt any stigma because of your diagnosis?"

194. The nurse discusses a birth plan with a pregnant couple. They have decided they would like to have a music playlist for the labour and delivery. What is an appropriate response by the nurse?
    1. "That is a good idea, but music is not allowed in the delivery room."
    2. "I like that idea—may I suggest appropriate musical selections?"
    3. "It would be more effective for you to do relaxation exercises together."
    4. "Put your playlist together on your preferred devices and we will help you set it up"

195. A nurse working at a summer camp instructs the children and counsellors about tick-bite safety. Which of the following would be teaching points? **Select all that apply.**
    1. Wear long-sleeved shirts and pants tucked into long socks.
    2. Take prophylactic antibiotics for Lyme disease.
    3. Apply insect repellents containing DEET.
    4. If a tick is found, crush it between two fingers.
    5. If a tick is found on the body, save it for later identification.
    6. To remove a tick grasp close to the skin with tweezers and pull up.

196. An older person lives alone in their own house. The nurse must assess the appropriateness of the living conditions. Which of the following questions should the nurse ask first?
    1. "What support do you have from family, friends, and the community?"
    2. "Do you want to move to an assisted-living facility?"
    3. "Are you concerned to be living by yourself?"
    4. "Do you live in a two-story house?"

197. Post myocardial infarction, a client is started on "bridge therapy" of heparin sulphate and warfarin prior to discharge. The nurse advises the client that once at home, they will require weekly blood tests to monitor the INR. The client asks for an explanation of INR. What would the nurse respond?
    1. "This is a measurement to determine appropriate levels of anticoagulants, or blood thinners."
    2. "This is a test to see if the platelets in your blood are clotting properly."
    3. "This test monitors your cardiac enzymes, which have been elevated since your heart attack."
    4. "This test will warn us if you might have another heart attack."

198. A client has just been told that he has approximately 6 months to live and asks about advance directives. Which statements by the nurse give the client correct information? **Select all that apply.**
    1. "You have the right to refuse treatment at any time."
    2. "If you want certain procedures or actions taken or not taken, and you might not be able to tell anyone at the time, you need to complete documents ahead of time that give your health care provider this information."
    3. "You will be resuscitated at any time to allow you the longest length of survival."
    4. "You might want to think about choosing someone who will make medical decisions for you in the event that you are unable to make your desires known."
    5. "If you travel to another province, your advance directive should cover your wishes."

199. Which of the following is most effective as a smoking cessation aid?
    1. Nicotine patches
    2. Nicotine gum
    3. e-cigarettes, also called *vaping*
    4. Varenicline (Chantix/Champix)

200. Which of the following are normal serum electrolyte values?
    1. Na 137 mmol/L, K 3.8 mmol/L
    2. Na 151 mmol/L, K 5.9mmol/L
    3. Na 142 mmol/L, K 3.2mmol/L
    4. Na 129mmol/L, K 5.0mmol/L

201. The health care provider has ordered a serum creatinine test for a client. What condition is this test ordered for?
    1. Liver function
    2. Circulating tumour factors
    3. Renal function
    4. Diverticulitis

202. A nurse has provided care to a client. Which entries are appropriate for the nurse document in the client's health record? **Select all that apply.**
    1. Client seems to be in pain and states, "I feel uncomfortable."
    2. "Status unchanged, doing well."
    3. "Left abdominal incision 5 cm in length without redness, drainage, or edema."
    4. "Client is hard to care for and refuses all treatments and medications. Family present."
    5. "Skin on lower legs pale and cool."

203. It is determined that a confused client needs to have restraints applied to prevent them from pulling out their Foley catheter because all other alternatives have proven unsuccessful. Which of the following options can the nurse delegate under supervision to an unregulated care provider (UCP)?
    1. Applying restraints
    2. Obtaining a physician's order to restrain the client
    3. Documenting the events that led to restraining the client
    4. Evaluating the effectiveness of the restraints

204. A client goal is to remain free from falls. However, the client fell just before shift change. What is the nurse's

priority action when evaluating the client's plan of care?

1. Counsel the unregulated care provider who was on duty when the client fell.
2. Identify factors interfering with goal achievement.
3. Place the "fall risk" sign in a more prominent position.
4. Request that the more experienced charge nurse complete a revised plan of care.

205. During a blood transfusion, a client begins to report chills and back pain. Which action is appropriate for the nurse to take?

1. Observe for other symptoms.
2. Slow the infusion rate and monitor vital signs.
3. Discontinue the infusion immediately and notify the health care provider.
4. Tell the client that the symptoms are a normal reaction to the blood product.

206. The nurse provides education for a client receiving external beam radiation therapy for breast cancer. Which of the following would the nurse include in teaching? **Select all that apply.**

1. Fatigue is the most common side effect.
2. Use emollient creams at the radiation site.
3. Expose area to the sun if possible.
4. Wash the irradiated area daily with warm water.
5. Take care not to remove the markings that indicate radiation beam focus.
6. Advise there is a risk of emitting radiation.

207. The staff nurse observes a nursing student perform tracheostomy suctioning with a client. Which of the following actions by the student requires the staff nurse to intervene?

1. The student preoxygenates the client for 1 minute before suctioning.
2. The student puts on clean gloves and uses a sterile catheter to suction.
3. The student inserts the catheter about 15 cm into the tracheostomy tube.
4. The student applies suction for 7 seconds while withdrawing the catheter.

208. A client returns to the unit following a cardiac catheterization using the antecubital site in the right arm. The client reports numbness and tingling in their right hand. The nurse observes the hand is cool, with absent radial pulse. What is the priority action by the nurse?

1. Apply a warm compress to the insertion site.
2. Notify the health care provider in charge of the client.
3. Assess the left arm and hand for pulses and perfusion.
4. Have the client flex their right hand repeatedly to improve circulation.

209. When the nurse is giving a scheduled morning medication, the client states, "I haven't seen that pill before. Are you sure it's correct?" The nurse checks the medication administration record and sees that medication is listed. Which of the following is the nurse's best response to the client?

1. "It's listed here on the medication sheet, so you should take it."
2. "Go ahead and take it, and then I'll check with your doctor about it."
3. "It wouldn't be listed here if it wasn't ordered for you!"
4. "I'll check on the order first, before you take it."

210. A client is being placed on a calcium channel blocker. What should the nurse inform the client with regard to this medication. **Select all that apply.**

1. The medication may cause peripheral edema.
2. The medication may cause hypertension.
3. The medication may interact with grapefruit juice, increasing its effect.
4. The medication may cause cold extremities.
5. The medication may cause constipation.
6. The medication may cause flushing of the face.

211. A client with second-degree burns has been receiving morphine through a patient-controlled analgesia (PCA) pump for a week. The client wakes up frequently during the night complaining of pain. Which of the following actions should the nurse implement?

1. Administer a dose of morphine every 1–2 hours from the client-controlled analgesia machine while the client is sleeping.
2. Consult with the health care provider about using a different treatment protocol to control the client's pain.
3. Request that the health care provider order a bolus dose of morphine to be given when the client awakens with pain.
4. Teach the client to push the button every 10 minutes for an hour before going to sleep, even if the pain is minimal.

212. A nurse gives an incorrect medication to a client without doing all of the mandatory checks, but the client has no ill effects from the medication. What actions should the nurse take after reassessing the client? **Select all that apply.**

1. Notify the primary health care provider of the situation.
2. Document in the client's health record than an incident report was filed.
3. Document in the client's health record why the omission occurred.
4. Continue to monitor the client for any untoward effects from the medication.
5. Send an incident report to risk management.

213. Parents of a 24-month-old child ask the nurse when they should start toilet learning because many of the other children in the day care centre are trained. What should the nurse respond?

1. "When your child can tell you they have a need to urinate or defecate, that indicates a readiness."
2. "At 24 months the child not yet ready for urinary toilet training."
3. "There are some theories that infants can start toilet learning by frequently holding them on the toilet so you could try that strategy."
4. "Don't worry about the other children, they are probably quite advanced."

214. The nurse is preparing to administer a barbiturate. Which condition(s) or disorder(s) are contraindications to the use of these drugs? **Select all that apply.**
    1. Pregnancy
    2. Epilepsy
    3. Severe chronic obstructive pulmonary disease
    4. Advanced liver disease
    5. Current use of an opioid analgesic
    6. Alcohol dependency

215. After receiving change-of-shift report for the following four clients with neutropenia, which client should the nurse assess first?
    1. 66-year-old who has white pharyngeal lesions
    2. 35-year-old who has a fever of 38.2°C
    3. 56-year-old who has frequent explosive diarrhea
    4. 23-year-old who is complaining of severe fatigue

216. Which of the following nursing activities is appropriate for the home care nurse caring for a client newly diagnosed with type 2 diabetes to delegate to an unregulated care provider? **Select all that apply.**
    1. Assist the client to choose an appropriate diet.
    2. Check the client's feet for signs of breakdown.
    3. Help the client with a daily bath and oral care.
    4. Teach the client how to monitor blood glucose.
    5. Measure the client's oral intake.

217. A 25-year-old client tells the nurse about feeling quite anxious and stressed due to the COVID-19 pandemic but does not want to take any antianxiety medications. What strategy might the nurse suggest to the client that might be of immediate help?
    1. Take a variety of vitamin and mineral supplements.
    2. Encourage a healthy diet.
    3. Stress-reduction exercises
    4. Watching uplifting online streaming productions

218. Which of the following assessment findings is of most concern in a client who is currently being restrained with mechanical wrist restraints?
    1. Angry, loud crying
    2. Urinary incontinence
    3. Reddened areas on wrists
    4. Hands cool to the touch

219. The nurse is administering a unit of blood to a client. What are the signs and symptoms of a transfusion reaction? **Select all that apply.**
    1. Chills
    2. Shaking
    3. Flank pain
    4. Hypothermia
    5. Sudden severe headache
    6. Hyperthermia (fever)

220. The client is to receive phenytoin (Dilantin) at 0900 hours. The nurse knows that the ideal time to measure the trough level is when?
    1. 0800 hours
    2. 0830 hours
    3. 0900 hours
    4. 0930 hours

221. The client is in severe pain and is requesting a prn medication before the prn time interval has elapsed. What is the nurse's priority?
    1. Give the medication early for any pain score greater than 8.
    2. Call the prescriber and request a stat order.
    3. Explain to the client why they will have to wait for the medication.
    4. Document the client's request and pain score.

222. Which of the following statements leads a nurse to determine that a child's caregiver understands information related to tick bites? **Select all that apply.**
    1. "I'll have my son wear dark clothing on his hike."
    2. "We should all get the Lyme disease vaccine before our trip."
    3. "We will wear long pants and long-sleeved shirts in the woods."
    4. "If a tick is found attached to the skin, we will use tweezers to remove it."
    5. "We will use an insect repellant containing DEET to deter ticks."

223. A client at the family practice unit tells the nurse: "I am definitely not getting the influenza vaccine this year. Last year I got the flu the very next day and had body aches and a temperature of 38 degrees!" How would the nurse respond to the client?
    1. "Those are serious symptoms so it is wise for you not to have the vaccine."
    2. "That is just an allergic response to last year's vaccine."
    3. "Those signs are not the flu, but the body's immune system is gearing up to fight the influenza virus, which is a serious disease."
    4. "These are not serious symptoms; you have likely been listening to vaccine misinformation on social media."

224. A 4-year-old child asks tearfully if the intramuscular (IM) injection will hurt. What is a nurse's most effective response?
    1. "No. It is over before you know it."
    2. "Yes. It will sting a little."
    3. "No. Would you like to see the syringe?"
    4. "Yes. Your mom and I are going to hold you to help you be still."

225. The nurse is caring for a terminally ill client. The client states, "I have always been unsure if there was a God or life after death. Do you think there is?" The nurse states, "Yes, absolutely there is life after death." What has the nurse attempted to do?
    1. Strengthen the client's religion.
    2. Impose their beliefs on the client.
    3. Support the client's agnostic beliefs.
    4. Support the clients' spiritual beliefs.

226. How would the nurse best prevent postsurgical thrombophlebitis prior to surgery? **Select all that apply.**
    1. Teach deep breathing and coughing techniques.
    2. Instruct the client about ambulation after surgery.
    3. Ensure antiembolism stockings are applied 12 hours prior to surgery.
    4. Administer anticoagulants as ordered.

5. Teach client range of motion exercise.

6. Inform the client they will be required to dangle their legs from the bed post surgery.

227. When preparing to administer nasal spray, what should the nurse tell the client?

1. "You will need to blow your nose before I give you this medication."

2. "You will need to blow your nose after I give you this medication."

3. "When I give you this medication, you will need to hold your breath."

4. "You should sit up for 5 minutes after you receive the nasal spray."

228. The nurse has administered a dose of epinephrine intro muscularly to a 12-month-old infant. For which adverse reactions of epinephrine should the nurse monitor? **Select all that apply.**

1. Nausea

2. Tremors

3. Irritability

4. Bradycardia

5. Hypotension

6. Sleepiness

229. A nurse works in a long-term care facility. One of the clients has not passed urine for 12 hours. What action will assist the nurse to determine if urine is being retained in the bladder?

1. Bladder ultrasonography (bladder scanner)

2. An 'in and out' catheterization

3. Crede manoeuvre

4. Pour warm water over the perineum to see if this stimulates urination

230. At the family practice clinic, the nurse instructs the client on collecting a midstream urine test. What would teaching include?

1. Start urinating then stop, place sterile collection container under urethra, resume urinating into the container.

2. Place sterile collection container close to the urethra, catch first 20 mL of urine.

3. Provide the client with a sterile urinal, the nurse will collect the urine from the urinal.

4. Begin to urinate, move collection container into the stream of urine.

231. The nurse assesses an irregular radial pulse on a newly admitted client who has a previous history of cardiac disease. What would be the nurse's next action?

1. Notify the health care provider.

2. Wait for 5 minutes, then retake the radial pulse.

3. With a stethoscope, auscultate the apical pulse.

4. Palpate the carotid artery

232. The nurse takes a client's blood pressure and obtains a reading of 132/85 mmHg. What is the client's pulse pressure? Fill in the blank.

233. The nurse in a geriatric clinic suspects one of the clients is a victim of family abuse. The client presents with finger mark bruises on their arms, a swollen eye, flat affect, and a dishevelled appearance. The client denies any suggestions by the nurse that abuse is occurring. What is the nurse's responsibility?

1. Report suspected abuse to the appropriate authorities.

2. Discuss with the family possible causes for the client injuries.

3. Make a note in the client record to monitor for further abuse.

4. Tell the client it is obvious abuse has occurred and warn that it will escalate.

234. Acetaminophen 650 mg by gastrostomy tube is prescribed every 4 hours prn for a client with shoulder pain following a stroke. The nurse prepares to administer how many millilitres to the client? Refer to the figure **Record your answer using one decimal place.**

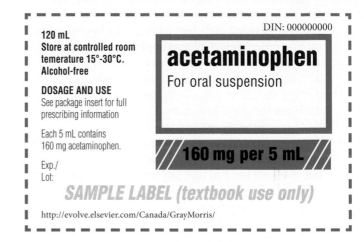

SAMPLE LABEL (textbook use only)

http://evolve.elsevier.com/Canada/GrayMorris/

Answer: _____ mL

235. Which of the following is a risk factor for cardiovascular disease?

1. Diabetes, type 1 or 2

2. High fibre diet

3. Caucasian heritage

4. Blood pressure 124/82

236. A health care provider prescribes Synthroid 0.3 mg PO daily for an adult with hypothyroidism. The medication label states: "Synthroid 0.15 mg/1 tablet." The nurse prepares to administer one dose. How many tab(s) should the nurse prepare to administer one dose? **Record your answer using a whole number. Fill in the blank.**

Administer _____ tablets

237. The nurse works as the psychiatric resource in the emergency department of a hospital. Which is the most common substance abuse condition encountered in the community?

1. Alcohol

2. Cannabis

3. Cocaine

4. Prescription drugs

238. A home care nurse assesses a client with chronic obstructive pulmonary disease (COPD). The nurse speaks with the spouse, who provides care. The spouse says, "I don't

need much sleep anymore. I might need to help during the night." Select the nurse's most therapeutic response.

1. "It sounds like you are very devoted to your spouse."
2. "I noticed you fell asleep while I was assessing your spouse. I'm concerned about you."
3. "Your spouse is lucky to have you to provide care rather than being placed in a long-term care facility."
4. "If you keep going like this, your health will be impaired also. Then who will take care of both of you?"

239. Which of the following nursing actions would most increase a client's risk for developing a health care-associated infection?
1. Use of surgical aseptic technique to suction an airway
2. Placement of a urinary catheter drainage bag below the level of the bladder
3. Clean technique for inserting a urinary catheter
4. Use of a sterile bottled solution more than once within a 24-hour period

240. Which of the following is a normal value for glycolysated haemoglobin (HgA1C)?
1. 1 to 3%
2. 4 to 6 %
3. 7 to 9%
4. 10 to 12%

241. A 65-year-old female client is distressed because she is developing a larger waist size. She has always been slim, with what she calls a "good figure" and doesn't understand why this is happening. What should the nurse tell her?
1. "You are probably eating too many carbohydrates. I will help you with a healthier diet."
2. "Perhaps you have osteoporosis, I will arrange for you to have a bone density test."
3. "All postmenopausal women of your age become heavier."
4. "You lose height as you age because of thinner vertebral discs, this leads to thickening of the torso."

242. A nursing colleague confesses to watching pornography during breaks at work. Watching pornography may be classed as which of the following?
1. Physical dependency
2. Compulsive behaviour
3. Psychological dependency
4. Addiction

243. Shown is a picture of a double lumen urinary catheter. When should a double lumen catheter be used?

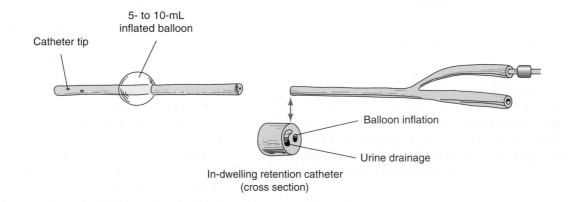

5- to 10-mL inflated balloon
Catheter tip
Balloon inflation
Urine drainage
In-dwelling retention catheter (cross section)

1. When the nurse has to perform intermittent urinary catheterization
2. When the client requires aspiration of the catheter
3. When the catheter will need to be irrigated
4. When it is to be an in-dwelling urinary catheter

244. During the night shift, a client's total parenteral nutrition (TPN) infusion finishes, but no TPN solution is on hand. Which condition does the nurse know may occur if the TPN infusion is discontinued abruptly?
1. Fluid overload
2. Hyperglycemia
3. Dumping syndrome
4. Rebound hypoglycemia

245. The nurse is caring for a client who becomes nauseated and vomits on the nurse without warning. The nurse now has contaminated hands. What is the nurse's best next step?
1. Cleaning hands with wipes from the bedside table
2. Washing hands with an antimicrobial soap and water
3. Using an alcohol-based waterless hand gel
4. Instructing the client to wash their face and hands

246. A 14-month-old infant has vomiting with diarrhea caused by rota virus. Which of the following would indicate the infant is dehydrated? **Select all that apply.**
1. Sunken anterior fontanelle
2. Less than 8 wet diapers a day
3. Clear, pale urine
4. Dry lips and mucous membranes
5. Oliguria
6. Elevated heart rate

247. The client tells the nurse they are thinking of starting a vegetarian diet. What should be the nurse's priority response?
1. "Tell me what you know about maintaining optimum nutrition with a vegetarian diet."

2. "That is a very good choice. Let's review some menus."

3. "Vegetarianism might be a good choice, but you will have to be careful to take vitamin and mineral supplements."

4. "Is this a religious or ethical choice?"

248. The nurse works in an endoscopy clinic where same-day procedures are performed on an outpatient basis. A client arrives for a barium swallow. There are many clients scheduled, and the nurse does not have much time to spend with each client. What would be the most effective action to ensure this client is educated appropriately about the procedure?

1. Tell the client what will happen in the procedure.

2. Ask the client what they understand about the procedure.

3. Ensure the client has completed the informed consent.

4. Check the health record for documentation about client education.

249. The nurse reviews laboratory values for an adolescent client.

Blood glucose	7 mmol/L
White Blood cell (WBC)	7 000 mm³
Cholesterol	3 mmol/L
Hemoglobin (Hgb)	98 g/L

Which of the above values would the nurse bring to the attention of the health care provider?

1. Blood glucose

2. WBC

3. Cholesterol

4. Hgb

250. The client is to receive oral furosemide (Lasix) every day; however, because the client is unable to swallow, they cannot take medication orally as ordered. The nurse needs to contact the health care provider. What type of problem is this?

1. A "right time" problem

2. A "right to refuse" problem

3. A "right route" problem

4. A "right medication" problem

ANSWERS AND RATIONALES FOR REX-PN PRACTICE EXAM BOOK ONE

The correct answer is set off in boldface.

1. **Client Needs: Safe and Effective Care Environment; T: Application**
   1. This option puts the child's welfare at risk.
   2. As in choice 1.
   3. As in choice 1.
   4. **All individuals in Canada who suspect child abuse are required to report it to the proper child protection agencies as mandated by law. First Nations peoples also have access to specific child protection agencies.**

2. **Client Needs: Physiological Integrity; T: Application**
   1. This is inappropriate and may be embarrassing for the client.
   2. **There are female urinals which may be offered; most female clients prefer a bedpan.**
   3. This is inappropriate and unnecessary.
   4. As in choice 3.

3. **Client Needs: Physiological Integrity; T: Knowledge**
   1. This is incorrect placement.
   2. As in choice 1
   3. As in choice 1
   4. **The correct placement of a pulse oximeter is on a vascular, pulsatile area, such as the fingertip, earlobe, toe, or nose.**

4. **Client Needs: Physiological Integrity; T: Application**
   1. Bisphosphonates should be taken on an empty stomach, not after eating.
   2. Leg cramps are not an adverse effect of a bisphosphonate.
   3. **To avoid esophageal erosions, the client taking bisphosphonates should be upright for at least 30 minutes after taking the medication.**

4. Bisphosphonates should be taken on an empty stomach, not after taking other medications.

5. **Client Needs: Safe and Effective Care Environment; T: Knowledge**
   1. A promotion is not a direct result of research.
   2. **Nursing research is a way to identify new knowledge.**
   3. **Nursing research is a way to improve professional practice.**
   4. **Nursing research is a way to use resources effectively**
   5. Nursing research does not always result in lower budget expenditures.

6. **Client Needs: Health Promotion and Maintenance; T: Critical Thinking**
   1. This disregards the parent's wishes.
   2. The nurse has the capability to answer the parent's question.
   3. The nurse may not be able to arrange for the circumcision, as it is no longer standard in most agencies. This is something the parents must arrange.
   4. **Circumcision, or bris, is a ritual in the Jewish religion. Because it is no longer recommended by the Canadian Paediatric Society, it is not as common a neonatal procedure. However, some health care providers and Jewish rabbis will perform circumcisions. The nurse has a responsibility to the family to facilitate a referral.**

7. **Client Needs: Psychosocial Integrity; T: Application**
   1. This statement is punitive.
   2. This statement is punitive.
   3. **When the nurse is respectful and empathetic, the client will be more accepting to listen without feeling embarrassed.**
   4. This is authoritative.

8. Client Needs: Safe and Effective Care Environment; T: Application
   1. **By placing colour-coded stickers and keep a thermometer near the tub the client is able to safely avoid hot water injury.**
   2. Asking the nurse to test the water does not promote independence, although it does promote safety.
   3. Zipper and Velcro clothing is easier for a client with a tactile impairment to wear but does not promote safety.
   4. Placing all medication together causes difficulty for the client to identify and select the correct pills.

9. Client Needs: Physiological Integrity; T: Application
   1. **Menstrual blood may invalidate the test.**
   2. **Red meat may invalidate the test.**
   3. **Testing instructions may be specific to the test. The client should thoroughly read the instructions just prior to doing the test.**
   4. There is no need to stop antihypertensive medications for this test.
   5. The stool should be caught in a container or paper provided, do not allow it to fall into the toilet.
   6. **A smear in each of two places should be taken and applied to the enclosed test paper or slide.**

10. Client Needs: Physiological Integrity; T: Application
    1. Parental visiting is not dependent on transfusion.
    2. There is no evidence that the child is currently infected.
    3. **When the number of circulating RBCs is increased, tissue hypoxia decreases, cardiac function is improved, and the child will have more energy.**
    4. Forming a clot is the function of platelets.

11. Client Needs: Psychosocial Integrity; T: Critical Thinking
    1. This may have to be done, but the first action is to find out more information from the caregiver.
    2. It is reasonable to inquire about other care giving resources, but the first option would be to explore the caregiver's discomfort.
    3. The discharge may have to be delayed, but not until there is discussion with the caregiver and until home care services are contacted.
    4. **Discharge planning with a family involves an accurate assessment of what will be needed for care at the time of discharge. The first action is to assess the cause of the caregiver's discomfort. Perhaps they have not been taught how to do the dressings.**

12. Client Needs: Physiological Integrity; T: Critical Thinking
    1. The formula may be warmed or at room temperature.
    2. This is not necessary.
    3. The client should be in a semi-upright angle, but this is not the most important.
    4. **Checks for placement, aspiration of stomach contents, testing the pH, and measurement of length of tube are vitally important to make sure the formula is infused into the stomach, and not the esophagus or airway.**

13. Client Needs: Health Promotion and Maintenance; T: Application
    August 27 of the following year.
    Add 7 days to the first day of the last menstrual period and count forward 9 months. Alternatively subtract 3 months and add 7 days to the first day of the last menstrual period (LMP) then add a year. November 20 + 7 days = November 27. Count forward 9 months = August 27 of the following year.

14. Client Needs: Safe and Effective Care Environment; T: Application
    1. **The SBAR (situation, background, assessment, recommendation) format is a useful tool when there is a change in a client's health status and is a best practice protocol. During the situation component of SBAR, the nurse identifies themselves, the person, and the problem.**
    2. During the recommendation component of SBAR, the nurse tells what is needed.
    3. The client's allergies are a component of the client's background.
    4. During the background component of SBAR, the nurse relates the client's background.

15. Client Needs: Physiological Integrity; T: Application
    1. **This is the correct action. The bowel must remain moist until the client is assessed by a surgeon.**
    2. This is not a safe option as it may cause torsion or compression of the bowel.
    3. As in choice 2.
    4. The client should be placed in low Fowler's position.

16. Client Needs: Psychosocial Integrity; T: Application
    1. The child is not hearing impaired. People with autism refrain from making eye contact.
    2. Children with autism generally do not engage in imaginative play.
    3. **Children with autism require routine and consistency.**
    4. **Some children with autism display self-injurious behaviour, such as head banging.**
    5. Autism is partly a communication disorder there is abnormal nonverbal communication.
    6. **Each person with autism spectrum disorder is first an individual. As such, each child's communication patterns must be individually assessed.**

17. Client Needs: Safe and Effective Care Environment; T: Application
    1. **The nurse should devise a plan of care that accommodates the client's visual impairment. Placing a sticker on the call light allows the client to find it and page the nurse for assistance as needed.**
    2. Yelling loudly is stressful for the client and for surrounding clients.
    3. Making hourly rounds is not sufficient; the nurse needs to ensure that the client can get in touch with them at any time.
    4. The client will may not be able to visualize the cellphone keypad.

18. **Client Needs: Health Promotion & Maintenance; T: Application**
    1. This may be reassuring but is not helpful.
    2. **Referral to a breastfeeding clinic provides her with a concrete and helpful resource.**
    3. The mother may not have any friends that can help
    4. The mother is asking for help with breastfeeding. Breastfeeding is recommended.

19. **Client Needs: Physiological Integrity; T: Critical Thinking**
    1. This may relax the client but may not help them to sleep. It could add more stimuli.
    2. Turning the monitor alarms off is unsafe.
    3. Opioid medications should not be the first option; however antianxiety medications and sleep aids may be considered.
    4. **Earplugs should block out the monitor noise and provides the client with control over the sensory stimuli.**

20. **Client Needs: Physiological Integrity; T: Application**
    1. **Urine will be pink tinged due to slight bleeding from the biopsy site and irritation to the bladder mucosa.**
    2. **Urine should be observed for clots, tissue as a result of the scraping of bladder mucosa.**
    3. There is no dye injected with this type of cystoscopy and biopsy.
    4. **Bladder spasms are likely to occur.**
    5. There should be no frank bleeding.
    6. **The client should be aware a burning sensation, particularly during urination, is expected.**

21. **Client Needs: Psychosocial Integrity; T: Application**
    1. Telling the client not to worry is dismissive.
    2. This is incorrect and dismissive.
    3. This is dismissive.
    4. **Asking about the client understanding and experience of being gender fluid in a nonjudgemental fashion establishes trust with the nurse.**

22. **Client Needs: Health Promotion and Maintenance; T: Application**
    1. **All vital signs are within normal limits for a marathon runner.**
    2. While the pulse is low, this is normal for an athlete or runner.
    3. Respirations is normal.
    4. Blood pressure is normal.

23. **Client Needs: Safe and Effective Care Environment; T: Application**
    1. **Safety is the highest priority for this client. Sleep deprivation causes psychomotor impairments. Driver drowsiness and fatigue lead to many automobile injuries and fatalities.**
    2. Sleep deprivation should be evaluated and treated; a 1-year delay is too long.
    3. This strategy may help but is not the highest priority.
    4. Alcohol compounds problems associated with sleep deprivation.

24. **Client Needs: Physiological Integrity; T: Application**
    1. Carbonated beverages are gas producing and not appropriate.
    2. The infant will become more dehydrated.
    3. **This will maintain the infant fluid and electrolyte balance until the vomiting stops.**
    4. There is no indication for this.

25. **Client Needs: Safe and Effective Care Environment; T: Application**
    1. **Sterile objects held below the waist are considered contaminated.**
    2. To open sterile supplies, the sides of the package are carefully separated and peeled apart; this prevents the sterile contents from accidentally opening and touching contaminated objects.
    3. **Gloving the dominant hand helps improve dexterity.**
    4. Touching the outside of the glove surface will contaminate the sterile item.
    5. **Slipping the fingers underneath the second glove cuff helps protect the gloved fingers. Sterile touching sterile prevents glove contamination.**
    6. **Interlocking fingers ensures a smooth fit over the fingers.**

26. **Client Needs: Safe and Effective Care Environment; T: Application**
    1. Private health information cannot be shared without the client's specific permission.
    2. This response reflects poor communication techniques.
    3. **Private health information may be shared if the client gives permission.**
    4. Private health information may be shared if the client gives permission.

27. **Client Needs: Physiological Integrity; T: Application**
    1. The nurse should teach parents that acetylsalicylate acid (Aspirin) is inappropriate for children, teenagers or young adults with chickenpox, influenza, or flulike symptoms because of the risk for Reye's syndrome.
    2. Indomethacin is a prescription medication that is not used as an antipyretic.
    3. Ketorolac is a prescription medication that is not used as an antipyretic.
    4. **Ibuprofen is available in many preparations as an over-the-counter antipyretic.**

28. **Client Needs: Physiological Integrity; T: Application**
    65 kg divided by 1.65 metres (2) = 23.87
    This is a normal, healthy BMI.

29. **Client Needs: Physiological Integrity; T: Application**
    1. The suture is snipped distal to the knot.
    2. The skin should not be pinched as it causes the skin to be injured.
    3. Never snip both ends of the suture; there will be no way to remove the part of the suture situated below the surface.
    4. **This is the correct procedure. The suture should be gently pulled with the forceps.**

30. **Client Needs: Physiological Integrity; T: Knowledge**

1. Scope of practice for the speech-language pathologist includes comprehensive assessments for swallowing.
2. The nurse may be able to observe swallowing ability but is not educated to provide complex swallowing assessments.
3. As in choice 2.
4. As in choice 2.

31. **Client Needs: Physiological Integrity T: Application**
Answer: 20
Rationale: Formula for calculating intravenous flow rate

Formula:

$$\text{Flow Rate } \frac{mL}{hr} = \frac{\text{Amount of solution } (mL)}{\text{Time } (hr)}$$

Solution:

$$\text{Time } (hr) = \frac{\text{Amount of solution } (mL)}{\left(\text{Flow Rate } \left(\frac{mL}{hr}\right)\right)}$$
$$= \frac{1000 \ mL}{50 \ mL/hr} = 20 \ hr$$

32. **Client Needs: Safe and Effective Care Environment; T: Critical Thinking**
1. Monthly in-service education places emphasis on education, not on action.
2. Biohazard bags are appropriate but cannot be used on every item that *C. difficile* comes in contact with.
3. Mandatory cultures are expensive and unnecessary and would not prevent the spread of bacteria.
4. **Proper hand hygiene is the best way to prevent the spread of bacteria.**

33. **Client Needs: Physiological Integrity; T: Critical Thinking**
1. **All actions are important, but this is the priority action. The client is demonstrating signs of preeclampsia, a hypertensive disorder of pregnancy which may have serious consequences. The health care team needs to know the client's BP.**
2. This should occur but is not the priority action. The health care provider will need to know the blood pressure.
3. This will occur but is not the priority action.
4. Proteinuria is no longer a diagnostic test for preeclampsia.

34. **Client Needs: Safe and Effective Care Environment; T: Application**
1. **Nurses follow health care providers' orders unless they believe the orders are in error or may harm clients. Therefore, the nurse needs to assess all orders. If an order seems to be erroneous or harmful, further clarification from the health care provider is necessary. If the health care provider confirms an order and the nurse still believe that it is inappropriate, the nurse should inform the** designated nursing authority or follow the established chain of command.
2. **The nurse should follow the established chain of command policy for such situations.**
3. Harm to the infant could occur if the medication dosage was too high.
4. The nurse may not change an order. Only the health care provider who wrote the order or their substitute can change the order.
5. Although the pharmacy is an excellent resource, only the health care provider can change the order.

35. **Client Needs: Health Promotion and Maintenance; T: Knowledge**
1. Echinacea has no reported value in promoting sleep.
2. **Some research suggests that melatonin supplements might be helpful in treating sleep disorders. This should be used with caution, under the advice of a HCP, as there may be adverse effects.**
3. As in choice 1.
4. As in choice 1.

36. **Client Needs: Physiological Integrity; T: Knowledge**
1. Misoprostol is not used to reduce the symptoms of arthritis.
2. Misoprostol does not potentiate the action of an NSAID.
3. Misoprostol does not reduce mucous secretions in the stomach.
4. **Misoprostol inhibits gastric acid secretions and stimulates mucous secretions and has proved successful in preventing the gastric ulcers that may occur in clients taking NSAIDs.**

37. **Client Needs: Physiological Integrity; T: Knowledge**
1. **This is sinus bradycardia with a regular rhythm and rate less than 60 beats/minute.**
2. This is incorrect.
3. As in choice 2.
4. As in choice 2.

38. **Client Needs: Physiological Integrity; T: Application**
1. **This indicates a healthy stoma.**
2. The stool, if present, will be liquid or soft.
3. The stoma may bleed a bit if touched, but there should be no passage of frank blood.
4. Flatus may be present; this indicates a return of peristalsis.

39. **Client Needs: Safe and Effective Care Environment; T: Application**
1. The drainage bag should be emptied and output recorded every 8 hours or when needed. This does not increase risk for a urinary tract infection (UTI).
2. Urine specimens are obtained by temporarily kinking the tubing; a prolonged kink could lead to bladder distension, not a UTI.
3. **Placing the drainage bag on the side rail of the bed could allow the bag to be raised above the level of the bladder and urine to flow back into the bladder. The urine in the drainage bag is a medium for bacteria; its re-entrance into the bladder can cause infection.**

4. Failure to secure the catheter to the client's thigh places the client at risk for tissue injury, not UTI from catheter dislodgement.

40. **Client Needs: Health Promotion and Maintenance; T: Critical Thinking**
    1. This is not necessary.
    2. **Condoms will help to protect her from sexually transmitted diseases.**
    3. This appears to be judgemental and possibly not realistic.
    4. **She needs to discuss sexual history to assess the risk for transmission of disease.**
    5. She should be tested for STD if she has symptoms, twice a year is not necessary.
    6. A barrier foam is poor protection against STD, the spermicide is not necessary.

41. **Client Needs: Physiological Integrity; T: Critical Thinking**
    1. This is not necessary: this is not an emergency.
    2. **The symptoms are of a fracture, which needs to be diagnosed by an X-ray, then casted at the fracture clinic.**
    3. This is a possibility, but the client would then have to be sent to the hospital for X-ray and casting.
    4. This is not the correct action for a possible fracture. If the foot is fractured, it needs to have a cast.

42. **Client Needs: Safe and Effective Care Environment; T: Knowledge**
    1. Tasks should be delegated to UCPs who are capable, not necessarily to those who are willing.
    2. **When delegating, the nurse should always provide unambiguous and clear directions by describing the task, the desired outcome, and the period within which the task should be completed.**
    3. A laissez-faire style of leadership is not a requirement for delegation.
    4. The nurse does not necessarily have to supervise the UCP, unless it is required by policy or unless the nurse is unsure of the UCP's ability to perform the task.

43. **Client Needs: Safe and Effective Care Environment; T: Knowledge**
    1. To reduce the risk of needlesticks, the nurse should never recap needles.
    2. **Needleless systems or sharps with engineered sharps injury protections (SESIP) safety devices should be used when available.**
    3. To reduce the risk of needle sticks, use one hand to dispose of sharps into the disposal.
    4. **Needles should not be forced into the sharps disposal box.**
    5. **Receptacles should be marked clearly to warn of danger.**

44. **Client Needs: Physiological Integrity; T: Application**
    1. An increased RBC count is not an expected effect of antibiotic therapy.
    2. An increased WBC count is an indication of progression of infection and may indicate that the antibiotic therapy is not effective.

3. **A decreased WBC count is an indication of the reduction of infection and the therapeutic effect of antibiotic therapy.**
4. A decreased platelet count is not an expected effect of antibiotic therapy.

45. **Client Needs: Physiological Integrity; T: Application**
    1. Povidone-iodine is cytotoxic and may damage tissue.
    2. Woven gauze may leave fibres in the wound bed.
    3. Tight packing of a wound will result in pressure to the walls of the wound, slowing down the healing process.
    4. **Lightly filling all the wound dead space with moistened packing material allows healing to occur.**

46. **Client Needs: Physiological Integrity T: Application**
    Answer: 19
    Rationale: Formula for calculation for intravenous drip rate.

    $$\frac{\text{Amount of solution to administer}}{\text{Time for infusion in hours}} \times \frac{\text{Drip factor of tubing}}{60 \text{ min}} = \text{Drip rate (gtt/min)}$$

    Solution:

    $$\frac{\text{mL}}{1 \text{ hr}} \times \frac{15}{60 \text{ min}} = 18.75 = 19 \text{ gtt/min}$$

47. **Client Needs: Safe and Effective Care Environment; T: Application**
    1. Holding the client will shift the nurse's centre of gravity and may lead to a back injury.
    2. **If the client has a fainting episode or begins to fall, assume a wide base of support with one foot in front of the other, thus supporting the client's body weight. Then extend one leg and let the client slide against the leg, and gently lower the client to the floor, protecting the client's head.**
    3. Allowing the client to fall could lead to head injury for the client.
    4. Moving the client against the wall could also cause the client to hit their head and cause injury.

48. **Client Needs: Safe and Effective Care Environment; T: Application**
    1. The shelter will provide this referral as necessary.
    2. As in choice 1.
    3. **Because the person has no safe place to go, referral to a shelter is necessary.**
    4. As in choice 1.

49. **Client Needs: Physiological Integrity; T: Application**
    1. **If the drainage device is half full, empty the chamber and measure the drainage.**
    2. **The vacuum seal is disconnected in order to measure the drainage.**
    3. This is applicable for a straight, or Penrose, drain.
    4. **Tubings must be patent in order to collect wound drainage.**
    5. **Wound drainage is part of the client intake and output.**
    6. The health care provider or surgeon will state what type of drainage device is required.

50. **Client Needs: Physiological Integrity; T: Knowledge**
   1. **This is the correct procedure for cleansing a drain site.**
   2. Up and down strokes are not correct.
   3. This is incorrect, the principle is clean to dirty.
   4. A specific order is not necessary.

51. **Client Needs: Health Promotion and Maintenance; T: Knowledge**
   1. **These are the recommended immunizations for ages 50 to 59 years.**
   2. Pneumococcal polysaccharide is not required.
   3. Rotavirus is not required, influenza is annual.
   4. Measles-mumps-rubella and pneumococcal polysaccharide are not required.

52. **Client Needs: Physiological Integrity T: Critical Thinking**
   1. Anaphylactic shock would present with urticaria, dyspnea, and hypotension.
   2. Septicemia would include a fever.
   3. **The signs and symptoms are concurrent with fluid volume overload.**
   4. A hemolytic reaction would consist of flank pain, chills, and fever.

53. **Client Needs: Physiological Integrity; T: Critical Thinking**
   1. The client may not be telling the truth.
   2. **All criteria may be used to evaluate the plan, however the most important is proof that the client has been able to maintain weight.**
   3. Group therapy is important but is not the most important factor.
   4. This is important, but maintaining weight is most important.

54. **Client Needs: Physiological Integrity T: Application**
   Answer: 50
   Rationale: Formula for calculation of oral and parenteral doses of medications
   Formula:

   $$\frac{\text{Dosage ordered}}{\text{Dosage available}} \times \text{Drug form}$$
   $$= \text{Amount of drug to administer}$$

   Solution: 2000/20000×500=50 mL

55. **Client Needs: Safe and Effective Care Environment; T: Critical Thinking**
   1. **A visual disturbance poses great risk for injury from falling as a result of impaired depth perception and inability to see obstacles.**
   2. *Body image disturbance* does not address the greatest risk for injury.
   3. *Social isolation* does not address the greatest risk for injury.
   4. *Fear* does not address the greatest risk for injury.

56. **Client Needs: Psychosocial Integrity; T: Application**
   1. This is a punitive response.
   2. This is vague.
   3. **This is encouraging the client to be specific and encourage them to discuss their problems.**
   4. This does not encourage the client to open up.

57. **Client Needs: Physiological Integrity; T: Application**
   1. **Polyethylene glycol is a very potent laxative that induces total cleansing of the bowel and is most commonly used before diagnostic or surgical bowel procedures.**
   2. Lactulose is a laxative most commonly used to treat constipation.
   3. Mineral oil is a laxative most commonly used to treat constipation associated with hard stools or fecal impaction.
   4. Milk of magnesia is a laxative most commonly used to evacuate the bowel rapidly in preparation for endoscopic examination.

58. **Client Needs: Psychosocial Integrity; T: Knowledge**
   1. **These are behaviour characteristics in children ages 2 to 5 years.**
   2. **As in choice 1.**
   3. **As in choice 1.**
   4. **As in choice 1.**
   5. This is a response for a child 1 to 2 years.
   6. This is a response for a child 5 to 9 years.

59. **Client Needs: Health Promotion and Maintenance; T: Knowledge**
   1. **There is a proven identified risk of thrombosis and myocardial infarction in female smokers who use oral contraceptives.**
   2. Bladder cancer is a risk related to smoking only.
   3. As in choice 2.
   4. Liver disorders are not increased with either.

60. **Client Needs: Safe and Effective Care Environment; T: Application**
   1. This client has an issue that can be handled with less restrictive alternatives than hospitalization.
   2. As in choice 1.
   3. As in choice 1.
   4. **Admission to the hospital would be justified by the risk of client danger to self or others.**

61. **Client Needs: Safe and Effective Care Environment; T: Application**
   1. Nurses often delegate some interventions to unregulated care providers. Unregulated care providers may perform such tasks as turning and positioning clients, applying elastic stockings, and helping client use the incentive spirometer.
   2. Occupational therapists are a resource for planning ADLs that clients need to modify or relearn.
   3. **The nurse should collaborate with other health care team members such as physiotherapists or occupational therapists when considering mobility needs.**
   4. Many times, actual problems such as pressure injuries are addressed only after they develop. They should be addressed before they develop.

62. **Client Needs: Physiological Integrity; T: Critical Thinking**
    1. The client may have a fever, or this may be the client's normal temperature.
    2. The client may have a normal temperature, but the nurse needs to determine the client's normal baseline.
    3. **An acceptable temperature range for adults depends on age, gender, and range of physical activity. The nurse must determine the client's baseline temperature, and monitor for any changes**
    4. This may be true, but it is not the most important consideration. An alternative site may be selected if the nurse believes the tympanic temperature was not performed correctly.

63. **Client Needs: Health Promotion and Maintenance; T: Knowledge**
    1. Babinski reflex occurs when the sole of the foot is firmly stoked. The big toe moves upward.
    2. Rooting reflex is when the newborn's lip cheek is touched by the nipple, the newborn will turn its head towards the nipple and begin to suck.
    3. The startle reflex is in response to a loud noise the newborn's arms adduct while the elbows flex.
    4. **Tonic neck reflex occurs when the infant's head is turned to one side, the same-side arm and leg extend outward while the opposite arm and leg flex.**

64. **Client Needs: Physiological Integrity; T: Application**
    1. This would be embarrassing for the client.
    2. **This is a general question that might help the nurse to discuss hygiene and incontinence.**
    3. As in choice 1.
    4. Personal hygiene needs to be addressed with this client; it cannot be ignored.

65. **Client Needs: Physiological Integrity; T: Application**
    1. **Rinsing of the mouth after using an inhaler or nebulizer is recommended in order to prevent fungal infections.**
    2. Nebulizer tubings and mouthpieces should be cleaned with soap, water, and white vinegar.
    3. With intranasal dosage forms, the medication should be inhaled with the head tipped slightly forward.
    4. Instruct the client to hold the breath for approximately 10 seconds, then remove the inhaler.

66. **Client Needs: Safe and Effective Care Environment; T: Application**
    1. **Hypersensitivity reactions may be manifested by wheezing.**
    2. Diarrhea can be a adverse effect of antibiotics, but it is not an indication of a hypersensitivity reaction.
    3. **Hypersensitivity reactions may be manifested by shortness of breath.**
    4. **Hypersensitivity reactions may be manifested by swelling of the face, tongue, or hands (angioedema).**
    5. **Hypersensitivity reactions may be manifested by itching or rash.**

67. **Client Needs: Physiological Integrity; T: Application**
    1. Unopened vials should be refrigerated and are good until the expiration date on the label.
    2. **Insulin should not be left in a hot environment.**
    3. Freezing renders insulin inactive.
    4. **Insulin vials that have been "opened" (i.e., the stopper has been punctured) should be stored for up to 28 to 30 days. After 1 month, these vials should be discarded.**
    5. **Insulin vials that have been opened should be stored at room temperature or refrigerated.**

68. **Client Needs: Health Promotion and Maintenance; T: Critical Thinking**
    1. A Mediterranean diet will be helpful to lose weight but may not improve his general mood.
    2. His blood glucose is a bit high but may not require home monitoring.
    3. His BP is borderline high and will likely respond to lifestyle changes.
    4. **All options may be required for this client; however, the best and easiest strategy is to start walking. Walking has been proven to improve mood, reduce blood pressure, help reduce weight, and therefore may lower blood sugar.**

69. **Client Needs: Physiological Integrity; T: Application**
    1. If there is an anaphylactic event, the epi pen must be immediately available.
    2. The adolescent needs to be responsible for both the Benadryl and the epi pen.
    3. **Benadryl may help, but if there is an anaphylactic event, the epi pen must be immediately available with the adolescent.**
    4. There is no indication the adolescent is not taking responsibility but possibly has not understood the teaching.

70. **Client Needs: Physiological Integrity; T: Critical Thinking**
    1. This is important but is not the priority.
    2. As in choice 1.
    3. **These are signs of cardiogenic shock and must be medically treated immediately.**
    4. As in choice 1.

71. **Client Needs: Safe and Effective Care Environment; T: Application**
    1. *C. difficile* **is a spore-forming organism that can be transmitted through direct and indirect client contact. Because** *C. difficile* **is a spore-forming organism, hand sanitizer is not effective in preventing its transmission. Hands must be washed with soap and water to prevent transmission.**
    2. This organism is not transmitted via the droplet route; therefore, droplet precautions are not needed.
    3. An N95 respirator is used primarily for providing care to clients with airborne illness.
    4. All clients should be taught cough etiquette; this action is not one specific to a client who has *C. difficile* infection.

72. **Client Needs: Physiological Integrity; T: Application**
   1. Pain should be controlled. The child will need human contact, particularly with the family.
   2. The need for fluids decreases in the dying client.
   3. **Research indicates hearing is the last sense to stop functioning in the dying client. Family should be encouraged to speak with their child.**
   4. Family will want and need to provide care for the child

73. **Client Needs: Psychosocial Integrity; T: Critical Thinking**
   1. There are likely no additional staff to hire.
   2. Gifts will be appreciated but will not alleviate stress.
   3. **All of these options will help nurses manage stress. The best option under the circumstance is to facilitate collegial support networks with plans for addressing the various stressors in a manageable and positive manner.**
   4. This will increase the problem of being short staffed, thus creating more stress for nursing caregivers.

74. **Client Needs: Health Promotion and Maintenance; T: Knowledge**
   1. **Tuberculosis is an identified health problem that is more prevalent in the Indigenous than non-Indigenous population.**
   2. **As in choice 1.**
   3. **As in choice 1.**
   4. **As in choice 1.**
   5. Arthritis has a similar or lower prevalence than in the non-Indigenous population.
   6. Bowel disorders have a similar or lower prevalence than in the non-Indigenous population.

75. **Client Needs: Physiological Integrity; T: Application**
   1. **Saline-based oral rinses and those with prescribed local anesthetics can prevent or decrease the severity of the mucositis and treat the pain.**
   2. Alcohol-based mouth washes may irritate the mucosa.
   3. Due to the risk of bleeding with chemotherapy, Aspirin is to be avoided.
   4. Dental floss may irritate the mouth sores.

76. **Client Needs: Safe and Effective Care Environment; T: Application**
   1. The nurse may instruct a UCP to select the appropriate route and device to measure temperature.
   2. The UCP may obtain the temperature measurements at the ordered frequency.
   3. The nurse may make the UCP aware of the usual values for the client.
   4. **The nurse is responsible for assessing and evaluating changes in body temperature.**

77. **Client Needs: Physiological Integrity T: Application**
   Answer: 8
   Rationale: Formula for calculation for intravenous drip rate. PRBCs can be split by the blood bank, allowing for one-half of a unit to be given over at time frame of up to 4 hours.

Formula:

$$\frac{\text{Amount of solution to administer}}{\text{Time for infusion in hours}} \times \frac{\text{Drip factor of tubing}}{60 \text{ min}} = \text{Drip rate (gtt/min)}$$

Solution:

$$\text{mL/4 hr} \times 15/60 \text{ min} = 7.8 = 8 \text{ gtt/min}$$

78. **Client Needs: Physiological Integrity; T: Application**
   1. There is no radiation with an MRI.
   2. An MRI does not routinely require contrast medium.
   3. **Conventional MRI scanners can generate noise in excess of 110 decibels, requiring ear protection.**
   4. Clients will not routinely feel cold nor require a warming blanket during an MRI.

79. **Client Needs: Safe and Effective Care Environment; T: Application**
   1. **Anticipatory guidance to prevent aspiration for a 4-month-old infant considers that the infant will begin to be more active and place objects in the mouth. Buttons and other small objects should be kept out of reach.**
   2. **Anticipatory guidance to prevent aspiration for a 4-month-old infant considers that the infant will begin to be more active and place objects in the mouth. Toys should be checked for removable parts.**
   3. The infant should not go to bed with a bottle.
   4. Teething biscuits should be used with caution because large chunks may be broken off and aspirated.
   5. **Anticipatory guidance to prevent aspiration for a 4-month-old infant considers that the infant will begin to be more active and place objects in the mouth. Hard candy, nuts, and foods with pits should be avoided.**

80. **Client Needs: Health Promotion and Maintenance; T: Application**
   1. This sounds punitive.
   2. As in choice 1.
   3. **Addresses the need to provide education to his daughter.**
   4. This does not solve the problem.

81. **Client Needs: Physiological Integrity; T: Application**
   1. There is no need to obtain a venous specimen for comparison.
   2. Slowing the rate of the infusion is beyond the nurse's scope of practice and will decrease the client's nutritional intake.
   3. **Mild hyperglycemia is expected during the first few days after TPN is started and requires ongoing monitoring.**
   4. Because the glucose elevation is small and expected, notification of the health care provider is not necessary.

82. **Client Needs: Safe and Effective Care Environment; T: Application**

1. The nurse should introduce themselves, provide relevant information, and assist in role clarification by explaining the skills they can contribute, such as initiation of intravenous (IV) treatment or medication administration. It is the nurse's responsibility as the client's primary nurse to provide the information and skills they have to offer in this situation.

2. To function best as a group, the team members need to be aware of each other's roles. If the nurse were to immediately assist with the airway without introducing themself, the team may not know who they are or what their role is.

3. The nurse is not being an active team member by standing back and waiting for a role during the code.

4. The nurse is not being an active team member by leaving the room during the code.

83. **Client Needs: Physiological Integrity; T: Application**

1. This option does not properly reassure the client or build trust. It is telling the client what to do.

2. **Crisis intervention is a type of brief therapy that is more directive than typical psychotherapy or counselling. It focuses on problem solving and involves only the problem created by the crisis. The goal of crisis intervention is to create stability for the person involved in the crisis while promoting self-reliance.**

3. This is dismissive and patronizing.

4. There is no indication the family needs to communicate better.

84. **Client Needs: Safe and Effective Care Environment; T: Application**

1. The nurse should not change the order without the prescriber's consent.

2. **If the nurse is concerned about the drug, dose, route, or reason for a medication, the nurse must call the prescriber to clarify.**

3. The nurse can be held responsible for administering an incorrect medication.

4. If the prescriber is unwilling to change the order and does not justify the order in a reasonable and evidence-informed manner, the nurse may refuse to give the medication and notify their supervisor.

85. **Client Needs: Safe and Effective Care Environment; T: Application**

1. Respect for autonomy grants clients the right to expect that information shared for the purposes of competent and compassionate care will remain confidential and will only be shared within the parameters included in the consent to care.

2. **Respect for autonomy includes respecting a client's refusal of treatment for an infected wound.**

3. **Respect for autonomy includes respecting a client's request to stop a treatment midway through a procedure.**

4. Respect for autonomy includes respecting the client's right not refuse a blood transfusion for religious reasons.

5. Respect for autonomy includes respecting a client's refusal to take a prescribed medication.

6. This may be true, but it does not foster client autonomy.

86. **Client Needs: Physiological Integrity; T: Application**

1. Generally time taken to find a pulse on an infant is not recommended. If a pulse is taken, the brachial should be used.

2. Two fingers are used, up to 100 per minute.

3. Rescue breaths are given after the first 30 compressions; the mouth is place over the mouth and nose providing a tight seal.

4. **This is the recommended ratio of compressions and breaths.**

87. **Client Needs: Physiological Integrity; T: Application**

1. The residual should be refed.

2. This volume is too large a flush.

3. This is dependent on the volume of the feed.

4. **To prevent regurgitation and aspiration, the adolescent is place' in the Fowler's position on the right side to promote gastric emptying after a gastrostomy tube feeding.**

88. **Client Needs: Safe and Effective Care Environment; T: Application**

1. Assessment of the client requires nurse education and cannot be delegated to a UCP.

2. Client teaching cannot be delegated to a UCP.

3. **UCP education varies according to the type of worker; however, unregulated care providers are able to measure vital signs.**

4. Assessment of the client's ability to increase activity needs to be done by the nurse and cannot be delegated.

89. **Client Needs: Physiological Integrity; T: Application**

1. Based on the information provided, this medication can be safely administered.

2. As in choice 1.

3. **The glyburide should be held since the blood glucose level is 2.9 mmol/L. The nurse should provide the client with 15–20 g of simple carbohydrate and notify the health care provider of the situation.**

4. As in choice 1.

90. **Client Needs: Physiological Integrity; T: Application**

1. The nurse is responsible for knowing the indicated times for tubing and filter changes.

2. **All TPN solutions are changed at 24 hours. Changing the IV tubing and filter more frequently than required will unnecessarily increase costs.**

3. TPN solutions containing dextrose and amino acids require a change in tubing and filter every 72 hours rather than daily.

4. The client has been receiving TPN for 24 hours and the solution should be changed. Infusion of the additional 50 mL will increase client risk for infection.

91. **Client Needs: Safe and Effective Care Environment; T: Application**

1. **The older person who moves to a different location needs a thorough orientation to the environment. The unit should foster client orientation by displaying large-print clocks, avoiding complex or visually confusing wall designs, clearly**

designating doors, and using simple bed and nurse-call systems.

2. There is no indication chemical restraints may be necessary.

3. There is no indication physical restraints may be necessary.

4. There is no indication that the client needs observation at this time.

92. **Client Needs: Psychosocial Integrity; T: Application**

1. This is not a medical or psychiatric emergency, calling 9-1-1 is not necessary.

2. **A health care provider can help to reduce situational stress factors for individuals. Providing the student with a list of resources is one way to begin this process, as part of secondary prevention strategies.**

3. Not everyone who has sadness needs medications; some need only counselling.

4. Not enough information is given to indicate whether leaving the university is the best solution for the student.

93. **Client Needs: Safe and Effective Care Environment; T: Application**

1. **Post-sedation the client may feel dizzy and unsteady walking. The nurse must assess there is no danger of a fall.**

2. **Post-sedation the client may feel difficulty returning to full consciousness.**

3. This would only be necessary if a general anaesthetic were used.

4. This is not necessary post colonoscopy.

5. The preparation for a colonoscopy involves a complete bowel cleanse, passing stool will not occur.

6. **The client may not be capable of safely and independently travelling to their home.**

94. **Client Needs: Physiological Integrity; T: Critical Thinking**

1. **Kinking the tube prevents gastric contents from being aspirated into the respiratory tract, a serious complication.**

2. This is true but is not the priority rationale.

3. As in choice 2.

4. As in choice 2.

95. **Client Needs: Safe and Effective Care Environment; T: Application**

1. **The goal of pain management in a terminally ill client is adequate pain relief even if the effect of pain medications could hasten death.**

2. Administration of analgesics on a prn basis will not provide the consistent level of analgesia the client needs.

3. Clients usually do not require so much pain medication that they are oversedated and unaware of stimuli.

4. Adequate pain relief may require a dosage that will result in a decrease in respiratory rate.

96. **Client Needs: Safe and Effective Care Environment T: Knowledge**

1. **It is important to assess the person's level of understanding, exploring their perceptions and**

feelings about their health conditions and discussing issues that may interfere with self-care.

2. Clients should be involved in the decision-making process in establishing mutual health care goals and information needed to go home from the day of admission, not on the day of discharge.

3. It is important to use language that the client can understand, not medical terminology.

4. **Empowerment involves accepting the client's values.**

5. **Empowerment involves encouraging client autonomy in the decision-making process.**

97. **Client Needs: Safe and Effective Care Environment; T: Application**

1. This action does not support the principles of infection control.

2. As in choice 1.

3. **The mask should be changed as soon as possible because moisture encourages the growth of microorganisms.**

4. As in choice 1.

98. **Client Needs: Physiological Integrity; T: Application**

1. Pacemakers are surgically implanted. It would be impossible for the client to change the battery.

2. This may not be true.

3. **Lithium batteries have an average lifespan of 10 years, nuclear powered for 20 years, or may be designed to recharge externally. This should be reassuring to the client.**

4. This may not reassure the client as much as factual information.

99. **Client Needs: Safe and Effective Care Environment; T: Critical Thinking**

1. This action occurs after the client has given permission.

2. As in choice 1.

3. **The case manager must respect the client's right to privacy and confidentiality, which extends to discussions with family. Talking to family members is part of the case manager's role, with the client's consent.**

4. As in choice 1.

100. **Client Needs: Psychosocial Integrity; T: Application**

1. **This is a sign of moderate-stage Alzheimer's disease.**

2. **As in choice 1.**

3. This is a behavioural characteristic of normal age-related memory difficulties.

4. **As in choice 3.**

5. **As in choice 1.**

6. **As in choice 1.**

101. **Client Needs: Physiological Integrity; T: Critical Thinking**

1. The protein is necessary for wound healing, but inadequate for nutritional needs.

2. The calories are required for energy, but inadequate for nutritional needs.

3. **High protein and calories will aid in wound healing and energy needs. Fluids may be more readily tolerated than solids.**

4. Carbonated water would likely be tolerated and would provide necessary fluids but would not fulfill nutritional needs.

102. **Client Needs: Physiological Integrity; T: Application**
   1. Elevated blood glucose is a common adverse effect of antiretroviral therapy (ART).
   2. Fatigue is a common adverse effect of ART.
   3. The nurse should discuss medication adverse effects with the client, but this is not as important as addressing the skipped doses of AZT.
   4. **Since missing doses of ART can lead to drug resistance, this client statement indicates the need for interventions such as teaching or changes in the drug scheduling.**

103. **Client Needs: Physiological Integrity T: Application**
   800 calories (325 + 80 + 470 +125 = 1000. 1800 − 1000 = 800)

104. **Client Needs: Safe and Effective Care Environment; T: Application**
   1. Urine or feces do not have any radioactivity and do not require special precautions.
   2. **Because clients with temporary implants emit radioactivity while the implants are in place, exposure to the client is limited.**
   3. Laundry does not have any radioactivity and does not require special precautions.
   4. Cervical radiation will not affect the oral mucosa, and alcohol-based mouthwash is not contraindicated.

105. **Client Needs: Psychological Integrity; T: Application**
   1. This is not an open-ended question, and shows concern for sleep, rather than for PTSD.
   2. This is not an open-ended question and is not an appropriate question at this time.
   3. As in choice 2.
   4. **People who have PTSD often have flashbacks, re-experiencing the trauma through dreams. All other options will likely need to be explored by the nurse, however asking an open-ended description of the dreams provides an opportunity for the client to discuss.**

106. **Client Needs: Safe and Effective Care Environment T: Application**
   1. **As occurs with other needle-sharing activities, using the same unsterilized needle to tattoo body parts of multiple individuals presents a risk of hepatitis C virus.**
   2. **Using the same unsterilized needle on multiple individuals presents a risk of hepatitis B virus transmission.**
   3. The hepatitis E virus is transmitted via the fecal–oral route, principally via contaminated water, not by contaminated needles.
   4. **Using the same unsterilized needle on multiple individuals presents a risk of human immunodeficiency virus (HIV) transmission.**
   5. **Contaminated tattoo ink can cause nontuberculous *M. chelonae* skin infections.**

107. **Client Needs: Physiological Integrity; T: Knowledge**
   1. **This is the definition of a bronchoscope. It is fibre-optic and may have a camera. Occasionally bronchoscopes are rigid for suction of foreign bodies, or for obtaining a biopsy.**
   2. The tube does not go into the lungs. Saying large and stiff may scare the client.
   3. The tube does not go into the esophagus.
   4. The tube is inserted orally and goes through the trachea into the bronchi.

108. **Client Needs: Physiological Integrity; T: Critical Thinking**
   1. Thoroughly shaking the medication mixes the medication before administration but does not affect absorption.
   2. Flushing the medications ensures that all were administered.
   3. Clients with nasogastric tubes should never be positioned supine but instead should be positioned at a 30- to 90-degree angle to prevent aspiration, provided no contraindication to such positioning is known.
   4. **Absorption time for a medication administered through a nasogastric tube is the same as for an oral medication: 30 to 60 minutes. Therefore, the nurse would need to hold the suction for that amount of time to let the medication absorb.**

109. **Client Needs: Health Promotion and Maintenance; T: Application**
   1. **After a warm shower the scrotal skin is moist and relaxed, making the testicles easy to feel.**
   2. The exam should be performed once a month.
   3. **Each testicle should feel like an egg, firm but not hard and smooth with no lumps.**
   4. Testicular cancer is most prevalent between the ages of 15 to 29 years.
   5. **Cryptorchidism is a risk factor for testicular cancer.**
   6. **Any changes from month to month should be reported to the health care provider for follow up and testing.**

110. **Client Needs: Physiological Integrity; T: Critical Thinking Application**
   1. The health care provider probably does not have any pediatric ibuprofen if there is a shortage.
   2. This is not an emergency and does not require going to the hospital.
   3. This may help the child's comfort level but is not the best option.
   4. **This child's dose of ibuprofen would be 100 mg. Adult ibuprofen is 200 mg. The parent may easily crush half a tablet and administer to the child in jam or preferred solution. Many parents during the widespread shortage of pediatric ibuprofen and acetaminophen used this strategy.**

111. **Client Needs: Safe and Effective Care Environment; T: Application**
   1. Evaluative data that show signs of effective coping will help the nurse determine whether the client

has met the outcome. Feeling better after talking to family and friends is a positive sign of coping.

2. This behaviour does not indicate successful progress toward meeting the client's goal.

3. As in choice 2.

4. As in choice 2.

112. **Client Needs: Safe and Effective Care Environment; T: Application**

1. This order is appropriate.

2. **Restraints may be imposed but the nurse should question the indications for use with this client as well as the time frame of use.**

3. As in choice 1.

4. As in choice 1.

113. **Client Needs: Physiological Integrity; T: Application**

1. This is a normal value.

2. As in choice 1.

3. As in choice 1.

4. **This is a low value for white blood cells and indicates neutropenia. The client is at risk for infection.**

114. **Client Needs: Safe and Effective Care Environment; T: Application**

1. This action is appropriate but can be accomplished after contact precautions are implemented.

2. As in choice 1.

3. As in choice 1.

4. **The client's history and new onset diarrhea suggest a *C. difficile* infection, which requires implementation of contact precautions to prevent spread of the infection to other clients.**

115. **Client Needs: Physiological Integrity; T: Application**

1. This is a nursing responsibility as it is the initial assessment post surgery.

2. This is a nursing responsibility.

3. **Comfort measures may be safely provided by the UCP.**

4. Pain assessments are a nursing responsibility.

116. **Client Needs: Safe and Effective Care Environment T: Application'**

1. **By the wife's admission, the family has deficient knowledge of parenting practices.**

2. **Anger management counselling for the father is appropriate.**

3. **Support for this family will be an important component of treatment.**

4. Physical abuse is not suspected, so a safety plan would not be a priority at this time.

5. Whenever possible, the goal of intervention should be to keep the family together; thus, removing the children from the home should be considered as a last resort. The nurse would have a duty to report to children's services but cannot place the child in foster care.

117. **Client Needs: Safe and Effective Care Environment; T: Application**

1. The nurse, as an advocate, may not force the medication.

2. **Clients with mental illness retain their right to refuse treatment unless there is clear, cogent, and convincing evidence of harming themselves or harming others. The client in this situation presents no evidence of harm. The nurse should seek more information about the client's decision.**

3. As in choice 1.

4. As in choice 1.

118. **Client Needs: Psychosocial Integrity; T: Critical Thinking**

1. **Providing the client with resources such as local self-help groups will provide the client with supports in the community.**

2. Trying to avoid *all* triggers that can result in addictive behaviours is not realistic.

3. Recognizing that triggers will arise and the client will need to have a plan to avoid the triggers not to never be tempted.

4. This will have been explored during the residential program. It would be important also to identify areas of strength.

119. **Client Needs: Safe and Effective Care Environment T: Knowledge**

1. Balance is enhanced by keeping the body's centre of gravity low.

2. **Balance is enhanced by maintaining a wide base of support.**

3. **Balance is enhanced by keeping the body's centre of gravity low.**

4. **Balance is enhanced by maintaining correct body posture.**

5. Prolonged immobility leads to impaired balance.

120. **Client Needs: Safe and Effective Care Environment; T: Application**

1. Facilitating early discharge is not in the client's best interests before exploring the reason for the request.

2. As in choice 1.

3. **A voluntarily admitted client has the right to decide to leave the hospital. However, as a client advocate, the nurse is responsible for weighing factors related to the client's wishes and best interests. By asking for information, the nurse may be able to help the client reconsider the decision.**

4. A voluntarily admitted client has the right to decide to leave the hospital.

121. **Client Needs: Physiological Integrity; T: Critical Thinking**

1. **The client likely has a pneumothorax caused by the hockey injury. All actions are important, but administering oxygen is the priority**

2. This is important, but not the priority.

3. As in choice 2.

4. As in choice 2.

122. **Client Needs: Physiological Integrity T: Application**

1. Treatment may eventually be stopped in some, but others will experience repeated seizures unless AED therapy continues.

2. **Clients need to be aware that AED therapy is usually lifelong.**
3. **Adherence to consistent dosing is important for effective seizure control.**
4. Skipped doses may precipitate rebound seizure activity.
5. **Antiepileptic drugs must never be abruptly discontinued as it may precipitate rebound seizure activity.**

123. Client Needs: Psychosocial Integrity; T: Application
    1. This may not be a belief of the parents depending on their culture or religion. It may be offensive.
    2. Grief is individual for everyone. There is no absolute timeline.
    3. **Talking and reminiscing about a loved one aid in the grief process.**
    4. This is not true.

124. Client Needs: Safe and Effective Care Environment; T: Application
    1. This is important but not fundamental to this particular problem.
    2. As in choice 1.
    3. As in choice 1.
    4. **The ability of the client to get to the clinic is of paramount importance to the success of the plan.**

125. Client Needs: Physiological Integrity; T: Application
    1. This medication is a nonsedating antihistamine, which may be preferred for daytime pruritus relief.
    2. As in choice 1.
    3. As in choice 1.
    4. **Because pruritis increases at night, a mildly sedating antihistamine such as diphenhydramine (Benadryl) may be preferred.**

126. Client Needs: Safe and Effective Care Environment T: Critical Thinking
    1. **This can be considered an intentional tort, because the nurse is aware that they should not be breaching confidentiality and violated the client's rights.**
    2. This action is an example of an intentional tort, not an unintentional tort, because the nurse is aware that this is a breach of confidentiality.
    3. **This action is an example of invasion of privacy and occurs if a client's medical information is discussed without the consent of the client.**
    4. This action is not an example of negligence.
    5. This action is not an example of battery.

127. Client Needs: Safe and Effective Care Environment; T: Application
    1. **When a client does not wish to breastfeed, a snug bra worn around the clock can help alleviate discomfort from engorgement.**
    2. A warm shower will help milk flow.
    3. Breast stimulation is not encouraged when a client does not wish to breastfeed.
    4. As in choice 3.

128. Client Needs: Safe and Effective Care Environment; T: Application
    1. This situation does not lend itself to this nursing diagnosis.

2. As in choice 1.
    3. **Risk for low self-esteem is the appropriate diagnosis because the client was previously independent.**
    4. As in choice 1.

129. Client Needs: Physiological Integrity; T: Knowledge
    1. This is not part of the medication reconciliation process.
    2. As in choice 1.
    3. **When admitting a client to any health care setting, the nurse should compare the medications the client took in the previous setting (e.g., at home or in another nursing unit) with the client's current medication orders.**
    4. The nurse is comparing the medication taken while the client was on the previous unit, not the medications taken at home.

130. Client Needs: Physiological Integrity; T: Application
    1. This is a normal pH.
    2. This is a normal pO_2 for an 85-year-old male.
    3. This is a normal pCO_2.
    4. **All values are within normal limits for an 85-year-old male.**

131. Client Needs: Safe and Effective Care Environment; T: Application
    1. **The priority nursing diagnosis is *risk for injury*. This client could cause harm to themselves by interrupting the oxygen therapy or by damaging the urethra by pulling the urinary catheter out. Before restraining a client, it is important to implement and exhaust alternative strategies. Such strategies can include distraction and providing companionship or supervision. If these and other strategies fail, the client may need restraints; in this case, an order must be obtained for the restraint.**
    2. This client may have deficient knowledge and educating the client about treatments could be considered as an alternative to restraints; however, the highest priority is preventing injury.
    3. This scenario does not indicate that the client has a disturbed body image.
    4. This scenario does not indicate that the client's caregiver is strained.

132. Client Needs: Safe and Effective Care Environment; T: Critical Thinking
    1. This option reflects an important partner in care.
    2. As in choice 1.
    3. **The client is the expert in the management of their illness.**
    4. As in choice 1.

133. Client Needs: Physiological Integrity; T: Application
    1. ECT does not cure depression.
    2. This may have no importance in decreasing client anxiety.
    3. **Clients are often disoriented, confused, and have memory loss post-ECT. This will help decrease client anxiety by reassuring them this is normal**
    4. There should be no pain from ECT.

134. **Client Needs: Physiological Integrity; T: Application**
    1. **AIDS is a viral disease caused by the human immunodeficiency virus.**
    2. AIDS is not curable.
    3. **With the newer antiviral drug cocktails it is considered to be a chronic illness.**
    4. **This is the action of the virus.**
    5. It often has a very long incubation period.
    6. **High-risk groups include IV drug users, those with sexual contact with HIV-positive individuals, persons receiving blood products (prior to strict screening of blood donors), health care workers, and babies of infected mothers.**

135. **Client Needs: Physiological Integrity; T: Application**
    1. This does not allow for evaluation of the client's technique.
    2. As in choice 1.
    3. As in choice 1.
    4. **Return demonstrations allow the nurse to evaluate the client's newly learned skills.**

136. **Client Needs: Safe and Effective Care Environment; T: Knowledge**
    1. A primary health care provider's order for restraints must have a limited time frame.
    2. Restraints are not to be ordered as needed.
    3. The use of restraints must be part of the client's treatment and must be ordered according to provincial or territorial legislation and agency policy.
    4. **Restraints must be periodically removed, and the nurse must reassess the client to determine whether the restraints continue to be needed.**

137. **Client Needs: Physiological Integrity; T: Application**
    1. **Black is used to describe necrotic or desiccated tissue.**
    2. Yellow, not black tissue may indicate the presence of an infection.
    3. This is unlikely.
    4. Black tissue is not normal healing. Healthy, healing tissue would be pinkish.

138. **Client Needs: Psychosocial Integrity; T: Application**
    1. 60 to 80% of dementias are AD.
    2. **Lewy Body, frontotemporal, vascular, and traumatic brain injuries are types of dementia.**
    3. **Dementia is a collection of symptoms with different etiologies.**
    4. **Dementia manifests as a progressive deterioration in cognitive function.**
    5. Dementias cause other cognitive problems, such as a decline in executive function and problem solving in addition to memory loss.
    6. **If mild, the individual may be able to function independently and perform ADLs with occasional assistance.**

139. **Client Needs: Safe and Effective Care Environment; T: Application**
    1. **Clients have the right to use a telephone for communication with family members or to secure counsel.**

2. Clients have the right to send and receive mail and be present during package inspection.
    3. The client should be protected against possible harm to self or others.
    4. Clients have the right to refuse treatment.

140. **Client Needs: Safe and Effective Care Environment; T: Knowledge**
    1. **A dysfunctional IV pump can cause an equipment-related accident, such as too-rapid infusion of IV fluids.**
    2. Measuring devices used by the nurse to measure urine can break but are not used directly on a client.
    3. Computer-based documentation can malfunction but is not used directly on a client.
    4. A manual medication-dispensing device can break or malfunction but is not used directly on a client.

141. **Client Needs: Safe and Effective Care Environment T: Knowledge**
    1. **Clinical decision making for groups of clients should begin with identifying the nursing diagnosis of each client in order to prioritize care.**
    2. **Care is prioritized based on the urgency and complexity of problems.**
    3. Client- and family-centred care should not be delayed; clients and families should be involved in decision making and participants in care at all times.
    4. **Combining activities can be an effective use of time, if used appropriately.**
    5. **Basic care activities can be delegated to unregulated care providers so that the nurse can spend time on activities requiring professional nursing knowledge.**

142. **Client Needs: Physiological Integrity; T: Application**
    1. **These are signs of an infection. The nurse will need to take a sample to determine the causative organism for appropriate antibiotic therapy**
    2. Antibiotics may be administered in the home.
    3. Dialysis should not be discontinued unless there is an order from the health care provider.
    4. Reassurance is necessary, but this infection may be serious.

143. **Client Needs: Safe and Effective Care Environment; T: Application**
    1. Comments about hygiene are not necessarily required in nursing documentation of restraints.
    2. **Attempts at alternative strategies are documented in the health record.**
    3. **The time a client is restrained is documented in the health record.**
    4. **Assessments related to oxygenation, orientation, skin integrity, circulation, and position are documented in the health record.**
    5. **The release from restraints and the client response are documented in the health record.**

144. **Client Needs: Health Promotion and Maintenance; T: Critical Thinking**
    1. Nausea is a normal finding in the first trimester.
    2. As in choice 1.

3. Major concerns related to adolescent pregnancy include poor nutritional status, likelihood of smoking, lack of support system, lack or readiness for parenthood, low birth weight infants, and cephalopelvic disproportion.

4. Hemoglobin levels decline during gestation as a result of increased plasma volume; however, a hemoglobin of 90 g/L indicates anemia.

5. As in choice 1.

6. Genital warts may enlarge during pregnancy and affect urination, defecation, and fetal descent. Caesarean birth may be required if obstructions are too large.

145. Client Needs: Physiological Integrity; T: Application
1. Infants would not be sedated.
2. This is not family-centred care, and would likely further upset the infant.
3. While an oxygen mist tent may be necessary treatment for the bronchiolitis, the tent is upsetting the infant. Crying may cause further laryngospasm. It may be more effective for the parents to comfort the infant and provide oxygen and mist via a face mask.
4. The infant is in respiratory distress and must be observed in a well-lit room.

146. Client Needs: Physiological Integrity; T: Knowledge
1. There is no evidence light therapy is helpful with digestive disorders.
2. Light therapy has proven effective in the treatment of persons with seasonal affective disorders.
3. As in choice 1.
4. As in choice 1.

147. Client Needs: Physiological Integrity; T: Application
1. This is a sign of dehydration.
2. This is a sign of fluid volume excess.
3. As in choice 1.
4. This is a sign of fluid volume excess.
5. As in choice 1.
6. As in choice 1.

148. Client Needs: Safe and Effective Care Environment; T: Knowledge
1. Clients cannot automatically be placed in restraints. The restraint process consists of many steps, including thorough assessment and exhausting of alternative strategies.
2. Locking the bed and wheelchairs when the client is transferred helps prevent these pieces of equipment from moving during transfer and will assist in the prevention of falls.
3. All mats and rugs should be secured to help prevent falls.
4. Silencing alarms upon the request of family is not appropriate and could endanger the client.

149. Client Needs: Psychosocial Integrity; T: Application
1. Palliative care may be initiated at any point in care when there are no curative options.
2. This alienates the family.
3. Many people believe that palliative care only occurs when death is imminent. Palliative services by a skilled, dedicated team are focused on improving

symptoms and quality of life, part of which is pain control. It does not mean that death is imminent.
4. This implies the family is being selfish.

150. Client Needs: Physiological Integrity; T: Application
1. High ammonia levels due to liver failure is an indication for laxative use.
2. Laxatives should be used with caution in the presence of undiagnosed abdominal pain.
3. Laxatives are not recommended in the presence of nausea and vomiting.
4. Certain laxatives may be used to treat constipation during pregnancy.
5. Laxatives should not be used if an acute surgical abdomen is suspected.
6. This is not a contraindication for laxative use.

151. Client Needs: Safe and Effective Care Environment; T: Application
1. A verbal order involves the health care provider giving orders to a nurse while they are standing near each other.
2. A telephone order may be required when significant events or changes in a client's condition have occurred. Because the primary care provider is not present, the nurse will need to call the primary care provider for a telephone order.
3. As in choice 1.
4. Reading an order that is correctly written in the chart does not require a telephone order.

152. Client Needs: Physiological Integrity; T: Application
1. The client should be positioned on the left side, not the right.
2. Have the client take a deep breath and exhale through the mouth during rectal suppository insertion.
3. The suppository should be lubricated with a small amount of water-soluble lubricant.
4. For rectal suppository insertion, the client should be positioned on the left side of the body and then remain lying on the left side for 15 to 20 minutes to allow absorption of the drug.

153. Client Needs: Safe and Effective Care Environment; T: Knowledge
1. Hand hygiene interrupts the chain of infection.
2. Washing hands can assist in decreasing the incidence of health care–associated infection.
3. Washing hands can assist in protecting the nurse from the transfer of microorganisms.
4. Washing hands can assist in decreasing the transmission of microbes to other clients.
5. Proper hand hygiene does not decrease the drying effects of soap; in fact, in increases the drying effect of soap.

154. Client Needs: Physiological Integrity; T: Knowledge
1. In guided imagery, focusing on a specific image may reduce stress.
2. This is not the definition of guided imagery.
3. As in choice 2.
4. As in choice 2.

155. Client Needs: Safe and Effective Care Environment; T: Knowledge

1. This choice reflects evidence-informed practice rather than evidence-informed practice.
2. **In Canada, the term evidence-informed practice (EIP) is more often used than *evidence-based*, in recognizing that health care providers need to not only be knowledgeable about evidence coming from research but also take into consideration clinical experience and judgement as 'well as persons' preferences, values, and beliefs, and the context of the situation.**
3. As in choice 1.
4. As in choice 1.

156. **Client Needs: Psychosocial Integrity; T: Critical Thinking**
   1. These are all necessary assessments for this client and family.
   2. **Safety of the client within the home is the priority assessment.**
   3. As in choice 1.
   4. As in choice 1.

157. **Client Needs: Safe and Effective Care Environment; T: Application**
   1. **Physiotherapists are a resource for planning range-of-motion or strengthening exercises.**
   2. **Occupational therapists are a resource for planning activities of daily living that clients need to modify or relearn.**
   3. Because the client exhibits good respiratory function, respiratory therapy is probably not needed at this time.
   4. Cardiac rehabilitation is probably not needed at this time since he has not cardiac issues.
   5. **Referral to psychology services to assist with coping or other psychosocial issues is appropriate.**

158. **Client Needs: Physiological Integrity; T: Application**
   1. **The parents should notify the health care provider if the tube falls out. They will need to recognize what the tubes look like.**
   2. The child should not blow their nose for 7 to 10 days after tube insertion.
   3. The ears should be kept dry.
   4. The child may swim and shower but should wear earplugs.

159. **Client Needs: Safe and Effective Care Environment; T: Critical Thinking**
   1. The nurse should assess the situation and not turn the client alone if this cannot be done safely.
   2. This is not a one-person task: the nurse must not pull from the head of the bed.
   3. **The nurse must assess and determine the number of people needed; to prevent injury, the task should not be started until it can be completed safely.**
   4. The nurse's trunk should be erect and the knees bent, so that multiple muscle groups (not just the arms) work together in a coordinated manner.

160. **Client Needs: Physiological Integrity; T: Application**
   1. Hypodermoclysis is commonly used for clients at risk for or with mild dehydration.

2. **Marked edema is a contraindication for the use of hypodermoclysis.**
3. **Renal failure is a contraindication for the use of hypodermoclysis.**
4. **Fluid overload is a contraindication for the use of hypodermoclysis.**
5. Hypodermoclysis is commonly used for clients with limited IV access.

161. **Client Needs: Psychosocial Integrity; T: Application**
   1. This is valid in certain psychiatric diagnoses, but not with dementia.
   2. Questioning the client with dementia will only make them more agitated.
   3. The confused client will not accept that they are confused, and it will lead to further agitation. "Truth" is not the goal.
   4. **Confused clients may frequently be distracted from whatever is upsetting to them, this will decrease stress for the client and also the family.**

162. **Client Needs: Physiological Integrity; T: Application**
   1. The client should wait 1 to 2 minutes between puffs.
   2. **To administer a metered-dose inhaler, the client presses down on the inhaler to release the medication while inhaling slowly.**
   3. This technique is incorrect.
   4. The client should position the inhaler at the open mouth with the inhaler 3 to 5 cm away from the mouth, attach a spacer to the mouthpiece of the inhaler, or place the mouthpiece in the mouth.

163. **Client Needs: Safe and Effective Care Environment T: Application**
   1. **Evidence-informed practice involves using research finding to provide the most effective nursing care.**
   2. **Evidence-informed practice involves using Standards of Nursing Practice to provide the most effective nursing care.**
   3. Evidence is continuously emerging, so nurses cannot rely solely on experience.
   4. Trial and error is an unsystematic approach to care.
   5. Intuition is an unsystematic approach to care.

164. **Client Needs: Safe and Effective Care Environment; T: Application**
   1. **A quiet, shadow-free room offers an environment that produces the fewest sensory perceptual distortions for a client with cognitive impairment associated with delirium.**
   2. This option has the potential to produce increased perceptual alterations.
   3. As in choice 2.
   4. As in choice 2.

165. **Client Needs: Safe and Effective Care Environment; T: Application**
   1. **The nurse should not attempt to restrain a competent client or ask security to do so.**
   2. If the client is competent and not at risk of harming others there is no reason to alert the police.

3. The nurse cannot legally withhold a client's personal effects.

4. **The nurse should alert the team because others may be able to persuade the client to stay. However, ultimately, there is nothing hospital staff can do to prevent a competent client from leaving. The nurse should give the client their personal effects and allow them to leave. If a competent client refuses to sign the waiver, the fact that they are leaving against medical advice should be carefully documented in the chart.**

166. **Client Needs: Physiological Integrity; T: Application**
    1. Tolerance may occur, but addiction to opioids will not develop in the acute postoperative period.
    2. **Monitoring for pain relief and adverse effects is an appropriate action when administering opioids for acute pain.**
    3. The client should use the opioids to achieve adequate pain control, and so the nurse should not emphasize the adverse effects.
    4. **Teaching the client about how opioid use will improve postoperative outcomes is an appropriate action when administering opioids for acute pain.**
    5. Although postoperative clients usually need decreasing amounts of opioids by the second postoperative day, each client's response is individual.

167. **Client Needs: Safe and Effective Care Environment; T: Application**
    1. **When the role of the nurse and the role of the client shift, boundary blurring may arise. In this situation the nurse is becoming over-involved with the client.**
    2. This situation does not describe sexual harassment.
    3. The data does not suggest positive regard.
    4. This is not an example of advocacy.

168. **Client Needs: Safe and Effective Care Environment; T: Knowledge**
    1. When the number of cases of a communicable disease exceeds the normal expected occurrence during a given period, it is referred to as an epidemic.
    2. **When a communicable disease occurs among a cluster of individuals, it is referred to as an outbreak.**
    3. If transmission of the disease is widespread and affects large numbers of people across several countries or continents or globally, it is considered to be a pandemic.
    4. Mitigation, also called *prevention*, is a critical first step to emergency management that occurs in the pre-incident phase of the disaster management continuum.

169. **Client Needs: Safe and Effective Care Environment; T: Application**
    1. **Prevention of falls requires alterations in the environment, including keeping call light and desired items within reach.**
    2. The bed should be in the lowest position possible with tall the side rails up.
    3. At least a dim light should be left on at night.

4. Personal belongings and clutter should not be on the floor—they should be in a cabinet.
5. **Having the child wear an appropriate-size gown and nonskid footwear is a falls prevention strategy.**

170. **Client Needs: Psychosocial Integrity; T: Application**
    1. This is not an appropriate response.
    2. **Information about cultural beliefs and practices should be obtained from clients when they enter health care facilities. To provide holistic and culturally sensitive care, the nurse should take into account the biological, psychological, social, cultural, and spiritual needs of clients.**
    3. Although it is true that client information is kept confidential, and that the client must be informed of confidentiality, this does not answer the client question
    4. It is important for the nurse to inform the client that they are obtaining information to ensure sensitivity to the client's needs and give the client the opportunity to communicate his cultural needs.

Multiple Response
171. **Client Needs: Safe and Effective Care Environment T: Application**
    1. Waiting is not appropriate as the dressing is saturated and needs to be changed now.
    2. **Because the dressing is saturated, the nurse must revise the plan of care and change the dressing now.**
    3. As in choice 1.
    4. There is no data to support discontinuing the plan of care.

172. **Client Needs: Safe and Effective Care Environment; T: Critical Thinking**
    1. **A registered dietitian works with the nurse to determine a meal plan that will support wound healing.**
    2. **An enterostomal or wound care nurse specializes in caring for the needs of the client with wounds.**
    3. **Physiotherapy can assist an immobile client to progress toward mobility and decrease the risk for pressure injury.**
    4. **Pressure injuries take a long time to heal and usually require continued therapy in the home. Case management personnel are useful in obtaining care for the client outside the home.**
    5. If the client has a need associated with medications, the pharmacist can assist however pharmacists usually are not part of the wound care multidisciplinary team, unless a special need arises.

173. **Client Needs: Physiological Integrity; T: Application**
    1. Clients are infectious during only the early part of the treatment.
    2. Medication therapy for TB may last up to 24 months and client adherence to the drug therapy is key; if symptoms become severe, the prescriber should be contacted for an adjustment of drug therapy.

3. **Because of potential liver toxicity, clients on this drug therapy should not drink alcohol.**

4. Discoloration of the urine is an expected adverse effect, which the client should be warned about.

5. **This is an appropriate teaching statement for anti-tubercular drug therapy**

174. **Client Needs: Psychosocial Integrity; T: Critical Thinking**

1. **Apraxia is a common symptom whereby a person with moderate-stage dementia needs repeated instructions and directions to perform the simplest tasks. For the individual with Alzheimer's disease, the world is very frightening and nothing makes sense.**

2. This denies the client the positive feelings of competence.

3. This reminds the client they have forgotten and might be distressing. They want to brush their teeth.

4. Clients with dementia may become upset if they are tasked with trying to remember.

175. **Client Needs: Safe and Effective Care Environment; T: Knowledge**

1. *Responsibility* refers to respecting one's professional obligations and following through on promises.

2. **Nurses advocate for clients by supporting the client's cause. A nurse's ability to advocate adequately for a client is based on the unique relationship that develops between the nurse and the client and on the opportunity to better understand the client's point of view.**

3. *Confidentiality* refers to privacy issues.

4. *Accountability* refers to owning one's actions.

176. **Client Needs: Safe and Effective Care Environment; T: Application**

1. Results should not be described simply as "good" or "poor"; they should be specific. The description "no complaints" assumes the client would be complaining and is not specific.

2. Critical comments about the client's or family's behaviour are considered idle gossip and should not be mentioned.

3. **Significant changes in the way therapies are to be given such as a new medication should be described to staff.**

4. This information is not relevant and should not be mentioned.

5. **This is significant information that should be described to staff.**

177. **Client Needs: Safe and Effective Care Environment; T: Knowledge**

1. *Advocacy* refers to the support of a particular cause.

2. *Responsibility* **refers to one's willingness to respect and adhere to one's professional obligations. One of the obligations of nurses is to protect clients and communities, including other nurses. If narcotics are missing, this may indicate that clients have not received medications ordered for their care, or it may suggest that a health care provider may be working under the influence of these drugs.**

3. *Confidentiality* involves protecting clients' personal health information and privacy.

4. *Accountability* refers to the ability to answer for one's actions.

178. **Client Needs: Physiological Integrity; T: Critical Thinking**

1. **The immediate priority is to perform CPR until the AED is available. An AED may be used for pre-hospital cardiac arrest. Voice prompts direct the user to safe and effective use.**

2. As in choice 1.

3. This is important, but not the priority.

4. This is important, but not the priority.

179. **Client Needs: Safe and Effective Care Environment; T: Application**

1. This is an acceptable nursing practice and does not constitute a breach of the client's right to privacy.

2. **Release of information without client authorization violates the client's right to privacy.**

3. As in choice 1.

4. As in choice 1.

5. **Nurses may not divulge client information to police unless there is a specific court order, or unless the client provides permission.**

180. **Client Needs: Psychosocial Integrity; T: Application**

1. **Most clients will not spontaneously provide information about family violence because of fear, guilt, and embarrassment; however, many clients will often disclose if asked.**

2. **Abuse is a life-threatening public health concern that affects many clients and their children.**

3. **Confirming confidentiality will reassure the client they are safe to speak.**

4. If a partner is present, they should be encouraged to leave the room because the client may not disclose experiences of abuse in their presence, or the partner may try to answer questions for the client to protect themselves.

5. Intimate partner violence tends to increase during pregnancy.

6. Threatening is considered abuse, and often escalates.

181. **Client Needs: Physiological Integrity; T: Application**

1. Documentation of the client's refusal to take the medication is an inadequate response by the nurse.

2. The Aspirin is not ordered to prevent aches and pains.

3. **Acetylsalicylic acid can reduce platelet aggregation. It is ordered to prevent stroke in clients who have experienced TIAs. The 81-mg tablets (traditionally thought of as "children's" Aspirin) and the 325-mg pills appear to be equally beneficial for the prevention of thrombotic events.**

4. There is no need to clarify the order with the health care provider.

182. **Client Needs: Physiological Integrity; T: Application**

1. The nurse may not know if this is the plan by the health care provider.

2. This may be appropriate, but accessing diagnostic results via a health care portal is a more effective and efficient strategy.

3. As in choice 2.

4. **Most labs across Canada now have digital health portals so clients can access their diagnostic results. Abnormal results will be flagged for the health care provider's attention.**

183. **Client Needs: Safe and Effective Care Environment; T: Application**

1. This situation may be resolved with education.

2. This is acceptable practice.

3. **The nurse has a duty to intervene and report if a team member tries to provide client care in an alcohol-impaired state as it jeopardizes client safety.**

4. **Violation of relationship boundaries jeopardizes client safety. The nurse has a duty to intervene and report this situation.**

5. The client has the right to refuse medication.

6. **This is a violation of client confidentiality.**

184. **Client Needs: Safe and Effective Care Environment; T: Application**

1. A transfer belt maintains stability of the client during transfer and reduces risk for falls.

2. If the client can bear weight and move to a sitting position independently, they should be allowed to do so, and the nurse may offer assistance.

3. **Careful assessment of the client's ability to assist in the positioning technique to be used is extremely important. The use of a mechanical lift should be considered.**

4. The nurse must ensure that the client has stable non-skid shoes, not socks, on the feet.

185. **Client Needs: Health Promotion and Maintenance; T: Critical Thinking**

1. **Sit facing the client so that they can lip read and watch facial expressions.**

2. **Speaking loudly may be perceived by the client as yelling or anger.**

3. **Older people can hear low frequency rather than high-frequency sounds.**

4. **To help the client concentrate, focus on a single topic.**

5. It is a myth that all older persons have difficulty learning.

6. The older person may not need or have a family member to join the discussion. There must be approval by the older person to have another person join the discussion.

186. **Client Needs: Physiological Integrity; T: Knowledge**

1. The ear canal needs to be straightened when administering eardrops.

2. Pulling on the lobe will not straighten the ear canal.

3. **For an infant or a child younger than 3 years, straighten the ear canal by pulling the pinna down and back.**

4. For adults, pull the pinna up and outward.

187. **Client Needs: Physiological Integrity; T: Application**

1. The pulse is increased.

2. A 5-year-old child will have a closed fontanelle.

3. **The child will be irritable.**

4. **Mucous membranes, particularly in the mouth and eyes, will be dry.**

5. **With decreased blood volume there will be less perfusion of the kidneys and less urine output.**

6. **Capillary refill over 4 seconds is sluggish due to decreased blood volume.**

188. **Client Needs: Safe and Effective Care Environment; T: Application**

1. Until the policy is changed the nurse is obligated to follow hospital procedure.

2. **As a result of their finding, the nurse should meet with the policy and procedure committee to recommend routine use of transparent dressings.**

3. Until the policy is changed or the nurse receives approval to conduct a pilot study, the nurse is obligated to follow hospital procedure.

4. If the nurse has information that can lead to better client care, the nurse has an obligation (moral and professional) to bring it to the attention of policymakers.

189. **Client Needs: Physiological Integrity; T: Application**

1. **The Braden Scale is a valid and reliable tool that provides guidance for effective interventions.**

2. **The Norton Scale is a valid and reliable tool that provides guidance for effective interventions.**

3. The client, depending on the assessment, may require turning more frequently than ever 6 hours.

4. **Clinical judgement decreases the potential for pressure injury development.**

5. **Critical thinking decreases the potential for pressure injury development.**

6. **Targeted interventions decreases the potential for pressure injury development.**

190. **Client Needs: Health Promotion & Maintenance; T: Critical Thinking**

1. The nurse does not need to know, at this point, if there is a new partner.

2. This shows disregard for the client.

3. **While all of the responses by the nurse may be discussed in the conversation, the nurse's priority is to help the resident feel comfortable with the topic of sex, and indicate they are accepted as a sexual being. It is a common myth that older persons are no longer capable nor interested in sexual relations.**

4. The client did not ask about sexually transmitted diseases.

191. **Client Needs: Psychosocial Integrity; T: Application**

1. Initiating confinement measures is inappropriate at this point.

2. **During the escalation period the client's behaviour is moving toward loss of control. Acknowledging the client's behaviour helps to de-escalate the situation.**

3. **This helps to de-escalate the situation.**

4. **This provides safety for the nurse.**

5. It is the nurse who needs to take control of the situation.

6. Contacting security is inappropriate at this point.

192. **Client Needs: Safe and Effective Care Environment; T: Critical Thinking**
   1. A family member or acquaintance who speaks a client's language should not interpret health information. Privacy regarding the client's condition, assessment, and other medical matters must be protected. There is no way to confirm that the family member is translating exactly what the nurse is saying.
   2. After consent is obtained for treatment, the health care provider would be notified because little can be done without consent. The health care provider needs to have the translator available during the history and physical examination, as well as other times, but the first step is to get a translator to obtain informed consent because this is not an emergency situation.
   3. **An official interpreter must be present to explain the terms of consent to a client who speaks only a foreign language. Privacy must be ensured and accurate information must be provided to the client.**
   4. Using hand gestures and medical equipment is inappropriate when communicating with a client who does not understand the language spoken because (1) certain hand gestures may be acceptable in one culture and not appropriate in another, (2) the medical equipment may be unknown and frightening to the client, and (3) the client still does not understand what is being said.

193. **Client Needs: Psychosocial Integrity; T: Critical Thinking**
   1. **The first step in the nursing process is assessment, gathering data. The nurse needs first to know the client symptoms.**
   2. This is important. but not as important as gathering data on symptoms.
   3. As in choice 2.
   4. As in choice 2.

194. **Client Needs: Physiological Integrity; T: Application**
   1. Although the nurse should check hospital policy, it is likely music would be allowed.
   2. Music should be preferred choices by the parents, not the nurse.
   3. Relaxation exercises are effective, but music is effective as well.
   4. **Music therapy has been shown to be an effective relaxation strategy. This answer provides helpful assistance for the couple.**

195. **Client Needs: Physiological Integrity; T: Application**
   1. **Clothing protects the skin from tick bites.**
   2. Antibiotics are only necessary if a person is bitten by a tick and is suspected of borrelia bergdoferi.
   3. **This is an effective repellent. It should be used with caution in infants and young children.**
   4. Ticks can be killed by freezing for several hours or in rubbing alcohol. They are difficult to kill by crushing.
   5. **The tick should be sealed in a container and brought to the primary health care provider to inspect the tick and determine its type.**
   6. **With tweezers, slowly pull out the tick without crushing it.**

196. **Client Needs: Health Promotion and Maintenance; T: Critical Thinking**
   1. **This is an open-ended question which will provide more information. Assessing support to the individual will help to determine safety and appropriateness of the living situation and is a nonthreatening initial question.**
   2. This may be discussed later on in the conversation. Most older people do not want to leave their homes.
   3. This could possibly be true but is not the priority question.
   4. This is important for risk of falls but is not the most immediate concern.

197. **Client Needs: Physiological Integrity; T: Knowledge**
   1. **This is the definition of an INR. The INR must be within normal range to determine therapeutic effects of the anticoagulants.**
   2. INR is not a measure of platelets.
   3. This is not a test of cardiac enzymes.
   4. The INR does not predict myocardial infarction.

198. **Client Needs: Safe and Effective Care Environment; T: Application**
   1. **The ethical doctrine of autonomy ensures the client the right to refuse medical treatment.**
   2. **Advance directives are written documents that direct treatment in accordance with a client's wishes in the event of a terminal illness or condition. With this legal document, the client is able to declare which medical procedures they want or do not want when terminally ill or in a persistent vegetative state.**
   3. Legally competent adult clients can consent to a do not resuscitate (DNR) order verbally or in writing after receiving appropriate information from the health care provider.
   4. **An advance directive is a legal document that designates a person or persons of one's choosing to make health care decisions when the client is no longer able to make decisions on their own behalf. This agent makes health care treatment decisions based on the client's wishes.**
   5. Differences among the provinces have been noted regarding advance directives, so the client should check provincial/territorial laws to see if a province/territory will honour an advance directive that was originated in another province/territory.

199. **Client Needs: Psychosocial Integrity; T: Critical Thinking**
   1. A meta-analysis found varenicline to be twice as effective as the nicotine patch.
   2. A meta-analysis found varenicline to be more than two thirds more likely to assist a person to stop smoking than using nicotine gum.
   3. E-cigarettes deliver nicotine to the blood. Presently much still needs to be learned about these devices, and their use as an option in nicotine replacement therapy and smoking cessation is undetermined.

4. **Varenicline (Chantix/Champix), a nicotine receptor partial agonist that affects the CNS to reduce cravings and withdrawal symptom by weakly stimulating nicotine receptors.**

200. **Client Needs: Physiological Integrity; T: Application**
    1. **Normal sodium (Na) is 136 to 144 mmol/L, normal potassium (K) is 3.7 to 5.1 mmol/L. These electrolytes are all within normal limits.**
    2. The Na is high; the K is normal.
    3. The Na is normal; the K is low.
    4. The Na is normal; the K is low.

201. **Client Needs: Physiological Integrity; T: Knowledge**
    1. Creatinine is not a measure of liver function.
    2. Creatinine does not assess tumour factors.
    3. **Serum creatinine reflects the glomerular filtration rate, an indication of renal function.**
    4. Creatinine does not assess for diverticulitis.

202. **Client Needs: Safe and Effective Care Environment; T: Application**
    1. Vague terms such as *appears, seems,* or *apparently* convey opinion rather than fact, do not accurately communicate facts, and do not inform another caregiver of details regarding behaviours exhibited by the client.
    2. The nurse should avoid using generalized, uninformative phrases such as "Status unchanged" or "Doing well."
    3. **Use of exact measurements establishes accuracy. The client's record should include objective data to support subjective data, so that charting is as descriptive as possible.**
    4. A statement such as "Client is hard to care for" is a personal opinion and should be avoided. It is also a critical comment that can be used as evidence of nonprofessional behaviour or poor quality of care.
    5. **A factual record contains descriptive, objective information about what a nurse sees, hears, feels, and smells.**

203. **Client Needs: Safe and Effective Care Environment; T: Application**
    1. **A UCP may apply restraints under the nurse's direction.**
    2. Physicians' orders cannot be taken by a UCP.
    3. Documenting the events that led to restraining the client cannot be done by the UCP.
    4. A UCP cannot evaluate the effectiveness of the restraints.

204. **Client Needs: Safe and Effective Care Environment; T: Application**
    1. The fall may not have been due to an error by the unregulated care provider; therefore, counselling should be reserved until after the cause has been determined.
    2. **After a change in the client's condition or an untoward event, the nurse attempts to identify factors interfering with goal achievement. In this case, the nurse identifies the factors that interfered with goal achievement to determine the cause of the fall.**

3. This may be one component of the re-evaluation of the plan of care.
4. The charge nurse can be consulted to review the plan, but it is the nurse's responsibility.

205. **Client Needs: Physiological Integrity; T: Application**
    1. This choice is incorrect because the infusion needs to be discontinued.
    2. As in choice 1.
    3. **Because of the possibility of a transfusion reaction, the infusion should be discontinued immediately and the health care provider notified.**
    4. This is not a normal reaction to a blood transfusion.

206. **Client Needs: Physiological Integrity; T: Application**
    1. **Fatigue is the most common side effect of radiation.**
    2. Creams and ointments are not to be used unless prescribed by the radiologist.
    3. Sun exposure should be avoided.
    4. **This keeps the area clean and helps prevent irritation.**
    5. **The markings need to be clearly visible to focus the radiation.**
    6. The client will not emit radiation with external beam.

207. **Client Needs: Safe and Effective Care Environment; T: Application**
    1. Although the client may not need 1 minute of preoxygenation, this would not be unsafe.
    2. **Sterile gloves and a sterile catheter are used when suctioning a tracheostomy.**
    3. The length of the catheter that should be inserted depends on the length of the tracheostomy tube, but the range is 13 to 15 cm for most adult clients.
    4. Suctioning for 7 seconds is appropriate.

208. **Client Needs: Physiological Integrity; T: Critical Thinking**
    1. There is a possible clot, a warm compress will not be effective.
    2. **These signs could indicate clot formation and constitute an emergency. The health care provider must be notified immediately.**
    3. The procedure was in the right arm, pulses in the left arm can be monitored for comparison but there is no right radial pulse.
    4. This will not improve the circulation if there is a clot.

209. **Client Needs: Safe and Effective Care Environment; T: Application**
    1. This response does not demonstrate listening to the client and could potentially lead to a medication error.
    2. As in choice 1.
    3. As in choice 1.
    4. **When giving medications, the nurse must always listen to and honour any concerns or doubts expressed by the client. If the client doubts an order, the nurse should check the written order, check with the prescriber, or both.**

210. **Client Needs: Physiological Integrity; T: Application**
    1. **Calcium channel blockers may cause peripheral edema.**

2. Calcium channel blockers may cause hypotension, not hypertension.

3. **Calcium channel blockers may interact with grapefruit juice, increasing the bioavailability of the medication.**

4. Betablockers can cause cold extremities, but calcium channel blockers do not cause this potential adverse effect.

5. **Calcium channel blockers may cause constipation.**

6. **Calcium channel blockers may cause facial flushing.**

211. **Client Needs: Physiological Integrity; T: Application**
    1. It is illegal for the nurse to administer the morphine for a client through a client-controlled analgesia device.
    2. **Patient-controlled analgesia devices are best for controlling acute pain; this client's history indicates chronic pain and a need for a pain management plan that will provide adequate analgesia while the client is sleeping.**
    3. Administering a dose of morphine when the client already has severe pain will not address the problem.
    4. Teaching the client to administer unneeded medication before going to sleep can result in oversedation and respiratory depression.

212. **Client Needs: Safe and Effective Care Environment T: Application**
    1. **Errors should be discussed only with those who need to know, such as the client, health care provider, appropriate administrative personnel, and risk management.**
    2. The report is confidential and separate from the health record. The fact that an incident report was completed is not documented in the client's health record.
    3. No discussion of why the omission in procedure occurred should be documented in the client's health record.
    4. **It is important to continue to monitor the client for any untoward effects of the medication.**
    5. **The risk management department of the institution also requires complete documentation.**

213. **Client Needs: Health Promotion and Maintenance; T: Application**
    1. **A child's recognition of the urge to urinate and defecate is a crucial component in the child's mental readiness for toilet learning.**
    2. This readiness appears at various ages, not necessarily by age 24 months.
    3. Infant toileting is training the parents, not the children.
    4. This does not answer the parent's question.

214. **Client Needs: Physiological Integrity T: Application**
    1. **Pregnancy is a contraindication to barbiturates.**
    2. Barbiturates may be used in the treatment of epilepsy.
    3. **Significant respiratory difficulty is a contraindication to barbiturates.**
    4. **Severe liver disease is a contraindication to barbiturates.**
    5. **Coadministration of barbiturates with opioids, alcohol, benzodiazepines, and some medications from other drug groups can result in additive CNS depression.**

6. **Effects and dangers of barbiturates are increased greatly if they are taken with alcohol.**

215. **Client Needs: Safe and Effective Care Environment; T: Application**
    1. This client also needs to be assessed but is not exhibiting symptoms of a potentially life-threatening problem.
    2. **Any fever in a neutropenic client indicates infection and can quickly lead to sepsis and septic shock. Rapid assessment and (if prescribed) initiation of antibiotic therapy within 1 hour are needed.**
    3. As in choice 1.
    4. As in choice 1.

216. **Client Needs: Safe and Effective Care Environment T: Application**
    1. Instructing the client in this new skill is within nursing scope of practice.
    2. Assessment of the client is a complex skill that is within nursing scope of practice.
    3. **Assisting with client hygiene is included in the unregulated care provider's scope of practice.**
    4. As in choice 1.
    5. **Measuring the client's oral intake is an appropriate task to delegate to the unregulated care provider.**

217. **Client Needs: Health Promotion and Maintenance; T: Critical Thinking**
    1. Advice regarding supplements needs to be more specific.
    2. Advice about diet needs to be more specific.
    3. **All options may be of assistance, but immediate help is best achieved by performing relaxation exercises.**
    4. Too much screen time may actually increase anxiety and stress.

218. **Client Needs: Safe and Effective Care Environment; T: Critical Thinking**
    1. This is a concern, but it is not the most critical concern.
    2. As in choice 1.
    3. As in choice 1.
    4. **Coolness of the client's hands would indicate poor circulation, which can result in permanent damage.**

219. **Client Needs: Physiological Integrity T: Application**
    1. **Chills are a symptom of a transfusion reaction.**
    2. **Shaking is a sign of a transfusion reaction.**
    3. **Flank pain is a symptom of a transfusion reaction.**
    4. Hyperthermia, not hypothermia occurs.
    5. **Sudden severe headache is a symptom of a transfusion reaction.**
    6. **Hyperthermia is a sign of a transfusion reaction.**

220. **Client Needs: Physiological Integrity; T: Knowledge**
    1. This time would be too early to ensure the lowest concentration of the drug in the body.
    2. **Trough levels are the lowest concentration of a drug reached in the body after it falls from its peak level and are generally measured 30 minutes before the drug is administered. If the medication is to be administered at 0900 hours, the trough should be measured at 0830 hours.**

3. Measurement of the trough level would be done prior to, not at the same time as, administration of the medication.

4. Measurement of the trough level would be done prior to the administration of the medication, not after.

221. **Client Needs: Physiological Integrity; T: Critical Thinking**
   1. The nurse cannot give a medication without an order because this violates the "right time" portion of the Ten Rights of Medication Administration.
   2. **The nurse should use clinical judgement to advocate for the client by requesting a stat order for the client's breakthrough pain.**
   3. If a nurse determines that a client is in severe pain, they must use clinical judgement to find that client a means of pain relief.
   4. Although the nurse should document the client's request and pain score, this is not the priority.

222. **Client Needs: Safe and Effective Care Environment T: Application**
   1. Light-coloured clothing is preferred as it makes the tick more noticeable.
   2. There is currently no Lyme disease vaccine available.
   3. **In the prevention of Lyme disease, individuals should keep the skin covered by wearing protective clothing in wooded areas to prevent tick bites.**
   4. **Attached ticks should be removed with tweezers (not fingers).**
   5. **Insect repellant containing DEET should be used to prevent tick bites.**

223. **Client Needs: Physiological Integrity; T: Application**
   1. The influenza vaccine cannot cause influenza. These are not serious symptoms.
   2. These are not allergic symptoms.
   3. **This is correct information. Many people believe they should not have the vaccine because it gives them "the flu," but it is the body's inflammatory response to building the immune system. These symptoms are mild and rarely last more than 24 to 48 hours. Influenza is a highly contagious viral infection which causes a higher fever, muscle aches, fatigue, weakness, sore throat, and cough. It can lead to death.**
   4. This may be partly true but is patronizing and will not encourage the client to have the vaccine.

224. **Client Needs: Safe and Effective Care Environment; T: Application**
   1. This is not a truthful answer.
   2. **Truthful answers will give a child a realistic expectation and help establish trust in the nurse.**
   3. As in choice 1.
   4. The child may not need to be held to be kept still.

225. **Client Needs: Psychosocial Integrity; T: Application**
   1. Religion is the system of organized beliefs and worship that a person practices to outwardly express spirituality. This is not evident here. Agnostics do not know whether God or another ultimate reality exists and are uncertain whether there is life after death.

   2. The client is agnostic and the nurse has differing religious beliefs. The emphasis that there is life after death does not support the client beliefs.
   3. As in choice 2.
   4. This denies the client's spiritual beliefs.

226. **Client Needs: Physiological Integrity; T: Application**
   1. This does not prevent thrombophlebitis.
   2. **Early ambulation is preventative.**
   3. These may be applied after, not before surgery.
   4. **Anticoagulants help prevent clot formation.**
   5. **Range-of-motion exercises are preventative.**
   6. Dangling legs from the bed is contraindicated.

227. **Client Needs: Physiological Integrity; T: Application**
   1. **The client will need to blow their nose before the medication is administered, because the nasal passages should be cleared before receiving nasal spray.**
   2. Blowing the nose after receiving the medication will remove the medication from the nasal passages.
   3. The client should receive the spray while inhaling through the open nostril.
   4. Afterwards, the client should remain in a supine position for 5 minutes.

228. **Client Needs: Physiological Integrity T: Application**
   1. **Epinephrine increases activation of the sympathetic nervous system. Nausea is an adverse effect.**
   2. **Tremors are an adverse effect of epinephrine.**
   3. **This medication can cause irritability.**
   4. Tachycardia would occur, not bradycardia.
   5. Hypertension, not hypotension would occur.
   6. Epinephrine may cause agitation, not sleepiness.

229. **Client Needs: Physiological Integrity; T: Knowledge**
   1. **A bladder scanner is a noninvasive method for measuring the volume of urine in the bladder.**
   2. This may not be necessary.
   3. Crede manoeuvre (exerting pressure over the bladder) is no longer recommended.
   4. This may not be necessary nor effective.

230. **Client Needs: Physiological Integrity; T: Application**
   1. **This is the correct procedure for midstream urine. The client should cleanse the area first with a bacteriostatic solution.**
   2. The container should not touch the urethra.
   3. The client does not void into a sterile urinal.
   4. The client would likely get urine on their hands.

231. **Client Needs: Physiological Integrity; T: Critical Thinking**
   1. This is not necessary at this time, only if the apical rate is irregular.
   2. There is no need nor rationale to wait for 5 minutes.
   3. **The apical pulse is the assessment of the actual heartbeat; thus it is the most reliable.**
   4. The carotid pulse is a possible option, but the apical rate is preferred.

232. **Client Needs: Physiological Integrity; T: Application**
   47 mmHg

   Pulse pressure is the difference between systolic and diastolic blood pressure readings. 132 − 85 = 47mmHg

233. Client Needs: Psychosocial Integrity; T: Critical Thinking
1. **By law, any cases of suspected abuse must be reported by registered health care professionals to the appropriate authorities according to provincial or territorial guidelines.**
2. The family will likely deny allegations of abuse.
3. Making a note does not protect the client.
4. This approach will likely be ignored by the client, who is in denial and does not fulfill legal requirements.

234. **Client Needs: Physiological Integrity T: Application**
Answer: 20.3
Rationale: Formula for calculation of oral and parenteral doses of medication
Formula:

$$\frac{\text{Dosage ordered}}{\text{Dosage available}} \times \text{Drug form}$$
$$= \text{Amount of drug to administer}$$

Solution: $650\,\text{mg}/160\,\text{mg} \times 5\,\text{mL} = 20.3\,\text{mL}$

235. **Client Needs: Health Promotion and Maintenance; T: Knowledge**
1. **Diabetes is a known risk factor for developing cardiovascular disease.**
2. A low-fibre diet may be a risk factor.
3. South Asian, African, and Indigenous heritage are risk factors.
4. BP of 124/82 mm Hg is considered to be normal.

236. **Client Needs: Physiological Integrity T: Application**
Answer: 2
Rationale: Formula for calculation of oral and parenteral doses of medications

Formula:

$$\frac{\text{Dosage ordered}}{\text{Dosage available}} \times \text{Drug form}$$
$$= \text{Amount of drug to administer}$$

Solution:

$$0.3/0.15 \times 1 = 2 \text{ tablets of Synthroid}$$

237. **Client Needs: Psychosocial Integrity; T: Application**
1. **Alcohol abuse is the most prevalent of the substance abuse conditions. Therefore alcohol-related medical conditions are the comorbidities most commonly seen in medical settings.**
2. Cannabis use is common but has not been found to be as addictive as alcohol.
3. Cocaine is harmful, but not as prevalent as alcohol.
4. As in choice 3.

238. **Client Needs: Safe and Effective Care Environment; T: Application**
1. This does not invite further dialogue with the spouse.
2. **Sleep deprivation can cause accidents. This answer makes an observation, gives important** information about safety, and communicates care and compassion for the spouse.
3. As in choice 1.
4. As in choice 1.

239. **Client Needs: Safe and Effective Care Environment; T: Critical Thinking**
1. Sterile technique should be used in suctioning an airway because the airway is considered a sterile body cavity.
2. Keeping the urinary catheter drainage bag below the bladder helps decrease the risk of developing a health care–associated infection because it prevents reflux of urine from the bag back into the bladder.
3. **Using clean technique (medical asepsis) to insert a urinary catheter would place the client at risk for a health care–associated infection. Placing a catheter into a sterile body cavity such as the bladder necessitates sterile technique.**
4. Bottled solutions may be used repeatedly during a 24-hour period; however, special care is needed to ensure that the solution in the bottle remains sterile. After 24 hours, the solution should be discarded.

240. **Client Needs: Physiological Integrity; T: Knowledge**
1. This is not a normal value.
2. **Normal reference interval is 4 to 6%.**
3. As in choice 1.
4. As in choice 1.

241. **Client Needs: Health Promotion and Maintenance; T: Application**
1. That she is eating too many carbohydrates is an assumption.
2. Osteoporosis is more likely to cause kyphosis.
3. Although there is a tendency to gain weight after menopause, the weight would be distributed throughout the body, not just the torso.
4. **This is the physiological reason for thickening torsos in aging adults.**

242. **Client Needs: Psychosocial Integrity; T: Knowledge**
1. Physical dependency is cellular adaptation such that the person physically needs a substance to function or to avoid the physical pain of withdrawal.
2. **Although sometimes labeled as addictions, compulsive behaviours do not have the biological element but only the psychological and social elements. This is not to diminish the severity of these issues, but they simply do not have direct biological risk of overdose or physical harm.**
3. Psychological dependence occurs when a substance becomes so important to an individual's thoughts and actions that the person believes that they cannot manage without the substance.
4. Addiction must include three elements: biological, psychological, and social

243. **Client Needs: Physiological Integrity; T: Application**
1. A straight catheter is used for intermittent catheterization.

2. The second lumen is not required for aspiration.

3. A triple lumen catheter is used for irrigation.

4. **The second lumen is used to inflate a balloon which keeps the catheter positioned in the bladder.**

244. **Client Needs: Physiological Integrity; T: Critical Thinking**

   1. Fluid overload is not a risk of abrupt discontinuation of TPN.

   2. Hyperglycemia is not a risk of abrupt discontinuation of TPN.

   3. Dumping syndrome is not a risk of abrupt discontinuation of TPN.

   4. **Rebound hypoglycemia may occur if TPN is discontinued abruptly and may be prevented with the infusion of 5 to 10% glucose when TPN must be stopped abruptly.**

245. **Client Needs: Safe and Effective Care Environment; T: Application**

   1. Cleaning hands with wipes does not meet the recommended standard.

   2. **Infection control guidelines recommend that when hands are visibly soiled, the health care provider should wash with a plain soap or with antimicrobial soap.**

   3. Using an alcohol-based waterless hand gel should not be used when the hands are visibly soiled.

   4. The client may need to wash their face and hands, but this is not the best next step.

246. **Client Needs: Physiological Integrity; T: Application**

   1. The anterior fontanelle is closed at 14 months.

   2. A 14-month-old infant will urinate less than eight diapers per day.

   3. Dehydration causes strong-smelling, dark yellow urine.

   4. **The lips and mucous membranes become dry with dehydration.**

   5. **Oliguria means low urine output, a sign of dehydration.**

6. **The heart rate will increase with low circulating blood volume caused by dehydration.**

247. **Client Needs: Health Promotion and Maintenance; T: Critical Thinking**

   1. **The first step of the nursing process is assessment, finding out what the client understands about vegetarian diets.**

   2. This may be discussed but is not the priority response.

   3. As in choice 2.

   4. As in choice 2.

248. **Client Needs: Physiological Integrity; T: Critical Thinking**

   1. This is not client-centred care and is not efficient use of time. There may be too much or too little information.

   2. **This is client centred and efficient. The nurse can address gaps in knowledge about the procedure.**

   3. If the client has completed the informed consent the nurse could possibly assume they have an understanding of the procedure, but the better option is to speak with the client.

   4. As in choice 3.

249. **Client Needs: Physiological Integrity T: Knowledge**

   1. This is a normal value.

   2. As in choice 1.

   3. As in choice 1.

   4. **This level of hemoglobin is low, indicating anemia.**

250. **Client Needs: Physiological Integrity; T: Knowledge**

   1. This is not a "right time" problem because the ordered frequency has not changed.

   2. This is not a "right to refuse" problem because the client is unable, not unwilling, to take the medication.

   3. **This is a "right route" problem: the nurse cannot assume the route and must clarify the route with the prescriber.**

   4. This is not a "right medication" problem because the medication ordered will not change, just the route.

1. After receiving change-of-shift report, which of the following four clients should the nurse assess first?
   1. A 31-year-old with Cushing's syndrome and a blood glucose level of 13.7 mmol/L
   2. A 22-year-old admitted with syndrome of inappropriate antidiuretic hormone (SIADH) who has a serum sodium level of 130 mmol/L
   3. A 70-year-old who recently started taking levothyroxine and has an irregular pulse of 134
   4. A 53-year-old who has Addison's disease and is due for a scheduled dose of hydrocortisone

2. After administering an intradermal injection for a skin test, the nurse notices a small bleb at the injection site. What is the proper action for the nurse to take?
   1. Apply heat.
   2. Massage the area.
   3. Report the bleb to the health care provider.
   4. No action is required.

3. The nurse greets a client on the memory unit of a long-term care facility. "Good morning, how was your weekend?" The client replies: "Well, you know yesterday was Monday, so I did all the laundry and cooked a curry for dinner." What is this response by the client an example of?
   1. Confabulation
   2. Lying
   3. Denial
   4. Perseveration

4. Interpret this test:

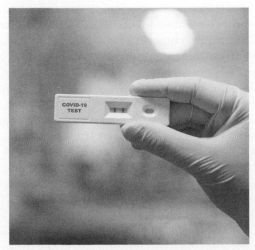

1. A positive rapid antigen test for COVID-19
2. A negative rapid antigen test for COVID-19
3. A false positive antigen test for COVID-19
4. A false negative rapid antigen test for COVID-19

5. When does a nurse begin discharge planning measures with a hospitalized client?
   1. Near the time of discharge
   2. At the time of admission
   3. Three days into the hospital stay
   4. On the day before discharge

6. By middle adolescence, ages 15 to 17 years, which developmental task is expected?
   1. Behavioural standards are set by the peer group.
   2. Emotional and physical separation from parents is completed.
   3. The person has a strong desire to remain dependent on parents.
   4. The person is preoccupied with rapid body changes.

7. A client is admitted to hospital with an acute severe asthma attack. The nurse administers intravenous steroid medication, fluids, and nebulized bronchodilators. Which of the following assessments would most concern the nurse?
   1. No air entry nor wheezing heard on chest auscultation
   2. Respiratory rate of 20 breaths per minute
   3. The client is sleepy
   4. There is mild substernal and suprasternal indrawing

8. The nurse is preparing to complete documentation on a client's chart. Which should be included in documentation of nursing care? **Select all that apply.**
   1. Reassessments
   2. Incident reports
   3. Initial assessments
   4. Nursing care provided
   5. Client's response to care provided

9. What is the term for the removal of nonviable tissue from a wound or burn?
   1. Debridement
   2. Scaling
   3. Escharotomy
   4. Peeling

10. The nurse has completed a preoperative assessment for a client about to undergo surgery. Of the following, which would be the most important next step?

1. Notify the operating suite that the client has a latex allergy.
2. Document that the client had a bath at home this morning.
3. Ask the unregulated care provider to obtain vital signs.
4. Administer the ordered preoperative intravenous antibiotic.

11. The nurse educates a parent's group about safety for toddlers and preschoolers. Which of the following are injury prevention actions for this age group? **Select all that apply.**
    1. Do not allow children lollipops when they are walking or running.
    2. Do not allow children to walk up or down stairs.
    3. Teach child to never go anywhere with a stranger.
    4. Do not place child on their stomach to sleep.
    5. Do not call medications or edible cannabis products candy.
    6. Turn pot handles to the back of the stove.

12. A client has a 9-year history of a seizure disorder that has been managed well with phenytoin therapy. The client is to receive nothing by mouth because they have surgery in the morning. What should the nurse do about the client's morning dose of phenytoin?
    1. Give the same dose intravenously.
    2. Give the morning dose with a small sip of water.
    3. Contact the health care provider for another dosage form of the medication.
    4. Notify the operating room that the medication has been withheld.

13. An adolescent client with an eating disorder participates in a behaviour-modification program to increase daily nutritional intake and increase weight. How would the nurse best evaluate the success of the of the program?
    1. Schedule weekly appointments to weigh the client.
    2. Have the client repeat back to the nurse an understanding of the behaviour-modification program.
    3. Ask the client to telephone the nurse each morning to report daily weight.
    4. Have the client keep a daily food diary.

14. A health care provider has prescribed amoxicillin 40 mg/kg a day divided q8hr by mouth for a 6-month-old infant with otitis media. The infant weighs 7.5 kg. The medication label states: "Amoxicillin 125 mg/5 mL." The nurse is preparing to administer the 1 400 dose. The nurse prepares to administer how many millilitres to the infant? **Record your answer using one decimal place. Fill in the blank.**
    Answer: _____ mL

15. For a client currently experiencing a panic attack, which nursing intervention should be implemented first?
    1. Teach relaxation techniques.
    2. Administer an anxiolytic medication.
    3. Prepare to implement physical controls.
    4. Provide calm, brief, and directive communication.

16. What is the term for a state which occurs in clients with some dementias late afternoon and early evening, causing behaviours such as an anxiety, aggression, and pacing?
    1. Lewy body disorder
    2. Confusion
    3. Sundowning
    4. Delirium

17. A client with insulin dependent diabetes has been NPO since midnight for 0800 surgery. What is the most important lab value for the nurse to check prior to the client going to the operating room?
    1. HgA1C
    2. Electrolytes
    3. CBC
    4. Blood glucose/sugar

18. What should the teaching plan include about infant fall precautions? **Select all that apply.**
    1. Remove all unsteady furniture.
    2. Use a baby walker to improve balance when walking.
    3. Steady infant with hand when on changing table.
    4. Use tray attachment on high chair as restraint.
    5. Keep infant seat on the floor while indoors.

19. The nurse cares for a client who has experienced a stroke and needs to relearn self-care skills such as dressing and self-feeding. Which referral is most appropriate?
    1. Dietitian
    2. Speech-language pathologist
    3. Physiotherapist
    4. Occupational therapist

20. What drug is usually given first in the emergency treatment of an acute, severe asthma episode?
    1. Ephedrine
    2. Theophylline
    3. Aminophylline
    4. Salbutamol

21. An immobilized client requires an ankle splint. How would the nurse prevent skin breakdown at the ankle?
    1. Apply a pressure-reduction dressing to the ankle.
    2. Inspect skin under the splint at routine intervals.
    3. Remove the splint at routine intervals.
    4. Apply talc to the skin under the splint.

22. To be able to meet the needs of assigned clients and professional responsibilities, nurses must be aware of time-management techniques. Time-management skills for the nurse include which of the following? **Select all that apply.**
    1. Meeting all of the clients' needs in the early morning hours
    2. Planning effectively and being aware of competing priorities
    3. Completing the activities started with one client before moving on to another
    4. Leaving each day unplanned to allow for adaptations in treatments
    5. Reflecting on how time is used

23. The nurse is evaluating the crutch-walking technique of a client who is to have no weight bearing on the right leg.

Which of the following observations indicates that the client can safely ambulate independently?

1. The client keeps the padded area of the crutch firmly in the axillary area when ambulating.
2. The client advances the right leg and both crutches together and then advances the left leg.
3. The client moves the left crutch with the left leg and then the right crutch with the right leg.
4. The client uses the bedside chair to assist in balance as needed when ambulating in the room.

24. While discussing attention-deficit/hyperactivity disorder (ADHD) with parents and school officials, the nurse encourages which of the following to reduce stress in ADHD children regarding homework assignments?

1. Time-management skills
2. Reduction in take-home assignments
3. Employment of an education assistant to assist with schoolwork
4. Speech articulation skills

25. As seen in this picture, this condition is a permanent shortening of a muscle or joint, usually in response to prolonged spasticity or loss of movement of a joint. The nurse may prevent this condition by providing range-of-motion exercises. What is this condition called?

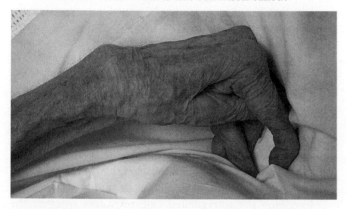

1. Contracture
2. Clonus
3. Tetanus
4. Repetitive strain injury

26. When teaching clients about over-the-counter (OTC) and natural health products which of the following statements should the nurse include? **Select all that apply.**

1. Natural health products and OTC drugs cannot be safely administered to infants, children, and pregnant or lactating clients without first checking with the health care provider.
2. Use of OTC drugs may delay treatment of more serious ailments.
3. Drug interactions are rare with OTC product because OTC drugs are natural.
4. Manufacturers of natural health products are required to provide evidence of safety and effectiveness; therefore, check the labels carefully.
5. OTC drugs are indicated for long-term treatment of conditions.

6. Natural health products are nontoxic and safer than prescription medications.

27. The nurse receives change-of-shift report about the following four clients. Which of the following clients should the nurse assess first?

1. A client who has malnutrition associated with 4+ generalized pitting edema
2. A client whose parenteral nutrition has 10 mL of solution left in the infusion bag
3. A client whose gastrostomy tube is plugged after crushed medications were given through the tube
4. A client who is receiving continuous enteral feedings and has new-onset crackles throughout the lungs

28. A person who escaped to Canada from a country at war is assessed at a refugee health centre. The client speaks no French and a bit of English but states, "I not speak English too good." Which of the following actions is most appropriate for the nurse?

1. Arrange to have a translator when planning the client's care.
2. Ask the client about any special cultural beliefs or practices.
3. Avoid upsetting the client by discussing the war.
4. Involve the client's family in making health care decisions.

29. The nurse must administer a medication via gastrostomy tube. The medication is not available in a solution, only as a pill. What steps should the nurse take to administer this medication?

1. Crush the pill and mix with a small amount of water.
2. Crush the pill and mix with enteral feeding formula.
3. Administer the crushed medication then flush the tube with air.
4. Check the placement of the tube before administering the crushed medication.

30. Parents ask the nurse about safety concerns giving herbal supplements to children. Which of the following products are considered safe for the pediatric population? **Select all that apply.**

1. Ephedra
2. Ginger
3. Fish oil
4. Chamomile
5. Aloe vera
6. Belladonna

31. The nurse is caring for a client with conductive hearing loss in one ear resulting from prolonged cerumen impaction. Which intervention by the nurse is most important in establishing effective communication with the client?

1. Speaking in a loud voice, enunciating every syllable
2. Having conversation with the client directed toward his affected ear
3. Repeating the phrase if the client does not hear what the nurse is saying
4. Speaking with hands, face, and expressions

32. The nurse is about to start a peripheral intravenous (IV) line on an adult client. How should the nurse determine an optimum site for the IV?
    1. Recognize that veins in the antecubital fossa are the most common and safest sites for an IV line.
    2. Assess the veins of both arms closely before selecting a site.
    3. Choose a site proximally on a limb rather than distally.
    4. Prioritize legs and feet over hands and arms.

33. An older client diagnosed with Alzheimer's disease lives with family and attends a day program. The nurse at the program observes the client has poor hygiene and speaks with the caregiver who becomes upset and says, "It takes all my energy to care for my parent. I am awake all night with them, I never get any sleep." Which nursing intervention has priority?
    1. Reassure the caregiver they are doing the best they can in a difficult situation.
    2. Secure additional resources for the parent's evening and night care.
    3. Support the caregiver to grieve the loss of the parent's cognitive abilities.
    4. Teach the family how to give physical care more effectively and efficiently.

34. A client has been discharged home with heart failure following a myocardial infarction (MI). The home health care nurse visits the client to discuss strategies for managing the condition. Which of the following would be included in the client-caregiver teaching guide? **Select all that apply.**
    1. Provide individually tailored information about heart failure and how it is treated.
    2. Discuss how the client will have a chronic debilitating disease that will alter their self-image.
    3. Discuss the benefits of participation in a cardiac rehabilitation exercise program.
    4. Review with client prescribed medications, adverse effects, and administration guidelines.
    5. Educate the client about signs of worsening heart failure such as weight gain, breathing difficulties, and increased fatigue.
    6. Discuss the need for complete bed rest, with trips to the bathroom as necessary.

35. A young client has a thyroidectomy for precancerous nodules of the thyroid. Which of the following would be a priority assessment by the nurse when the client returns to the unit after surgery?
    1. Signs of respiratory distress
    2. Indications of hemorrhage
    3. Puffiness and edema around the eyes
    4. Level of pain

36. A client has been prescribed a rapid-acting insulin. What important information should the nurse give this client about taking this type of insulin?
    1. It should be taken within 15 minutes of beginning a meal.
    2. It should be taken after the meal.

3. Dosing is once daily at the midday meal.
4. It is taken only in the evenings with a snack before bedtime.

37. The staff nurse observes a student nurse caring for a client with a urinary catheter. Which of the following actions require the staff nurse to intervene?
    1. Taping the catheter to the skin on the client's upper inner thigh
    2. Cleaning around the client's urinary meatus with soap and water
    3. Using an alcohol-based hand cleaner before performing catheter care
    4. Disconnecting the catheter from the drainage tube to obtain a specimen

38. Parents of a 1-year-old child ask the nurse which method is best for taking their child's temperature. What is the nurse's response?
    1. Orally using a glass thermometer
    2. Rectally using a digital thermometer
    3. Fever sticker strips
    4. Forehead temporal artery thermometer

39. A client asks the nurse about research related to hearing and development of dementia, saying "I am over 80 years old and think I might not hear very well anymore. Is it true that poor hearing might be linked to getting dementia? What should I do?" How would the nurse respond?
    1. "You should make an audiology appointment to have your hearing tested."
    2. "You probably need to get hearing aids."
    3. "I will refer you to an ears nose and throat (ENT) physician."
    4. "Don't worry, I find that you hear quite well, and the link with dementia is not proven."

40. The nurse is caring for a client who has an open wound. Which should be included in the evaluation of the progress of wound healing? **Select all that apply.**
    1. Asking the unregulated care providers whether the wound looks better
    2. Documenting the progress of wound healing as "better" in the client's chart
    3. Measuring the wound's length, depth, and width
    4. Observing the wound for redness, swelling, or drainage
    5. Leaving the dressing off the wound for easier access and more frequent assessments

41. A pediatric outpatient clinic nurse is floated to the orthopedic trauma unit. What actions should the nurse in charge of the orthopedic unit take to enable this floated nurse to give safe care?
    1. Provide a complete orientation to the functioning of the unit.
    2. Determine the acuity of clients and the care that the nurse can safely provide.
    3. Allow the nurse to read all unit policies prior to beginning client care.
    4. Assign unregulated care providers to assist with the floated nurse with care.

42. A client has a peripheral intravenous line for hydration and medication administration. The nurse performs hourly checks and assesses that there has been infiltration of the IV solution. What should the nurse do?
   1. Clamp the intravenous line.
   2. Massage the site of infiltration after IV removal.
   3. Remove the IV device immediately.
   4. Slow the intravenous rate and monitor for any further signs of infiltration.

43. A nurse is caring for a client with cancer who presents with anorexia, blood pressure of 100/60, elevated white blood cell count, and oral candidiasis. The nurse knows that the purpose of starting total parenteral nutrition (TPN) is which of the following?
   1. Replaces fluid, electrolytes, and nutrients in the client
   2. Stimulates the client's appetite to eat
   3. Provides medication to raise the client's blood pressure
   4. Delivers antibiotics to fight off infection

44. A client has been providing care for their terminally ill partner. Which of the following may indicate caregiver strain?
   1. Contacting the palliative care team routinely for support
   2. Telling the nurse they have "not gotten around to" having their routine PSA testing
   3. Displaying emotion when discussing their partner's death
   4. Increasing interest in attending religious services

45. A nurse is caring for an older client with arthritis in both hips. Based on the information provided, which of the following ordered PRN medications should the nurse prepare to administer prior to ambulation?

Nurse's note:	Alert and oriented
	Reports pain 5/10 both hips when ambulating
Vital signs:	Temperature: 37°C
	Pulse (beats per minute): 90
	Respirations (breaths per minute): 14
	Blood pressure: 110/70
	Oxygen saturation: 98%
Allergy:	Sulfa drugs

   1. Acetylsalicylic acid 650 mg orally
   2. Naproxen 200 mg orally
   3. Oxycodone 5 mg orally
   4. Acetaminophen 650 mg orally

46. A nurse is preparing to discharge a client home from hospital whose care plan has been focused on improving impaired physical mobility. Prior to discharge the nurse reviews the plan of care. Before discontinuing the client's plan of care, what does the nurse need to do?
   1. Determine whether the client has transportation to get home.
   2. Evaluate whether the client goals and outcomes have been met.

   3. Establish whether the client has a follow-up appointment scheduled.
   4. Ensure that the client's prescriptions have been filled.

47. A client has a body mass index (BMI) of 38, high blood pressure, shortness of breath, and high cholesterol. The treatment plan includes a diet incorporating fruits, vegetables and whole grains and decreasing intake of fast foods such as French fries, hamburgers, cookies, and ice cream. At the clinic appointment the client admits they have not adhered to the new diet. What should the nurse say to the client?
   1. "This is very serious; you must start to eat properly."
   2. "I understand the new diet is not as tasty as your usual foods."
   3. "What is there about the new diet that stops you from eating these foods?"
   4. "That is OK, just cut down a bit on the amounts of fast foods you eat."

48. While pouring cleansing solutions onto a dressing tray, one of the solutions splashes into the nurse's eye. The eye immediately becomes extremely painful, with stinging and tear production. What should be the nurse's first action?
   1. Identify the chemicals in the cleansing solution.
   2. Call for help.
   3. Wipe the eye with a sterile compress.
   4. Flush the eye with water, or saline if available.

49. A new client assessed by the nurse at the street health clinic appears agitated, reports chronic aches and pains with "bad nerves," and requests "something for the pain." What is the most appropriate statement by the nurse?
   1. "Do you abuse drugs or alcohol?"
   2. "Can you describe your symptoms and tell me what you take for the pain?"
   3. "Have you ever been in rehab for substance use disorder?"
   4. "We do not prescribe pain medication at this clinic for new clients."

50. A nurse is caring for a client with cancer pain. The client is ordered hydromorphone 1.5 mg by subcutaneous injection every 6 hours. The medication label states: "Hydromorphone 2 mg/mL." The nurse prepares to administer one dose. How many millilitres will the nurse prepare to administer one dose. **Record your answer using two decimal places. Fill in the blank.**
   Answer: _____mL

51. Which of the following demonstrates a nurse utilizing self-reflection to improve clinical decision making?
   1. Using an objective approach in all situations
   2. Obtaining data in an orderly manner
   3. Improving a plan of care while thinking back on interventions performed
   4. Providing evidence-informed explanations for all nursing interventions

52. A client presents to the emergency department with the complaint of vomiting and diarrhea for the past 48 hours. The nurse anticipates which fluid therapy initially?
   1. 0.9% sodium chloride
   2. Dextrose 10% in water

3. Dextrose 5% in water

4. 0.45% sodium chloride

53. The nurse evaluates any adverse effects of diabetes therapy with a client. What question would the nurse ask the client?

1. Have you had any hypoglycemic episodes?

2. How is your appetite?

3. Do you take your insulin at the same time every day?

4. Do you have any problems giving yourself the injections?

54. A nurse works in a first aid clinic at a country fair. A 6 year old child has sustained a 4 cm × 2 cm abrasion on the leg. The nurse applies an adhesive transparent film dressing. What instructions would the nurse provide to the parents?

1. Do not remove the dressing as this will be painful.

2. The dressing is not waterproof, so it needs to be kept dry.

3. Take the child to the health care provider tomorrow for an alginate dressing.

4. Observe the abrasion through the transparent film for signs of infection.

55. Which scenario places a toddler at risk for injury? **Select all that apply.**

1. The toddler playing with their school-aged sibling's toy

2. A mop and a bucket of clean water in the kitchen

3. A cup of hot coffee on the kitchen counter

4. A 12-kg toddler sitting in a forward-facing car seat in the back seat of a car

5. A home entertainment centre with the remote control on the top shelf

56. When an appreciative family offers the nurse a box of chocolates, what action is most appropriate for the nurse to take?

1. Accept all gifts offered to avoid embarrassing the person and family receiving care.

2. Politely refuse to accept the chocolates.

3. Consider the agency policies, and professional standards.

4. Inform the family that the candy will be shared among staff and clients receiving care.

57. The nurse performs an initial antenatal assessment with a young primigravida client and her partner. The client tells the nurse she and her partner live "off the grid," with no running water nor electricity, in a remote area of the province. What further information is important for the nurse to find out from the client?

1. What support services and relationships there are within their community

2. If the clients belong to a cult or commune

3. Whether clients practise alternative or homeopathic health care

4. What sanitation facilities the clients have access to

58. Choose all recommended health screening tests for a 25-year-old client.

1. Total cholesterol

2. Once-a-year blood pressure

3. Digital rectal or prostate specific antigen (PSA) for men

4. Annual Papaniculou (Pap) test for sexually active women

5. Yearly chest X-ray

6. Annual or twice annual dental examinations

59. A female client is concerned about personal hygiene in her perineal area. She has severe arthritis and finds that she is unable to wipe herself sufficiently after urinating or having a bowel movement. What might the nurse suggest?

1 Have a trusted caregiver provide perineal care for her.

2. Wear adult incontinence underwear to prevent the hygiene problem.

3. Pour water over her perineum or purchase a portable bidet for use after urination or bowel movement.

4. Use prepackaged moist sanitary towelettes.

60. A nurse is educating a group of parents of preschoolers about the importance of safety. Which statement by a parent indicates the need for further education?

1. "I continue to provide a great deal of indirect supervision for my child."

2. "My stairway is always free of clutter."

3. "I only leave my child in the car for brief moments."

4. "Medications are kept in a locked cabinet."

61. After leaving work, a nurse realizes documentation of administration of a PRN medication was omitted. The off-duty nurse phones the nurse on duty and says, "Please document administration of the medication for me. My password is alpha1." The nurse receiving the call should do which of the following?

1. Fulfill the request promptly.

2. Document the caller's password and document the medication administration.

3. Make a notation in the medication record of missed documentation and advise the nurse to make a late entry when next on shift.

4. Report the request to the nurse manager to determine the correct action.

62. A client has had a peripherally inserted central catheter (PICC) line inserted via the basilic vein in the left arm. Which of the following would be postprocedure nursing actions? **Select all that apply.**

1. Monitor the radial pulse on the left wrist.

2. Assess for evidence of bleeding at the insertion site.

3. Fasten the catheter as per unit policy.

4. Ensure catheter placement is verified according to protocol.

5. Monitor blood pressure on both arms.

63. A 62-year-old client receives an elevated result of 8 ng/mL on a prostate specific antigen (PSA) test. Their previous PSA level 2 years ago was 2 ng/mL The client asks the nurse what this means. How would the nurse respond?

1. "This is an indication that you have prostate cancer, and you will need a biopsy."
2. "Cancerous and noncancerous conditions can increase the PSA; your health care provider will discuss this with you."
3. "There is a lot of controversy about PSA tests and they are often no longer recommended."
4. "Let's sit down and talk about symptoms you may have of prostate cancer and the required treatment."

64. A 46-year-old client is devastated to be diagnosed with early-onset Alzheimer's disease (AD). The client asks the nurse 'Why is this happening to me? Why did I get Alzheimer's?' What would the nurse respond?
    1. "Has anyone in your family ever been diagnosed with early-onset Alzheimer's, before age 60?"
    2. "You must have had an undiagnosed brain injury at some point in your life."
    3. "I know you are upset but don't think about that now."
    4. "Have you ever been diagnosed with a psychiatric condition?"

65. A client being treated for a myocardial infarction (MI) has been transferred to a medical unit from the Critical Care Unit. The client uses the call bell as often as every 15 minutes. Each time a staff member responds, the client complains about the care or makes seemingly small requests. Several staff tell the primary nurse that the client is "obnoxious." The primary nurse can be most helpful by doing which of the following?
    1. Meet with the client to reassure them and develop coping strategies for their anxiety.
    2. "Laying down the law" to the client, limiting use of the call light to once per hour.
    3. Rotating caregivers to give each person a much-needed respite from the client's complaints.
    4. Asking the client's family to sit with them and help meet their need for attention.

66. The health care provider has prescribed ondansetron (Zofran) 0.1 mg/kg as needed for nausea for a child admitted for vomiting. The child weighs 55 pounds. Calculate the correct dose of Zofran in milligrams. **Record your answer using one decimal place. Fill in the blank.**
    Answer: _____ mg

67. What is the most effective evaluation of a client's response to previous teaching about self-care for their diabetes?
    1. A fasting blood sugar at this visit reading of 6 mmol/L.
    2. The client states they are following a diabetes diet.
    3. The client demonstrates effective insulin injection.
    4. HgA_{1C} has decreased to 6% from 7.2%.

68. A client with dementia has been admitted to the long-term care facility. The client uses a wheelchair during the day. What should the nurse implement for this client to protect against skin breakdown?
    1. Use an appropriate pressure-reduction cushion.
    2. Advise the client to change position every 15 minutes.

3. Encourage the client to stand up and walk whenever possible.
4. Apply medicated pressure dressings to bony prominences.

69. When listening to a client's breath sounds, the nurse is unsure about a sound that is heard. The nurse should take which of the following actions?
    1. Notify the client's health care provider immediately.
    2. Document the sound exactly as it was heard.
    3. Validate the data by asking a colleague to listen to the breath sounds.
    4. Assess again in 20 minutes to note whether the sound is still present.

70. A nurse is preparing a change-of-shift report for a client who had chest pain. Which information is critical for the nurse to include? **Select all that apply.**
    1. "Pupils equal and reactive to light."
    2. "The family is 'difficult.'"
    3. "Had poor results from the pain medication."
    4. "Sharp pain of 8 on a scale of 1 to 10."
    5. "Pain resolved 5 minutes after prn nitroglycerin 0.4 mg sublingual given."

71. A client with COVID-19 has been intubated and ventilated in the Critical Care Unit for 2 weeks. After the client is extubated, they are transferred to a COVID-19 step-down unit. The client is very weak and complains about a sore throat. What should the nurse explain to the client about the probable cause of the sore throat?
    1. "Your sore throat is due to the dry air in the CCU."
    2. "Your sore throat is most likely due to the tube used when you were on the ventilator."
    3. "The medications given to you when you were so sick damage the skin in your throat."
    4. "This is something we see in all clients with COVID-19, but we are not sure why it happens."

72. A 75-year-old woman is admitted to hospital after being hit by a car while on her bicycle. She was wearing a helmet but has significant cuts, bruises, and facial swelling. CT and MRI scans are unremarkable. She has staples in her forehead. She says to the nurse 'Will I need plastic surgery?' What should the nurse respond?
    1. "I can't answer that, you will have to speak with the doctors."
    2. "Yes, but just concentrate on getting better now."
    3. "Perhaps, but you were very lucky to not have any major injuries."
    4. "When the swelling goes down you can be assessed for plastic surgery."

73. A nurse is overheard by a client's family member discussing the condition of the client. The nurse is in violation of which of the following?
    1. Client's informed consent
    2. Right to competent care
    3. *Employment Equity Act*

4. *Personal Information Protection and Electronic Documents Act*

74. The health care provider asks a client to draw a clock showing 10 minutes after 11:00. The client draws the following clock.

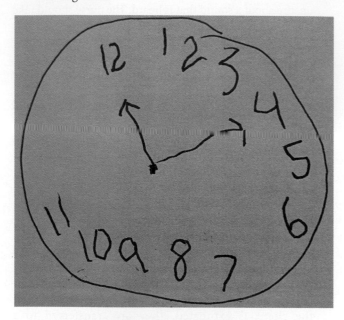

The nurse understands this picture of the clock by the client indicates which of the following?
1. An unreliable test for dementia
2. A score of 1, which indicates the client has Alzheimer's type of dementia
3. Difficulty with the task, suggesting the client may have dementia
4. The test should be repeated several times before a score is determined

75. A client with a new prescription for furosemide (Lasix) is being discharged. What should the nurse say to this client concerning this new prescription?
1. "Keep a weekly journal or log of your weight."
2. "Avoid foods high in potassium, such as bananas, oranges, fresh vegetables, and dates."
3. "If you experience weight gain, such as 2.3 kg or more a week, be sure to tell your health care provider during your next routine visit."
4. "Be sure to change your body position slowly and rise slowly after sitting or lying. This will prevent dizziness and possible fainting because of blood pressure changes."

76. The nurse is working at a COVID-19 vaccination clinic. A client wishes to speak with the nurse about vaccine concerns. Which of the following statements would indicate that a client understands information concerning the COVID-19 mRNA vaccine?
1. "I understand that the vaccine will provide 100% immunity against getting covid."
2. "I know this vaccine is not safe because it was developed too quickly."

3. "I believe having the vaccine is risky because it may alter my DNA."
4. "Having the COVID vaccine will protect me and others from serious COVID disease."

77. The nurse counsels a client on strategies to promote sleep at bedtime. Which of the following would the nurse recommend?
1. Discuss with the client's health care provider use of sleeping pills such as zoplicone (Imovane).
2. Schedule a late evening workout at the gym three times per week.
3. Turn off electronic devices at least an hour before bedtime.
4. Watch an interesting television program in bed.

78. A person with a history of angina experiences chest pain while playing tennis. This person carries sublingual nitroglycerin. The tennis partner is a nurse. Which of the following actions are appropriate in this situation? **Select all that apply.**
1. Stop the activity and advise the person to lie down or sit down.
2. Call 9-1-1 immediately.
3. Place a tablet in the space between the person's gum and cheek.
4. Advise the person to take another sublingual tablet if chest pain is not relieved after 5 minutes.
5. Call 9-1-1 if the pain is not relieved within 5 minutes after taking one sublingual tablet.
6. Remain close by.

79. A nurse would teach a family who have a child with a gluten intolerance that the child should not eat flours made from which of the following?
1. Corn
2. Wheat
3. Rice
4. Soybean

80. A 72-year-old client with a history of moderate heart failure comes to the family practice clinic because of "being awakened from sleep with shortness of breath." Which of the following is the most appropriate first action by the nurse?
1. Advise the client to sleep in an upright position to improve breathing.
2. Refer the client to a sleep clinic for possible sleep apnea.
3. Obtain a history of allergies and asthma.
4. Assess for signs and symptoms of paroxysmal nocturnal dyspnea.

81. The nurse is planning to transfuse a client with a unit of packed red blood cells (PRBCs). Which is the only solution with which PRBCs can be administered?
1. 5% dextrose in water
2. 0.9% sodium chloride
3. 5% dextrose in 0.9% sodium chloride
4. 5% dextrose in lactated Ringer's solution

82. A school nurse suspects one of the adolescent students has undiagnosed social anxiety disorder. The student

avoids groups, is very quiet and shy, and is absent frequently from school. How might the nurse best assist the student?

1. Call the parents to discuss their child's behaviours.
2. Discuss with the student their behaviours and implement referral for counselling.
3. Report the presumed diagnosis to the student's teachers.
4. Speak with other students about how they can help this shy student.

83. A client is in a cardiac rehabilitation program after having myocardial infarction. The client tells the nurse they know they need to exercise but it is just "not for me. I don't like exercise and I don't have the money to join a gym." The nurse suggests exercise activities can be incorporated into activities of daily living (ADLs). Which of the following activities might the nurse suggest? **Select all that apply.**

1. Shovelling snow
2. Vacuuming
3. Dancing
4. Gardening
5. Ironing
6. Climbing stairs

84. A febrile 22-year-old with autism is brought to the clinic by their parents, who are the client's primary caregivers and guardians. They report that although the client can make wishes known the client has limited communication skills, responding with only "yes" or "no" answers to questions. What should the nurse do?

1. Request that the parents leave the interview room to provide client privacy for their adult child.
2. Ask the client: "Do you feel sick today?"
3. Use facial expressions and eye contact to improve understanding.
4. Limit the conversation to just the parents in order to determine correct information.

85. A 3-year-old child has a diagnosis of otitis media. What would the nurse advise to the parents for symptom relief?

1. Warm baths
2. Children's acetaminophen (Tylenol)
3. Cold compresses
4. Saline nasal drops

86. A new parent relates to the nurse that the family has many known food allergies. Which is considered a primary strategy for feeding the infant with many family food allergies?

1. Using soy formula for feeding
2. Breastfeeding to avoid use of cow's milk protein
3. Exclusive breastfeeding for 4 to 6 months
4. Delaying the introduction of highly allergenic foods for 6 months

87. There is an outbreak of tuberculosis in a northern community. The nurse performs tuberculin testing on the children. One child has a positive skin test showing 15 mm induration. What are the immediate implications of this positive test?

1. The child has active tuberculosis.
2. The child will require immediate isolation.
3. The child will be prescribed a 9-month course of isoniazid (INH).
4. The child will require sputum cultures and a chest X-ray.

88. An 85-year-old client who is taking antihypertensive medication tells the nurse about the dizziness they experience getting out of bed in the morning. The nurse suspects orthostatic hypotension. What advice would the nurse suggest to the client? **Select all that apply.**

1. Get up slowly from bed in the morning.
2. Sit on the side of the bed for a few minutes.
3. Stand slowly.
4. Sit down if dizziness occurs.
5. Drink 550 mL of water or juice before getting out of bed.
6. Purchase a home blood pressure monitor; take BP before and after getting out of bed.

89. A client who has been treated for lung cancer for 3 years has noticed that over the past few months the opioid analgesic that is being used is not helping as much and says that taking more medication is needed for the same pain relief. What is this client experiencing?

1. Opioid toxicity
2. Addiction
3. Opioid tolerance
4. Abstinence syndrome

90. A 92-year-old client in a long-term care facility has chronic obstructive pulmonary disease (COPD) requiring long-term supplemental oxygen therapy. Which of the following is the most appropriate delivery system for this client?

1. Simple face mask
2. Low-flow nasal cannula
3. Venturi mask
4. Nonrebreather mask

91. A client is hospitalized due to psychosis as a result of schizoaffective disorder. The client's partner had been attempting to manage them at home because in their culture mental illness is an embarrassment. The client was stabilized on medication and psychotic behaviour disappeared. What would the nurse suggest to the client and partner to assist them in managing this condition in the future?

1. Referral to a cultural healer to help them integrate beliefs within their adopted culture
2. Refrain from discussing the mental health disorder with friends and family
3. Ensure care giving is restricted to the client's partner
4. Advocate for the client to attend self-help groups with people of various cultures.

92. When assessing a client who is receiving a loop diuretic, the nurse assesses for the manifestations of potassium deficiency. Which symptoms are indicative of hypokalemia? **Select all that apply.**
    1. Dyspnea
    2. Anorexia
    3. Tinnitus
    4. Muscle weakness
    5. Mental confusion
    6. Decreased blood pressure

93. Parents call the clinic to ask for advice about their 2-week-old infant, who they say appears to be in pain. The child had a very red diaper rash for 3 days, with open areas oozing blood. There are also white spots in the infant's mouth. What would the nurse advise?
    1. Apply a commercial barrier cream obtained at the pharmacy.
    2. Take the child to the emergency department.
    3. Wash the area with warm water and leave open to air.
    4. Bring the infant to the clinic for diagnosis and possible medication.

94. The nurse participates in a family conference concerning care for an adult child who has a severe disability from an accident. Which of the following is an appropriate initial assessment statement by the nurse?
    1. "Which family members will be primarily responsible for providing care?"
    2. "I assume the mother will be the primary caregiver."
    3. "This must have been a horrible accident. How did it happen?"
    4. "Any family member who will not be providing care does not have to participate in the meeting."

95. A confused client with a urinary catheter, a nasogastric tube, and an intravenous line keeps picking at these items. The nurse has tried to explain to the client that they should not touch them, but the client continues. What is the best action by the nurse at this time?
    1. Apply restraints loosely on the client's dominant wrist.
    2. Try restraint-free approaches to prevent the client from touching these care items.
    3. Notify the health care provider that restraints are needed immediately to maintain the client's safety.
    4. Allow the client to pull out lines to prove that the client needs to be restrained.

96. A nurse begins infusing a 250-mL bag of IV fluid at 0600 hrs and programs the pump to infuse at 20 mL/hr. At what time should the infusion be completed? **Record your answer in international time. Fill in the blank.**
    Answer: ____hr

97. Which allergy would contraindicate the use of silver sulfadiazine as a topical agent for burns?
    1. Penicillin
    2. Iodine
    3. Tetanus immunizations
    4. Sulfa

98. A 48-year-old client is diagnosed with metabolic syndrome and is started on metformin (Glucophage). The client asks the nurse why they need this drug. The nurse would explain that metformin performs which of the following actions?
    1. Increases the pancreatic secretion of insulin
    2. Decreases glucose production by the liver
    3. Increases intestinal absorption of glucose
    4. Decreases the pancreatic secretion of insulin

99. A nurse is shopping in a grocery store on a day off. The nurse observes an infant sitting in a cart eating grapes. The infant suddenly appears acutely distressed, with a weak cough, then turns cyanotic. The nurse understands these are signs of severe airway obstruction. What should the nurse do?
    1. Deliver five back slaps between the infant's shoulder blades, then five chest thrusts.
    2. Sweep the mouth with two fingers to dislodge the aspirated grape.
    3. Circle the infant's chest placing a fist under the sternum and perform rapid abdominal thrusts.
    4. Place the infant on the floor, then administer 5 to 10 rapid chest compressions.

100. The health care provider has prescribed an antihypertensive medication for a client with a BP of 162/91 mm Hg. The client is instructed to purchase a home blood pressure monitor. The nurse instructs the client on proper technique for home monitoring. Which of the following actions should be included in this instruction?
    1. Take BP in the morning before breakfast.
    2. Sit with arm raised and fist closed tightly.
    3. Position cuff in the middle of the upper arm over clothing.
    4. Keep a record of daily readings.
    5. Wait for 1 to 3 minutes after the first reading, then take again to check accuracy.
    6. Measure BP twice daily.

101. A client who has a thriving business as a house cleaner is diagnosed with repetitive strain injury. The client will be unable to continue with their profession, even after surgery and physiotherapy. The client tearfully says to the nurse, "What am I going to do?" How should the nurse respond?
    1. "Do you financially need to work?"
    2. "Cleaning houses is hard work; you will be glad to find something else to do."
    3. "Let's look at what you can do."
    4. "Perhaps in the future you will be able to return to your profession."

102. A client with an end-stage terminal illness says, "I don't have enough energy for many visitors anymore, and I am embarrassed about how I look. I only want to see my parents and sister." What action should the nurse take?

1. Support the client to share the request with the parents and sister. Suggest that they inform the client's friends of the request.
2. Encourage the client to reconsider this decision. Interested and caring friends can be a source of support.
3. Suggest that the client discuss these wishes with the health care provider.
4. Place a "No Visitors" sign on the client's door.

103. A pregnant person comes to the birthing centre in obvious distress and in advanced labour. Which of the following actions represent the best example of culturally appropriate nursing care?
    1. Ask permission before performing a physical assessment.
    2. Consider the person's ethnicity as the most important factor in planning the birth experience.
    3. Ask the person for their birthing plan.
    4. Involve the family members in the assessment interview.

104. When administering morning medications for a newly admitted client, the nurse notes that the client has an allergy to sulfa drugs. The client has an order for sulfonylurea gliclazide (Diamicron). What is the best action for the nurse to take?
    1. Give the drug as ordered 30 minutes before breakfast.
    2. Hold the drug and check the order with the health care provider.
    3. Give the drug and monitor for adverse effects.
    4. Give a reduced dose of the drug with breakfast.

105. Utilizing *Canada's Food Guide* plate, choose the most nutritious lunch to send in a school lunch box for a 6-year-old child.

1. Hot dog in a bun, cheese sticks, sunflower seeds, bottled juice
2. Peanut butter and jelly sandwich, dried cranberries, Jell-O, vitamin water
3. Pizza, fruit bottom yogourt, granola bar, chocolate milk
4. Vegetable slices, whole-wheat crackers and cheese, hard-boiled egg, strawberries, and water

106. A toddler is being sent to the operating room for surgery at 0900. As the nurse prepares the child, what is the priority action?
    1. Administering preoperative antibiotic
    2. Verifying that the child and procedure are correctly identified
    3. Ensuring that the toddler has been NPO since midnight
    4. Informing the parents where they can wait during the procedure

107. Which of the following are indications for negative pressure wound therapy (NPWT)?
    1. Necrotic tissue with eschar present
    2. Osteomyelitis
    3. Older clients with sensitive skin
    4. Chronic and dehisced wounds

108. The nurse performs a nasal swab for methicillin-resistant *Staphylococcus aureus* (MRSA) on a client prior to cardiac bypass surgery. Why is this necessary screening test before surgery?
    1. MRSA can be spread by droplet causing severe respiratory infections.
    2. MRSA can be prevalent in hospitals, causing postoperative infection.
    3. MRSA is a rare infection with a high mortality rate.
    4. All clients are presumed to carry MRSA.

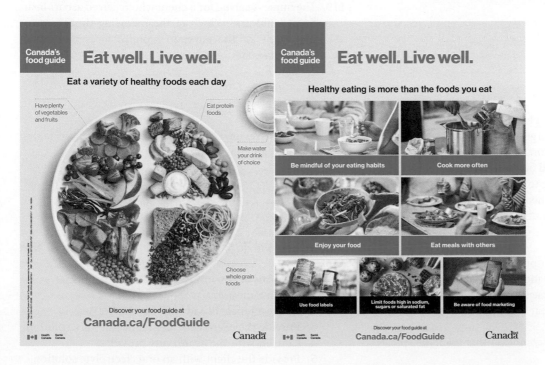

109. Which communicable diseases must be reported in all provinces and territories? **Select all that apply.**
    1. Gonorrhea
    2. Human immunodeficiency virus (HIV)
    3. Herpes simplex virus 2 (HSV-2)
    4. Chlamydia
    5. Infectious syphilis

110. A nurse receives a call at a suicide telephone hotline from a person who says they are going to kill themselves, and they have the gun in their hand to "do it." What is the nurse's priority action?
    1. Notify the supervisor.
    2. Find out more about the gun and suicide plan.
    3. Contact emergency services.
    4. Stay engaged with the person, providing support and counselling.

111. Which general dietary measure should the nurse include in a teaching plan for the child with type 1 diabetes?
    1. Limit intake of carbohydrates and eat fewer calories.
    2. Focus on complex carbohydrates and eat foods high in fibre.
    3. Obtain most calories from proteins and fats.
    4. Eat a low fat and low carbohydrate diet.

112. A parent tells the nurse that they do not want their infant immunized because of the pain associated with injections. What should the nurse explain?
    1. The pain cannot be prevented but it is brief.
    2. Infants do not feel pain as adults do.
    3. This is not a good reason for refusing immunization.
    4. A topical anaesthetic can be applied before injections are given.

113. A client sits in a wheelchair. Where are the potential areas for pressure ulcers and skin breakdown? **Select all that apply.**
    1. Scapula
    2. Occiput
    3. Sacrum
    4. Coccyx
    5. Elbow
    6. Achilles tendon

114. A client arrives at the ambulatory surgery centre for a scheduled outpatient surgery. Which of the following information is of most concern to the nurse?
    1. The client has not had outpatient surgery before.
    2. The client is planning to drive home after surgery.
    3. The client provincial health insurance does not cover the scheduled procedure.
    4. The client had a glass of water a few hours before arriving.

115. A 9-year-old child hospitalized for neutropenia is placed in protective isolation. What is the most appropriate response for a nurse to make when the child asks, "Why do you have to wear a gown and mask when you are in my room?"
    1. "Because you have a condition that could be spread to others."
    2. "To protect you because you could get an infection very easily."
    3. "I'm wearing this because there are a lot of bacteria in the hospital."
    4. "I won't need to wear this after you have had medication for 24 hours."

116. Which of the following would be most important to support wound healing in a 94-year-old malnourished and debilitated client?
    1. Liquid high protein nutritional supplements
    2. High-calorie electrolyte drinks
    3. Servings of red meat at every meal
    4. Vegetable-based soups and purees

117. A client in hospital has died unexpectedly. Which of the following postmortem actions should be performed by the nurse? **Select all that apply.**
    1. Ensure correct identification prior to transfer to the morgue.
    2. Contact next of kin as indicated in the health record.
    3. Prepare the body for family viewing.
    4. Remove all tubes and dressings.
    5. Contact the designated responsible health care provider.
    6. Notify the police as the death was unexpected.

118. Which of these clients should the nurse refer for home health nursing care services?
    1. A 71-year-old with dementia who needs 24-hour care to prevent injury
    2. An 82-year-old whose family has asked for help to organize pills into a pill box
    3. A 67-year-old who requires assistance with shopping, housework, and cooking
    4. A 79-year-old with terminal cancer who needs hospice palliative care

119. The nurse is caring for a client who received aspart insulin at 0800 hrs. Which of the following times is most important for the nurse to monitor for symptoms of hypoglycemia?
    1. 0900 hrs
    2. 1130 hrs
    3. 1600 hrs
    4. 2000 hrs

120. The nurse reviews blood work on a client who is taking diuretics and has been vomiting

Sodium (Na)	128 mmol/L
Potassium (K)	3.0 mmol/L
Magnesium	0.68 mmol/L

What action should be taken by the nurse? **Select all that apply.**
    1. Administer an intravenous bolus of normal saline with magnesium.
    2. Request repeat bloodwork for electrolytes.
    3. Provide the client with an oral magnesium solution.
    4. Consult with the health care provider.
    5. Provide the client with an oral electrolyte solution.

121. The nurse is admitting a female client for an outpatient surgery procedure. Which of the following information is most important to report to the anaesthesiologist before surgery?
    1. The client's lack of knowledge about postoperative pain control measures
    2. The client's statement that their last menstrual period was 8 weeks previously
    3. The client's history of a postoperative infection following a prior cholecystectomy
    4. The client's concern that they will be unable to care for their children postoperatively

122. A nurse works in a long-term care facility. As part of the plan of care, the nurse is preparing to transfer an obese and immobile client to a bedside chair. The nurse says to the client: "We are ready to transfer you to the chair. Do you remember what you can do to help?" The client appears to be unable to comprehend what the nurse is saying. What should the nurse do?
    1. Leave the client in bed as the client does not wish to sit in the chair.
    2. Obtain the assistance of another staff member to transfer the client.
    3. Consider the use of a hydraulic lift.
    4. Reposition the client and turn every 2 hours.

123. The nurse is to insert a nasogastric (NG) tube in an adult client. Which of the following is correct procedure for measurement of the tube?
    1. Measure distance from tip of nose to earlobe to xiphoid process of sternum. Mark this distance on tube with indelible ink.
    2. Measure distance from tip of nose to earlobe to mid-umbilicus. Mark the distance with waterproof tape.
    3. Measure distance from the tip of the nose to the tip of the ear to midsternum. Add 20 cm.
    4. Measure distance from the bridge of the nose to the lower earlobe to midabdomen. Pinch the tube at this spot.

124. The nurse is discussing thyroid replacement therapy and establishing treatment goals with a client. What important adverse effects should the nurse discuss with the client? **Select all that apply.**
    1. Tachycardia
    2. Edema
    3. Dysrhythmias
    4. Weight loss
    5. Fever
    6. Nervousness

125. The nurse is performing a urinary catheterization on a female client. After inserting it 7 cm, there is no urine flow. What should be the next action by the nurse?
    1. Leave the catheter in place. Open another sterile catheter and insert this catheter in the orifice above the in situ catheter.
    2. Remove the catheter and try again to insert it into the urinary meatus.
    3. Advance the catheter another 2 cm.

    4. Flush the catheter with normal saline to determine if there are any obstructions.

126. Psychotropic medications can cause a parasympathetic and/or sympathetic response in the autonomic nervous system. Which of the following is considered a sympathetic response?
    1. Pupil dilation
    2. Increased saliva production
    3. Decreased heart rate
    4. Constricted airway

127. A nurse visits an older person during the summer. The client does not have air conditioning. Which of the following items would help prevent heat stroke in the client?
    1. Fan
    2. Porch chair
    3. Synthetic blend clothing
    4. Atmospheric thermometer

128. A nurse works in an immigrant aid clinic. A recent unemployed refugee to Canada reports being chronically malnourished for the past 10 years while living in a displaced persons' camp. What actions would the nurse take to assist the client accomplishing optimum nutrition? **Select all that apply.**
    1. Ask the client their cultural food preferences.
    2. Determine financial resources for purchasing food.
    3. Referral to local immigrant and refugee food banks.
    4. Give the client a *Canada's Food Guide* pamphlet.
    5. Discuss with the client various diets, including ketogenic, Mediterranean, and paleo.

129. A client has been diagnosed with early-stage dementia. The family wants the client to move into an assisted living facility, but the client refuses, saying "I can look after myself. And I don't want to live with a bunch of sick old people." What is the best approach by the nurse to assist this family?
    1. Refer the family to a social worker who will help them find living accommodation or supports acceptable to the client.
    2. Encourage the family to complete a Power of Attorney form for personal and financial care so they may make accommodation plans for the client.
    3. Discuss with the client that the diagnosis means that assisted living will be needed in the near future.
    4. Accept that the client has the right of self-determination and may live where they wish.

130. A client arrives at the emergency department experiencing a probable fractured arm, rating the pain as 7 out of 10. Which of the following nonpharmacological interventions should the nurse implement for this client while waiting for orders for pain medication from the health care provider?
    1. Frequently reassessing the client's pain score
    2. Reassuring the client they will receive pain medication as soon as the health care provider sees them
    3. Assisting the client to listen to music with their phone and ear buds
    4. Teaching the client how to do relaxation exercises

131. A 23-year-old university student has just been diagnosed with multiple sclerosis. The student wishes to learn about the disease. What would the nurse first advise?
    1. Speak with other people who have multiple sclerosis.
    2. Access reputable websites, for example, the Multiple Sclerosis Society.
    3. Compile a list of question for their next clinic visit.
    4. Go to the university library for specific resources.

132. Which clients meet criteria for hospice services? **Select all that apply.**
    1. A 92-year-old with pneumonia and late-stage Alzheimer's disease
    2. A 74-year-old with advanced COPD self-managed at home
    3. A 54-year-old with glioblastoma and life expectancy of 8 to 10 weeks
    4. A 16-year-old with type 1 diabetes, multiple infections, and substance use disorder
    5. A 36-year-old with multiple sclerosis complicated by depression and pain associated with muscle spasms

133. The nurse observes an unregulated care provider performing the following activities when caring for a client with a pulmonary embolism. Which of the following actions should cause the nurse to intervene with the client's care?
    1. Lowering the head of the client's bed to 10 degrees.
    2. Splinting the client's chest during coughing.
    3. Helping the client ambulate to the bathroom.
    4. Assisting the client to a bedside chair for meals.

134. A man walks into the emergency department and tells the triage nurse that he has severe jaw pain and shortness of breath. The man has come to the emergency department for medication for the pain, which he assumes is a toothache. The nurse applies an ECG and calls the on-duty health care provider. The man asks: "Why all this just for a toothache?" What should the nurse respond?
    1. "This is routine for any person who comes to the emergency department with jaw pain."
    2. "You are likely having a heart attack."
    3. "The jaw pain and shortness of breath are possible symptoms of a cardiac problem, so we need to check this."
    4. "It probably isn't necessary; I am just following protocol for our emergency department."

135. The nurse performs perineal care on an uncircumcised male client. Which of the following describes the correct procedure? **Select all that apply.**
    1. Grasp the shaft firmly but gently.
    2. Pull back the foreskin.
    3. If the client has an erection wait briefly for it to subside.
    4. Wash the penis at the base of the shaft first.
    5. Wash the tip of the penis at the urethral meatus first.
    6. Using an up and down motion, cleanse from the meatus to the base.

136. A new parent is installing a car seat for an infant. Which of the following information should be given to the client by the nurse?
    1. The infant should be in a rear-facing car seat in the front seat.
    2. The infant should be in a rear-facing car seat in the back seat.
    3. The infant should be in a front-facing car seat in the front seat.
    4. The infant should be in a front-facing car seat in the back seat.

137. The nurse counsels a family at a pediatric obesity clinic. The child, age 8 years, is significantly overweight. The mother tells the nurse that the father "gives in" to the child, allowing the child to eat sugary snacks. The father feels the mother is rigid, not allowing the child any treats. How would the nurse respond?
    1. Refer the parents for marriage counselling.
    2. Support the mother in her firm approach to diet.
    3. Support the father in his approach to parenting.
    4. Discuss role modelling healthy eating and having no sugary snacks in the house.

138. The nurse has received a change-of-shift report about the following clients with chronic obstructive pulmonary disease (COPD). Which client should the nurse assess first?
    1. A client with a respiratory rate of 38
    2. A client with loud expiratory wheezes
    3. A client with neck vein distension and peripheral edema
    4. A client who has a cough productive of thick, green mucus

139. Which of the following symptoms indicate a too-high dose of thyroid replacement hormone? **Select all that apply.**
    1. Bradycardia
    2. Insomnia
    3. Weight loss
    4. Dry skin
    5. Anxiety

140. An infant born at 36 weeks' gestation is now 2 hours old. The nurse monitors the infant's vital signs and obtains a temperature of 35.0°C axilla. The nurse understands that this temperature means which of the following?
    1. A sign of neonatal hyperbilirubinemia
    2. A normal value
    3. A need to perform an oral temperature
    4. A sign of cold stress

141. A nurse in a rural farming community visits a family who has been ill with food poisoning. To lower the risk of another episode of food poisoning, the nurse would caution them against eating which of the following?
    1. Unpasteurized dairy products
    2. Packaged deli meat
    3. Cooked eggs
    4. Raw vegetables

142. A client with atopic dermatitis has been using a high-potency topical corticosteroid ointment for several weeks. Which of the findings by the nurse indicates a possible adverse effect of the medication?
    1. Thinning of the affected skin
    2. Alopecia of the affected areas
    3. Reddish-brown discoloration of the skin
    4. Dryness and scaling in the areas of treatment

143. Which electronic health records (EHR) practices are considered to be best practice? **Select all that apply.**
    1. Changing personal EHR password frequently
    2. Charting in a quiet location free of distractions
    3. Sharing passwords only among unit staff involved in client care
    4. Delaying charting until the end of a shift to save time
    5. Logging out whenever not actively engaged in charting

144. In a hospital setting, what is the priority practice by a nurse to ensure administration of the correct medication to the correct client?
    1. Check each client's identification bracelet.
    2. Address each client by their last name prior to administering the medication.
    3. Check each client's health card or hospital identification card.
    4. Check the names that are posted above the client's bed or attached to the bottom of the bed.

145. After assessing the client and identifying the need for headache relief, the nurse administers acetaminophen (Tylenol) for the client's headache. What is the nurse's next priority action?
    1. Determine from the client health history if there are pathological reasons for the headache.
    2. Direct the unregulated care provider to ask if the client's headache is relieved.
    3. Reassess the client's pain level in 30 minutes.
    4. Revise the plan of care.

146. What is the term for the form of behaviour therapy, often used with pedophiles, in which negative reinforcement is used to change behaviour?
    1. Aversion therapy
    2. Conversion therapy
    3. Cognitive behavioural therapy
    4. Biofeedback

147. Which of the following should the nurse do when using electronic health records? **Select all that apply.**
    1. Review the data prior to entering it.
    2. Enter notes in real time.
    3. Provide eye contact with the client.
    4. Cut and paste from previous nursing notes.
    5. Create shortcuts.

148. The nurse admits a client to the rehabilitation unit who has had a stroke. Orders for the client include "ROM as required." What does the nurse understand about this situation?
    1. The nurse should move all the client's extremities.
    2. The client is unable to move their extremities.
    3. Further assessment of the client is required.
    4. The client needs to restrict mobility as much as possible.

149. An 84-year-old client expresses concern about skin bruising and tears, particularly on the arms. What should the nurse advise?
    1. Use tape or adhesive on areas of skin breakdown.
    2. Referral to a dermatologist for treatment.
    3. Restrict exposure to direct sunlight.
    4. Ensure adequate hydration and nutrition.

150. A healthy low-risk person at 38 weeks' gestation who is experiencing regular contractions comes to the prenatal clinic in a small northern Indigenous community. The nurse performs fetal heart monitoring. Which of the following is the correct action by the nurse?
    1. Obtain consent for internal fetal monitoring.
    2. Perform Leopold manoeuvres to determine the correct placement of the external fetal heart rate (FHR) monitor.
    3. Obtain the FHR at the height of contractions with a fetoscope.
    4. Position the client in a supine position if the FHR is below 120 bpm.

151. A client has ophthalmic surgery for a detached retina. Postsurgery, the client must be at home for 2 weeks in a face-down position round the clock, except for brief trips to the washroom. What assistive devices would the nurse recommend? **Select all that apply.**
    1. A padded massage table with opening for the face
    2. A lift chair recliner
    3. A portable hydraulic lift
    4. Periscope type glasses
    5. Straws
    6. An elevated toilet seat

152. What is the priority intervention for a client diagnosed with delirium who has fluctuating levels of consciousness, disturbed orientation, and perceptual alterations?
    1. Distraction using sensory stimulation
    2. Careful observation and supervision
    3. Avoidance of physical contact
    4. Activation of the bed alarm

153. During assessment of a client with decreased renal function, which of the following medications taken by the client at home is of most concern to the nurse?
    1. Ibuprofen
    2. Warfarin
    3. Folic acid
    4. Penicillin

154. Why should the nurse advise parents to have their children receive this vaccine?

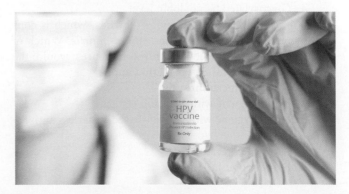

1. It will prevent COVID-19.
2. It will prevent some types of cancer.
3. It is prophylactic against HIV.
4. It will prevent herpes 2.

155. Which of the following best describes the expectations of a nurse caring for an Indigenous client?
1. The nurse should ask an Indigenous colleague to care for this client.
2. Nurses must be knowledgeable about all Indigenous cultures and customs.
3. Nurses should identify client's unique Indigenous cultural practices and plan nursing care accordingly.
4. Nurses must provide care to all clients regardless of their culture.

156. Following total hip replacement surgery, how would the nurse best position the legs of the client?
1. Internally rotated
2. Externally rotated
3. In adduction
4. In abduction

157. The nurse educator conducting an in-service for staff nurses about the importance of client-centred care will discuss which characteristics? **Select all that apply.**
1. Promoting dependence of clients on staff
2. Allowing the client time for questions
3. Supporting the client in making informed decisions
4. Respecting clients' cultural values and needs
5. Incorporating effective teaching methods as appropriate

158. A client has a temporary two-lumen nasogastric tube to decompress the stomach until peristalsis resumes following surgery. The main lumen of the Salem sump tube is connected to suction. Which of the following are correct nursing actions for this client?
1. Clamp off the air vent when indicated.
2. Monitor the abdomen for distension and bowel sounds.
3. Attach the tube to low constant suction.
4. Provide continuous nasogastric feeds via a feeding pump.

159. Which of the following tests will a nurse schedule to assess the effectiveness of treatment for a client with type 2 diabetes?
1. Urine dipstick for glucose
2. Oral glucose tolerance test
3. Fasting blood glucose level
4. Glycosylated hemoglobin level

160. A hospitalized client develops diarrhea, which is confirmed to be caused by *Clostridium difficile*. Which of the following infection control measures would the nurse implement? **Select all that apply.**
1. Contact precautions
2. Hand hygiene with soap and water
3. Hand hygiene with alcohol-based waterless antiseptic
4. Airborne precautions
5. Droplet precautions

161. The nurse takes the health history on four clients in the sleep clinic. Which client information is most important to communicate to the health care provider?
1. A 21-year-old student takes melatonin to assist in sleeping when travelling from Canada to Europe.
2. A 32-year-old who is experiencing a stressful week uses diphenhydramine for several nights.
3. A 41-year-old with a body mass index (BMI) of 42 kg/m^2 says that their spouse complains about the client's snoring.
4. A 64-year-old nurse who works the night shift reports drinking hot chocolate before going to bed in the morning.

162. Why might clients from diverse cultural backgrounds be at risk in a health care setting?
1. Language barriers always interfere with care.
2. Clients' food preferences may not be available.
3. Clients may feel marginalized and not important.
4. There may not be a shared understanding of what is meaningful to the client.

163. When teaching parents how to administer eye drops to their child, where should the nurse tell the parents to place them?
1. At the lacrimal duct
2. On the sclera while the child looks to the side
3. In the conjunctival sac when the lower eyelid is pulled down
4. Carefully under the eyelid while it is gently pulled upward

164. The nurse obtains the following pulse assessments for a 3-month-old infant:

Rate	132 bpm
Rhythm	Irregular
Strength	4+

Evaluate these findings.
1. Normal for age
2. High rate for age
3. Abnormal irregular
4. Too strong, indicating possible cardiac condition

165. A client in the psychiatric emergency department becomes angry, begins to throw objects, and waves a knife in front of the nurse. He insists on leaving against medical advice. What should the nurse do?
1. Call security.
2. Let the client go but call police.
3. Refuse to give the client their personal effects.
4. Allow the client to leave.

166. Near-miss situations, such as a potential medication error, need to be reported for which of the following reasons?
1. Better understanding of communication breakdowns
2. Identifying individuals making errors
3. Identifying improved processes
4. Addressing leadership issues

167. Which of the following statements are true regarding selective serotonin reuptake inhibitors (SSRIs)? **Select all that apply.**
    1. Therapeutic effects may not be seen for about 6 weeks after the medication has started.
    2. SSRIs are associated with fewer adverse effects than are the older first-generation antidepressants.
    3. St. John's Wort is often recommended to reduce the adverse effects that may occur with SSRIs.
    4. A potentially hazardous effect called serotonin syndrome may occur.
    5. They may cause sexual dysfunction.
    6. SSRIs have a relatively high adverse effect profile.

168. Which of the following actions should the nurse take when assisting a totally blind client to walk to the bathroom?
    1. Take the client by the arm and lead the client slowly to the bathroom.
    2. Have the client place a hand on the nurse's shoulder and guide the client.
    3. Stay beside the client and describe any obstacles on the path to the bathroom.
    4. Walk slightly ahead of the client and allow the client to hold the nurse's elbow.

169. The nurse is caring for a client who is taking prednisone 40 mg daily for an exacerbation of rheumatoid arthritis (RA). Which of these assessment data obtained by the nurse indicates that the client is experiencing an adverse effect of the medication?
    1. The client's blood glucose is 9.2 mmol/L.
    2. The client has no improvement in symptoms.
    3. The client has experienced a recent 2.5 kg weight loss.
    4. The client's erythrocyte sedimentation rate (ESR) has increased.

170. Which of the following will help ensure the dignity of older clients, regardless of their cognitive abilities?
    1. Use very simple terms such as "pee pee" for urine.
    2. Engage in conversation with older persons about their lives.
    3. Impose control as much as possible to decrease the stress of decision making.
    4. Call older clients by their first name to promote friendship.

171. The pediatric nurse educator is planning a staff education program about infection control practices. Which of the following disease processes would require contact isolation? **Select all that apply.**
    1. Rotavirus
    2. Hepatitis A
    3. Streptococcal pharyngitis
    4. Mycoplasma pneumonia
    5. Respiratory syncytial virus

172. Because of a COVID-19 outbreak among the nursing staff, a nurse has been moved from the ophthalmology unit to the general surgery unit. The nurse feels inexperienced in this specialty. What should the nurse do?

    1. Politely refuse to move, take the day off, and go home.
    2. Ask to work with an experienced general surgery nurse.
    3. Submit a report noting their dissatisfaction.
    4. Notify the Canadian Nurses Association (CNA) of the issue.

173. The health care provider has written admission orders which the nurse transcribes. The nurse is having difficulty transcribing one order because of the physician's handwriting. The best action for the nurse to take is which of the following?
    1. Ask a colleague what the order says.
    2. Contact the health care provider to clarify the order.
    3. Contact the pharmacy to clarify the order.
    4. Ask the client what medications are being taken at home.

174. A client with terminal stage 4 lung cancer has refused palliative care, informing the nurse they wish to have medical assistance in dying (MAiD). The client's family are very upset and wish treatment, in addition to palliative care, to be continued. What is the best action by the nurse?
    1. Refer the client to the MAiD team.
    2. Discontinue all treatment and palliative care.
    3. Tell the family the client has the right to determine their end of life.
    4. Inform the client they should discuss this with their family before they meet with the MAiD team.

175. Which injection type does the following graphic depict?

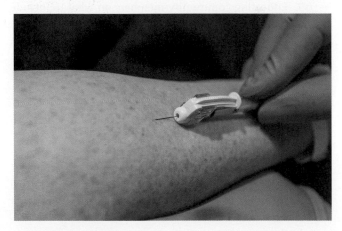

    1. Intramuscular
    2. Intradermal
    3. Subcutaneous
    4. Intravenous

176. The nursing management team in a facility is researching a nursing care delivery model that involves staff members working under the direction of an RN leader. What does this model reflect?
    1. Team nursing
    2. Primary nursing
    3. Functional nursing
    4. Total client care

177. What equipment will the nurse require to perform oropharyngeal suctioning on an adult client?
    1. Sterile saline solution
    2. Yankauer suction catheter
    3. Manual self-inflating resuscitation bag
    4. Flexible # 8 French suction tubing

178. Parents of a toddler with a brain injury who is ventilated have been advised to sign a Do Not Resuscitate (DNR) order for their child. They ask the nurse what this means. What is the best response by the nurse?
    1. This means the health care team will not provide any care
    2. This means the child will be allowed to have a natural death.
    3. This means the child will be removed from the ventilator.
    4. This means the health care team and parents will decide exactly what care will be provided in a terminal situation.

179. A nurse is participating in disaster preparedness planning for the local community. Which of the following would be an appropriate responsibility for the nurse? **Select all that apply.**
    1. Working to reduce hazards in the home and work settings
    2. Implementing strategies to decrease post-traumatic stress disorder (PTSD)
    3. Participating in drills and training exercises
    4. Evaluating the economic impact of the disaster
    5. Educating community members on what to include in an emergency preparedness kit

180. The student nurse practices blood pressure monitoring using an electronic device. The student nurse is aware that too loose a cuff may cause which of the following errors?
    1. False low systolic reading
    2. False low diastolic reading
    3. False high systolic reading
    4. False low systolic and diastolic reading

181. A young woman is brought to the emergency department by police. She is hysterical and crying, saying she has been raped at a party. Using the principles of crisis management, what is the nurse's first action?
    1. Reassure the client she is safe now.
    2. Place her in a private room apart from other emergency room clients.
    3. Console her, reassuring her that everything will be okay.
    4. Ask her exactly what happened to her.

182. The nurse is preparing an airborne infection isolation room for a client. Which of the following communicable diseases does the client likely have?
    1. Varicella
    2. Pertussis
    3. Influenza
    4. Scarlet fever

183. The nurse performs a physical assessment on an 80-year-old client, and observes the posture as seen in the picture below. What is the term for this posture?

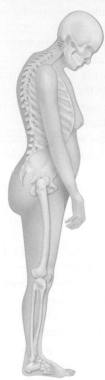

    1. Scoliosis
    2. Kyphosis
    3. Lordosis
    4. Normal age-related posture

184. The nurse is changing linens for a postoperative client and feels a needlestick in their hand. A non-activated safe needle is noted in the linens. In this scenario, the nurse may be at risk for which of the following infections?
    1. Hepatitis B
    2. *C. difficile*
    3. Methicillin-resistant *S. aureus* (MRSA)
    4. Diphtheria

185. Which of the following sensory changes are normal with aging?
    1. Impairment of night vision
    2. Difficulty hearing low-pitch sounds
    3. Increase in sense of taste
    4. Heightened sense of smell

186. Choose recommended methods to decrease the incidence, prevalence, and morbidity of COVID-19. **Select all that apply.**
    1. Wear a securely fitting mask in public.
    2. Maintain a distance of 3 metres from others.
    3. Choose open spaces, preferable outdoors, over inside spaces.
    4. Always cough into your hand.
    5. Stay home if you feel unwell.
    6. Clean hands frequently only with alcohol-based sanitizer.

187. The nurse is helping a client take their medications; however, the medication cup falls to the floor, spilling the contents. Which of the following is the appropriate action for the nurse to take?
    1. Discard the medications and repeat the preparation.
    2. Document the client's refusal of the medications.
    3. Wait until the next dosage time, then give the medications.
    4. Retrieve the medications and administer them to avoid waste.

188. An older person is being placed on an ACE inhibitor. What should the nurse inform the client with regard to this medication? **Select all that apply.**
    1. Avoid rapid position changes.
    2. Increase intake of potassium.
    3. Adverse effects may include cough.
    4. Take the medication with meals.
    5. Stay well hydrated.

189. The nurse visits a bedridden client and the caregiver spouse. The caregiver says that looking after their spouse is an expected duty but is exhausting, as expected. The couple's children help out whenever they are in town. The caregiver appears thin, weak, and exhausted, and the nurse notices that several of the client's prescription medication bottles are empty. This situation is best described by which term?
    1. Physical abuse
    2. Financial neglect
    3. Psychological abuse
    4. Unintentional neglect

190. An 82-year-old client makes an appointment at the family practice clinic because they have noticed increased bruising and bleeding when they brush their teeth. The client tells the nurse they have been taking a "children's Aspirin" because they have read it is helpful to prevent heart attacks and strokes. What should the nurse advise the client?
    1. "These are symptoms of a blood cancer, and you must see your health care provider."
    2. "The bruising and bleeding may be caused by the acetylsalicylate acid (Aspirin), you should speak with the health care provider about whether it is necessary for you."
    3. "You should not take any medication, even if it is over the counter, without consulting your health care provider."
    4. "Bruising of the skin and bleeding gums are normal at your age because the skin and mucous membranes are thinner."

191. A family has removed their parent from a long-term care facility because they are concerned about an unsafe level of care and worry their parent might contract COVID-19. The client is currently well. What would the nurse advise them about COVID-19 precautionary care of the parent? **Select all that apply.**
    1. Perform rapid antigen tests every 2 to 3 days, or if symptomatic.

    2. Monitor for signs and symptoms of COVID-19.
    3. Ensure they have polymerase chain reaction (PCR) testing every 2 days, performed by a lab.
    4. Purchase an oxygen saturation monitor.
    5. Maintain strict isolation precautions.
    6. Monitor vital signs every 4 hours.

192. A new nurse says, "My client has Lewy body disease. What should I do about assessing for pain?" Select the best response by the nurse educator.
    1. "Ask the client's family if they think the client is experiencing pain."
    2. "Use a visual analogue scale to help the client determine the presence and severity of pain."
    3. "There are special scales for assessing pain in clients with dementia. Let's review how to use them."
    4. "The perception of pain is diminished by this type of dementia. Focus your assessment on the client's mental status."

193. A nurse volunteers in the first aid centre at a marathon race. A runner is brought to the centre, having collapsed on route. The runner is conscious, but the nurse assesses signs of dehydration: increased pulse, low blood pressure and confusion. Which of the following interventions is the most important for the nurse to implement?
    1. Ask another volunteer to find a health care provider immediately.
    2. Start an intravenous (IV) with normal saline.
    3. Administer oral rehydration therapy.
    4. Monitor vital signs.

194. Which of the following chemical substances produced in the body act as natural pain relievers?
    1. Adrenaline
    2. Endorphins
    3. Cortisol
    4. Insulin

195. Which of the following are components of physical care with the terminally ill client? **Select all that apply.**
    1. Restrain the client if they become agitated.
    2. Provide favourite foods.
    3. Do not force food or fluids.
    4. Advocate for alternate routes if oral pain medications are not effective.
    5. Ensure the client does not mobilize.
    6. Ensure pain medications are administered on a strict schedule.

196. An 8-year-old child is 12 hours post–cardiac surgery. The nurse notices the child is holding themselves rigid, has perspiration on their forehead, and is grimacing. When the nurse asks if they would like medicine for pain, the child refuses. What would be the next action by the nurse?
    1. Ask the child to complete a pediatric pain scale assessment.
    2. Respect the child's wishes.
    3. Tell the child they may have a pill, not a needle, to help with their pain.
    4. Ask the parents to convince their child to have pain medication.

197. What security measure should a nurse implement when bringing an infant from the neonatal unit to the child-bearing parent?
    1. Ask the child-bearing parent, "Is this your ID bracelet number?"
    2. Confirm room number of the child-bearing parent.
    3. Ask the child-bearing parent to identify themselves verbally.
    4. Check the ID bracelet number of the infant with that of the child-bearing parent.

198. Which of the following assessments would indicate infiltration of a client's IV line? **Select all that apply.**
    1. Edema of the extremity near the insertion site
    2. Skin discoloured or bruised in appearance
    3. Skin cool to the touch
    4. Reddish streak proximal to the insertion site
    5. Numbness or loss of sensation
    6. No blood return when briefly disconnected

199. Which of the following may be a risk factor for Alzheimer's disease (AD)
    1. Lyme disease
    2. Depression
    3. Obesity
    4. Low vitamin D levels

200. Clients who are placed on spironolactone (Aldactone) should be assessed continuously for which condition?
    1. Hypokalemia
    2. Hyperkalemia
    3. Hyponatremia
    4. Hypercalcemia

201. A nurse performs a preoperative assessment with a client. The client states they are allergic to penicillin. Which of the following is the best response to this information?
    1. Are you allergic to any other drugs?
    2. How often have you received penicillin?
    3. I will make note of your allergy in the chart so that you will not receive any.
    4. What happens to you when you have penicillin?

202. A client with type 2 diabetes, obesity, and cardiovascular disease must plan a low-fat low sodium approximate 500-calorie lunch. Of the following menu items, which foods should the client choose for lunch? **Select all** foods that would be included to meet the caloric and nutritional goals for lunch.
    1. Macaroni and cheese – 425 calories
    2. Orange juice – 120 calories
    3. Tuna salad – 225 calories
    4. Carrot and cucumber sticks with dipping sauce – 130 calories
    5. Canned vegetable soup – 325 calories
    6. Two servings of raspberries and blueberries – 110 calories

203. A nurse discusses child-proofing the home for safety with the parent of a 9-month-old infant. Which statement made by the parent would indicate an unsafe behaviour?
    1. "I put covers on all of the electrical outlets."
    2. "In the car, she rides in a front-facing car seat."
    3. "There are locks on all of the cabinets in the house."
    4. "I have a gate at the top and bottom of the stairs."

204. The quality improvement (QI) committee has been alerted to an increased number of falls in the hospital. Most of these falls have occurred at night and have involved clients who were trying to crawl over bed rails. The committee created a practice change stating that bed rails should be left in the down position, and hourly nursing rounds should be conducted. What is the committee's next step?
    1. Evaluate the changes in 1 month.
    2. Wait a month before implementing the changes.
    3. Implement the changes as a pilot study.
    4. Communicate the planned practice change to staff.

205. The nurse has just received a change-of-shift report about the following four clients. Which client should the nurse assess first?
    1. 38-year-old who has pericarditis and is complaining of sharp, stabbing chest pain
    2. 45-year-old who had a myocardial infarction (MI) 4 days ago and is anxious about the planned discharge
    3. 51-year-old with unstable angina who has just returned to the unit after having a percutaneous coronary intervention (PCI)
    4. 60-year-old with variant angina who is to receive a scheduled dose of nifedipine (Adalat)

206. A newly hired but experienced nurse is preparing to change a client's abdominal dressing. The nurse has not done performed this procedure at this hospital before. Which action by the nurse is appropriate?
    1. Ask another nurse to do it so the correct method can be viewed.
    2. Check the policy and procedure manual for the agency's method.
    3. Change the dressing using the method taught in nursing school.
    4. Ask the client how the dressing change has been recently done.

207. A nurse is creating a plan to reduce data entry errors in the electronic health record and maintain client confidentiality. Which guidelines should the nurse include? **Select all that apply.**
    1. Create a password with just letters.
    2. Bypass the firewall.
    3. Use a programmed speed-dial key when faxing.
    4. Implement an automatic sign-off.
    5. Impose disciplinary actions for inappropriate access.
    6. Shred papers containing personal health information.

208. A client's plan of care includes the goal of increasing mobility. As the client is ambulating to the bathroom at the beginning of the shift, the client experiences a fall. How should the nurse first revise the plan of care?
    1. Ask physiotherapy to assist the client because of the new injuries.
    2. Disregard all previous diagnoses and establish a new plan of care.

3. Reassess the client.

4. Set new priorities for the client.

209. A client arrives in the emergency department of a small community hospital. The client gestures to the nurse they are deaf and cannot speak. The client is not accompanied by any friend or family and appears to be in pain. Which of the following would be the first action for the nurse to obtain relevant information regarding the client's need for emergency services?

1. Provide the client with an electronic device to type out a message.

2. Obtain the services of a deaf interpreter.

3. Face the client and speak slowly and carefully to enable lip reading.

4. Demonstrate to the client to use hand gestures to illustrate symptoms.

210. An unconscious client with a head injury needs immediate life-saving surgery. The client's family speaks only French, and the health care providers, who are not fluent in French, are having a difficult time explaining the client's condition to them. In this situation, what must the nurse know?

1. Two registered health care workers should witness and sign the preoperative consent form indicating that they heard an explanation of the procedure given in English.

2. An ethical review board must be contacted to give its emergency advice on the situation.

3. A friend of the family may act as an interpreter, but the explanation cannot contain details of the client's accident because of confidentiality laws.

4. The health care team should continue with the surgery after providing information in the best possible manner.

211. The nurse is providing anticipatory guidance to the parents of a 1-month-old infant on preventing a suffocation injury. Which should the nurse include in the teaching? **Select all that apply.**

1. Do not place pillows in the infant's crib.

2. Crib slats should be 10 cm or less apart.

3. Keep all plastic bags stored out of the infant's reach.

4. Plastic over the mattress is acceptable if it is covered with a sheet.

5. A pacifier should not be tied on a string around the infant's neck.

212. The nurse assesses a client's ability to manage home oxygen care for chronic obstructive pulmonary disease (COPD) postdischarge from hospital. What would be the priority assessment?

1. Client's physical and cognitive ability to perform home oxygen monitoring

2. Client's preference for an oxygen concentrator or liquid oxygen system

3. Client's ability to obtain home oxygen services via insurance or government programs

4. Client's access to community resources such as respiratory therapists

213. A client with dementia is receiving oxygen at 4 litres per minute via nasal prongs. Which of the following are nursing considerations for this client? **Select all that apply.**

1. Monitor frequently as the cannula is easily dislodged.

2. Ensure the prongs are positioned correctly in the nares.

3. Do not use with a portable oxygen canister.

4. Assess nasal mucosa for irritation and drying effects of oxygen.

5. Monitor oxygen saturation levels as per agency policy.

6. Apply mittens or hand restraints to prevent dislodging of the cannula.

214. A hospitalized client has a temperature of 39.5°C. In addition to administering antipyretics, what actions should be taken by the nurse to reduce the fever?

1. Place the client in a cool bath.

2. Reduce external covering on client's body.

3. Provide an alcohol sponge bath.

4. Give the client ice chips.

215. A nurse visits a relative in a long-term care facility. The nurse observes that hygiene standards, infection control, and cleanliness have deteriorated, and the relative appears to be neglected. What should the nurse do?

1. Speak with the manager of the long-term care home.

2. Provide hygienic care to the relative.

3. Ask other visitors to the home if they have the same concerns.

4. Complain to the Ministry of Health and Long Term Care about this facility.

216. A woman has just given birth to her first child. She tells the nurse, in her culture babies are not breastfed. What is the appropriate action for the nurse?

1. Explain to the woman the benefits of breastfeeding.

2. Ask the woman what culture has this practice.

3. Encourage the woman to put the child to breast to develop a sucking reflex, which will be necessary for bottle feeding.

4. Assist the woman to apply a snug-fitting bra and apply ice packs for engorgement.

217. A nurse works at an esthetician's office, providing services to clients requesting anti-aging procedures. Which of the following are skills that may be expected of the nurse in this setting? **Select all that apply.**

1. Intake interview to assess client wishes concerning anti-aging procedures

2. Assessment of client overall general health

3. List of prescription and over-the-counter medications

4. Discussing with potential clients financial cost of various procedures

5. Obtaining consent for any surgical procedures

6. Initiating anaesthesia for procedures

218. Before the administration of preoperative medications, a client says, "I do not really understand what the doctor said about my operation." Which of the following actions is best for the nurse to take?

1. Provide an explanation of the planned surgical procedure.

2. Notify the surgeon that the informed-consent process is not complete.

3. Administer the prescribed preoperative antibiotics and withhold any ordered sedative medications.

4. Notify the operating room staff that the surgeon needs to give a more complete explanation of the procedure.

219. A nurse is conducting a community health education program about osteoporosis with a group of older persons. Which of the following individuals in attendance is at greatest risk for developing osteoporosis? **Select all that apply.**

1. A 65-year-old Asian woman who smokes one pack of cigarettes per week

2. An 81-year-old White man who drinks three glasses of wine per day

3. A 74-year-old White woman on daily oral prednisone for emphysema

4. A 68-year-old Black man who has a sedentary lifestyle

5. A 72-year-old Indigenous man who regularly hunts in cold, damp weather

220. A client returns to the unit after a cardiac catheterization via the femoral artery. How should the nurse position the client?

1. High semi-Fowler's with leg elevated

2. Side-lying, recovery position with leg on pillows

3. Flat, with leg extended

4. Recumbent, with legs flexed

221. The nurse is caring for a client who has pneumonia and is prescribed gentamicin 60 mg IV. Which of the following parameters should the nurse monitor to evaluate the client for adverse effects of the medication?

1. Urine osmolality

2. Serum potassium

3. Blood glucose level

4. Blood urea nitrogen (BUN) and creatinine

222. A client tells the nurse they have been taking laxatives three times a day to lose weight. After stopping the laxative, the client had difficulty with constipation, and wonders if they should resume taking laxatives. Which of the following teaching points should the nurse discuss with the client?

1. Long-term laxative use causes the bowel to become less responsive to normal evacuation stimuli, and constipation may occur so laxatives should be avoided.

2. Laxatives can cause trauma to the intestinal lining, causing scarring which decreases peristalsis.

3. Natural laxatives such as mineral oil are safer than chemical laxatives for relieving constipation.

4. Laxatives cause the body to become malnourished so when they are stopped, the body absorbs all the food, and no waste products are produced.

223. The nurse is preparing to admit a client who has been treated for status epilepticus in the emergency department. Which of the following equipment should the nurse have available in the room? **Select all that apply.**

1. Side rail pads

2. Tongue blade

3. Oxygen mask

4. Suction tubing

5. Nasogastric tube

224. The charge nurse observes a new nurse providing discharge teaching for a client who is hypertensive and has a new prescription for enalapril (Vasotec). Which of the following instructions to the client by the new nurse should cause the charge nurse to intervene in the client's care?

1. Check your BP with a home BP monitor every day.

2. Move slowly when changing position from lying to standing.

3. Increase your dietary intake of high-potassium foods.

4. Make an appointment with the dietitian for teaching.

225. A client who is receiving chemotherapy develops a *Candida albicans* oral infection. Which of the following actions should the nurse anticipate?

1. Hydrogen peroxide rinses

2. The use of antiviral agents

3. Referral to a dentist for professional tooth cleaning

4. Administration of nystatin oral rinse

226. The nurse manager recognizes a need to take steps to promote conflict resolution among health care team members on a nursing unit. What intervention will promote conflict resolution most effectively?

1. Soliciting the perspectives of the nurses

2. Encouraging socializing among group members

3. Promoting certain individuals within the group

4. Depersonalizing conflict situations

227. What are some of the characteristics of systemic corticosteroid drugs? **Select all that apply.**

1. Inhibits inflammatory and allergic reactions

2. Effective vasodilator

3. Prolonged use could suppress a child's growth

4. Dosage should be gradually tapered

5. Possess antimicrobial properties

6. May cause edema and weight gain

228. A client has refused to undergo an invasive procedure that could possibly extend their life by a few months. The nurse supports the client's decision based on which essential value?

1. Equality

2. Truth

3. Human dignity

4. Autonomy

229. The elderly partner of a client with Alzheimer's disease states that their spouse seems to wander aimlessly from room to room placing things in incorrect places, such as kitchen utensils in the bedroom and laundry detergent in the kitchen. The partner asks the nurse for suggestions of what they can do to help. What is the nurse's best response?

1. "Keep rooms well lit."

2. "Keep the home environment simple and user friendly for her."

3. "Have clocks and calendars with large letters in several rooms of the house."

4. "Place large signs on doors or entryways that identify the room."

230. A client has experienced a massive stroke and is no longer able to chew or swallow foods or fluids. Insertion of a gastric tube is discussed with the family as the client is not able to communicate. Which of the following is the priority to be considered in this situation?

1. The gastric tube will offer life-sustaining nutrition.

2. The gastrostomy tube will not be able to replace the social and symbolic benefits of sharing meals.

3. The gastric tube will enhance the quality of life for the client.

4. The cultural, spiritual, psychological, and advance directives by the client should be considered.

231. A preceptor is supervising a new nurse on documentation. Which situation will cause the preceptor to intervene? **Select all that apply.**

1. The new nurse charts consecutively on every other line.

2. The new nurse documents a medication given by another nurse.

3. The new nurse uses a black ink pen to chart.

4. The new nurse keeps the password secure.

5. The new nurse ends each entry with signature and title.

232. A client has a PEG tube inserted. The nurse provides postoperative instructions to the client before discharge. The client asks the nurse: "Can I eat and drink by mouth with a PEG tube?" How should the nurse respond?

1. "Most people receive food and liquid only through the tube."

2. "You will not be allowed to take food or liquids by mouth."

3. "You may still eat and drink small amounts through the mouth."

4. "You will need to speak with your health care provider about eating and drinking restrictions."

233. The nurse is preparing to administer a measles, mumps, rubella, and varicella (MMRV) vaccine. Which of the following is a contraindication associated with administering this vaccine?

1. The child has recently been exposed to an infectious disease.

2. The child has symptoms of a cold but no fever.

3. The child is having intermittent episodes of diarrhea.

4. The child has a disorder that causes a deficient immune system.

234. The nurse is caring for a client with expressive aphasia caused by a traumatic brain injury. What should be the desired outcome in the plan of care?

1. Client will recover full use of speech by discharge.

2. Client will use pen and paper for communication.

3. Client will thicken drinks to prevent aspiration.

4. Client will learn nonverbal communication strategies.

235. The nurse is counselling an older person on ways to prevent falls. Which of the following information should the nurse include?

1. Purchase heavyweight throw rugs.

2. Most falls happen outside the home.

3. Buy shoes that provide good support and are comfortable to wear.

4. Range-of-motion exercises should be taught by a physiotherapist.

236. A nurse volunteered to work at the site of a recent natural disaster. A 26-year-old male victim, who has experienced trauma, cries almost constantly and says, "Why did this happen to me? I have nothing left." Which of the following questions should the nurse ask to determine if the victim has suicide ideation?

1. "Tell me about your life."

2. "What do you do for work? How has your work been affected by this disaster?"

3. "Have you thought of harming yourself?"

4. "Have you seen your friends since the disaster?"

237. The nurse is teaching a client about using hydrochlorothiazide. The nurse should ensure that the client knows to be cautious when taking which medication with hydrochlorothiazide?

1. Digitalis

2. Antacids

3. Potassium supplements

4. Over-the-counter acetylsalicylate (Aspirin) preparations

238. A health care provider has prescribed gentamicin 6 mg/kg a day divided q8h intravenously for a child with a urinary tract infection. The child weighs 20.5 kg. The medication label states: "Gentamicin 20 mg/2 mL." The nurse is preparing to administer the 0600 dose. How many millilitres will the nurse prepare to administer one dose? **Record your answer using one decimal place. Fill in the blank.**

Answer: _____ mL

239. A friend of a nurse says they have heard about wastewater testing for COVID-19 and insists it is more fake news from the government. What factual response would be appropriate by the nurse?

1. "It is true, you cannot screen for COVID-19 in sewer water."

2. "People infected with SARS-CoV-2 can shed the virus in their feces, which then gets into the public sewer system."

3. "This was a hypothesis by the COVID-19 researchers but was proved untrue."

4. "COVID-19 can only be tracked by positive rapid or PCR tests."

240. The nurse provides postoperative teaching for a client who has just had bilateral cataract surgery with lens implantation. Which statement by the client demonstrates understanding of the health teaching?

1. I should sleep face down, on my stomach.

2. I should not cough, or strain when having a bowel movement.

3. I should only use the eye drops if my eyes feel irritated.

4. I should wear my glasses at night when in bed.

241. A 12-year-old child has just been diagnosed with type 1 diabetes. The child tells the nurse they don't understand diabetes. How would the nurse initially best explain diabetes to a 12-year old?

1. "Insulin is a hormone produced by the beta cells in the islets of Langerhans of the pancreas. Insulin transports glucose across the cell membrane into the body."

2. "A special organ in your body called a *pancreas* makes insulin, which helps your body use the food you eat. If the pancreas does not make enough insulin, you cannot use the food you eat, and you develop a disease called *diabetes*."

3. "Diabetes is a very serious disease. You get too much sugar in the blood and will need to have insulin needles for your entire life."

4. "Diabetes is a multisystem disease related to abnormal insulin production, impaired insulin utilization, or both. It is a serious health problem throughout the world, particularly in Indigenous populations like yours."

242. A client is recovering from an intestinal volvulus which has caused an obstruction. The nurse receives orders to remove the nasogastric (NG) tube. What assessment should the nurse perform prior to removal of the NG tube?

1. The colour of the NG drainage is yellow or light green.

2. Bowel sounds are audible in all four quadrants.

3. The client has stopped vomiting.

4. The client has passed stool.

243. A pregnant client has an abdominal ultrasound at 20 weeks' gestation. What is the most important reason for this test?

1. To assess fetal well-being

2. To determine if the fetus is a boy or girl

3. To assess the need for amniocentesis

4. To confirm the gestational age

244. Which situation will cause the nurse to intervene and follow up on the unregulated care provider's behaviour?

1. The unregulated care provider is calling the older client "honey."

2. The unregulated care provider is facing the older client when talking.

3. The unregulated care provider cleans the older client's glasses.

4. The unregulated care provider allows time for the older client to respond.

245. A postsurgical client has an intravenous line for fluids and medication administration and nasogastric tube for enteral feedings. Calculate the fluid volume excess or deficit for an 8-hour time frame.

Intake

IV	400 mL
NG	600 mL
Sips of water	30

Output

Urine	350
Wound drainage	85
Emesis	120

246. A 37-week pregnant client in a remote community calls the nursing station. The client tells the nurse they have gained 3 kg weight in the past few days, have a terrible headache that started this morning, and are "seeing stars." What would the nurse advise?

1. Find transport to the nursing station immediately.

2. Check well-being of the baby by performing a fetal kick count test.

3. Go to the nearest pharmacy to take their blood pressure.

4. Lie down, restrict fluids, take acetaminophen (Tylenol) for the headache. Call back to the nursing station in 6 hours.

247. A client with dysphagia is to have a percutaneous endoscopic gastrostomy (PEG) tube inserted. Although the surgeon has obtained informed consent, the nurse reinforces teaching with the client. What will the nurse explain to the client about the procedure?

1. "The surgeon will make a small incision in your upper abdomen and place the tube through the incision into your stomach."

2. "The PEG tube is inserted via a stab wound through the abdominal musculature to the jejunum then sutured in place."

3. "A long gastrostomy tube is threaded down your esophagus to your stomach."

4. "A small flexible feeding tube is tunnelled through your skin and into your intestine."

248. A health care provider has prescribed phenobarbital for a child with seizures. The child weighs 16 kg. The recommended dosage is 6 to 8 mg/kg/24 hr. What is the safe dosage range of this medication for the child?

1. 96 mg/day to 128 mg/day

2. 144 mg/day to 192 mg/day

3. 6 mg/day to 8 mg/day

4. 22 mg/day to 24 mg/day

249. The bed position shown in the picture below, where the head of the bed is raised to an angle of 45 to 90 degrees, is used when clients are eating and promotes lung expansion. What is the term for this position?

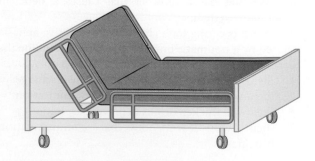

1. Trendelenberg
2. Fowler's
3. Recovery
4. Supine

250. The nurse assesses capillary refill in a cardiac client. Which of the following is the correct procedure and result?

1. Grasp the client's fingernail, apply forceful pressure, observe colour change after 2 minutes.
2. Exert firm pressure on the nail, observe time for blanching to occur.
3. Apply gentle, firm pressure to nail bed, release quickly, colour should return in 2 seconds.
4. Squeeze nail bed tightly, release, pink colour should return in 10 seconds.

ANSWERS AND RATIONALES FOR REX-PN PRACTICE EXAM BOOK TWO

The correct answer is set off in **boldface**.

1. **Client Needs: Safe and Effective Care Environment T: Critical Thinking**
   1. This client also requires nursing assessment but is not at risk for life-threatening complications.
   2. As in choice 1.
   3. **Initiation of thyroid replacement in older persons may cause angina and cardiac dysrhythmias. The client's high pulse rate needs rapid investigation by the nurse to assess for and intervene with any cardiac problems.**
   4. As in choice 1.

2. **Client Needs: Physiological Integrity T: Knowledge**
   1. Application of heat is not required.
   2. It is not recommended to massage the area.
   3. There is no need to report the bleb to the physician.
   4. **The formation of a small bleb is expected after an intradermal injection for skin testing if correct technique is used.**

3. **Client Needs: Psychosocial Integrity T: Knowledge**
   1. **Confabulation (the creation of stories or answers in place of actual memories, in an attempt to maintain self-esteem); it is not the same as lying because it is done unconsciously.**
   2. Lying is deliberately not telling the truth.
   3. Denial is refusing to believe something is true.
   4. Perseveration is the repetition of phrases or behaviour.

4. **Client Needs: Health Promotion and Maintenance; T: Knowledge**
   1. **Two red lines are indicative of a positive rapid antigen test for COVID-19**
   2. This is not correct.
   3. As in choice 2.
   4. As in choice 2.

5. **Client Needs: Safe and Effective Care Environment T: Knowledge**
   1. This choice would not allow sufficient time to make the necessary arrangements for discharge.
   2. **Discharge planning should be initiated as soon as possible after the client is admitted so that ample time is allowed to make necessary plans for sending the client home or discharging them to another facility.**
   3. As in choice 1.
   4. As in choice 1.

6. **Client Needs: Health Promotion and Maintenance; T: Knowledge**
   1. **This is an expected developmental task for the middle adolescent.**
   2. This is a task for late adolescence.
   3. This is a task for early adolescence.
   4. As in choice 3.

7. **Client Needs: Physiological Adaptation; T: Critical Thinking**
   1. **This is called a "silent chest" and is an ominous sign that the airway is so inflamed air is not able to move.**
   2. This is a slightly elevated respiratory rate, as expected during an asthma episode.
   3. Asthma attacks are quite tiring for the client; sleepiness is to be expected.
   4. Mild, rather than pronounced, indrawing may be a sign the treatment is effective.

8. **Client Needs: Safe and Effective Care Environment T: Application**
   1. **Reassessments should be included in the client's health record.**
   2. Incident reports are not documented in the client's chart.
   3. **Initial assessments should be included in the client's health record.**
   4. **Nursing care provided should be included in the client's health record.**
   5. **The client's response to care provided should be included in the client's health record.**

9. **Client Needs: Physiological Integrity T: Knowledge**
   1. **This is the correct term.**
   2. This is not the correct term.
   3. As in choice 2.
   4. As in choice 2.

10. **Client Needs: Safe and Effective Care Environment T: Application**
    1. **Many products that contain latex are used in the operating suite and the postanaesthesia care unit (PACU). For a client with this allergy, special considerations are required for preparation of the room and the types of tubes, gloves, drapes, and instruments utilized. Ensuring that the client has a safe environment takes time, and if the correct supplies are not available, awaiting their arrival may cancel or delay the surgery.**

2. This is part of the process and should be done with the latex allergy in mind however, making sure that the operating suite and PACU are safe environments is the first step.
3. As in choice 2.
4. As in choice 2.

11. **Client Needs: Health Promotion and Maintenance; T: Application**
    1. **Lollipops may cause injury if the child falls.**
    2. Toddlers and preschoolers are capable of navigating stairs.
    3. **Children need to be taught stranger-danger.**
    4. This is a safety strategy for infants.
    5. **Children are curious and love candy; they may view harmful medications or parent's edible cannabis as something sweet to eat.**
    6. **Children like to reach heights; they could pull boiling foods on top of themselves.**

12. **Client Needs: Physiological Integrity T: Critical Thinking**
    1. The route should not be changed without a health care provider's order.
    2. The morning dose should not be given with a small sip of water.
    3. **The health care provider should be contacted for an order of the appropriate dosage form of the medication.**
    4. Withholding the medication may lead to seizure activity during the surgical procedure.

13. **Client Needs: Health Promotion and Maintenance; T: Critical Thinking**
    1. **All of the answers may provide some follow-up. With clients with eating disorders, the most appropriate evaluation activity is to monitor if weight gain is actually occurring.**
    2. This may help but does not assure the nurse of compliance and achievement of goals.
    3. As in choice 2; the client may not accurately report daily weight.
    4. As in choice 2.

14. **Client Needs: Physiological Integrity T: Application**
    Answer: 4.0
    Rationale:
    Step 1: Use the formula for calculations for pediatric dosages of oral and parenteral medications.
    Step 2: Use the formula for calculation of oral and parenteral doses of medications.
    Formula:
    Step 1:

    $$\frac{\text{Drug dosage per}}{\text{kg of body weight}} \times \text{Weight of child (kg)}$$
    $$= \text{Dosage to administer}$$

Step 2:

$$\frac{\text{Dosage ordered}}{\text{Dosage available}} \times \text{Drug form}$$
$$= \text{Amount of drug to administer}$$

Solution:
Step 1:

$$40 \text{ mg} \times 7.5 \text{ kg} = 300 \text{ mg of amoxicillin daily}$$
$$(3 \text{ doses})$$
$$300 \text{ mg} \div 3 = 100 \text{ mg per dose of amoxicillin}$$

Step 2:

$$100 / 125 \times 5 = 4.0 \text{ mL}$$

15. **Client Needs: Safe and Effective Care Environment T: Application**
    1. Clients experiencing panic-level anxiety are unable to focus on reality; thus, learning relaxation techniques is virtually impossible.
    2. Administering anxiolytic medication should be considered if providing calm, brief, and directive communication is ineffective.
    3. Although the client is disorganized, violence may not be imminent, ruling out the intervention of preparing for physical control until other less restrictive measures are proven ineffective.
    4. **Calm, brief, and directive verbal interaction can help the client gain control of overwhelming feelings and impulses related to anxiety.**

16. **Client Needs: Psychosocial Integrity; T: Knowledge**
    1. This is a type of dementia; people with Lewy body dementia may demonstrate sundowning.
    2. People with sundowning are confused, but this is not the correct term.
    3. **Sundowning is the correct term for the particular behaviours which occur late afternoon and evening with some people who have dementia.**
    4. Delirium is generally a temporary state causing confusion and disorientation. It can occur in people who do not have dementia.

17. **Client Needs: Reduction of Risk Potential; T: Critical Thinking**
    1. HgA_{1C} determines blood sugar levels over time. An acute reading is necessary prior to surgery.
    2. This is necessary but is not expected to differ after NPO for 12 hours.
    3. As in choice 2.
    4. **The client has been NPO, so the nurse needs to check the morning blood glucose to determine if morning insulin should be administered.**

18. **Client Needs: Safe and Effective Care Environment T: Application**
    1. **Removing all unsteady furniture helps prevent an infant from falling.**

2. Infant walkers are illegal as they increase the risk of falling down stairs.

3. **Steadying the infant with a hand when on a change table helps prevent an infant from falling.**

4. The tray attachment to a high chair is an inadequate restraint.

5. **Keeping the infant seat on the floor while indoors helps prevent an infant from falling.**

19. **Client Needs: Safe and Effective Care Environment T: Knowledge**
    1. Dietitians assist with nutritional choices.
    2. Speech-language pathologists assist with speech and swallowing needs.
    3. Physiotherapists assist with strengthening, transferring, and ambulation.
    4. **Occupational therapists assist clients with self-care skills.**

20. **Client Needs: Physiological Integrity T: Application**
    1. This medication is not helpful in acute asthma exacerbations.
    2. This medication is not necessary for treating asthma exacerbations.
    3. As in choice 3.
    4. **Short-acting beta$_2$-agonists such as salbutamol are the first treatment in an acute asthma exacerbation.**

21. **Client Needs: Physiological Integrity T: Application**
    1. This is not necessary
    2. **Inspection of the areas where the splint comes in contact with the skin identifies any areas of potential skin breakdown. Interventions can be implemented prior to breakdown.**
    3. Removal of the splint may be contraindicated.
    4. Talc should never be used under a splint or cast. Inspect skin under the splint at routine intervals.

22. **Client Needs: Safe and Effective Care Environment T: Application**
    1. Meeting all of the clients' needs in the early morning hours would be an unrealistic and possibly unnecessary goal.
    2. **Time management skill for nurses includes planning effectively and being aware of competing priorities.**
    3. **The nurse should complete the activities started with one client before moving on to another unless a priority occurs with another client.**
    4. The nurse, in reviewing the care requirements, organizes their time so the activities of care and client goals can be achieved.
    5. **Time management skills for nurses include reflecting on how time is used.**

23. **Client Needs: Safe and Effective Care Environment T: Application**
    1. The client is taught to place weight on the hands, not in the axilla, to avoid nerve damage.
    2. **When using crutches, clients are usually taught to move the assistive device and the injured leg forward at the same time and then to move the unaffected leg.**

3. If the two- or four-point gaits are to be used, the crutch and leg on opposite sides move forward, not the crutch and same-side leg.

4. Clients are discouraged from using furniture to assist with ambulation.

24. **Client Needs: Psychosocial Integrity; T: Critical Thinking**
    1. **Time-management skills are most helpful in reducing homework-related stress because the child will be able to better manage workload.**
    2. This may be necessary, but the first option is to assist the child to manage time.
    3. This may be necessary, but the first option is to provide self-skills for the child.
    4. Speech and other developmental aspects need to be addressed if the child is to be successful, but skill development will not directly reduce homework-related stress.

25. **Client Needs: Physiological Integrity T: Knowledge**
    1. **This is the correct term for the condition in the picture.**
    2. This is not the correct term.
    3. This is not the correct term.
    4. Repetitive strain injury is caused by repeated use of a body part, not loss of movement or joint.

26. **Client Needs: Physiological Integrity T: Knowledge**
    1. **Natural health products and OTC drugs are not necessarily safe for infants, children, and pregnant or lactating clients; the health care provider should be contacted before use.**
    2. **OTC drugs may delay treatment of more serious ailments and this information should be included when clients are being taught about their use.**
    3. Drug interactions may indeed occur with prescription medications, other OTC drugs, and natural health products.
    4. This statement is false.
    5. Normally, OTC drugs are intended for short-term treatment of minor ailments.
    6. **Natural and OTC products can be toxic and are not always safer.**

27. **Client Needs: Safe and Effective Care Environment T: Critical Thinking**
    1. This client also should be assessed as quickly as possible, but the data about them do not suggest any immediately life-threatening complications.
    2. As in choice 1.
    3. As in choice 1.
    4. **The client data suggest aspiration has occurred and rapid assessment and intervention are needed.**

28. **Client Needs: Health Promotion and Maintenance; T: Critical Thinking**
    1. **Optimum communication requires fluency if the examination is conducted in English or French. A translator will be required.**
    2. Further assessment of the client's health care preferences is required for culturally appropriate care but is not the priority action.

3. This may not be appropriate to the health assessment situation.

4. Family should not be used to translate private health information unless no translator is available and the client gives permission.

29. **Client Needs: Physiological Integrity T: Application**
    1. **Pills may be crushed and mixed with small amounts of water but not with other liquids, such as formula or elixir medications, because these may act together to form a sludge that can interfere with gastrostomy tube function.**
    2. **As in choice 1.**
    3. The tube should not be flushed with air.
    4. Placement does not need to be checked because it is directly into the stomach.

30. **Client Needs: Physiological Integrity T: Critical Thinking**
    1. Ephedra may cause palpitations, myocardial infarction, and possible death.
    2. **Ginger is considered to be safe for stomach upsets.**
    3. **Fish oil is safe as a nutritional supplement.**
    4. **Chamomile is safe as an anti-inflammatory and sedative.**
    5. **Aloe vera is safe as a soothing ointment.**
    6. Belladonna could cause cardiac, bleeding, and sedative complications.

31. **Client Needs: Safe and Effective Care Environment T: Application**
    1. Speaking in loud tones can distort a client's ability to hear; the nurse should speak in normal, low tones.
    2. The nurse can direct conversation toward the client's unaffected ear.
    3. If the client does not understand the first time, the nurse should try rephrasing instead of repeating the message.
    4. **Using gestures other than just speaking helps the client understand what the nurse is saying and makes it a meaningful stimulus.**

32. **Client Needs: Reduction of Risk Potential; T: Critical Thinking**
    1. While the antecubital fossa is a common site, there is a risk for occlusion when the elbow is bent.
    2. **A full assessment of all intravenous sites leads the nurse to the most appropriate site.**
    3. Intravenous lines should be place distally rather than proximally.
    4. Sites on the lower extremities are not suitable as they are a risk for thrombus formation.

33. **Client Needs: Safe and Effective Care Environment T: Application**
    1. Reassurance is supportive but will not ease the workload of the caregiver.
    2. **The family needs respite care during the evening and night care. Caregivers require sleep in order to be able to cope with the demands of caring for the client.**
    3. Support for grieving may be reassuring but will not ease the workload of the caregiver.

4. This may help, but the caregiver requires respite assistance.

34. **Client Needs: Physiological Integrity T: Application**
    1. **It is important that the client understand their heart failure as it relates to them individually.**
    2. With incomplete information of the severity of this client's heart failure, the nurse should not assume their condition will be debilitating and life altering.
    3. **Cardiac rehabilitation programs provide physiotherapy, tailored exercise, dietary advice, and group support.**
    4. **A key component of heart failure treatment is individualized medications: antihypertensives, blood thinners, statins, potassium supplements, and diuretics.**
    5. **The client needs to be aware of worsening symptoms with guidelines for contacting their health care provider.**
    6. There is likely no need for complete bed rest. In fact, this may be detrimental.

35. **Client Needs: Physiological Adaptation; T: Application**
    1. **The thyroid gland is located in the anterior neck region. Swelling at the surgical site may cause respiratory distress.**
    2. This is of obvious importance, but respiratory distress is the primary concern.
    3. Puffiness and eye edema are signs of hypothyroidism and are not a prime concern postoperatively.
    4. As in choice 2.

36. **Client Needs: Physiological Integrity T: Application**
    1. **Rapid-acting insulins are able to closely mimic the body's natural rapid insulin output after a meal. For this reason, both are usually dosed within 15 minutes of beginning a meal.**
    2. This is not the best time to take a rapid-acting insulin.
    3. As in choice 2.
    4. As in choice 2.

37. **Client Needs: Safe and Effective Care Environment T: Application**
    1. This action is appropriate and does not require any intervention.
    2. As in choice 1.
    3. As in choice 1.
    4. **The catheter should not be disconnected from the drainage tube because this increases the risk for urinary tract infection (UTI).**

38. **Client Needs: Health Promotion and Maintenance; T: Application**
    1. Oral temperatures are not recommended for young children, and mercury glass thermometers are prohibited.
    2. Rectal temperatures are invasive.
    3. Skin strips are useful for fever screening but may not be accurate.
    4. **Temporal artery thermometers are rapid, noninvasive, and comfortable for the child.**

39. **Client Needs: Physiological Integrity; T: Application**
   1. **This is the first step in assessing if there hearing loss and a need for hearing aids. There is some evidence that hearing loss influences dementia.**
   2. The nurse does not know if the client needs hearing aids.
   3. The client does not need an ENT physician unless there is an identified problem at audiology.
   4. This is patronizing and does not provide help for the client.

40. **Client Needs: Safe and Effective Care Environment T: Application**
   1. Nurses do not delegate assessment to unregulated care providers.
   2. Documenting "better" is subjective and does not objectively describe the wound.
   3. **The nurse performs evaluative measures, such as assessing the size of the wound to evaluate wound healing.**
   4. **Observing the wound for redness, swelling, or drainage is an evaluative measure of the progress of wound healing.**
   5. Leaving the dressing off for the nurse's benefit of easier access is not a part of the evaluation process.

41. **Client Needs: Safe and Effective Care Environment T: Application**
   1. A complete orientation to the functioning of the entire unit would take a period of time that would exceed what the nurse has to spend on orientation.
   2. **The nurse assigning client care must ensure they give a staff nurse an assignment that they can safely handle.**
   3. The nurse is required to research unit policies associated with the particular client, not for the entire unit. This is not an effective use of time.
   4. Unregulated care providers may help the nurse complete basic tasks such as hygiene and turning, but their help does not enable safe nursing care, for which the nurse is ultimately responsible.

42. **Client Needs: Reduction of Risk Potential; T: Application**
   1. The intravenous device must be removed immediately to prevent further tissue irritation.
   2. The infiltration site must not be massaged; this can cause a hematoma or further tissue irritation depending on the IV solution.
   3. **The device must be removed immediately, and the nurse must elevate the extremity and apply compresses to the site.**
   4. As in choice 1.

43. **Client Needs: Physiological Integrity T: Application**
   1. **TPN is an intravenous (IV) solution composed of nutrients and electrolytes to replace the ones the client is not eating.**
   2. TPN does not stimulate the client's appetite to eat.
   3. TPN does not contain blood pressure medication.
   4. TPN does not contain antibiotics.

44. **Client Needs: Psychosocial Integrity; T: Application**
   1. This is appropriate behaviour.
   2. **Sacrificing their own health to care for the identified client places caregivers at risk for becoming ill themselves. A nurse will identify a caregiver's lack of self-care as a potential example of caregiver role strain. If caregivers jeopardize their own health, they may not be able to care for the actual client. In all of the other options, the caregiver is handling caregiver stress appropriately.**
   3. This is appropriate behaviour.
   4. This is common behaviour during times of grief.

45. **Client Needs: Physiological Integrity T: Application**
   1. Acetylsalicylic acid is associated with a high incidence of gastrointestinal bleeding in elderly clients.
   2. NSAIDs are associated with a high incidence of gastrointestinal bleeding in elderly clients.
   3. Nonopioid analgesics are used first for mild to moderate pain, although opioids may be used later.
   4. **Acetaminophen is the best first-choice medication. The principle of "start low, go slow" is used to guide therapy when treating older persons because the ability to metabolize medications is decreased and the likelihood of medication interactions is increased.**

46. **Client Needs: Safe and Effective Care Environment T: Application**
   1. The client needs transportation, but that does not address the client's mobility status.
   2. **The nurse needs to evaluate whether goals and outcomes have been met before revising, continuing, or discontinuing a plan of care.**
   3. Whether the client has a follow-up appointment is not immediately relevant to the mobility impairment.
   4. Ensuring that prescriptions are filled is not immediately relevant to the mobility impairment.

47. **Client Needs: Psychosocial Integrity; T: Application**
   1. This is a punitive response.
   2. The client has not said that the foods are not as tasty. This response shuts down the conversation.
   3. **This encourages the client to discuss the problems with the new diet. It could be that these foods are too expensive or that the client does not know how to cook them.**
   4. The diet of fast foods is not all right; it is unhealthy regardless of the amounts eaten.

48. **Client Needs: Physiological Integrity; T: Critical Thinking**
   1. This is appropriate but is not the first action.
   2. As in choice 1.
   3. As in choice 1.
   4. **The priority is to flush the eye to wash out the chemicals before they can seriously damage the eye. Sterile saline is ideal, but water is also appropriate—whatever can be accessed quickly.**

49. **Client Needs: Health Promotion and Maintenance; T: Application**

1. This assumes substance use disorder without sufficient information.
2. **The client should be approached in a caring non-judgemental way. The nurse requires more information to make an assessment of substance use disorder or drug-seeking behaviour.**
3. As in choice 1
4. As in choice 1

50. **Client Needs: Physiological Integrity T: Application**
Answer: 0.75
Rationale: Use the formula for calculation of oral and parenteral doses of medications.

Formula:

$$\frac{\text{Dosage ordered}}{\text{Dosage available}} \times \text{Drug form}$$

= Amount of drug to administer

Solution: 1.5/2 ×1 = 0.75 mL

51. **Client Needs: Safe and Effective Care Environment T: Knowledge**
1. This choice represents good nursing practice but is not the best example of self-reflection. This choice does not involve purposefully thinking back to discover the meaning or purpose of a situation.
2. As in choice 1.
3. **In self-reflection, the nurse utilizes critical thinking in evaluating the effectiveness of interventions and how they were performed.**
4. Providing evidence-informed explanations for nursing interventions does not always involve thinking back to discover the meaning of a situation.

52. **Client Needs: Physiological Integrity T: Application**
1. **Clients with prolonged vomiting and diarrhea become hypovolemic. The best solution to replace extracellular volume is 0.9% sodium chloride, which is an isotonic solution.**
2. Dextrose 10% in water acts as a hypotonic solution in the body.
3. Dextrose 5% in water acts as a hypotonic solution in the body.
4. 0.45% sodium chloride acts as a hypotonic solution in the body.

53. **Client Needs: Physiological Adaptation T: Knowledge**
1. **A hypoglycemic episode is an adverse reaction to insulin or oral hypoglycemic therapy.**
2. This is not related to adverse reactions.
3. As in choice 2.
4. As in choice 2.

54. **Client Needs: Reduction of Risk Potential; T: Application**
1. The dressing should not be painful to remove. Soak with saline if it sticks to the abrasion.
2. The dressing should be waterproof.
3. This is not necessary.
4. **The dressing is transparent so the wound may be visualized. Signs of infection need to be monitored.**

55. **Client Needs: Safe and Effective Care Environment T: Application**

1. Toys are a common source of injury, especially toys intended for older children.
2. **Toddlers can drown in water just deep enough to cover their noses and mouths, including pails of water.**
3. **Hot water, boiling water, coffee, tea, and food are the most common sources of injury and should not be kept within reach of the child.**
4. Once children reach 10 kg, they should be switched to a forward-facing child safety seat, and preferably be placed in the rear seat to avoid injury risk from air bags in the front seat.
5. **Trying to reach the remote control on the top shelf of the home entertainment centre puts the child at immediate at risk because of the potential for the entertainment centre to fall on the child while they are trying to climb it.**

56. **Client Needs: Safe and Effective Care Environment T: Application**
1. In general, nurses should not accept money or gifts of significant material value.
2. Depending on agency policy, some token gifts such as chocolates or flowers may be acceptable.
3. **Each nursing regulatory body and agency has standards and policies regarding gifts. The nurse must adhere to these regulations.**
4. If the chocolate is allowed by agency policy to be accepted, it should be considered a communal gift, for all of the team. It may not be appropriate for clients.

57. **Client Needs: Health Promotion and Maintenance; T: Critical Thinking**
1. **The nurse may need information from all of these options, but the most important at this visit is to find out supportive relationships for the new parents. Being socially and environmentally isolated may be of concern for the health and safety of the baby and parents. There may be informal networks providing necessary services important for the new baby and parents.**
2. This sounds prejudiced, although it may be of some importance.
3. This is not important information at this time.
4. This is important for the safety of the infant and mother but is not the most important information at this initial assessment.

58. **Client Needs: Health Promotion and Maintenance; T: Knowledge**
1. Cholesterol does not need to be monitored until age 40.
2. **Annual blood pressure testing is recommended.**
3. PSA is not required until age 50 unless there are risk factors.
4. **Pap test is a recommended screening test for this age group.**
5. Annual chest X-ray is not necessary unless specifically indicated.
6. **Dental exams are recommended screening tests for this age group.**

59. **Client Needs: Physiological Integrity T: Application**
1. This is not appropriate nor necessary.
2. This may increase the problem with perineal hygiene and is not necessary.
3. **Portable bidets available for purchase will cleanse the perineal area. If the client cannot afford a bidet, even with her arthritis, the client should be able to pour water over her perineum while on the toilet.**
4. The client's arthritis would prevent use of the towelettes.

60. **Client Needs: Safe and Effective Care Environment T: Application**
1. Preschool children still require a great deal of indirect supervision.
2. Stairways should be kept free of clutter.
3. **Children must never be left alone, even for a brief moment, in the car.**
4. Medications should be kept out of reach.

61. **Client Needs: Safe and Effective Care Environment T: Application**
1. This would be considered fraudulent documentation, grounds for discipline by provincial/territorial nursing associations or colleges.
2. Nurses should not provide passwords nor document for others.
3. **This is the correct action for missed documentation. The off-shift nurse will need to make a "late entry" in the client medication administration record. In the meantime, the on-duty nurse can note the conversation as per hospital policy.**
4. The nurse is responsible for their own documentation and complying with hospital policies. The nurse manager may be informed but does not need to make a decision.

62. **Client Needs: Physiological Integrity; T: Application**
1. **The left radial must be monitored for potential arterial occlusion.**
2. **A small amount of bleeding may occur at the insertion site.**
3. **The catheter must be firmly fastened to prevent slipping.**
4. **Catheter placement is verified via radiography.**
5. Blood pressure may not be taken on the left arm.

63. **Client Needs: Reduction of Risk Potential; T: Critical Thinking**
1. This may be true, but the high level is not necessarily an indication of prostate cancer. This statement will alarm the client.
2. **This test measures the level of PSA in the blood, produced by both cancerous and noncancerous tissue. It is also elevated in enlarged and inflamed prostate tissue. The health care provider will need to further assess the client.**
3. There is conflicting advice regarding PSA tests; however, they are still routinely used as a screening tool for prostate cancer, and it has been ordered by the client's health care provider.

4. While the nurse may discuss symptoms with the client, this statement will alarm the client unnecessarily at this stage.

64. **Client Needs: Psychosocial Integrity; T: Application**
1. **With some cases of early-onset Alzheimer's there is a genetic link, thus family history is important.**
2. Traumatic brain injury can be a cause of early-onset AD but is not a definitive cause.
3. This is patronizing and does not address the client's concern.
4. Although depression is a factor in AD, it is not causal in early-onset AD.

65. **Client Needs: Safe and Effective Care Environment T: Application**
1. **The primary nurse should focus on interventions to reduce the client's anxiety, which should reduce the number of calls.**
2. Setting limits on calling for staff does not help the cause of the behaviour and will only increase the client's distress and desperation.
3. This action benefits the staff but not the client.
4. As in choice 3.

66. **Client Needs: Physiological Integrity T: Application**
Answer: 2.5
Rationale: Formula for calculation of oral and parenteral doses of medications
Formula:
Covert the weight to kg: 2.2 lb = 1 kg

$$\frac{\text{Drug dosage per}}{\text{kg of body weight}} \times \text{Weight of child (kg)}$$
$$= \text{Dosage to administer}$$

Solution:
55 pounds/2.2 kg = 25 kg
mg × 25 = 2.5 mg

67. **Client Needs: Health Promotion and Maintenance; T: Critical Thinking**
1. This is a good level, but is not an indication of long-term blood sugar control.
2. The client may feel they are following a beneficial diet, but the proof of diabetic control is in the HgA_{1C} value.
3. Ability to inject insulin does not necessarily mean there is optimum diabetic control.
4. **All options may indicate effective actions by the client in controlling their diabetes. HgA_{1C} is the most effective indication of optimum blood glucose levels over time and is not affected by short-term fluctuations. If it has increased, there has not been effective control.**

68. **Client Needs: Physiological Integrity; T: Application**
1. **Clients who sit for long periods in a wheelchair or chair should have an appropriate and functional pressure-reduction cushion.**
2. The client has dementia and likely will not remember to change position.

3. The client has dementia and requires a wheelchair. Standing and walking may not be possible nor safe.

4. This is not necessary as a preventative step.

69. **Client Needs: Safe and Effective Care Environment T: Application**

1. Notifying the client's health care provider immediately would be unnecessary as the nurse needs to validate the data.

2. The nurse should validate the data before documenting the sound.

3. **The nurse must validate any data to ensure accuracy. If the nurse has less experience in an area, a colleague may be consulted.**

4. The nurse should not wait to assess the sound as a nursing intervention may be required.

70. **Client Needs: Safe and Effective Care Environment T: Application**

1. Report elements do not include normal findings.

2. Report elements do not include derogatory or inappropriate comments about the client or family.

3. Results should not be described simply as "good" or "poor"; they should be specific.

4. **Elements in change-of-shift report include identification of significant changes in measurable terms such as a pain scale and by observation.**

5. **Significant medication administration and the specific results should be described.**

71. **Client Needs: Physiological Adaptation; T: Application**

1. Clients do complain about dry air in a CCU; however, this would no likely be the cause of the sore throat.

2. **Intubation and pressure from the ventilator cause irritation to the mucosa of the larynx and bronchus.**

3. This is not likely.

4. This does not answer the client.

72. **Client Needs: Psychosocial Integrity; T: Application**

1. This is not a professional response. The nurse is capable of addressing client concerns.

2. The nurse does not know for certain that plastic surgery will be required; the answer is patronizing.

3. This does not answer the client concern.

4. **Swelling does need to decrease before the client can be assessed for a need for plastic surgery.**

73. **Client Needs: Safe and Effective Care Environment T: Knowledge**

1. *Informed consent* refers to giving appropriate information to the client such that they can make informed decisions regarding their care.

2. The *right to competent care* refers to the right of the client to receive care from an individual who is knowledgeable and skilled in providing care.

3. The *Employment Equity Act* refers to the rights of persons with disabilities.

4. **The nurse has violated the client's right to privacy and confidentiality. Health care providers in Canada are expected to comply with federal privacy rules. The *Personal Information Protection and Electronic Documents Act* (PIPEDA) provides the** national standards for protecting the privacy of an individual's health information and regulates how personal health information is disclosed and used by the private sector. The basic obligation of health care providers is to protect the client's privacy.

74. **Client Needs: Psychosocial Integrity T: Application**

1. The clock drawing test is considered to be a reliable screening tool for early dementia.

2. The clock test cannot predict the type of dementia.

3. **The clock drawing test is able to detect cognitive decline as people with dementia often have problems reading traditional clocks. Although very simple, it can often detect early dementia before the mini mental state exam or Montreal Cognitive Assessment can.**

4. The test is scored at the time of the clock drawing. The test may be repeated on different occasions.

75. **Client Needs: Physiological Integrity T: Application**

1. A daily log of weight should be kept.

2. Foods high in potassium should be eaten more often.

3. A weight gain of 2.3 kg or more a week should be reported immediately not at the next visit.

4. **Orthostatic hypotension is a possible problem with diuretic therapy.**

76. **Client Needs: Health Promotion and Maintenance; T: Application**

1. The vaccines provide approximately 90% protection from the SARS-CoV-2 infection and its variants.

2. Vaccine trials were conducted with all safety measures.

3. The mRNA vaccines cannot enter the nucleus of the cell, thus cannot alter DNA.

4. **All COVID-19 vaccines provide protection from serious disease and decreased transmission to others. Options 1, 2, and 3 contain common misinformation about the mRNA COVID-19 vaccines.**

77. **Client Needs: Physiological Integrity; T: Application**

1. Sleeping pills are not to be used routinely, only short term in acute situations.

2. This will not promote sleep.

3. **Turning off all electronic devices—smartphones, electronic tablets, computers, televisions—is recommended to promote relaxation and sleep.**

4. As in choice 2.

78. **Client Needs: Physiological Integrity T: Application**

1. **Stopping the activity and lying or sitting down is a correct action.**

2. Calling 9-1-1 immediately is an incorrect action because 9-1-1 should be called only after one tablet has been taken and there is no relief within 5 minutes apart.

3. This describes buccal administration. The correct action for sublingual administration is to place the tablet under the tongue.

4. **Taking another sublingual tablet if chest pain is not relieved after 5 minutes is a correct action.**

5. **Call 9-1-1 if the pain is not relieved within 5 minutes after taking one sublingual tablet.**

6. The nurse should stay close by in case a 9-1-1 call is required.

79. **Client Needs: Safe and Effective Care Environment T: Knowledge**
    1. Gluten is not in this flour.
    2. **Gluten is in wheat flour.**
    3. As in choice 1.
    4. As in choice 1.

80. **Client Needs: Physiological Adaptation; T: Critical Thinking**
    1. This will likely help but the nurse requires more information.
    2. The client may have sleep apnea, but with a history of heart failure, the nurse requires more information.
    3. The shortness of breath could be due to postnasal drip, but the nurse needs more information of possible paroxysmal nocturnal dyspnea.
    4. **This is the nurse's primary assessment. Being awakened from sleep with shortness of breath is a sign of paroxysmal nocturnal dyspnea, a sign of heart failure.**

81. **Client Needs: Physiological Integrity T: Knowledge**
    1. A solution of 5% dextrose in water will cause hemolysis of the blood product.
    2. **Blood products should be given only with 0.9% sodium chloride.**
    3. A solution of 5% dextrose in 0.9% sodium chloride will cause hemolysis of the blood product.
    4. A solution of 5% dextrose in lactated Ringer's solution will cause hemolysis of the blood product.

82. **Client Needs: Psychosocial Integrity T: Application**
    1. This is a breach of confidentiality.
    2. **The nurse should speak with the student with empathy and understanding. Referral for counselling is action oriented.**
    3. This is a breach of confidentiality, and the diagnosis is presumed.
    4. This is a breach of confidentiality.

83. **Client Needs: Psychosocial Integrity T: Application**
    1. This is not safe exercise for a client post–myocardial infarction.
    2. **These activities can be considered appropriate for cardiac rehabilitation and for general fitness.**
    3. As in choice 2.
    4. As in choice 2.
    5. Ironing is not active enough and will not improve fitness levels.
    6. **As in choice 2.**

84. **Client Needs: Health Promotion and Maintenance; T: Application**
    1. If the parents are asked to leave, this may upset the client. Parents are the substitute decision makers/guardians thus are allowed client information.
    2. **Parents have said the client is able to make the client's wishes known and is able to answer yes or no answers.**

3. The autistic person finds it difficult to filter out information and interpret sensory or visual clues.
4. All clients, regardless of disability, should participate in their health care.

85. **Client Needs: Physiological Integrity; T: Application**
    1. The child likely has a temperature; warm baths would be contraindicated.
    2. **Otitis media is a common ear infection in children. It causes fever and pain. Acetaminophen (Tylenol) will reduce the fever and help with the pain.**
    3. Cold compresses to the ear will not be effective for fever or pain.
    4. As in choice 3.

86. **Client Needs: Safe and Effective Care Environment T: Critical Thinking**
    1. Studies have shown that soy formula does not prevent allergic disease in infants.
    2. There is no evidence that child-bearing clients' avoidance (during pregnancy or lactation) of cow's milk protein or other dietary products known to cause food allergy will prevent food allergy in children.
    3. **Exclusive breastfeeding for 4 to 6 months is now considered a primary strategy for avoiding atopy in families with known food allergies.**
    4. Researchers indicate that delaying the introduction of highly allergenic foods past 4 to 6 months of age may not be as protective for food allergy as previously believed.

87. **Client Needs: Physiological Integrity; T: Application**
    1. This is a sign the child has been infected by the tubercle bacillus but does not confirm the presence of active disease.
    2. Isolation is not required unless the child has active tuberculosis.
    3. This is not determined until the results of the chest X-ray and sputum cultures.
    4. **A definitive diagnosis is made by showing presence of mycobacteria in the culture. Chest X-rays are supplemental to sputum culture.**

88. **Client Needs: Physiological Integrity T: Application**
    1. **Orthostatic hypotension occurs with older persons, especially those taking antihypertension medications, when there is a postural change. Getting up slowly helps to prevent the drop in blood pressure.**
    2. **This helps to prevent the drop in blood pressure.**
    3. **As in choice 2.**
    4. **As in choice 2.**
    5. It would likely be too difficult for the older client to drink this much fluid in the morning.
    6. This might be diagnostic for orthostatic hypotension but is not necessary.

89. **Client Needs: Physiological Integrity T: Knowledge**
    1. The client is not experiencing opioid toxicity.
    2. This is not addiction.
    3. **Opioid tolerance is a common physiological result of long-term opioid use. Clients with opioid**

tolerance require larger doses of the opioid agent to maintain the same level of analgesia.

4. This is not abstinence syndrome.

90. **Client Needs: Physiological Integrity T: Application**
    1. This is most appropriate for short-term oxygen administration in an emergency.
    2. **This is used for long-term use at lower flows of oxygen. It is easily tolerated.**
    3. A venturi mask is used for higher flows and is not appropriate for long-term use.
    4. As in choice 3.

91. **Client Needs: Psychosocial Integrity T: Application**
    1. **This action will assist both the client and the partner integrate the beliefs and resources of their original and adopted cultures, reducing their guilt and distress.**
    2. This reinforces the belief that mental health conditions are an embarrassment.
    3. As in choice 2.
    4. This could possibly be helpful, but the more immediate need is to accept the condition within their own culture.

92. **Client Needs: Physiological Integrity T: Application**
    1. Dyspnea is not a symptom of hypokalemia.
    2. **Anorexia is a symptom of hypokalemia.**
    3. Tinnitus is not a symptom of hypokalemia.
    4. **Muscle weakness is a symptom of hypokalemia.**
    5. **Mental confusion is a symptom of hypokalemia.**
    6. Decreased blood pressure is a sign of hyperkalemia.

93. **Client Needs: Physiological Integrity; T: Critical Thinking**
    1. This may be effective but the rash needs to be seen first by a health provider.
    2. This is not an emergency.
    3. As in choice 1.
    4. **The rash is likely a candida/thrush yeast infection, especially as there are white plaques in the mouth. The area needs to be seen by a health care provider to provide a diagnosis, prescribe an oral or topical antifungal, and ensure the rash is not bacterial.**

94. **Client Needs: Health Promotion and Maintenance; T: Application**
    1. **The nurse needs to establish who will provide care for the child.**
    2. Assuming the mother will be the primary caregiver may be erroneous; the nurse should never assume.
    3. This is not the goal of the meeting.
    4. All family members will require knowledge and expertise in care giving.

95. **Client Needs: Safe and Effective Care Environment T: Application**
    1. The risks associated with the use of restraints are serious. The inappropriate or unjustified use of restraints (e.g., by confining a person to an area or by using physical or chemical restraints) may also be viewed as false imprisonment.

2. **A restraint-free environment is the first goal of care for all clients. Many alternatives to the use of restraints are available.**
3. The health care provider needs to know the situation but also needs to ensure that all approaches possible are used before restraints are ordered.
4. Allowing the client to pull out any of these items could cause harm to the client.

96. **Client Needs: Physiological Integrity T: Application**
    Answer: 1830
    Rationale: Formula for calculating intravenous flow rate
    Formula:

    $$\text{Flow Rate} \frac{mL}{hr} = \frac{\text{Amount of solution (mL)}}{\text{Time (hr)}}$$

    Solution:

    $$\text{Time (hr)} = \frac{\text{Amount of solution (mL)}}{\left(\text{Flow Rate}\left(\frac{mL}{hr}\right)\right)}$$

    $$= \frac{250\ mL}{20\ mL/hr} = 12.5\ hr$$

    0.5 hr × 60 min = 30 min
    0600 + 12 hours and 30 min = 1830 hrs

97. **Client Needs: Safe and Effective Care Environment T: Knowledge**
    1. This allergy is not a contraindication for the use of silver sulfadiazine.
    2. As in choice 1.
    3. As in choice 1.
    4. **The use of silver sulfadiazine cream on burns is contraindicated if the client has a sulfa allergy.**

98. **Client Needs: Physiological Integrity T: Application**
    1. Metformin does not alter the pancreatic secretion of insulin.
    2. **Metformin works by decreasing glucose production by the liver. It may also decrease intestinal absorption of glucose and improve insulin receptor sensitivity. This results in increased peripheral glucose uptake and use and in decreased liver production of triglycerides and cholesterol.**
    3. Metformin may decrease intestinal absorption of glucose, not increase it.
    4. As in choice 1.

99. **Client Needs: Physiological Integrity T: Application**
    1. **These are Heart and Stroke and Canadian Red Cross recommended actions for treating a choking infant.**
    2. The nurse should not perform blind finger sweeps.
    3. This is the procedure for an older child or adult.
    4. This will not dislodge the foreign body.

100. **Client Needs: Health Promotion and Maintenance T: Application**
    1. **The first measurement should be in the morning before eating or taking medications.**
    2. The arm should be rested and raised to the level of the heart.

3. The cuff should be placed on bare skin, not over clothing.

4. **BP readings should be tracked by hand or inputted into a personal mobile device, to be shared with the health care provider.**

5. **Wait for 1 to 3 minutes after the first reading, and then take another to check accuracy.**

6. **The second should be in the evening.**

101. **Client Needs: Psychosocial Integrity T: Application**

1. This does not answer the client's question and is dismissive.

2. As in choice 1.

3. **This is a positive response and helps the client to focus on their capabilities.**

4. As in choice 1.

102. **Client Needs: Safe and Effective Care Environment T: Application**

1. **This response empowers the client.**

2. In the stage of acceptance, many clients are exhausted, and interactions of a social nature are a burden.

3. It is not necessary for the client to discuss these wishes with the health care provider.

4. The client wishes to have visits from family members.

103. **Client Needs: Health Promotion and Maintenance T: Application**

1. **Many cultures consider it disrespectful and inappropriate for touch to occur without permission.**

2. This may be appropriate, but not necessarily across all cultural groups for all clients.

3. As in choice 2.

4. As in choice 2.

104. **Client Needs: Physiological Integrity T: Knowledge**

1. There is a risk of allergy and this drug should not be administered.

2. **There is an increased risk of cross-allergy when a client who is allergic to sulfa drugs takes a sulfonylurea drug for diabetes. Therefore, the drug should be held and the order checked with the health care provider.**

3. As in choice 1.

4. As in choice 1.

105. **Client Needs: Physiological Integrity T: Application**

1. This is appealing to a 6-year-old and contains some nutritious foods, but there are some items which are not recommended.

2. As in choice 1.

3. As in choice 1.

4. **This provides fruits and vegetables, protein, and whole grains and makes water the drink of choice.**

106. **Client Needs: Safe and Effective Care Environment T: Critical Thinking**

1. If an antibiotic is ordered, administering it is important, but correct identification is a priority.

2. **The most important intervention is to ensure that the correct child is going to the operating room for the identified procedure. It is the nurse's responsibility to verify identification of the child and what procedure is to be done.**

3. Clear liquids can be given up to 2 hr before surgery. If the child was NPO (taking nothing by mouth) since midnight, intravenous fluids should be administered.

4. Parents should be encouraged to accompany the child to the preoperative area. Many institutions allow parents to be present during induction.

107. **Client Needs: Physiological Integrity; T: Application**

1. This is contraindicated.

2. As in choice 1.

3. As in choice 1.

4. **Negative pressure wound therapy helps with removing wound exudates and maintain a moist wound surface with chronic and dehisced wounds.**

108. **Client Needs: Physiological Integrity; T: Application**

1. MRSA is spread by direct contact.

2. **MRSA can be hospital or community acquired and may cause severe postoperative infections. Clients with a positive culture should be isolated.**

3. MRSA is not rare. Death is a possibility but is not common.

4. This is not factual.

109. **Client Needs: Safe and Effective Care Environment T: Knowledge**

1. **Gonorrhea is a reportable communicable disease in all provinces and territories.**

2. **HIV is a reportable communicable disease in all provinces and territories.**

3. This is not a reportable disease.

4. **Chlamydia is a reportable communicable disease in all provinces and territories.**

5. **Infectious syphilis is a reportable communicable disease in all provinces and territories.**

110. **Client Needs: Psychosocial Integrity; T: Critical Thinking**

1. This is important but is not the priority action.

2. As in choice 1.

3. **This is the priority action, to get emergency services to the person to prevent the suicide or harm to others from the gun.**

4. As in choice 1.

111. **Client Needs: Physiological Integrity; T: Application**

1. The calorie allotment for the child with diabetes is essentially the same as that of the nondiabetic child.

2. **Intake of complex carbohydrates and high-fibre foods helps to reduce blood glucose levels.**

3. Nutritional needs include carbohydrates as well as protein and fats.

4. The diet does not need to be low in fat.

112. **Client Needs: Physiological Integrity T: Application**

1. Pain associated with many procedures can be prevented.

2. Numerous research studies have indicated that infants perceive and react to pain in the same manner as children and adults.

3. The parent should be allowed to discuss their concerns and the alternatives available.

4. **To minimize the discomfort associated with intramuscular injections, a topical anaesthetic agent such as eutectic mixture of local anaesthetic (EMLA) can be used on the injection site.**

113. **Client Needs: Physiological Integrity; T: Knowledge**
   1. **The most common sites for pressure injuries are over bony prominences. That includes the scapula.**
   2. The back of the head should not be in contact with the wheelchair.
   3. **The sacrum is a bony prominence under pressure in a wheelchair**
   4. **The coccyx is a bony prominence receiving pressure in a wheelchair.**
   5. The elbow will not be immobilized in a wheelchair.
   6. The Achilles tendon is not a bony prominence and should not be immobilized in a wheelchair.

114. **Client Needs: Safe and Effective Care Environment T: Application**
   1. The client's experience with outpatient surgery is assessed, but it does not have much application to the client's physiological safety.
   2. **After outpatient surgery, the client should not drive home and will need assistance with transportation and home care.**
   3. Some outpatient procedures are not covered by provincial universal health care plans. This is not a concern for the nurse.
   4. Having clear liquids a few hours before surgery does not usually increase risk for aspiration as the guideline indicates that clear fluids can be taken up to 2 hr before surgery.

115. **Client Needs: Safe and Effective Care Environment T: Application**
   1. Neutropenia is not a communicable condition.
   2. **Clients with neutropenia have reduced immunity and are highly susceptible to infection. Neutropenic clients require protective isolation. Visitors and caregivers must wear gown, mask, and other forms of personal protective equipment (PPE) as required.**
   3. Protective isolation is used to protect the client from all pathogens in the environment.
   4. Increased resistance to infection would not occur after being on a medication for 24 hours.

116. **Client Needs: Physiological Integrity T: Application**
   1. **Wound healing requires additional consumption of protein and calories, particularly in the older population. Nutritional supplement drinks provide easily digestible sources of proteins, calories, vitamins, and minerals.**
   2. These do not provide the necessary protein.
   3. Red meat will provide protein for wound healing, but the older client may not be able to digest the meat and they may not have the appetite to consume enough meat.

4. Vegetables do not provide enough protein.

117. **Client Needs: Physiological Integrity; T: Application**
   1. **The body must have correct identification prior to transport to the morgue or funeral parlour.**
   2. **Next of kin will need to be notified.**
   3. **The body is prepared if family will be viewing.**
   4. As this was an unexpected death, tubes and dressings are not to be removed until the coroner has been notified.
   5. **The responsible physician or health care provider must be notified.**
   6. This is not necessary unless directed by the coroner.

118. **Client Needs: Safe and Effective Care Environment T: Application**
   1. Institutional care is required for clients who need 24 hour care.
   2. Medication assistance can be achieved through the client's pharmacy; when filling medications, request bubble packs.
   3. Services such as shopping, housework, and cooking are not skilled nursing services and do not require home health care.
   4. **Hospice palliative care is one aspect of home health care services.**

119. **Client Needs: Physiological Integrity T: Knowledge**
   1. **The rapid-acting insulins peak in 60 to 90 minutes.**
   2. The client is not at high risk for hypoglycemia at this time, although hypoglycemia may occur.
   3. As in choice 2.
   4. As in choice 2.

120. **Client Needs:**
   1. This is not the correct action. In addition, it is not within the scope of practice to independently administer an IV bolus.
   2. The nurse must consult the health care provider to order new bloodwork.
   3. That may occur but is at the direction of the health care provider.
   4. **These values demonstrate an electrolyte imbalance. They require assessment and treatment decisions by the health care provider.**
   5. This may occur but is at the direction of the health care provider.

121. **Client Needs: Safe and Effective Care Environment T: Critical Thinking**
   1. Although this information may also be communicated with the surgeon and anaesthesiologist, they will affect postoperative care and do not indicate a need for further assessment before surgery.
   2. **This statement suggests that the client may be pregnant, and pregnancy testing is needed before administration of anaesthetic agents.**
   3. As in choice 1.
   4. As in choice 1.

122. **Client Needs: Physiological Integrity; T: Application**
   1. The client may not comprehend the instructions but still requires transfer to the chair.

2. This is possible, but not ideal.

3. **A hydraulic lift is the safest option and should be available in a long-term care facility.**

4. This is not appropriate care.

123. **Client Needs: Physiological Integrity; T: Application**

1. **This is the correct measurement to approximate from the nose to the stomach. The length should be marked with indelible ink.**

2. This is the correct measurement for a pediatric NG tube. Tape is not to be used to mark the spot, as it may occlude the nares or be aspirated into the nasopharynx.

3. This is an approximate measure for a nasojejunal (NJ) tube.

4. This is incorrect.

124. **Client Needs: Physiological Integrity T: Critical Thinking**

1. **One of the more serious adverse effects of thyroid drugs is tachycardia.**

2. Edema is not an adverse effect of thyroid drugs.

3. **Dysrhythmias are a serious adverse effect of thyroid drugs.**

4. **Weight loss is an important adverse effect the client should be made aware of.**

5. **Fever is one of the more serious adverse effects of thyroid drugs.**

6. **Nervousness is an adverse effect of thyroid replacement therapy.**

125. **Client Needs: Physiological Integrity; T: Application**

1. **Insertion of a urinary catheter into the vagina is a common unexpected outcome. Leaving the catheter in situ prevents the next catheter from entering the vagina, making it easier to find the urinary meatus.**

2. The catheter should not be removed until after another catheter has been successfully inserted into the urinary meatus. The catheter must not be reused.

3. If there is no urinary flow at 7 cm, it is not likely the catheter is in the bladder. Advancing the catheter will only cause discomfort for the client.

4. This is a new sterile catheter. There would be no obstructions.

126. **Client Needs: Physiological Integrity T: Knowledge**

1. **Pupil dilation is a sympathetic response.**

2. This is an example of a parasympathetic response.

3. As in choice 2.

4. As in choice 2.

127. **Client Needs: Safe and Effective Care Environment T: Application**

1. **A fan will help cool the ambient air.**

2. A porch may be quite hot, depending on ambient temperature.

3. Clothing, whether light weight or synthetic, is unlikely to prevent heat stroke.

4. An atmospheric thermometer will not prevent heat stroke.

128. **Client Needs: Physiological Integrity; T: Application**

1. **The client needs to increase dietary intake and will likely prefer foods familiar to their culture.**

2. **The client is not employed. The nurse needs to determine if the client has money to purchase food.**

3. **Many charities and communities operate local and culturally focused food banks to provide assistance for those who require food supplements to what they can afford.**

4. This is not an effective strategy.

5. These are North American diets, whose focus is not on re-establishing optimal nutrition following malnourishment.

129. **Client Needs: Psychosocial Integrity T: Application**

1. **The role of the social worker includes assisting clients with appropriate living accommodations or home supports. The social worker may be able to find a place that is safe and allows the client to have input into decisions.**

2. The client is in the beginning stages of dementia and does not yet need Powers of Attorney.

3. This may be discussed, but this is an early stage, and the client is not yet feeling ready for assisted living.

4. This is true, but the nurse still has the professional responsibility to assist the client and family with a social work referral.

130. **Client Needs: Psychosocial Integrity T: Application**

1. The client's pain scores are reassessed during evaluation.

2. Building the client's expectation of the provider's arrival does not address the client's pain.

3. **The appropriate nonpharmacological pain management intervention is to quietly play music that the client finds relaxing in a quiet environment. Music diverts a person's attention away from pain and creates relaxation.**

4. Relaxation techniques are effective when a client is not experiencing acute pain. Because the client is having acute pain, this is not an appropriate time to provide client teaching.

131. **Client Needs: Health Promotion and Maintenance; T: Critical Thinking**

1. This is a possible option, but for this client and age group, accessing internet resources is the initial step.

2. **Health literacy is an important health determinant for many health outcomes. Health literacy requires the client to be able to access information, process that information to understand it, and act on that information to make good health decisions. Young university student would be most familiar with web-based resources but should be cautioned to only use reputable sources.**

3. As in choice 1.

4. As in choice 1.

132. **Client Needs: Safe and Effective Care Environment T: Application**
    1. **Hospice care is appropriate for this client.**
    2. The client is managed at home and does not require hospice care.
    3. **Due to the limited lifespan, hospice care is appropriate.**
    4. There are no indications for hospice care for this client.
    5. As in choice 4.

133. **Client Needs: Safe and Effective Care Environment T: Application**
    1. **Positioning the client with the head of the bed lowered will decrease ventilation.**
    2. This action is appropriate for a client with a pulmonary embolism.
    3. As in choice 2.
    4. As in choice 2.

134. **Client Needs: Physiological Integrity; T: Application**
    1. This will not reassure the client.
    2. This will likely frighten the client and may not be true.
    3. **This is a clear and truthful response, educating the client about emergency procedures.**
    4. This is patronizing. The client requires a clear and truthful answer.

135. **Client Needs: Physiological Integrity T: Application**
    1. **Correct technique for male perineal care involves grasping the shaft of the penis.**
    2. **The foreskin is pulled back gently if uncircumcised.**
    3. If an erection occurs, defer the procedure to another time.
    4. The tip, not the base, is washed first.
    5. **The tip and meatus are washed first.**
    6. An up and down motion is not used.

136. **Client Needs: Safe and Effective Care Environment T: Application**
    1. This is not the correct use of an infant car seat.
    2. **The Canadian Paediatric Society (CPS) recommends rear-facing car safety seats for most infants up to 2 years of age. The back seat is recommended because of the danger posed by air bags.**
    3. As in choice 1.
    4. As in choice 1.

137. **Client Needs: Psychosocial Integrity T: Application**
    1. There is no indication the parents require marriage counselling.
    2. This is inappropriate.
    3. As in choice 2.
    4. **These are action-oriented realistic approaches. If there are no sugary snacks, there is not the issue of what each parent will allow. Parental modelling of a healthy lifestyle increases the chances that good health practices will be retained throughout the child's life.**

138. **Client Needs: Safe and Effective Care Environment T: Critical Thinking**
    1. **A respiratory rate of 38 indicates severe respiratory distress, and the client needs immediate assessment and intervention to prevent possible respiratory arrest.**
    2. This client also needs assessment as soon as possible, but they do not need to be assessed as urgently as the client with tachypnea.
    3. As in choice 2.
    4. As in choice 2.

139. **Client Needs: Physiological Integrity T: Application**
    1. This is not a symptom of overdose of thyroid replacement hormone.
    2. **The adverse effects of thyroid medication are usually the result of overdose. Insomnia is a common adverse effect.**
    3. **Weight loss is a common adverse effect of a too-high dose of thyroid replacement hormone.**
    4. As in choice 1.
    5. **Anxiety is a common adverse of thyroid replacement hormone overdose.**

140. **Client Needs: Physiological Integrity; T: Application**
    1. A low body temperature is not a sign of neonatal jaundice.
    2. This is not a normal temperature.
    3. Oral temperatures are not performed on infants.
    4. **This is a low temperature for a neonate, indicating cold stress. Cold stress can cause serious metabolic and physiological problems. The nurse must take action to prevent and correct heat loss.**

141. **Client Needs: Health Promotion and Maintenance; T: Application**
    1. **Pasteurization kills potentially harmful organisms.**
    2. If the package of deli meat is sealed, it should be safe.
    3. Cooking will likely kill any microorganisms.
    4. As long as they are washed, raw vegetables should be safe.

142. **Client Needs: Physiological Integrity T: Application**
    1. **Thinning of the skin indicates that atrophy, a possible adverse effect of topical corticosteroids, is occurring. The prescriber should be notified so that the medication can be changed or tapered.**
    2. This is not an adverse effect of topical corticosteroid use.
    3. As in choice 2.
    4. As in choice 2.

143. **Client Needs: Safe and Effective Care Environment T: Application**
    1. **Frequently changing passwords is important for the security of EHR.**
    2. **Documenting care in quiet, low stimulus areas helps to avoid distractions that may lead to errors.**
    3. Passwords are never to be shared.
    4. Documentation should be done frequently and in real time rather than waiting until the end of a shift.

5. Breaches of confidentiality are avoided by logging out of the computer system when not actively engaged in documenting.

144. Client Needs: Safe and Effective Care Environment T: Critical Thinking
   1. **Checking the client's identification bracelet is the safest method to ensure the "right client."**
   2. Clients may have similar names.
   3. Some clients may not have access to their health card or hospital identification card.
   4. Clients may not be in the correct bed.

145. Client Needs: Safe and Effective Care Environment T: Application
   1. This should have been assessed prior to administration of the acetaminophen.
   2. Assessment is the nurse's responsibility and is not to be delegated to an unregulated care provider.
   3. **The nurse's next priority action for this client is to evaluate whether the nursing intervention of administering acetaminophen was effective.**
   4. The nurse does not have enough evaluative data to determine whether the client's plan of care needs to be revised.

146. Client Needs: Psychosocial Integrity; T: Knowledge
   1. **Aversion therapy is a form of behaviour therapy utilizing negative reinforcement to change behaviour.**
   2. This is not correct.
   3. Aversion therapy is a type of cognitive behavioural therapy but is more specific.
   4. This is not correct.

147. Client Needs: Safe and Effective Care Environment T: Critical Thinking
   1. **Nurses should review the data prior to entering it when using electronic health record systems.**
   2. **Documentation in the electronic health record should be done frequently and in real time rather than waiting until the end of a shift.**
   3. **Providing eye contact periodically with the client when entering data is a strategy to manage communication rapport.**
   4. Nurses must use their own words in the narrative section, not what another nurse documented.
   5. To avoid work burden and allow for task completion, some nurses create shortcuts to bypass aspects of the computerized system, known as "workarounds." These shortcuts raise safety concerns and may alter a system that is designed to improve safety, making it less safe.

148. Client Needs: Physiological Integrity T: Application
   1. This is not necessarily true; the client may be able to move some extremities.
   2. As in choice 1.
   3. **The client must be individually assessed. They may be able to move some joints actively or require assistance from the nurse with others.**
   4. Mobility should not be restricted.

149. Client Needs: Health Promotion and Maintenance; T: Application
   1. Tape may precipitate skin tears.
   2. Skin bruising and tears do not require referral to a dermatologist
   3. Caution should be taken against exposure to direct sunlight without a sunscreen; however, unless the skin is burned, this should not lead to bruising or tears.
   4. **Skin breakdown and bruising are common in the older population. Dehydration and improper nutrition are recognized risk factors.**

150. Client Needs: Physiological Integrity; T: Application
   1. Internal fetal monitoring is not indicated. It requires rupturing of the membranes and attachment of an electrode to the fetus.
   2. **The fetal back is determined by Leopold manoeuvres. The ultrasound transducer, or fetoscope, is placed over this area.**
   3. A fetoscope may be used for FHR monitoring but should be measured between contractions.
   4. This is a normal FHR. Positioning supine is contraindicated as it may lead to maternal supine hypotensive syndrome.

151. Client Needs: Physiological Integrity; T: Critical Thinking
   1. **The client must remain face down. A massage table provides comfort, enabling the client to remain in position.**
   2. The client does not need a recliner; they must be face down.
   3. The client does not need a lift; they are able to mobilize.
   4. **Periscope glasses will allow the client to see above the table.**
   5. Straws are useful as the client cannot sit up to drink.
   6. The client does not require an elevated toilet seat.

152. Client Needs: Safe and Effective Care Environment T: Application
   1. This has the potential to produce increased perceptual distortions.
   2. **Careful observation and supervision are of ultimate importance because an appropriate outcome would be that the client will remain safe and free from injury.**
   3. Physical contact during care cannot be avoided.
   4. Activating a bed alarm is only one aspect of providing for the client's safety.

153. Client Needs: Physiological Integrity T: Application
   1. **The nonsteroidal anti-inflammatory drugs (NSAIDs) are nephrotoxic and should be avoided in clients with impaired renal function.**
   2. The nurse should ask the reason the client is taking this medication, but the medication of most concern is ibuprofen.
   3. As in choice 2.
   4. As in choice 2.

154. **Client Needs: Health Promotion and Maintenance; T: Application**
   1. The HPV vaccine will not protect against SARS-CoV-2.
   2. **Infections from most common types of HPV can be prevented with the HPV vaccine. Some types of HPV can cause genital warts and cancer, such as anal, cervical, and penile.**
   3. The HPV vaccine will not protect against HIV.
   4. The HPV vaccine will not protect against herpes.

155. **Client Needs: Psychosocial Integrity T: Application**
   1. The nurse must care for this client without involving another nurse.
   2. It is impossible for nurses to be knowledgeable about the cultural backgrounds and values of all clients.
   3. **Nurses should perform a cultural assessment of their clients to plan care consistent with client values and beliefs.**
   4. This is true, but care should involve cultural perspectives.

156. **Client Needs: Physiological Integrity T: Knowledge**
   1. Internal rotation is to be avoided.
   2. External rotation is to be avoided.
   3. Adduction is to be avoided.
   4. **Positioning following a total hip replacement depends on the surgical technique, the method of implantation, the prosthesis, and the primary health care provider's preference. However, in most cases, abduction is to be maintained.**

157. **Client Needs: Safe and Effective Care Environment T: Application**
   1. Promoting dependence on staff is not a characteristic of client-centred care.
   2. **Client-centred care involves providing information and allowing the time for the client to ask questions.**
   3. **A characteristic of client-centred care is to support the client in making informed decisions. The decision-making process starts with providing each client with enough information, tailored to their unique circumstances, to make an informed decision.**
   4. **Respecting the client's cultural values and needs is a characteristic of client-centred care.**
   5. **Incorporating effective teaching methods as appropriate is a characteristic of client-centred care. Some clients value knowing as much as possible; others want just the basic facts. Others may need to have essential information developed in steps and spread over several encounters to allow for better processing and formulation of related questions.**

158. **Client Needs: Physiological Integrity; T: Application**
   1. The air vent is never to be clamped.
   2. **Distension of the abdomen indicates nasogastric suction is not effective. Assessing for bowel sounds is an indication peristalsis has resumed.**

3. The tube should be connected to a drainage bag or intermittent suction.
   4. Feeds are not to be started with a nasogastric tube attached to suction.

159. **Client Needs: Physiological Integrity T: Application**
   1. Urine glucose testing is not an accurate reflection of blood glucose level and does not reflect the glucose over a prolonged time.
   2. Oral glucose tolerance testing is done to diagnose diabetes but is not used for monitoring glucose control once diabetes has been diagnosed.
   3. A fasting blood level indicates only the glucose level at one time.
   4. **The glycosylated hemoglobin (HbA$_{1C}$) test shows the overall control of glucose over 90 to 120 days.**

160. **Client Needs: Safe and Effective Care Environment T: Application**
   1. **Placing the client on contact precautions is an infection control measure to prevent transmission of *C. difficile*.**
   2. **Good hand hygiene, preferably with soap and water, for clients who have diarrhea is an infection control measure to prevent transmission of *C. difficile*.**
   3. Hand hygiene with soap and water is more effective in preventing transmission of *C. difficile* in clients who have diarrhea.
   4. This precaution will not prevent the transmission of *C. difficile*.
   5. As in choice 4.

161. **Client Needs: Safe and Effective Care Environment T: Critical Thinking**
   1. Melatonin is safe to use as a therapy for jet lag.
   2. Short-term use of diphenhydramine in young adults, although not recommended, is not an immediate concern.
   3. **The client's BMI and snoring suggest possible sleep apnea, which can cause complications such as cardiac dysrhythmias, hypertension, and right-sided heart failure.**
   4. Hot chocolate contains only 5 mg of caffeine and is unlikely to be affecting this client's sleep quality.

162. **Client Needs: Psychosocial Integrity; T: Application**
   1. Language barriers may be an issue, but do not always interfere with care.
   2. Family members may provide food, and this may be a short-term issue.
   3. This may be true but is a generalization.
   4. **Nurses should attempt to understand cultural norms of the client in order to provide meaningful care.**

163. **Client Needs: Physiological Integrity T: Application**
   1. The lacrimal duct is not the appropriate placement for the eye medication. It will drain into the nasopharynx, and the child will taste the drug.
   2. The medication should not be administered directly on the eyeball.

3. The lower eyelid is pulled down, forming a small conjunctival sac. The solution or ointment is applied to this area.

4. As in choice 2.

164. **Client Needs: Physiological Integrity; T: Application**
   1. **These are normal finding for a 3-month-old infant.**
   2. This is not a high pulse for a 3-month old. Normal pulse is 120 to 140 bpm.
   3. Pulse rate should be regular, but depending on activity, temperature, and crying, infants can demonstrate fluctuations of heart rate.
   4. 4+ is a normal pulse strength.

165. **Client Needs: Psychosocial Integrity T: Application**
   1. **The nurse's safety is a priority. Calling security protects the safety of the nurse and may prevent the client from harming others.**
   2. The client can go if security cannot prevent this, in which case the police may be notified.
   3. This will increase client anger and violence.
   4. The nurse may have to allow the client to leave if calling security is not effective.

166. **Client Needs: Safe and Effective Care Environment T: Knowledge**
   1. Communication breakdowns can cause near-miss situations, but there are other processes that can also cause near misses.
   2. This is not a reason to report near-miss situations.
   3. **Each time an error or near miss occurs, team members should get together and discuss it in a nonjudgemental way in order to determine improved processes to help decrease future errors.**
   4. As in choice 2.

167. **Client Needs: Physiological Integrity T: Critical Thinking**
   1. **SSRIs take about 6 weeks to reach maximum clinical effectiveness.**
   2. **Second-generation antidepressants are generally considered superior to tricyclic antidepressants (TCAs) and monoamine oxidase inhibitors (MAOIs).**
   3. St. John's Wort is contraindicated when a client is taking an SSRI.
   4. **Serotonin syndrome is a rare collection of symptoms from elevated levels of the neurotransmitter serotonin that can occur in clients taking an SSRI.**
   5. **SSRIs may cause sexual issues such as lack of interest and erectile dysfunction.**
   6. There is a relatively low adverse-effect profile compared with older antidepressants.

168. **Client Needs: Safe and Effective Care Environment T: Application**
   1. This technique is not safe in assisting a blind client.
   2. As in choice 1.
   3. As in choice 1.
   4. **When using the sighted-guide technique, the nurse walks slightly in front and to the side of the client and has the client hold the nurse's elbow.**

169. **Client Needs: Physiological Integrity T: Application**
   1. **Corticosteroids have the potential to cause diabetes mellitus. The finding of an elevated blood glucose reflects this adverse effect of prednisone.**
   2. No improvement in symptoms would indicate that the prednisone was not effective but would not be an adverse effect of the medication.
   3. Corticosteroids increase appetite and lead to weight gain, not weight loss.
   4. An elevated ESR would indicate that the prednisone was not effective but would not be an adverse effect of the medication.

170. **Client Needs: Psychosocial Integrity T: Application**
   1. This may be disrespectful and demeaning to older persons.
   2. **Engaging in conversation with older persons helps them feel valued. Older persons need stimulation, socialization, and respect.**
   3. Giving older persons as much control as possible allows them to feel valued and maintains dignity.
   4. Depending on the client's background, this may be perceived as disrespectful. When possible, the nurse should ask the client how they wish to be addressed.

171. **Client Needs: Safe and Effective Care Environment T: Critical Thinking**
   1. **Rotavirus is easily transmitted by direct client contact or by contact with items in the client's environment. Contact precautions will reduce the risk of transmission.**
   2. **Hepatitis A is transmitted by direct client contact and requires contact precautions.**
   3. Streptococcal pharyngitis requires droplet precautions.
   4. Mycoplasma pneumonia requires droplet precautions.
   5. **Respiratory syncytial virus is easily transmitted by direct client contact or by contact with items in the client's environment. Contact precautions will reduce the risk of transmission.**

172. **Client Needs: Safe and Effective Care Environment T: Application**
   1. Refusing to accept an assignment may be considered insubordination, and clients will suffer if the number of available staff drops.
   2. **Nurses who are temporarily reassigned to another unit (i.e., float) should inform the nurse manager of their lack of experience in caring for clients on a particular nursing unit. They also should request, and be given, basic orientation to the unit. Asking to work with an experienced general surgery nurse would be an appropriate action.**
   3. The nurse can make a written protest to nursing administrators, but it should not be the nurse's initial recourse.
   4. Notifying the CNA should not be the nurse's initial recourse.

173. Client Needs: Safe and Effective Care Environment T: Application
    1. The nurse should not ask a colleague what the order says because the colleague did not write the order.
    2. **If a prescriber writes an order that is illegible, the nurse should contact the prescriber for clarification.**
    3. The nurse should not contact the pharmacy to clarify the order because this action would delay implementation of the order.
    4. Asking the client what medications are taken at home is incorrect because this question will not clarify the current order.

174. Client Needs: Psychosocial Integrity; T: Application
    1. **The client has expressed their end-of-life wishes, and it is the nurse's responsibility to comply with these wishes.**
    2. It is the health care provider's responsibility to discontinue treatment, not the nurse's.
    3. The nurse may facilitate a family meeting; it is not up to the nurse to tell the family.
    4. The nurse may suggest discussing MAiD with the family, but the referral to the MAiD team should not be delayed.

175. Client Needs: Physiological Integrity T: Application
    1. Intramuscular injections are inserted at a 90-degree angle.
    2. **This image depicts an intradermal injection.**
    3. Subcutaneous injections are inserted at a 45- to 90-degree angle.
    4. The graphic depicts insertion of an injection into the dermis, not a vein.

176. Client Needs: Safe and Effective Care Environment T: Knowledge
    1. **In team nursing, an RN leads a team that is composed of other RNs, registered psychiatric nurses or licensed and registered practical nurses (LPNs and RPNs), and unregulated care providers (UCPs). The team members provide direct client care to groups of clients, under the direction of the RN team leader.**
    2. Primary nursing is a model of care delivery whereby an RN assumes responsibility for a caseload of clients over time. Typically, the RN selects the clients for their caseload and cares for those clients during their hospitalization or stay in the health care setting. When a primary nurse is off duty, other team members, including RPNs, LPNs, or other RNs, follow the care plan.
    3. Functional nursing is task focused, not client focused; in a functional nursing model, tasks are divided, with each nurse assuming responsibility for specific tasks.
    4. In a total client care model, an RN is responsible for all aspects of care for one or more clients. The RN may delegate aspects of care but retains accountability for care of all assigned clients.

177. Client Needs: Physiological Integrity T: Knowledge
    1. This is not a sterile procedure.

    2. A Yankauer suction catheter is made of rigid, minimally flexible plastic with one large and several small openings through which the mucus enters with application of negative pressure.
    3. A resuscitation bag should not be required.
    4. The catheter should not be flexible; #8 is too small for an adult.

178. Client Needs: Psychosocial Integrity T: Application
    1. The child will continue to receive care according to the parent's wishes.
    2. The child may be allowed to have a natural death, but this is to be determined.
    3. The child will not be removed from the ventilator without the parent's permission.
    4. **A DNR is specific to individual clients and situations. The health care team and parents will determine what care the child is to receive—for example, cardiac compressions if the child's heart stops.**

179. Client Needs: Safe and Effective Care Environment T: Application
    1. **The role of the nurse concerning disaster preparedness includes working within communities to reduce hazards in the home and work settings.**
    2. Implementing strategies to decrease PSTD would come after a given disaster occurs and the needs of the community have been identified in this regard.
    3. **The role of the nurse in disaster preparedness includes participating in drills and training exercises.**
    4. Evaluating the economic impact of a disaster would also occur after the disaster has occurred and would not be a nursing responsibility.
    5. **Nurses play an important role in preparedness by educating individuals and communities on disaster preparedness.**

180. Client Needs: Physiological Integrity T: Knowledge
    1. This is not correct.
    2. As in choice 1.
    3. **Too loose a blood pressure cuff may cause a false high systolic reading.**
    4. As in choice 1.

181. Client Needs: Psychosocial Integrity T: Critical Thinking
    1. **The first action in crisis intervention is to reassure the client they are safe.**
    2. This is appropriate but not the first action.
    3. Consoling the client is appropriate, but saying everything will be okay is not necessarily true.
    4. As in choice 2.

182. Client Needs: Safe and Effective Care Environment T: Critical Thinking
    1. **Measles, varicella, or tuberculosis are infectious diseases transmitted via the airborne route.**
    2. Pertussis requires droplet transmission precautions.
    3. Influenza requires droplet transmission precautions.
    4. Scarlet fever requires droplet transmission precautions.

183. **Client Needs: Physiological Integrity T: Knowledge**
   1. Scoliosis is a lateral spinal curvature, sometimes seen in adolescents.
   2. **This picture is of kyphosis, an exaggerated posterior curvature of the thoracic spine, sometimes called "dowager's hump."**
   3. Lordosis is increased lumbar curvature sometimes called "swayback."
   4. This is not normal posture.

184. **Client Needs: Safe and Effective Care Environment T: Knowledge**
   1. **Bloodborne pathogens such as those associated with hepatitis B and C are most commonly transmitted by contaminated needles.**
   2. *C. difficile* is spread by contact with and ingestion of this microbe.
   3. MRSA is spread by contact.
   4. Diphtheria is spread by droplets when a person is within 1 m (3 feet) of the client.

185. **Client Needs: Psychosocial Integrity; T: Knowledge**
   1. **Night vision becomes impaired as physiological changes in the eye occur.**
   2. Older persons lose the ability to distinguish high-pitched noises and consonants.
   3. Sense of taste is decreased.
   4. Sense of smell is decreased.

186. **Client Needs: Health Promotion and Maintenance T: Application**
   1. **Wearing a mask has been proven to decrease viral transmission.**
   2. Physical distancing needs to be only 2 metres.
   3. **Well-ventilated spaces reduce the likelihood of inhaling virus particles.**
   4. People should cover their nose and mouth with a bent elbow or tissue when coughing or sneezing.
   5. **Staying home will prevent an infected person from transmitting the virus to others.**
   6. Clean hands often with soap and water or hand sanitizer.

187. **Client Needs: Physiological Integrity T: Application**
   1. **Medications that fall onto the floor need to be discarded, and the procedure must be repeated with new medications.**
   2. The client has not refused the medications.
   3. Waiting until the next dosage time would result in the client missing the required doses of the prescribed medications.
   4. The medications need to be discarded since they have fallen to the floor.

188. **Client Needs: Physiological Integrity T: Application**
   1. **The client should be instructed to avoid rapid position changes (due to risk of postural hypotension caused by drug).**
   2. ACE inhibitors do not deplete potassium.
   3. **Adverse effects may include a cough when on an ACE inhibitor.**

   4. ACE inhibitors should be taken 1 hr before meals to increase absorption.
   5. **The client should be instructed to drink plenty of water to avoid dehydration (which could worsen hypotension).**

189. **Client Needs: Safe and Effective Care Environment T: Application**
   1. This option does not describe the situation.
   2. As in choice 1.
   3. As in choice 1.
   4. **Despite the caregiver's good intentions, the older client may experience profound unintentional neglect. Unintentional neglect is usually not viewed as a crime, but it must be addressed.**

190. **Client Needs: Physiological Adaptation; T: Critical Thinking**
   1. This possibly could be true but is not the most likely cause. Saying this to the client will frighten them.
   2. **A common adverse effect of acetylsalicylate acid (Aspirin), which has blood thinning properties, is bleeding into the skin and mucous membranes.**
   3. This is true but is not the most appropriate answer.
   4. This is partly true but needs to be assessed by the health care provider.

191. **Client Needs: Physiological Integrity; T: Application**
   1. **While the rapid antigen tests are not 100% conclusive, they may display a positive result even without symptoms.**
   2. **Symptoms may include shortness of breath, cough, runny nose, sneezing, decreased consciousness, decreased appetite.**
   3. This is not necessary nor reasonable.
   4. **There are many home oxygen saturation monitors available for purchase at a reasonable price. They may show a decreasing oxygen level in the blood, an indication of COVID-19 infection.**
   5. Strict isolation is not necessary unless the client becomes COVID-19 positive or develops symptoms.
   6. This is not necessary in a home environment.

192. **Client Needs: Safe and Effective Care Environment T: Critical Thinking**
   1. The family may be able to help the nurse gain perspective about pain, but this strategy alone is inadequate.
   2. A client with dementia would be unable to use a visual analogue scale.
   3. **Lewy body disease is a form of dementia. There are special scales to assess the presence and severity of pain in clients with dementia. The Pain Assessment in Advanced Dementia Scale (PAINAD) evaluates breathing, negative vocalizations, body language, and consolability.**
   4. This type of dementia does not include a diminished perception of pain.

193. **Client Needs: Physiological Adaptation; T: Critical Thinking**
   1. This might be appropriate, but the runner is not in a life-threatening situation at this time.

2. This might be necessary if the runner does not respond to oral therapy.
3. The first line of treatment is to replace fluids and electrolytes with an oral solution. There is no indication that the client is not able to take fluids by mouth.
4. Vital signs must be monitored, but this is not the priority action.

194. Client Needs: Physiological Integrity; T: Knowledge
 1. Adrenaline does not act as a natural pain reliever.
 2. **Endorphins are body substances that are similar to morphine and may provide natural pain relief.**
 3. As in choice 1.
 4. As in choice 1.

195. Client Needs: Psychosocial Integrity T: Application
 1. Clients should never be restrained.
 2. **Small portions of the client's favourite foods will provide comfort.**
 3. **There is no need to force food or fluids; this increases discomfort and nausea.**
 4. **Oral medications may not be tolerated. It is a nursing responsibility to advocate for alternate routes.**
 5. The client should mobilize if they feel able.
 6. Adhering to a strict administration schedule may not adequately manage pain. Pain levels should be continually assessed, regardless of the schedule.

196. Client Needs: Psychosocial Integrity; T: Critical Thinking
 1. This is not necessary, although it can be done. Visual assessment provides information the child is in pain.
 2. The child is in pain; this does not provide optimum care for the child.
 3. **Children of this age are very afraid of needles. The child may be more afraid of having a needle than in receiving pain relief.**
 4. This may be necessary if the child refuses the pill.

197. Client Needs: Safe and Effective Care Environment T: Application
 1. This is not an effective security measure.
 2. As in choice 1.
 3. As in choice 1.
 4. **The nurse should check the ID bracelet number of the infant with that of the child-bearing parent.**

198. Client Needs: Physiological Integrity T: Knowledge
 1. Infiltration causes skin near the IV insertion site to become edematous.
 2. **Infiltration may cause the skin near the IV insertion site to be bruised or discoloured.**
 3. **Infiltration causes skin near the IV insertion site to be cool to the touch.**
 4. A reddish streak proximal to the insertion site is a symptom of phlebitis.
 5. **Infiltration may cause the client to experience some numbness.**
 6. **If an IV is in situ, there should be blood return.**

199. Client Needs: Psychosocial Integrity; T: Application
 1. Lyme disease has not been found to be associated with AD.

2. Depression has been found to have a causal relationship with Alzheimer's disease.
3. As in choice 1.
4. As in choice 1.

200. Client Needs: Physiological Integrity T: Comprehension
 1. Hyperkalemia, not hypokalemia, may occur.
 2. **Hyperkalemia may occur with administration of potassium-sparing diuretics.**
 3. This is not an adverse effect of this medication.
 4. As in choice 3.

201. Client Needs: Physiological Adaptation; T: Critical Thinking
 1. This may be necessary information; however, the nurse needs to know more about the penicillin allergy.
 2. As in choice 1.
 3. This is a necessary action, but the nurse must first determine if this is a true allergy.
 4. **The nurse requires a description of client symptoms to determine if this is a true allergy, a sensitivity, or an adverse effect of another agent.**

202. Client Needs: Physiological Integrity; T: Critical Thinking
 1. This is high fat, not appropriate for this client's needs.
 2. Orange juice is high in sugar and glycemic index, not appropriate with type 2 diabetes.
 3. **Tuna salad provides appropriate nutrients and is low calorie.**
 4. **Carrot and cucumber provide appropriate nutrients; dipping sauce is low calorie.**
 5. Canned vegetable soup is high in sodium.
 6. **Raspberries and blueberries provide appropriate nutrients.**
 All correct menu selections add up to 465 calories, within the 500-calorie limit.

203. Client Needs: Safe and Effective Care Environment T: Critical Thinking
 1. This is an effective strategy to increase safety when child-proofing the home.
 2. **By law a rear-facing infant car seat should be used for infants who weighs less than 10 kg (usually about 1 year of age or more).**
 3. As in choice 1.
 4. As in choice 1.

204. Client Needs: Safe and Effective Care Environment T: Application
 1. Once communicated, changes should be put in place as the committee deems reasonable (i.e., either fully or as a pilot study) and as soon as practical; this should be followed by re-evaluation.
 2. As in choice 1.
 3. As in choice 1.
 4. **The QI committee must communicate the practice change to staff before it is implemented.**

205. **Client Needs: Safe and Effective Care Environment T: Critical Thinking**
   1. This client should also be assessed as quickly as possible, but assessment of this client is not the highest priority.
   2. As in choice 1.
   3. **This client is at risk for bleeding from the arterial access site for the PCI, so the nurse should assess the client's blood pressure, pulse, and the access site immediately.**
   4. As in choice 1.

206. **Client Needs: Safe and Effective Care Environment T: Application**
   1. The nurse being observed may not be doing the procedure according to the agency's policy or procedure.
   2. **The Canadian Council on Health Services requires accredited hospitals to have written nursing policies and procedures. These agency standards of care are specific and need to be accessible on all nursing units. For example, an agency policy/procedure would outline specific steps to follow in changing a dressing.**
   3. The procedure taught in nursing school may not be consistent with the policy or procedure for this agency.
   4. The client is not responsible for maintaining the standards of practice; client input is important, but it's not what directs nursing practice.

207. **Client Needs: Safe and Effective Care Environment T: Application**
   1. Strong passwords are combinations of letters, numbers, and symbols that are difficult to guess.
   2. A firewall is a combination of hardware and software that protects private network resources (e.g., the information system of the hospital) from outside hackers, network damage, and theft or misuse of information and should not be bypassed.
   3. **In faxing, programmed speed-dial keys should be used to eliminate the chance of a dialing error and misdirected information.**
   4. **An automatic sign-off is a safety mechanism that logs a user off the computer system after a specified period of inactivity; it is used in most client care areas and other departments that handle sensitive data.**
   5. **Disciplinary action, including loss of employment, occurs when nurses or other health care personnel inappropriately access client information.**
   6. **All papers containing private health information must be destroyed. Most agencies have shredders or locked receptacles for shredding and later incineration.**

208. **Client Needs: Safe and Effective Care Environment T: Application**
   1. Asking physiotherapy to assist the client is premature before the client is reassessed and before prescriber orders have been made.

   2. The nurse may not need to disregard all previous diagnoses.
   3. **The nurse needs to reassess the client after any type of change of health status.**
   4. Setting new priorities is not recommended before assessment and establishing diagnoses.

209. **Client Needs: Physiological Integrity T: Critical Thinking**
   1. **Use of an electronic device, a smartphone, or electronic tablet will enable the client to fully describe their symptoms.**
   2. This may be helpful, but it is unlikely for a deaf interpreter to be on staff at a small community hospital. Use of the electronic device is an immediate solution.
   3. This may assist the client to understand the nurse but will not enable the client to describe their symptoms.
   4. The client may not be able to adequately describe symptoms by gestures alone.

210. **Client Needs: Safe and Effective Care Environment T: Critical Thinking**
   1. Two witnesses are usually required when telephone consents are involved. This is not the case in this situation.
   2. In an emergency, it is not necessary to contact the institutional review board; doing so would take up valuable time.
   3. An official interpreter must be available to explain the terms of consent except in an emergency situation. A family interpreter is not necessary as emergency consent policies apply.
   4. **In emergency situations, if it is impossible to obtain consent from the client or an authorized person, the beneficial or life-saving procedure may be undertaken without liability for failure to obtain consent. In such cases, according to the law, the health care team would assume that the client would wish to be given the treatment.**

211. **Client Needs: Safe and Effective Care Environment T: Application**
   1. **Pillows should not be placed in the infant's crib. Anticipatory guidance for a 1-month-old infant to prevent a suffocation injury considers that the infant will have increased eye–hand coordination and a voluntary grasp reflex as well as a crawling reflex that may propel the infant forward or backward.**
   2. Crib slats should be 6 cm or less apart; 10 cm is too wide.
   3. **Plastic bags should be kept out of reach.**
   4. The mattress should not be covered with plastic even if a sheet is used to cover it.
   5. **A pacifier should not be tied on a string around the infant's neck.**

212. **Client Needs: Health Promotion and Maintenance; T: Critical Thinking**
   1. **Clients requiring home oxygen need extensive teaching to be able to continue oxygen therapy at home efficiently and safely. Assessment of their**

cognitive and physical abilities determines if teaching will be effective.

2. This is a consideration but not the priority.

3. As in choice 2

4. As in choice 2

213. **Client Needs: Physiological Integrity; T: Application**

1. **This is appropriate, particularly as the client has dementia.**

2. **The prongs must be positioned appropriately to deliver the required flow.**

3. The cannula may be used with portable oxygen tanks. Wall oxygen may not be available in long-term care settings.

4. **Particularly if the oxygen is not adequately humidified, it is drying to the nasal mucosa. Also, the prongs may irritate the mucosa.**

5. **Any time oxygen is administered, its effects on oxygen saturation must be assessed.**

6. Restraints are not to be routinely applied.

214. **Client Needs: Physiological Integrity T: Application**

1. This is contraindicated as it may induce shivering.

2. **The client should be loosely covered with light bed linens.**

3. This is contraindicated, as it may induce shivering and will dry the skin.

4. Ice chips will not reduce the client temperature, although may show a falsely low reading if an oral temperature is taken.

215. **Client Needs: Psychosocial Integrity T: Critical Thinking**

1. **This is the first action. The manager needs to answer questions concerning the decreasing standards at the home and if there is a plan to correct the problems.**

2. The nurse might have to help with some care for the relative, but this will not correct the status of care in the home.

3. The nurse may speak with other families to gather information, but this will not correct the status of care in the home.

4. If speaking with the nurse manager does not provide satisfactory answers, then the Ministry of Health and Long Term Care may need to be contacted.

216. **Client Needs: Health Promotion and Maintenance; T: Application**

1. It is not the responsibility of the nurse to convince the woman to breastfeed; her choice must be respected.

2. This statement may appear to be disapproving and culturally insensitive

3. This action will stimulate the nipple and encourage the flow of milk.

4. **These actions will help to manage breast engorgement for a nonbreastfeeding infant.**

217. **Client Needs: Health Promotion and Maintenance; T: Application**

1. **This action is within the scope of practice for a nurse, regardless of the setting.**

2. As in choice 1.

3. As in choice 1.

4. As in choice 1.

5. The nurse is not permitted to obtain consent for a procedure performed by another health care provider.

6. The nurse is not allowed to initiate anaesthesia.

218. **Client Needs: Safe and Effective Care Environment T: Application**

1. It is not within the nurse's legal scope of practice to explain the surgical procedure.

2. **The surgeon is responsible for explaining the surgery to the client. The nurse needs to contact the surgeon for client clarification.**

3. No preoperative medications should be administered until the client signs the consent form.

4. The nurse should communicate directly with the surgeon about the consent form rather than asking other staff to pass on the message.

219. **Client Needs: Safe and Effective Care Environment T: Application**

1. **Because of the higher risk of osteoporosis in the older population, a fall can result in a fracture. This choice depicts a client with two risk factors for osteoporosis, including Asian ancestry and smoking cigarettes.**

2. **This choice depicts a client with three risk factors for osteoporosis, including White ancestry, drinking alcohol, and age over 80.**

3. **This choice depicts a client with three risk factors for osteoporosis, including White ancestry, age over 70, and daily oral prednisone.**

4. This choice describes a client with no risk factors for osteoporosis.

5. As in choice 4.

220. **Client Needs: Physiological Integrity; T: Application**

1. The client is to lie flat, with leg extended.

2. As in choice 1.

3. **The client will need to lie flat for about 6 hours, depending on unit protocol, and the extremity should be extended and immobilized.**

4. As in choice 1.

221. **Client Needs: Physiological Integrity T: Application**

1. This would not be useful in assessing for an adverse effect of the gentamicin.

2. As in choice 1.

3. As in choice 1.

4. **An adverse effect of gentamicin is impaired renal function. Renal function including BUN and creatinine levels should be monitored.**

222. **Client Needs: Physiological Integrity; T: Application**

1. **Long-term laxative use can lead to constipation. Increasing fluid and fibre can help with this problem; further laxative use should be avoided.**

2. Laxatives do not cause scarring.

3. Natural laxatives such as mineral oil have risks, such as rendering the body unable to absorb fat-soluble vitamins.

4. Even if malnourished, the body will produce wastes if food is consumed.

223. **Client Needs: Safe and Effective Care Environment T: Application**
    1. **The bed's side rails should be padded to minimize the risk for client injury during a seizure.**
    2. Use of a tongue blade during a seizure is contraindicated.
    3. **The client is at risk for further seizures, and oxygen may be needed after any seizures to maximize oxygenation.**
    4. **Suctioning may be needed after any seizures to clear the airway.**
    5. Insertion of a nasogastric (NG) tube is not indicated because the airway problem is not caused by vomiting or abdominal distension.

224. **Client Needs: Safe and Effective Care Environment T: Application**
    1. This is appropriate teaching by the new nurse for a client with newly diagnosed hypertension who has just started therapy with enalapril.
    2. As in choice 1.
    3. **The ACE inhibitors cause retention of potassium by the kidneys, so hyperkalemia is a possible adverse effect. The client should not consume a high-potassium diet.**
    4. As in choice 1.

225. **Client Needs: Physiological Integrity T: Application**
    1. Hydrogen peroxide rinses are not indicated for *Candida* infection. Oral saltwater rinses may be used but will not cure the infection.
    2. Antiviral agents are used for viral infections such as herpes simplex.
    3. Referral to a dentist is indicated for gingivitis but not for *Candida* infection.
    4. ***Candida albicans* is treated with an antifungal agent such as nystatin.**

226. **Client Needs: Safe and Effective Care Environment T: Application**
    1. It is important to solicit the perspectives of all members of the health care team on the nursing unit, not just the nurses.
    2. This intervention would not be beneficial in the promotion of conflict resolution.
    3. As in choice 2.
    4. **Depersonalization of conflict situations is an effective intervention to promote conflict resolution.**

227. **Client Needs: Physiological Integrity T: Application**
    1. **Systemic corticosteroids are valuable in the treatment of severe skin disorders because of their capacity to inhibit inflammatory and allergic reactions.**
    2. Vasoconstriction, not vasodilation, is a possible effect of systemic steroids.
    3. **Prolonged use may temporarily suppress the child's growth.**

4. **The dose is carefully adjusted and gradually tapered to the minimum dosage that is effective.**
    5. Corticosteroids do not possess antimicrobial activity.
    6. **Corticosteroids often cause edema and weight gain.**

228. **Client Needs: Safe and Effective Care Environment T: Application**
    1. This is not the essential value described in this situation.
    2. As in choice 1.
    3. As in choice 1.
    4. **Clients need to be in control of their own destiny. Advocacy should support client autonomy, even when the decision reached is not what the nurse would recommend for the client's health and well-being.**

229. **Client Needs: Safe and Effective Care Environment T: Critical Thinking**
    1. This will assist the client in keeping orientation to the environment but is not the most helpful strategy for wandering.
    2. As in choice 1.
    3. As in choice 1.
    4. **Because the client is wandering to the wrong rooms to look for items, signs on the doors and entryways would be most helpful to assist with searches for the appropriate room.**

230. **Client Needs: Physiological Integrity; T: Critical Thinking**
    1. This is true but is not the priority.
    2. As in choice 1.
    3. This depends on the client's perception of quality of life.
    4. **The client's advance directives or known stated wishes priority must be known to the interprofessional team and family team prior to any treatment decision.**

231. **Client Needs: Safe and Effective Care Environment T: Application**
    1. **Charting should be consecutive, line by line (not every other line); if space is left, a line should be drawn horizontally through it, and the nurse's name should be signed at the end.**
    2. **Nurses must not document a medication given by another nurse.**
    3. All entries should be written legibly and in blue or black ink as per agency policy.
    4. For computer documentation, the nurse should keep the password secure.
    5. Each entry should end with the nurse's signature and title.

232. **Client Needs: Physiological Integrity T: Application**
    1. This does not answer the question.
    2. This may not be correct.
    3. As in choice 2.
    4. **People require PEG tubes for various conditions. They may not be able to chew and swallow, they**

may not tolerate liquids, they may have a risk of aspiration. It is the responsibility of the health care provider to determine what is allowed.

233. **Client Needs:** Safe and Effective Care Environment **T:** Application
    1. Exposure to an infectious disease is not a contraindication to receiving live vaccine.
    2. Symptoms of a cold are not a contraindication to receiving a live vaccine.
    3. Intermittent episodes of diarrhea are not a contraindication to receiving a live vaccine.
    4. **The MMRV (measles, mumps, rubella, and varicella) vaccine is an attenuated live virus vaccine. Children with deficient immune systems should not receive the MMRV vaccine because of a lack of evidence of its safety in this population.**

234. **Client Needs:** Psychosocial Integrity; **T:** Application
    1. Clients with expressive aphasia may take a prolonged time to regain speech function, depending on the severity of the brain injury.
    2. This is a communication strategy but is not the overall goal.
    3. Thickening drinks prevents aspiration but does not need to be in the plan of care for this client.
    4. **To adapt to expressive aphasia, the nurse and the client need to develop nonverbal communication strategies such as pointing and gestures.**

235. **Client Needs:** Safe and Effective Care Environment **T:** Application
    1. Throw rugs should be eliminated, not replaced with heavily weighted rugs.
    2. Falls inside the home are responsible for many injuries.
    3. **Comfortable shoes with good support will help decrease the risk for falls.**
    4. Activities of daily living provide range-of-motion exercise; these do not need to be taught by a physiotherapist.

236. **Client Needs:** Safe and Effective Care Environment **T:** Application
    1. This could possibly encourage the client to discuss his problems but is not the immediate need.
    2. As in choice 1.
    3. **Direct questioning about the intent to harm oneself is appropriate for the nurse to ask during screening or counselling sessions. Even with education of the public and health care providers about the incidence of suicide in the young adult population, suicide continues to be a major health problem, and annual rates, especially for young men, remain high. Direct questioning is required to screen for suicidal ideation.**
    4. As in choice 1.

237. **Client Needs:** Physiological Integrity **T:** Application
    1. **Hydrochlorothiazide therapy may lead to hypokalemia, which can put the client at an increased risk of digitalis toxicity.**

    2. This medication does not require extra caution when taken with hydrochlorothiazide.
    3. As in choice 2.
    4. As in choice 2.

238. **Client Needs:** Physiological Integrity **T:** Application
    Answer: 4.1
    Rationale:
    Step 1: Formula for calculations for pediatric dosages of oral and parenteral medications
    Step 2: Formula for calculation of oral and parenteral doses of medications
    Formula:
    Step 1:

    $$\frac{\text{Drug dosage per}}{\text{kg of body weight}} \times \text{Weight of child (kg)}$$

    $$= \text{Dosage to administer}$$

    Step 2:

    $$\frac{\text{Dosage ordered}}{\text{Dosage available}} \times \text{Drug form}$$

    $$= \text{Amount of drug to administer}$$

    Solution:
    Step 1:

    $$6 \text{ mg} \times 20.5 \text{ kg} = 123 \text{ mg of gentamicin daily (3 doses)}$$
    $$123 \text{ mg} \div 3 = 41 \text{ mg per dose of gentamicin}$$

    Step 2: $41/20 \times 2 = 4.1$ mL

239. **Client Needs:** Physiological Integrity; **T:** Application
    1. Screening for SARS-CoV-2 can be determined by wastewater testing.
    2. **The virus can be shed in feces by people even if they don't have symptoms and then detected in the sewer system. Wastewater surveillance can serve as an early warning that COVID-19 is spreading in a community.**
    3. It was a hypothesis that was proved true.
    4. Specific number of cases can be tracked by rapid and PCR tests, but community levels can be determined in wastewater.

240. **Client Needs:** Reduction of Risk Potential; **T:** Application
    1. Sleeping face down would increase intraocular pressure.
    2. **The client should not cough or bend or strain during defecation as this will increase intraocular pressure.**
    3. Eye drops are to be used routinely as directed.
    4. Glasses should be worn during the day; they are not necessary at night in bed.

241. **Client Needs:** Psychosocial Adaptation; **T:** Critical Thinking
    1. Although true, this is too complicated an explanation for a 12-year old.
    2. **This is an appropriate, clear, and correct definition of diabetes.**
    3. Although true, saying "sugar" in the blood may be confusing, and focus on needles may scare the child.

    4. As in choice 1.

242. **Client Needs: Reduction of Risk Potential; T: Application**
    1. This is normal colour drainage from an NG tube. It does not affect whether the tube should be discontinued.
    2. **If bowel sounds are heard, then normal intestinal function has resumed and the tube may be safely removed.**
    3. This is not necessarily an indication for removal of the NG tube.
    4. After a bowel obstruction stool may not be passed immediately. This should not delay removal of the tube.

243. **Client Needs: Reduction of Risk Potential T: Critical Thinking**
    1. **Fetal ultrasound at 20 weeks identifies fetal and maternal structures, assists in confirming gestational age, identifies fetal anomalies, and evaluates amniotic fluid levels, if 'real-time' ultrasound can monitor movements and breathing.**
    2. This often is possible, but is not the primary reason for fetal ultrasound.
    3. Amniotic fluid volume can be assessed, but not necessarily the need for amniocentesis.
    4. This can be determined, but is only part of assessing fetal well-being.

244. **Client Needs: Safe and Effective Care Environment T: Application**
    1. **Health care providers should communicate with older persons on an adult level and avoid patronizing or speaking in a condescending manner. Terms of endearment such as "honey," "dear," "grandma," or "sweetheart" should be avoided.**
    2. This action by the unregulated care provider facilitates communication with older clients and should be encouraged, not stopped.
    3. As in choice 2.
    4. As in choice 2.

245. **Client Needs: Physiological Integrity T: Critical Thinking**
    Intake: 400 + 600 + 30 = 1 030 mL
    Output: 350 + 85 + 120 = 555 mL
    Calculation of fluid balance: 1030 – 555 = 475 mL excess

246. **Client Needs: Physiological Integrity T: Critical Thinking**

    1. **These are ominous symptoms and require immediate assessment by a health care provider. The client may need stabilization and transport to the nearest medical facility to deliver the baby.**
    2. Fetal activity does need to be monitored; this will occur after the client arrives in the nursing station.
    3. A blood pressure test is necessary, but the client cannot wait to go to a pharmacy. It is a remote community, and there may not be a pharmacy close by.
    4. The priority is to obtain medical intervention as this is likely a pre-eclamptic crisis.

247. **Client Needs: Physiological Integrity T: Application**
    1. **This is the correct procedure. The nurse uses plain language that is understandable to the client.**
    2. Saying "stab wound" and suturing the tube may alarm the client; they may not understand the term PEG tube.
    3. This is not the correct procedure.
    4. This is not the correct procedure, and the tube does not go into the intestine.

248. **Client Needs: Physiological Integrity T: Application**
    1. **Use the following formula to determine the dosage range:**

$$\frac{\text{Drug dosage per}}{\text{kg of body weight}} \times \text{Weight of child (kg)}$$

$$= \text{Dosage to administer}$$

    6 mg × 16 = 96 mg/day
    8 mg × 16 = 128 mg/day
    1. **The safe dosage range is 96 mg/day to 128 mg/day**
    2. This is not the recommended dosage range.
    3. As in choice 2.
    4. As in choice 2.

249. **Client Needs: Physiological Integrity T: Knowledge**
    1. This is not correct.
    2. **This is the correct term for the head of the bed at a 45- to 90- degree angle.**
    3. As in choice 1.
    4. As in choice 1.

250. **Client Needs: Physiological Integrity; T: Knowledge**
    1. Forceful pressure is not applied. Colour change should occur in 2 seconds.
    2. Capillary refill does not measure blanching.
    3. **This is the correct procedure. Brisk capillary refill should occur in 2 seconds.**
    4. Colour change should occur in 2 seconds; 10 seconds is sluggish.

Entry-Level Competencies for Licensed (or Registered) Practical Nurses in Canada

THE CPNRE COMPETENCIES

Assumptions

The following set of assumptions are understood to apply to the practice of practical nursing in Canada and to the entry-level competencies that follow.

- The foundation of practical nursing is defined by:
  - entry-level competencies
  - professional nursing **Standards of Practice** of the **regulatory authority**
  - nursing code(s) of ethics and ethical standards
  - scope of nursing practice applicable in the jurisdiction
  - provincial or territorial and federal legislation and regulations that direct practice
- Licensed practical nurse (LPN, also referred to as registered practical nurses in some jurisdictions) practice is built upon the four concepts of person, environment, health, and nursing and is grounded within the context of the current Canadian health care system, primary health care, and emerging health trends.
- LPNs possess competencies that are transferable across all areas of **responsibility** (e.g., direct care, administration, education, and **research**).
- LPNs are active participants in health promotion, illness prevention, and harm reduction activities.
- LPNs practise in any setting or circumstance where health care is delivered.
- Requisite skills and abilities are required to attain the LPN entry-level competencies.
- LPNs practise **autonomously**, safely, **competently,** and ethically along the continuum of care in situations of health and illness across a client's lifespan.
- LPNs practise in situations of varying complexity and work collaboratively with the **health care team** to maximize client outcomes.
- LPNs demonstrate **leadership** by fostering continued self-growth to meet the challenges of an evolving health care system.
- LPNs follow a systematic approach by using the nursing process to deliver safe, **competent,** and ethical care.
- LPNs **advocate** for the implementation and utilization of **evidence-informed practice.**

Professional Practice

Licensed practical nurses adhere to **Standards of Nursing Practice** and an ethical framework. They are responsible and accountable for safe, **competent,** and ethical nursing practice. They are expected to demonstrate professional conduct as reflected through personal attitudes, beliefs, opinions, and actions. Licensed practical nurses focus on personal and professional growth. Licensed practical nurses are expected to utilize knowledge, **critical thinking**, **critical inquiry,** and **research** to build an **evidence-informed practice**.

1. Demonstrates **accountability** and accepts **responsibility** for own decisions and actions.
2. Practises **autonomously** within legislated **scope of practice.**
3. Displays self-awareness and recognizes when to seek assistance and guidance.
4. Adheres to regulatory requirements of jurisdictional legislation.
5. Practises within own level of **competence.**
6. Initiates, maintains, and terminates the **therapeutic nurse–client relationship.** For example:
   6.1. The duty to provide care.
7. Provides **client** care in a nonjudgemental manner.
8. Adapts practice in response to the **spiritual beliefs** and cultural practices of **clients.** For example:
   8.1. Adapts practice to what the client finds meaningful.
9. Supports **client**s in making informed decisions about their health care and respects their decisions.
10. Engages in self-reflection and continuous learning to maintain and enhance **competence.**
11. Integrates relevant evidence into practice.
12. Collaborates in the analysis, development, implementation and evaluation of practice and policy. For example:
   12.1 Understands the importance and currency of policies, how they are evaluated, and how they apply to practice.
13. Integrates continuous **quality improvement** principles and activities into nursing practice.
14. Demonstrates a professional presence, honesty, integrity, and respect in all interactions.
15. Demonstrates **fitness to practise.**
16. Maintains current knowledge about trends and issues that impact the **client,** the licensed practical nurse, the **health care team,** and the delivery of health services.
17. Identifies and responds to inappropriate behaviour and incidents of **professional misconduct.**
18. Recognizes, responds and reports own and others' **near miss**es, errors and **adverse event**s.
19. Distinguishes between the mandates of **regulatory bodies**, professional associations, and unions.

Ethical Practice

Licensed practical nurses use ethical frameworks (e.g., Code of Ethics, ethical standards) when making professional judgements and practice decisions. They engage in **critical thinking** and **critical inquiry** to inform decision-making and use self-reflection to understand the impact of personal values, beliefs, and assumptions in the provision of care.

20. Establishes and maintains **professional boundaries.**
21. Takes action to minimize the impact of personal values and assumptions on interactions and decisions.
22. Demonstrates respect for the values, opinions, needs and beliefs of others.
23. Applies ethical frameworks and reasoning to identify and respond to situations involving moral and ethical conflict, dilemma, or distress.
24. Obtains knowledge of and responds to the *Calls to Action of the Truth and Reconciliation Commission of Canada.*[1]
25. Preserves the dignity of **client**s in all personal and professional contexts.
26. **Advocate**s for **equitable** access, treatment, and allocation of resources, particularly for vulnerable and **diverse cli**ents and populations.
27. **Advocate**s for **client**s or their representatives especially when they are unable to **advocate** for themselves.

Legal Practice

Licensed practical nurses adhere to applicable provincial or territorial and federal legislation and regulations, professional standards, and employer policies that direct practice. They engage in professional regulation by enhancing their **competence**, promoting safe practice, and maintaining their **fitness to practise**. Licensed practical nurses recognize that safe nursing practice includes knowledge of relevant laws and legal boundaries within which the licensed practical nurse must practise.

28. Practises according to legislation, **Standards of Nursing Practice**, ethics, and organizational policies.
29. Practises according to relevant mandatory reporting legislation.
30. Recognizes, responds, and reports questionable orders, actions or decisions made by others. For example:
    30.1 Initiate contact and receive, transcribe, and verify orders.
31. Adheres to the **duty to report.**
32. Protects **client**s' rights by maintaining confidentiality and privacy in all personal and professional contexts.
33. Respond to the **client**s' right to health care information in accordance with relevant privacy legislation.
34. Documents according to established legislation, **practice standards**, ethics, and organizational policies.
35. Obtains **informed consent** to support the **client**'s informed decision-making.

Foundations of Practice

Licensed practical nurses use **critical thinking**, reflection, and evidence integration to assess **client**s, plan care, implement interventions, and evaluate outcomes and processes. Foundational knowledge includes nursing theory, health sciences, humanities, pharmacology, and ethics.

36. Completes comprehensive **health assessment**s of **client**s across the lifespan.
37. Selects and utilizes **information and communications technologies** in the delivery of **client** care.
38. **Researches** and responds to relevant **clinical data.**
39. Engages in **evidence-informed practice** by considering a variety of relevant sources of information.
40. Comprehends, responds to, and reports assessment findings.
41. Formulates **clinical decisions** consistent with **client** needs and priorities. For example:
    41.1 Organize and manage multiple priorities.
    41.2 Respond appropriately to changing situations.
    41.3 Develop individualized nursing interventions.
    41.4 Set priorities that reflect individual client needs.
42. Identifies nursing diagnoses.
43. Develops the plan of care with the client, health care team, and others.
44. Implements nursing interventions based on assessment findings, client preferences, and desired outcomes.
45. Responds to clients' conditions by organizing competing priorities into actions.
46. Assesses clients' health literacy, knowledge, and readiness to learn.
47. Assesses, plans, implements, and evaluates the teaching and learning process.
48. Provides information and access to resources to facilitate health education.
49. Evaluates the effectiveness of health education.
50. Applies principles of client safety.
51. Engages in quality improvement and risk management to promote a quality practice environment.
52. Evaluates the effectiveness of nursing interventions by comparing actual outcomes to expected outcomes.
53. Reviews and revises the plan of care and communicates accordingly.
54. Assesses implications of own decisions.
55. Uses critical thinking, critical inquiry, and clinical judgement for decision-making.
56. Demonstrates professional judgement in utilizing information and communications technologies and social media.
57. Recognizes high-risk practices and integrates mitigation strategies that promote safe care. For example:
    57.1 Apply knowledge of pharmacology and principles of safe medication practice.
    57.2 Implement strategies to optimize medication safety.
    57.3 Implement strategies to promote safe transitions of care (e.g., change in provider, shift change, change in care setting, which includes discharge).
    57.4 Recognize when a nurse's approach to practice and communication needs to evolve based on client needs, nursing competence or **practice context.**

---

[1]See *Truth and Reconciliation Commission of Canada: Calls to Action,* http://trc.ca/assets/pdf/Calls_to_Action_English2.pdf

58. Applies strategies to prevent, de-escalate and manage disruptive, aggressive, or violent behaviour. For example:
    58.1 Involving the client and others, not limited to family, friends, visitors, coworkers, and team members.
59. Recognizes and responds immediately when a **client**'s condition is deteriorating.
60. Demonstrates knowledge of nursing theory, pharmacology, health sciences, humanities, and ethics. For example:
    60.1 Engage in safe medication practices.
    60.2 Engage in safe infusion therapy practices (e.g., infusion therapy, central lines, pain management systems).
    60.3 Apply standards and principles when administering blood and blood products.
    60.4 Use the nursing process in the plan of care.

Collaborative Practice

Licensed practical nurses work collaboratively with **client**s and other members of the **health care team**. They recognize that collaborative practice is guided by shared values and **accountability**, a common purpose or care outcome, mutual respect, and effective communication.

61. Engages **clients** in identifying their health needs, strengths, capacities, and goals.
62. Communicates collaboratively with the **client** and the **health care team.**
63. Provides essential **client** information to the **client** and the **health care team.**
64. Promotes effective interpersonal interaction.
65. Uses **conflict resolution** strategies to promote healthy relationships and optimal **client** outcomes.
66. Articulates own role based on legislated **scope of practice**, individual **competence,** and care context including employer policies.
67. Determines own professional and **interprofessional** role within the team by considering the roles, responsibilities, and **scope of practice** of others.
68. **Advocate**s for the use of Indigenous health knowledge and healing practices in **collaboration** with the **client.**
69. Demonstrates **leadership**, direction, and supervision to **unregulated health workers** and others.
70. Participates in emergency preparedness and disaster management.
71. Participates in creating and maintaining a quality **practice environment** that is healthy, respectful, and psychologically safe.
72. Fosters an environment that encourages questioning and exchange of information.
73. Initiates and fosters mentoring relationships. For example:
    73.1 Seek, provide, and reflect on constructive feedback.
74. Applies the principles of **team dynamics** and group processes in **interprofessional** team **collaboration.**
75. Demonstrates **formal** and **informal leadership** in practice.
76. Organizes workload, assigns and coordinates nursing care, sets priorities, and demonstrates effective time management skills.

BIBLIOGRAPHY

Yardstick Assessment Strategies. (2019). *Canadian practical nurse registration examination blueprint (Appendix C).*

REx-PN CLIENT CARE NEEDS

Assumptions

Certain assumptions about people and nursing are integral to the content being tested on the practical nurse (PN) exam, including:

- People are unique; live according to their own set of values, motives, and lifestyles; and are able to function in society to varying capacities.
- People have the right to make decisions regarding their health care needs and to participate in meeting those needs. The nurse-client relationship is the foundation of nursing practice across all practice settings. It is always client-focused, based on clients' care needs, and maintains professional boundaries.
- A client's right to safe, competent, and ethical care is of the highest importance.
- Nurses advocate for and educate their clients.
- PNs must have the knowledge, skills, and judgement (competencies) required to provide clients with safe, competent, ethical, and compassionate care.
- Graduates of PN education programs achieve the competencies required for entry-level practice through a variety of learning experiences including theory courses, labs, simulations, and practice placements.
- PNs provide care across the lifespan and continuum of clients' care as members of a health care team. Client care is consistent with the client's unique cultural and spiritual preferences, and adheres to provincial standards, regulations, legislation, and employer policies.
- Nursing is a dynamic, continually evolving discipline. PNs must think critically to integrate complex knowledge, skills, technologies, and client care activities into evidence-informed nursing practice.
- The goals of nursing in client care are:
  - preventing illness and potential complications.
  - protecting, promoting, restoring, and facilitating comfort, health, and dignity in dying.

SAFE AND EFFECTIVE CARE ENVIRONMENT

The nurse promotes achievement of client outcomes by providing and directing nursing care that enhances the care delivery setting in order to protect clients and health care personnel.

Management of Care

- **Management of Care** – the nurse provides and directs nursing care that enhances the care delivery setting to protect the client and health care personnel.
  Management of Care. See the Related Activity Statements from the *2019 REx-PN Practice Analysis* available at https://www.ncsbn.org/public-files/2022_RExPN_FINAL.pdf.

Related content includes, but is **not limited** to:
Advance Directives, Self-Determination, and Life Planning
- Integrate advance directives into client plan of care*
Advocacy
- Advocate for client rights and needs*
Assignment, Delegation and Supervision
- Delegate and supervise care of client provided by others (e.g., unregulated care providers)*
- Organize workload to manage time effectively*
Case Management
- Initiate, evaluate, and update client plan of care*
Client Rights
- Provide education to clients and staff about client rights and responsibilities*
- Involve client in care decision-making*
Collaboration with Interprofessional Team
- Collaborate with interprofessional team members when providing client care*
Concepts of Management
- Provides support and facilitates learning to new staff and health care students*
- Participates in conflict resolution*
Confidentiality and Information Security
- Maintain client confidentiality and privacy*
Continuity of Care
- Provide and receive hand-off of care (report) on assigned clients*
- Use approved abbreviations and standard terminology when documenting care*
- Perform procedures necessary to safely admit, transfer, or discharge a client*
Establishing Priorities
- Prioritize the delivery of client care*
Ethical Practice
- Recognize ethical dilemmas and take appropriate action*
- Practice in a manner consistent with a code of ethics for nurses*
- Assess and develop professional competence (e.g., self-reflection, professional activities) *
Informed Consent
- Obtain consent for nursing care and procedures and provide appropriate client education*
Information Technology
- Receive and transcribe health care provider orders*
- Use resources to enhance client care (e.g., evidence-informed research, information technology, policies and procedures)*
Legal Rights and Responsibilities
- Provide care within the legislated scope of practice*
- Recognize limitations of one's competence and seek assistance when needed*
- Report client information as required by law (e.g., abuse or neglect and communicable disease)*
- Respond to the unsafe practice of a health care provider (e.g., intervene, report)*
Quality Improvement

- Participate in performance improvement projects and quality improvement processes*
Referrals
- Assess the need for referrals or consults and obtain necessary orders*

Safety and Infection Control

- **Safety and Infection Control – the nurse protects clients and health care personnel from health and environmental hazards.**
  Related content includes, but is **not limited** to:
  Accident, Error, and Injury Prevention
- Assess client for allergies and sensitivities and intervene as needed*
- Promote and educate client on safety and injury prevention (e.g., falls, electrical hazards)*
- Ensure proper identification of client when providing care*
- Verify appropriateness and accuracy of health care provider order*
  Emergency Response Plan
- Participate in internal and external emergency response plans*
  Ergonomic Principles
- Use ergonomic principles when providing care (e.g., safe client handling, proper lifting)*
  Handling Hazardous and Infectious Materials
- Follow procedures for handling biohazardous and hazardous materials*
- **Home Safety**
  Reporting of Incident, Event, Irregular Occurrence, or Variance
- Identify practice errors and near misses and intervene*
  Safe Use of Equipment
- Safely and appropriately use equipment*
  Security Plan
- Adhere to security procedures (e.g., newborn nursery security, controlled access)*
  Standard Precautions/Routine Practices, Transmission-Based Precautions, Surgical Asepsis
- Apply principles of infection control (e.g., hand hygiene, aseptic technique, universal precautions)*
- Educate client and staff regarding infection control measures*
  Use of Restraints or Safety Devices
- Follow policies and procedures for use of restraints*

Health Promotion and Maintenance

- **Health Promotion and Maintenance – the nurse provides and directs nursing care of the client that incorporates knowledge of expected growth and development; prevention and early detection of health conditions, and strategies to achieve optimal health.**
  Health Promotion and Maintenance. See the Related Activity Statements from the *2019 REx-PN Practice Analysis*

- **Perform comprehensive health assessments**
  Related content includes, but is **not limited** to:
  Aging Process
- **Provide care and education for the newborn, infant, and toddler client from birth to 2 years***
- **Provide care and education for the preschool, school age, and adolescent client ages 3 yo 17 years***
- **Provide care and education for the adult client ages 18 to 64 years***
- **Provide care and education for the adult client ages 65 years and over***
  Ante-, Intra-, and Postpartum and Newborn Care
- **Provide prenatal care and education***
- **Provide care and education to an antepartum client***
- **Provide care and education to a client in labour***
- **Provide postpartum care and education***
  Community Resources
- **Identify and facilitate access to community resources for clients***
  Developmental Stages and Transitions
- **Assess client's growth and development throughout the lifespan***
- **Identify barriers to communication***
  Health Promotion and Disease Prevention
- **Assess client about determinants of health and implement interventions***
- **Assess client's readiness to learn, learning preferences and barriers to learning***
- **Plan and participate in health care activities for clients in community setting***
- **Educate client about health promotion and maintenance recommendations (e.g., physician visits, immunizations)***
  Health Screening
- **Perform preventative screening assessments (e.g., vision, hearing, cognitive, nutrition)***
  High-Risk Behaviours
- **Educate client about prevention and treatment of high-risk health behaviours (e.g., smoking cessation, safe sexual practice, needle exchange)***
  Lifestyle Choices
  Self-Care
- **Assess client ability to manage care in home environment and plan care accordingly***
  Techniques of Physical and Psychosocial Assessment
- **Perform comprehensive health assessments***

Psychosocial Integrity

- **Psychosocial Integrity** – the nurse provides and directs nursing care that promotes and supports the emotional, mental, and social well-being of the client experiencing stressful events, as well as clients with acute or chronic mental illness.
  Psychosocial Integrity. See the Related Activity Statements from the *2019 REx-PN Practice Analysis*
  Related content includes, but is **not limited** to:
  Abuse or Neglect
- **Assess client for abuse or neglect and intervene***

Behavioural Interventions
- **Manage and support clients with emotional or behavioural issues***
  Coping Mechanisms
- **Assess client's ability to cope with life changes and provide support***
- **Assist client to cope and adapt to stressful events and changes in health status***
  Crisis Intervention
- **Assess the potential for violence and aggression and use safety precautions***
  Cultural Awareness and Cultural Influences on Health
- **Incorporate client cultural practices and beliefs when planning and providing care***
- **Incorporate the use of Indigenous health knowledge and practices when planning and providing care to Indigenous clients***
  End-of-Life Care
- **Provide end-of-life care to clients***
  Family Dynamics
- **Assess family dynamics to determine care plan***
  Grief and Loss
- **Provide care for a client experiencing grief or loss***
  Mental Health Concepts
- **Provide care of the cognitively impaired client***
- **Provide care and support to clients with acute and chronic mental health disorders***
- **Explore reasons for client nonadherence with treatment plan***
  Religious and Spiritual Influences on Health
  Sensory or Perceptual Alterations
- **Provide care for a client experiencing sensory or cognitive distortions***
  Stress Management
- **Recognize client stressors that affect care***
- **Recognize nonverbal cues to physical and psychological stressors***
- **Recognize health care provider stressors that affect client care***
  Substance Use and Other Disorders and Dependencies
- **Assess client for substance misuse, dependency, withdrawal or toxicities, and intervene***
  Support Systems
  Therapeutic Communication
- **Use therapeutic communication techniques***
  Therapeutic Environment

PHYSIOLOGICAL INTEGRITY

The nurse promotes physical health and wellness by providing care and comfort, reducing client risk potential, and managing health alterations.

Basic Care and Comfort

- **Basic Care and Comfort** – the nurse provides comfort and assistance in the performance of activities of daily living.

Basic Care And Comfort. See the Related Activity Statements from the *2019 REx-PN Practice Analysis*

Related content includes, but is **not limited** to:

Assistive Devices

- Educate and assist client to compensate for a physical or sensory impairment (e.g., assistive devices, positioning, compensatory techniques)*

Elimination

- Assess client elimination and intervene*

Mobility and Immobility

- Apply, maintain, or remove orthopedic devices (e.g., traction, splints, braces)*
- Perform skin assessment and implement measures to maintain skin integrity*
- Implement measures to promote circulation and venous return (e.g., active or passive range of motion, anti-embolic stockings, sequential compression devices, positioning and mobilization)*

Nonpharmacological Comfort Interventions

- Provide nonpharmacological comfort measures*
- Assess client for pain and intervene*
- Perform irrigations (e.g., bladder, wound, eye)*
- Identify use of client alternative therapies and potential contraindications (e.g., aroma-therapy, acupressure, supplements)*

Nutrition and Oral Hydration

- Monitor the client's nutritional status*
- Provide enteral nutrition*
- Assess and maintain site care for client with enteral tubes*
- Assess client intake and output and intervene*

Personal Hygiene

- Assess client ability to perform activities of daily living and intervene*

Postmortem Care

- Perform postmortem care*

Rest and Sleep

- Assess client sleep and rest pattern and intervene*

Pharmacological and Parenteral Therapies

- **Pharmacological and Parenteral Therapies** – the nurse provides care related to the administration of medications and parenteral therapies.

Pharmacological and Parenteral Therapies. See the Related Activity Statements from the *2019 REx-PN Practice Analysis*

Related content includes, but is **not limited** to:

Adverse Effects, Contraindications, Adverse Effects, and Interactions

Blood and Blood Products

- Administer blood products and evaluate client response*

Expected Actions and Outcomes

- Evaluate client response to medication*

Medication Administration

Parenteral and Intravenous Therapies

- Access peripheral venous access devices*
- Monitor intravenous infusion and maintain site*
- Calculate and monitor intravenous flow rate*

Pharmacological Pain Management Devices

- Maintain pain control devices (e.g., epidural, client control analgesia, peripheral nerve catheter)*

Total Parenteral Nutrition (TPN)

- Administer parenteral nutrition and evaluate client response *

Reduction of Risk Potential

- **Reduction of Risk Potential** – the nurse reduces the likelihood that clients will develop complications or health conditions related to existing conditions, treatments, or procedures.

Reduction of Risk Potential. See the Related Activity Statements from the *2019 REx-PN Practice Analysis*

Related content includes, but is **not limited** to:

Changes or Abnormalities in Vital Signs

Diagnostic Tests

Laboratory Values

Potential for Alterations in Body Systems

Potential for Complications of Diagnostic Tests, Treatments, and Procedures

- Use precautions to prevent injury or complications associated with a procedure or diagnosis*
- Evaluate responses to procedures and treatments and intervene*
- Insert a nasal or oral gastrointestinal tube*
- Maintain or remove a nasal or oral gastrointestinal tube*
- Monitor continuous or intermittent suction of nasogastric (NG) tube*
- Insert, maintain, or remove a urinary catheter*
- Insert a peripheral intravenous line*
- Maintain or remove a peripheral intravenous line*
- Maintain percutaneous feeding tube*

System Specific Assessments

- Perform focused assessments*
- Recognize trends and changes in client condition and intervene*

Therapeutic Procedures

- Educate client about treatments and procedures*
- Provide preoperative or postoperative education*
- Provide preoperative care*
- Manage client following a procedure with moderate sedation*

Physiological Adaptation

- **Physiological Adaptation** – the nurse manages and provides care for clients with acute, chronic or life-threatening physical health conditions.

Physiological Adaptation. See the Related Activity Statements from the *2019 REx-PN Practice Analysis*

Related content includes, but is **not limited** to:

Alterations in Body Systems

- Assist with invasive procedures (e.g., central line, thoracentesis, bronchoscopy)*
- Maintain optimal temperature of client*

- Monitor and maintain devices and equipment used for drainage (e.g., surgical wound drains, chest tube suction, negative pressure wound therapy)*
- Perform suctioning (oral, tracheal, nasopharyngeal)*
- Perform wound care and dressing change*
- Perform wound drainage device removal*
- Remove wound sutures or staples*
- Provide ostomy care and education (e.g., tracheal, enteral)*
- Provide postoperative care*
  Fluid and Electrolyte Imbalances
- Manage the care of the client with a fluid and electrolyte imbalance*
  Hemodynamics
- Manage the care of a client with alteration in hemodynamics, tissue perfusion, or hemostasis*
- Manage the care of a client with a permanent pacing device*
  Illness Management
- Educate client regarding an acute or chronic condition*
- Manage the care of a client with impaired ventilation or oxygenation*

- Evaluate the effectiveness of the treatment plan for a client with an acute or chronic diagnosis*
  Medical Emergencies
- Perform emergency care procedures (e.g., cardiopulmonary resuscitation, respiratory support, automated external defibrillator)*
  Pathophysiology
- Identify pathophysiology related to an acute or chronic condition*
  Unexpected Response to Therapies
- Recognize signs and symptoms of client complications and intervene*

REFERENCES

Meazure Learning-Yardstick. (2019). *Canadian practical nurse registration examination blueprint (2022–2026)*.

National Council of State Boards of Nursing. (2022). *Test plan for the Regulatory exam–practical nurse*.

Terminology

An understanding of the distinct language used in the health sciences is of critical importance for safe nursing practice. Medical terminology can be simplified and better understood by analyzing the structural characteristics of the words.

Understanding the meaning of the basic prefixes and suffixes, and the definition of the root word, will allow you to derive the meaning of specific terms and greatly enhance your vocabulary.

ROOT WORD: The foundation word; directs us to the general, fundamental meaning of the word; e.g. cardio (pertaining to the heart) = cardiology (the study of the heart)

PREFIX: Added to the beginning of a word to specify a particular meaning of the root word; e.g. endo (within or inside) = endocardium (inner lining of the heart)

SUFFIX: Added to the end of a word to specify a particular meaning of the root word; e.g. itis (inflammation of) = endocarditis (inflammation of the inner lining of the heart)

Commonly Used PREFIXES in Medical Terminology

Prefix	Meaning	Example
a-	without/not	**a**pnea: absence of breathing
ab-	away from	**ab**duction (of arm): moving arm away from the centre of the body
ad-	toward	**ad**duction (of arm): bringing arm toward the centre of the body
ante-	before	**ante**natal: before birth
anti-	against	**anti**histamine: against (opposes) histamine
auto-	self	**auto**graft: grafting tissue from one part of the body to another part
brady-	slow	**brady**cardia: slow heart rate
contra-	against	**contra**ceptive: against conception
dorsi-	back	**dorsi**flexion: flexing a joint backward
dys-	faulty/difficult/abnormal	**dys**pnea: difficulty in breathing
ecto-	outside	**ecto**pic pregnancy: embryo growing outside the uterus
endo-	Inside/within/in	**endo**cardium: inner lining of the heart
exo-	outside	**exo**crine gland: gland that secretes onto an outside surface
eu-	normal	**eu**pnea: normal breathing
hemi-	half	**hemi**plegia: paralysis of half the body
hyper-	above normal/excessive	**hyper**tension: abnormally high blood pressure
hypo-	below/deficient/under	**hypo**thermia: below normal body temperature
infra-	below/beneath/under	**infra**mandibular: below the jaw
inter-	between	**inter**cellular: between the cells
intra-	inside, within/in	**intra**venous: inside the veins
macro-	large	**macro**cyte: an enlarged erythrocyte
mal-	bad	**mal**absorption: faulty absorption
micro-	small	**micro**cytic: small blood cell
neo-	new	**neo**plasm: new tumour growth
noct-	night	**noct**uria: urination during the night
para-	beside, near, resembling	**para**plegia: paralysis of the lower half of the body
peri-	around	**peri**cardium: around (outer layer of) the heart
pneum-	breathing	**pneum**onia: condition of abnormal breathing due to infection of the lungs
poly-	many, much	**poly**uria: excessive urine
post-	after, behind	**post**operative: after surgery
pre-	before, in front of	**pre**ganglionic: before a ganglion
pro-	in front of, before	**pro**dromal: beginning, initial stages
retro-	behind, backward	**retro**peritoneal: behind the peritoneum

Continued

Commonly Used PREFIXES in Medical Terminology—cont'd

Prefix	Meaning	Example
sub-	below, under	**sub**chondral: below the cartilage
super-	above/excessive	**super**sensitive: extra sensitivity
supra-	above/excessive	**supra**pubic: above the pubic region
tachy-	fast/rapid	**tachy**cardia: fast heart rate
trans-	across/through	**trans**membrane: across a membrane

Commonly Used SUFFIXES in Medical Terminology

Suffix	Meaning	Example
-ac	pertaining/relating to	cardi**ac**: pertaining to the heart
-al	"	abdomin**al**: pertaining to the abdomen
-ar	"	ventricul**ar**: pertaining to a ventricle
-eal	"	perin**eal**: pertaining to the perineum
-ic	"	opt**ic**: pertaining to the eye
-ose	"	adip**ose**: pertaining to fatty tissue
-ous	"	cutane**ous**: pertaining to skin
-algia	pain	neur**algia**: neural pain
-cele	sac/pouch/hernia, swelling	cysto**cele**: herniation of the bladder
-centesis	puncture into a cavity	thora**centesis**: puncture wound into thorax to remove fluid
-clasia	breaking up, division, fracture	osteo**clasia**: intentional fracture of a bone to correct abnormality
-ectomy	removal of, excision	append**ectomy**: removal of appendix
-emia	condition of the blood	leuk**emia**: cancer of the white blood cells (WBCs)
-genic	begin/generate/produce/formation	patho**genic**: producing disease
-gram	a drawing or recording	cardio**gram**: a recording of the electrical activity of the heart
-graph	recording instrument	cardio**graph**: recording device that registers the electrical activity of the heart
-graphy	recording process	cardio**graphy**: recording and study of the electrical activity of the heart
-ia	condition/abnormal state	anem**ia**: condition of reduced red blood cells (RBCs)
-ian/ist	specialist in field of study	pediatric**ian**: physician who specializes in the care of children
-iasis	formation/condition of/morbid condition	nephrolith**iasis**: formation of calculi (stones) in the kidney
-ism	condition of	alcohol**ism**: condition of excess alcohol intake
-itis	inflammation of	dermat**itis**: inflammation of the skin
-logist	specialist in area of study	patho**logist**: physician who specializes in the study of disease
-logy	study of	cyto**logy**: the study of cells
-lysis	breaking down, dissolution	hemo**lysis**: breaking down of blood cells
-megaly	enlargement	cardio**megaly**: enlargement of the cells
-oma	neoplasm or tumour	sarc**oma**: cancerous tumour of connective tissue
-parous	bearing or giving birth to	multi**parous**: pertaining to multiple births
-pathy	disease, suffering	nephro**pathy**: disease of the kidney
-penia	pathological reduction/reduced amount, deficiency	erythrocyto**penia**: abnormal decrease in the number of RBCs
-phile, -philia	an attraction to or abnormal tendency toward	lipo**philic**: attracted to fats
-phobia	fear of	hydro**phobia**: fear of water
-plasia	formation, growth	hyper**plasia**: excessive formation of new cells
-plasm	a material that forms cells, growth	neo**plasm**: new growth/tumour
-plasty	repair of/reconstruction, mold, shape	rhino**plasty**: reconstruction of the nose
-pnea	breathing	ortho**pnea**: difficulty breathing in recumbent position
-poiesis	formation of, production	erythro**poiesis**: formation of RBCs
-scope	instrument for visual examination	broncho**scope**: instrument that visualizes the bronchial tree
-scopy	examination using a scope	cysto**scopy**: procedure that uses a cystoscope to visualize the urinary bladder
-stasis	constancy, stillness, or stagnation, stop	hemo**stasis**: arrested or halted blood flow

Commonly Used SUFFIXES in Medical Terminology—cont'd

Suffix	Meaning	Example
-stenosis	narrowing, stricture	pyloric **stenosis**: narrowing of the pyloric valve
-stomy	creation of artificial opening	colo**stomy**: an opening from the colon to the surface of the body
-therapy	treatment	cryo**therapy**: treatment of diseased body tissues by using extreme cold
-trophy	development; a certain type of growth, nourishment	hyper**trophy**: increase in the size of a body structure or organ
-uria	condition of the urine	olig**uria**: abnormally low urine output

Commonly Used ROOT WORDS in Medical Terminology

Root Word	Meaning	Example
amnio-	amnion	**amnio**centesis: aspiration of fluid from the amniotic sac
angi-	vessel	**angi**ogram: X-ray of blood vessel
arter-	artery	**arter**iosclerosis: hardening of the arteries
arth-	joint	**arth**rectomy: removal of a joint
ather-	fatty material/plaque	**ather**osclerosis: fatty deposit causing hardening of an artery
audi-	hearing	**audi**ogram: a graphic recording of hearing
bronch-	bronchus	**bronch**oscopy: examination of the bronchi
carcin-	cancer	**carcin**ogen: cancer-producing substance
cardi-	heart	**cardi**ologist: heart specialist
cephal-	head	**cephal**opathy: disease involving the brain
cerebr-	brain	**cerebr**ovascular: blood vessel of brain
cervic-	neck of body or uterus	**cervic**itis: inflammation of uterine cervix
chem-	chemical	**chem**otherapy: drug therapy (for cancer)
cholecyst-	gallbladder	**cholecyst**ectomy: removal of gallbladder
chondr-	cartilage	**chondr**oma: tumour of cartilage
col-	colon	**col**onoscopy: examination of the colon
crani-	skull	**crani**otomy: opening in cranium
cutane-	skin	**cutane**ous: pertaining to the skin
cyst-	bladder	**cyst**ectomy: removal of the bladder
cyt-	cell	**cyt**ology: study of cells
derm-	skin	**derm**atitis: inflammation of the skin
dipl-	double	**dipl**opia: double vision
encephal-	brain	**encephal**opathy: disease of the brain
enter-	intestines	**enter**itis: inflammation of small intestine
erythr-	red	**erythr**ocyte: red blood cell
esophag-	esophagus	**esophag**itis: inflamed esophagus
gastr-	stomach	**gastr**ectomy: removal of stomach
gloss-	tongue	**gloss**itis: inflammation of the tongue
gly-	sugar	**gly**cosuria: sugar in the urine
gynec-	woman	**gynec**ology: study of diseases of women
hem-	blood	**hem**atoma: blood clot
hepat-	liver	**hepat**omegaly: enlarged liver
hydr-	water	**hydr**ophobia: fear of water
hyster-	uterus	**hyster**ectomy: removal of uterus
lapar-	abdomen	**lapar**oscopy: endoscopic examination of abdomen
laryng-	larynx	**laryng**itis: inflammation of larynx
leuk(c)-	white	**leuk**ocytosis: increased number of WBCs
lingu-	tongue	**lingu**al: pertaining to the tongue
mamm-	breast	**mamm**ogram: X-ray of the breasts
muc-	mucus	**muc**olytic: substance that breaks down mucus
my-	muscle	**my**opathy: muscle disease
myel-	spinal cord	**myel**ogram: X-ray of spinal cord
necr-	death	**necr**osis: tissue death
nephr-	kidney	**nephr**itis: inflammation of the kidney

Continued

Commonly Used ROOT WORDS in Medical Terminology—cont'd

Root Word	Meaning	Example
neur-	nerve	**neur**ectomy: removal of a nerve
onc-	tumour	**onc**ology: study of tumours
ophthalm-	eye	**ophthalm**ologist: eye specialist
oste-	bone	**oste**oporosis: loss of calcium from the bones
ot-	ear	**ot**ic: pertaining to the ear
path-	disease	**path**ogen: disease-causing organism
p(a)ed-	child	**ped**iatrics: study of medical care and treatment of children
periton-	peritoneum	**periton**itis: inflammation of the peritoneum
pleur-	pleura	**pleur**al: pertaining to the pleura
pneum-	air, lungs	**pneum**onia: infection of the lungs
proct-	anus, rectum	**proct**itis: inflammation of the rectum
pulmon-	lung	**pulmon**ary artery: blood vessel leading to the lungs
ren-	kidney	**ren**al: pertaining to the kidneys
rhin-	nose	**rhin**oplasty: plastic surgery on the nose
seps-	infection	a**seps**is: absence of infection
thorac-	thorax	**thorac**otomy: surgical opening into the thorax
thromb-	clot	**thromb**us: blood clot attached to side of blood vessel obstructing blood flow
tox-	toxin	**tox**icology: study of poisons (toxins)
trache-	trachea	**trache**otomy: surgical opening into the trachea
ur-	urine	**ur**ology: study of the urinary system
ven-	vein	intra**ven**ous: into a vein

Common Directional Terms and Body Positions Relating to Medical Terminology

Term	Meaning
abduction	moving a body part away from the midline of the body
adduction	moving a body part toward the midline of the body
anterior	toward the front of the body
bilateral	both sides of the body
coronal (frontal)	lengthwise plane of the body; dividing the body into front and back halves
deep	interior of the body
distal	away from the centre of the body
dorsal recumbent	lying supine with knees bent
eversion	turning a body part outward
extension	straightening out a joint
flexion	bending a joint
inferior	lower; toward the feet
inversion	turning inward
lateral	to the side of the body
medial	toward the midline of the body
palmar	relating to the palm of the hand
plantar	relating to the sole of the foot
posterior	toward the back of the body
prone	lying on the stomach with legs extended
proximal	close to the centre of the body
sagittal	lengthwise plane dividing the body into front and back halves
modified left lateral recumbent position/modified left prone position	lying on left side, left arm extended along back, chest forward, left knee slightly flexed, right knee highly flexed
superficial	on or near the surface of the body
superior	toward the head
supine	lying on the back, with legs extended
transverse (horizontal)	cross-section of body dividing it into upper and lower parts
Trendelenburg position	lying supine with the head lower than the feet
unilateral	applying to one side of the body

BIBLIOGRAPHY

Chabner, D. (2022). *Medical terminology—A short course* (9th ed.). Elsevier Canada.

Perry, A., Potter, P., Corbett, S., Ostendorf, W., & Laplante, N. (2020). *Canadian clinical nursing skills & techniques* (1st ed.). Elsevier.

C APPENDIX

Approved List of Abbreviations - CPNRE

Abbreviation	Meaning	Abbreviation	Meaning
BMI	body mass index	kg	kilogram(s)
BP	blood pressure	kJ	kilojoule(s)
BUN	blood urea nitrogen	L	litre(s)
°C	degrees Celsius	mcg	microgram
cc	cubic centimetre	mEq	milliequivalent
cm	centimetre(s)	mg	milligram(s)
ECG	electrocardiogram	min	minute(s)
EEG	electroencephalogram	mL	millilitre(s)
EENT	ear, eye, nose, throat	mmol/L	millimoles per litre
h	hour	mm Hg	millimetres of mercury
Hgb	hemoglobin	pH	hydrogen ion concentration;
HIV	human immunodeficiency virus		potential of hydrogen
HR	heart rate (beats/min)	p.r.n	as needed
HR	pulse	RR	respiratory rate (breaths/min)
IM	intramuscular	stat.	immediately
IV	intravenous	T	temperature
g	gram(s)	t.i.d.	three times a day

BIBLIOGRAPHY

Adapted from Meazure Learning-Yardstick. (2021). *Canadian practical nurse registration examination (CPNRE) prep guide* (6th ed.). (p. 14). Appendix A.

Common Laboratory and Diagnostic Tests

LABORATORY VALUES ABBREVIATIONS

Abbreviation	Meaning	Abbreviation	Meaning	Abbreviation	Meaning
<	less than	kPa	kilopascal	mm	millimetre
>	greater than	L	litre	mm Hg	millimetres of mercury
≤	less than or equal to	mcg	microgram	mmol	millimole
≥	greater than or equal to	mcL	microlitre	mOsm	milliosmole
cc	cubic centimetre	mcmol	micromole	ng	nanogram
dL	decilitre	microU	microunit	nmol	nanomole
fL	femtolitre	mEq	milliequivalent	pg	picogram
g	gram	mg	milligram	pmol	picomole
IU	international unit	mL	millilitre	U/L	units per litre

HEMATOLOGY

- Involves tests on whole blood
- Tests focus on the examination of the blood cells

Test	Normal Value	Interpretation
Complete Blood Count and Differential (CBC and diff.)	Screening of all blood cells, including Hgb, Hct, platelets, and breakdown of white blood cells (WBCs)	
Erythrocyte Count (red blood cell [RBC])	Male: $4.7–6.1 \times 10^{12}$/L Female: $4.2–5.4 \times 10^{12}$/L	• The number of circulating RBCs
Hematocrit (Hct)	Male: 42–52% Female: 37–47%	• Percentage of RBCs to whole blood
Hemoglobin (Hgb)	Male: 140–180 g/L Female: 120–160 g/L	• Measures hemoglobin on RBC of venous blood

Test	Normal Value	Interpretation
Red Blood Cell (RBC) Indices		
• Mean Corpuscular Volume (MCV)	80–95 fL	• Average size of RBC
• Mean Corpuscular Hemoglobin (MCH)	27–31 pg	• Average Hgb weight of RBC
• Mean Corpuscular Hemoglobin Concentration (MCHC)	32–36 g/dL	• % of Hgb on RBC
• Erythrocyte Sedimentation Rate (ESR)	Male: ≤15 mm/hr Female: ≤20 mm/hr	• Measures the time it takes RBC to settle out on standing • Indicative of systemic inflammatory disease
White Blood Cell (WBC) Count	5 000–10 000⁹/L	• WBCs in venous blood

Test	Normal Value	Interpretation
Differential WBC Count		
• Neutrophils	$2.5–7.5 \times 10^9$/L	• Bacterial infections
• Monocytes	$0.1–0.7 \times 10^9$/L	• Infection, inflammation
• Eosinophils	$0.00–0.5 \times 10^9$/L	• Allergic reactions, parasites
• Basophils	$0.02–0.05 \times 10^9$/L	• Inflammation
• Lymphocytes	$1.0–4.0 \times 10^9$/L	• Immune response

Test	Normal Value	Interpretation
Coagulation Tests		
Prothrombin Time (PT)	11–12.5 sec	• Used to measure degree of anticoagulation, therapeutic level; 2–3 min
International Normalization Ratio (INR)	0.81–1.20	• Standardized PT for clients on coumadin
Activated Partial Thromboplastin Time (aPTT)	30–40 sec	• Used for clients on heparin to measure degree of anticoagulation
Partial Thromboplastin Time (PTT)	60–70 sec	• Therapeutic level: 46–76 sec
Platelets (Thrombocytes)	$150–400 \times 10^9$/L	• Necessary for normal clotting of blood in the early stages of the clotting process

BLOOD CHEMISTRY

• Measures noncellular components of the blood

Test	Normal Value	Interpretation
Arterial Blood Gases (ABGs)		
• Arterial pH	7.35–7.45	• Evaluates respiratory, cardiac, and renal functioning and determines acid–base balance
• Arterial PaO_2	80–100 mm Hg	
• Arterial $PaCO_2$	35–45 mm Hg	
• Bicarbonate (HCO_3^-)	21–28 mmol/L	
• O_2 Saturation	95–100%	
Cardiac Markers		
Cholesterol	<5 mmol/L	• ↑ Risk of coronary artery disease (CAD)
High-Density Lipoproteins (HDL)	>1.55 mmol/L	• "Good cholesterol"
Low-Density Lipoproteins (LDL)	<2.59 mmol/L	• "Bad cholesterol"
Triglycerides	Male: 0.45–1.81 mmol/L	• Storage form of lipids
	Female: 0.40–1.52 mmol/L	• ↑ Risk of CAD
Transaminases		
• Aspartate Aminotransferase (AST)	0–35 IU/L	• ↑ Liver disease, pulmonary and myocardial infarctions
• Alanine Aminotransferase (ALT)	4–36 IU/L	• ↑ Liver disease, shock
• Troponin T (TnT)	<0.1 mcg/L	• Cardiac damage, renal failure
• Troponin I (TnI)	<0.35 mcg/L	• ↑ 3 hours following damage
• Creatine Kinase (CK)	Male: 55–170/mcL	• ↑ Cardiac muscle, skeletal muscle, brain damage
	Female: 30–135 mcL	• ↑ 6 hours following damage
Lactic Dehydrogenase (LDH)	100–190 U/L	• Tissue damage, heart failure, myocardial infarction (MI), liver disease, muscle damage
Gamma-Glutamyl Transpeptidase (GGT)	Male: 8–38 U/L	• ↑ MI; liver disease, pancreatic disease, cytomegalovirus infections
	Female: 5–27 U/L	
Folic Acid	11–57 mmol/L	• ↑ Pernicious anemia, vegan diet
		• ↓ Alcoholism, deficiency, malnutrition, renal disease
Diabetic Markers		
• Fasting Blood Glucose (FBG)	4–6 mmol/L	• ↑ Indicates hyperglycemia (diabetes mellitus)

Test	Normal Value	Interpretation
Two-Hour Oral Glucose Tolerance Test (OGTT)		
• After 1 hour postintake	<11.1 mmol/L	• Evaluates absorption of glucose into cells, assesses for diabetes mellitus or excess insulin secretion
• After 2 hours postintake	<7.8 mmol/L	
Glycosylated Hemoglobin (HbA$_{1c}$)	<6%	• Measures the average blood glucose levels over approx. 2 months. A high value indicates blood glucose level fluctuations (unbalanced diet).
• Glycohemoglobin		
Electrolytes		
• Sodium (Na$^+$)	135–145 mmol/L	• Required for normal fluid and electrolyte balance, acid–base balance, nerve impulse conduction, muscle contraction
• Potassium (K$^+$)	3.5–5 mmol/L	
• Chloride (Cl$^-$)	98–106 mmol/L	
• CO$_2$ content	21–28 mmol/L	
Calcium		
• Total Calcium	2.25–2.755 mmol/L	• Osteoporosis, hypo-, and hyperparathyroidism
• Ionized Calcium	1.05–1.30 mmol/L	
Serum Magnesium	0.74–1.07 mmol/L	• Required for adenosine triphosphate (ATP) production, neuromuscular functioning
		• ↓ Malnutrition, alcoholism
		• ↑ Mg^{++} antacids, renal disease
Serum Phosphorus	Adult: 0.97–1.45 mmol/L	• ↑ P = ↓ Ca^{++}
		• ↓ Hypercalcemia; chronic P-containing antacids, low dietary intake, alcoholism
		• ↑ Renal and liver failure, hypocalcemia, bone cancer
Iron		
• Serum Iron	Male: 14–32 mcmol/L	• ↓ Inadequate dietary intake, malabsorption, blood loss, neoplasms
	Female: 11–29 mcmol/L	
• TIBC (total iron-binding capacity)	45–82 mcmol/L	
• Ferritin	Male: 26–674 pmol/L	• ↑ Liver disease, hemochromocytosis, hemolytic anemias
	Female: 22–337 pmol/L	

Test	Normal Value	Interpretation
Liver and Renal Disease Markers		
Protein		
• Total	64–83 g/L	• Malnutrition, renal disease, liver disease, burns
• Albumin	35–50 g/L	
• Globulin	23–34 g/L	
Bilirubin		
• Total	5.1–17 mcmol/L	• Elevated with impaired liver functioning
• Indirect	3.4–12 mcmol/L	
• Direct	1.7–5.1 mcmol/L	
Blood Urea Nitrogen (BUN)	3.6–7.1 mmol/L	• Liver and renal disease, protein catabolism
Creatinine	15.3–76.3 mcmol/L	• Secreted by kidneys, result of creatine metabolism

Test	Normal Value	Interpretation
Uric Acid	Male: 240–501 mcmol/L	• End product of purine metabolism
	Female: 160–430 mcmol/L	• High-protein diet, alcoholism, tissue destruction
Serum Amylase	100–300 U/L	• Assess for pancreatitis
		• ↑ Bowel obstruction and perforation, mumps
Thyroxine (T$_4$) Free	10–36 pmol/L	• Diagnosis of hypo- or hyperthyroidism
Triiodothyronine (T$_3$)	1.7–5.2 pmol/L	
Viral Testing for AIDS		
Enzyme Immunoassay Assay (EIA)	Negative	• Identifies antibodies to HIV, not viral antigens; usually takes 2–12 weeks to develop

Continued

Test	Normal Value	Interpretation
Western Blot Test **Viral Load**	Negative Undetected	• Used to verify positive EIA test, presence of viral genetic material in blood, viral load of less than 500 copies/mL is indicative of effective treatment
Polymerase Chain Reaction (PCR)	Negative	• Detects presence of virus

URINE CHEMISTRY

- Measures components of the urine
- General characteristics: clear, amber yellow, aromatic odour

Test	Normal Value	Interpretation
pH	4.6–8.0	• Alkaline urine: vegetarian diet, renal failure • Acidic urine: acidosis, starvation, diarrhea, fever
Specific Gravity (SG)	1.005–1.030	• ↑ (meaning a high specific gravity, above the high range given): dehydration, glycosuria, syndrome of inappropriate antidiuretic hormone (SIADH) • ↓ (meaning a low specific gravity, below the low range given): overhydration, diabetes insipidus
Bilirubin	5.1–16 mcmol/L	• Presence indicative of liver disease
Catecholamines		
• Epinephrine	<109 nmol/day	• ↑ Indicative of heart failure, pheochromocytoma
• Norepinephrine	<590 nmol/day	• 24-hour specimen
Chloride (Cl⁻)	110–250 mmol/day	• 24-hour specimen • ↑ Addison's disease • ↓ Dehydration, perspiration, burns, vomiting

Test	Normal Value	Interpretation
Creatinine	Male: 53–106 mcmol/L Female: 44–97 mcmol/L	• 24-hour specimen • ↓ Renal disease • ↑ Anemia, leukemia, atrophy
Creatinine Clearance	1.42–2.25 mL/sec	• 24-hour specimen • ↓ Renal disease
Glucose	Negative	• Presence indicative of diabetes mellitus, stress, infection; low renal threshold for reabsorption of glucose
Ketone Bodies	Negative	• Presence indicative of diabetes mellitus, excess protein in diet, starvation
Protein (Single Specimen)	Negative	• Presence indicative of heart disease, stress, renal disease
Protein (24-hr Specimen)	<0.15 g/day	• Renal disease
Sodium (Na⁺)	40–250 mmol/day	• 24-hour specimen • ↑ Renal disease • ↓ Hyponatremia
Uric Acid	1.48–4.43 mmol/day	• 24-hour specimen • ↑ Gout, leukemia • ↓ Renal inflammation
Urobilinogen	0.5–4.0 mmol/day	• 24-hour specimen • ↑ Liver disease, hemolytic disease • ↓ Biliary obstruction
Microscopic Examination		
• Red blood cells	0–2	• Presence indicative of infection, renal disease, trauma
• White blood cells	0–4	• ↑ Indicative of infection

Test	Normal Value	Interpretation
• Casts	Negative	• ↑ Glomerulonephritis
• Crystals	Negative	• ↑ Infections, renal calculi
• Bacteria	Negative	• ↑ Infections

STOOL

Test	Normal Value	Interpretation
Occult Blood	Negative	• Intestinal bleeding that cannot be visualized directly • May indicate tumours, diverticulitis, ulcers, inflammatory bowel disease, oral or nasopharyngeal bleeding
Ova and Parasites	Presence of pathogenic organisms	• Intestines normally contain bacteria (e.g. *Escherichia coli*, *Staphylococcus aureus*, *Clostridium*) • Overgrowth due to imbalance may cause disease • Ova = parasitic eggs

MISCELLANEOUS

Test	Normal Value	Interpretation
Cerebrospinal Fluid (CSF)	Clear, colourless RBC: negative WBC: 0–5 cells/L (adult) Organisms: negative Pressure: <20 cm H_2O	• Change → infection, tumour, hemorrhage, trauma
Sweat Chloride Test	<50 mmol/L	• ↑ Used to diagnose cystic fibrosis

DIAGNOSTIC PROCEDURES

Abdominal Paracentesis

This is a sterile procedure in which accumulated fluid from within the abdominal cavity is removed for client comfort or for analysis. The client first voids to avoid bladder injury and is then, in most instances, placed in a supine position for the procedure. A large-bore needle is inserted into the peritoneal cavity, and fluid is withdrawn into a syringe or drained into a vacuum bottle. Following the procedure, pressure to the inserting site is applied for several minutes, followed by a sterile dressing. Monitor for signs of hypovolemia.

Amniocentesis

This sterile test involves the insertion of a needle transabdominally to remove a sample of amniotic fluid from the amniotic sac. The woman voids and is placed in a supine position with a towel under the right buttock to displace the uterus. A fetal monitor assesses the fetus during the procedure, and a sonogram is used to direct the needle. The test is used to detect certain defects, such as chromosomal abnormalities, ABO and Rh incompatibilities, and disorders such as fetal anemia.

Angiography (Arteriogram)

An angiogram is an X-ray of blood vessels following the injection of a radio-opaque contrast medium. The contrast medium is injected via a percutaneous catheter. Images of the area being examined are visualized on a monitor and may be recorded on film. The contrast medium will outline abnormalities and obstructions.

Arthroscopy

This test is an invasive surgical procedure involving the insertion of a fibre-optic arthroscope into a joint space for the purpose of directly visualizing the internal structures of the joint. Abnormalities caused by injury or disease can be identified. In addition, boney debris can be removed and specimens obtained for laboratory examination.

Barium Enema (Lower GI Series)

This test is an X-ray of the lower bowel following the insertion of a radio-opaque barium contrast medium enema. Preparation of the bowel with laxatives or enemas is required on the day prior to the examination to ensure that the lower bowel is clear of stool. The patient is put on clear liquid diet the evening before the procedure. Keep patient NPO (nothing by mouth) for 8 hours before the test. The examination identifies any gross abnormalities, such as growths or obstructions.

Barium Swallow (Upper GI Series)

X-rays are taken as the client swallows a radio-opaque contrast barium drink. X-rays can identify abnormalities of structure and motility in the pharynx, esophagus, and stomach. The client needs to be on NPO 8 to 12 hours prior to the test, and all metal objects must be removed. Instruct the patient to avoid smoking after midnight the night before the test. To promote excretion of the barium, the client is encouraged to drink plenty of fluids following the test.

Bone Marrow Aspiration

This sterile test involves the removal of bone marrow cells from sites such as the iliac crest or sternum, for laboratory examination. Bone marrow cells are responsible for the production of blood cells (hematopoiesis), and, consequently, laboratory examination can identify defects in the cells and their formation. Specimens may be taken for the diagnosis of such conditions as anemias, blood carcinomas, lymphomas, and effects of chemotherapy. Pressure applied to the site following post procedure.

Colposcopy

This procedure is used to locate suspicious areas of the cervix requiring biopsy. A colposcope is a microscope containing a light source and magnifying glass that allows the physician to see abnormal areas of the cervix that would not be visible to the naked eye. It directs the physician more accurately to areas of tissue that need to be biopsied. After the specimen for cytological examination has been obtained, the cervix is cleansed with 3% acetic acid to remove cellular debris. Changes in epithelial tissues can more clearly be observed. Following the procedure, the client should be advised that a small amount of bleeding may occur if a biopsy was taken. Abstinence from intercourse is recommended until biopsy results have been obtained.

Bone Mineral Density (BMD)

The dual-energy X-ray absorptiometry (DEXA) procedure measures the mass of bone density per unit volume. Two X-rays of different energy levels measure the density of the bones being examined. The procedure measures the density of the bone in the specific areas of the hips, spine, and forearm. This test is commonly done on menopausal women to assess for osteoporosis.

Bronchoscopy

Direct visualization of the upper respiratory passageways (tracheobronchial tree) is done through the use of a bronchoscope. The bronchoscope may be rigid or flexible. Specimens may be taken during the procedure for laboratory examination. The procedure may also be used for therapeutic purposes, such as removal of foreign bodies or obstructions. The client requires sedation and local anaesthesia to prevent activation of the choking reflex. Patient instructed to be NPO 6 to 12 hours prior to the test. Keep patient NPO until their gag reflex returns post procedure.

Cardiac Catheterization

This test is a sterile, invasive procedure that involves the insertion of a catheter through a vein or artery that is then passed into the heart chambers. Following injection of a radio-opaque dye through the catheter, X-ray images of the gross cardiac structures and coronary arteries can be visualized. For right-sided catheterization, the catheter is inserted into the femoral, brachial, or subclavian vein and passed into the structures of the right side of the heart. For left-sided heart catheterization, the catheter is inserted into the right femoral or brachial artery and then passed into the aorta and left heart chambers.

Cardiac catheterization is used to determine pressures within the heart structures, narrowing of coronary arteries, congenital abnormalities, and ventricular aneurysms and to perform angioplasty surgery. Clients require sedation and should be NPO for at least 8 hours. An intravenous line is inserted for access should medications be required during the procedure. The client should void prior to the procedure.

Following the procedure, the client remains on bed rest for 8 hours; a pressure dressing is applied to the catheter insertion site and monitored carefully for hemorrhage; the affected extremity remains extended and immobilized to ensure effective clotting at the catheter insertion site; and vital signs are monitored carefully.

Cardiac Exercise Stress Test

This noninvasive test is used to evaluate cardiac functioning under physical stress. The client undertakes controlled exercise on a stationary bicycle or treadmill while an electrocardiography (ECG, EKG), the heart rate, blood pressure, and development of chest pain are monitored. At regular intervals, the intensity of the exercise is increased in order to identify any abnormal changes that may occur as the exercise increases. The degree of intensity of the exercise is predetermined by the cardiologist based on the client's health, physical condition, and age. Abnormal changes in the ECG, heart rate, blood pressure, and development of pain indicate the inability of the coronary arteries to meet the demands of the heart, as in coronary artery disease. Stress testing is contraindicated in clients suffering from conditions such as unstable angina, severe congestive heart failure, recent myocardial infarction (MI), certain chronic lung diseases, and so on.

Colonoscopy

Direct visualization of the colon is observed through the use of an endoscope. The endoscope is long and flexible and is inserted through the rectum, back through the colon to the cecum. The physician is able to visualize the lining of the colon for abnormalities and growths. On the day prior to the test, complete cleansing of the bowel is required through the prescription of strong cleansing laxatives or enemas. The client is also restricted to clear fluids. This ensures that the bowel can be visualized clearly.

Computed Tomography Scan (CT Scan)

A CT scan is a noninvasive, specialized computerized scanner that X-rays the body from different angles, providing a three-dimensional picture of the specific body part to identify abnormalities. The procedure uses ionized radiation as an energy source. Assess patient for Shellfish (iodine) allergy if a CT scan with contrast material is ordered.

Cystoscopy

Direct visualization of the urethra and inner lining of the urinary bladder is observed through the use of a cystoscope. The procedure is usually performed with the use of a local anaesthetic. Abnormalities in the urethra, prostate, and bladder lining can be identified.

Biopsy

A biopsy involves the removal of a small sample of tissue for macroscopic and microscopic pathological examination. Biopsies may be taken by a needle inserted into the tissue and withdrawing a sample, excision of a small piece of tissue, a scraping from a surface of the tissue to be biopsied, or a punch that when placed on top of the tissue excises a sample. In some instances, local anaesthesia may be used to reduce discomfort. Tissue for biopsy is also commonly taken during surgical procedures under general anaesthetic.

Echocardiogram (Heart Sonogram)

This noninvasive ultrasound test uses sound waves to assess the structures of the heart and how they function. A transducer is moved over the chest wall emitting high-frequency sound waves that reflect off the heart structures and back to the transducer. The waves are then displayed on an oscilloscope, allowing for direct visualization of the heart shape, size, and thickness; activity of the heart valves; and related structures. Structural and functional abnormalities can be identified, such as atrial septal defects, valve disease, and aortic stenosis.

Electrocardiogram (ECG, EKG)

This noninvasive test provides a graphic recording of the cardiac cycle during depolarization and repolarization of the heart. Electrodes (leads) are placed on each of the client's limbs and at specific regions of the chest. The electrodes detect the activity of the heart from a variety of regions and can detect abnormalities in the electrical conduction of the intrinsic cardiac conducting system, such as cardiac arrhythmias or damage to myocardial tissue. An individual ECG using 12 leads provides a comprehensive recording of myocardial currents in two different planes. ECG monitoring may be continuous at the bedside, allowing for constant monitoring of cardiac activity, as in critical care units. In this situation, either three or five leads are usually applied to the chest.

Electroencephalography (EEG)

This test is a noninvasive electrophysiological procedure that evaluates the electrical activity within the brain. With the client in a sitting or supine position, approximately 10 electrodes are placed in specific positions around the head. Electrical records are then taken and produced on paper for analysis. Specific wave patterns indicate certain disorders, such as seizure activity, the presence of lesions, effects of certain toxic substances, inflammation, increased intracranial pressure, and the determination of death.

Endoscopy

The direct visualization of a hollow organ or a tubular structure within the body is achieved using a flexible fibre-optic scope or an inflexible scope. Endoscopy can be used to examine the bronchi, esophagus, stomach, colon, bladder, and so on. See the sections on bronchoscopy, gastroscopy, and cystoscopy

Endoscopic Retrograde Cholangiopancreatography (ERCP)

This test uses a fibre-optic endoscope to provide direct visualization of the pancreatic and biliary ducts. Injection of radio-opaque dye into the area allows for X-ray visualization of the pancreatic, common bile, and hepatic ducts. With the client sedated, the endoscope is inserted down the esophagus, through the stomach, and into the duodenum for examination of the area.

The endoscopic procedure also allows for gallstones to be removed from the common bile duct, drainage of bile in jaundiced clients, insertion of stents in areas that have become narrowed, and widening of the bile duct. Specimens of tissue may also be taken for pathological examination.

The client is on NPO from midnight of the day before and is administered sedation just prior to the procedure. Following the procedure, the client remains on NPO until the gag reflex returns.

Gastroscopy

Direct visualization of the lining of the stomach is observed through the use of an endoscope. The esophagus is also visualized during the procedure. Sedation is required to prevent choking.

Intravenous Pyelogram (IVP)

Following the intravenous injection of a radio-opaque contrast medium, a series of X-rays are taken as the dye is excreted in the urine, passing through the kidneys, ureters, and bladder. Obstructions and abnormalities can be identified. Care needs to be taken when using the dye as clients may have adverse reactions. The dye can also be nephrotoxic to the kidneys. Encourage fluids (if permitted) after the procedure, to flush out contrast medium.

Laparoscopy

This procedure involves the insertion of a scope into the abdomen to directly observe the abdominal and pelvic organs. It is used to identify pathological conditions that are manifested by acute and chronic abdominal pain, such as cancerous lesions. Certain surgical procedures may also be performed using a laparoscope, such as cholecystectomy, appendectomy, tubal ligation, and hernia repair.

This procedure is performed under general anaesthetic and requires all the pre- and postoperative care precautions and nursing care.

Lumbar Puncture

This invasive test involves the insertion of a cannular needle into the subarachnoid space of the spinal column at the 3_4 lumbar space. The client is side-lying, the back rounded, and knees flexed toward the abdomen. The client should be directed to remain still during the procedure and, following completion of the procedure, remain flat for approximately 8 hours. Patient may logroll according to health care provider's prescriptions. Observe for excessive drainage at the site. Fluid loss can predispose patient to infection and headache.

This test allows for measurement of cerebrospinal fluid (CSF) pressure by attaching a manometer to the needle. It also allows the removal of CSF for examination (colour, clarity, presence of RBCs, bacteria, malignant cells, protein, glucose, etc.). Medications can also be administered via this route, such as antimicrobials or anaesthetics.

Magnetic Resonance Imaging (MRI)

MRI is a noninvasive examination of a particular area of the body using magnetic and radio waves. A three-dimensional picture of the area is created, and abnormalities can then be identified. MRI does not use ionized radiation. All loose metal objects need to be removed from the client and procedure room. Contraindicated for pregnant clients.

Mammography

This test is a low-dose X-ray that reveals images and views of the breast from different angles. The breast is placed between two plastic plates that then gently compress and flatten the breast to provide a clearer image of the breast tissue. No preparation is required for this X-ray. Based on research, the Canadian Cancer Society suggests that under normal circumstances, women over the age of 40 have a yearly mammogram. Between the ages of 50 and 69, a mammogram every two years is suggested. The rationale for this change is based on the different types of breast cancer that develop in the different age groups.

Nuclear Imaging Scans (Scintigraphy)

This test scans different areas of the body and involves the injection of a radionucleotide that is taken up by specific tissues. Gamma rays are emitted by the radionucleotide and detected by a scintillator. The scintillator converts the rays to an image of the body part. Inform the patient that substance to be ingested contains only traces of radioactivity and poses little to no danger. Patient lies flat during the procedure.

Bone Scan

A bone scan is a nuclear medicine procedure used in the examination of bones. A radioactive contrast medium is injected and then a scanner visualizes the condition of the bone. Abnormal bone tissue absorbs greater quantities of radionucleotide, producing areas of concentration (hot spots). The procedure is used in the diagnosis of such conditions as tumour growth, osteomyelitis, and arthritis. The procedure requires 1 hour while the patient lies supine. Increased fluid postprocedure helps excrete isotopes from the body within 6 to 24 hours.

Nuclear Cardiology

A radiological study with radioactive isotope (technetium-99m sestamibi) identifies myocardial contractibility, acute cell injury, and myocardial perfusion. Intravenous line insertion for the injection of isotopes. Radioactive uptake is counted over the heart by scintillation camera.

Lung Scan

This test identifies changes in blood perfusion through the lungs, as well as pulmonary emboli.

Gallium Scan

Gallium is the radionucleotide used for scanning the entire body. The body is scanned at 24, 48, and 72 hours following the injection of the radionucleotide. Gallium scan is used to identify tumours (benign and malignant), inflammation, infection, and abscesses.

Positron Emission Tomography (PET) Scan

This type of scanning procedure is commonly used for evaluation of the brain and heart and in oncology. Radioactive chemicals are administered to the client that in turn become part of the normal metabolic processes of the particular organ.

Positrons are emitted from the radioactive chemicals and detected and converted by sensors and computed tomography to two- or three-dimensional images indicating a particular metabolic process at a particular site.

Pelvic Ultrasonography

A noninvasive procedure to confirm pregnancy and evaluate whether it is normal, abnormal, or multiple; the stage of development of the fetus; fetal position; or whether a tumour exists instead of a pregnancy.

A transducer is passed over the abdomen above the uterus, reflecting sound waves off the structures within the uterus back to the transducer. The waves are translated into pictures on an oscilloscope. Ectopic pregnancies, placenta previa, abruptio placentae, and tubal pregnancies can be identified.

Pulmonary Function Tests

These tests are prescribed to determine respiratory functioning to assess for the presence and degree of lung disease, identify the type of lung disease, or assess for the effectiveness of therapeutic interventions for lung disease.

Tests include spirometry, lung volume and capacity, rates of airflow, and gas exchange. For the airflow rates and spirometry, the client breathes through a sterile mouthpiece, inhaling deeply and then forcibly exhaling several times. Calculations are made to assess for the following:

- Forced vital capacity (FVC)
- Forced expiratory volume in one second (FEV_1)
- Peak inspiratory and expiratory flow rates (PIFR/PEFR)
- Maximum mid-expiratory flow (MMEF)
- Maximal volume ventilation (MVV) is calculated by having the client breathe deeply and frequently for 15 seconds.
- Expiratory reserve volume (ERV) is calculated by having the client breathe normally into the spirometer and then exhale forcibly.
- Inspiratory capacity (IC) is calculated by having the client breathe normally into the spirometer and then inhale forcibly.
- Total lung capacity (TLC) is calculated by having the client breathe normally into the spirometer.
- Gas exchange of the lungs is usually evaluated by having the client inhale CO and then determining the difference between the amount of CO inhaled and exhaled.

For these tests to be successful, the cooperation of the client is important. Directions given to the client need to be clear. For 6 hours prior to the test, the client should refrain from taking any bronchodilators or smoking tobacco.

Thoracentesis

This sterile test involves the insertion of a needle into the pleural cavity for the purpose of removing fluid that has accumulated within the pleural space. With the client sitting upright, a large-bore needle is inserted into the pleural space and fluid is then aspirated. Assist the patient to remain immobile during the procedure to prevent injury to the visceral pleura.

Following removal of the needle, pressure is applied to the insertion site followed by a chest X-ray to check for pneumothorax. Monitor blood pressure for hypotension if a large quantity of fluid is removed.

Transcranial Magnetic Stimulation

This is noninvasive procedure in which a changing magnetic field is introduced into the brain to influence the brain's activity. The field is generated by passing a large electrical current through a wire stimulation coil over a brief period. After assessing a patient's resting motor threshold to determine dosing, an insulated coil is placed on or close to a specific area of the patient's head, allowing the magnetic field to pass through the skull and into target areas of the brain. Used in psychiatry for treatment of mood disorders.

Tuberculin Skin Testing

This test is used to identify a tuberculosis infection. It does not, however, detect whether the infection is active or dormant. An intradermal injection of purified protein derivative (PPD) of the tubercle bacillus is administered into the arm. An individual who is infected will produce a reaction at the injection site as lymphocytes that have been activated by the original infection will react to the PPD. A reaction (induration, not redness) at the injection site of greater than 5 mm in diameter read 48 to 72 hours following the injection indicates a positive result. A second injection may be administered to an individual who is suspected as having been infected but was negative for the first injection.

Individuals who received bacille Calmette-Guérin (BCG) vaccine in the past will show a positive result even though they have not been infected with the tubercle bacillus.

Ultrasonography

High-frequency sound waves are passed into the body, echo off body organs, and are then translated into a picture. Ultrasonography helps identify abnormalities. Depending on the area of the body being examined, certain preparation of the client may be required, such as NPO.

Ultrasonography can be performed on many areas of the body, such as the cardiac, abdominal, and pelvic regions, as well as the breast, to identify abnormalities in structure and function.

Virtual Colonoscopy

Combines MRI or CT scanning with computer virtual reality software to detect colon and lower bowel diseases and conditions, such as polyps, lower GI bleeding, colorectal cancer, and diverticulosis. Air is introduced via a tube into the rectum to enlarge colon for improved visualization. Bowel preparation similar to colonoscopy. Requires less sedation and no endoscope for this procedure. Take about 15 to 20 minutes to perform the test.

BIBLIOGRAPHY

Astle, B., & Duggleby, W. (2024). *Potter and Perry's Canadian fundamentals of nursing* (7th ed.). Elsevier.

Bard, B., MacMullin, E., Williamson, J., & Morrison-Valfre, M. (2022). *Morrison-Valfre's foundations of mental health care in Canada*. Elsevier.

Pagana, K. D., Pagana, T. J., & Pike MacDonald, S. A. (2019). *Mosby's Canadian manual of diagnostic and laboratory tests* (2nd Cdn). Elsevier.

Tyerman, J., & Cobbett, W. (2023). *Lewis's medical-surgical nursing in Canada: Assessment and management of clinical problems* (5th ed.). Elsevier.

Mathematical Formulae Related to the Practice of Nursing

CALCULATION OF ORAL AND PARENTERAL DOSES OF MEDICATIONS

The **dosage ordered** refers to the dosage of the drug that has been prescribed for the client, for example, 500 mg, 2 g, or 30 UI. The **dosage available** is the dosage of the drug that is on hand, such as 250 mg or 0.5 g. The **drug form** is the form in which the available dosage is supplied, for example, tablets, capsules, or liquid.

Formula

$$\frac{\text{Dosage ordered}}{\text{Dosage available}} \times \text{Drug form}$$
$$= \text{Amount of drug to administer}$$

Example 1

Your client is ordered digoxin (Lanoxin) 0.125 mg by mouth daily. You have Lanoxin available in 0.25 mg tablets. How many tablets should you administer daily to your client?

Solution using the Formula Method:

$$\frac{0.125 \text{ mg}}{0.25 \text{ mg}} \times 1 \text{ tablet} = 0.5 \text{ tablet of Lanoxin}$$

Solution using Dimensional Analysis:

$$x \text{ tab} = \frac{1}{0.25 \text{ mg}} \times \frac{0.125 \text{ mg}}{1}$$

$$x \text{ tab} = \frac{1 \times 0.125}{0.25}$$

$$x = \frac{0.125}{0.25}$$

$$x = 0.5 \text{ tablet of Lanoxin}$$

Example 2

Your client is ordered furosemide (Lasix) oral solution 40 mg daily for edema due to renal failure. The label on the container indicates 20 mg per 5 mL. How many millilitres should you administer daily to your client?

Solution using the Formula method:

$$\frac{40 \text{mg}}{20 \text{mg}} \times 5 \text{mL} = 10 \text{mL of Lasix}$$

SOLUTION USING DIMENSIONAL ANALYSIS

$$x \text{ mL} = \frac{5 \text{ mL}}{20 \text{ mg}} \times \frac{40 \text{ mg}}{1}$$

$$x \text{ mL} = \frac{5 \times 40}{20} = 10$$

$$x = 10 \text{ mL}$$

CALCULATIONS FOR PEDIATRIC DOSAGES OF ORAL AND PARENTERAL MEDICATIONS

Medications prescribed for infants and children require adjustments in the dosages to accommodate the differences in their weights and body surface areas; gastro-intestinal, liver, and kidney functions; and metabolic activities. Much smaller doses of medications are required to avoid overdosage and toxicity. The child's weight and height are often used to calculate the correct dosage for a child. In addition, dosages for young children are usually ordered in liquid form.

Calculating Pediatric Dosage Based on Body Weight

Formula

$$\frac{\text{Drug dosage per}}{\text{kg of body weight}} \times \text{Weight of child (kg)}$$
$$= \text{Dosage to administer}$$

Example

A 2-month-old infant with septicemia is ordered ampicillin (Ampicin) 100 mg/kg/day every 8 hours intravenously. The infant weighs 4 kg. How many milligrams should be administered with each dose?

$$100 \text{ mg} \times 4 \text{ kg} = 400 \text{ mg of ampicillin daily (3 doses)}$$
$$400 \text{ mg} \div 3 = 133.3 \text{ mg per dose of ampicillin}$$

CALCULATIONS FOR INTRAVENOUS DROP RATE

The **amount of solution to administer** is the quantity of fluid in millilitres that is to be administered during the shift. Intravenous tubing is selected according to the amount of fluid to be administered. The **drop factor** is the amount of fluid delivered by the specific tubing being used.

Formula:

$$\frac{\text{Amount of solution to administer}}{\text{Time for infusion in hours}} \times \frac{\text{Drop factor of tubing}}{60 \text{ min}}$$
$$= \text{Drop rate (gtt/min)}$$

Example 1

The client is receiving 1 200 mL of 2/3 and 1/3 per 8-hr shift. At what rate should you set the drop rate if the intravenous tubing delivers 10 drops per minute?

Solution using the Formula Method:

$$\frac{1\,200\ mL}{8\ hr} \times \frac{10}{60\ min} = 25\ gtt/min$$

Solution using Dimensional Analysis:

$$\frac{x\ gtt}{min} = \frac{10\ gtt}{1\ mL} \times \frac{1200\ mL}{8\ hr} \times \frac{1\ hr}{60\ min}$$

$$x = \frac{10 \times 1200}{8 \times 60} = 25$$

$$x = 25\ gtt/min$$

Example 2

The client is receiving 50 mL of 5% dextrose in water per hour. At what rate should you set the drop rate if the intravenous tubing delivers 60 drops per minute?

Solution using the Formula Method:

$$\frac{50\ mL}{1\ hr} \times \frac{60}{60\ min} = 50\ gtt/min$$

Solution using Dimensional Analysis:

$$\frac{x\ gtt}{min} = \frac{60\ gtt}{1\ mL} \times \frac{50\ mL}{1\ hr} \times \frac{1\ hr}{60\ min} = 50$$

$$x = \frac{60 \times 50}{1 \times 60} = 50$$

$$x = 50\ gtt/min$$

UNITS OF MEASUREMENT

Canada adopted the international system of units (called *Système Internationale d'Unités* in French and abbreviated as *SI*), or the metric system of measurement, in 1970. It is used by most countries of the world.

Although this system of measurement has been universally adopted throughout the healthcare system, the household system of measurement occasionally appears due to long-term habit. It is therefore important for the nurse to be aware of the more common equivalents.

Liquid Measure

3 teaspoons (tsp)	=	1 tablespoon (tbsp)
2 tablespoons (tbsp)	=	1 fluid ounce (fl oz)
8 fluid ounces (fl oz)	=	1 cup (C)
2 cups (C)	=	1 pint
2 pints	=	1 quart
4 quarts	=	1 gallon (gal)

Mass Measure

16 ounces (oz)	=	1 pound (lb)

Linear Measure

12 inches (in)	=	1 foot (ft)
3 feet (ft)	=	1 yard (yd)

Conversion of Household Measure to SI Measure

Liquid Measure

1 teaspoon (tsp)	=	5 mL
1 tablespoon (tbsp)	=	15 mL
1 ounce (oz)	=	30 mL
1 cup (C)	=	240/250 mL
1 pint	=	500 mL
1 quart	=	1 000 mL (1 L)
1 gallon (gal)	=	4 000 mL

Mass Measure

2.2 pounds (lb)	=	1 kg

Linear Measure

1 inch	=	2.54 cm
39.4 inches	=	1 m

Measurement of Temperature

To Convert Celsius to Fahrenheit

°Celsius × 1.8 + 32	=	°F

To Convert Fahrenheit to Celsius

°Fahrenheit − 32 ÷ 1.8	=	°Celsius

ANSWERS AND RATIONALES FOR PRACTICE QUESTIONS

CHAPTER 4

The correct answer is set off in boldface.

1. **C: Professional, Ethical, and Legal Practice CN: Safe and Effective Care Environment T: Application**
   1. Abbreviations must be approved by the organization or agency.
   2. The Canadian Nurses Association does not approve abbreviations for documentation.
   3. **Abbreviations must be approved by the organization or agency.**
   4. Abbreviations must be approved by the organization or agency, not the individual unit.

2. **C: Professional, Ethical, and Legal Practice CN: Safe and Effective Care Environment T: Critical Thinking**
   1. The person most involved in the procedure must obtain client consent. Nurses do not obtain consent for procedures performed by others.
   2. **The person most involved in the procedure and the one who can explain the procedure fully should obtain client consent.**
   3. Verbal consent is acceptable for some procedures, but surgery usually requires written consent.
   4. Consent can be withdrawn at any time during investigation or treatment, even if a signed consent had previously been obtained.

3. **C: Professional, Ethical, and Legal Practice CN: Safe and Effective Care Environment T: Application**
   1. **Verbal orders are not telephone orders and should not be utilized unless in an emergency situation.**
   2. Verbal orders are not equivalent to telephone orders.
   3. Verbal orders may need to be accepted in emergency situations.
   4. There are no regulations that define which kind of nurse can accept verbal orders.

4. **C: Professional, Ethical, and Legal Practice CN: Safe and Effective Care Environment T: Application**
   1. The dose is not correct, and the frequency is not identified.
   2. **The dose is accurate, the route is identified, the frequency is identified, and the qualifier is identified.**
   3. The dose is not correct, and the frequency is not identified.
   4. The dose is not correct, and the route is not identified.

5. **C: Professional, Ethical, and Legal Practice CN: Safe and Effective Care Environment T: Knowledge**
   1. Evidence-informed care does not relate to government funding.
   2. **Evidence-informed care is founded in the transfer of current research into practice.**
   3. Evidence-informed care is described after research has been completed.

4. Not all evidence-informed care focuses on assessment skills.

6. **C: Professional, Ethical, and Legal Practice CN: Safe and Effective Care Environment T: Knowledge**
   1. This is not correct.
   2. This is not correct.
   3. This is not correct.
   4. **A nurse practitioner is usually educated at the master's level.**

7. **C: Collaborative Practice CN: Safe and Effective Care Environment T: Application**
   1. Different learning styles require different teaching approaches.
   2. Learning is easier when the material is connected to what the learner already knows.
   3. **Learning occurs best when the learner identifies a learning need.**
   4. It is best to offer a variety of options to learners because some individuals learn best in the morning, whereas others learn best in the afternoon or evening.

8. **C: Collaborative Practice CN: Safe and Effective Care Environment T: Application**
   1. "I" statements should be utilized with clients and colleagues.
   2. **When genuineness and warmth are utilized, the communication is more effective.**
   3. Communication is better facilitated by open-ended questions.
   4. Self-disclosure should be utilized minimally and only to build a therapeutic nurse–client relationship, not to share the nurse's point of view.

9. **C: Collaborative Practice CN: Safe and Effective Care Environment T: Critical Thinking**
   1. Differences may contribute to conflict, but the conflict must then be acknowledged and resolved rather than the differences suppressed.
   2. Team collaboration is the most effective method of conflict resolution, even more effective than introducing a third party.
   3. **Team collaboration is the most effective method of conflict resolution. The team is required to work together to resolve the conflict.**
   4. At times there must be imposed guidelines, but team collaboration is most effective.

10. **C: Professional, Ethical, and Legal Practice CN: Safe and Effective Care Environment T: Critical Thinking**
    1. This may not be practical or applicable in every client situation.
    2. **This is the primary consideration prior to the decision to apply restraints.**
    3. This is not a consideration.

4. Consent may be required, but it may be verbal, or it may be from a substitute decision maker. It does not necessarily have to be a signed consent.

11. **C: Professional, Ethical, and Legal Practice CN: Safe and Effective Care Environment T: Application**
    1. This is an assumption rather than factual documentation and does not note the exact time.
    2. As in choice 1.
    3. **This is factual documentation.**
    4. As in choice 1.

12. **C: Professional, Ethical, and Legal Practice CN: Safe and Effective Care Environment T: Critical Thinking**
    1. Standards may help the nurse identify learning gaps, but this is not the most important purpose.
    2. **Standards of nursing practice define the expectation for nurses in various practice settings and situations and generally guide nursing practice.**
    3. While standards of nursing practice focus on defining expectations for acceptable practice, they do not focus on malpractice.
    4. The primary purpose of nursing practice and health professions acts, and thereby standards of nursing practice, is to protect the public's (not the nurse's) health, safety, and welfare.

13. **C: Professional, Ethical, and Legal Practice CN: Safe and Effective Care Environment T: Knowledge**
    1. **The primary mandate of a health regulatory organization is protection of the public.**
    2. Labour organizations have the mandate of protecting nurses.
    3. The employer has a responsibility to serve the clients to whom they provide service.
    4. The nursing regulatory body protects the public from unsafe, unethical nursing care—it cannot be generalized to any other regulated profession.

14. **C: Professional, Ethical, and Legal Practice CN: Safe and Effective Care Environment T: Application**
    1. Analysis and grouping of data are part of the nursing process, not the Best Practice Guidelines.
    2. Advance directives are individualized to specific clients; they cannot be generalized as best practice for whole groups.
    3. **Evidence-informed guidelines are tools that improve client, nurse, and organizational outcomes. They involve care that is based on actual observed and proven outcomes, not tradition-based care.**
    4. A code of ethics provides guidelines for compassionate care, educates about ethical responsibilities, and informs about moral commitments.

15. **C: Professional, Ethical, and Legal Practice CN: Safe and Effective Care Environment T: Critical Thinking**
    1. This is a generally accepted interpretation, but it is not the most correct answer as the health care team has the responsibility to determine the client's exact wishes.
    2. Do Not Resuscitate may be open to interpretation and not involve only cardiac compressions.

3. This is too vague an interpretation.
4. **The client or substitute decision maker must decide what, if any, resuscitation is desired. The nurse has the responsibility to comply with the stated wishes of the capable client, whether they are written as a DNR or not.**

16. **C: Collaborative Practice CN: Safe and Effective Care Environment T: Application**
    1. **During the situation component of I-SBAR-R the nurse states the problem.**
    2. During the assessment component of I-SBAR-R, the nurse states a conclusion that is based on what they think is wrong.
    3. **During the recommendation component of I-S-BAR-R, the nurse states an informed suggestion for the continued care of the person by proposing an action and stating what is needed and in what time frame it needs to be completed.**
    4. During the identification component of I-SBAR-R, the nurse identifies themselves and their role.
    5. During the background component of I-SBAR-R, the nurse related the person's background.

17. **C: Professional, Ethical, and Legal Practice CN: Safe and Effective Care Environment T: Application**
    1. **When administering medications in accordance with a prescriber's prescription the nurse is responsible for knowing the purpose of the medication.**
    2. **When administering medication in accordance with a prescriber's prescription the nurse is responsible for knowing the effect of the medication.**
    3. The nurse is not expected to know the cost of the medications they are giving.
    4. **When administering medication in accordance with a prescriber's prescription the nurse is responsible for knowing the potential adverse effects of the medication they are giving.**
    5. **When administering medication in accordance with a prescriber's prescription the nurse is responsible for knowing the contraindications of the medication they are giving.**

18. **C: Professional, Ethical, and Legal Practice CN: Safe and Effective Care Environment T: Application**
    1. This does not ensure that client care is provided. The nurse has an ethical obligation to provide the required client care or find a substitute to provide the care.
    2. **The nurse has an ethical obligation to provide client care since no one else is available to provide the care.**
    3. The nurse must first provide the care (the referral to the gynecologist) or find a substitute to provide the care.
    4. The client's care cannot be deferred until next week. The nurse has an ethical obligation to provide the required care.

19. **C: Professional, Ethical, and Legal Practice CN: Safe and Effective Care Environment T: Critical Thinking**

1. The client may not accurately recall what was said or may be afraid to discuss the event for fear of reprisal from the unregulated care provider.
2. This action does not deal with the issue of verbal abuse. Situations of abuse must be addressed as close to the time of the incident as possible.
3. **It is the professional responsibility of the nurse to stop the abuse immediately and notify the manager in order to ensure client safety.**
4. This action does not deal with the issue of verbal abuse.

20. **C: Professional, Ethical, and Legal Practice CN: Safe and Effective Care Environment   T: Application**
   1. The nurse is not accountable for the actions of the unregulated care provider (UCP); the UCP is accountable for her own actions.
   2. The nurse is not accountable for the actions of the UCP despite being on her lunch break.
   3. The nurse is not accountable for the actions of the UCP despite being the only registered/licensed staff on duty at the time of the fall.
   4. **UCPs are accountable for their care, including any actions or inactions taken that relate to the resident falling.**

21. **C: Professional, Ethical, and Legal Practice CN: Safe and Effective Care Environment   T: Application**
   1. The nurse's decision to work the additional hours is their choice.
   2. The nurse's involvement of the labour union is separate from the nurse's accountability to provide safe and effective care.
   3. Payment of overtime is not the primary concern for the nurse; they must be competent to provide care.
   4. **The nurse's first priority is to provide high-quality client care. They must determine if they are too tired to provide competent care.**

22. **C: Professional, Ethical, and Legal Practice CN: Safe and Effective Care Environment   T: Knowledge**
   1. **The consent must be voluntary.**
   2. **The consent may also be given verbally.**
   3. **The client must be legally capable.**
   4. **The consent must be specific to the proposed treatment or procedure.**
   5. **The client must be told of the risks and benefits of the proposed procedure.**

23. **C: Professional, Ethical, and Legal Practice CN: Safe and Effective Care Environment   T: Critical Thinking**
   1. **ASA is contraindicated for clients who are receiving Coumadin. The nurse must clarify the order with the physician.**
   2. The client may not have accurate knowledge of his medications.
   3. The pharmacist cannot change the prescribed medication order.
   4. The nurse does not need to consult with colleagues.

24. **C: Professional, Ethical, and Legal Practice CN: Safe and Effective Care Environment   T: Knowledge**

1. **Chemical restraints include medications.**
2. **Physical restraints include side rails, extremity restraint, etc.**
3. **"Hazardous" is not a restraint category.**
4. **Environmental restraints include a locked ward or room.**
5. **"Natural" is not a restraint category.**

25. **C: Professional, Ethical, and Legal Practice CN: Safe and Effective Care Environment T: Application**
   1. Passwords should never be shared, even if client care is provided.
   2. The student nurse who provided the care should document the care.
   3. **Passwords should not be shared. Anyone who will be documenting client care should be provided with a password.**
   4. The student nurse should take responsibility for retrieving a forgotten password.

26. **C: Professional, Ethical, and Legal Practice CN: Safe and Effective Care Environment T: Application**
   1. **The client has withdrawn consent; the nurse cannot force treatment.**
   2. The client has expressed her wishes. This does not require intervention from the charge nurse.
   3. The diagnosis of depression does not mean the client is unable to provide informed consent for treatments.
   4. It is not ethical nor therapeutic for the nurse to insist that the client take the medication.

27. **C: Professional, Ethical, and Legal Practice CN: Safe and Effective Care Environment   T: Application**
   1. **A tort is a civil wrong against a person that violates their rights. Threatening to insert a urinary catheter without consent is a tort.**
   2. **Giving unnecessary medication for the convenience of staff, controls behaviour in a manner similar to secluding a client; thus, false imprisonment is a possible charge.**
   3. This does not exemplify a tort.
   4. **Starting an IV line without client consent is a tort.**
   5. As in choice 3.

28. **C: Professional, Ethical, and Legal Practice CN: Safe and Effective Care Environment   T: Application**
   1. The client may not have accurate knowledge of the obstetrician's orders for postpartum pain relief.
   2. **Nurses must have the original prescriber clarify the order.**
   3. Clarification must be obtained from the prescriber, not other health care providers.
   4. As in choice 2.

29. **C: Professional, Ethical, and Legal Practice CN: Safe and Effective Care Environment   T: Application**
   1. This is acceptable nursing practice and does not constitute a breach of the client's right to privacy of information (confidentiality).
   2. **Release of information without client authorization violates the client's right to privacy.**

3. As in choice 1.
4. As in choice 1.
5. **To dispose of confidential client information without risk of a breach of confidentiality, it is important to place papers in a secure bin marked for shredding.**

CHAPTER 5

The correct answer is set off in boldface.

1. C: **Professional, Ethical, and Legal Practice CN: Psychosocial Integrity T: Application**
   1. Nurses should always address the person by the last name, as some older persons may resent being called by their first names by younger persons.
   2. If Mrs. Sloane was hard of hearing, it is best for the nurse to face her directly so that her mouth and face are visible. Speaking loudly or shouting may distort speech.
   3. **It is important to adjust the pace of the interview to allow older persons sufficient time to report background historical information. Also, it may take the older person a greater amount of response time to interpret the question and process the answer.**
   4. Touch is a nonverbal skill that is very important to older people. Touch communicates empathy and understanding.

2. C: **Foundations of Practice CN: Health Promotion and Maintenance T: Critical Thinking**
   1. Older persons do lose muscle mass as they age, but this is not the cause of shortened stature.
   2. **With age, the intervertebral discs become thinner, thus shortening the spinal column and leading to shortened stature.**
   3. Many older persons develop osteoporosis leading to decreased height, but this is not the primary reason.
   4. Kyphosis mostly occurs as a result of osteoporosis.

3. C: **Foundations of Practice CN: Health Promotion and Maintenance T: Knowledge**
   1. Systolic, but not diastolic, pressures tend to increase.
   2. As in choice 1.
   3. Blood pressure does not become variable due to age.
   4. **As the heart pumps against a stiffer aorta, the systolic pressure increases, leading to a widened pulse pressure.**

4. C: **Foundations of Practice CN: Health Promotion and Maintenance T: Knowledge**
   1. **Skin tags are overgrowths of normal skin that form a stalk and are polyplike. They occur frequently on the eyelids, cheeks, neck, axillae, and trunk of the older person.**
   2. Edema is an abnormal finding and may indicate a circulatory or cardiac condition.
   3. There is often increased hair on the chin, upper lip, and eyebrows of older females due to unopposed androgens.

4. Older persons have thinner skin on the backs of their hands, forearms, lower legs, and dorsa of feet and over bony prominences.

5. C: **Foundations of Practice CN: Health Promotion and Maintenance T: Application**
   1. This greyish-white arc is called *arcus senilis*. It is not related to cataracts.
   2. **Arcus senilis is commonly seen around the cornea and is due to deposition of lipid material. Although the cornea may appear thickened and raised, it does not affect vision.**
   3. Although arcus senilis may cause the cornea to look thickened, it does not affect vision.
   4. Xanthelasma are soft raised yellow plaques occurring on the lids at the inner canthus and are more frequent in women. They are found with both high and normal blood levels of cholesterol.

6. C: **Foundations of Practice CN: Health Promotion and Maintenance T: Application**
   1. **Impacted cerumen ("ear wax") is a common but reversible cause of hearing loss in older people. Ear canal irrigation can remove the impacted cerumen and will be performed more easily if the cerumen is softened. Application of a cotton ball will help to seal the oil in the ear canal and soften the cerumen.**
   2. Although coarse ear hairs may increase the accumulation of cerumen, application of a cotton ball is the appropriate action.
   3. This is not necessary unless the cerumen cannot be removed by irrigation.
   4. It is likely that use of a cotton swab will push the cerumen farther into the ear canal and could cause damage to the canal and eardrum.

7. C: **Foundations of Practice CN: Health Promotion and Maintenance T: Critical Thinking**
   1. It is normal for many older persons to temporarily forget the day of the week, especially due to the lack of structure or routine of not going out to a job. While a person may not provide the precise date, Mrs. Sloane would be considered oriented if she knew generally the present period of time and place.
   2. Scores of 24 to 27 indicate no cognitive impairment. A slight decline to 25 may be a normal variable.
   3. Most people temporarily misplace articles. It would be of concern if Mrs. Sloane were placing her belongings in inappropriate places, such as putting her hearing aid in the refrigerator.
   4. **This indicates confusion, loss of orientation, and impairment of short-term memory and is an indication of dementia.**

8. C: **Foundations of Practice CN: Health Promotion and Maintenance T: Critical Thinking**
   1. This would be the second assessment.
   2. This would be done early in the assessment provided that the infant was not crying.

3. This would disturb the infant and should be left until after the general assessment, heart rate, and respirations.

4. **Prior to the nurse disturbing the infant, she should develop an overall impression: body symmetry, spontaneous position, flexion of limbs, spontaneous movement, and any obvious facial abnormalities.**

9. C: Foundations of Practice CN: Health Promotion and Maintenance T: Application

1. Although the baby needs to be examined while naked, there may be concerns about heat regulation if the environment is not warm. In addition, particularly for male babies, the diaper should be left on until the genitalia and anus are examined.

2. The parents should be present so they may be reassured by the examination, so they may learn about the normal growth and development of their infant, and so the infant is calmed by their presence.

3. **The baby responds to a soft, soothing tone of voice.**

4. The exam should be scheduled 1 to 2 hours after feeding, when the baby is not hungry or drowsy.

10. C: Foundations of Practice CN: Health Promotion and Maintenance T: Application

1. **An infant's respirations are primarily diaphragmatic rather than thoracic; thus, the abdomen is watched to count and evaluate respirations.**

2. The normal respiratory rate for a newborn is 30 to 60 breaths per minute. A rate of 70 is tachypnea.

3. Infants display a respiratory pattern that is irregular, from rapid breaths to short periods of apnea.

4. Young infants are obligatory nose-breathers up to the age of 3 months, at which point they become nose- and mouth-breathers, so mouth-breathing would be an abnormal finding.

11. C: Foundations of Practice CN: Health Promotion and Maintenance T: Application

1. This may be visually assessed and is rarely clinically important.

2. Head circumference is not part of the Apgar score.

3. **The newborn's head measures about 32 to 38 cm and is about 2 cm larger than the chest. The measurement is plotted on a standard growth chart. An enlarged head circumference may be an indication of increased intracranial pressure, such as in hydrocephalus. A smaller than normal head circumference is an indication of microcephaly resulting from genetic or congenital conditions.**

4. Fontanelles are assessed visually and by palpation.

12. C: Foundations of Practice CN: Health Promotion and Maintenance T: Critical Thinking

1. **This is the most reliable and least invasive determination of a patent rectum and anus. It guarantees that the intestine is sufficiently patent to allow the passage of stool.**

2. This is the anal reflex and is used to check sphincter tone.

3. This is not a recommended practice as there is danger of harming the rectal mucosa.

4. This should not be necessary, and even the fifth finger may be too large for the size of the newborn rectum.

13. C: Foundations of Practice CN: Health Promotion and Maintenance T: Knowledge

1. This elicits the Babinski reflex.

2. **This will elicit the Moro reflex, as will placing the infant on a flat surface and hitting the surface sharply.**

3. This will elicit the startle reflex.

4. This will elicit the stepping reflex.

14. C: Collaborative Practice CN: Health Promotion and Maintenance T: Application

1. Depending on the age of the teenager, it may not be appropriate to involve the parents. Most adolescents need to feel in control of their bodies and their lives and may not want parents involved unless a serious condition is identified.

2. Adolescents may not respond positively to authority, particularly in a health assessment situation. It is more important for the nurse to obtain their trust.

3. **With this approach, the nurse will be able to gain the trust of the adolescent.**

4. Future health conditions will not be of interest or concern to the adolescent.

15. C: Foundations of Practice CN: Health Promotion and Maintenance T: Application

1. Alcohol has no effect on menstruation.

2. Family history of ovarian cancer has no relation to the onset of menstruation.

3. **Because Hilary is thin, she may have anorexia and be malnourished. Onset of menstruation is affected by nutritional status.**

4. Sleep has no effect on menstruation.

16. C: Collaborative Practice CN: Health Promotion and Maintenance T: Critical Thinking

1. This does nothing to reassure Bradley and may sound patronizing.

2. It is normal for boys of Bradley's age to be short prior to a growth spurt at puberty. Evaluation by a physician is necessary only if Bradley is extremely short.

3. While some exercises may help to increase muscle size, they will not affect Bradley's height. It is more important to reassure him that this will occur at puberty.

4. **This is a factual answer that will reassure Bradley that he is normal and that he will grow and be more like his friends when he reaches puberty.**

17. C: Foundations of Practice CN: Health Promotion and Maintenance T: Application

1. **This is called the forward bend test. The spine should appear vertical. If there is unequal height of scapulae, shoulders, or iliac crests, scoliosis is suspected.**

2. Kyphosis is common during adolescence because of chronic poor posture. This is not a test for scoliosis.

3. This will not identify scoliosis.

4. This will not help to identify a curvature of the spine seen in scoliosis.

18. **C: Foundations of Practice CN: Safe and Effective Care Environment T: Application**
   1. This question may solicit information about the parent–child relationship, but it is not the most important safety-related question.
   2. This question is directed at finding information concerning Sheldon's ability to manage the stress of balancing sports and school demands, but it is not the most important safety-related question.
   3. This question may lead to an assessment of Sheldon's goals and aspirations for his future, but it is not the most important safety-related question at this time.
   4. **Adolescents playing football are at particular risk of injury. The nurse needs to obtain information regarding protective equipment.**

19. **C: Foundations of Practice CN: Psychosocial Integrity T: Critical Thinking**
   1. This obtains information about his cognitive function and compliance with academic expectations, not thought processes.
   2. This is a question that may obtain information about mood and affect.
   3. This is a test of a person's ability to remember new learning. It is more useful in assessing for dementia.
   4. **Paranoia and auditory and visual hallucinations occur with psychiatric and organic brain disease and with psychedelic drugs.**

20. **C: Foundations of Practice CN Health Promotion and Maintenance T: Knowledge**
   1. This is a common inflammatory condition of the skin, but it is not the most common skin condition in adolescence.
   2. **All teens have some form of acne, although with some, it is in the milder form of open comedones (blackheads).**
   3. Eczema is a type of dermatitis with various forms. It is not specific to the adolescent.
   4. Rosacea is a type of acne found primarily in persons.

21. **C: Foundations of Practice CN: Physiological Integrity T: Critical Thinking**
   1. **A third heart sound is an abnormal finding.**
   2. Palpation of the apical pulse is a normal finding.
   3. Capillary refill less than 3 seconds is a normal finding.
   4. Calf circumferences within 1 cm is a normal finding.

22. **C: Foundations of Practice CN: Physiological Integrity T: Application**
   1. **When assessing cerebellar function, the nurse assesses the client's coordination and balance by observing them while they are heel-to-toe tandem walking.**
   2. **When assessing cerebellar function, the nurse assesses the client's coordination and balance by observing them while they are walking normally.**

3. **When assessing cerebellar function, the nurse assesses the client's coordination and balance by observing them while they are performing knee bends.**
4. **When assessing cerebellar function, the nurse assesses the client's coordination and balance by observing them while complete the Romberg test.**
5. Checking for PERRLA (pupils Equal, Round, React to Light and Accommodation) is completed as part of cranial nerve testing.

23. **C: Foundations of Practice CN: Physiological Integrity T: Application**
   1. This is a normal heart rate for a 2-month-old infant.
   2. This is a normal heart rate for a child this age after exercise.
   3. Although lower than the textbook normal heart rate, 50 is not abnormal in a young, well-conditioned athlete.
   4. **This is bradycardia in a 5-day-old infant. Although there are wide variations published as normal neonatal heart rates that range from approximately 100 to 160, this rate, especially after crying, is below normal.**

24. **C: Foundations of Practice CN: Physiological Integrity T: Critical Thinking**
   1. This is a common but not ominous sign in a client who has had a head injury.
   2. **This is of concern as it implies that there has been some injury to the brain with loss of memory and cognitive function.**
   3. This is a normal finding postinjury and implies superficial rather than brain injury.
   4. The blood pressure presently remains within normal limits. It may become elevated due to pain, or there may be later deviations indicative of shock or brain swelling.

25. **C: Foundations of Practice CN: Health Promotion and Maintenance T: Knowledge**
   1. As a person ages, salivation decreases.
   2. As a person ages, esophageal emptying is delayed.
   3. As a person ages, peristalsis is thought to remain fairly constant. Decreased peristalsis may result from a decreased amount of bulk in a person's diet.
   4. **As a person ages, gastric acid secretion decreases.**

26. **C: Foundations of Practice CN: Psychosocial Integrity T: Application**
   1. This tests abstract reasoning, not judgement and decision making.
   2. This is a test of cognitive function and does not evaluate judgement.
   3. **This requires the client to apply judgement and decision-making abilities to develop a wise course of action.**
   4. This tests abstract reasoning.

27. **C: Foundations of Practice CN: Physiological Integrity T: Knowledge**

1. Wheezes are abnormal or adventitious sounds.
2. Crackles are abnormal or adventitious sounds.
3. **Tracheal breath sounds are normal breath sounds found over the trachea.**
4. **Bronchovesicular breath sounds are normal breath sounds found over the bronchi.**
5. **Vesicular breath sounds are normal breath sounds found over the rest of the chest.**

28. C: Foundations of Practice CN: T: Knowledge
    1. **A normal finding in the physical assessment of the auditory system is the ability to hear low whisper at 30 cm.**
    2. Rhinc's test result for a normal finding is that air conduction is better than bone conduction.
    3. **A normal finding is 'no lateralization' Weber's test result.**
    4. A red tympanic membrane indicates infection in the middle ear.
    5. **A normal finding is ears symmetrical in location and shape.**

29. C: Foundations of Practice CN: Safe and Effective Care Environment T: Application
    1. **The mnemonic OPQRSTUV will help you remember the crucial characteristics that must be assessed. This question reflects R: "region".**
    2. **This question reflects S: "severity".**
    3. **This question reflects T: "timing".**
    4. **This question reflects P: "palliative".**
    5. This question reflects family history.
    6. **This question reflects U: "understanding".**

30. C: Foundations of Practice CN: Safe and Effective Care Environment T: Critical Thinking
    1. **Closed or direct questions are helpful in obtaining specific details. This is an appropriate direct question to ask as part of an elder abuse assessment screening.**
    2. The nurse does not ask this question because the client may not consider what is happening to them to be abuse.
    3. **This is an appropriate direct question to ask as part of an elder abuse assessment screening.**
    4. **This is an appropriate direct question to ask as part of an elder abuse assessment screening.**
    5. **This is an appropriate direct question to ask as part of an elder abuse assessment screening.**

CHAPTER 6

The correct answer is set off in boldface.
1. C: Foundations of Practice CN: Safe and Effective Care Environment T: Application
   1. **The health sector uses a significant amount of electrical energy by burning nonrenewable fossil fuels. This process produces greenhouse gases and significantly contributes to global climate change. Hospital waste and incineration practices contribute emissions of dioxins, mercury, and other heavy metals, which are toxic to human health.**
   2. Although hospital practices often lead to waste that could otherwise be recycled or avoided, any landfill runoff is not directly associated with hospital practices.
   3. The energy used and the waste produced affect the quality of the outdoor environment—the air, food, soil, and water.
   4. Although wind energy may be an alternative source of energy, it is not the result of the energy used and the waste produced by the health sector.

2. C: Collaborative Practice CN : Health Promotion and Maintenance T. Application
   1. This assumes that there is a conflict, which may not be true.
   2. **For effective and sustainable change, it is critical to build a community of people within the organization who understand and are motivated to work on the issues.**
   3. Focus groups may be used to facilitate discussion and input on the issues but are only mechanisms for the advocacy process and community building.
   4. Community promotion is not an actual process.

3. C: Collaborative Practice CN: Safe and Effective Care Environment T: Critical Thinking
   1. Administrators are not likely to support policy changes without first understanding the rationale for and significance of the problem.
   2. Assessing clients for exposure to environmental contaminants would not increase awareness of environmentally responsible behaviours within the organization.
   3. **Implementing educational sessions on environmentally responsible health care would help to increase awareness of the issues among staff and administrators.**
   4. Promoting environmentally friendly products in the hospital gift store would not be the most effective strategy for increasing awareness of environmentally responsible behaviours in the health sector.

4. C: Foundations of Practice CN: Health Promotion and Maintenance T: Critical Thinking
   1. Calorie-rich foods provide energy but often lack other essential nutrients.
   2. **Nutrient-rich foods are best to correct and prevent malnutrition-related diseases.**
   3. Inexpensive foods may not necessarily provide the nutrients required for a population that is malnourished.
   4. Some canned foods are nutrient-rich, but canned foods are not the only source of nutrient-rich foods.

5. C: Foundations of Practice CN: Health Promotion and Maintenance T: Critical Thinking
   1. This improves health but is a long-term goal that may not be achieved.

2. **Studies have shown that stable housing is the most important determinant for homeless clients to improve their socio-economic status and health.**

3. This is a long-term goal but is unlikely to be achieved if there is no stable housing.

4. This will improve general health, but stable housing has a greater influence.

6. **C: Foundations of Practice CN: Physiological Integrity T: Critical Thinking**

1. Most cases of tuberculosis may be treated in the community. Unless the person is a danger to others due to the communicability of the tuberculosis, the client cannot be forced into hospital.

2. **Directly observed therapy is recommended for clients, such as those at a shelter for the homeless, known to be at risk for noncompliance.**

3. The medications do not come in sustained-release formulations.

4. This may improve compliance but is not the best method to ensure treatment. Medications that have the fewest adverse effects may not be the most effective for the particular strain of tuberculosis.

7. **C: Foundations of Practice CN: Physiological Integrity T: Critical Thinking**

1. While it is true that homeless people are more likely to be reinjured on the streets, if they are adequately nourished, the injuries would not likely become chronic.

2. This may cause skin breakdown and injuries; however, with adequate nutrition, the lesions would not necessarily be chronic.

3. Communicability of pathogens is possible; however, improved nutrition would strengthen the immune system to fight the pathogens.

4. **Major complications of protein–calorie malnutrition are delayed wound healing and increased susceptibility to infection from a compromised immune system.**

8. **C: Professional, Ethical, and Legal Practice CN: Safe and Effective Care Environment T: Application**

1. Complementary therapies may be controversial, but fully informed clients may request them, and nurses can become trained and certified.

2. **Reiki is a complementary therapy. Such therapies may be integrated into the scope of professional practice provided that the practitioners have the requisite knowledge, skill, and competency; the client has made an informed decision, and it is sanctioned by agency policies and procedures.**

3. The nurse does not need to schedule Reiki treatments outside of her scheduled shift.

4. Olga is asking for Reiki treatment now, not after discharge.

9. **C: Foundations of Practice CN: Physiological Integrity T: Knowledge**

1. **Complementary therapies are those therapies used in addition to and in conjunction with conventional, or traditional, Western medicine.**

2. Therapies that are used instead of traditional or conventional medicine are called *alternative therapies*. Many of the same interventions can be complementary and alternative therapies.

3. Homeopathic remedies are a type of alternative or complementary therapy.

4. Most complementary therapies are considered to be natural; however, this is not the definition.

10. **C: Foundations of Practice CN: Psychosocial Integrity T: Application**

1. Mrs. Broadfoot has not stated that this is how she wishes to be treated. This is not individualized care.

2. **This is client-centred, individualized care.**

3. Mrs. Broadfoot—not the family—should be providing information about her plan of care.

4. Clients should not all be treated the same. They should be treated as individuals.

11. **C: Foundations of Practice CN: Psychosocial Integrity T: Application**

1. While there are many Indigenous dialects, most Indigenous people speak and understand English.

2. There is no indication from her admission diagnosis that she would be too weak to talk.

3. There is no indication that she is in denial.

4. **Use of silence is a common communication phenomenon among members of Indigenous communities.**

12. **C: Foundations of Practice CN: Physiological Integrity T: Application**

1. **Red meats have high iron content that is well absorbed by the body. There is no indication that Mrs. Broadfoot is vegetarian and will not eat a meat-containing diet.**

2. Plant sources of iron are not as well absorbed as those in meat.

3. As in choice 2.

4. As in choice 2.

13. **C: Professional, Ethical, and Legal Practice CN: Psychosocial Integrity T: Critical Thinking**

1. This may be neither practical nor possible as it is not known how long it will take the family to arrive. Also, it is not known if they wish to view the body.

2. There will likely be an autopsy as this is an unexpected death, but consent is not required.

3. There is no indication that this is necessary. If it were, it would be included in specific cultural death rites.

4. **This is the most inclusive answer. The nurse should obtain information by telephone from the family or consult other cultural resources.**

14. **C: Foundations of Practice CN: Safe and Effective Care Environment T: Application**

1. The Canadian Paediatric Society recommends that babies be positioned "back to sleep" to reduce the risk of sudden infant death syndrome (SIDS).
2. Research has found associations between SIDS and the prone position for sleep.
3. There is controversy regarding co-sleeping. While some studies do suggest it is a factor in SIDS, it is not as important as positioning infants on their backs.
4. Hats and booties are required only when babies are exposed to cold.

15. **C: Foundations of Practice CN: Health Promotion and Maintenance   T: Application**
   1. Early detection is secondary prevention.
   2. Megavitamin therapy is controversial, and in this situation, "postdiagnosis" of disease.
   3. Surgical treatment (appendectomy) is tertiary-level prevention.
   4. **Research has shown that remaining out of direct sunlight contributes to primary risk reduction of skin cancers.**
   5. **Eating a variety of healthy foods each day contributes to primary risk reduction of diseases such as heart disease, type 2 diabetes, and some cancers etc.**

16. **C: Professional, Ethical, and Legal Practice CN: Health Promotion and Maintenance   T: Critical Thinking**
   1. Although assisting a client with discussing their health conditions with their family is a nursing action, it is not an example of providing culturally competent care.
   2. **It is very important for nurses to be aware of how people interpret their health issues or illnesses to be capable of providing culturally competent care. A culturally competent nurse should be able to consistently and thoroughly recognize and understand the differences in their own culture and that of the person or an individual, to respect the person's values and beliefs, and adjust the approach of delivering care to meet each person's needs and expectations. Asking the person to describe their traditional healing methods demonstrates the nurse is seeking input from the person into the care that is received.**
   3. While encouraging a client to take their medications as prescribed is a nursing action, it is not an example of providing culturally competent care.
   4. Demonstrating the proper way to administer an insulin injection is a nursing action, but it is not an example of providing culturally competent care.
   5. **The nurse who assists the family of a Puerto Rican client to light candles is providing culturally attuned care. Latin American culture provides for religious rituals including the lighting of candles especially within the context of Catholicism.**

17. **C: Foundations of Practice CN: Health Promotion and Maintenance   T: Application**
   1. **Cancer-smart nutrition includes a diet high in antioxidant-rich fruits and vegetables. Antioxidants** have been shown to neutralize free radicals that cause damage to cells.
   2. **Maintaining body weight in a healthy range can reduce the risk of developing some types of cancer.**
   3. Cancer-smart nutrition includes a diet low, not high, in smoked, cured, and barbecued meats.
   4. **Reducing alcohol intake can reduce the risk of developing some types of cancer.**
   5. Cancer-smart nutrition includes reducing dietary fat to no more than 25 to 30% fat and no more than 10% as saturated fat.

18. **C: Foundations of Practice CN: Safe and Effective Care Environment   T: Application**
   1. Research has shown that good body mechanics alone are insufficient to prevent back injuries among nurses.
   2. This is not the safest way to move the client and could cause injury to the unregulated care providers and the client.
   3. **Use of a mechanical lift is the only safe way to accomplish this transfer.**
   4. Explaining the procedure will not change the client's limited ability to stand even if using a support aid. Both client and nurse could sustain injuries.

19. **C: Foundations of Practice CN: Health Promotion and Maintenance   T: Application**
   1. Some herbal remedies are safe, but pregnant clients need full information.
   2. Ginger is known to have many medicinal properties.
   3. **Although knowledge about herbal remedies is incomplete, research about the pharmacology of ginger is available and can be shared with clients to enable their informed decision making.**
   4. The first trimester is a time of organogenesis; however, clients need to be able to differentiate between benign, helpful, and harmful exposures.

20. **C: Professional, Ethical, and Legal Practice CN: Psychosocial Integrity   T: Critical Thinking**
   1. This statement assumes that the nurse knows what the client is feeling and may elicit an answer based on bravado.
   2. Initially, the client may not want to reveal information about their sexual relationships.
   3. **This sentence assures the client that they are not unique in their possible concerns and opens up the discussion about sexuality.**
   4. While nerve-sparing surgery is effective, this is not a conclusion that can be definite.

21. **C: Foundations of Practice CN: Health Promotion and Maintenance   T: Application**
   1. Family history is a nonmodifiable risk factor for the development of CAD.
   2. Male gender is a nonmodifiable risk factor for the development of CAD.
   3. Age is a nonmodifiable risk factor for the development of CAD.

4. Decreases in LDL will help reduce the client's risk for developing CAD.

22. **C: Foundations of Practice CN: Health Promotion and Maintenance   T: Application**
    1. The food pyramid is a nutrition resource used by Americans, not Canadians. In Canada. the *Eat Well Plate* is used.
    2. **In the Canadian population, 58% of all persons and 72% of children between the ages of 4 and 13 years consumed sodium above the recommended limit.**
    3. **In Canada, the intake of vegetables and fruits remains consistently low.**
    4. **In 2015, sugary drinks were the main source of total sugars in the diet of Canadians, with children and adolescents (ages 9–18 years) having the highest average intake.**
    5. One in two Canadians consume saturated fat above the recommended limit. Increasing daily intake of unsaturated fats is recommended.

23. **C: Foundations of Practice CN: Health Promotion and Maintenance   T: Critical Thinking**
    1. Because of Canada's geographical location, the client is not likely to obtain adequate vitamin D all year round. There is also the danger of skin cancer as a result of being exposed to direct sunlight.
    2. Milk is a source of vitamin D, but it is not likely that the client will be able to drink enough to achieve 1 000 IU per day.
    3. **Although in most cases it is best to achieve optimum nutrition through the diet, in the case of vitamin D, an intake of 1 000 IU can best be achieved by taking a supplement.**
    4. Fortified cereals contain vitamin D, but it is not likely that the client will be able to eat a sufficient amount to achieve 1 000 IU per day.

24. **C: Collaborative Practice CN: Health Promotion and Maintenance   T: Application**
    1. **All people, regardless of age, handicap, or life choices, are sexual beings. Sexuality involves one's inner sense of being male, female, or some combination; gender role; and biological identity.**
    2. Many parents would disagree with this statement, preferring that their children learn about sexuality in the home.
    3. The purpose of teaching children about sexuality is not to prepare them for sexual intercourse. This may be what the parents are concerned about.
    4. This is not necessarily a Canadian value. All cultures must be respected with discussions about sexuality.

25. **C: Foundations of Practice CN: Health Promotion and Maintenance   T: Knowledge**
    1. Reading a light novel can help a person to relax, which can be helpful at bedtime.
    2. Listening to music can help a person to relax, which can be helpful at bedtime.

3. A client should not try to resolve family problems before bedtime.
4. Eating a large meal before bedtime can interfere with sleep.
5. A dairy snack such as warm milk, contains L-tryptophan and may be helpful in promoting sleep.

26. **C: Foundations of Practice CN: Psychosocial Integrity T: Application**
    1. **Music is an example of alternative or complementary therapy.**
    2. **Aromatherapy is an example of alternative or complementary therapy.**
    3. Taking chemotherapy recommended by a physician trained in conventional medicine is not an example of alternative or complementary therapy.
    4. **Prayer is an example of alternative or complementary therapy.**
    5. **Movement therapy is an example of alternative or complementary therapy.**

27. **C: Foundations of Practice CN: Health Promotion and Maintenance   T: Application**
    1. Cigarette smoking is not associated with increased breast cancer risk.
    2. **Menarche prior to the age of 12 is a risk factor for the development of breast cancer because of the prolonged exposure to estrogen that occurs.**
    3. Fibrocystic breast changes are not associated with increased breast cancer risk.
    4. Breast trauma is not associated with increased breast cancer risk.
    5. **Heavy alcohol use is a risk factor for the development of breast cancer.**

28. **C: Foundations of Practice CN: Health Promotion and Maintenance   T: Knowledge**
    1. Research indicates that restraints do not actually prevent falls and injury and may even increase the severity of injury.
    2. **Household items that are easy to trip over, such as throw rugs, are a risk factor for falls.**
    3. **Locking beds and wheelchairs when transferring clients reduces the risk of falls.**
    4. **Promoting the wearing of skid-free footwear reduces the risk of falls.**
    5. **Installing grab rails near the toilet and tub reduces the risk of falls.**

29. **C: Collaborative Practice CN: Health Promotion and Maintenance   T: Application**
    1. **One way in which poverty adversely affects health is the inability to purchase needed medications. Asking an open-ended question invites the person to share thoughts and feelings about the medication expense. The nurse needs to determine whether the parent is able to buy the child's medications. If not, the nurse may be able to access alternate means of obtaining the necessary medications.**

2. This is not a therapeutic approach, particularly if the parent does not have the financial resources to purchase the medications.

3. It is not within the scope of nursing practice, nor is it ethical, to tell a parent which medications are not important for the child.

4. It is not within the scope of nursing practice or legal to change a health care provider's prescription.

30. **C: Foundations of Practice CN: Health Promotion and Maintenance   T: Critical Thinking**

1. The most effective teaching and learning is experiential. A computer game, while it may be a good supplement, is not as effective as actual practice.

2. Rewards may work to reinforce learned behaviours but are not as effective as role-modelling as a teaching tool.

3. Role-modelling and actual practice are more effective.

4. **Children learn best from role-modelling and practice.**

31. **C: Foundations of Practice CN: Health Promotion and Maintenance   T: Application**

1. Asking if someone wears sunscreen may increase awareness but does not screen for disease.

2. **The process of screening is part of secondary prevention. Screenings are done by oneself, or can be clinical, procedural, or lab-based. Performing testicular self-examination is an example of screening.**

3. **Obtaining a mammogram is an example of screening.**

4. Undergoing a needle biopsy would be diagnostic.

5. **Screening for skin cancer during regular client assessments is an example of screening.**

6. Creating an exercise program for women with osteoporosis is an example of tertiary prevention.

CHAPTER 7

The correct answer is set off in boldface.

1. **C: Foundations of Practice CN: Physiological Integrity T: Knowledge**

1. An auscultatory gap is more common in older clients or clients with hypertension, but it does not always occur in these populations.

2. Normal pulse pressure is 40 mm Hg.

3. Orthostatic hypertension is measured by recording blood pressure (BP) and pulse with the client in three positions: supine, sitting, and standing.

4. **This statement is correct. The nurse might make the mistake of recording the last sound at the beginning of the auscultatory gap as diastolic BP or the last sound at the end of the auscultatory gap as systolic BP.**

2. **C: Foundations of Practice CN: Physiological Integrity T: Knowledge**

1. **Rectal is the correct site for core temperatures.**

2. Oral is only a surface temperature.

3. Axillary is a surface temperature.

4. Skin is only a surface temperature.

3. **C: Foundations of Practice CN: Physiological Integrity T: Application**

1. The pain and tingling are from poor circulation to the left foot because the elastic bandage is applied too tight. No blood flow is getting to the toes. The dressing will need to be removed.

2. Administration of the analgesia will not decrease the pain if the poor circulation is the result of the elastic bandage being too tight.

3. **First the nurse needs to assess the circulation, sensation, and movement of the toes and foot to help determine if the dressing is too tight and affecting the blood flow to the foot. Then the nurse can remove the dressing once they have made the appropriate assessment.**

4. Elevation will not decrease the pain and tingling in the foot if the elastic bandage is on too tight.

4. **C: Foundations of Practice CN: Safe and Effective Care Environment T: Application**

1. Giving the injection quickly may increase client discomfort, and putting it into the sharps container without using the safety shield needles could still cause a needle-stick injury.

2. **Safety-engineered needles retract after the injection is given and reduce the risk of needle-stick injuries.**

3. This is not appropriate in this case.

4. Wearing gloves prevents the nurse from coming in contact with any blood that oozes from the injection site. It does not prevent needle-stick injuries. It might prevent the needle from entering the nurse's skin as deeply or decrease the amount of blood entering the nurse's skin from the needle tip.

5. **C: Foundations of Practice CN: Physiological Integrity T: Application**

1. It is not correct to slow down the intravenous (IV) line if the nurse needs it to finish within the 8-hour time limit.

2. It is not correct to slow down the IV line if the nurse needs it to finish within the 8-hour time limit.

3. The IV line would normally be running at 125 mL/hr, but that rate must be increased slightly as there is 100 mL extra in the IV bag at 1500 hours.

4. **The IV line is 100 mL behind schedule, and there is 600 mL to be infused over the next 4 hours. To calculate the new rate, divide the volume remaining over the time remaining: 600 mL ÷ 4 hr = 150 mL/hr. Although agency policies should be consulted, it is acceptable to increase the IV rate (25 mL/hr over the ordered rate) in this situation as the client is not an older person, has no apparent cardiac history, is not at risk for fluid overload, and does require the fluid volume as ordered.**

6. **C: Foundations of Practice CN: Physiological Integrity T: Application**

1. Transdermal patches or discs should not be applied to hairy areas. They do not stick well to hairy areas, and that could affect the amount of medication absorbed.
2. Transdermal medications can stay in place from 1 to 7 days, depending on what drug is being used.
3. All old patches and discs of the same medication must be removed prior to applying a new transdermal medication or an overdose could occur.
4. **The nurse should wear gloves when applying transdermal medications as they can be absorbed through the skin during application.**

7. **C: Foundations of Practice CN: Physiological Integrity T: Critical Thinking**
   1. **Mrs. Gupta may have a baseline blood pressure of 90/60. The nurse needs to check the health record for previous baseline vital signs. If Mrs. Gupta is feeling faint or lightheaded, she could be symptomatic from the hypotension and needs treatment. The other vital signs are all within the normal range.**
   2. The nurse needs more information before calling the physician. The doctor will want to know the baseline vital signs, and the nurse will want to recheck the client's blood pressure prior to calling the physician.
   3. Dehydration or decreased circulating blood volume can cause the blood pressure to be lower, but that cannot be assumed before checking the urine output, asking the client how she feels, and looking at the baseline vital signs.
   4. Modified Trendelenburg is a position in which the legs are elevated to promote venous return to the heart and thus increase cardiac output and blood pressure. That is not necessary unless Mrs. Gupta is going into shock, which her vital signs do not indicate.

8. **C: Foundations of Practice CN: Physiological Integrity T: Application**
   1. Porridge is only allowed on a full fluid diet. Broth and apple juice would be permitted on a clear fluid diet.
   2. None of these foods are part of a clear fluid diet but can be eaten with a full fluid diet.
   3. Broth and Popsicles are part of a clear fluid diet, but orange juice would only be permitted on a full fluid diet.
   4. **All these foods would be allowed on a clear fluid diet.**

9. **C: Foundations of Practice CN: Physiological Integrity T: Application**
   1. Limited mobility and exercise can be contributing factors, but they are not the cause of paralytic ileus in this situation.
   2. Eating too much too soon after surgery is much more likely to contribute to paralytic ileus. In a postoperative client, it is advised to wait until bowel sounds return after surgery before advancing to the postoperative diet.
   3. **Paralytic ileus in a postoperative client is most often caused by the action of narcotics and anaesthetics, delayed gastric emptying, slowed peristalsis resulting from the handling of the bowel during surgery, and resumption of the oral intake too soon after surgery.**
   4. Mrs. Gupta might need a rectal suppository (often on postoperative day 2 or later) to stimulate peristalsis and expulsion of the flatus; however, not giving it on postoperative day 1 would not have caused a paralytic ileus.

10. **C: Foundations of Practice CN: Physiological Integrity T: Critical Thinking**
    1. **The nurse's first priority is to do a further assessment, which should include looking for redness or swelling in the calf area, measuring calf circumference in both legs, asking Mrs. Gupta if she has any pain in that area, and possibly gently palpating the area.**
    2. It is possible that Mrs. Gupta has a clot in her leg (thrombophlebitis), so it is best not to put the TED stocking back on until the medical team does a further assessment. It is appropriate to place the leg on a pillow to promote venous return to the heart.
    3. The calf circumference should be measured, but both legs should be measured to compare results. This is done after the area is assessed for redness and pain and the client is asked about the history of the present swelling. The health care provider would be notified after the nurse has done their assessment.
    4. The nurse should not wash the client's leg or encourage her to exercise the leg until she is sure that there is no clot in her leg. Clots from the leg can travel to the lungs and cause a pulmonary embolism.

11. **C: Foundations of Practice CN: Physiological Integrity T: Application**
    1. Measuring from the tip of the nose to the earlobe to the xiphoid process is the correct measurement to determine length of insertion.
    2. The client should not have too much water as this may cause aspiration. The client can dry swallow or sip on water (if allowed) while the nurse advances the tube. The client swallows to the predetermined length.
    3. Radiography is the most reliable way to check placement of nasogastric tubes. Many health care settings only insist on radiography to check the placement of small-bore feeding tubes prior to the start of enteral feeds. Some agencies may require X-ray confirmation of the placement of all nasogastric tubes prior to enteral feeds. In this scenario, a placement X-ray is not necessary as the tube is being used for decompression.
    4. **As the nasogastric tube is to be used for decompression, a reliable way of assessing tube placement is by aspirating gastric contents and testing pH. Gastric pH should be less than 4.**

12. **C: Foundations of Practice CN: Physiological Integrity T: Application**

1. This is the hourly flow rate for the replacement intravenous line (IV) (640 mL ÷ 8 hr = 80 mL/hr).
2. This is the hourly flow rate for the main IV.
3. **This rate is correct, using the following formula:**

$$\frac{80 \text{ mL} \times 15 \text{ gtt/mL}}{60 \text{ min}} = 20 \text{ gtt/min}$$

4. This is using an hourly flow rate of 100 mL/hr for the calculations rather than 80 mL.

13. **C: Foundations of Practice CN: Physiological Integrity T: Application**
    1. All intravascular delivery system components up to the hub are changed every 24 to 72 hours according to agency policy, to prevent infection.
    2. When total parenteral nutrition (TPN) infusions are started, serum glucose levels are checked frequently at the bedside as some elevation of blood glucose is expected. Weights are taken daily to monitor the client's hydration status and weight gain with therapy.
    3. More frequent monitoring of the temperature is required as infection is the most common TPN complication. At least monitor the temperature every 4 hours, not daily.
    4. **Speeding up the rate can cause hyperglycemia, and slowing the rate can cause hypoglycemia. TPN is almost always managed with an infusion pump.**

14. **C: Collaborate Practice CN: Physiological Integrity T: Critical Thinking**
    1. It is not necessary to isolate a client for a catheter-related infection and septicemia.
    2. **A blood culture will determine if the infection is from the total parenteral nutrition (TPN) site. Other common sources of infection are the bladder or lung, thus the urine and sputum tests.**
    3. The TPN is not held. If the blood cultures are positive, the central line might be removed and a new one started elsewhere. Antibiotics would be prescribed, but TPN would not be stopped abruptly.
    4. There is no reason to stop the TPN and run dextrose 10%. The central line might need to be relocated, however, if it is thought to be the cause of the infection.

15. **C: Foundations of Practice CN: Safe and Effective Care Environment T: Application**
    1. This does not interfere with sterile technique as the saline has already been poured.
    2. This is correct procedure and does not compromise sterile technique.
    3. This is medical asepsis and correct procedure prior to doing a dressing change.
    4. **This compromises sterile technique. If the normal saline was already open and not labelled, the nurse cannot assume that it is still sterile. It is considered sterile for only 24 hours after opening.**

16. **C: Foundations of Practice CN: Safe and Effective Care Environment T: Critical Thinking**

1. Overuse of antibiotics predisposes clients to health care–associated infections (HAIs) such as MRSA (methicillin-resistant *Staphylococcus aureus*), although this is not likely to be the most significant factor with Mr. Roustas.
2. Spinal cord injury could lead to skin breakdown and the decubitus ulcer, but the actual skin breakdown is the most significant factor.
3. Mr. Roustas is only 42, which is generally not an age that predisposes him to decreased immunity, poorer nutrition, inadequate circulation, or skin breakdown.
4. **With skin breakdown, pathogens are able to enter the body, making this the most significant factor in the development of his HAI.**

17. **C: Foundations of Practice CN: Safe and Effective Care Environment T: Critical Thinking**
    1. A colonized or infected health care worker may disseminate the organism, but this is not the principal mode of transmission. The most frequently colonized site is the anterior nares.
    2. **The principal mode of transmission is transfer from client to client on the hands of hospital personnel.**
    3. Environmental contamination is uncommon.
    4. Droplet transmission may occur during the care of a client with MRSA (methicillin-resistant *Staphylococcus aureus*) pneumonia, but this is not common.

18. **C: Foundations of Practice CN: Physiological Integrity T: Application**
    1. Slowing the rate will not help to correct the tissue irritation.
    2. **These are signs that the vancomycin is irritating the intravenous (IV) site and it needs to be changed.**
    3. It is not necessary to notify the physician.
    4. The infusion will be stopped briefly while the IV site is changed.

19. **C: Foundations of Practice CN: Physiological Integrity T: Knowledge**
    1. Iodine should not be used on a wound bed as this solution is toxic to cells involved in wound healing.
    2. **Moist, interactive wound healing promotes faster healing, better tissue quality, and less pain than other methods. Other methods, such as wet-to-dry dressings for pressure injury, are no longer recommended as they cause mechanical debridement that is not selective and can damage healthy tissue.**
    3. Moist dressings often require more supplies than simple dry dressings.
    4. There is no current research to indicate increased bacteria in a moist dressing.

20. **C: Foundations of Practice CN: Physiological Integrity T: Application**
    1. It is important to chart findings, but initially the nurse needs to respond and treat the hypoxia.
    2. Deep breathing and coughing will not provide the oxygen the CN first for hypoxia.

3. Elevating the head of the bed and administering oxygen will relieve the client's symptoms of hypoxia.

4. It is important to treat the client's breathing difficulties first, before calling the health care provider.

21. **C: Foundations of Practice CN: Physiological Integrity   T: Application**

1. The nurse needs to perform an assessment prior to administering any analgesia and find out why the client is feeling prickling and itchiness sensations. Pain analgesia may not be the appropriate action.

2. **The nurse needs to perform a proper assessment. They must look at the incision to determine the cause of the prickling and itchiness sensations. They could be caused by the type of dressing used, infection, or other reasons.**

3. This is not a normal sensation to have at the incision site after surgery.

4. The nurse needs to perform a proper assessment before calling the health care provider.

22. **C: Foundation of Practice CN: Physiological Integrity   T: Critical Thinking**

1. To validate pain relief, the nurse needs to ask the client to rate the pain before and after administration of analgesics. The words "mild" and "severe" may not be specific enough.

2. Facial expressions do not always reflect the amount of pain that a client is experiencing.

3. Vital signs may or may not change when clients are in pain or after they receive analgesics. It is important to ask clients to rate their pain before and after analgesics as pain is subjective. Only the client knows the level of pain and pain relief.

4. **An effective way to rate pain relief in most adults is to use a numeric rating scale from 0 to 10 (0 being no pain; 10 being the most severe pain) before and after the administration of analgesics. For clients unable to respond to other pain intensity scales (such as children and older person), a series of faces ranging from "smiling" to "crying" can be used. The rating scale has been shown to be ineffective in some studies, but it remains the most effective tool at present.**

23. **C: Foundations of Practice CN: Physiological Integrity   T: Application**

1. **Clients with peripheral neuropathy are at greater risk for developing serious foot conditions due to the inability to feel pain and pressure. Clients with peripheral neuropathy require special nail and foot care.**

2. **Clients with peripheral vascular disease are at greater risk for developing serious foot conditions due to reduced blood flow to the extremities. Clients with peripheral neuropathy require special nail and foot care.**

3. Clients with pancreatitis are not at a greater risk for developing serious foot conditions and do not require special nail and foot care.

4. **Clients with diabetes are at greater risk for developing serious foot conditions due to the risk of peripheral neuropathy and peripheral vascular disease. Clients with diabetes require special nail and foot care.**

5. Clients with pancreatitis are not at a greater risk for developing serious foot conditions and do not require special nail and foot care.

24. **C: Foundations of Practice CN: Physiological Integrity   T: Application**

1. The inner cannula is removed and is placed in a basin of normal saline to loosen secretions.

2. As in choice 1.

3. **After the inner cannula is thoroughly cleaned, it is rinsed with normal saline.**

4. The exposed outer cannula surfaces at the stoma are dried with a 4 × 4 gauze to prevent a moist environment and prohibit microorganism growth and skin excoriation.

25. **C: Foundations of Practice CN: Physiological Integrity   T: Application**

1. The client should not sit in a bathtub of warm water as she has just given birth and infection is a possibility.

2. **The bladder needs to be emptied via catheterization. An intermittent catheterization carries less risk of infection.**

3. The client should not go home until her bladder has been emptied. The full bladder would interfere with uterine contractions that are necessary to expel blood and any remaining uterine contents.

4. An in-dwelling catheter is not necessary. It might be a source of a health care-associated infection (nosocomial infection).

26. **C: Foundations of Practice CN: Physiological Integrity   T: Application**

1. Urinary catheterization is an example of surgical asepsis or sterile technique. This includes all procedures used to eliminate all micro-organisms from an area.

2. Surgical asepsis or sterile technique is used to change a dressing on nonintact skin immediately postoperatively.

3. **Cleaning the hospital environment and equipment routinely with approved solutions is used to reduce and prevent the spread of micro-organisms. This is an example of *medical asepsis* or *clean technique*.**

4. An intramuscular injection is given using surgical asepsis. A sterile needle is used to perforate the client's skin.

5. **Hand hygiene will reduce and prevent the spread of micro-organisms. This is an example of *medical asepsis* or *clean technique*.**

27. **C: Foundations of Practice CN: Physiological Integrity   T: Application**
Answer: 10.4 = 10 gtt/min
Rationale: Using the following formula:

$$\frac{\text{Amount of solution to administer}}{\text{Time for infusion in hours}} \times \frac{\text{Drip factor of tubing}}{60 \text{ min}}$$

$$= \text{Drip rate (gtt/min)}$$

$$\frac{250 \text{ mL}}{4 \text{ hr}} \times \frac{10 \text{ gtt}}{60 \text{ min}} = 10.4 = 10 \text{ gtt/min}$$

28. **C: Foundations of Practice CN: Physiological Integrity T: Application**

    Answer: 2 000 mg/day. Rationale: **The infant's weight must first be converted from pounds to kilograms (1 kg = 2.2 pounds). The infant weighs 11 pounds, which is 11 lb. ÷ 2.2 lb. = 5 kg. The maximum dosage is 400 mg × 5 kg = 2 000 mg/day.**

29. **C: Foundations of Practice CN: Physiological Integrity T: Application**
    1. **Pinching the skin elevates the subcutaneous tissue and may desensitize the area. Alternatively, for an average-sized person, the skin can be spread tightly across the injection site since the needle will penetrate tight skin easier than loose skin.**
    2. The site of a heparin injection should not be massaged, as this can cause bruising.
    3. This is the method for giving an intradermal injection. For a subcutaneous injection, the medication should be injected at a 45- to 90-degree angle.
    4. **Aspiration for subcutaneous injections is not necessary, as adipose tissue is not very vascular and injection into a blood vessel is rare.**
    5. **Only 0.5 to 1.0 mL should be given subcutaneously as subcutaneous injections can cause discomfort.**

30. **C: Professional, Ethical, and Legal Practice CN: Safe and Effective Care Environment T: Critical Thinking**
    1. Restraints might possibly make him more agitated, but this is not the most appropriate explanation.
    2. Most health care facilities are either restraint-free or advocate minimum restraints. This statement makes the nurse appear to be basing action on rules rather than professional judgement.
    3. **Restraints should be a last resort. The presence of a family member may prevent him from trying to get out of bed. If a family member could be present around the clock, it might be a good short-term solution until his confusion clears.**
    4. It is true that the doctor must order restraints, but this is not the best answer. It is better to use restraints as a last resort.

31. **C: Collaborative Practice CN: Physiological Integrity T: Application**
    1. With stomatitis, it is important to continue gentle flossing and brushing with a soft toothbrush or toothette to keep the mouth, teeth, and gums clean and prevent infection.
    2. Commercial mouthwashes contain alcohol, which stings and dries mucous membranes. Commercial mouthwashes such as Listerine are not recommended.

3. **Normal saline mouthwashes are recommended as often as every 2 hours if necessary for clients with stomatitis.**
4. Regular oral hygiene is important for clients with stomatitis to prevent infections. It is recommended that the client use a mild analgesic if necessary for pain so that mouth care can be done.

32. **C: Foundations of Practice CN: Physiological Integrity T: Application**
    1. Chest tubes can remove air and fluid from the pleural space, not the lungs.
    2. **Turning in bed or ambulating can shift the position of the chest tube in the pleural space slightly and promote drainage. Lying on the side of the unaffected lung can expand the affected lung more fully as well.**
    3. Chest tubes are not commonly clamped, as clamping can cause a tension pneumothorax. Air pressure builds up in the pleural space, collapsing the lung and creating a life-threatening emergency. Clamping chest tubes requires an order from the physician.
    4. The chest tube drainage system should remain below the chest to aid gravity by drainage and to prevent reflux of drainage back into the chest cavity.

33. **C: Foundations of Practice CN: Physiological Integrity T: Application**
    1. Initiation of a blood transfusion cannot occur in the radiology department.
    2. Blood is stored in the blood bank.
    3. **If the blood cannot be started within 30 minutes of the time of release from the blood bank, immediately return the blood to the blood bank and retrieve it when it can be administered.**
    4. Initiation of the blood transfusion needs to occur within 30 minutes of the time of release from the blood bank.

34. **C: Professional, Ethical, and Legal Practice CN: Safe and Effective Care Environment T: Critical Thinking**
    1. The nurse follows agency policy about disclosure, but this is not the first priority.
    2. The nurse informs the manager and prescriber (physician, extended role nurse, dentist, chiropractor), but that is not the first responsibility.
    3. The nurse must complete an incident report with the details after ensuring the client is not in danger and has informed the appropriate agency personnel.
    4. **The nurse's first responsibility is to assess the client and make sure they are not in immediate danger.**

35. **C: Professional, Ethical, and Legal Practice CN: Safe and Effective Care Environment T: Application**
    1. This is not appropriate unless the nurse knows why the client is restrained and the cost of a sitter has been negotiated with the unit manager or family.
    2. Restraints should be tied with a quick-release tie rather than a knot for safety reasons.

3. **Proper placement of the restraint, skin integrity, pulses, colour, and sensation of the restrained part should be assessed every hour or according to agency policy.**

4. Reviewing the order for restraints should be done frequently but varies from agency to agency. Restraints may need to be reordered on a daily or weekly basis.

5. **It is important that the client and their family or substitute decision maker are informed and involved in the plan of care.**

36. C: Foundations of Practice CN: Physiological Integrity T: Knowledge

1. **Normal oral temperature for an older person tends to be lower.**

2. **Infections in older person may not present typically as they tend to have lower body temperatures, decreased pain sensation, and less immune response to infection. Older person can often have advanced infection before it is identified.**

3. The older person has decreased pain sensation.

4. Constipation can be a common complaint in older persons due to a combination of many factors, such as impaired general health, use of medication, and decreased bowel motility and physical activity.

5. Assess functional status to see if the older person will need help in taking the medications.

37. C: Foundations of Practice CN: Safe and Effective Care Environment T: Application

1. It is not possible, nor is there any reason, to restrain someone during a seizure.

2. Nothing should be inserted into the mouth of someone having a seizure.

3. **Placing a pillow or folded blanket under their child's head will protect them from traumatic injury.**

4. **It is most important to protect the client from traumatic injury. They should make sure their child is safe and protect them from injury by putting them on a flat surface and clearing the area of hazards.**

5. **Following the seizure, placing the client in the recovery position will prevent aspiration. During a seizure, only put the client in a side-lying position if it is possible. This is usually possible only at the beginning of a seizure.**

38. C: Foundations of Practice CN: Physiological Integrity T: Application

1. **The Braden Scale measures sensory perception, moisture, activity, mobility, nutrition, and friction and shear, in an attempt to identify clients most at risk for pressure injuries.**

2. The Braden Scale is a risk-assessment tool and does not identify interventions.

3. The Braden Scale is a risk-assessment tool and does not classify the stage of pressure injuries.

4. The Braden Scale is a risk-assessment tool and does not identify preventive measures.

39. C: Foundations of Practice CN: Physiological Integrity T: Application

1. Incentive spirometry is used to prevent or treat atelectasis in the postoperative client and should be used hourly while awake.

2. **Leg exercises, including foot circles, dorsiflexion and plantar flexion, quadriceps setting, and hip and knee exercises, should be performed at least every 2 hours for five successive times while awake.**

3. All postoperative clients are encouraged to use controlled rather than vigorous coughing to loosen and expectorate mucus that will have collected during and postsurgery in their lungs. Vigorous coughing may disturb the surgical site.

4. The client will likely have a chest tube but will probably not be on bed rest for long. Movement in bed as well as ambulation is encouraged to promote drainage from the pleural space and lung expansion.

40. C: Foundations of Practice CN: Physiological Integrity T: Application

1. **Answer: 25 gtt/min Rationale using the following formula:**

$$\frac{\text{Amount of solution to administer}}{\text{Time for infusion in hours}} \times \frac{\text{Drip factor of tubing}}{60 \text{ min}}$$
$$= \text{Drip rate (gtt/min)}$$

$$\frac{1000 \text{ mL}}{10 \text{ hr}} \times \frac{15 \text{ gtt}}{60 \text{ min}} = 25 \text{ gtt/min}$$

CHAPTER 8

The correct answer is set off in boldface.

1. C: Foundations of Practice CN: Physiological Integrity T: Application

1. It is not within the role of the nurse to make an adjustment to a medication dosage. Concerns need to be reported to the physician, who will make changes as necessary.

2. It is the physician's role to decide whether medications are to be given. Nurses do not withhold medications unless an order is written or they have a concern. If there is a concern, nurses consult with the physician or prescriber of the medication.

3. As a general rule, digoxin is withheld and reported if the heart rate is less than 60 beats per minute.

4. **Withholding digoxin and reporting is the established procedure if the heart rate is less than 60 beats per minute. The physician will then determine whether the client is to receive the medication at that time.**

2. C: Foundations of Practice CN: Physiological Integrity T: Application

1. Furosemide will start to work within an hour, causing the client to awaken to void during the night and therefore to lose sleep.

2. While doses of furosemide should be spaced to maintain therapeutic levels, the medication should be administered in the morning to avoid nocturnal diuresis.

3. **This is the correct time to administer a diuretic in order for diuresis to take place during the day prior to bedtime. This permits a restful sleep.**

4. It is not necessary to take furosemide with meals.

3. **C: Foundations of Practice CN: Physiological Integrity T: Knowledge**

1. **Diuretics remove electrolytes, including potassium, putting the client at risk of developing hypokalemia. Supplements prevent this from occurring.**

2. Potassium supplements do not facilitate the action of diuretics.

3. Although potassium plays a major role in the generation of a nerve impulse, potassium supplementation in this case is not for that purpose.

4. Potassium supplementation plays no significant role in preventing the adverse effects of digoxin.

4. **C: Foundations of Practice CN: Physiological Integrity T: Application**

1. Patches should remain on the skin until a new dose is applied. The purpose of a dermal patch is to provide continuous, slow absorption of the medication throughout the day. Occasionally, patches may be removed overnight to reduce the development of tolerance.

2. Skin areas should be rotated to avoid skin irritation. Absorption will naturally occur in all areas of skin.

3. **The patch should be removed and the skin cleansed to remove medication left on the skin; then the new patch is applied to a different area. Leaving the skin uncleansed may produce added dosage of the medication when added to the new dosage, causing undesirable effects.**

4. This is incorrect, as the patch is applied to provide slow, natural absorption. By massaging the site, absorption will occur more quickly, with the possibility of undesirable adverse effects.

5. **C: Foundations of Practice CN: Physiological Integrity T: Application**

1. Only a maximum of three sprays should be taken. If pain persists, medical attention should be obtained immediately as a myocardial infarction may be occurring.

2. One spray may not be sufficient. Up to three sprays may be taken at 5-minute intervals. Sublingual forms of nitroglycerin are destroyed by gastric secretions and will not be absorbed.

3. One spray may not be enough to relieve the pain. Up to three sprays may be administered. Patches are used as a preventive and have no effect on acute pain due to their slow absorption.

4. **This is the correct method of using sublingual nitroglycerin sprays to relieve anginal pain. Three** successive doses are acceptable, but persistent pain may indicate a myocardial infarction, and medical attention is required if the pain is not relieved in five minutes (client or family must call 911 immediately).

6. **C: Foundations of Practice CN: Physiological Integrity T: Application**

1. At noon, regular insulin is peak action, so no additional insulin is required.

2. At mid-morning (about 1000 hours), regular insulin is near the peak level and NPH insulin is above the minimum effective concentration; therefore, no new dose is required.

3. At mid-afternoon (1500 hours) regular insulin has reached its minimum effective concentration level, but NPH insulin is at peak; therefore, no new dose is required.

4. **By bedtime (2100–2200 hours), NPH insulin is present but will fall below the MEC soon after midnight.**

7. **C: Foundations of Practice CN: Physiological Integrity T: Application**

1. Between 0.5 and 1 hours and 2 to 3 hours after administering the insulins, the minimum effective concentration is reached for both types of insulin and blood levels are too low to cause adverse effects (hypoglycemia).

2. **Between 2 to 4 hours and 5 to 8 hours after administering the insulins, the peak is reached for both types of insulin and the adverse effects occur at these peak levels.**

3. Between 5 to 8 hours and 18 hours after administering the insulins, the minimum effective concentration is reached and adverse effects are unlikely.

4. After 18 hours, no adverse effect is likely because the MEC is passed.

8. **C: Foundations of Practice CN: Physiological Integrity T: Knowledge**

1. H_2 receptor antagonists do not act as bases. Only bases neutralize acids.

2. **By blocking the receptor sites, H_2 receptor antagonists prevent histamine from binding to the surface of parietal cells, which prevents the cells from producing H^+.**

3. H_2 receptor antagonists have no effect on digestive enzymes.

4. Acid plus base converts to salt and water, but H_2 receptor antagonists are not bases.

9. **C: Foundations of Practice CN: Physiological Integrity T: Knowledge**

1. Stimulation of peristalsis is helpful in the presence of constipation, but it does not relieve gas.

2. **Simethicone changes the surface tension of gas bubbles in the gastro-intestinal tract, resulting in collection of one large gas bubble. This enables the individual to eructate or pass flatus.**

3. Simethicone is not an antidiarrheal medication. Although simethicone relieves gaseous distension, it has no effect on the intestinal lining to prevent diarrhea.

4. Simethicone is not an absorbent. It does not absorb excess HCl.

10. **C: Foundations of Practice CN: Physiological Integrity T: Knowledge**
   1. If an antimicrobial affects only bacteria, it is simply called an *antibiotic*.
   2. The therapeutic index has to do with the safety of administration of a drug. A drug with a narrow therapeutic index means the therapeutic dose is very close to the toxic dose.
   3. Spectrum is not related to toxicity.
   4. **The spectrum of microbial activity is the range of distinctly different types of microbes affected by an antimicrobial drug. Narrow-spectrum antibiotics treat effectively only a limited number of types of bacteria.**

11. **C: Foundations of Practice CN: Physiological Integrity T: Application**
   1. Chlamydia is a bacterium that can be treated with antibiotics.
   2. *E. coli* is a bacterium that can be treated with antibiotics.
   3. Gonorrhea is caused by a bacterium and can be treated with antibiotics.
   4. **Influenza A and B are viral infections. They are not susceptible to antibiotics but can be treated with antiviral drugs.**

12. **C: Foundations of Practice CN: Physiological Integrity T: Application**
   1. The client will possibly require lower doses of their medications, but it is not a nursing responsibility to independently change the dose.
   2. The client will likely need lower, not higher, doses.
   3. **Due to the renal failure, there is likely to be reduced excretion of some of the medications. It is the responsibility of the health care provider and pharmacist to decide if altered doses are required, depending on the particular medication and the client's condition.**
   4. It is not within the role of the nurse, in this situation, to independently withhold medications for the client.

13. **C: Foundations of Practice CN: Physiological Integrity T: Application**
   1. **Opioid analgesics are known to cause nausea and vomiting. Administration of antiemetics at the same time as administration of the morphine may prevent this adverse effect.**
   2. With the severe pain of colon cancer, this is an inappropriate choice. If the morphine is ordered with a range of dosing, the amount given should be based on the pain as rated by the client and previous doses that have resulted in therapeutic effects.

3. While a history of previous abuse is a nursing consideration in many cases of morphine administration, this is neither an important nor necessary assessment with a client who has severe pain from terminal cancer.
4. The morphine may need to be held if the client has a respiratory rate of less than 10 respirations per minute.

14. **C: Foundations of Practice CN: Physiological Integrity T: Knowledge**
   1. Antacids interfere with the absorption of oral iron.
   2. **Iron tablets should be taken with meals in order to reduce gastrointestinal distress.**
   3. Milk interferes with absorption of oral iron.
   4. **It is recommended to take oral iron with orange juice because vitamin C helps the body to absorb more iron.**
   5. **Stools may become black and tarry in clients who are on iron supplements.**
   6. Iron tablets should be taken whole, not crushed.

15. **C: Foundations of Practice CN: Physiological Integrity T: Knowledge**
   1. CNS stimulants increase alertness and are not indicated for the treatment of insomnia.
   2. CNS stimulants are not indicated for the treatment of Alzheimer's disease.
   3. **CNS stimulants are indicated for the treatment of narcolepsy.**
   4. **CNS stimulants are indicated for the treatment of ADHD.**
   5. CNS stimulants suppress the appetite and are not indicated for appetite enhancement.

16. **C: Foundations of Practice CN: Physiological Integrity T: Knowledge**
   1. Partial opioid agonists are not used for mild pain.
   2. **Partial opioid agonists are used for moderate to severe pain.**
   3. Opioid antagonists (e.g., naloxone) are the medication of choice for reversing the effects of opioids in cases of overdose.
   4. **They are sometimes chosen for clients who have a history of opioid addiction since they have a lower potential for abuse.**
   5. **Adverse effects of partial opioid agonists are similar to those of opioid agonists.**

17. **C: Foundations of Practice CN: Physiological Integrity T: Knowledge**
   1. Renal insufficiency is not a contraindication for taking an opioid analgesic.
   2. **Respiratory insufficiency, as in severe chronic obstructive pulmonary disease, would be a contraindication for giving an opioid analgesic due to the potential for respiratory depression.**
   3. Liver disease is not a contraindication for taking an opioid analgesic.
   4. Diabetes mellitus is not a contraindication for taking an opioid analgesic.

5. **Allergy is a contraindication for taking an opioid analgesic.**

18. C: Foundations of Practice CN: Physiological Integrity T: Critical Thinking
    1. **Salbutamol (a β_2-agonist) is used for acute bronchospasms**.
    2. Ipratroprium bromide is an inhaled anticholinergic used for asthma prophylaxis.
    3. **Aminophylline can be used for mild to moderate asthma attacks.**
    4. Zafirlukast is an antileukotriene medication used for asthma prophylaxis.
    5. Fluticasone is an inhaled corticosteroid used for asthma prophylaxis.

19. C: Foundations of Practice CN: Physiological Integrity T: Knowledge
    1. **Diarrhea is a symptom of digitalis toxicity.**
    2. **Visual disturbances (yellow-green distortion) are a symptom of digitalis toxicity.**
    3. **Nausea and vomiting are symptoms of digitalis toxicity.**
    4. Insomnia is not a symptom of digitalis toxicity.
    5. Urinary retention is not a symptom of digitalis toxicity.

20. C: Foundations of Practice CN: Physiological Integrity T: Knowledge
    1. The rate of excretion may be decreased because drugs metabolized by the liver may not be water soluble and therefore cannot be excreted in the urine.
    2. The duration of action of the drug will increase due to the failure of the medication to be metabolized for excretion.
    3. Only antagonist drugs, not liver disease, block receptors to produce no response.
    4. **When a drug is metabolized by the liver, inactive or active metabolites are produced. Inactive metabolites are usually removed by excretory organs, thus preventing drug accumulation. Active metabolites go to target cells and are subsequently inactive or excreted. If the drug is not metabolized by the liver because of cirrhosis, higher levels remain in the body for longer periods and produce actions and effects similar to a drug overdose.**

21. C: Foundations of Practice CN: Physiological Integrity T: Application
    1. Routine adult doses can cause toxicity, since liver metabolism and renal excretion decline with age.
    2. The frequency of medication administration is dependent on the drug's half-life, not the age of the recipient.
    3. **Body organs have fewer cells and reduced function with age; hence, the body requires a lower amount than the routine adult dose to produce the therapeutic effect.**
    4. Oral administration is easier, safer, and more practical than parenteral administration.

22. C: Foundations of Practice CN: Physiological Integrity T: Knowledge
    1. Barbiturates promote drowsiness, which is not therapeutic for depression.
    2. Antianxiolytics are used to treat anxiety, not depression.
    3. **Depressive symptoms are related to insensitivity of receptors and low serotonin levels. Selective serotonin reuptake inhibitors work to promote the continued presence of serotonin in the synaptic cleft by inhibiting its uptake.**
    4. Cholinergic agonists have no effect on serotonin receptors.

23. C: Foundations of Practice CN: Physiological Integrity T: Knowledge
    1. Although cortisone limits the activity of white blood cells (WBCs), it does not attract microbes.
    2. **Higher than normal physiological levels of cortisone promote protein breakdown. Antibodies are composed of proteins. In addition, cortisone impairs the ability of antibodies to bind to cell surface receptors and so reduces cell-mediated response. The net result is lowering of the immune response.**
    3. Cortisone has no direct or indirect antibiotic activity.
    4. Cortisone reduces cellular factors that lead to vascular permeability.

24. C: Foundations of Practice CN: Physiological Integrity T: Application
    1. **Naloxone, an opioid reversal agent, is used to reverse the effects of acute opioid overdose and is the medication of choice for reversal of opioid-induced respiratory depression.**
    2. Opioid tolerance is not a priority concern.
    3. An agonist opioid would further depress the respirations.
    4. This action is not in the scope of the nurse and is not required.

25. C: Foundations of Practice CN: Physiological Integrity T: Knowledge
    1. B-complex vitamins produce orange-coloured urine. INH may cause vitamin B deficiency.
    2. **INH is hepatotoxic, and liver function must be monitored carefully. Alcohol is not permitted while on INH, a factor that causes nonadherence in many cases.**
    3. While INH is used to treat and prevent tuberculosis, monthly X-rays are not necessary. If the disease is active, the client will be monitored by collecting sputum cultures.
    4. Antacids interfere with the absorption of INH and should never be taken concurrently.

CHAPTER 9

The correct answer is set off in boldface.

1. **C: Foundations of Practice CN: Physiological Integrity T: Critical Thinking**
   1. The throat is a vascular area, and even with laser surgery, there is a recognized danger of hemorrhage. It may occur quickly and is the most immediately life-threatening postsurgical complication.
   2. It is expected that the throat will be very sore after surgery. Around-the-clock analgesia with acetaminophen (Tylenol), rather than ASA (Aspirin), is administered. An ice collar may provide relief.
   3. This is a normal postoperative finding.
   4. Oral pharyngeal edema is a common postoperative complication from throat surgery resulting from trauma to the site. It may lead to a gradual increase in airway obstruction. The nurse must monitor Mr. Kingsley's airway status but, more immediately, must be alert for sudden signs of hemorrhage.

2. **C: Foundations of Practice CN: Physiological Integrity T: Application**
   1. This position would encourage pooling of the secretions in the mouth and possibly cause choking, coughing, or aspiration.
   2. This position would not encourage drainage of secretions out of the mouth.
   3. **Positioning the client in a semi-Fowler's with the neck flexed helps prevent pooling of secretions in the mouth and allows easier breathing and less chance of choking, coughing, and aspirating. Clients often put themselves into the high Fowler's position for comfort and ease of breathing.**
   4. This position would be uncomfortable and impossible for the client to remain in for very long.

3. **C: Foundations of Practice CN: Physiological Integrity T: Application**
   1. Clients are given cool, not warm, fluids once they are able to swallow. The coolness helps soothe the sore throat and decrease the chance of swelling. Coolness also reduces spasms in the muscles surrounding the throat.
   2. Aspirin or any other medication that alters bleeding time is not given to postoperative clients.
   3. **Acetaminophen (Tylenol) elixir or pills is the analgesic of choice and should be given around the clock. Sometimes rinsing the mouth out with viscous lidocaine is effective to decrease pain in the throat.**
   4. Ice collars rather than heating pads are used to help decrease swelling and pain. Heat may cause increased swelling and bleeding.

4. **C: Foundations of Practice CN: Physiological Integrity T: Application**
   1. Active disease is diagnosed by sputum cultures for acid-fast bacilli. Three consecutive sputum specimens collected on different days are obtained and sent for smear and culture. Material obtained from gastric washing, cerebrospinal fluid, and pus from an abscess may also be examined.
   2. This is a positive reaction. It indicates the presence of a tuberculosis (TB) infection but does not show whether the infection is active or dormant. People who have been vaccinated with bacille Calmette-Guérin will have positive skin tests due to exposure to the vaccine.
   3. Further studies need to be done before treatment is started. The health care provider needs to know if, in fact, the client has TB before initiating treatment.
   4. Two-step testing is generally recommended only for initial testing for health care workers who require repeated testing and for those who have a decreased response to allergens. For these people, a second purified protein derivative (PPD) test later may cause an accelerated response (booster effect), misinterpreted as a new PPD conversion.

5. **C: Foundations of Practice CN: Physiological Integrity T: Critical Thinking**
   1. Although the findings of a chest X-ray are important, it is not possible to make a diagnosis of tuberculosis (TB) solely on the basis of the X-ray. Other diseases can mimic the X-ray appearance of TB.
   2. **The demonstration of tubercle bacilli bacteriologically is essential for establishing a diagnosis.**
   3. This is a new rapid diagnostic test for TB that provides results within a few hours. It does not replace the routine sputum smears and cultures, but it offers a health care provider increased confidence in the diagnosis.
   4. Repeated Mantoux testing will only show that the person has either been vaccinated with bacille Calmette-Guérin or exposed to the mycobacterium. It does not mean that the person has contracted the disease.

6. **C: Foundations of Practice CN: Physiological Integrity T: Application**
   1. Adverse effects of ethambutol include skin rash, gastro-intestinal (GI) disturbances, malaise, peripheral neuritis, and optic neuritis.
   2. Adverse effects of isoniazid include peripheral neuritis, hepatotoxicity, skin rash, optic neuritis, and vitamin B_6 neuritis.
   3. Adverse effects of rifampin include hepatitis, GI disturbances, and peripheral neuritis.
   4. **Adverse effects of streptomycin include ototoxicity (affecting the eighth cranial nerve), nephrotoxicity, and hypersensitivity.**

7. **C: Foundations of Practice CN: Physiological Integrity T: Application**
   1. This is too short a time.
   2. As in choice 1.
   3. As in choice 1.
   4. **A problem with adherence to therapy for tuberculosis has been the length of time medication must be taken. Six to 9 months of therapy have proven to be effective.**

8. **C: Foundations of Practice CN: Physiological Integrity T: Knowledge**

1. Primary hypertension may be managed by medications, but lifestyle modifications will often be attempted initially to bring the pressure within normal range.
2. **Primary hypertension has no identifiable cause.**
3. This answer refers to secondary hypertension, in which an identifiable cause can be determined.
4. Research has shown that blood pressure is related to obesity and that if Ms. Mathias were to decrease her weight, her blood pressure could be lowered.

9. C: **Foundations of Practice CN: Physiological Integrity T: Knowledge**
   1. **HydroDIURIL may cause loss of potassium. Clients are encouraged to eat foods containing potassium, such as bananas, and monitor serum potassium levels.**
   2. While this is advised for clients who are hypertensive, it is not related to the HydroDIURIL.
   3. High-sodium diets are contraindicated.
   4. This may cause hypokalemia.

10. C: **Foundations of Practice CN: Physiological Integrity T: Application**
    1. Calcium channel blockers may cause polyuria in some clients.
    2. Calcium channel blockers may cause skin rash, dermatitis, pruritus, and urticaria, but they do not cause hair loss.
    3. Calcium channel blockers may cause hypotension, not hypertension.
    4. **Cardiovascular effects from the use of calcium channel blockers may include peripheral edema, hypotension, palpitations, bradycardia, tachycardia, and arrhythmias that may induce orthostatic hypotension.**

11. C: **Foundations of Practice CN: Physiological Integrity T: Application**
    1. **Clients with Cushing's syndrome may have thin, fragile skin, purplish red striae, petechial hemorrhages, bruises, facial plethora, acne, and poor wound healing.**
    2. There is usually increased axilla and pubic hair. Hirsutism is commonly found with Cushing's syndrome.
    3. Tachycardia and bulging eyes suggest hyperthyroid disease.
    4. Hypertension and hyperglycemia are found with Cushing's syndrome.

12. C: **Collaborative Practice CN: Physiological Integrity T: Application**
    1. This statement is patronizing and ineffective.
    2. This statement does not address Ms. Hynes's concern.
    3. Her appearance will change after surgery, but it will take time for all the physical and mental changes to occur.
    4. **The statement addresses Ms. Hynes's concern and gives accurate information.**

13. C: **Foundations of Practice CN: Physiological Integrity T: Application**
    1. Because the client is unable to open their mouth after surgery, the client must be closely monitored for airway obstruction and aspiration of vomitus. Lying on the stomach will not facilitate this.
    2. **Brian should be positioned on his side with his head slightly elevated to help drain secretions and prevent airway obstruction.**
    3. Lying on his back will not facilitate drainage of secretions and could result in airway obstruction.
    4. Having the head slightly below the chest will encourage secretions to drain into the mouth, causing a potential for aspiration and choking.

14. C: **Foundations of Practice CN: Physiological Integrity T: Critical Thinking**
    1. Adequate nutrition is important but is not the priority postoperatively.
    2. The jaw is immobilized by wiring the jaws together during surgery; therefore, it is not the nursing priority.
    3. Oral hygiene is another important intervention but is not the priority immediately postoperatively.
    4. **Two major potential problems in the immediate postoperative period are airway obstruction and aspiration of vomitus. The nurse must observe for signs of respiratory distress.**

15. C: **Foundations of Practice CN: Physiological Integrity T: Critical Thinking**
    1. Suctioning should be necessary only if the client vomits or chokes. The nasopharyngeal or oral route may be used, depending on the extent of injury and the type of repair. A nasogastric tube may be needed to remove fluids and gas from the stomach.
    2. This is one method of suctioning if needed.
    3. **Wire cutters or scissors (for rubber bands) must be taped to the head of the bed and sent with Brian on all appointments and examinations away from the bedside. These may be used to cut the wires and elastic bands in case of an emergency.**
    4. Oxygen is required only if Brian experiences any respiratory distress.

16. C: **Foundations of Practice CN: Physiological Integrity T: Application**
    1. This is not necessary. Mrs. Cheng may use a slipper bedpan.
    2. **A trapeze suspended over Mrs. Cheng's bed will allow her to lift herself if she is uncomfortable or for use with the bedpan.**
    3. This would encourage a twisting motion, and the limb and joint must be maintained in alignment.
    4. Mrs. Cheng will not be allowed to sit in a chair until after surgery. Moving her into a chair would cause pain and would not keep the leg in alignment.

17. C: **Foundations of Practice CN: Health Promotion and Maintenance T: Application**

1. **Bisphosphonate medication, such as risedronate (Actonel), inhibits bone resorption and absorbs calcium–phosphate crystals in bone. Bisphosphonates are "front-line" medications in the treatment of osteoporosis. Calcium supplements are required to increase available calcium to the bone.**

2. Weight-bearing exercises are recommended for osteoporosis as they help strengthen muscles around the bone and increase the strength of the bones.

3. Vitamin D is needed for regulation of calcium. Recommended levels for women of Mrs. Cheng's age are 1 000 IU or greater; 200 IU is not sufficient.

4. This is a premature recommendation. There is no indication that Mrs. Cheng may require any assistance with activities of daily living postrehabilitation.

18. **C: Foundations of Practice CN: Physiological Integrity T: Application**

    1. Symptoms for urinary tract infection may include dysuria, frequency of urination, urgency, and suprapubic discomfort or pressure.

    2. Pyelonephritis may manifest with symptoms of cystitis, flank pain, fever, chills, vomiting, and malaise.

    3. Nephrotic syndrome may manifest with peripheral edema, massive proteinuria, dyslipidemia, and hypoalbuminemia.

    4. **Acute glomerulonephritis may present with a variety of signs and symptoms, including edema, hypertension, oliguria, hematuria, and proteinuria. Fluid retention is usually first found in the low-pressure tissues, such as those around the eyes. Acute poststreptococcal glomerulonephritis develops 5 to 21 days after an infection of the pharynx or skin by group A beta-hemolytic *Streptococcus*.**

19. **C: Foundations of Practice CN: Physiological Integrity T: Application**

    1. Management for acute glomerulonephritis focuses on symptomatic relief. If Ms. Procinski has a high potassium level, she will be instructed to eat foods low in potassium and to stay away from foods high in potassium. In some instances, the client will be given polystyrene sulfonate (Kayexalate) to remove potassium from the body.

    2. **For all cases of glomerulonephritis, rest is recommended until the signs of the glomerular inflammation subside.**

    3. If Ms. Procinski is hypertensive, she may be started on a short-term course of antihypertensives.

    4. Glomerulonephritis is an antigen–antibody immune situation resulting from a previous infection. Antibiotics will not correct the glomerulonephritis, although some health care providers do prescribe antibiotics prophylactically.

20. **C: Foundations of Practice CN: Physiological Integrity T: Critical Thinking**

    1. International normalized ratio is used to measure warfarin (Coumadin) action in the body.

    2. Partial thromboplastin time is used to measure heparin action in the body.

    3. Platelet function assay is used to detect platelet dysfunction.

    4. Prothrombin time is used to measure Coumadin action in the body.

21. **C: Foundations of Practice CN: Physiological Integrity T: Critical Thinking**

    1. Heparin should not be stopped until a therapeutic level of Coumadin is attained.

    2. As in choice 1.

    3. Five milligrams of Coumadin is an appropriate dose.

    4. **A therapeutic level of Coumadin must be attained before heparin is stopped to maintain anticoagulant blood levels.**

22. **C: Foundations of Practice CN: Physiological Integrity T: Knowledge**

    1. This refers to adduction.

    2. **This is the definition of *abduction*.**

    3. This refers to external rotation.

    4. This refers to internal rotation.

23. **C: Foundations of Practice CN: Physiological Integrity T: Application**

    1. **Diminished or absent pedal, popliteal, or femoral pulses are frequently noted in clients with peripheral arterial disease (PAD) due to obstruction of the artery.**

    2. The foot will become pale on elevation. Clients with PAD will have reddened feet when they are in a dependent position.

    3. Lower leg edema may be seen in venous, not arterial, obstruction.

    4. Assessment requires more than just a blood pressure measurement at the thigh. Segmental blood pressures are taken at the thigh, below the knee, and at ankle level while the client is supine. A fall-off in segmental pressure of more than 30 mm Hg indicates PAD.

24. **C: Foundations of Practice CN: Physiological Integrity T: Application**

    1. Heating devices should not be used on the feet of clients with vascular conditions as the client may not be able to feel a burn injury.

    2. Support stockings are used for venous conditions.

    3. **Walking promotes the development of collateral circulation.**

    4. Feet should be inspected daily for redness.

25. **C: Foundations of Practice CN: Physiological Integrity T: Knowledge**

    1. These are manifestations of hypernatremia.

    2. **Severe diarrhea can lead to excessive loss of potassium. Hypokalemia can lead to rapid arrhythmias, which, in turn, can lead to a cardiac arrest. Other symptoms include muscle fatigue and weakness, leg cramps, nausea, and vomiting, polyuritis, and hyperglycemia.**

    3. These are manifestations of hyperphosphatemia.

4. These are manifestations of hypocalcemia.

26. **C: Foundations of Practice CN: Physiological Integrity T: Application**
    1. The rectal packing helps stop bleeding in the perineal area. It should not be removed right after surgery unless it is saturated with serosanguinous drainage.
    2. Feeding of any kind would not be established until peristalsis has returned and drainage appears in the ileostomy bag.
    3. **In the first 24 to 48 hours after surgery, the amount of drainage from the stoma may be negligible. An ileostomy causes a loss of absorptive functions provided by the colon. Once peristalsis returns, there may be a period of high-volume bilious output, up to 1 200 to 1 800 mL per day. Fluid and electrolyte imbalance is a potential problem.**
    4. The nasogastric tube would not be removed until peristalsis has returned.

27. **C: Foundations of Practice CN: Physiological Integrity T: Application**
    1. **Clients are encouraged to cook fruits and vegetables and limit their amounts in the initial postoperative period, as there is the potential for these foods to cause obstruction.**
    2. Beans and legumes are gas forming.
    3. Eggs are odour producing.
    4. Strong cheese is gas forming.

28. **C: Foundations of Practice CN: Health Promotion and Maintenance T: Application**
    1. There is no reason Mrs. O'Brien cannot have sharp utensils. The aide should help Mrs. O'Brien locate the utensils on the meal tray.
    2. Mrs. O'Brien does not require finger foods. She is able to use utensils. Finger foods would be more appropriate for the person who has dementia and experiences difficulty managing a knife and fork.
    3. **At mealtime, Mrs. O'Brien can be oriented to her meal by comparing her plate to a clock. This visual image will help her easily locate each item of food.**
    4. There is no indication that Mrs. O'Brien needs assistance with eating. She just needs assistance in finding food she cannot see.

29. **C: Foundations of Practice CN: Physiological Integrity T: Application**
    1. **The nurse could offer a stool softener to prevent constipation. Straining at stool increases intraocular pressure and must be avoided post cataract surgery.**
    2. There is no need to either increase or decrease fluids after cataract surgery.
    3. Some physicians may restrict showers after cataract surgery, but there is no contraindication to baths.
    4. Mrs. O'Brien's right eye will likely be patched, making watching TV or reading difficult. However, there are no contraindications to reading or watching TV provided that there are no rapid head or eye movements.

30. **C: Foundations of Practice CN: Physiological Integrity T: Application**
    1. A prone position would encourage fluid buildup in the lungs, which is what is causing her shortness of breath.
    2. A semi-Fowler's position is not adequate to help decrease fluid buildup in the lungs. In this position, the legs are level with the sacrum and encourage fluid return from the lower limbs.
    3. This position would simply magnify the shortness of breath while encouraging fluid return from the extremities.
    4. **A high Fowler's position, sitting upright with legs dependent, promotes fluid retention in the legs, decreasing the fluid return to the heart and keeping the fluid in the bases of the lungs.**

31. **C: Foundations of Practice CN: Physiological Integrity T: Critical Thinking**
    1. The electrolytes will need to be monitored but will not significantly change as quickly as the blood pressure (BP).
    2. **Although all assessments are important, the priority of care is BP. Once Mrs. Gardner starts to diurese volume from the intravascular space, BP can decrease drastically and result in hypotension.**
    3. Hourly output tells the nurse how much volume the client is voiding, but the more important determination is the effect the decreased volume has on the lungs. The nurse would monitor lung sounds to evaluate the decrease in crackles, signifying the loss of fluid in the lungs.
    4. Monitoring the respiratory rate is important as a decreased rate will indicate improvement. Mrs. Gardner may have clear lung fields but be hypotensive; therefore, BP is the priority.

32. **C: Foundations of Practice CN: Physiological Integrity T: Knowledge**
    1. This is a manifestation of left-sided heart failure.
    2. As in choice 1.
    3. As in choice 1.
    4. **Fluid in the lungs is symptomatic of left-sided heart failure.**

33. **C: Foundations of Practice CN: Physiological Integrity T: Application**
    1. Clients with gout, not renal failure, are encouraged to limit purine in their diet. Purine is found in red meat, particularly organ meat and shellfish.
    2. **Failing kidneys do not excrete potassium efficiently; thus, a renal diet is low in potassium. Potatoes and citrus fruit such as oranges, grapefruit, and strawberries are high in potassium and should be avoided.**
    3. Cookies and cake are high in calories and low in nutritive value. Mrs. Gardner will be allowed to eat these but will be encouraged to include more complex carbohydrates.

4. Mrs. Gardner may need to limit protein; however, protein is necessary for tissue repair and maintenance of the immune system.

34. **C: Foundations of Practice CN: Physiological Integrity T: Comprehension**
   1. Thrombus is a complication of immobility, but it is not prevented with proper body alignment.
   2. **Positioning of clients to maintain correct body alignment is essential in preventing complications such as pressure injuries.**
   3. Kyphosis is a chronic condition that complicates proper body alignment.
   4. **Contractures can occur within a few days when muscles, tendon, and joints become less flexible because of lack of mobility and incorrect alignment.**
   5. Incontinence is not a complication of incorrect body alignment.

35. **C: Foundations of Practice CN: Physiological Integrity T: Knowledge**
   1. Prothrombin time, partial thromboplastin time, and international normalized ratio are all tests that evaluate clotting time, not heart damage.
   2. **Troponin I and cardiac troponin T are proteins in myocardial tissue. When cardiac muscle is damaged, this protein is released into the blood within an hour of injury. CK-MB is one of the three isoenzymes that can be separated from creatine kinase (CK). CK-MB is released into the blood when cardiac tissue has been damaged. LDH refers to lactate dehydrogenase, which is released into the blood when tissues are damaged.**
   3. Sodium and potassium levels are important in that abnormal levels may hinder conduction, but they do not detect heart muscle damage. CK-BB is an isoenzyme separated from CK and shows when brain tissue has been damaged.
   4. Blood urea nitrogen and creatinine are kidney function tests. Elevated levels show that the kidneys are not functioning optimally. CK-MM is an isoenzyme separated from CK and shows when skeletal muscle tissue has been damaged.

36. **C: Foundations of Practice CN: Physiological Integrity T: Critical Thinking**
   1. This is a good strategy to provide immobilization to the neck injury and can be done while the guest is still in the pool. However, breathing is the priority.
   2. This is a possibly appropriate first aid measure but is not as urgent as providing rescue breathing.
   3. This is appropriate as people who have sustained a spinal cord injury while swimming should not be lifted out of the pool until there is experienced help. Moving the guest may cause further damage. However, it is not as important as breathing.
   4. **Spinal cord injuries above C3 may cause respiratory paralysis. The priority action must be to provide rescue breathing until the paramedics arrive.**

37. **C: Foundations of Practice CN: Physiological Integrity T: Critical Thinking**
   1. While this is true, it is in language that she may not understand.
   2. This is true, but it does not answer the client's question.
   3. **This describes the action and the rationale in language that the client will be able to understand.**
   4. This is true but does not answer the client's question.

38. **C: Collaborative Practice CN: Psychosocial Integrity T: Critical Thinking**
   1. This is an encouraging but not helpful comment. The nurse cannot predict how fast his Parkinson's disease will progress or whether medications will be effective.
   2. **This is the first step of the nursing process: data collection. The nurse needs to find out, by using an open-ended question, what the client has been told by the physician and whether the client understands what was discussed. Once the nurse has this information, they may gauge the client's level of readiness for clarification of information and teaching about the disease.**
   3. This is true, but it is not the appropriate response at this time. It may downplay the client's worries and may not invite dialogue between the client and the nurse.
   4. While this may be an appropriate action in some situations, it is not likely to be helpful initially with the client. If the client indicates to the nurse that they are neither able nor willing to talk at present, then the nurse might offer to sit with them quietly.

39. **C: Foundations of Practice CN: Physiological Integrity T: Knowledge**
   1. **With anemia, the body must work hard to get what oxygen it has to all tissues. Clients frequently complain of weakness, malaise, and being unable to accomplish normal activities.**
   2. Bradycardia is not a manifestation of anemia. Tachycardia and palpitations occur even in mild anemia as the body attempts to compensate for the decrease in oxygen in the blood.
   3. The eyes and skin are not affected until the anemia is severe. Then the client may experience pallor, jaundice, pruritus, icteric conjunctiva and sclera, retinal hemorrhage, and blurred vision.
   4. **Palpitations are a manifestation of mild anemia.**
   5. Neurological symptoms do not develop until the anemia is severe. Then the client may experience headaches, vertigo, irritability, depression, or impaired thought processes.

40. **C: Foundation of Practice CN: Physiological Integrity T: Knowledge**
   1. Hypermagnesemia usually occurs only in renal insufficiency or failure.
   2. Hypocalcemia can be caused by any condition that results in a decrease in the production of parathyroid hormone. Diarrhea does not cause hypocalcemia.

3. **Hypokalemia, or low potassium, can result from abnormal losses of potassium due to a shift of potassium from extracellular fluid to intracellular fluid or, rarely, from a dietary deficiency of potassium. The most common causes of hypokalemia are abnormal losses via either the kidneys or the gastrointestinal tract.**

4. Hypernatremia, or high sodium, can be caused by an increase in insensible water loss, such as in diabetes insipidus, or osmotic diuresis. Hypernatremia is not a result of diarrhea.

41. **C: Foundations of Practice CN: Physiological Integrity T: Application**
    1. Peppermint will lower LES pressure and increase the chance for reflux.
    2. Small, frequent meals are recommended to avoid abdominal distention.
    3. **Pyrosis (heartburn) is the most common manifestation of gastroesophageal reflux disease (GERD) and can be soothed by antacid preparations prior to H$_2$ antagonist treatment.**
    4. **Elevating the head of the bed will reduce the incidence of reflux while the client is sleeping.**
    5. There is no need to make changes in physical activities because of GERD.

42. **C: Foundations of Practice CN: Physiological Integrity T: Critical Thinking**
    1. This is a priority for bleeding from esophageal varices, not peptic ulcer disease.
    2. Establishing an intravenous line is important so the nurse has access to a vein if volume replacement is required. However, it is not the priority.
    3. **A nasogastric tube will be established, followed by saline or water lavages until the returns are clear and the bleeding has stopped.**
    4. In many situations, oxygen is the priority. However, in this situation, the priority is to stop the bleeding. There is no indication that the client is in respiratory distress.

43. **C: Foundations of Practice CN: Physiological Integrity T: Application**
    1. Bulk-forming laxatives, rather than stool softeners, are usually given, and these will be implemented later in the hospitalization.
    2. **The client with acute diverticulitis will be given parenteral fluids to maintain fluid and electrolyte balance while NPO.**
    3. A diet high in fibre and fluids will be implemented before discharge.
    4. **The client with acute diverticulitis will be NPO to allow the colon to rest and the inflammation to subside.**
    5. The client with acute diverticulitis will not have a colonoscopy because of the risk for perforation and peritonitis.

44. **C: Foundations of Practice CN: Physiological Integrity T: Application**

1. **The client's clinical manifestations are consistent with appendicitis. The client should be NPO in case immediate surgery is needed.**
2. The client will need to know how to cough and deep breathe postoperatively, but coughing will increase pain at this time.
3. **The O$_2$ saturation is only 90%, therefore administration of oxygen is required.**
4. The client should be NPO in case immediate surgery is needed.
5. Checking for rebound tenderness frequently is unnecessary and uncomfortable for the client.

45. **C: Foundations of Practice CN: Physiological Integrity T: Knowledge**
    1. The liver does not store vitamin C or E, so these would not be affected by hepatitis.
    2. **The liver may not be able to produce albumin. Therefore, albumin levels may be decreased.**
    3. **The liver may not be able to produce prothrombin and other factors essential for blood clotting. Therefore, the prothrombin time may be prolonged.**
    4. Calcium is not stored in the liver.
    5. Potassium levels are not affected by hepatitis.

46. **C: Foundations of Practice CN: Physiological Integrity T: Application**
    1. A high-fibre diet helps reduce fat absorption.
    2. A high-fibre diet helps decrease the risk of constipation.
    3. A high-fibre diet does not affect potassium absorption.
    4. **A high-fibre diet helps trap ammonia in the gut before it is absorbed into the bloodstream.**

47. **C: Foundations of Practice CN: Physiological Integrity T: Critical Thinking**
    1. Postoperative pain should be expected.
    2. Low-grade fever is expected.
    3. **Stridor is a serious finding as it could indicate that inflammation is compressing the trachea. The client should be placed in a semi-Fowler's position to decrease edema and limit tension on the suture line.**
    4. Serosanguinous drainage is expected initially.

48. **C: Foundations of Practice CN: Physiological Integrity T: Knowledge**
    1. **This is a manifestation of Addison's disease.**
    2. This is a manifestation of Cushing's syndrome.
    3. **This is a manifestation of Addison's disease.**
    4. This is a manifestation of Cushing's syndrome.
    5. This is seen in Grave's disease or hyperthyroidism.

49. **C: Foundations of Practice CN: Physiological Integrity T: Knowledge**
    1. This describes tension-type headache.
    2. This describes migraine headache.
    3. This describes tension-type headache.
    4. **These are manifestations of cluster headaches.**

50. **C: Professional, Ethical, and Legal Practice CN: Physiological Integrity T: Application**
    1. Valuables left in the client's room may be lost or stolen.

2. **Inventory the items and give them to the family members or the client's caregiver or have security lock them up. Document a list of items and their locations in a preoperative checklist or in the nurses' notes per employer policy.**
3. Items not secured could be misplaced or lost.
4. As in choice 3.

51. **C: Foundations of Practice CN: Physiological Integrity T: Application**
    1. The client is to be taught to wipe from front to back.
    2. Diaphragm use should be discouraged temporarily, rather than suggested as an option.
    3. **Advise the client to report cloudy urine, as well as pain, frequency, and urgency.**
    4. **The nurse would teach the client to avoid constipation.**
    5. **The nurse would teach the client to empty the bladder regularly.**

52. **C: Foundations of Practice CN: Physiological Integrity T: Application**
    1. **The client is taught to avoid high heels and that leather shoes are preferred.**
    2. The feet should be washed, but not soaked, in warm water daily.
    3. The client should have someone else inspect the feet due to poor eyesight.
    4. Commercial callus and corn removers should be avoided.

53. **C: Foundations of Practice CN: Physiological Integrity T: Knowledge**
    1. This refers to possible gastro-intestinal upset such as gastroesophageal reflux disease (GERD). People with abdominal aortic aneurysm (AAA) do not usually complain of pain.
    2. This refers to heartburn, experienced by clients with GERD.
    3. **Abdominal bruit is symptomatic of AAA.**
    4. This refers to aortic dissection.
    5. **A pulsating periumbilical mass is symptomatic of AAA.**

54. **C: Foundations of Practice CN: Physiological Integrity T: Application**
    1. The client is extremely lethargic and will not be able to drink enough fluids to bring the sodium level to within normal limits.
    2. A 10% dextrose solution is a hypertonic solution that will draw fluid from the tissues and increase diuresis in an already dehydrated client.
    3. **Establishing an intravenous line of an isotonic solution will help rehydrate the client and bring the hematocrit and sodium levels within their normal limits.**
    4. Inserting a nasogastric tube will not bring the sodium and hematocrit to within normal limits.

55. **C: Foundations of Practice CN: Physiological Integrity T: Knowledge**

1. Adenocarcinomas are malignant tumours arising from glandular organs.
2. **Basal cell carcinoma is the most common human cancer, a malignancy typically found on skin exposed to sun or other forms of ultraviolet light.**
3. The client is also at risk for malignant melanoma. Although the incidence is increasing, it is not as common as basal cell carcinoma.
4. Spongioblastoma is a glioma of the brain (a neoplasm or tumour composed of neuroglial cells) derived from spongioblasts.

56. **C: Foundations of Practice CN: Psychosocial Integrity T: Knowledge**
    1. **Delirium is a disturbance of consciousness that develops over a short period of time.**
    2. Apraxia (inability to use objects properly) is not a characteristic of delirium.
    3. **Memory impairments may occur with delirium.**
    4. **Delirium may be due to a medical condition.**
    5. Agnosia (loss of the ability to recognize sensory inputs) is not a characteristic of delirium.

57. **C: Foundations of Practice CN: Physiological Integrity T: Application**
    1. Weight-bearing exercises are recommended for osteoporosis. Swimming is not a weight-bearing exercise.
    2. **The best exercises for osteoporosis are weight-bearing ones. The client will be able to walk using their walker.**
    3. While aerobics are beneficial for older person for increased muscle strength, coordination, and osteoporosis, it is unlikely that if the client requires a walker, they would be able to participate in aerobic exercise.
    4. This is not a weight-bearing exercise.

58. **C: Foundations of Practice CN: Physiological Integrity T: Application**
    1. **Multiple sclerosis is a chronic, progressive, degenerative disorder of the central nervous system characterized by disseminated demyelination of nerve fibres of the brain and spinal cord. The initial manifestations are often vague and inconsistent but include sensory disturbances such as blurred vision and tinnitus.**
    2. This refers to Parkinson's disease.
    3. This refers to myasthenia gravis.
    4. This refers to restless legs syndrome.

59. **C: Foundations of Practice CN: Physiological Integrity T: Application**
    1. This is a component of postsurgical care and is not directly related to the manifestations of abdominal pain and bladder distension.
    2. **Post transurethral resection of the prostate with continuous bladder irrigation, it is common for blood clots to block the catheter, requiring the nurse to flush the catheter.**
    3. The catheter is likely blocked by clots. Decreasing the flow will not solve this problem.

4. The physician does not need to be notified unless flushing does not solve the problem.

60. C: Foundations of Practice CN: Physiological Integrity T: Application
    1. **Citrus fruits such as oranges are a good source of potassium.**
    2. **Potatoes are a good source of potassium.**
    3. **Green leafy vegetables such as spinach are a good source of potassium.**
    4. Pasta is not high in potassium.
    5. Corn is not high in potassium.

CHAPTER 10

1. C: Foundations of Practice CN: Physiological Integrity T: Application
   1. Early postpartum hemorrhage is most often associated with failure of the uterus to remain contracted and poor uterine tone on palpation.
   2. There are no apparent signs of infection.
   3. **A full bladder will push the uterus higher in the abdomen and cause it to deviate away from the expected midline position. It is common for the bladder to become full in the first 24 to 48 hours postpartum due to swelling and trauma from birth and elimination of excess intravascular volume.**
   4. A normal uterine involution would mean that the top of the uterus could be found midline in the abdomen and about two fingerbreadths below the umbilicus.

2. C: Foundations of Practice CN: Health Promotion and Maintenance T: Application
   1. The newborn should feed on demand and not on a timed schedule.
   2. Six to eight wet diapers in 24 hours indicate adequate hydration and nourishment.
   3. **Frequent audible swallows ensure the newborn is feeding well.**
   4. The newborn should gain at least 20 g per day.

3. C: Foundations of Practice CN: Physiological Integrity T: Application
   1. **Breastfed infants need vitamin D supplementation of 400 IU/day, available in infant drops.**
   2. The breastfed newborn has adequate iron stores for the first 6 months of life.
   3. Vitamin A supplementation is not recommended or required.
   4. Breast milk contains all the necessary essential fatty acids.

4. C: Foundations of Practice CN: Psychosocial Integrity T: Application
   1. While the partner might be tired, this answer ignores his question and does not provide useful information about the process of taking in the experience of labour and birth.
   2. Referral for counselling is not indicated in this situation.

3. Attachment is a process that takes place over time. No one event or behaviour is essential. The term *bonding* is avoided as it implies a short-term process that may fail or succeed if feelings and behaviours are not quickly established.
4. **Ms. Viraj's behaviour is a normal part of adaptation to parenting. Providing information to the partner about this expected behaviour would help address his concerns.**

5. C: Foundations of Practice CN: Health Promotion and Maintenance T: Knowledge
   1. Moulding is a temporary overlapping of the cranial bones. The head appears pointed and elongated in shape.
   2. **Caput succedaneum is soft scalp swelling commonly due to pressure on the head from the cervix. It is poorly defined and crosses the suture lines of the skull. It appears at or shortly after birth and resolves within a few days.**
   3. Cephalohematoma appears after 24 hours, is localized on one side of the head, and does not cross the suture lines of the skull. It is a collection of blood under the periosteum and takes several weeks to be reabsorbed.
   4. Congenital dermal melanocytosis is a darkened pigmentation of the skin located over the lumbar spine area.

6. C: Foundations of Practice CN: Health Promotion and Maintenance T: Application
   1. Circumcision is most often practised to comply with religious or cultural beliefs but may also be a personal preference and choice made by the parents.
   2. The nurse's responsibility is to provide current, evidence-informed information so the parents can make an informed decision.
   3. **Routine circumcision is not recommended.**
   4. The evidence supporting or refuting the need for circumcision is not absolute or definitive in supporting routine circumcision in infancy.

7. C: Foundations of Practice CN: Physiological Integrity T: Critical Thinking
   1. Fetal well-being in this situation would be better assessed with the use of fetal heart monitoring.
   2. Detecting fetal abnormalities by ultrasound would be part of an ultrasound assessment early in the pregnancy and is not a priority in this situation.
   3. **Ultrasound would be used to locate and confirm the position of the placenta to determine whether it is implanted near the cervix.**
   4. These determinations are made in early ultrasonograms and would not be a priority in this situation.

8. C: Foundations of Practice CN: Physiological Integrity T: Application
   1. **Placenta previa is manifested by painless red vaginal bleeding in the third trimester. Ms. Smitherman's advanced maternal age is also a known risk factor.**
   2. Placental abruption more often occurs during labour and is manifested by concealed or apparent vaginal

bleeding and pain, with the uterus feeling hard, tense, and painful.

3. Spontaneous abortion (miscarriage) occurs prior to 20 weeks' gestation.

4. Rh incompatibility is not indicated by these manifestations. The hemolytic process would affect the newborn only and does not result in painless vaginal bleeding in the third trimester.

9. **C: Foundations of Practice CN: Health Promotion and Maintenance T: Application**

1. Women have been able to give birth vaginally after having a Caesarean birth.

2. It is not possible to predict whether a vaginal birth will be an option with the next delivery.

3. It takes longer to recover from a Caesarean surgery than a vaginal birth.

4. **There are parameters the physician will use as a guide to help make the decision for a vaginal birth after Caesarean birth (VBAC). It will be based on the next pregnancy and labour experience.**

10. **C: Foundations of Practice CN: Physiological Integrity T: Critical Thinking**

1. **The priority assessment is ensuring spontaneous respirations so that the infant may be adequately oxygenated. If the infant is not breathing adequately, the infant will require supplemental oxygen, bagging, and possibly intubation with mechanical ventilation.**

2. This would be an important assessment, but breathing is the priority.

3. Colour is part of the assessment related to breathing. A newborn at birth will likely be cyanosed, becoming pink centrally after spontaneous respirations or supplemental bagging is initiated.

4. This is part of the neonatal assessment but is not the priority assessment.

11. **C: Foundations of Practice CN: Physiological Integrity T: Application**

1. **Pathological jaundice associated with liver damage would occur at birth or in the first 24 hours. Physiological jaundice in a full-term, otherwise healthy infant occurs after 24 hours, peaks within 3 to 4 days, and resolves within a week.**

2. The bruising and blood from the cephalohematoma may have contributed to the elevated bilirubin levels but are not the cause. An immature liver and limited ability to conjugate bilirubin lead to physiological jaundice.

3. Pathological hyperbilirubinemia occurs at birth or in the first 24 hours of life and requires investigation.

4. A blood exchange transfusion is not always required, especially for physiological jaundice.

12. **C: Foundations of Practice CN: Physiological Integrity T: Application**

1. Fluid requirements increase by 10%, and more frequent breastfeeding should be supported.

2. Stools become looser and more frequent.

3. The baby will be drowsier and lethargic.

4. **Skin exposure is important to maximize the benefit of the ultraviolet lights. Eyes must always be covered for protection.**

13. **C: Foundations of Practice CN: Safe and Effective Care Environment T: Application**

1. This is not a safe option. In many cases, the membranes do not rupture until shortly before delivery.

2. **Regular painful contractions are an indication of labour. It is not known how quickly the client's labour will progress; therefore, they should be assessed by a nurse or physician at the hospital.**

3. Suggesting the pregnant client walk when they feel contractions is often advised to distinguish between true and false labour. The client has indicated that the contractions are regular, so it is not likely that this is false labour. The client should be assessed at the hospital.

4. As it is not known how quickly the labour will progress, the client should not delay being assessed.

14. **C: Foundations of Practice CN: Physiological Integrity T: Knowledge**

1. Infants do not possess the ability to shiver at birth.

2. **Nonshivering thermogenesis uses the chemical breakdown of brown fat stores to generate heat.**

3. Cold, stress, and heat production increase oxygen demands and consumption.

4. An extended body posture increases heat loss.

15. **C: Foundations of Practice CN: Physiological Integrity T: Knowledge**

1. Weight is not used to assess gestational age as infants may be small, large, or average weight independent of their gestational age.

2. Head circumference is not a reliable indicator of gestational age. A newborn may be small, large, or average in growth regardless of gestational age.

3. **Absence of ear cartilage is seen in prematurity, while the presence of ear cartilage is a sign of full-term gestational maturity.**

4. Body length is influenced by growth patterns, and infants may be average, below, or above average in length regardless of gestational age.

16. **C: Foundations of Practice CN: Physiological Integrity T: Knowledge**

1. Increased oxygen levels cause the ductus arteriosus to constrict.

2. Clamping of the umbilical cord closes the ductus venosus.

3. **When the pulmonary vessels open, more blood flows into the left atrium, increasing pressure and volume. This pressure becomes greater than the pressure in the right atrium, and the foramen ovale functionally closes.**

4. During transition, the pulmonary blood vessels dilate and pulmonary blood pressure decreases.

17. **C: Foundations of Practice CN: Safe and Effective Care Environment T: Application**
    1. This is more frequent than required for an uncomplicated pregnancy.
    2. **Monthly visits are scheduled up to 28 weeks, and then visits increase to every 2 weeks through 36 weeks. From 36 weeks until birth, visits are weekly.**
    3. Visits are scheduled every 2 weeks after 28 weeks.
    4. As in choice 1.

18. **C: Foundations of Practice CN: Physiological Integrity T: Application**
    1. Rh immune globulin (Rhogam) is administered to Rh-negative mothers who give birth to an Rh-positive newborn. There will not be an immune response if the newborn is also Rh-negative; therefore, prophylaxis is not required.
    2. **Rh immune globulin (Rhogam) is given in this situation in case the embryo or fetus was Rh-positive and isoimmunization has occurred.**
    3. Rh immune globulin (Rhogam) is administered to Rh-negative mothers who give birth to an Rh-positive newborn or in situations where the Rh factor of the embryo or newborn is unknown, including ectopic pregnancies and spontaneous or induced abortions. Blood type is not a consideration.
    4. Rh immune globulin (Rhogam) is not required in this situation as the incompatibility occurs with an O-positive mother who has anti-A and anti-B antibodies. Rh immune globulin (Rhogam) will not affect blood type incompatibilities.

19. **C: Foundations of Practice CN: Physiological Integrity T: Application**
    1. The fundus should stay firm.
    2. **An increase in lochia or a return to bright red bleeding after the lochia has become pink indicates a complication.**
    3. The lochia should decrease in amount over time.
    4. Large clots after discharge are a sign of a complication and should be reported.

20. **C: Foundations of Practice CN: Physiological Integrity T: Knowledge**
    1. **The full-term infant is born with the Moro (startle) reflex.**
    2. **The full-term infant is born with the Babinski reflex (when the sole of the foot is stroked upward, the toes extend outward).**
    3. **The full-term infant is born with the rooting reflex (turns head toward stroked cheek).**
    4. **The full-term infant is born with the stepping reflex (held upright, legs move as if stepping).**
    5. Pincer grasp does not occur until between 8 and 12 months (grasps object between the thumb and index finger).
    6. **The full-term infant is born with the tonic neck reflex (head turned to one side, same side arm and leg extend, opposite arm and leg flex).**

21. **C: Foundations of Practice CN: Physiological Integrity T: Knowledge**
    1. **There is an increased risk of hypoglycemia as the child-bearing client's glucose supply stops at birth, the newborn's pancreas continues to produce large amounts of insulin, and the infant, particularly if the child is large for gestational age (LGA), uses up glucose stores quickly.**
    2. Infants of child-bearing clients with gestational diabetes are at risk of being LGA due to the additional child-bearing client's glucose supply. Small for gestational age is a risk for people with type 1 diabetes who may experience chronic urinary tract infections.
    3. There is an increased risk of hypoglycemia, not hyperglycemia. See rationale 1.
    4. The fetal pancreas responds to increased glucose from the child-bearing client by producing large amounts of insulin in the first few days of life, resulting in temporary hyperinsulinism, not insulin resistance.

22. **C: Foundations of Practice CN: Physiological Integrity T: Knowledge**
    1. **An overdistended uterus (e.g., polyhydramnios) is a risk factor for a postpartum hemorrhage**.
    2. Tachycardia is not a risk factor for postpartum hemorrhage.
    3. **Trauma such as lacerations of the genital tract, lacerations during Caesarean birth, uterine rupture, and uterine inversion are risk factors for postpartum hemorrhage.**
    4. **Urinary atony is marked hypotonia of the uterus and is the leading cause of postpartum hemorrhage.**
    5. Thromboembolism is not a risk factor for postpartum hemorrhage.

23. **C: Foundations of Practice CN: Physiological Integrity T: Application**
    1. Encourage fluid intake of 2 to 3 litres of fluid a day.
    2. **Frequent breastfeeding or use of a breast pump is important to empty the breast.**
    3. **Taking a warm shower prior to feeding helps to stimulate milk flow.**
    4. **Wearing a supportive bra is a supportive measure.**
    5. Warm packs rather than ice packs help to stimulate milk flow.
    6. Antibiotics may be prescribed and are taken until the full prescribed course is completed. They are not stopped when symptoms improve.

24. **C: Foundations of Practice CN: Physiological Integrity T: Knowledge**
    1. **Toxoplasmosis is a TORCH infection.**
    2. **This is not a TORCH infection.**
    3. **Cytomegalovirus is a TORCH infection.**
    4. **Rubella is a TORCH infection.**
    5. **Herpes simplex is a TORCH infection.**

25. **C: Foundations of Practice CN: Physiological Integrity T: Knowledge**

1. The amniotic fluid provides maintenance of even temperature
2. The amniotic fluid allows fetal movement
3. The amniotic fluid prevents the amniotic sac from adhering to fetal skin
4. Although the fetus does swallow amniotic fluid, it has no nutritional value
5. **The amniotic fluid acts as a cushion for the fetus.**

CHAPTER 11

The correct answer is set off in boldface.

1. **C: Foundations of Practice CN: Physiological Integrity T: Application**
   1. **The child adopts this position in an attempt to facilitate the use of accessory muscles of respiration. If the child is able to lie down, the asthma attack is not likely to be severe.**
   2. This is a manifestation of laryngotracheobronchitis (croup).
   3. Children with asthma try to breathe deeply. There are rarely periods of apnea, unless the child is progressing to respiratory arrest.
   4. This is a manifestation of laryngotracheobronchitis (croup).
2. **C: Foundations of Practice CN: Physiological Integrity T: Application**
   1. This is a recognized adverse effect of salbutamol. The inhalation should not be stopped.
   2. **Shaking is a recognized adverse effect of salbutamol and occurs especially with increased frequency of inhalations. Simon should be reassured that it is normal.**
   3. The shakes are not due to Simon being cold. A blanket will not help.
   4. Air flow does not influence the adverse effect of shaking with salbutamol.
3. **C: Foundations of Practice CN: Physiological Integrity T: Application**
   1. Milk products tend to increase mucus secretions in the airways and so should be avoided in clients with respiratory distress.
   2. Solid foods are not recommended during respiratory distress as they may increase the risk of vomiting and aspiration.
   3. It is appropriate to have clear fluids, but a child would not be likely to choose beef soup.
   4. **Children with respiratory distress should have diets consisting of clear fluids. These are better tolerated, provide recommended fluids to help liquefy mucus secretions, and do not pose a risk for aspiration. Ice pops would be an attractive choice for a child.**
4. **C: Foundations of Practice CN: Health Promotion and Maintenance T: Critical Thinking**
   1. **Research has shown that children who have developed a comprehensive plan for asthma management**

with their health care provider have the best management of symptoms and the fewest hospitalizations.
   2. This may be true, but it is not the most helpful answer.
   3. This is true, but an asthma plan will help identify triggers.
   4. While this is true for some children with asthma, it is not known if Simon will require this level of medication.
5. **C: Foundations of Practice CN: Health Promotion and Maintenance T: Critical Thinking**
   1. This may be necessary but would be distressing for Simon. Removal of pets should not be considered unless allergen testing proves Simon is allergic to dog dander.
   2. **Second-hand smoke is a definite trigger for asthma. Several Canadian provinces have enacted legislation preventing adults from smoking in cars with children.**
   3. This is a valuable strategy to help clean the air in Simon's home but is not the most important, immediate strategy.
   4. Wet dusting is necessary to remove dust accumulation but is not as important or immediate as not smoking in the car.
6. **C: Foundations of Practice CN: Health Promotion and Maintenance T: Application**
   1. A visit to a physician for a "cold" is not necessary. She will need to see a physician if the fever continues for a week or if the illness becomes worse.
   2. Aspirin should not be given to children due to the risk of Reye's syndrome.
   3. **Pediatric acetaminophen and ibuprofen are appropriate analgesics and antipyretics for minor childhood conditions such as teething, colds, immunizations, and so on.**
   4. These medications are not recommended for infants and children and in some cases have been removed from pharmacies.
7. **C: Foundations of Practice CN: Health Promotion and Maintenance T: Application**
   1. Infant walkers are unsafe and not allowed for sale in Canada.
   2. A baby rattle is more appropriate for an infant of 1 to 3 months.
   3. Reading, while an excellent method of promoting bonding, literacy, and reading readiness, does not develop motor skills.
   4. **Manipulating these objects will assist in the development of fine motor skills.**
8. **C: Foundations of Practice CN: Safe and Effective Care Environment T: Application**
   1. Provided that the finger foods are not hard and large (such as peanuts or carrots), finger foods are nutritious, help develop motor skills, and are well liked by older infants and toddlers.

2. This is not necessary. If the sides of the crib are in the raised position, Leah will not fall.

3. This is not realistic. Other closures such as zippers and snaps are safe.

4. **Small movable parts may become dislodged from the toy and are a hazard to infants and toddlers**.

9. **C: Professional, Ethical, and Legal Practice CN: Psychosocial Integrity T: Application**

1. Leah is exhibiting stranger anxiety, which is developmentally normal at 9 months. Removing Leah from her father will frighten her.

2. This should not be necessary if the right approach is taken and Leah is given time to get used to the nurse.

3. **This is the recommended approach as the soft voice is comforting and meeting the child at eye level makes the stranger appear smaller**.

4. This is intrusive and is likely to frighten Leah.

10. **C: Foundations of Practice CN: Health Promotion and Maintenance T: Application**

1. This is an appropriate developmental milestone for a 9-month-old infant.

2. **This would be expected to be achieved by 7 months.**

3. This becomes evident at 6 months of age.

4. This is appropriate to a developmental age of 12 months.

11. **C: Foundations of Practice CN: Safe and Effective Care Environment T: Critical Thinking**

1. **Peanuts may be used in many ingredients that may not be evident. A ban on all homemade foods (such as cakes and ice cream) will prevent inadvertent sources of peanut by-products from being ingested by the children. Many daycare centres have enacted this practice.**

2. This will communicate the peanut allergy to the parents but may not prevent food substances that contain peanuts from being available to the children. Parents may not be aware of which foods are likely to have traces of peanuts.

3. This will help the staff identify children at risk but will do nothing to prevent foods containing peanuts from being in the daycare centre.

4. All sources of peanut, for example, peanut oil, may not be easily identifiable.

12. **C: Foundations of Practice CN: Health Promotion and Maintenance T: Critical Thinking**

1. This is a safe practice but should be performed before changing diapers as well. It may not be effective in preventing airborne transmission of micro-organisms.

2. Hand hygiene is the best infection control practice, but several times a day is not frequent enough to prevent transmission.

3. This is not practical in most daycare settings.

4. **Children with obvious signs of infection should be cared for at home. However, if they develop symptoms during the day, they should be isolated from the rest of the children.**

13. **C: Foundations of Practice CN: Physiological Integrity T: Application**

1. This is too frequent and will tire Jayden unnecessarily. There will not be sufficient rest time between feedings.

2. **Feeding of the infant with heart failure is similar to exercise in an adult. The infant often tires and may need frequent rest periods.**

3. Infants with a congenital heart defect require feedings with increased caloric density in the formula or breast milk.

4. This may be necessary if it is found Jayden cannot tolerate bottle feedings. There may not be trained staff at the daycare centre to competently gavage-feed infants.

14. **C: Foundations of Practice CN: Health Promotion and Maintenance T: Knowledge**

1. **Varicella-zoster virus is the name of the herpes virus that causes the disease varicella, or chicken pox.**

2. MMR is the vaccine that protects the child from measles, mumps, and rubella.

3. Hib is the *Haemophilus influenzae* type b (Hib) vaccine and protects the child primarily against bacterial meningitis and epiglottitis.

4. DTaP is a combination vaccine that provides immunity to diphtheria, tetanus, and pertussis.

15. **C: Foundations of Practice CN: Health Promotion and Maintenance T: Application**

1. This is a breach of confidential information. The child with pediculosis (lice) does not have to be specifically identified. Shobana may not be the only child with head lice.

2. **This alerts the families to the condition and provides practical information to examine and treat their children. Treatment at home will prevent transmission of the head lice at the child care centre.**

3. It is not practical to examine the hair of every child on arrival and then to send the child home without prior notice to the parents. A useful alternative would be to screen all children early in the day, isolate those found to have lice, and then notify the families.

4. This is not the responsibility of the child care centre. Treatment should be provided in the home.

16. **C: Foundations of Practice CN: Physiological Integrity T: Application**

1. Absent bowel sounds are not a clinical manifestation of intussusception.

2. **The passage of red currant jelly-like stools is a clinical manifestation of intussusception.**

3. Anorexia is not a clinical manifestation of intussusception.

4. **A tender, distended abdomen is a clinical manifestation of intussusception.**

5. Hematemesis is not a clinical manifestation of intussusception.

6. **Sudden acute abdominal pain is a clinical manifestation of intussusception.**

17. **C: Foundations of Practice CN: Physiological Integrity T: Knowledge**
    1. Flushing, not pallor would occur.
    2. **A characteristic of diabetic ketoacidosis is acidosis.**
    3. Respirations are rapid (Kussmaul respirations), not slow.
    4. **A characteristic of diabetic ketoacidosis is dehydration.**
    5. **A characteristic of diabetic ketoacidosis is hyperglycemia.**

18. **C: Foundations of Practice CN: Safe and Effective Care Environment T: Application**
    1. **Infants with Down syndrome often have difficulty with feedings due to their large tongues and poor muscle control and coordination.**
    2. There can be decreased immunity with Down syndrome, but it is not a common finding.
    3. Down syndrome infants and children are very receptive to affection.
    4. There is a gradual increase, not deterioration, in developmental functioning.

19. **C: Foundations of Practice CN: Physiological Integrity T: Application**
    1. **A high-pitched cry is a clinical manifestation of increased ICP in an infant.**
    2. **Poor feeding is a clinical manifestation of increased ICP in an infant.**
    3. **Setting-sun sign is a clinical manifestation of increased ICP in an infant.**
    4. The infant would have a tense, bulging fontanel.
    5. **Distended scalp veins are a clinical manifestation of increased ICP in an infant.**
    6. The infant would have an increased head circumference.

20. **C: Foundations of Practice CN: Physiological Integrity T: Critical Thinking**
    1. **This is the first step in the nursing process: data collection. The nurse needs more information about the diet and pattern of discomfort. The infant likely has colic, and the detailed history will assist the nurse to provide potential therapeutic measures to ease the infant's discomfort.**
    2. This is a possibility, but a thorough history is required initially.
    3. Re-establishing breast milk may not be possible at this stage. Breastfed infants also develop colic.
    4. This may be true, but in order to develop individualized and appropriate comfort measures, the nurse requires more information.

21. **C: Foundations of Practice CN: Physiological Integrity T: Application**
    1. **The initial action the nurse should take is to position the client on their side to prevent aspiration.**
    2. This may be an appropriate action but is not the priority.

    3. The health care provider needs to be notified once the client has been positioned on their side.
    4. Although pain management will be required, this would not be the priority action.
    5. **Muscle weakness is a symptom of anemia.**

22. **C: Foundations of Practice CN: Physiological Integrity T: Application**
    1. This is a sign of hypertonic dehydration.
    2. **Slightly moist mucous membranes are a clinical manifestation of hypotonic dehydration.**
    3. **Absent tears are a clinical manifestation of hypotonic dehydration.**
    4. **A very rapid pulse is a clinical manifestation of hypotonic dehydration.**
    5. Hyperirritability is a sign of hypertonic dehydration.

23. **C: Foundations of Practice CN: Physiological Integrity T: Application**
    1. This is not true. There are a variety of pain rating scales and behavioural indicators that are useful for assessing pain in children. Children by the age of four can accurately point to the body area where they have pain.
    2. Narcotics can be successfully and safely used with children. They are no more dangerous for children than for adults.
    3. **Several research studies have examined the pattern of pain medication in children compared with adults and have found consistently that many children are not medicated appropriately for their degree of pain.**
    4. Children may not admit having pain to avoid an injection or may not ask for analgesia because they believe adults know how they feel.

24. **C: Foundations of Practice CN: Physiological Integrity T: Application**
    1. **Having the parent assist may help calm the child and achieve compliance with taking the prednisone. The child is more likely to trust the parent than the nurse.**
    2. Prednisone does not come in suppository form. A suppository is inappropriate and invasive.
    3. Children should never be restrained unless there is a medical order. Restraints would be frightening for the child.
    4. This may sound like an attractive option, but the bitter taste of the prednisone would not be masked by the applesauce, and it is unlikely that the child would eat a sufficient amount to receive all of the prednisone. The child may be offered applesauce or another favourite food after the prednisone to help clear the mouth of the bitter taste.

25. **C: Professional, Ethical, and Legal Practice CN: Safe and Effective Care Environment T: Critical Thinking**
    1. **The family is included to collaborate with all levels of care. Family-centred care values the family as the spokespersons for their children during health care discussions and decisions.**

2. The family will need guidance in understanding the lab values and how it will affect treatment. They will need this understanding in order to make informed decisions about the care of their child.

3. Most facilities do have Internet access, which is used for a variety of reasons. Although resources for completing school work are often offered in pediatric care settings, they are not an integral part of family-centred care.

4. It is encouraged that parents continue to follow bedtime routines that have been established at home rather than have the agency establish these routines.

CHAPTER 12

The correct answer is set off in boldface.

1. C: **Foundations of Practice CN: Psychosocial Integrity T: Knowledge**
   1. **This is the definition of *psychosis*.**
   2. This is the definition of *neurosis*.
   3. This is the definition of *delirium*.
   4. Schizophrenia is a psychotic illness but is not synonymous with psychosis. Psychosis may also occur in manic phases of bipolar disorder, substance use disorder, delirium, organic mental health disorders, posttraumatic stress disorder, and major depression.

2. C: **Foundations of Practice CN: Safe and Effective Care Environment T: Application**
   1. Emergency involuntary admission is permitted when a person is deemed in need of psychiatric treatment, presents a danger to self or others, or is unable to meet his basic needs.
   2. Depending on the province or territory, there are different ages for consent. Many have an age of consent that is 16 years or younger. Regardless of his age or the age of consent of the jurisdiction, Jason has rights.
   3. **Under law, Jason may apply to a review board to review the involuntary admission.**
   4. Jason does have legal rights.

3. C: **Professional, Ethical, and Legal Practice CN: Safe and Effective Care Environment T: Application**
   1. Quiet seclusion may help some clients. Chemical restraints may not always be preferable.
   2. In many cases, physical restraints increase violent behaviour and chemical restraints are preferable.
   3. **The policy of least restraint and guidelines for use of restraints apply equally to physical and chemical restraints.**
   4. The setting of an emergency department still requires a physician order for a chemical restraint as it is a medication.

4. C: **Foundations of Practice CN: Psychosocial Integrity T: Application**
   1. **This is an honest and truthful response, which helps identify the voices as a unique experience for Jason but does not involve arguing reality with him.**

2. Although it may be useful for the nurse to find out more about the hallucinations, it is not helpful to Jason to pretend to believe in them.
3. It is not helpful to Jason to argue with him about reality. The voices are real to him.
4. Hallucinations are a symptom of psychosis. It is neither helpful nor therapeutic to explore why Jason is hearing voices.

5. C: **Foundations of Practice CN: Psychosocial Integrity T: Application**
   1. This is a good suggestion but does not answer Jason's mother's question.
   2. This may not be true.
   3. This is a vague response and implies that the nurse is not competent to provide an answer.
   4. **This is the most complete and most correct response to Jason's mother's question.**

6. C: **Foundations of Practice CN: Psychosocial Integrity T: Knowledge**
   1. People who exhibit narcissistic behaviour feel superior to everyone else and lack empathy for others. This is evident in narcissistic behaviour disorder.
   2. People who exhibit schizoid behaviour, found in schizoid personality disorder, are loners. They display very little emotion and tend to be indifferent to the feelings of others.
   3. **Mr. Steele displays splitting behaviour, setting one person up against another. It is a type of manipulative behaviour common in people with borderline personality disorder and some other personality disorders.**
   4. People with dependent personality disorder are very dependent on others. They lack self-confidence and would be unlikely to say anything negative about Sarah or anyone else for fear of losing that person's support and approval.

7. C: **Foundations of Practice CN: Psychosocial Integrity T: Application**
   1. **People with borderline personality disorder are impulsive. Self-injury and suicide threats are common with this disorder. The nurse must assess for suicidal or homicidal thoughts, as ensuring the safety of the client and others is a nurse's first priority.**
   2. Hallucinations are a sign of psychosis. Borderline personality disorder is not a psychotic illness.
   3. While personality disorders may develop from a socially disrupted childhood, the nurse would not probe for such information until they are confident that the client is safe and until a relationship has been established.
   4. Sexual orientation is unrelated to personality disorders, although some symptoms, such as low self-esteem, fear of rejection, and sensitivity to criticism, that are common in personality disorders may also be

present in people if they are confused or not accepting of their sexual orientation.

8. **C: Foundations of Practice CN: Physiological Integrity T: Application**
   1. People with both anorexia and bulimia suffer complications in many body systems. In extreme cases, death can result from cardiac, gastro-intestinal, metabolic, or central nervous system complications.
   2. Although eating disorders are much more common in women than men, men do suffer from both anorexia and bulimia.
   3. **About half the women with anorexia display bulimic behaviours or develop bulimia later in their lives.**
   4. People with bulimia may feel intense hunger and binge to satisfy this hunger.

9. **C: Foundations of Practice CN: Physiological Integrity T: Critical Thinking**
   1. Skin breakdown may occur secondary to inadequate nutrition but is not as important as blood pressure.
   2. While constipation may occur with eating disorders, it is more logical to ask Tiffany about her bowel pattern rather than perform an abdominal palpation.
   3. People with an eating disorder often develop dental caries. While the nurse may examine Tiffany's mouth, it may not be possible to determine dental caries on inspection. It would be more efficient to refer Tiffany to a dentist or dental hygienist.
   4. **People with an eating disorder often have a lower-than-normal blood volume, leading to hypotension.**

10. **C: Professional, Ethical, and Legal Practice CN:Psychosocial Integrity T: Application**
    1. **This is an example of clarification. It helps clients clarify their own thoughts and maximizes mutual understanding.**
    2. This is the therapeutic technique of exploring, which examines experiences more fully.
    3. This is reflecting, directing feelings and ideas back to the client.
    4. This is focusing, which concentrates attention on a single point.

11. **C: Foundations of Practice CN: Psychosocial Integrity T: Application**
    1. **Young women with eating disorders, particularly anorexia, may attempt to mask their weight loss by drinking excessive water (water loading) or hiding articles within their clothing prior to weighing.**
    2. Generally, most young women with anorexia are superficially compliant with weight monitoring.
    3. It is more important that Tiffany be weighed wearing the same clothes on each occasion. It is preferable not to wear shoes or clothing where heavy articles may be hidden.
    4. Depending on the provincial law, there may be no legal imperative to inform Tiffany's parents. This needs to be discussed between Tiffany and the nurse, and parental involvement should be encouraged.

12. **C: Foundations of Practice CN: Physiological Integrity T: Application**
    1. People with anorexia are not able to tolerate large meals. They should be offered small meals and frequent nutritious drinks and snacks, paying special attention to their likes and dislikes.
    2. **The nurse must record intake and output carefully as a measure of adequate hydration. Other indicators to be monitored are skin turgor and colour and moistness of oral mucous membranes.**
    3. Mealtimes should be time limited. To decrease stress while eating, ensure a pleasant atmosphere and conversation about topics other than food.
    4. Adolescents with eating disorders generally respond well to group therapy. In addition, isolating the client provides more opportunities for secretive purging.

13. **C: Foundations of Practice CN: Safe and Effective Care Environment T: Application**
    1. Clients are at risk immediately on admission as medications are not effective yet.
    2. Clients are at risk on discharge when the reality that things are the same as before. They return home to find that the things caused the depression have not changed.
    3. **As depression deepens, the client has less motivation and physical energy to follow through on suicidal action.**
    4. Clients are at high risk for suicide for the first few days following initiation of treatment. Energy levels and motivation have improved as now the person is less apathetic. Thus, early in treatment, the client is still severely depressed but may now have the energy necessary to follow through with suicidal thoughts

14. **C: Professional, Ethical, and Legal Practice CN: Psychosocial Integrity T: Application**
    1. This is not a therapeutic response. It does not address Ms. Balkan's present feelings, and she may not feel better the next day.
    2. This is not a therapeutic response as it does not invite Ms. Balkan to discuss her feelings.
    3. **This recognizes Ms. Balkan's feelings and invites her to discuss these feelings.**
    4. This is not therapeutic as it may appear to belittle Ms. Balkan's feelings, and it may not be true that the feeling is temporary.

15. **C: Foundations of Practice CN: Physiological Integrity T: Knowledge**
    1. **Therapeutic effects may take up to 4 weeks to be achieved.**
    2. Although there have been reports of an increase in suicide after starting Prozac (fluoxetine hydrochloride), there is not a large body of research to substantiate this. It is possible that in early treatment, there is an increased risk of suicide due to the fact that the clients are beginning to feel better.

3. Anxiety and nervousness are adverse effects of Prozac and may increase.
4. Herbal preparations (such as St. John's wort) may have an additive effect with Prozac and should not be taken.

16. **C: Foundations of Practice CN: Physiological Integrity T: Application**
    1. This is an adverse effect that usually disappears after several weeks.
    2. **The yellow skin and conjunctiva indicate jaundice, which is a sign of liver damage. The medication should be stopped.**
    3. As in choice 1.
    4. Extrapyramidal signs usually indicate that the dose of Haldol should be reduced. The Haldol is not stopped unless the extrapyramidal symptoms persist at the lower dose.

17. **C: Foundations of Practice CN: Safe and Effective Care Environment   T: Application**
    1. **One-on-one observation at arm's length is necessary for anyone who has limited or unreliable control over suicidal impulses.**
    2. **This ensures the client does not have access to a potential means of self-harm.**
    3. **Finger foods allow the client to eat without silverware; "no silver or glassware" orders restrict access to a potential means of self-harm.**
    4. Vision impairment requires eyeglasses (or contacts); although they could be used dangerously, watching the client from arm's length at all times would allow enough time to interrupt such an attempt and would prevent the disorientation and isolation that uncorrected visual impairment could create.
    5. Every-15-minute checks are inadequate to assure the safety of an actively suicidal person.

18. **C: Foundations of Practice CN: Psychosocial Integrity T: Knowledge**
    1. This characteristic is not seen in a usual case of gender dysphoria.
    2. **People with gender dysphoria, prior to gender reassignment, medical and/or psychological support, suffer from a pervasive and sustained low mood.**
    3. As in choice 1.
    4. As in choice 1.

19. **C: Foundations of Practice CN: Psychosocial Integrity T: Application**
    1. This is more pertinent to a client with suspected social phobia.
    2. This is more pertinent to a client with suspected psychosis.
    3. This is more pertinent to a client with suspected post-traumatic stress disorder.
    4. **This question refers to obsessive thinking which is a clinical manifestation of obsessive-compulsive disorder.**

5. **This question refers to compulsive behaviours which is a clinical manifestation of obsessive-compulsive disorder.**

20. **C: Foundations of Practice CN: Psychosocial Integrity T: Knowledge**
    1. Touching the client may precipitate aggressive behaviour.
    2. Leading a community meeting would be appropriate when the client's behaviour is less grandiose.
    3. **People with mania are hyperactive, grandiose, and distractable. Structure will support a safe environment.**
    4. **People with mania need reminders to eat and drink.**
    5. Activities that require concentration will produce frustration.

21. **C: Professional, Ethical, and Legal Practice CN: Psychosocial Integrity   T: Application**
    1. Individual expressions of culture vary according to the persons characteristics and experiences. Clients should be first treated as individuals and then consider their culture preferences in order to provide culturally competent care.
    2. **In some cultures, mental health disorders are considered shameful or frightening.**
    3. In some cultures, a discussion of feelings is neither acceptable nor comfortable. The nurse must interview in accordance with the comfort level of the client.
    4. Manifestations of stress may vary from one culture to another.

22. **C: Collaborative Practice CN: Physiological Integrity T: Application**
    1. It is not likely that the family will be able to distinguish between dementia and delirium. This question will not elicit the most important information.
    2. **Delirium tends to be of short duration and may be triggered by a specific condition. Dementia is a progressive cognitive disorder, occurring gradually over a period of time.**
    3. This may be an important question if it is determined that the client has dementia.
    4. Violent behaviour does not help distinguish between delirium and dementia.

23. **C: Foundations of Practice CN: Psychosocial Integrity T: Knowledge**
    1. People with antisocial personality disorder are more extroverted than reclusive.
    2. **People with antisocial personality disorder tend to be impulsive with poor self-control.**
    3. People with this disorder are more likely to be impulsive than to be perfectionists.
    4. **People with this disorder characteristically demonstrate aggressive behaviours.**
    5. People with antisocial personality disorder rarely demonstrate clinging behaviours.
    6. People with antisocial personality disorder rarely show anxiety.

24. **C: Professional, Ethical, and Legal Practice CN: Safe and Effective Care Environment T: Application**
    1. **There are situations where the therapeutic plan includes monitoring and assistance in a social situation. If the outing is part of the agreed-upon care plan, it is appropriate. The nurse must take care to keep the outing strictly professional.**
    2. It is not appropriate for a nurse to have a social relationship with a mental health client.
    3. It is appropriate if it is decided upon by the health care team and is part of the care plan.
    4. As in choice 3.
25. **C: Collaborative Practice CN: Psychosocial Integrity T: Application**
    1. **The child has moderate anxiety. A calm manner will calm the child.**
    2. **A simple, structured, predictable environment is desirable to decrease anxiety and reduce stimuli.**
    3. Repetition is often needed when the individual is unable to concentrate because of elevated levels of anxiety.
    4. Opportunities for play and exercise should be provided as avenues to reduce anxiety. Physical movements help channel and lower anxiety. Play helps by allowing the child to act out concerns.
    5. **Calm, simple explanations that reinforce reality validate the environment.**

CHAPTER 13

Answers and Rationales for End of Chapter 13 Questions
The correct answer is set off in boldface.
1. **C: Foundations of Practice CN: Health Promotion and Maintenance T: Application**
    1. **Palliative care is supportive treatment designed to relieve or reduce uncomfortable symptoms such as pain, nausea, and shortness of breath.**
    2. Palliative care should be supportive rather than curative. It should not postpone or delay death. Enteral feeds would postpone death.
    3. Both client and family needs are the focus of any interventions.
    4. The palliative care team offers bereavement support to families after the death of a client.
2. **C: Foundations of Practice CN: Psychosocial Integrity T: Application**
    1. Visitors are encouraged to be "present" with the client, talking softly and making physical contact in a way that does not demand a response from the client.
    2. **Withdrawal is a normal psychosocial response to approaching death.**
    3. Stimulation will tire the client and is not an appropriate response to withdrawal on this circumstance.
    4. Dying clients may maintain the ability to hear while not being able to respond.

3. **C: Foundations of Practice CN: Physiological Integrity T: Application**
    1. **As death approaches, the skin becomes cool, clammy, and mottled due to diminished circulation.**
    2. Respirations are often rapid and shallow, progressing to Cheyne-Stokes respirations.
    3. The pulse becomes weak, but the rate does not increase.
    4. Although the skin feels cool to touch, body temperature often increases prior to death.
4. **C: Foundations of Care CN: Psychosocial Integrity T: Application**
    1. **The nurse's initial action should be to assess Mrs. Dain's wishes at this time.**
    2. This action may be implemented if Mrs. Dain or her family express a desire to discuss this topic, but it should not be implemented until the assessment indicates that it is appropriate.
    3. As in choice 2.
    4. As in choice 2.
5. **C: Foundations of Practice CN: Psychosocial Integrity T: Application**
    1. **Mr. Dain's behaviour and statements indicate the absence of anticipatory grieving, which may lead to impaired adjustment as Mrs. Dain progresses toward death.**
    2. Mr. Dain does not appear to feel anxious about Mrs. Dain's impending death.
    3. Mr. Dain does not appear to feel overwhelmed by caregiving.
    4. Mr. Dain does not appear to feel hopeless about the current situation.
6. **C: Foundations of Practice CN: Psychosocial Integrity T: Application**
    1. The client's behaviour and verbalization are not an example of social isolation.
    2. Hopelessness is more reflective of the comment, "I have no future" than of "What does it matter?"
    3. The client's behaviour and verbalization does not indicate denial.
    4. **A defining characteristic for the nursing diagnosis of *Powerlessness* may include a statement by the client such as "What does it matter?" when offered choices or information concerning him or her.**
7. **C: Foundations of Practice CN: Psychosocial Integrity T: Application**
    1. Stating that no one feels ready for death fails to address Mrs. Dain's concerns.
    2. **Staying at the bedside and listening allows her to discuss any unresolved issues or physical discomforts that should be addressed.**
    3. Family members may not feel comfortable staying at her bedside; the nurse should not insist they remain there.
    4. Telling Mrs. Dain that everything is being done does not address her fears about dying, especially since she is likely to die soon.

8. **C: Foundations of Practice CN: Psychosocial Integrity T: Application**
   1. If the nurse tells the family what is best, this removes the decision making from the parents. It also increases pressure on the nurse to be the expert. The nurse is in a supportive role.
   2. The nurse should not leave the family alone to deal with their tragedy.
   3. Becoming involved is an objective, deliberate choice. Ideally, the nurse achieves detached concern, which allows sensitive, understanding care because the nurse is sufficiently detached to make objective, rational decisions.
   4. **The nurse can enhance the quality of life for Krish and his family by advocating for and implementing pain and symptom relief measures.**

9. **C: Foundations of Practice CN: Psychosocial Integrity T: Application**
   1. After the death of a child, the parent recognizes the responsibilities to the rest of the family but needs to be able to experience the grief of the loss.
   2. **Acknowledging that the family has been through a very tough time validates the loss that the parents have experienced. It is nonjudgmental.**
   3. Telling the parents what they should do is giving advice. The parent would not be happy that the child has died and stating so is argumentative.
   4. The parents may be angry with God, or their religious beliefs may be unknown, so the nurse should not provide false reassurance by talking to them about God.

10. **C: Foundations of Practice CN: Health Promotion and Maintenance T: Critical Thinking**
    1. Adolescent children are abstract thinkers.
    2. **Games, art, and play provide children a way to use their natural expressive means to stimulate dialogue.**
    3. Children may not understand the implication of facts just because they can recite them.
    4. The assessment is more complete when children's questions direct the conversation.

11. **C: Foundations of Practice CN: Psychosocial Integrity T: Application**
    1. If Krish has built a tolerance to the opioids, adverse effects are not likely.
    2. At this time, many children do begin to comfort their families and tell them that they are not afraid and are ready to die, but the visions usually precede this stage.
    3. There is no evidence of tissue hypoxia.
    4. **Near the time of death, many children experience visions of "angels" or people and talk with them. The children mention that they are not afraid and that someone is waiting for them.**

12. **C: Professional, Ethical and Legal practice CN: Psychosocial Integrity T: Critical Thinking**
    1. Burnout is a state of physical, emotional, and mental exhaustion. It results from prolonged involvement with individuals in situations that are emotionally demanding. Attending the funeral of a child can be an effective coping measure.
    2. Attending funerals does not detract from the professionalism of care.
    3. Although it is important to consider the family's expectations, the act of attending the funeral provides a sense of closure with the family and facilitates the grief process for the nurse.
    4. **Some nurses find shared remembrance rituals useful in resolving grief. Attending funeral services can be a supportive act for both the family and the nurse.**

13. **C: Professional, Ethical, and Legal Practice CN: Safe and Effective Care Environment T: Application**
    1. Nurses do not have the right to share their views on MAID with their clients.
    2. Determining the eligibility of a client for MAID is not the responsibility of the nurse. This falls under the scope of practice of the NP or physician.
    3. The law does not require that all health care professionals participate.
    4. **The nurse has a duty to inform their employer about personal conscientious objection in advance so that the organization can ensure that they are not involved in the process.**
    5. **One of the roles of the nurse in MAID is to provide bereavement care to the family of the person receiving MAID.**

14. **C: Professional, Ethical, and Legal Practice CN: Psychosocial Integrity T: Knowledge**
    1. **Listening is an appropriate intervention for unresolved grief.**
    2. **Providing emotional support is an appropriate intervention for unresolved grief.**
    3. Forcing a client to eat is not a therapeutic intervention for unresolved grief.
    4. **Referring to appropriate resources is an appropriate intervention for unresolved grief.**
    5. The client with unresolved grief is unable to shift their attention from the loss and would have difficulty functioning effectively at work.

15. **C: Foundations of Practice CN: Health Promotion and Maintenance T: Critical Thinking**
    1. An adolescents' concept of death is a mature understanding of death.
    2. **A school-aged child concept of death includes responding to logical explanations of death.**
    3. **A school-aged child personifies death as the devil or bogeyman.**
    4. **A school-aged child has a deeper understanding of death in a concrete sense.**
    5. **A school-aged child fears mutilation and punishment associated with death.**

16. **C: Professional, Ethical, and Legal Practice CN: Psychosocial Integrity T: Application**

1. Although coursework on death and dying may add to the nurse's knowledge base, it does not best prepare the nurse for caring for a dying patient.
2. The death of a patient can raise many emotions. Being able to control one's own emotions is important; however, it is unlikely that the nurse would be able to do so if they have not first acknowledged their own feelings about death.
3. The death of a loved one is not a prerequisite to caring for a dying patient. The experience of caring for a dying patient may help a nurse mature in dealing with loss, or it may bring up many negative emotions if complicated grief is present.
4. **When caring for patients experiencing grief, it is important for the nurse to assess their own emotional well-being and to understand their own feelings about death. The nurse who is aware of their own feelings will be less likely to place personal situations and values before those of the patient.**

17. C: **Foundations of Practice CN: Physiological Integrity T: Knowledge**
    1. **Mottling of skin is a physical sign of approaching death.**
    2. Sleeping increases, not decreases as death approaches.
    3. **Cheyne-Stokes respirations is a physical sign of approaching death.**
    4. Hearing is the last sense to fail.
    5. **There is a tendency for dying clients to take in less food and fluid.**

18. C: **Foundations of Practice CN: Psychosocial Integrity T: Application**
    1. Restlessness is frequently a behaviour associated with an inability to express emotional or physical distress, but this client does not express distress and is able to communicate clearly.
    2. There is no indication that the client is manifesting this.
    3. **The client's statement indicates that there is some unfinished family business that the client would like to address before dying.**
    4. As in choice 2.

19. C: **Foundations of Practice CN: Safe and Effective Care Environment T: Application**
    1. The nurse should identify the least invasive alternative routes of administration for medications needed for symptom management for a client experiencing dysphagia at the end of life. Although medications may be given subcutaneously, there are other choices such as rectal, buccal, and transdermal medication routes.
    2. **The client should be suctioned orally as required.**
    3. **Elevating the head of the bed for meals and for 30 minutes after is an appropriate nursing intervention for the client with dysphagia.**
    4. **The nurse should not force the client to eat or drink.**
    5. The nurse should modify diet as tolerated and as desired by the client. A pureed diet, or chopped meats,

not just a soft diet, are all potential dietary modifications that could be chosen.

20. C: **Foundations of Practice CN: Physiological Integrity T: Application**
    1. **If the client wore dentures, reinsert them. Dentures maintain the client's natural facial expression.**
    2. Elevation of the head of the bed prevents pooling of blood in the face and subsequent discolouration.
    3. Placing one hand on top of the other can lead to discolouration of the skin.
    4. Changing dressings helps control odours caused by microorganisms and creates a more acceptable appearance.

21. C: **Foundations of Practice CN: Psychosocial Integrity T: Application**
    1. **When death is imminent, care should be limited to interventions for palliative care.**
    2. Music may be used to provide comfort to the client.
    3. Vital signs do not need to be measured frequently.
    4. The nurse should speak to the client in a clear, distinct voice.

22. C: **Professional, Ethical, and Legal Practice CN: Safe and Effective Care Environment T: Critical Thinking**
    1. There are many strategies that can be employed to allow this practice while ensuring safety.
    2. Although it is important that nurses have a foundational knowledge of the values and beliefs of various cultures, not all persons of those cultures hold those values.
    3. It is inappropriate for nurses to impose their values on others.
    4. **It is not possible to know in advance the beliefs and rituals of all cultures; therefore, it is important to ask the patient and family what is most significant to them.**

23. C: **Foundations of Practice CN: Physiological Integrity T: Application**
    1. Poor circulation may cause temperature changes in the extremities. Keep the client warm.
    2. An indwelling catheter provides client comfort in the final stages of dying.
    3. **Poor circulation of body fluids, immobilization, and inability to expectorate secretions may cause rattling. Elevate the head of the bed and turn the head to the side to drain secretions.**
    4. Do not force the client to eat or drink. Offer ice chips, soft drinks or juice as tolerated.

24. C: **Foundations of Practice CN: Safe and Effective Care Environment T: Knowledge**
    1. **Addiction is not an issue when care is provided for the terminally ill. The goal is to make the client comfortable and pain free.**
    2. Addiction is not an issue when providing end-of-life care to a client.
    3. As in choice 2.
    4. As in choice 2.

INDEX

Page numbers followed by "*f*" indicate figures, "*t*" indicate tables, and "*b*" indicate boxes.